Handbuch der inneren Medizin

Begründet von L. Mohr und R. Staehelin

Herausgegeben von
H. Schwiegk

Siebter Band: Stoffwechselkrankheiten

Fünfte, völlig neu bearbeitete und erweiterte Auflage

Teil 3

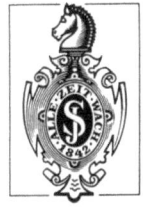

Springer-Verlag Berlin Heidelberg New York 1976

Gicht

Bearbeitet von

A. Göb · A. Griebsch · W. Gröbner · P. U. Heuckenkamp · E. W. Holmes
R. R. Howell · W. Kaiser · W. N. Kelley · H. Lydtin · M. Marshall · P. May
D. P. Mertz · W. M. Mikkelsen · A. Rauch-Janßen · L. B. Sorensen
M. Schacherl · M. Schattenkirchner · F. Schilling · U. Trabert · E. Uehlinger
G. Wolfram · J. B. Wyngaarden · N. Zöllner

Herausgegeben von

N. Zöllner und W. Gröbner

Mit 205 zum Teil farbigen Abbildungen

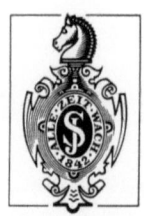

Springer-Verlag Berlin Heidelberg New York 1976

Herausgeber Professor Dr. N. Zöllner und Privatdozent Dr. W. Gröbner
Pettenkoferstraße 8a, D-8000 München 2

ISBN-13: 978-3-642-66139-6   e-ISBN-13: 978-3-642-66138-9
DOI: 10.1007/978-3-642-66138-9

Library of Congress Cataloging in Publication Data. Gicht. (Handbuch der inneren Medizin: Bd. 7. Stoffwechselkrankheiten; T. 3) Bibliography; p. Includes index. 1. Gout. I. Göb. A., 1918— II. Zöllner, Nepomuk and Gröbner, Wolfgang. III. Series. RC41.H342 Bd. 7. T3 [RC629] 616'.026'08s [616.3'99] 75-12747

Das Werk ist urheberrechtlich geschützt. Die dadurch begründeten Rechte, insbesondere die der Übersetzung, des Nachdruckes, der Entnahme von Abbildungen, der Funksendung, der Wiedergabe auf photomechanischem oder ähnlichem Wege und der Speicherung in Datenverarbeitungsanlagen bleiben, auch bei nur auszugsweiser Verwertung, vorbehalten. Bei Vervielfältigung für gewerbliche Zwecke ist gemäß § 54 UrhG eine Vergütung an den Verlag zu zahlen, deren Höhe mit dem Verlag zu vereinbaren ist.

© by Springer-Verlag Berlin · Heidelberg 1976

Softcover reprint of the hardcover 5th edition 1976

Die Wiedergabe von Gebrauchsnamen, Handelsnamen, Warenbezeichnungen usw. in diesem Werk berechtigt auch ohne besondere Kennzeichnung nicht zu der Annahme, daß solche Namen im Sinne der Warenzeichen- und Markenschutz-Gesetzgebung als frei zu betrachten wären und daher von jedermann benutzt werden dürften.

Gesamtherstellung Brühlsche Universitätsdruckerei, Gießen.

Vorwort

Die Gicht ist eine klassische Krankheit. Sie war schon im Altertum genau bekannt, und Thomas Sydenham lieferte bereits im Jahre 1717 eine heute noch nosologisch mustergültige Beschreibung des Gichtanfalles. Die Aufklärung der Zusammenhänge zwischen Harnsäure und Gicht ist ein klassisches Beispiel früher Zusammenarbeit zwischen Klinikern und Chemikern. Scheele hatte die Harnsäure 1776 beschrieben und bereits 20 Jahre später konnte WOLLASTON nachweisen, daß die Ablagerungen bei der Gicht großenteils aus dieser Substanz bestehen. 1848 führte A. B. GARROD den Nachweis der Harnsäurevermehrung im Blut von Gichtkranken.

Im Jahre 1960 war es möglich, eine Übersicht über moderne Probleme der Gicht anhand von weniger als 300 Literaturstellen zu geben, heute bedarf es dazu eines Handbuches. Offensichtlich hat die Krankheit viele Forscher fasziniert. Diese Faszination ist erklärlich, denn es gibt kaum ein Gebiet der Inneren Medizin, welches in so breiter Front Angriffsflächen und Möglichkeiten für den Fortschritt geboten hat. Aus der klinischen Nosologie sind die Beschreibung der Gichtniere, die Definition der sekundären Gicht und die Abgrenzung der verschiedenen Formen der juvenilen Gicht zu nennen. Neue und genauere pathologische Beschreibungen der Gichtniere und der Gelenkgicht sind erfolgt. Man hat gelernt, den Gichtanfall im Experiment zu erzeugen und seine Voraussetzungen zu untersuchen. Über die Mechanismen, welche die Hyperuricämie hervorrufen, besteht grundsätzliche Klarheit: Die Biosynthese der Purine und ihre Regelung ist weitgehend bekannt, die Rolle der Nahrungspurine ist quantitativ faßbar und im Bereich der Nierenphysiologie besteht weitgehende Einigung darüber, daß Filtration im Glomerulum, Rückresorption und Sekretion im Tubulus in einem komplexen Zusammenspiel die Harnsäureausscheidung bestimmen.

Seit Ende des letzten Weltkrieges sind große Fortschritte im Bereich der Therapie gemacht worden. Uricosurica, Allopurinol, gute Colchicinpräparate und hochwirksame Antiarthritica lassen zusammen mit klaren Vorstellungen über die Diätetik der Gicht eine in nahezu allen Fällen erfolgreiche Behandlung zu. Die Suche nach dem molekularen Defekt bei der Gicht hat nicht nur zu Fortschritten in der Biochemie geführt, sondern auch zur Aufklärung mehrerer Stoffwechseldefekte, die zur Hyperuricämie führen. Ihre Bearbeitung in Fibroblastenkulturen von Patienten hat außerdem nennenswerte Fortschritte in der Genetik mit sich gebracht, ebenso wie die Erkenntnis, daß Stoffwechsel- und Ernährungskrankheiten an Zellkulturen bearbeitet werden können.

So groß die Fortschritte sind, so viele neue Fragen haben sie aufgeworfen. Dieser Band des Handbuches der Inneren Medizin zeigt beides, den Stand des Wissens und den Stand der Problematik, der teils in den einzelnen Kapiteln, teils aber auch durch Unterschiede in den Meinungen, die in den einzelnen Kapiteln vertreten werden, zu ersehen ist. Dem Herausgeber war die Gewinnung der Autoren des Handbuches darüber hinaus eine erfreuliche Erfahrung in der internationalen Zusammenarbeit.

Handbücher wenden sich an viele. Wir haben versucht, die notwendige Mischung von Beiträgen für den Internisten ebenso wie für den Grundlagenforscher zusammenzustellen.

N. ZÖLLNER

Mitarbeiterverzeichnis

Göb, Albert, Prof. Dr., Orthopädische Poliklinik der Universität, Pettenkoferstr. 8a, D-8000 München 2

Griebsch, Anton, Dr., Internist, Rosenstr. 2, D-8023 Großhesselohe-Pullach

Gröbner, Wolfgang, Privatdozent Dr., Medizinische Poliklinik der Universität, Pettenkoferstr. 8a, D-8000 München 2

Heuckenkamp, Peter-Uwe, Privatdozent Dr., Würmstr. 37, D-8032 Gräfelfing

Holmes, E. W., M. D., Assistant Professor of Medicine, Duke University, Medical Center, Durham, N.C. 27706/U.S.A.

Howell, R., Rodney, M. D., Professor and Chairman, Department of Pediatrics, University of Texas, Medical School at Houston, 6400 West Cullen, Texas Medical Center, Houston, Texas 77025, U.S.A.

Kaiser Wolfram, Privatdozent Dr., Medizinische Poliklinik der Universität, Pettenkoferstr. 8a, D-8000 München 2

Kelley, William, N., M. D., Professor of Medicine, University of Michigan, University Hospital, 1405 E. Ann Street, Ann Arbor, Mich. 48104/U.S.A.

Lydtin, Helmut, Prof. Dr., Kreiskrankenhaus, D-8130 Starnberg

Marshall, Markward, Dr., Medizinische Poliklinik der Universität, Pettenkoferstr. 8a, D-8000 München 2

May, Peter, Prof. Dr., Urolog. Klinik d. Allgem. Krankenhauses, D-8600 Bamberg

Mertz, Dieter, P., Prof. Dr., Kurklinik am Park, D-4934 Horn-Bad Meinberg 2

Mikkelsen, William, M., M. D., Professor of Medicine, University of Michigan, Medical School, 1405 E. Ann Street, Ann Arbor, Michigan 48109, U.S.A.

Rauch-Janssen, Angelika, Dr., Medizinische Poliklinik der Universität, Pettenkoferstr. 8a, D-8000 München 2

Sorensen, Leif, B., M. D., Ph. D., Professor of Medicine, University of Chicago, 950 East 59th Street, Chicago, Illinois 60637/U.S.A.

Schacherl, Martin, Dr., Röntgenabteilung der Klinik für Rheumakranke, Saarstr. 1, D-6550 Bad Kreuznach

Schattenkirchner, Manfred, Privatdozent Dr., Medizinische Poliklinik der Universität, Pettenkoferstr. 8a, D-8000 München 2

Schilling, Fritz, Prof. Dr., Dozent für Rheumatologie, Zentrum für Rheuma-Pathologie, Kleine Windmühlenstr. 2 1/10, D-6500 Mainz

Trabert, Ulrich, Dr., Friedrich-Rottra-Str. 32, D-7859 Efringen-Kirchen

UEHLINGER, ERWIN, Prof. Dr., Pathologisches Institut der Universität, Kantonsspital, Schmelzbergstr. 12, CH-8091 Zürich

WOLFRAM, GÜNTHER, Privatdozent Dr., Medizinische Poliklinik der Universität, Pettenkoferstr. 8a, D-8000 München 2

WYNGAARDEN, JAMES B., M. D., Professor of Medicine, Duke University, Medical Center, Durham, N.C. 27710/U.S.A.

ZÖLLNER, NEPOMUK, Prof. Dr., Medizinische Poliklinik der Universität, Pettenkoferstr. 8a, D-8000 München 2

Inhaltsverzeichnis

I. Einführung

Einleitung. N. ZÖLLNER und W. GRÖBNER 3

II. The Epidemiology of Hyperuricemia and Gout

The Epidemiology of Hyperuricemia and Gout. W. M. MIKKELSEN. With 2 Figures 9

Introduction 9
Measurements of Uric Acid 9
   Methods 9
   Effects of Drugs on Serum Uric Acid 10
   Effects of the Other Disease States on Serum Uric Acid 10
   Hypouricemia 11
Distribution of Serum Uric Acid Values in the General Population Mean Values; Age and Sex Influences 12
   The "Normal Range" 13
Correlation of Serum Uric Acid with Other Population Characteristics 14
   Diabetes Mellitus 15
   Lipid Disorders 16
   Hypertension 16
   Psychosocial Factors 17
   Comment 18
Diagnostik Criteria for Gout 18
Geographic and Ethnic Differences in Serum Uric Acid Levels and Gout 19
   Pacific Population 19
   Filipinos 24
   Chinese 24
   Japanese 25
   Caucasian Populations 25
   American Indians 25
Relationship of Hyperuricemia to Clinical Manifestations 25
   Acute Gouty Arthritis 25
   Tophaceous Deposits 26
   Nephrolithiasis 27
   Gouty Nephropathy 28
   Coronary Heart Disease 28
Genetic Aspects of Hyperuricemia and Gout 29
   Family Studies 29
   Population Studies 30
   Twin Studies 30

Identified Genetic Defects Associated with Hyperuricemia and Gout 31
Programs for Preventation of Gout 32
References 33

III. Ätiologie und Pathogenese der Hyperuricämie

1. The Etiology and Pathogenesis of Gout. J. B. WYNGAARDEN and W. N. KELLEY.
With 20 Figures 43

    Definition and Significance of Hyperuricemia 43
    Potential Pathophysiologic Mechanisms of Hyperuricemia 45
    Genetics 45
        Familial Incidence of Gout 45
        Asymptomatic Hyperuricemia in Families of Gouty Patients 45
        Hypothesis of an Autosomal Dominant Gene 46
        Hypothesis of Multifactorial Inheritance 47
        Hyperuricemia in Population Studies 47
        Genetic Control of Uric Acid Excretion 49
        X-linked Hyperuricemia 49
            Complete and Partial Deficiencies of Hypoxanthine-Guanine Phosphoribosyl-
transferase (PRT) 49
        Hyperuricemia in Autosomally Inherited Conditions 50
            Glucose 6-Phosphatase Deficiency 50
            Glutathione Reductase Variants 50
            Adenine Phosphoribosyltransferase (A-PRT) Deficiency 51
            Deficiency of an $\alpha_1 - \alpha_2$ Urate Binding Globulin 51
            Indiopathic Uric Acid Nephrolithiasis 52
        Subtypes of Uncertain Genetic Patterns 52
            PP-ribose-P Synthetase Variants 52
            Hyperuricemia and Hyperlipoproteinemia 52
    Biochemistry of Purine Compounds 53
        Biosynthesis of the Purine Ring 53
        Biosynthesis of Other Nucleotides 56
        Salvage Pathways 57
        Economy of Purine Biosynthesis in the Mammal 59
        Nucleic Acid Catabolism 59
        Catabolism of Ingested Nucleoproteins 60
        Formation of Uric Acid 60
        Uric Acid Ribonucleoside 61
    Regulation of Purine Biosynthesis De Novo 62
        Rate-limiting Step 62
        Substrates 62
            5-phosphoribosyl-1-pyrophosphate 62
            L-Glutamine 63
        Glutamine Phosphoribosylpyrophosphate Amidotransferase 64
        End-Product Inhibition 65
    Production of Uric Acid in Gout 65
        Chemical Balance 65
        The Miscible Pool of Uric Acid and Its Turnover 66
        Incorporation of Labeled Precursors into Uric Acid 68
            Incorporation of Labeled Glycine into Urinary Uric Acid 68
            Incorporation of Labeled Glycine into Total Body Uric Acid 70
            Incorporation of Ammonium-^{15}N into Urinary Uric Acid 71
            Incorporation of Formate-^{14}C into Urinary Uric Acid 72

Incorporation of Glycine, 5-Aminoimidazole-4-Carbox-amide, Hypoxanthine or Adenine into Urinary Uric Acid and Purine Bases 72
Overproduction of Uric Acid in Gout 73
Gout Associated with Specific Enzymatic Defects 74
  Glucose-6-Phosphatase Deficiency in Gout 74
  Hypoxanthine-guanine Phosphoribosyltransferase Deficiency in Gout 76
    Other Enzyme Abnormalities 79
    Purine Metabolism in Heterozygotes 79
    Relationship of PRT Defiency to Accelerated Purine Biosynthesis 79
  Increased PP-Ribose-P Synthetase Activity in Gout 81
Primary Gout 82
  The Role of L-Glutamine in Gout 83
    Amino Acids and Urinary Ammonia Production in Gout 83
    Intramolecular Distribution of ^{14}C or ^{15}N in Urinary Uric Acid 84
    Hypothesis of Abnormal Glutamine Metabolism in Primary Gout 84
    The Kinetic Hypothesis 85
  The Role of Phosphoribosylprophosphate in Gout 86
    Phosphoribosylpyrophosphate Turnover in Gout 86
    Phosphoribosylpyrophosphate Concentration in Gout 87
    Glutathione Reductase Variants and Gout 88
    Role of Abnormal Properties of Glutamine-PP-ribose-P Amidotransferase 88
    Role of Inhibitor Ribonucleotides in Gout 89
    Xanthine Oxidase Activity in Gout 89
  Renal Mechanisms of Uric Acid Excretion in Gout 90
  Ethanol 93
  Excretion of Purine Bases in Gout 93
  Extrarenal Disposal of Uric Acid in Gout 94
    Uricolysis in Normal Man 94
    Sites of Uricolysis 94
    Uricolysis in Gout 95
    Dietary Factors in Primary Gout 95
Secondary Hyperuricemia and Gout 96
  Hematologic Disorders 97
  Drug-induced Hyperuricemia 98
    Diuretics 98
  Saturnine Gout 99
References 100

2. Spezielle Probleme 115

a) Genetik der Gicht: W. Kaiser 115

Literatur 122

b) Einfluß exogener Purine auf den Harnsäurestoffwechsel. A. Griebsch und W. Kaiser. Mit 3 Abbildungen 123

Geschichtliches 123
Wirkung purinarmer und purinfreier Diät 124
Einfluß verschiedener exogener Purine 127
  Auswirkungen bei Normalpersonen 127
  Wirkung exogener Purine auf Personen mit vorbestehender Hyperuricämie 127
Einfluß der Nahrungsproteine auf den Harnsäurestoffwechsel 129
Ausmaß und Mechanismen der Resorption von Nahrungspurinen 135
Literatur 135

c) Harnsäureabbau im menschlichen Organismus. W. KAISER 138

   Literatur 141

d) Excretion of Uric Acid in Health and in Disease. L. B. SORENSEN. With 6 Figures 142

   Renal Excretion of Uric Acid 142
      Normal Values for Renal Excretion of Uric Acid 142
      Normal Mechanism of Renal Excretion of Urate in Man 143
      Renal Mechanism for Urate Homeostasis 146
      The Effect of Drugs and Intermediary Metabolites on the Renal Excretion of Uric Acid 149
      Excretion of Uric Acid in Chronic Renal Disease 152
      The Role of the Kidney in the Pathogenesis of Primary Gout 153
      Excretion of Uric Acid during Excessive Hyperuricemia in Myeloproliferative Diseases . 155
      Urate Spillage in Renal Tubular Dysfunction 156
   Extrarenal Elimination of Uric Acid 156
      Excretion of Uric Acid into the Intestinal Tract 156
      Excretion of Uric Acid in Sweat 159
      Uricolytic activity in human tissues 160
   References 160

e) Sekundäre Hyperuricämie und sekundäre Gicht. N. ZÖLLNER. Mit 2 Abbildungen 164

   Geschichtliches und Definitionen 164
   Wichtige Beispiele sekundärer Hyperuricämien 169
      Blutkrankheiten 169
      Arzneimittel 171
      Blei 172
      Sarkoidose und Berylliose 172
      Fasten und Diabetes 173
      Hyperparathyreoidismus 173
      Psoriasis 173
      Schlußbemerkungen 173
   Literatur 174

IV. Pathogenese der Harnsäureablagerungen und des Gichtanfalles

1. Pathogenese der Harnsäureablagerungen und des Gichtanfalles. P.-U. HEUCKENKAMP.
Mit 4 Abbildungen 179

   Pathogenese der Harnsäureablagerungen 179
      Eigenschaften der Harnsäure 179
      Harnsäureablagerungen 179
         Die Bedeutung des Natriumurates für die Tophusbildung 180
      Die Bedeutung des pH, der Glykolyse, der Temperatur und der Milchsäure für die
      Uratablagerungen 184
      Bedeutung mechanischer Einflüsse auf die Tophusbildung 185
   Zusammenfassung 185
   Die Pathogenese des akuten Gichtanfalles 185
      Die Bedeutung der Harnsäure und ihrer Salze für die Pathogenese des akuten
      Gichtanfalles 185
      Die Bedeutung der Leukocyten und ihrer Enzyme 189

Kristallbildung und Auslösung des Gichtanfalles 191
Die Bedeutung der Kinine, des Hageman-Faktors (Faktor XII) und des Complementsystemes für die Pathogenese des akuten Gichtanfalles 192
    Kinine im akuten Gichtanfall 194
    Bedeutung des Hageman-Faktors 195
Bedeutung des Complements 198
Chemotaktische Eigenschaften der Uratkristalle 199
Faktoren, die einen Gichtanfall auslösen können 199
Die Bedeutung von ACTH und Steroiden für die Pathogenese des akuten Gichtanfalles . 201
Molekulare Grundlagen des akuten Gichtanfalles 202
Literatur 204

V. Die pathologische Anatomie der Gicht

1. Die pathologische Anatomie der Gicht. E. UEHLINGER. Mit 21 Abbildungen 213

Die Gelenkgicht 213
Die Gichtniere 223
Gicht und assoziierte Krankheiten 231
Literatur 232

VI. Klinik, Diagnose und Differentialdiagnose der Gicht

1. Klinische Wertigkeit der Hyperuricämie. Beziehung zu anderen Krankheiten. G. WOLFRAM . 237

Hyperuricämie und Übergewicht 237
Hyperuricämie und Fettleber 238
Hyperuricämie und Diabetes 241
Hyperuricämie und Hyperlipidämie 243
Hyperuricämie und Gicht als Risikofaktor 246
Literatur 249

2. Verlauf der Gicht 255

a) Gelenkgicht 255

aa) Der akute Gichtanfall. M. MARSHALL und M. SCHATTENKIRCHNER. Mit 6 Abbildungen . . 255

Die Klinik der akuten Gicht 255
Auslösende Momente des Gichtanfalls 256
Bevorzugte Lokalisationen 257
Klinische Symptomatik 259
Lokalsymptome 260
Begleitsymptome 260
Typische Laborbefunde 261
Verlauf des akuten Anfalls 261
Weiterer Verlauf der Gelenkgicht 261
    Kurze Differentialdiagnose des Gichtanfalles 262
Literatur 263

bb) Die chronische Gicht. M. SCHATTENKIRCHNER und N. ZÖLLNER. Mit 6 Abbildungen . . . 264

    Die Tophusbildung 269
    Literatur 274

cc) Die Differentialdiagnose der Gicht. F. SCHILLING. Mit 22 Abbildungen 276

    I. 276
    II. Die Differentialdiagnose des akuten Gichtanfalls 277
        A. Akute Synovitis, Arthritis und Paraarthritis 278
            1. Die CPPD-mikrokristallin induzierte Synovitis (Pseudogicht) der Chondrocalcinose-Pyrophosphat-Arthropathie 280
            2. Das rheumatische Fieber 291
            3. Andere akute Arthritiden und subakute Polyarthritiden 292
            4. Die psoriatische Arthritis (Arthritis psoriatica, chronische Polyarthritis psoriatica; Psoriasis arthropathica) 294
            5. Palindromer Rheumatismus 298
            6. Arthrosen 299
            7. Die eitrige Arthritis (Gelenkempyem, Pyarthros) 299
        B. Differentialdiagnose der extraarticulären Gichtanfälle 299
            1. Insertionsendopathien 299
            2. Periarthritiden 300
            3. Bursitiden 301
            4. Tenosynovitis (Tendovaginitis) 302
            5. Andere extraarticuläre anfallsartige Entzündungen 302
    III. Differentialdiagnose der chronischen Gicht (Tophus-Gicht) 302
        A. Die chronische Arthritis 303
            Die chronische (rheumatoide) Polyarthritis 305
            Arthrosen 308
        B. Subcutane Knoten 310
    Literatur 316

dd) Röntgendiagnostik der Gicht. M. SCHACHERL. Mit 36 Abbildungen 322

    Taktische und technische Hinweise 325
    Auswertung von Röntgenaufnahmen 325
    Röntgenbefunde an den einzelnen Gelenken 326
        Zehengelenke 328
        Sesambeine der Großzehengrundgelenke 332
        Finger- und Handgelenke 333
        Metatarsotarsalgelenke, Intertarsalgelenke und Sprunggelenke 334
        Kniegelenke 335
        Hüftgelenke 335
        Ellenbogengelenke 338
        Schultergelenke 338
        Wirbelsäule 338
        Iliosacralgelenke 339
    Radiologische Hinweis-Symptome 339
    Differentialdiagnose 344
        Chronische rheumatische Polyarthritis (rheumatoide Arthritis) 344
        Spondylitis ancylopoetica 348
        Arthritis psoriatica 348
        Polyarthrose und destruierende Form der Polyarthrose 351
        Weitere Erkrankungen, die differentialdiagnostisch eine Rolle spielen 352
    Literatur 354

b) Gichtniere 356

aa) Die Gichtniere. N. ZÖLLNER und W. GRÖBNER. Mit 9 Abbildungen 356

    I. Pathogenese 357
       1. Pathogenese der familiären Hyperuricämie 357
       2. Pathogenese sekundärer Hyperuricämieformen 359
       3. Pathogenese der Gichtniere 360
          a) Physiologie und Pathologie der renalen Harnsäureausscheidung 360
          b) Löslichkeit der Harnsäure 365
          c) Spezielle Fragen der Entstehung der Gichtniere 368
       4. Mutmaßlicher Verlauf der Gichtniere 370
    II. Symptomatologie und Diagnose 371
       1. Symptomatologie 371
          a) Häufigkeit der Nephrolithiasis bei Gicht 371
          b) Proteinurie 372
          c) Hämaturie 373
          d) Leukocyturie 373
          e) Cylindrurie 374
          f) Nierenfunktionsproben 374
          g) Symptome der akuten Pyelonephritis 375
          h) Hypertonie 375
       2. Diagnose 375
    III. Verlauf und Prognose 376
    IV. Therapie 377
       1. Erniedrigung der Harnsäurekonzentrationen im Plasma und Interstitium 377
          a) Einfluß der Diät auf den Harnsäurespiegel 377
          b) Uricosurische Maßnahmen zur Senkung der Plasmaspiegel 378
          c) Medikamente zur Hemmung der Harnsäurebildung 380
       2. Erniedrigung der tubulären Harnsäurekonzentration 382
          a) Einfluß von Diät oder Medikamenten, welche die Harnsäurebildung hemmen, auf die intratubuläre Harnsäurekonzentration 382
          b) Einfluß uricosurischer Medikamente auf die intratubuläre Harnsäurekonzentration 383
          c) Weitere Maßnahmen zur Verhütung der Harnsäureausfällung 383
       3. Erniedrigung der Harnsäurekonzentration im Harn und Maßnahmen zur Verhütung der Harnsäureausfällung 384
          a) Verringerung der Harnsäurekonzentration durch Verringerung der Harnsäurebildung 384
          b) Verringerung der Harnsäurekonzentration durch Diurese 385
          c) Beeinflussung der Harnsäurelöslichkeit durch Alkalizufuhr 385
       4. Vermeidung von Harnsäurespiegelerhöhungen in der Prophylaxe der Gichtniere . 386
    Literatur 386

bb) Harnsäurelithiasis. P. MAY. Mit 10 Abbildungen 391

    Vorkommen und Häufigkeit 391
    Die Pathogenese der Harnsäuresteinbildung 391
    Symptomatik 396
    Objektive Symptome 398
    Diagnostik 398
    Röntgenuntersuchungen 398
    Der klinisch-chemische Befund und seine Beurteilung 399
    Therapie 399
    Analyse der eigenen Behandlungsergebnisse bei Harnsäuresteinbildern mit und ohne Hyperuricämie 401
    Literatur 408

cc) Hyperuricämie und Hypertonie. H. LYDTIN 412

    Koincidenz von Gicht und Hochdruck 412
    Mögliche pathogenetische Zusammenhänge zwischen Hochdruck und Gicht bzw. Hyperuricämie 413
    Behandlung des Hochdrucks bei Gicht und Hyperuricämie 416
    Literatur 417

VII. Therapie und Prophylaxe der Gicht

1. Die Therapie des Gichtanfalles. M. SCHATTENKIRCHNER 423

    Colchicin 423
    Phenylbutazon 427
    Indomethacin 428
    Weitere Arzneimittel 428
    Literatur 429

2. Pharmakologie der Anfallsmittel. U. TRABERT 433

    Colchicin 433
        Einleitung 433
        Chemie 433
        Pharmakokinetik 435
        Wirkungsweise 438
        Toxikologie 444
        Zusammenfassung 445
    Antirheumatica 445
        Einleitung 445
        Phenylbutazon 445
            Chemie 445
            Pharmakokinetik 446
            Allgemeine Pharmakologie 448
        Indometacin 449
            Chemie 449
            Pharmakokinetik 450
            Allgemeine Pharmakologie 450
        Zur antiphlogistischen Wirksamkeit 451
    Literatur 455

3. Dauertherapie 461

a) **Einleitung.** N. ZÖLLNER 461

b) **Pharmakologische Hemmung der Purin- und Harnsäuresynthese.** W. KAISER. Mit 4 Abbildungen 462

    I. Analoge des Glutamins 465
    II. Analoge der Folsäure 465
    III. Analoge und Derivate von Purinbasen oder Nukleosiden 466

1. Allopurinol 468
   a) Klinik 469
   b) Metabolismus und Pharmakokinetik von Allopurinol 471
   c) Wirkungsmechanismus von Allopurinol auf die Purin- und Harnsäuresynthese . . 474
   d) Einfluß von Allopurinol auf die intestinale Absorption exogener Purine 478
   e) Einfluß von Allopurinol auf die Pyrimidinsynthese 479
   f) Einflüsse von Allopurinol auf andere Enzymsysteme 480
   g) Nebenwirkungen von Allopurinol 480
2. Hemmung der de novo-Purinsynthese durch verschiedene andere Purinanaloge . . . 482
   6-Mercaptopurin 482
   Azathioprin (6-[1-methyl-4-nitro-5-imidazolyl]-thiopurin 483
   6-Methylmercaptopurin-Ribonucleosid (6-Methyl-thioinosin) 483
   6-Thioguanin 483
   8-Azaguanin 484
   5-Aminoimidazol-4-Carboxamid (AICAR) 484
   Antibiotica 484
   Hadacidin (N-Formyl-Hydroxylamino-Essigsäure) 484
   Adenin 484
   Orotsäure 484
IV. Abbau der Harnsäure innerhalb des Körpers durch Injektion von Urikase 484
V. Stimulation der Purinbiosynthese durch Medikamente 485
Literatur 485

c) Uricosurica. W. GRÖBNER und N. ZÖLLNER. Mit 24 Abbildungen 491

Physiologie und Pathologie der Harnsäure 491
   Normaler Harnsäurespiegel und Hyperuricämie 491
Harnsäurebildung und -ausscheidung sowie deren Störung bei der familiären Hyperuricämie 492
Uricosurische Maßnahmen zur Senkung des Serumharnsäurespiegels 492
   Wasserdiurese 492
   Uricosurica 493
      Allgemeine Eigenschaften der Uricosurica 493
      Die einzelnen Uricosurica 496
      Benzofuranderivate 513
Komplikationen einer Uricosurischen Therapie und deren Prophylaxe 528
   Gichtanfälle 528
   Renale Komplikationen und deren Prophylaxe 528
Therapieverlauf 529
Literatur 530

d) Diät einschließlich experimenteller Grundlagen. A. GRIEBSCH. Mit 3 Abbildungen 536

Allgemeines 536
   Experimentelle Grundlagen 536
      Verwendung von Standard- und Formeldiäten für Ernährungsexperimente über den Harnsäurestoffwechsel 536
      Auswirkungen der Purinrestriktion 541
      Auswirkungen einzelner Harnsäurepräkursoren 542
      Auswirkungen von Alkohol, Fasten, Fett, Eiweiß und Kohlenhydraten auf den Harnsäurestoffwechsel 542
   Praktische Diätetik 548
      Einfache Diätempfehlungen bei Gicht 548
      Diät bei asymptomatischer Hyperuricämie 549
      Streng purinarme Diät 550
      Purinarme Kost 550
      Zusammenstellung von Diätplänen 557
Literatur 557

e) **Hyperuricämie durch therapeutische Maßnahmen.** D.P. Mertz. Mit 7 Abbildungen 560

  Allgemeine Gesichtspunkte 560
  Hyperuricämie durch Saluretica 562
  Sogenannte "Paradoxeffekte" uricosurischer Mittel 565
  Hyperuricämie durch cytostatische Therapie 566
  Hyperuricämie durch parenterale Infusionsbehandlung 566
    Lactat 566
    Äthylalkohol 566
    Fructose 567
  Hyperuricämie durch diätetische Maßnahmen 572
  Hyperuricämie durch respiratorische Acidose 574
  Verschiedenes 574
  Literatur 574

4. **Die chirurgische Behandlung der Gicht.** A. Göb. Mit 8 Abbildungen 579

  Schleimbeuteltophi an vorspringenden Körperregionen 579
  Deformierungen an Finger- und Zehengelenken 581
  Operationen am Großzehengrundgelenk 581
    Operation nach Brandes modifiziert 581
    Operation nach Hueter-Mayo 582
  Operation an den Fingergelenken 582
  Operationen bei Gelenkveränderungen mit Osteolysen an Fingern und Zehen, an Hand und
    Fuß 582
  Gicht an anderen Gelenken und ihre Behandlung 585
  Operationen am Kniegelenk 585
  Infizierte Tophi und Gelenkgicht 586
  Schluß 586
  Literatur 586

5. **Therapie der Gichtniere.** D.P. Mertz 587

  Prognose 590
  Literatur 591

VIII. Prognose der Gicht

Prognose der Gicht. A. Rauch-Janssen und A. Griebsch 595

  Prognose der Arthritis urica und der Uratnephrolithiasis 595
  Die Beurteilung der Berufsfähigkeit 596
  Die Prognose der Gicht quoad vitam 597
  Literatur 599

IX. The Lesch-Nyhan-Syndrome and Adult X-Linked Hyperuricaciduria

The Lesch-Nyhan Syndrome and Adult X-Linked Hyperuricaciduria. W.N. Kelley and
  J.B. Wyngaarden 603

Introduction 603
Enzyme Defect 604
Excessive Uric Acid Production 609
   Clinical description 609
   Pathogenesis 610
Central Nervous System Dysfunction 611
   Clinical description 611
   Pathology 614
   Pathogenesis 614
Hematologic Abnormalities 616
Genetics 616
Pharmacogenetics 617
Treatment 618
References 619

X. Xanthinuria

Xanthinuria. E.W. HOLMES and W.N. KELLEY. With 1 Figure 627

  Clinical Studies 635
    Case Report 635
  Metabolic Alterations 629
  Genetics 630
  Treatment 630
  References 631

XI. Hereditary Orotic Aciduria

Hereditary Orotic Aciduria. R.R. HOWELL. With 7 Figures 635

  Clinical Studies 635
    Case Report 635
    Crystalluria 637
    Summary of Clinical Features 639
  Nature of the Defect in Orotic Aciduria 639
  Treatment 642
    Vitamins, Iron 642
    Steroids 642
    Uridine and Pyrimidine Nucleotides 643
  Genetics 645
  The Possible Relationship of Orotic Aciduria and Gout 646
  Other Conditions Associated with Orotic Aciduria 646
  Orotic Aciduria Secondary to Other Genetic Defects 647
  Drug-Induced Orotic Aciduria 647
    6-Azauridine 647
    Allopurinol 648
  The Possibility of Prenatal Diagnosis 648
  Summary 648
  Acknowledgement 648
  References 649

Sachregister 651

I. Einführung

Einleitung

Von

N. ZÖLLNER und W. GRÖBNER

Die Gicht stellt in den meisten Fällen die klinische Manifestation einer angeborenen Stoffwechselstörung, nämlich der familiären Hyperuricämie dar. Weitere klinische Folgen dieses Stoffwechseldefektes sind Tophusbildung, chronische destruierende Gelenkveränderungen und Gichtgeschwüre einerseits, Gichtniere mit Niereninsuffizienz und Hypertonie sowie Harnsäurenephrolithiasis andererseits. Da gleichzeitig feststeht, daß das klinische Auftreten der Erkrankung in den meisten Fällen von einer reichlichen Zufuhr von Eiweiß und Purinen abhängt, haben wir das wichtige Beispiel einer sowohl endogenen als auch umweltbedingten Erkrankung vor uns. Schon den Ärzten aus früheren Jahrhunderten war bekannt, daß die Gicht in Zeiten der Not selten, in Zeiten des Wohlstandes häufig ist. So schrieb z.B. SYDENHAM, dem wir auf Grund eigenen Leidens und Erlebens die erste exakte Schilderung eines Gichtanfalls verdanken: „Die Gicht befällt meist diejenigen Leute, die in früheren Jahren üppig gelebt und bei reichlichen Mahlzeiten dem Wein und anderen Spirituosen stark zugesprochen haben." Von der primären Hyperuricämie unterscheidet man sekundäre Hyperuricämien, bei denen die Erhöhung des Harnsäurespiegels durch eine andere Erkrankung (meist eine Hämoblastose, z.B. Polycythaemia vera, myeloische Metaplasie, aber auch Nierenkrankheiten und Stoffwechselstörungen) bzw. durch langdauernde Medikamentenzufuhr (z.B. Saluretica) hervorgerufen wird.

In den vergangenen zwei Jahrzehnten wurden in der Erforschung der Epidemiologie, Vererbung, Pathogenese, Klinik und Therapie der Gicht bedeutende Fortschritte erzielt. Die Diagnostik ist durch genaue Definition der Kriterien präziser geworden, weitere Ursachen einer sekundären Hyperuricämie wurden erkannt sowie eigene Krankheitsbilder wie z.B. die Pseudogicht des Erwachsenen oder das Lesch-Nyhan-Syndrom von der eigentlichen Gicht abgegrenzt. Schließlich konnten mit Einführung der Xanthinoxydasehemmer vom Typ des Allopurinols neue Wege für die Therapie der Gicht eröffnet werden.

Gemeinsam mit Diabetes und den verschiedenen Hyperlipidämien gehört die Gicht zu den volksgesundheitlich bedeutsamen Stoffwechselkrankheiten des Erwachsenen. In Framingham erlitten 2,8% aller Männer vor dem 65. Lebensjahr einen Gichtanfall. Bei den Frauen lag die Häufigkeit bei 0,4%. Nierensteine wurden innerhalb der gesamten Gichtiker bei 13,2% der Patienten beobachtet. In unserem Krankengut liegt die Häufigkeit sogar bei 40%.

Der Serumharnsäurespiegel wird im wesentlichen von Alter, Geschlecht und Ernährung beeinflußt. In der im Jahre 1965 durchgeführten Tecumseh-Studie betrug der mittlere Serumharnsäurespiegel bei Männern 4,9 mg-%, bei Frauen 4,2 mg-%, in München lagen die Werte 1962 bei 4,9 mg-% bzw. 4,1 mg-%. Neuere Untersuchungen aus dem Jahr 1973 ergaben unter der Bevölkerung Süddeutschlands bei den Männern einen Mittelwert von 6,0 mg-%, während der mittlere Harnsäurespiegel bei den Frauen innerhalb des letzten Jahrzehnts praktisch keinen Anstieg zeigte. Geänderte Ernährungsgewohnheiten dürften die Ursache für den Anstieg des Serumharnsäurespiegels bei den Männern innerhalb der letzten acht bis zehn Jahre sein.

Über die Art der der familiären Hyperuricämie zugrundeliegenden Stoffwechselstörung bestand lange Zeit Meinungsverschiedenheit. So wurde eine Theorie der Überproduktion von Harnsäure einer Ausscheidungstheorie gegenübergestellt, die besagt, daß eine funktionelle Schwäche der Niere Ursache der Hyperuricämie sei. Aufgrund von neueren Untersuchungen aus den letzten Jahren wird heute allgemein akzeptiert, daß bei etwa 5% der Patienten mit primärer Gicht eine vermehrte Harnsäuresynthese vorliegt, während bei dem Rest eine Ausscheidungsstörung für Harnsäure als Ursache der Hyperuricämie angenommen werden muß. Ätiologisch ist also auch die primäre Gicht keine einheitliche Krankheit.

Für eine Vermehrung der Purinsynthese werden zur Zeit folgende Mechanismen am meisten diskutiert:

Eine Konzentrationsänderung der Schlüsselsubstrate der Glutamin-Phosphoribosylpyrophosphat-Amidotransferase, also des Enzyms, das den ersten geschwindigkeitsbestimmenden Schritt der Purinsynthese de novo katalysiert,

eine Änderung der Aktivität der Glutamin-Phosphoribosylpyrophosphat-Amidotransferase sowie

eine Änderung der intracellulären Konzentration von Adenyl-, Inosin- und Guanylsäure, der drei Nucleotide, die den ersten Schritt der Purinsynthese de novo hemmen können.

Schon Untersuchungen aus dem Jahre 1961 von JONES und Mitarb. ergaben Anhaltspunkte, daß bei einigen Gichtpatienten eine erhöhte Produktion von 5-Phosphoribosyl-1-pyrophosphat vorliegt. SPERLING und Mitarb. (1972) sowie BEKKER und Mitarb. (1973) beobachteten kürzlich je einen Gichtpatienten mit vermehrter Produktion von 5-Phosphoribosyl-1-pyrophosphat und Harnsäure sowie einer gesteigerten Aktivität der Phosphoribosyl-1-pyrophosphat-Synthetase, also des Enzyms, das die Bildung von 5-Phosphoribosyl-1-pyrophosphat aus Ribose-5-phosphat und Adenosintriphosphat katalysiert. Die Berichte lassen vermuten, daß eine Anomalie der Phosphoribosyl-1-pyrophosphat-Synthetase zu einer gesteigerten Harnsäuresynthese und auf diesem Wege zur Entwicklung einer Gicht führen kann.

In den letzten Jahren wurde mit dem Lesch-Nyhan-Syndrom eine weitere Erkrankung gefunden, die mit exzessiver Harnsäureproduktion einhergeht. Charakteristisch für dieses Syndrom sind eine an das X-Chromosom gebundene recessive Vererbung, die klinischen Zeichen einer Gicht mit Gichtarthritis, Gichttophi und Gichtniere sowie zentralnervöse und neurologische Störungen. Der augenfällige biochemische Defekt bei diesem Syndrom ist ein Fehlen der Hypoxanthinguaninphosphoribosyltransferase, des Enzyms, das aus Hypoxanthin und Guanin Inosinsäure bzw. Guanylsäure aufbaut, die wiederum Feed-Back-Inhibitoren der Purinsynthese de novo darstellen. Die Störung dieser Feed-back-Regulation sowie möglicherweise die erhöhte intracelluläre Konzentration von 5-Phosphoribosyl-1-pyrophosphat (infolge verminderten Verbrauchs) führen beim Lesch-Nyhan-Syndrom zu einer gesteigerten Purinsynthese. Seit der Aufklärung dieses Mechanismus wurden auch einige erwachsene Gichtpatienten mit gesteigerter Purinsynthese, aber ohne neurologische Symptome beschrieben, die einen partiellen Mangel an Hypoxanthinguaninphosphoribosyltransferase aufwiesen, sowie analog dazu Patienten mit einem Mangel an Adeninphosphoribosyltransferase.

Wie erwähnt sind Enzymdefekte, die zu vermehrter Purin- bzw. Harnsäuresynthese führen, selten, biochemische Kostbarkeiten. Bei der Mehrzahl der Gichtiker findet man dagegen Besonderheiten der renalen Harnsäureausscheidung, die sich in einer Verminderung der Harnsäureclearance ausdrücken, bzw. in einer im Vergleich zum Gesunden geringeren Harnsäureausscheidung bei (experimentell) gleich hohem Plasmaspiegel. Auch die Häufigkeit der Nephrolithiasis bei Gichtikern, der in der Regel keine vermehrte Harnsäureausscheidung zugrunde liegt, hatte auf Anomalien der renalen Ausscheidungsmechanismen hingewiesen.

Die Kontroversen um eine renale Pathogenese der Gicht in den Jahren nach dem Krieg zwischen THANNHAUSER in Boston (renale Theorie) und GUTMAN in New York (metabolische Theorie), die sich im Lichte späterer Ergebnisse auflösten, da sich sowohl renal als metabolisch verursachte Gichtfälle fanden, führten zu intensiver Bearbeitung der Mechanismen der Harnsäureausscheidung. GUTMAN und YÜ führten den Beweis, daß beim Menschen die Harnsäure nicht nur glomerulär filtriert, sondern auch tubulär secerniert wird. Die genaue Lokalisation der normalen tubulären Harnsäurerückresorption und -sekretion ist noch Gegenstand zahlreicher Forschungen.

Auf dem Gebiet der Therapie der Hyperuricämie wurde durch Einführung des Allopurinols ein wichtiger Fortschritt erzielt. Während noch vor Jahren lediglich Uricosurica zur Verfügung standen, wird heute vor allem bei Patienten mit Nierenfunktionseinschränkung dem Allopurinol Vorzug gegeben. Die Einführung weiterer Arzneimittel mit ähnlichen Angriffspunkten ist zu erwarten.

Forschungen in den letzten zwei Jahrzehnten haben aus der Gicht, einst einem scheinbar einfachen Stoffwechseldefekt mit vorwiegend articulären Manifestationen, eine vielfältige Krankheit gemacht — ätiologisch nicht mehr einheitlich, pathogenetisch enge Wechselbeziehungen zwischen Vererbung und Ernährung aufzeigend und klinisch von der Pädiatrie zur Neuropsychiatrie, Urologie und Nephrologie reichend. Der sehr einheitlichen Klinik der Gicht steht eine ätiologische bzw. pathogenetische Vielfalt gegenüber; die Forschung auf diesem Gebiet ist aber noch längst nicht abgeschlossen.

II. The Epidemiology of Hyperuricemia and Gout

The Epidemiology of Hyperuricemia and Gout

By

W. M. MIKKELSEN

With 2 Figures

Introduction

Although much remains to be learned, gout represents the best understood of the major rheumatic diseases at this time. The important advances which have been made in the past two decades in our understanding of this ancient disease have resulted largely from basic and clinical investigations, which have led to an improved understanding of the pathogenesis of the acute gouty attack and to a rediscovery of the key role of urate crystals in the primary clinical manifestations of the disease. The details of purine biosynthesis and its control have been clarified, and a better understanding of the complex renal handling of urates and the many factors which influence urinary uric acid excretion has been gained. A number of specific enzymatic defects leading to hyperuricemia and gout have been identified, although the precise defect in the great majority of cases of gout remains unidentified.

Epidemiologic studies have also contributed importantly to our increased knowledge of gout. They have led to a better understanding of the normal distribution of serum urate values in health, and to an appreciation of the arbitrary nature of the customary definitions of hyperuricemia. They have provided a basis for the assessment of the risk of development of clinical gout and/or uric acid nephrolithiasis in subjects with hyperuricemia of varying severity. They have increased our knowledge of the genetic aspects of hyperuricemia and gout, and have led to a clear appreciation of the fact that hyperuricemia as it is encountered in the general population is the result of the interaction of multiple hereditary and environmental factors.

Measurements of Uric Acid

Methods

An understanding of the many complexities associated with measurement of uric acid is essential to the proper interpretation of epidemiologic studies of hyperuricemia and gout. The methods employed for measurement of uric acid fall into 2 groups. In the older, colorimetric procedures uric acid reduces phosphotungstic acid to a bluish colored compound. A major disadvantage is nonspecificity; among the other substances contributing to or interfering with color development, is gentisic acid, a salicylate metabolite. A second problem is the need to deproteinize the sample, a process in which some uric acid may be lost by coprecipitation. The highly specific enzymatic spectrophotometric methods depend on the physical property of uric acid to maximally absorb light at 292 millimicrons in the ultraviolet range. The difference in optical density at this point before and after the action of purified uricase on the sample is therefore proportional to the concentration of uric acid.

Regardless of the method employed, it is obvious that much depends on the skill and care of the technician. It should also be realized that even with maximal care, absolute accuracy is an unattainable ideal and that pipettes, colorimeters, spectrophotometers and other laboratory devices all permit measurement only within a certain range of error. The introduction in recent years of automated equipment has made possible the rapid performance of large numbers of determinations with minimal variation in technical factors. It has been demonstrated that in routine use the automated colorimetric procedure entails less error than the manual colorimetric or spectrophotometric methods [33].

The nature of the sample also influences the outcome. Early methods which utilized whole blood have become obsolete because of the many interfering substances. The use of plasma rather than serum, the presence of anticoagulants used in collecting plasma samples, the occurrence of hemolysis, the presence of interfering drugs or metabolites, the duration and temperature of storage, and bacterial contamination of samples are among the many factors which will influence the result.

At the Third International Symposium on Population Studies of the Rheumatic Diseases in 1966 a subcommittee on standardization of serum uric acid methods recommended that the enzymatic spectrophotometric procedure be adopted as the reference method [42]. If other procedures are employed, it was suggested that a random subsample of sera also be assayed by the enzymatic spectrophotometric method. It was appreciated that, regardless of the method employed, it is important to evaluate its accuracy and reproducibility by appropriate recovery and quality control studies, which should be maintained to ensure continuity of satisfactory results.

Effects of Drugs on Serum Uric Acid

It has long been known that drug ingestion may interfere with satisfactory measurement of serum uric acid. Drugs are known which elevate the serum uric acid level by stimulating de novo production (the 2-substituted thiadiazoles) or depress levels by interfering with the metabolic pathway by which the oxypurines are degraded to uric acid (allopurinol, oxipurinol) [127]. However, the majority of drugs which influence serum urate levels do so by altering renal excretion of urate. It is presently believed that urate is virtually completely filtered at the glomerulus and that the filtered urate is then largely reabsorbed in the renal tubule [79]. The evidence is convincing that tubular secretion also occurs and that most of the urinary uric acid is thus derived [82]. Thus, if the major effect of a drug is to inhibit tubular reabsorption it will tend to reduce serum urate levels, whereas if it is to inhibit tubular secretion it will elevate them. It has been demonstrated that some drugs, including probenecid and salicylate, may exhibit a dual effect, depending on their greater inhibition of tubular reabsorption or secretion at different dose levels [201]. Thus, low doses of acetylsalicylic acid (1 to 2 g daily) tend to elevate serum urate levels, whereas higher doses (4 to 6 g daily) exert a uricosuric effect and lower levels. Among the major drugs which tend to promote hyperuricemia are the thiazides, furosemide, ethacrynic acid, and pyrazinamide. Among the drugs which tend to reduce serum urate content are acetohexamide, ethyl biscoumacetate, phenylindanedione, phenylbutazone, and corticosteroids, in addition to the major uricosuric agents, probenecid and sulfinpyrazone. In clinical situations it is advisable to discontinue any such medications for 3 to 5 days before attempting serum uric acid measurements. Such a course is generally not feasible in epidemiologic studies. Inquiry regarding recent ingestion of drugs, including those used therapeutically to lower serum urate levels, should be made, although interpretation in many cases will be difficult.

Effects of Other Disease States on Serum Uric Acid

Secondary hyperuricemia may occur in disorders associated either with increased synthesis or breakdown of cellular nucleic acids or with diminished renal excretion of urate. Included in the former category are psoriasis [56] and the myeloproliferative disorders [80], including leukemia, lymphoma, multiple myeloma, polycythemia (either primary or secondary), and myeloid metaplasia. Elevation of serum uric acid levels has also been reported in infectious mononucleosis [38], sickle cell anemia [74, 194], and thalassemia [158], although there is less available evidence to establish that this is the result of overproduction. Any chronic renal disease with decreased glomerular filtration is associated with hyperuricemia. Chronic lead nephropathy occurring as a sequela of acute or chronic lead poisoning, has long been recognized as a cause of hyperuricemia and gout, and in certain areas such as Queensland, Australia [57] and the southern United States [11] may still be a common etiologic factor. Hyperparathyroidism [145] and myxedema [132] have been associated with hyperuricemia, apparently on the basis of decreased urate clearance, although serum urate levels have often remained elevated after surgical correction of the hyperparathyroidism. Certain disorders and conditions are associated with hyperuricemia because of the presence of metabolites such as lactate, acetoacetate and β-hydroxybutyrate, which are known to inhibit tubular secretion of urate [31, 75]. Included in this category are diabetic acidosis [157], toxemia of pregnancy [85], acute alcoholism [138], starvation [39, 50, 131, 138], ingestion of a high fat diet [131], and von GIERKE's disease (type I). In the latter condition it has been clearly shown that increased de novo synthesis of uric acid occurs, as well as reduced renal excretion of uric acid, both mechanisms contributing to the hyperuricemia [5, 101, 118]. Hyperuricemia has been described in DOWN's syndrome (mongolism) [114, 159]; failure to demonstrate an increased rate of urate synthesis led one group of investigators to conclude that decreased uric acid excretion was responsible for the increased blood uric acid levels [37].

Although precise diagnosis of many disease states is not possible in large epidemiologic investigations, it seems reasonable to believe that the use of hemoglobin or hematocrit measurements, white blood cell counts, and estimation of the serum creatinine or blood urea nitrogen would serve, in many instances, to identify cases of secondary hyperuricemia. In one large population survey it was found that less than 3% of hyperuricemia could be regarded as secondary to renal disease, blood dyscrasia, or psoriasis [84]. Somewhat in contrast was the finding that of 51 hyperuricemic subjects in a Finnish rural community 19 had one or more factors which might have produced the hyperuricemia [99].

Hypouricemia

Abnormally low serum uric acid levels have been reported in a variety of disorders. Hypouricemia due to increased renal clearance of urates has been described in association with aminoaciduria in hepatolenticular degeneration (WILSON's disease) [14], HARTNUP disease [13], the FANCONI syndrome [195], and cancer of the lung [196]. It has also been reported without aminoaciduria in association with HODGKIN's disease [19] and as an apparently isolated renal tubular defect [78, 121, 164]. Very low serum urate levels are found in association with xanthinuria, in which uric acid production is markedly decreased as the

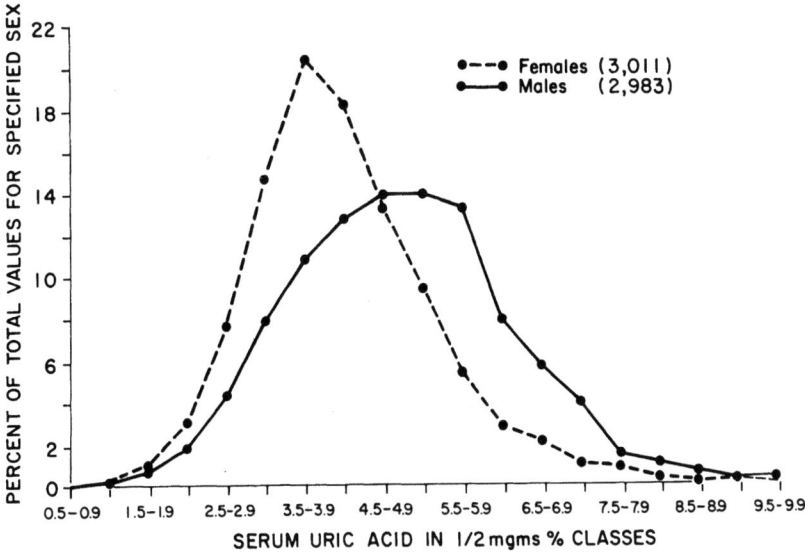

Fig. 1. Distribution of serum uric acid values (TECUMSEH, 1959—1960)

result of absence of the enzyme xanthine oxidase [27]. Hypouricemia (serum urate less than 2 mg/100 ml) was noted in 0.97% of 6629 consecutive serum urate measurements in two large hospitals [172]. In this setting, most cases of hypouricemia were due to drugs, including aspirin, allopurinol, x-ray contrast agents and glyceryl guaiacholate; nine cases of disseminated carcinoma were included, but the other diseases known to be associated with hypouricemia were not represented. Serum urate levels less than 2 mg/100 ml were present in 1% of more than 6000 apparently healthy subjects in one population survey [144]. Presumably, this would also reflect the effect of hypouricemic drugs in a majority of instances. It is clear that in clinical or epidemiologic situations hypouricemia is a significant finding demanding explanation.

Distribution of Serum Uric Acid Values in the General Population Mean Values; Age and Sex Influences

Investigation of the distribution of serum uric acid values in the general population provides the best basis for definition of the normal range of values and evaluation of the effects of age, sex and other characteristics on serum uric acid levels. In one such study, conducted in Tecumseh, Michigan in 1959 to 1960, serum uric acid determinations were made for 6000 subjects 4 years of age and over [144]. The distribution of serum uric acid values is indicated in Fig. 1. The mean serum uric acid value for males was higher than that for females, 4.9 mg/100 ml with a standard deviation of 1.4 as compared to 4.2 mg/100 ml with a standard deviation of 1.16. Essentially similar distribution curves have been reported from 3 additional studies, 2 in New England [84, 155] and 1 in Finland [99], although in several instances the mean serum uric acid values were somewhat higher, due mainly to the older age distribution of subjects selected for study. In each of the 4 studies the distribution curves were unimodal with skewing toward the upper end of the range.

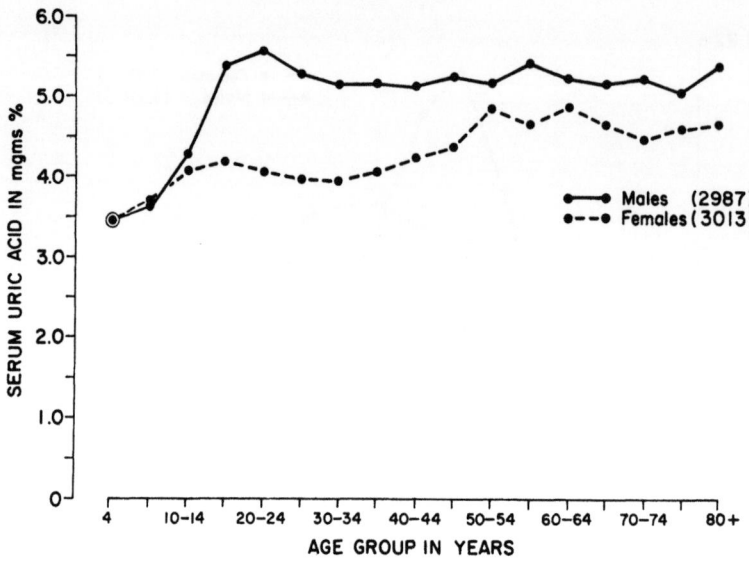
Fig. 2. Sex-age specific mean serum uric acid (TECUMSEH, 1959—1960)

The Tecumseh data serve to demonstrate the effect of age as well as sex on serum uric acid levels (Fig. 2). In childhood, mean levels were relatively low and there was no significant difference in male and female values. In both sexes the mean values rose, the increase being most marked during the pubertal years. The rise was more marked in males so that beginning at about age 12 there were appreciable sex differences. In males the peak mean levels were achieved in the early 20's, after which they declined slightly and then remained essentially unchanged throughout the remainder of the life span. In females mean levels remained 1.0 mg/100 ml or more below male values in the age range 20 to 40 years, after which they increased gradually in the age range 40 to 54 years and showed little change thereafter. This change in female levels at about the time of menopause was also apparent in the Sudbury study, in which premenopausal females age 15 years and over had a mean serum uric acid level of 4.15 mg/100 ml, as compared to mean levels of 4.47 for menopausal and 5.01 for postmenopausal females [155]. Although the causes of these age and sex differences are not entirely understood, it seems clear that hormonal influences play a major role. In this regard it is of interest to note that in the Tecumseh study the 68 females who were pregnant at the time of examination had a mean serum uric acid level significantly lower than that of nonpregnant women of the same age [144].

The "Normal Range"

Examination of the frequency distribution curves of serum uric acid levels obtained in these epidemiologic studies reveals no cutting point that can be used to separate "normal" from "abnormal" values. The range of normality for biochemical constituents is often defined as 2 standard deviations above and below the mean value of a large number of determinations on normal subjects. This approach is based on the mathematical properties of the normal frequency distribution curve; its application to characteristics which are not normally distributed will produce an erroneous estimate of the range of normality. A second statistical method for estimating the normal range, and one which makes no assumptions regarding the nature of the distribution, is the percentile method in which the 2.5 and 97.5 percentiles are calculated, thus setting off the lowest and highest 2.5% of measurements as abnormal (any other percentile can be utilized to delimit the desired proportion of extreme low and high values). Based on such statistical considerations and clinical experience the upper limits of normal for adult serum uric acid levels have usually been set at 6.0 mg/100 ml for men and 5.0 or 5.5 mg/100 ml for women for the colorimetric methods, 7.0 or 7.5 mg/100 ml for men and 6.0 or 6.5 mg/100 ml for women for the enzymatic spectrophotometric methods, and at somewhat higher levels, occasionally to as high as 8.5 mg/100 ml, for the automated colorimetric methods. The limits for females should take into consideration the significant increase in mean values which occurs at menopause. Objections have been voiced to the concept of hyperuricemia as an abnormal state defined by statistical techniques. While it must be acknowledged that any definition of hyperuricemia is largely arbitrary it should be observed that these upper limits as determined in epidemiologic studies have great physiologic significance in that, in males especially, they closely approach the theoretical limit of solubility of monosodium urate in serum. Inasmuch as more basic investigations have clearly related the major clinical manifestations of gout, acute arthritis and tophus formations, to local precipitation of urate crystals, it seems logical to consider a single definition of hyperuricemia, based on solubility limits, for both male and female subjects. On this basis, experimental evidence would suggest an upper limit of normal of about 7.0 mg/100 ml [178]. Such an approach clarifies, in part at least, the reasons for the observed sex ratio in gout.

Correlation of Serum Uric Acid with Other Population Characteristics

Epidemiologic studies have suggested significant correlations between serum uric acid and certain other population characteristics, in addition to age and sex. The most frequent association to be demonstrated has been with some measure of body mass, including, in various studies, weight, relative weight, ponderal index and body surface areas [3, 17, 32, 53, 61, 62, 84, 91, 92, 106, 123, 129, 142, 146, 154, 166, 173]. The nature of this association has not been clear, however, and the measure showing the strongest correlation with urate levels has varied from study to study. Indeed, not all studies have indicated such an association. Amongst male Australian aborigines [58] and a group of racially pure Hawaiians [90], for example, no significant correlation was found between serum uric acid concentration and height, weight, surface area or relative obesity. The Hawaiians were found to be as tall, heavy and obese as a previously reported group of Maoris in New Zealand, but had a mean serum urate level of 5.4 mg/100 ml as compared to 7.2 for the Maoris [90]. In contrast, Maoris living in the Cook Islands also had a high mean serum uric acid level although they lacked the obesity which characterized the New Zealand Maoris [167]. Similarly, New Guinea natives living in the rural highlands were found to be hyperuricemic in comparison to those employed in a nearby town and with a Caucasian control group, despite their lack of obesity, low protein diet and abstinence from alcohol [105].

Serum uric acid levels were correlated with hemoglobin levels in several studies [3, 62], but not in others [106, 204]. The former finding was consistent with the previously known association of hyperuricemia with polycythemia. Columbian army recuits revealed an association between serum uric acid and altitude of residence [2]. Study of a small group of Peruvian subjects living at an altitude of 14000 feet in the Andes indicated that serum uric acid levels were highly correlated with hematocrit values and higher than those of subjects living at sea level [186]. These studies tend to confirm the hypothesis that in certain populations elevation of serum uric acid may be the result of a physiological polycythemia related to altitude of residence [2]. Serum uric acid levels were significantly lower in Brazilian military recruits with blood type AB, but this finding was not confirmed for U.S. recruits or participants in the New Haven study [68]. Among recruits in Columbia significantly higher serum urate values were found for those with blood group B [2], while in recruits in Thailand there appeared to be an association of low serum uric acid levels with blood group A [67]. In the latter study, no association of serum uric acid with glucose-6-phosphate dehydrogenase deficiency or hemoglobin E was observed, but there was a strong association of low serum uric acid levels with presence of the thalassemia gene or increased osmotic resistence of erythrocytes.

Total serum protein values have shown correlation with serum uric acid levels in several studies [3, 204]. In this regard, it is of interest to recall that the incidence of acute gouty arthritis in Europe during the two World Wars was quite low, but rose after each as protein became available and general nutritional status improved [29, 205]. Although parallel information regarding temporal changes in serum uric acid levels in these populations is not available, the observation is consistent with the view that dietary factors and nutritional status are significant determinants of serum uric acid level. The suggestion of a secular trend for increasing serum urate levels in several American studies, if correct, might also be explained in part by nutritional factors [148]. The relatively high mean serum uric acid levels observed in several South Pacific Polynesian populations have been attributed in part to high caloric, high fat diets [167] and consumption of alcohol [61, 167]. Micronesian groups with relatively high serum uric acid values also revealed an association with total daily caloric intake [173]. In a number of studies there has been evidence of correlation between serum uric acid concentration and alcohol consumption [48, 62, 105, 106]. Smoking habits have also shown an association with serum uric acid levels. In the Tecumseh study smokers had lower mean levels than nonsmokers, exsmokers or pipe and cigar smokers [48]. Other studies revealed that smokers who inhaled had significantly lower serum uric acid levels than nonsmokers and noninhalers [133, 204]. There was no relationship in these studies between serum uric acid and the amount smoked.

Diabetes Mellitus

In several clinical series, patients with gout have been reported to have a low prevalence of clinical diabetes mellitus [104, 198]. With the application of biochemical screening for carbohydrate intolerance, however, latent or chemical diabetes has been found among gouty patients with considerable frequency [26, 46, 96, 197, 198]. In the great majority of cases the diabetes is mild, insulin-independent and readily controlled by diet. Clinical impression has suggested that the development of diabetes may have an ameliorative effect on gout, manifested by a decrease in frequency on severity of attacks. Diabetics have been found to have lower serum uric acid levels than nondiabetic controls, apparently as the result of the uricosuric action of hyperglycemia [16, 97, 142]. Epidemiologic studies have generally shown no evidence of association between gout and diabetes, as diagnosed clinically [84, 142], or between serum uric acid and blood sugar levels [84, 142, 173]. In one study, a strong negative correlation between fasting blood sugar and serum uric levels was demonstrated in both white and black females [123]. In several studies, an apparent relationship between serum uric acid and blood sugar levels [204] or a high prevalence of diabetes [167] was explained on the basis of obesity, illustrating the necessity of searching carefully for indirect relationships of this sort in seeking associations between hyperuricemia or gout and other variables.

Lipid Disorders

There is convincing evidence of a relationship between gout and hyperuricemia and lipid disorders. Most studies of this relationship have involved diseased patients, either with gout or hyperlipidemia. Early investigations suggested that hyperuricemia was frequent among patients with familial hypercholesterolemia [4, 87], although a recent, more comprehensive study failed to confirm this finding [103]. Hyperuricemia has been reported with an apparently increased frequency in patients with hyperlipoproteinemia type IV (common) as well as types III and V (uncommon) [120, 176]. Numerous studies of gouty patients have also emphasized the association with hypertriglyceridemia rather than hypercholesterolemia [12, 18, 21, 23, 41, 51, 141, 199]. A primary association between hypertriglyceridemia and decreased glucose tolerance was strongly suggested in a study of patients with hyperlipidemia or gout or both [22]. Impaired glucose tolerance was found in 72% of hypertriglyceridemic subjects, but in only 12% of subjects with essential hypercholesterolemia. Of 25 gouty patients, 19 had hypertriglyceridemia and, of these, 74% had abnormal glucose tolerance, as compared to only 1 of 6 normotriglyceridemic gouty subjects. Hypertriglyceridemic gouty subjects were shown to secrete significantly more insulin after oral but not after intravenous glucose administration; an accompanying relative insulin resistance raised the possibility of an excessive secretion of intestinal hormones in response to glucose ingestion in these patients [199]. Results were considered to indicate a direct relationship between primary gout and primary type IV hyperlipoproteinemia, independent of obesity and carbohydrate intolerance. It has been demonstrated that patients whose gout is secondary to chronic lead nephropathy do not share the hypertriglyceridemia of primary gout patients, indicating that this is not a regular consequence of hyperuricemia alone [59].

Among healthy subjects, these associations have been less pronounced. Study of healthy male executives [54] and of presumably healthy blood donors [18] failed to show such relationships. Relatively few epidemiologic studies of large population groups have reported results bearing on this matter. Most such studies have revealed no significant association between serum uric acid and cholesterol [90—92, 123, 142, 173]. There has been more evidence for an association of serum uric acid with triglycerides [91, 167, 173]. It seems not unlikely that this association, so striking in clinical studies, would be considerably masked in epidemiologic studies by the diluting effect of large numbers of individuals without abnormality of purine or lipid metabolism.

Hypertension

A number of associations between hyperuricemia and hypertension are recognized. Hypertension secondary to chronic renal disease is commonly associated with hyperuricemia. Antihypertensive drug therapy frequently produces hyperuricemia. Hyperuricemia has been reported in 27 to 38% of untreated hypertensive subjects [28, 34, 122], rates higher than reported for unselected populations [144]. Population studies have provided conflicting evidence regarding the relationship of hypertension and serum uric acid, but in general have not revealed a strong or consistent association [150]. In Framingham there was a trend for increasing systolic blood pressure with rising serum uric acid when subjects were grouped by the latter [83]. Similarly, in Evans County, Georgia, an increased prevalence of hypertension was observed in hyperuricemic subjects, a finding not attributable to cardiovascular drugs [123]. A statistically significant difference in blood pressure was demonstrated in Framingham between the gouty subjects and the total population. In several studies an apparent association between serum uric acid and blood pressure was found to be indirect and dependent on body weight, a situation similar to that earlier noted for diabetes [62, 106, 204]. The development of hypertension was reported in 6.3% of 124 asymptomatic hyperuricemic subjects during an observation of $4^1/_4$ years [65].

Psychosocial Factors

Numerous studies have suggested a relationship between serum uric acid and various social and psychological characteristics. A social class gradient in serum uric acid levels was demonstrated in a study involving executives, craftsmen, scientists, medical students and high school students [53]. A mean serum uric acid level of 5.73 mg/100 ml was found for executives as compared to 4.77 for craftsmen. A community study failed to reveal any clear, linear relationship between serum uric acid and the hierarchical classification of occupation used by the U.S. Census Bureau, although, among male heads of households, high mean levels were found for those in the professions or with business responsibilities, while the lowest levels were observed in agricultural and semiskilled workers [49]. A lack of correspondence between the urate levels of the males and their spouses or offspring suggested that the observed differences were not a reflection of different standards of living. Business executives attending a career development course had higher serum uric acid levels, as well as higher cholesterol levels, higher blood pressure, more obesity and more sedentary life patterns than were observed in an age-matched control population [146]. A similar study in Edinburgh revealed a mean plasma uric acid level of 6.0 mg/100 ml for business executives, compared to 4.5 for control subjects [8]. Among employees of the Paris Police Department, officers (predominantly of middle and upper middle class origin and with university education) had higher serum uric acid levels and a higher prevalence of gout than those in the lower ranks [204]. Several studies of more general population groups, however, have failed to reveal any obvious relationship between serum uric acid and occupation or social class [3, 163].

An association has also been suggested between serum uric acid and certain measures of intelligence or achievement. In a study of high school boys, a slight progressive rise in serum uric acid levels with increasing intelligence test scores was observed [53]. Medical students, however, showed no association of medical college aptitude test scores and serum uric acid. Among high school students, those with the most extracurricular activities, the greatest number of service awards and receiving the highest ratings from teachers for such characteristics as industry, leadership and responsibility had the highest serum uric acid levels. A subsequent re-evaluation of 62 male subjects who had had uric acid measurements as high school students revealed that those who attended college but failed had the highest levels [107]. Their high school grades were similar to those of students who did not attend college at all and it was suggested that what differentiated them was the motivation to attend college. Other investigators found no statistically significant relationships between serum uric acid and intelligence quotient or academic grades and no difference in serum uric acid between academic over- and underachievers [147].

An investigation of university professors suggested an association of serum uric acid levels with certain behavioural characteristics, including drive, achievement and leadership [30]. Edinburgh business executives displayed a positive correlation of plasma urate levels with drive and range of activities and a negative correlation with responsibility [8]. Study of white male state employees revealed an association of hyperuricemia with increased perception of change, decreased job stability, greater cigarette smoking, elevated blood pressure and lower ponderal index, suggesting that changing life patterns, particularly in persons of upward mobility, might be a contributing factor in hyperuricemia [130]. An investigation of adult brothers indicated that achievement-related variables could not be used to predict reliably which brother had the higher serum uric acid level, whereas information regarding obesity and dietary content provided a predictive accuracy significantly greater than chance [111].

In some longitudinal studies there has been evidence that certain psychological and physiological stresses may influence serum uric acid levels. Subjects undergoing underwater demolition team training were found to have elevated serum uric acid levels during periods of apparent anticipation of a demanding situation; subjects who withdrew from training had lower initial serum uric acid levels than those who ultimately succeeded [168, 169]. Trainees showed a positive correlation between serum uric acid and their estimate of their own motivation; consistently negative correlations were found between cholesterol and motivation and pleasant affect scores and no significant correlation was found between serum control levels and psychological variables [170]. Anticipation of job loss was found to be associated with higher serum uric acid levels, which dropped to normal if re-employment was rapidly found [108].

A recent review of the psychosomatic aspects of hyperuricemia and gout advanced the hypothesis that personality characteristics associated with hyperuricemia might render such subjects susceptible to certain types of psychosocial stress correlated with the onset of acute attacks of gout [110].

Comment

Epidemiologic investigations provide a valuable opportunity to examine the correlates and consequences of hyperuricemia. Although correlations between serum uric acid and various biochemical, physiological, psychological and social characteristics may be found, it should be cautioned that the demonstration of apparently "significant" correlation coefficients cannot prove a causal relationship and should be interpreted with appropriate regard for known biochemical and physiological facts.

Diagnostic Criteria for Gout

Effective diagnostic criteria are an essential requirement for the successful epidemiologic study of any disease. An attempt was made to modify the existing clinical diagnostic criteria for gout for use in epidemiologic studies in 1966 by a subcommittee of the Third International Symposium on Population Studies in the Rheumatic Diseases [42]. It was recommended that the diagnosis of gout be based on either:

1. "the presence of uric acid crystals in synovial fluid or of urate deposition in the tissues, demonstrated by chemical or microscopic examination; the demonstration of urate urinary calculi does not satisfy this criterion; or

2. the presence of two or more of the following four criteria:

a) a clear history and/or observation of at least two attacks of painful limb joint swelling; the attacks, at least in the early stages, must exhibit an abrupt onset of severe pain and complete clinical remission within a week or two;

b) a clear history and/or observation of podagra—an attack as described in criterion a) involving the great toe;

c) the presence of a tophus, observed clinically;

d) a clear history and/or observation of a good response to colchicine, defined as a major reduction in objective signs of inflammation within 48 hrs of the onset of therapy."

The subcommittee did not include hyperuricemia as a criterion, nor did it attempt any definition of hyperuricemia. It was assumed, however, that serum uric acid determinations would be included in population studies of gout, that frequency distribution curves of serum uric acid levels would be prepared, and that the serum uric acid levels of individuals with one or more of the criteria would be available.

Other clinical features which were considered but rejected as criteria included maleness, a positive family history of gout, a history of urinary calculi, radiographic changes, and precipitation of acute gouty arthritis by surgery, anesthesia, or catastrophic illness. The criteria did not attempt to distinguish between primary and secondary gout since it was felt that it would be difficult to do so and that in any event cases of secondary gout were likely to be rare in population surveys. In considering the problem of pseudogout the subcommittee concluded that it was probably quite rare in most populations and unlikely to be mistaken for gout. However, it should be noted that involvement of the great toe has been observed with pseudogout and that some cases may respond favorably to colchicine therapy. Among the other causes of acute episodic arthritis which might be confused with gout in epidemiologic studies are calcific tendinitis [139, 162, 192], and the arthritis and tendinitis associated with familial type II hyperlipoproteinemia [73, 120].

Geographic and Ethnic Differences in Serum Uric Acid Levels and Gout

Data concerned with mean serum uric acid levels, the prevalence of hyperuricemia, and the prevalence of clinical gout which are reasonably representative of various population groups are indicated in Table 1. While some of the observed differences are no doubt the result of technical factors, others, such as the increased frequency of hyperuricemia and gout amongst New Zealand Maoris and certain groups of Polynesians and Filipinos, seem highly significant. Such populations provide an opportunity for evaluation of genetic and environmental factors in the production of these disorders.

Pacific Population

New Zealand Maoris have been found to have a significantly greater prevalence of gout than non-Maoris [134]. Historical evidence indicating that gout was rare among the Maoris prior to the arrival of Europeans suggested that economic and dietary changes in the environment were responsible for the increased incidence of the disease in a race with a presumed latent genetic potential. Investigation of a more isolated and more racially pure group of Maoris revealed a remarkably high prevalence of ischemic heart disease in the women, and hyperuricemia, clinical gout, diabetes, and obesity in both sexes [166]. These investigations were extended by an epidemiologic survey of two additional Polynesian groups living outside of New Zealand, the Pukapukans and the Rarotongans, for comparison with the New Zealand Maoris [165]. Over 40% of men and women in each of the 3 groups were hyperuricemic. The prevalence of gout among males

Table 1. Geographic and ethnic studies of serum uric Acid levels, prevalence of hyperuricemia and prevalence of gout

Population	Age Range (years)	Males				Females			
		Total Number	Mean SUA; Std.Dev.	Percent Hyperuri- cemia[a]	Percent Gout	Total Number	Mean SUA; Std.Dev.	Percent Hyperuri- cemia[a]	Percent Gout
Europe									
Great Britain [163]									
Wensleydale[b]	15+	436	4.46	4.6 (>6.0)	0.0	475	3.70	1.26 (>6.0)	0.0
Leigh[c]	55—64	136	4.88	8.0 (>6.5)	2 cases	150	4.29	3.35 (>6.5)	0.0
Paris, France [203]	20—55	29923	5.88 ± 1.19	17.6	3.3[g]				
Sofia, Bulgaria [193]	15+	188	4.9	4.8	0.0	232	4.3	7.0	0.0
Finland [98, 99]	16+								
Saloinen[b]		737	5.0 ± 1.1	5.2	1 case	1048	4.0 ± 1.0	1.2 (>7.0)	0.0
Oulu[c]		52	5.2 ± 1.2	9.6		55	4.4 ± 1.2	5.5 (>7.0)	
Africa and West Asia									
Africa [49]	5+								
Ibgo-Ora[d]		30	3.9 ± 0.92	0.0		26	3.5 ± 0.92	0.0	0.0
Isheri[d]		30	4.8 ± 0.73	0.0		30	3.6 ± 0.70	0.0	0.0
Cavalla[d]		91	4.6 ± 0.93	2.2		85	3.8 ± 0.85	1.2	0.0
Brabant[e]		87	4.3 ± 0.85	1.1		85	3.8 ± 0.81	1.2	
South Africa [17]									
Phokeng, W. Transvaal	18–84	128	4.9 ± 1.09		0.0	242	4.46 ± 1.09		0.0
Israel [51]	30+								
Negev Bedouin		252	3.74 ± 0.70			139	3.12 ± 0.79		
Arab villagers		236	4.28 ± 0.98			227	3.60 ± 0.93		
Haifa Jewish port workers		192	4.26 ± 0.84			81	3.54 ± 0.75		
United States and Canada									
Tecumseh [143, 144]	4+	2987	4.91 ± 1.40	7.4	0.5	3013	4.18 ± 1.16	7.2	0.3
Framingham [84]	30—59	2069	5.12 ± 1.11	4.8	2.8	2488	4.00 ± 0.94	3.3	0.4
Sudbury [155, 156]	15+	2201	5.93 ± 1.17		0.66	1849	4.15 ± 0.88	(premenopause)	
						102	4.47 ± 1.17	(? menopause) 0.1	
						460	5.01 ± 1.17	(postmenopause)	

Table 1 (continued)

Population	Age Range (years)	Males Total Number	Mean SUA; Std.Dev.	Percent Hyperuricemia[a]	Percent Gout	Females Total Number	Mean SUA; Std.Dev.	Percent Hyperuricemia[a]	Percent Gout
New Haven [3]	21+	299	6.37 ± 1.33			380	4.75 ± 1.23		
Evans County, Ga. [123]	15+								
Caucasian		692	5.7	14.0		780	4.8	14.	
Black		313	5.6	19.0		427	4.9	21.	
American Indian [20]	30+								
Pima		473	4.56 ± 1.2		2 cases	475	3.85 ± 1.05	2.9	0.0
Blackfoot		587	5.21 ± 1.12		0.0	435	4.47 ± 1.16	9.1	0.0
British Columbia, Can. [69]	adult								
Caucasian		200	4.55 ± 1.02	1.0 (>7.2)					
Haida Indian		237	4.41 ± 0.99	0.0 (>7.2)					
Chinese		100	5.44 ± 1.08	3.0 (>7.2)					
Pacific and Orient									
Thailand [67]									
Recruits	20	710	4.96 ± 0.90	0.4 (>7.5)					
Prisoners	16—50	300	4.74 ± 0.97	0.4 (>7.5)					
Taiwan [52]	15—64								
Chinese		247	4.99 ± 0.91			120	3.87 ± 0.78		
Malaya [52]	15—64								
Chinese		298	6.11 ± 1.29			106	4.52 ± 0.98		
Malays		169	6.32 ± 1.25			9	4.21 ± 0.68		
Tamils		197	6.09 ± 1.22			18	4.20 ± 1.28		
Pacific and Orient, cont.									
Japan									
Akasaka-Chihaya [181]	20+	158	4.87 ± 1.09	12.7 (>6.5)	0.0	224	3.85 ± 0.96	5.8 (>5.5)	0.0
Shindo [181]	30+	220	4.22 ± 1.10	6.4 (>6.5)	0.0	210	3.41 ± 0.89	4.8 (>5.5)	0.0
Hiroshima [109]	15+	2636	5.67 ± 1.45		0.11	4813	4.23 ± 1.14		0.0
Nagasaki [109]	15+	1305	5.50 ± 1.39		0.15	1914	4.07 ± 1.02		0.0

Table 1 (continued)

Population	Age Range (years)	Males				Females			
		Total Number	Mean SUA; Std.Dev.	Percent Hyperuri-cemia[a]	Percent Gout	Total Number	Mean SUA; Std.Dev.	Percent Hyperuri-cemia[a]	Percent Gout
Australia									
Sydney [106]	19—59	500	6.28 ± 1.23	23.0	1.4				
Aborigines [58]	20+								
Aurukun		82	6.03 ± 1.25			135	4.78 ± 1.225		
Carpentaria		112	5.87 ± 1.24			170	4.80 ± 1.22		
New Zealand									
Maori [134]	adult								
Whanau-a-apanui		219			8.2	243			1.6
Arawa		83			6.0	103			0.0
NonMaori [134]	adult								
Rotorua		296			0.7	345			0.0
European [174]	20+								
Carterton		202	6.21 ± 1.21	23.3	2.0	228	4.98 ± 1.05	16.7	0.0
Maoris [174]	20+								
New Zealand		365	7.06 ± 1.54	47.1	10.4	382	5.77 ± 1.55	38.7	1.8
Pukapuka		188	7.04 ± 1.10	48.4	5.3	191	6.18 ± 1.05	49.2	0.0
Rarotonga		243	6.96 ± 1.35	44.	2.5	228	5.97 ± 1.20	42.5	0.0
Hawaii	adult								
pure Hawaiians [90]	(mean 44)	49	5.4 ± 1.1		0.0				
American Samoa [92]	adult	71	6.8 ± 1.2		"common"				
Mariana Islands									
Chamorros [32][f]	40+	160	6.23 ± 1.51	21.2		175	5.10 ± 1.41	21.2	
Carolinians [32][f]	40+	26	7.27 ± 1.67	32.7		29	5.70 ± 1.01	32.7	
Chamorros [173]	20+	559	6.9 ± 1.45	44.		655	5.3 ± 1.37	28. (>7.0)	
Palauans [173]	20+	219	6.7 ± 1.62	37. (>6.0)		291	5.3 ± 1.35	22. (>6.0)	
New Guinea [105]	adult								
Lufa highlanders		96	6.98 ± 0.83						
Gumine highlanders		100	6.79 ± 0.89						
Employed highlanders		110	6.55 ± 1.05						
Caucasians		99	6.48 ± 1.37						

Table 1 (continued)

Population	Age Range (years)	Males Total Number	Mean SUA; Std.Dev.	Percent Hyperuricemia[a]	Percent Gout	Females Total Number	Mean SUA; Std.Dev.	Percent Hyperuricemia[a]	Percent Gout
Filipinos									
Pacific Northwest, U.S. [44]									
Filipinos	40—67	113	6.3 ± 1.4						
Caucasians	40—69	88	5.0 ± 1.1						
Hawaii [190]	13+	334	6.23						
Institution [91]	adult								
Filipinos		60	6.1 ± 1.32						
Japanese		73	5.4 ± 1.18						
Caucasian		43	5.2 ± 1.31						
Philippine Islands [93]	21—87								
Manila		140	5.3 ± 1.4						
Cebu		146	5.1 ± 1.2						
Baenotan		115	5.3 ± 1.3						

[a] Using as the upper limit of normal 7.0 mg/100 ml for males and 6.0 mg/100 ml for females, unless otherwise indicated.
[b] Rural population sample.
[c] Urban population sample.
[d] Native African population samples.
[e] Dutch population sample.
[f] Using 7 mg-% for males and 6 mg-% for females, 21.2% of the Chamorros and 32.7% of the Carolinians were reported to be hyperuricemic.
[g] The prevalence of gout was 3.3% in a subsample of 4257 men between 46—52 years of age.

was 10.2% for the New Zealand Maoris, 2.5% for the Rarotongans, and 5.3% for the Pukapukans. A control group of Caucasian subjects living in Carterton were found to have lower mean serum uric acid levels and a much lower prevalence of hyperuricemia [167]. The demonstration of similar degrees of hyperuricemia in these racially similar groups living in different environments was thought to reflect strong genetic predisposition to gout [165]. Clinical gout was strongly associated with obesity and hypertension in the New Zealand Maoris but not in the other 2 groups. The New Zealand Maoris were noted to have a higher fat, alcohol, and calory intake than the other groups, possibly explaining their higher attack rate for gout.

Two Micronesian population groups living in the Mariana Islands in the Central Pacific and racially distinct from the Polynesians, the Chamorros and the Carolinians, have also been shown to have a high frequency of hyperuricemia and gout [32, 173].

These investigations led to the suggestion that the indigenous inhabitants of the Pacific area seemed to be "one large gouty family" [119]. It does not appear that this is entirely correct, however, since not all Pacific populations have been shown to share this high frequency of hyperuricemia and gout. For example, racially pure Hawaiian males, also a Polynesian people, were not found to be hyperuricemic, although they were as obese as the New Zealand Maoris [90]. Similarly, Australian aborigines were found to have mean serum uric acid levels which, although higher than those for a Caucasian population, were lower than those for the Maoris and unassociated with clinical gout [58].

Filipinos

Filipinos residing in the Hawaiian Islands and in the Pacific Northwest of the United States have been found to have both a statistically significantly higher mean serum uric acid level than non-Filipino control subjects and a greater prevalence of clinical gout [43, 44, 66, 91, 175, 190]. Filipinos being inducted into the army in Manila, however, were not found to have elevated serum uric acid levels, and the suggestion was made that hyperuricemia might be limited to Filipinos residing in or originating from the Ilocano provinces in northern Luzon, since most of the Hawaiian and U.S. Filipinos had emigrated from that region [189]. Subsequently, however, Filipinos from the Ilocano region, from Manila, and from Cebu were all found to have mean serum uric acid levels essentially the same as those of U.S. Caucasians [93]. These interesting studies have been interpreted to indicate the interaction of heredity and environment in the production of hyperuricemia. On the one hand, the high frequency of hyperuricemia and gout in Hawaiian and U.S. Filipinos in contrast to presumably racially identical Filipinos who have not left their homeland would appear to be the result of environmental factors. On the other hand, the demonstration that non-Filipino subjects sharing the same environment do not develop hyperuricemia suggests that hereditary factors are involved. The hypothesis has been advanced and supported that the affected Filipinos have a genetically determined renal tubular defect and are therefore incapable of increasing uric acid excretion in response to the higher purine loads imposed by the U.S. diet [89, 93].

Chinese

In a study undertaken because of the clinical impression that gout was unexpectedly common in the Chinese population of Vancouver, Chinese males were found to have a mean serum uric acid level significantly higher than that for Caucasians or Haida Indians [69]. In contrast, Chinese male patients in a mental hospital in Hawaii failed to show elevated serum uric acid levels in comparison with other ethnic groups [91]. Chinese subjects of Taiwan were found to have lower uric acid levels than Malayan Chinese, suggesting dietary or other environmental influences [52].

Japanese

In a comparative study, residents of Hiroshima and Nagasaki, Japan, were found to have mean serum uric acid levels similar to, although somewhat lower than, Caucasian residents of Tecumseh, U.S. [109]. Lower mean serum uric acid values were reported for residents of the Osaka region [181], probably as a result of differences in methods. Among male subjects the prevalence of gout was 0.19% in Hiroshima, 0.15% in Nagasaki, and 0.1% in the Osaka region.

Caucasian Populations

Epidemiologic studies of serum uric acid distribution and/or clinical gout in predominantly Caucasian population groups have shown generally good agreement [69, 84, 99, 144, 163]. The somewhat higher mean values obtained in several recent studies [3, 123, 155, 203] may be explained in part by methodologic differences but do provide some support for the hypothesis that there is a secular trend for increasing serum uric acid levels.

The estimated prevalence of clinical gout in Tecumseh was 0.5% for all male and 0.3% for all female subjects [143]. A similar prevalence, 0.66%, was reported for males over age 15 in the Sudbury study [156]. Somewhat higher prevalences have been reported for European subjects in Carterton, New Zealand [174] and for employees of the Paris Police Department [203], 2.0 and 3.3%, respectively. It should be recognized that the age distribution of the population under study has an important influence on the prevalence estimates obtained. Annual incidence rates have been estimated in several studies. In Sudbury the estimated annual incidence rate for gout was 0.1% for all subjects and 9.95% for hyperuricemic subjects [155]. A remarkably similar overall annual incidence rate of 0.09% was found in the Framingham study [84]. In this study, in which subjects were examined an average of seven times during a 12-year period, a cumulative prevalence rate of 2.8% was obtained for men. In a Finnish study, clinical gout appeared to be rare, only one case being observed among 737 men and none among 1048 women, although all subjects were not specifically examined for gout [99].

American Indians

Investigation of 2 tribes of American Indians revealed serum urate values comparable to those of the Caucasian groups just noted [20]. Mean values for Blackfoot subjects were somewhat higher than for the Pimas in both sexes. Hyperuricemia was uncommon and clinical gout was rare, being found in only two of 473 males in the Pima tribe. The Haida Indians of British Columbia had a low mean serum uric acid level and no hyperuricemia [69]. The Xavante Indians, a very primitive tribe living in the Brazilian interior, had relatively high serum uric acid levels [151].

Relationship of Hyperuricemia to Clinical Manifestations

Acute Gouty Arthritis

The most precise epidemiologic demonstration of the relationship of hyperuricemia to the clinical manifestations of gout is the Framingham study [84]. In this investigation, involving 5127 subjects ages 30 through 59 on entry into the study (mean age 44 years), the risk of development of acute gouty arthritis progressively rose with increasing degrees of hyperuricemia. Thus, gout developed in only 0.6% of males with a maximal serum uric acid level of less than 6 mg/100 ml and 1.9% of those with levels of 6 to 6.9; these figures rose to 16.7% for those with levels of 7 to 7.9, 25% for those with levels of 8 to 8.9, and 90% for those with levels of 9 and over.

Of subjects with clinical gout, 27.7% had serum uric acid levels of less than 6 mg/100 ml and 71% levels of less than 7 mg/100 ml. This finding should not be interpreted to mean that hyperuricemia is not a necessary precondition for the development of gout inasmuch as it is difficult in epidemiologic studies to exclude methodologic errors or the effect of drugs reducing serum urate levels. The differentiation of gout from pseudogout is also difficult in such a setting.

The average age at onset of gout was 47.7 years in males as compared to 51.1 years for females. In male subjects it appeared that the higher the serum uric acid level the earlier the onset of gout. The mean serum urate levels of male and female subjects developing gout was not statistically different, although the mean value for all females was 1.1 mg/100 ml lower than that for all males. The male to female ratio amongst subjects developing gout was 65 to 11, a lower ratio than is reported in most hospital derived statistics.

By the time the mean age of the population had reached 58 years, 1.5% (2.8% of males and 0.4% of females) had experienced one or more acute attacks of gout. The peak incidence of new attacks was about one case per 1000 subjects per year at the time when the mean age of the population was 48 years. Thereafter the incidence of new attacks declined despite the fact that at the time when the mean age of the population was 58 years only one-fifth of those with serum uric acid levels of 8 or over had developed gout. This observation was interpreted as suggesting that the development of gout might not be a function of hyperuricemia and time alone, but that other factors, as yet undefined, might also be involved. Among the possibilities to be further explored in this regard is that of urate-binding to serum proteins. The existence of a specific urate-binding α_{1-2} globulin, deficiency of which would tend to decrease urate solubility, has been described [7]. The isolation and partial characterization of this protein has recently been reported [1, 184]. Study of two gouty kindreds supported the hypothesis that deficiency of this urate-binding α_{1-2} globulin is inherited as an autosomal dominant trait [6]. Other investigations have confirmed the binding of urate to serum proteins, chiefly albumin [63, 125, 182, 183], but not the existence of a specific urate-binding globulin. Several studies have suggested that urate-binding in vivo is probably small and not physiologically significant [63, 182], but further information is needed on this point. It has also been demonstrated that the proteinpolysaccharide components of cartilage act in an as yet undetermined manner to enhance urate solubility, and that this ability is lost when the integrity of the proteinpolysaccharide molecule is destroyed by trypsin digestion, suggesting another mechanism by which urate crystals might be precipitated from saturated tissue fluids [112].

Tophaceous Deposits

In vitro investigations in which crystals of monosodium urate were incubated with sera of varying uric acid content from gouty and normal subjects have provided a model for the deposition of tophaceous deposits [178]. With initial serum urate levels greater than 7 mg/100 ml urate was precipitated from solution, whereas with initial values lower than this level sodium urate went into solution during incubation. From this study one would anticipate a clear relationship between hyperuricemia and tophi in epidemiologic studies. Clinical gout has been rare in most cross-sectional prevalence studies, however, and tophi have seldom been described. In the Framingham study, in which subjects were examined an average of 7 times during a 12-year period, tophi were observed in five men and one woman, all of whom had had acute gouty arthritis, except for one man [84]. Only 7% of the gouty patients had tophi, suggesting that gout as it occurs in the general population is probably milder than that seen in the hospital.

Nephrolithiasis

Uric acid nephrolithiasis is a well recognized manifestation of gout, occurring approximately 1000 times more frequently in gouty patients than in the general population [202]. This gross estimate was based on the report that of admissions to general hospitals, a diagnosis of urinary calculus was made in 9.47 persons per 10000 population [24], and on the assumption that in the United States about 10% of all stones are of uric acid composition. Thus, the prevalence of uric acid calculi in the population at large approximates 0.01%, as compared to 10 to 25% for patients with gout. In other geographic areas, a varying proportion of stones have been reported to be composed of uric acid; one of the highest ratios was reported from Israel where 34.6% of 1800 patients with urolithiasis were found to have uric acid stones [70].

Among the major factors in the pathogenesis of uric acid lithiasis are an increased urinary uric acid concentration, either because of hyperexcretion or reduced urine volume, and low urinary pH [10, 81, 202]. At lower urinary pH more uric acid is present in the undissociated free form, which is more sparingly soluble than the sodium salt. It has been estimated that the free uric acid concentration in a saturated solution of uric acid in urine would be approximately 60 mg/l at pH 5.0, 220 mg/l at pH 6.0, and 1580 mg/l at pH 7.0 [161]. It has been postulated that in gout there is a defect in renal production of ammonia from glutamine; as a result the buffering action of the ammonia is lost and the urine is unduly acid in reaction [81]. Idiopathic uric acid calculi have been reported in patients without either hyperuricemia or hyperuricosuria, both in a sporadic [140] and a familial [47] pattern. The major physiological abnormality in such patients is a low urinary pH [10, 81, 95].

Evidence for the existence of idiopathic uric acid lithiasis as an entity separate from gouty uric acid lithiasis is contained in the report that of 359 such patients followed for up to 12 years only 11 developed gout [70]. The great majority, 81.4%, were normouricemic when first seen and only 13.4% became hyperuricemic during subsequent observation. The male:female ratio was 2.7:1 in contrast to 12.3:1 for gouty uric acid lithiasis. Hyperuricosuria, uric acid excretion greater than 1000 mg per 24 hrs, was present in only 13.6%, but was also infrequent in the gouty group (19%), suggesting that in the subtropical climate of Israel low urinary pH, and perhaps low urinary volume, were decisive factors in stone formation. In this study it was noted that patients of European origin were more frequent than those of Near Eastern-Mediterranean origin, but whether this was a true ethnic difference or a result of bias in patient selection could not be determined.

In spite of the fact that it is the urinary uric acid concentration that is more significant in regard to nephrolithiasis, a relationship between serum levels and urinary calculi (not known to be of uric acid composition) was convincingly demonstrated in the epidemiologic study in Framingham [84]. Of male subjects with a maximal serum uric acid level of 7.0 mg/100 ml or more, 12.7% had a history of stone formation, of those with a maximal level of 8.0 or more, 22% gave such a history, while for those with levels of 9.0 or greater the figure rose to 40%. Of all gouty subjects 13.2% had renal stones, a figure virtually identical with that for all subjects with a maximal serum uric acid level of 7.0 mg/100 ml or greater (13.3%).

Gouty Nephropathy

Renal involvement occurs commonly in gout, and renal insufficiency is a critical development in 18 to 35% of cases [191]. Pathologic changes described in necropsy studies include varying degrees of arterionephrosclerosis, pylonephritis and tophus formation [136]. Changes are usually attributed to deposition of urates in the collecting tubules, resulting in local obstruction, atrophy and necrosis of proximal tubules, secondary fibrosis and bacterial pyelonephritis. Recent studies based on renal biopsy have indicated the early occurrence of glomerulosclerosis, vascular changes, tubular damage and interstitial inflammatory reaction, the latter change being regarded as noninfectious in nature [76, 77]. The precise role played by uric acid in the production of these lesions is obscure, although the early development of chronic renal disease in childhood hyperuricemic syndromes suggests that it may play a significant role [115].

Early attempts to study this problem were limited to acute experiments in which extremely large amounts of urate were infused intravenously, producing a situation more nearly analagous to that induced by cytolytic treatment of leukemia or lymphoma than to urate nephropathy in gout. Recent efforts to provide a more physiologic animal model have employed chronic administration of sodium oxonate, an inhibitor of uricase, to rats [124].

In epidemiologic studies it is obviously difficult, when gout or hyperuricemia coexist with chronic renal disease, to determine which is primary. As a result, there is very little information available in this area. In the Framingham study, however, two gouty subjects were identified who developed and died of renal disease in the course of the study [84]. This observation is at least consistent with the concept of gouty or urate nephropathy, although both subjects had hypertension as well as hyperuricemia on entry into the study and one had roentgenographic evidence of a renal stone.

Coronary Heart Disease

A number of major epidemiologic studies have helped to clarify the role of certain risk factors in the etiology of coronary heart disease, a risk factor being defined as an attribute which occurs more commonly among persons with the disease than among control subjects, although causality is not necessarily implied [60]. Evidence that gout and hyperuricemia constitute risk factors for arteriosclerotic disease is tenuous and difficult to interpret because of the multiple and poorly understood interrelationships with obesity, hypertension, diabetes mellitus, lipid disorders, and other attributes presently accepted as risk factors. An apparent increased prevalence of hyperuricemia in patients with myocardial infarction has been reported [72, 100, 126, 137]. Other investigators have also described an association of hyperuricemia with atherosclerotic conditions [9, 55, 86, 128, 160]. In a study of serum uric acid, cholesterol and triglyceride levels in blood donors, gouty subjects, myocardial infarction patients and cerebral thrombosis patients, it was found that all 3 components were elevated with increased frequency among the myocardial infarction group, whereas the results for the cerebral thrombosis group were identical to those of the blood donors, suggesting that these two major manifestations of arteriosclerosis might have a different metabolic basis [18].

Several epidemiologic studies have reported results concerning the association of serum uric acid levels or gout with coronary heart disease. In the Tecumseh study, males with coronary heart disease had a mean serum uric acid score (serum uric acid measurement adjusted for age, sex and relative weight) that was higher to a statistically significant degree than that of the total test population [150]. More comprehensive information has been reported from the Framingham study [83]. The incidence of coronary heart disease in those with serum uric acid levels over 7 mg/100 ml was twice as high as in those with levels under 4 mg/100 ml, and twice as high among gouty subjects as among the total population. When gouty subjects were removed from the population at risk, however, hyperuricemia no longer was associated with an increased risk of developing coronary heart disease. In this population, gouty subjects had the highest uric acid, blood pressure and cholesterol levels. They were also overweight and tended to consume more alcohol, but did not have higher blood sugar levels or smoke more than the total population at risk. Likewise, in the Evans County study there was a trend for increasing prevalence of coronary heart disease in hyperuricemic subjects, but this association was not significant when blood pressure, cardiovascular drugs and ponderosity were controlled [123]. Much of the accumulated epidemiologic evidence, from South Pacific and other population groups, supports the view that any association of hyperuricemia and gout with coronary heart disease is indirect, depending on the rather frequent occurrence in hyperuricemic subjects of other conditions which are accepted risk-factors for coronary heart disease. In keeping with this view was the demonstration that Pukapukans had as much hyperuricemia and clinical gout as the Maoris and Rarotongans, but almost no hypertension and less obesity, diabetes and ischemic heart disease [165].

Genetic Aspects of Hyperuricemia and Gout

Family Studies

The familial nature of gout has been recognized by physicians for centuries. Investigations of relatives of gouty patients have shown an average prevalence of gout of about 5% and of hyperuricemia of about 25%. In the late 1940s SMYTH et al. [185] suggested, on the basis of a study of 19 gouty families, that hyperuricemia was apparently due to a single autosomal dominant gene. STECHER et al. [188], in a similar study, reached much the same conclusion, although in some of their families hyperuricemia resembled an autosomal recessive trait. In both studies it was necessary to assume that the gene had incomplete penetrance, to a greater degree in the female. In both studies a key finding was the apparently bimodal distribution of uric acid levels. In 1955 HAUGE and HARVALD [88], reporting data regarding uric acid levels of siblings of gouty patients, found no evidence of bimodality and concluded that hyperuricemia was the result of the additive effect of multiple genes. In 1964 a report [152] based on re-examination [171] of the families in the original SMYTH et al. study after an average interval of 18 years also concluded that the evidence for bimodality was not convincing and that the hypothesis of multifactorial inheritance was "at least as tenable" as the one gene-hyperuricemia hypothesis. While these studies agree in suggesting a role for familial factors in the determination of uric acid levels, it has been repeatedly cautioned that not all familial factors are genetically determined; many infectious, nutritional or behavioral disorders, for example, demonstrate familial aggregation.

Population Studies

A number of population studies have been reported in which serum uric acid determinations were included. Some have purported to show a bimodal distribution curve, which would support the monogenic theory, while others have described a unimodal distribution which would be compatible with a polygenic basis for hyperuricemia. Of the studies describing a bimodal distribution most have been based on relatively small population samples and can quite probably be explained on the basis of sampling error. The larger studies are in generally good agreement in reporting a unimodal distribution which is skewed toward the higher values [84, 144, 155]. While such skewing may result from the superimposition of two normal distribution curves, this is a hypothesis which is most difficult to prove.

Analysis of data from the Pima and Blackfeet Indians in the U.S. revealed no evidence of a bimodal distribution either in the population as a whole or in the relatives of hyperuricemic probands [20]. The authors concluded that the uric acid level was a polygenic trait with a rather low degree of heritability; environmental factors were regarded as of major importance. Estimates of heritability in the Tecumseh study were similarly low and relatives of gouty or hyperuricemic probands showed no significant aggregation of gout or hyperuricemia [71]. An interesting observation in both of these studies was the higher degree of association of serum uric acid levels in mothers and daughters than in fathers and sons, raising the possibility of sex-linkage. No support for this possibility was found in more detailed analysis of the Tecumseh data and it was concluded that the serum uric acid phenotype resulted from the interaction of multifactorial inheritance with certain environmental factors.

Twin Studies

The twin-study approach is based on the fact that identical (or monozygotic) twins have identical genes; hence any differences in phenotype can be attributed to environmental factors. Fraternal (or dizygotic) twins, on the other hand, are not more alike than ordinary sibs; phenotypic differences between them thus reflect the influence of heredity as well as environment. Thus, in comparing monozygotic and like-sexed dizygotic twins, the finding of similar degrees of concordance in the two groups would suggest that the phenotypic trait under study was determined by environment. If monozygotic twins have a higher degree of concordance, it is an indication that genetic factors are involved.

Further information can be gained by comparing monozygotic twins raised together with those raised apart. A high degree of concordance in monozygous twins raised apart would indicate strong hereditary influence, whereas a high degree of discordance in this group would indicate strong environmental influences. Among the procedural problems encountered in such studies are the difficulties in collecting an adequate twin population, in accurately determining zygosity, and in classifying twins as concordant or discordant in the case of quantitative traits such as serum uric acid. The latter problem can be dealt with by studying intrapair differences in the various twin groups.

Only recently have such studies been reported which deal with serum uric acid. In 1965, JENSEN and others reported a study of serum lipids and uric acid in 67 pairs of twins [102]. In comparing mono- and dizygotic twins the intrapair difference was found to be significantly less for monozygotic than for dizygotic twins, indicating a genetic influence. It was also demonstrated that twins living apart had greater intrapair differences than twins living together, suggesting an environmental influence on serum uric acid level. The relative importance of environmental and hereditary influences on the serum uric acid phenotype could not be estimated from the authors' data. More recently BOYLE and others have reported a study of serum uric acid levels in 112 twin pairs, 51 of whom were monozygotic [25]. Intrapair variance in serum uric acid levels was significantly less for monozygotic twins than for dizygotic twins in the case of female subjects but not for the males. Intrapair variance for twins living apart was significantly greater than for twins living together in the case of monozygotic females; similar but less marked differences were present in the other groups except for the dizygotic male group which was very small: The authors concluded that their findings indicated a "fairly strong genetic control of the variation in serum uric acid levels in females. The failure to demonstrate a genetic control of the normal serum uric acid level in the male does not mean that such control does not exist but merely that it is likely to be weak and that there is a very strong environmental factor (or factors) operating in males in control of the serum uric acid level".

Identified Genetic Defects Associated with Hyperuricemia and Gout

Available evidence indicates that hyperuricemia may be the result of any one or more genetically or environmentally determined disorders producing either overproduction or decreased renal excretion of uric acid, and that acute gouty arthritis is a frequent complication of hyperuricemia, irrespective of its etiology. Once multifactorial inheritance has been demonstrated, as it clearly has for hyperuricemia, the challenge to the geneticist, clinical investigator, and epidemiologist is to identify the individual specific abnormalities and study their inheritance. Significant progress has been made in this regard. Soon after the clinical description of a childhood syndrome characterized by hyperuricemia, choreoathetosis, mental retardation and selfmutilation (the Lesch–Nyhan syndrome) [135] it was demonstrated that patients with this condition lacked the enzyme hypoxanthine-guanine phosphoribosyltransferase [179]. Subsequently it was found that some subjects with adult onset gout and with no or mild neurological and behavioral disorder had a partial deficiency of this same enzyme [117]. The properties of the mutant enzyme differed in two families studied, suggesting a different molecular alteration in each family. Family studies have indicated an X-linked pattern of inheritance for complete and partial deficiencies of this enzyme [94]. It is known that this defect accounts for only a small proportion of hyperuricemia, even among that subgroup characterized by overproduction of uric acid. There is no available information regarding the frequency of this enzyme defect in the general population, although it has been detected in 5 of 110 gouty patients in one center [115] and in 7 of 425 subjects with hyperuricemia and gouty arthritis or uric acid stone or both in another [200]. Screening tests for this condition have been described [35, 113], but have not been employed in broad epidemiologic studies.

Partial deficiency of a closely related enzyme, adenine phosphoribosyltransferase, has been described in patients without apparent abnormality of uric acid metabolism [116]. Evidence suggested that this defect was autosomally transmitted. As yet, subjects with the homozygous form of this enzyme deficiency have not been described. A single case has been reported of a 3-year-old boy with marked overproduction of uric acid, mild developmental retardation, dysplastic teeth and absence of tears when crying who had normal activity of hypoxanthine-guanine phosphoribosyltransferase [153]. The nature of the metabolic metabolic abnormality in this patient has not yet been elucidated.

Two pairs of brothers with hyperuricemia and clinical gout (and uric acid lithiasis in one pair) have been described in whom purine overproduction was associated with increased phosphoribosylpyrophosphate synthetase activity [15, 187]. This defect similarly appears to be heterogeneous and to account for only a small percentage of cases of hyperuricemia.

The occurrence of hyperuricemia and gout in association with glucose-6-phosphatase deficiency has been reported, and it has been demonstrated that both increased biosynthesis and decreased renal excretion of uric acid contribute to the hyperuricemia [5, 101, 118]. Hyperuricemia, apparently due to inhibition of renal urate excretion by the accumulated branched-chain keto acids, has also been described in a 20-month-old girl with a mild variant of maple syrup urine disease [177]. Deficiency of carboxylase activities for the keto acids of leucine, isoleucine and valine was demonstrated in this patient, and in cultured fibroblasts from one patient each with classic and intermittent maple syrup urine disease [40]. There seems little doubt but that with time additional specific enzymatic defects resulting in hyperuricemia and gout will be identified.

Programs for Prevention of Gout

The major goal of both basic medical research and epidemiologic studies is the acquisition of sufficient knowledge regarding etiology and pathogenesis to permit the application of effective therapeutic or preventive measures. Present knowledge permits contemplation of programs for the prevention of gout. It is now established that the acute gouty attack and the tophaceous deposit both result from precipitation of urate crystals from hyperuricemic body fluids. It is a reasonable assumption, though not yet proven on any substantial scale, that correction of hyperuricemia and maintenance of serum uric acid levels within the normal range will remove the risk of development of gouty arthritis and tophaceous deposits. Cobb [36] has suggested that a serum uric acid level of 8 mg/100 ml or above might serve as a manageable screening level for such a preventive program. The distribution of serum uric acid levels in the Tecumseh study would suggest that approximately 3% of the population might be selected for preventive therapy at this screening level [144]. Others have suggested that hypouricemic therapy be considered for asymptomatic patients with levels above 9 mg/100 ml.

A number of other considerations enter into any decision regarding preventive programs. Questions of inconvenience, expense and risk to the patient need to be evaluated. Patient motivation and education are of great importance since the individual with asymptomatic hyperuricemia feels no better and notices no change when he is made normouricemic. The natural history of gout and the present availability of effective therapeutic agents would argue against the routine introduction of preventive therapy. Individuals with hyperuricemia may remain asymptomatic for many years before developing an acute attack of gout, indeed some may never do so. Acute gout, when it occurs, can be effectively controlled by any of a number of available drugs. Fortunately, tophi rarely develop prior to an initial attack of gout. As a consequence, the risk of tophaceous deposit does not argue strongly for the early correction of asymptomatic hyperuricemia. The nature of the relationship between hyperuricemia and other disorders, including arteriosclerosis, coronary heart disease, hypertension, renal disease, diabetes mellitus and lipid disorders, has not been clearly established in each case and there is little evidence at present that correction of hyperuricemia by itself directly influences any of these conditions.

In dealing with asymptomatic hyperuricemia in otherwise healthy persons, whether identified through screening programs or individual examination it seems reasonable to pursue an intermediate course. Such persons should be informed of the abnormality and of the potential risks entailed. They should be carefully evaluated with respect to blood pressure, glucose tolerance, lipid disturbance, and evidence of arteriosclerosis. Where abnormalities are found, they should be treated appropriately. Occasionally, with an intelligent, cooperative patient with a strong positive family history, the decision may be made to institute treatment to lower the serum uric acid level. More often, perhaps, it will be to recommend periodic re-evaluation and to ensure prompt, effective treatment of any acute arthritis that may develop, as well as reconsideration of additional therapeutic measures thereafter.

References

1. AAKESSON, I., ALVSAKER, J. O.: The Urate-Binding α_{1-2} Globulin. Isolation and Characterization of the Protein from Human Plasma. Europ. J. clin. Invest. **1**, 281 (1971).
2. ACHESON, R. M.: Epidemiology of Serum Uric Acid and Gout: An Example of the Complexities of Multifactorial Causation. Proc. roy. Soc. Med. **63**, 193 (1970).
3. ACHESON, R. M., CHAN, Y. K.: New Haven Survey of Joint Diseases: The Prediction of Serum Uric Acid in a General Population. J. chron. Dis. **21**, 543 (1969).
4. ADLERSBERG, D.: Newer Advances in Gout. Bull. N.Y. Acad. Med. **25**, 651 (1949).
5. ALEPA, F. P., HOWELL, R. R., KLINENBERG, J. R., SEEGMILLER, J. E.: Relationships Between Glycogen Storage Disease and Tophaceous Gout. Amer. J. Med. **42**, 58 (1967).
6. ALVSAKER, J. O.: Genetic Studies in Primary Gout: Investigations on the Plasma Levels of the Urate-Binding $\alpha_1-\alpha_2$-Globulin in Individuals from Two Gouty Kindreds. J. clin. Invest. **47**, 1254 (1968).
7. ALVSAKER, J. O.: Uric Acid in Human Plasma. V. Isolation and Identification of Plasma Proteins Interacting with Urate. Scand. J. clin. Lab. Invest. **18**, 227 (1966).
8. ANUMONYE, A., DOBSON, J. W., OPPENHEIM, S., SUTHERLAND, J. S.: Plasma Uric Acid Concentrations Among Edinburgh Business Executives. J. Amer. med. Ass. **208**, 1141 (1969).
9. ASK UPMARK, E., ADNER, M. L.: Coronary Infarction and Gout. Acta med. scand. **139**, 1 (1950).
10. ATSMON, A., DEVRIES, A., FRANK, M.: *Uric Acid Lithiasis*, p. 55. Amsterdam: Elsevier Publishing 1963.
11. BALL, G. V., MORGAN, J. M.: Chronic Lead Ingestion and Gout. Sth. med. J. (Bgham, Ala.) **61**, 21 (1968).
12. BARLOW, K. A.: Lipid Metabolism in Gout. Proc. roy. Soc. Med. **59**, 325 (1966).
13. BARON, D. N., DENT, C. E., HARRIS, H., HART, E. W., JEPSON, J. B.: Hereditary Pellagra-like Skin Rash with Temporary Cerebellar Ataxia, Constant Renal Amino-Aciduric and other Bizarre Biochemical Features. Lancet **1956 II**, 421.
14. BEARN, A. G., YU, T. F., GUTMAN, A. B.: Renal Function in Wilson's Disease. J. clin. Invest. **36**, 1107 (1957).
15. BECKER, M. A., MEYER, L. J., SEEGMILLER, J. E.: Gout with Overproduction due to Increased Phosphoribosylpyrophosphate Synthetase Avtivity. Amer. J. Med. **55**, 232 (1973).
16. BECKETT, A. G., LEWIS, J. G.: Gout and the Serum Uric Acid in Diabetes Mellitus. Quart. J. Med. **29**, 443 (1960).
17. BEIGHTON, P., SOLOMON, L., SOSKOLNE, C. L., SWEET, B.: Serum Uric Acid Concentrations in a Rural Tiwana Community in Southern Africa. Ann. rheum. Dis. **32**, 346 (1973).
18. BENEDEK, T. G.: Correlations of Serum Uric Acid and Lipid Concentration in Normal, Gouty, and Athersclerotic Men. Ann. intern. Med. **66**, 851 (1967).
19. BENNETT, J. S., BOND, J., SINGER, I., GOTTLIEB, A. J.: Hypouricemia in Hodgkin's Disease. Ann. intern. Med. **76**, 751 (1972).
20. BENNETT, P. H., BURCH, T. A.: Serum Uric Acid and Gout in Blackfeet and Pima Indians. In: BENNETT, P. H., WOOD, P. H. N. (Eds.): Population Studies of the Rheumatic Diseases, pp. 358—362. Amsterdam: Excerpta Medica Foundation 1968.
21. BERKOWITZ, D.: Blood Lipid and Uric Acid Interrelationships. J. Amer. med. Ass. **190**, 856 (1964).
22. BERKOWITZ, D.: Gout, Hyperlipidemia, and Diabetes Interrelationships. J. Amer. med. Ass. **197**, 77 (1966).

23. BLUESTONE, R., LEWIS, B., MERVART, I.: Hyperlipoproteinaemia in Gout. Ann. rheum. Dis. **30**, 134 (1971).
24. BOYCE, W. H., GARVEY, F. K., STRAWCUTTER, H. E.: Incidence of Urinary Calculi Among Patients in General Hospitals, 1948 to 1952. J. Amer. med. Ass. **161**, 1437 (1956).
25. BOYLE, J. A., GRIEG, W. R., JASANI, M. K., DUNCAN, A., DIVER, M., BUCHANAN, W. W.: Relative Roles of Genetic and Environmental Factors in the Control of Serum Uric Acid Levels in Normouricaemic Subjects. Ann. rheum. Dis. **26**, 234 (1967).
26. BOYLE, J. A., MEKIDDIE, M., BUCHANAN, K. D., JASANI, M. K., GRAY, H. W., JACKSON, I. M. D., BUCHANAN, W. W.: Diabetes Mellitus and Gout. Blood Sugar and Plasma Insulin Responses to Oral Glucose in Normal Weight, Overweight and Gouty Patients. Ann. rheum. Dis. **28**, 374 (1969).
27. BRADFORD, M. J., KRAKOFF, I. H., LEEPER, R., BALIS, M. E.: Study of Purine Metabolism in a Xanthinuric Female. J. clin. Invest. **47**, 1325 (1968).
28. BRECKINRIDGE, A.: Hypertension and Hyperuricemia. Lancet **1966 I**, 15.
29. BRØCHNER-MORTENSEN, K.: Review of Diagnostic Criteria and Known Etiological Factors in Gout. In: The Epidemiology of Chronic Rheumatism, pp. 140—155. Oxford: Blackwell Scientific Publications; Philadelphia: F. A. Davis 1963.
30. BROOKS, G. W., MUELLER, E.: Serum Urate Concentrations Among University Professors; Relation to Drive, Achievement, and Leadership. J. Amer. med. Ass. **195**, 415 (1966).
31. BURCH, R. E., KURKE, N.: The Effect of Lactate Infusion on Serum Uric Acid. Proc. Soc. exp. Biol. (N.Y.) **127**, 17 (1968).
32. BURCH, T. A., O'BRIEN, W. M., NEED, R., KURLAND, L. T.: Hyperuricaemia and Gout in the Mariana Islands. Ann. rheum. Dis. **25**, 114 (1966).
33. BYWATERS, E. G. L., HOLLOWAY, V. P.: Measurement of Serum Uric Acid in Great Britain in 1963. Ann. rheum. Dis. **23**, 236 (1964).
34. CANNON, P. J., STASON, W. B., DEMARTINI, F. E., SOMMERS, S. C., LARAGH, H. J.: Hyperuricemia in Primary and Renal Hypertension. New Engl. J. Med. **275**, 457 (1966).
35. CHOW, D. C., KAWAHARA, F. S., SAUNDERS, T., SORENSEN, L. B.: A New Assay Method for Hypoxanthine-Guanine Phosphoribosyltransferase. J. Lab. clin. Med. **76**, 733 (1970).
36. COBB, S. (Editorial): The Prevention of Gout. Amer. J. publ. Hlth. **55**, 53 (1965).
37. COBURN, S. P., SIRLIN, E. M., MERTZ, E. T.: Metabolism of N^{15} Labeled Uric Acid in Down's Syndrome. Metabolism **17**, 560 (1968).
38. COWDREY, S. C.: Hyperuricemia in Infectious Mononucleosis. J. Amer. med. Ass. **196**, 107 (1966).
39. CRISTOFORI, F. C., DUNCAN, G. G.: Uric Acid Excretion in Obese Subjects During Periods of Total Fasting. Metabolism **13**, 303 (1964).
40. DANCIS, J., HUTZLER, J., COX, R. P.: Enzyme Defect in Skin Fibroblasts in Intermittent Branched-Chain Ketonuria and in Maple Syrup Urine Disease. Biochem. Med. **2**, 407 (1969).
41. DARLINGTON, L. G., SCOTT, J. T.: Plasma Lipid Levels in Gout. Ann. rheum. Dis. **31**, 487 (1972).
42. DECKER, J. L. (Chairman): Report from the Subcommittee on Diagnostic Criteria for Gout. In: BENNETT, P. H., WOOD, P. H. N. (Eds.): Population Studies of the Rheumatic Diseases, pp. 385—386. Amsterdam: Excerpta Medica Foundation 1968.
43. DECKER, J. L., LANE, J. L.: Gouty Arthritis in Filipinos. New Engl. J. Med. **261**, 805 (1959).
44. DECKER, J. L., LANE, J. L., REYNOLDS, W. E.: Hyperuricemia in a Male Filipino Population. Arthr. and Rheum. **5**, 144 (1962).
45. DECOEK, N. M.: Serum Urate and Urate Clearance in Diabetes Mellitus. Aust. Ann. Med. **14**, 205 (1965).
46. DENIS, G., LAVNAY, M. P.: Carbohydrate Intolerance in Gout. Metabolism **18**, 770 (1969).
47. DEVRIES, A., FRANK, M., ATSMON, A.: Inherited Uric Acid Lithiasis. Amer. J. Med. **33**, 880 (1962).
48. DODGE, H. J., MIKKELSEN, W. M.: The Relationship of Serum Uric Acid Scores to Occupation, Smoking Habits and Drinking Habits. Presented at the Annual Meeting of the Amer. Public Hlth. Assoc., New York 1964.
49. DODGE, H. J., MIKKELSEN, W. M.: Association of Serum Uric Acid Scores with Occupation: Male Heads of Households in Tecumseh Michigan 1959—1960. J. occup. Med. **10**, 402 (1968).
50. DRENICK, E. J.: Hyperuricemia, Acute Gout, Renal Insufficiency and Urate Nephrolithiasis Due to Starvation. Arthr. and Rheum. **8**, 988 (1965).
51. DREYFUSS, F., YARON, E., BALOGH, M.: Blood Uric Acid Levels in Various Ethnic Groups in Israel. Amer. J. med. Sci. **247**, 438 (1964).

52. DUFF, I. F., MIKKELSEN, W. M., DODGE, H. J., HIMES, D. S.: Comparison of Uric Acid Levels in Some Oriental and Caucasian Groups Unselected as to Gout or Hyperuricemia. Arthr. and Rheum. **11**, 184 (1968).
53. DUNN, J. P., BROOKS, G. W., MAUSNER, J., RODMAN, G. P., COBB, S.: Social Class Gradient of Serum Uric Acid Levels in Males. J. Amer. med. Ass. **185**, 431 (1963).
54. DUNN, J. P., MOSES, C.: Correlation of Serum Lipids with Uric Acid and Blood Sugar in Normal Males. Metabolism **14**, 788 (1965).
55. EIDLITZ, M.: Uric Acid and Arteriosclerosis. Lancet **1961 II**, 1046.
56. EISEN, A. Z., SEEGMILLER, J. E.: Uric Acid Metabolism in Psoriasis. J. clin. Invest. **40**, 1486 (1961).
57. EMMERSON, B. T.: The Clinical Differentiation of Lead Gout from Primary Gout. Arthr. and Rheum. **11**, 623 (1968).
58. EMMERSON, B. T., DOUGLAS, W., DOHERTY, R. L., FEIGL, P.: Serum Urate Concentrations in the Australian Aboriginal. Ann. rheum. Dis. **28**, 150 (1969).
59. EMMERSON, B. T., KNOWLES, B. R.: Triglyceride Concentrations in Primary Gout and Gout of Chronic Lead Nephropathy. Metabolism **20**, 721 (1971).
60. EPSTEIN, F. H.: The Epidemiology of Coronary Heart Disease: A Review. J. chron. Dis. **18**, 735 (1965).
61. EVANS, J. G., PRIOR, I. A. M., HARVEY, H. P. B.: Relation of Serum Uric Acid to Body Bulk, Haemoglobin, and Alcohol Intake in Two South Pacific Polynesian Populations. Ann. rheum. Dis. **27**, 319 (1968).
62. EVANS, J. G., PRIOR, I. A. M., MORRISON, R. B. I.: The Carterton Study: 5. Serum Uric Acid Levels of a Sample of New Zealand European Adults. N.Z. med. J. **70**, 306 (1969).
63. FARRELL, P. C., POPOVICH, R. P., BABB, A. L.: Binding Levels of Urate Ions in Human Serum Albumin and Plasma. Biochim. biophysica Acta (Amst.) **243**, 49 (1971).
64. FELDMAN, E. B., WALLACE, S. L.: Hypertriglyceridemia in Gout. Circulation **29**, 508 (1964).
65. FESSEL, W. J.: Hyperuricemia in Health and Disease. Seminars in Arthritis and Rheumatism **1**, 275 (1972).
66. FISHER, H. W.: The Diseases of Filipino Men. Hawaii med. J. **18**, 252 (1959).
67. FLATZ, G.: Genetic and Constitutional Influences on Serum-Uric-Acid in a Tropical Rural Population. Hum. Genet. **11**, 83 (1971).
68. FLOREY, C. DU V., ACHESON, R. M.: Serum Uric Acid in United States and Brazilian Military Recruits with a Note on ABO Blood Groups. Amer. J. Epidem. **88**, 178 (1968).
69. FORD, D. K., DEMOS, A. M.: Serum Uric Acid Levels of Healthy Caucasian, Chinese and Haida Indian Males in British Columbia. Canad. med. Ass. J. **90**, 1295 (1964).
70. FRANK, M., LAZEBNIK, J., DEVRIES, A.: Uric Acid Lithiasis—A Study of Six Hundred and Twenty-Two Patients. Urol. int. (Basel) **25**, 32 (1970).
71. FRENCH, J. G., DODGE, H. J., KJELSBERG, M. O., MIKKELSEN, W. M., SCHULL, W. J.: A Study of Familial Aggregation of Serum Uric Acid Levels in the Population of Tecumseh, Michigan, 1959—1960. Amer. J. Epidem. **25**, 117 (1966).
72. GERTLER, M. M., GARN, S. M., LEVINE, S. A.: Serum Uric Acid in Relation to Age and Physique in Health and in Coronary Heart Disease. Ann. intern. Med. **34**, 1421 (1951).
73. GLUECK, C. J., LEVY, R. I., FREDERICKSON, D. S.: Acute Tendinitis and Arthritis: A Presenting Symptom of Familial Type II Hyperlipoproteimia. J. Amer. med. Ass. **206**, 2895 (1968).
74. GOLD, M. S., WILLIAMS, J. C., SPIVACK, M., GRANN, V.: Sickle Cell Anemia and Hyperuricemia. J. Amer. med. Ass. **206**, 1572 (1968).
75. GOLDFINGER, S., KLINENBERG, J. R., SEEGMILLER, J. E.: Renal Retention of Uric Acid Induced by Infusion of β-Hydroxybutyrate and Acetoacetate. New Engl. J. Med. **272**, 351 (1965).
76. GONICK, H. C., RUBINI, M. E., GLEASON, I. O., SOMMERS, S. C.: The Renal Lesion in Gout. Ann. intern. Med. **62**, 667 (1965).
77. GREENBAUM, D., ROSS, J. H., STEINBERG, V. L.: Renal Biopsy in Gout. Brit. med. J. **1961 I**, 1502.
78. GREENE, M. L., MARCUS, R., AURBACH, G. D., KAZAM, E. S., SEEGMILLER, J. E.: Hypouricemia due to Isolated Renal Tubular Defect. Dalmation Dog Mutation in Man. Amer. J. Med. **53**, 361 (1972).
79. GUTMAN, H. B., YU, T. F.: A Three-Compartment System for Regulation of Renal Excretion of Uric Acid in Man. Trans. Ass. Amer. Phycns. **74**, 353 (1961).
80. GUTMAN, A. B., YU, T. F.: Secondary Gout. Ann. intern. Med. **56**, 675 (1962).
81. GUTMAN, A. B., YU, T. F.: Uric Acid Nephrolithiasis. Amer. J. Med. **45**, 756 (1968).

82. GUTMAN, A. B., YU, T. F., BERGER, L.: Tubular Secretion of Urate in Man. J. clin. Invest. **38**, 1778 (1959).
83. HALL, A. P.: Correlations Among Hyperuricemia, Hypercholesterolemia, Coronary Disease and Hypertension. Arthr. and Rheum. **8**, 846 (1965).
84. HALL, A. P., BARRY, P. E., DAWBER, T. R., MCNAMARA, P. M.: Epidemiology of Gout and Hyperuricemia; a Long-Term Population Study. Amer. J. Med. **42**, 27 (1967).
85. HANDLER, J. S.: The Role of Lactic Acid in the Reduced Excretion of Uric Acid in Toxemia of Pregnancy. J. clin. Invest. **39**, 1526 (1960).
86. HANSEN, O. E.: Hyperuricemia, Gout and Atherosclerosis. Amer. Heart J. **72**, 570 (1966).
87. HARRIS-JONES, J. N., JONES, E. G., WELLS, P. G.: Xanthomatosus and Essential Hypercholesterolemia. Lancet **1957 I**, 855.
88. HAUGE, M., HARVALD, B.: Heredity in Gout and Hyperuricemia. Acta med. scand. **152**, 247 (1955).
89. HEALEY, L. A., BAYANI-SIOSON, P. S. P.: A Defect in the Renal Excretion of Uric Acid in Filipinos. Arthr. and Rheum. **14**, 721 (1971).
90. HEALEY, L. A., CAMER, J. E. Z., BASSETT, D. R., DECKER, J. L.: Serum Uric Acid and Obesity in Hawaiians. J. Amer. med. Ass. **196**, 364 (1966).
91. HEALEY, L. A., CANER, J. E. Z., DECKER, J. L.: Ethnic Variations in Serum Uric Acid. I. Filipino Hyperuricemia in a Controlled Environment. Arthr. and Rheum. **9**, 288 (1966).
92. HEALEY, L. A., JONES, K. W.: Hyperuricemia in American Samoans. Arthr. and Rheum. **14**, 283 (1971).
93. HEALEY, L. A., SKEITH, M. D., DECKER, J. L., BAYANI-SIOSON, P. S.: Hyperuricemia in Filipinos: Interaction of Heredity and Environment. Amer. J. hum. Genet. **19**, 81 (1967).
94. HENDERSON, J. F., KELLEY, W. N., ROSENBLOOM, F. M., SEEGMILLER, J. E.: Inheritance of Purine Phosphoribosyltransferases in Man. Amer. J. hum. Genet. **21**, 61 (1969).
95. HENNEMAN, P. H., WALLACH, S., DEMPSEY, E. F.: The Metabolic Defect Responsible for Uric Acid Stone Formation. J. clin. Invest. **41**, 537 (1962).
96. HERMAN, J. B.: Gout and Diabetes. Metabolism **7**, 793 (1958).
97. HERMAN, J. B., MOUNT, F. W., MEDALIE, J. H., GROEN, J. J., DUBLIN, T. D., NEUFELD, N. H., RISS, E.: Diabetes Prevalence and Serum Uric Acid. Observations Among 10000 Men in a Survey of Ischemic Heart Disease in Israel. Diabetes **16**, 858 (1967).
98. ISOMÄKI, H.: Hyperuricaemia in Northern Finland. An Epidemiological Study of Serum Uric Acid in Rural, Urban and Hospital Populations. Ann. clin. Res., Suppl. 1, 1969.
99. ISOMÄKI, H. A., TAKKUNEN, H.: Gout and Hyperuricemia in a Finnish Rural Population. Acta rheum. scand. **15**, 112 (1969).
100. JACOBS, D.: Hyperuricaemia and Myocardial Infarction. S. Afr. med. J. **46**, 367 (1972).
101. JAKOVCIC, S., SORENSEN, L. B.: Studies of Uric Acid Metabolism in Glycogen Storage Disease Associated with Gouty Arthritis. Arthr. and Rheum. **10**, 129 (1967).
102. JENSEN, J., BLANKENHORN, D. H., CHIN, H. P., STURGEON, P., WARE, A. G.: Serum Lipids and Serum Uric Acid in Human Twins. J. Lipid Res. **6**, 193 (1965).
103. JENSEN, J., BLANKENHORN, D. H., KORNERUP, V.: Blood-Uric-Acid Levels in Familial Hypercholesterolaemia. Lancet **1966 I**, 298.
104. JOSLIN, E. P., ROTT, H. F., WHITE, P., MARBLE, A.: The Treatment of Diabetes Mellitus, Ninth Ed., p. 93. Philadelphia: Lea and Febiger 1952.
105. JEREMY, R., RHODES, F. A.: Studies of Serum Urate Levels in New Guineans Living in Different Environments. Med. J. Aust. **1**, 897 (1971).
106. JEREMY, R., TOWSON, J.: Serum Urate Levels and Gout in Australian Males. Med. J. Aust. **1**, 116 (1971).
107. KASL, S. V., BROOKS, G. W., COBB, S.: Serum Urate Concentrations in Male High School Students, A Predictor of College Attendance. J.A.M.A. J. Amer. med. Ass. **198**, 713 (1966).
108. KASL, S. V., COBB, S., BROOKS, G. W.: Changes in Serum Uric Acid and Cholesterol Levels in Men Undergoing Job Loss. J. Amer. med. Ass. **206**, 1500 (1968).
109. KATO, H., DUFF, I. F., RUSSELL, W. F., UDA, Y., HAMILTON, H. B., KAWAMOTO, S., JOHNSON, K. G.: Rheumatoid Arthritis and Gout in Hiroshima and Nagasaki, Japan: A Prevalence and Incidence Study. J. chron. Dis. **23**, 659 (1971).
110. KATZ, J. L., WEINER, H.: Psychosomatic Considerations in Hyperuricemia and Gout. Psychosom. Med. **34**, 165 (1972).

111. KATZ, J. L., WEINER, H., GUTMAN, A., YU, T. F.: Hyperuricemia, Gout, and the Executive Suite. J. Amer. med. Ass. **224**, 1251 (1973).
112. KATZ, W. A., SCHUBERT, M.: The Interaction of Monosodium Urate with Connective Tissue Components. J. clin. Invest. **49**, 1783 (1970).
113. KAUFMAN, J. M., GREENE, M. L., SEEGMILLER, J. E.: Urine Uric Acid to Creatinine Ratio—A Screening Test for Inherited Disorders of Purine Metabolism. J. Pediat. **73**, 583 (1968).
114. KAUFMAN, J. M., O'BRIEN, W. M.: Hyperuricemia in Mongolism. New Engl. J. Med. **276**, 953 (1967).
115. KELLEY, W. N., GREENE, M. L., ROSENBLOOM, F. M., HENDERSON, J. F., SEEGMILLER, J. E.: Hypoxanthine-Guanine Phosphoribosyltransferase in Gout. Ann. intern. Med. **70**, 155 (1969).
116. KELLEY, W. N., LEVY, R. I., ROSENBLOOM, F. M., HENDERSON, J. F., SEEGMILLER, J. E.: Adenine Phosphoribosyltransferase Deficiency: A Previously Undescribed Genetic Defect in Man. J. clin. Invest. **47**, 2281 (1968).
117. KELLEY, W. N., ROSENBLOOM, F. M., HENDERSON, J. F., SEEGMILLER, J. R.: A Specific Enzyme Defect in Gout Associated with Overproduction of Uric Acid. Proc. nat. Acad. Sci. (Wash.) **57**, 1735 (1967).
118. KELLEY, W. N., ROSENBLOOM, F. M., SEEGMILLER, J. E., HOWELL, R. R.: Excessive Production of Uric Acid in Type I Glycogen Storage Disease. J. Pediat. **72**, 488 (1968).
119. KELLGREN, J. H.: The Epidemiology of Rheumatic Diseases. Ann. rheum. Dis. **23**, 109 (1964).
120. KHACHADURIAN, A. K.: Migratory Polyarthritis in Familial Hypercholesterolemia (Type II Hyperlipoproteinemia). Arthr. and Rheum. **11**, 385 (1968).
121. KHACHADURIAN, A. K., ARSLANIAN, M. J.: Hypouricemia due to Renal Uricosuria: A Case Study. Ann. intern. Med. **78**, 547 (1973).
122. KINSEY, R., WALTHER, R., SISE, H. S., WHITLAW, G., SMITHWICK, R.: Incidence of Hyperuricemia in 400 Hypertensive Patients. Circulation **24**, 972 (1961).
123. KLEIN, R., KLEIN, B. E., CORNONI, J. C., MAREABY, J., CASSEL, J. C., TYROLER, H. A.: Serum Uric Acid. Its Relationship to Coronary Heart Disease Risk Factors and Cardiovascular Disease, Evans County, Georgia. Arch. intern. Med. **132**, 401 (1973).
124. KLINENBERG, J. R., BLUESTONE, R., SCHLOSSTEIN, L., WAISMAN, J., WHITEHOUSE, M. W.: Urate Deposition Disease. How is it Regulated and How Can it be Modified? Ann. intern. Med. **78**, 99 (1973).
125. KLINENBERG, J. R., KIPPEN, I.: The Binding of Urate to Plasma Proteins Determined by Means of Equilibrium Dialysis. J. Lab. clin. Med. **75**, 503 (1970).
126. KOHN, P. M., PROZAN, G. B.: Hyperuricemia—Relationship to Hypercholesterolemia and Acute Myocardial Infarction. J. Amer. med. Ass. **170**, 1909 (1959).
127. KRAKOFF, I. H.: Clinical Pharmacology of Drugs Which Influence Uric Acid Production and Excretion. Clin. Pharmacol. Ther. **8**, 124 (1967).
128. KRAMER, D. W., PERILSTEIN, P. K., DEMEDEINOS, A.: Metabolic Influences on Vascular Disorders with Particular Reference to Cholesterol Determinations in Comparison with Uric Acid Levels. Angiology **9**, 162 (1958).
129. KRIZEK, V.: Serum Uric Acid in Relation to Body Weight. Ann. rheum. Dis. **25**, 456 (1966).
130. LANESE, R. R., GRESHAM, G. E., KELLER, M. D.: Behavioral and Physiological Characteristics in Hyperuricemia. J. Amer. med. Ass. **207**, 1878 (1969).
131. LECOCG, F. R., MCPHAUL, J. J.: The Effects of Starvation, High Fat Diets, and Ketone Infusions on Uric Acid Balance. Metabolism **14**, 186 (1965).
132. LEEPER, R. D., BENVA, R. S., BRENER, J. L., RAWSON, R. W.: Hyperuricemia in Myxedema. J. clin. Endocr. **20**, 1457 (1960).
133. LELLOOCH, J., SCHWARTZ, D., TRAN, M. H.: The Relationships Between Smoking and Levels of Serum Urea and Uric Acid. Results of an Epidemiological Survey. J. chron. Dis. **22**, 9 (1969).
134. LENNANE, G. A. Q., ROSE, B. S., ISDALE, I. C.: Gout in the Maori. Ann. rheum. Dis. **19**, 120 (1960).
135. LESCH, M., NYHAN, W. L.: A Familial Disorder of Uric Acid Metabolism and Central Nervous System Function. Amer. J. Med. **36**, 561 (1964).
136. LICHTENSTEIN, L., SCOTT, H. W., LEVIN, M. H.: Pathologic Changes in Gout; Survey of Eleven Necropsied Cases. Amer. J. Path. **32**, 871 (1956).
137. LONDON, M., HUMS, M.: Distribution Patterns of Uric Acid in Coronary Artery Disease. Clin. Chem. **13**, 132 (1967).
138. MACLACHLAN, M. J., RODNAN, G. P.: Effects of Food, Fast and Alcohol on Serum Uric Acid and Acute Attacks of Gout. Amer. J. Med. **42**, 38 (1967).

139. McCarty, D. J., Gatter, R. A.: Recurrent Acute Inflammation Associated with Focal Apatite Crystal Deposition. Arthr. and Rheum. **9**, 804 (1966).
140. Melick, R. A., Henneman, P. H.: Clinical and Laboratory Studies of 207 Consecutive Patients in a Kidney-Stone Clinic. New Engl. J. Med. **259**, 307 (1958).
141. Mertz, D. P.: Dyslipoproteinemia in Primary Gout. Dtsch. med. Wschr. **98**, 1457 (1973).
142. Mikkelsen, W. M.: The Possible Association of Hyperuricemia and/or Gout with Diabetes Mellitus. Arthr. and Rheum. **8**, 853 (1965).
143. Mikkelsen, W. M., Dodge, H. J., Duff, I. F.: Estimates of the Prevalence of Rheumatic Diseases in the Population of Tecumseh, Michigan, 1959—60. J. chron. Dis. **20**, 351 (1967).
144. Mikkelsen, W. M., Dodge, H. J., Valkenburg, H. A., Himes, S.: The Distribution of Serum Uric Acid Values in a Population Unselected as to Gout or Hyperuricemia, Tecumseh, Michigan, 1959—1960. Amer. J. Med. **39**, 242 (1965).
145. Mintz, D. H., Canary, J. J., Carreon, G., Kyle, L. Y.: Hyperuricemia in Hyperparathyroidism. New Engl. J. Med. **265**, 112 (1961).
146. Montoye, H. J., Faulkner, J. A., Dodge, H. J., Mikkelsen, W. M., Willis, P. W., Block, W. D.: Serum Uric Acid Concentration Among Business Executives, with Observations on Other Coronary Heart Disease Risk Factors. Ann. intern. Med. **66**, 838 (1967).
147. Montoye, H. J., Mikkelsen, W. M.: Serum Uric Acid and Achievement in High School. Arthr. and Rheum. **16**, 359 (1973).
148. Mueller, E. F., Kasl, S. V., Brooks, G. W., Cobb, S.: Psychosocial Correlates of Serum Urate Levels. Psychol. Bull. **73**, 238 (1970).
149. Muller, A. S.: *Population Studies on the Prevalence of Rheumatic Diseases in Liberia and Nigeria*. The Hague: J. H. Pasmans 1970.
150. Myers, A. R., Epstein, F. H., Dodge, H. J., Mikkelsen, W. M.: The Relationship of Serum Uric Acid to Risk Factors in Coronary Heart Disease. Amer. J. Med. **45**, 520 (1968).
151. Neel, J. V., Mikkelsen, W. M., Rucknagel, D. L., Weinstein, E. D., Goyer, R. A., Abadie, S. H.: Further Studies of the Xavante Indiana. VIII. Some Observations on Blood, Urine, and Stool Specimens. Amer. J. Trop. Med. **17**, 474 (1968).
152. Neel, J. V., Rakic, M. T., Davidson, R. T., Valkenburg, H. A., Mikkelsen, W. M.: Studies on Hyperuricemia. II. A Reconsideration of the Distribution of Serum Uric Acid Values in the Families of Smyth, Cotterman, and Freyberg. Amer. J. hum. Genet. **17**, 14 (1965).
153. Nyhan, W. L., James, J. A., Teberg, A. J., Sweetman, L., Nelson, L. G.: A New Disorder of Purine Metabolism with Behavioral Manifestations. J. Pediat. **74**, 20 (1969).
154. O'Brien, W. M., Burch, T. A., Bunim, J. J.: Genetics of Hyperuricemia in Blackfeet and Pima Indians. Ann. rheum. Dis. **25**, 117 (1966).
155. O'Sullivan, J. B.: The Incidence of Gout and Related Uric Acid Levels in Sudbury, Massachusetts. In: *Population Studies of the Rheumatic Diseases* (Bennett, P. H., Wood, P. H. N., Eds.), p. 371—375. Amsterdam: Excerpta Medica Foundation 1968.
156. O'Sullivan, J. B.: Gout in a New England Town. A Prevalence Study in Sudbury, Massachusetts. Ann. rheum. Dis. **31**, 166 (1972).
157. Padova, J., Bendersky, G.: Hyperuricemia in Diabetic Ketoacidosis. New Engl. J. Med. **267**, 530 (1962).
158. Paik, C. H., Alavi, I., Dunea, G., Weiner, L.: Thalassemia and Gouty Arthritis. J. Amer. med. Ass. **213**, 296 (1970).
159. Pant, S. S., Moser, H. W., Krane, S. M.: Hyperuricemia in Down's Syndrome. J. clin. Endocr. **28**, 472 (1968).
160. Pearce, J., Aziz, H.: Uric Acid and Plasma Lipids in Cerebrovascular Disease. Part I. Prevalence of Hyperuricaemia. Brit. med. J. **1969 IV**, 78.
161. Peters, J. P., VanSlyke, D. D.: *Quantitative Clinical Chemistry*, Vol. 1, second Ed. Baltimore: Williams and Wilkins 1946.
162. Pinals, R. S., Short, C. L.: Calcific Periarthritis Involving Multiple Sites. Arthr. and Rheum. **9**, 566 (1966).
163. Popert, A. J., Hewitt, J. V.: Gout and Hyperuricaemia in Rural and Urban Populations. Ann. rheum. Dis. **21**, 154 (1962).
164. Praetorius, E., Kirk, J. E.: Hypouricemia with Evidence for Tubular Elimination of Uric Acid. J. Lab. clin. Med. **35**, 865 (1950).
165. Prior, I. A. M., Rose, B. S.: Uric Acid, Gout and Public Health in the South Pacific. N. Z. med. J. **65**, 295 (1966).

166. PRIOR, I. A. M., ROSE, B. S., DAVIDSON, F.: Metabolic Maladies in New Zealand Maoris. Brit. med. J. **1**, 1065 (1964).
167. PRIOR, I. A. M., ROSE, B. S., HARVEY, H. P. B., DAVIDSON, F.: Hyperuricaemia, Gout, and Diabetic Abnormality in Polynesian People. Lancet **1966 I**, 333.
168. RAHE, R. H., ARTHUR, R. J.: Stressful Underwater Demolition Training; Serum Urate and Cholesterol Variability. J. Amer. med. Ass. **202**, 1052 (1967).
169. RAHE, R. H., RUBIN, R. T., ARTHUR, R. J., CLARK, B. R.: Serum Uric Acid and Cholesterol Variability; A Comprehensive View of Underwater Demolition Team Training. J. Amer. med. Ass. **206**, 2875 (1968).
170. RAHE, R. H., RUBIN, R. T., GUNDERSON, E. K. E.: Measures of Subjects' Motivation and Affect Correlated with their Serum Uric Acid, Cholesterol, and Cortisol. Arch. gen. Psychiat. **26**, 357 (1972).
171. RAKIC, M. T., VALKENBURG, H. A., DAVIDSON, R. T., ENGELS, J. P., MIKKELSEN, W. M., NEEL, J. V., DUFF, I. F., HIMES, S.: Observations on the Natural History of Hyperuricemia and Gout. I. An Eighteen Year Follow-up of Nineteen Gouty Families. Amer. J. Med. **37**, 862 (1964).
172. RAMSDELL, C. M., KELLEY, W. N.: The Clinical Significance of Hypouricemia. Ann. intern. Med. **78**, 239 (1973).
173. REED, D., LABARTHE, D., STALLONES, R.: Epidemiologic Studies of Serum Uric Acid Levels Among Micronesians. Arthr. and Rheum. **15**, 381 (1972).
174. ROSE, B. S., PRIOR, I. A. M., DAVIDSON, F.: Gout and Hyperuricaemia in New Zealand and Polynesia. In: *Population Studies of the Rheumatic Diseases* (BENNETT, P. H., WOOD, P. H. N., Eds.), p. 358—362. Amsterdam: Excerpta Medica Foundation 1968.
175. ROSENBLATT, G., DECKER, J. L., HEALEY, L. A.: Gout in Hospitalized Filipinos in Hawaii. Pacif. Med. Surg. **74**, 312 (1966).
176. SANBAR, S. S.: *Hyperlipidemia and Hyperlipoproteinemia*, p. 142. Boston: Little, Brown and Company 1969.
177. SCHULMAN, J. D., LUSTBERG, T. J., KENNEDY, J. L., MUSELES, M., SEEGMILLER, J. E.: A New Variant of Maple Sugar Urine Disease (Branched Chain Ketoaciduria); Clinical and Biochemical Evaluation. Amer. J. Med. **49**, 118 (1970).
178. SEEGMILLER, J. E.: The Acute Attack of Gouty Arthritis. Arthr. and Rheum. **8**, 714 (1965).
179. SEEGMILLER, J. E., ROSENBLOOM, F. M., KELLEY, W. N.: Enzyme Defect Associated with a Sex-Linked Human Neurological Disorder and Excessive Purine Synthesis. Science **155**, 1682 (1967).
180. SHEIKH, M. I., MØLLER, J. V.: Binding of Urate to Proteins of Human and Rabbit Plasma. Biochim. biophys. Acta (Amst.) **158**, 456 (1968).
181. SHICHKAWA, K.: The Prevalence of Gout in Japan. In: *Population Studies of the Rheumatic Diseases* (BENNET, P. H., WOOD, P. H. N., Eds.), p. 354. Amsterdam: Excerpta Medica Foundation 1968.
182. SIMKIN, P. A.: Binding of Uric Acid in Normal Serum. Arthr. and Rheum. **11**, 117 (1968) (abstract).
183. SIMKIN, P. A.: Uric Acid Binding to Serum Proteins: Differences Among Species. Proc. Soc. exp. Biol. (N.Y.) **139**, 604 (1972).
184. SLETTEN, K., AAKESSON, I., ALVSAKER, J. O.: Presence of Ornithine in the Urate-Binding α_1—α_2 Globulin. Nature New Biology **231**, 118 (1971).
185. SMYTH, C. J., COTTERMAN, C. W., FREYBERG, R. H.: The Genetics of Gout and Hyperuricemia—An Analysis of Nineteen Families. J. clin. Invest. **27**, 749 (1948).
186. SOBREVILLA, L. A., SALAZAR, F.: High Altitude Hyperuricemia. Proc. Soc. exp. Biol. (N.Y.) **129**, 890 (1968).
187. SPERLING, O., BOER, P., PERSKY-BOOSH, S., KANAREK, E., DEVRIES, A.: Altered Kinetic Property of Erythrocyte Phosphoribosylpyrophosphate Synthetase in Excessive Purine Production. Europ. J. clin. biol. Res. **17**, 703 (1972).
188. STECHER, R. M., HERSH, A. H., SOLOMON, W. H.: The Heredity of Gout and Its Relationship to Familial Hyperuricemia. Ann. intern. Med. **31**, 595 (1949).
189. STEUERMANN, N.: Hyperuricemia in the Filipino Population of the Puna District of the Island of Hawaii. In: *The Epidemiology of Chronic Rheumatism*, p. 170—175. Oxford: Blackwell Scientific Publications, and Philadelphia: F. A. Davis 1963.
190. STEUERMANN, N., FARIAS, A. H.: Hyperuricemia in Filipinos. Hawaii med. J. **20**, 151 (1960).
191. TALBOTT, J. H., TERPLAN, K. L.: The Kidney in Gout. Medicine (Baltimore) **39**, 405 (1960).

192. THOMPSON, G. R., TING, Y. M., RIGGS, G. A., FENN, M. E., REYNOLDS, R. M.: Calcific Tendinitis and Soft-Tissue Calcification Resembling Gout. J. Amer. med. Ass. **203**, 464 (1968).
193. TZONCHEV, V. T., SHUBAROV, K., ILINOV, P.: Prevalence of Gout and Hyperuricemia in Bulgaria. In: *Population Studies of the Rheumatic Diseases* (BENNETT, P. H., WOOD, P. H. N., Eds.), p. 363. Amsterdam: Excerpta Medica Foundation 1968.
194. WALKER, B. R., ALEXANDER, F.: Uric Acid Excretion in Sickle Cell Anemia. J. Amer. med. Ass. **215**, 255 (1971).
195. WALLIS, L. A., ENGLE, R. L., JR.: The Adult Fanconi Syndrome. II. Review of Eighteen Cases. Amer. J. Med. **22**, 13 (1957).
196. WEINSTEIN, B., IRREVERRE, F., WATKIN, D. M.: Lung Carcinoma, Hypouricemia and Aminoaciduria. Amer. J. Med. **39**, 520 (1965).
197. WEISS, T. E., SEGALOFF, A., MOORE, C.: Gout and Diabetes. Metabolism **6**, 103 (1967).
198. WHITEHOUSE, F. W., CLEARY, W. J., JR.: Diabetes Mellitus in Patients with Gout. J. Amer. med. Ass. **197**, 73 (1966).
199. WIEDEMANN, E., ROSE, H. G., SCHWARTZ, E.: Plasma Lipoproteins, Glucose Tolerance and Insulin Response in Primary Gout. Amer. J. Med. **53**, 299 (1972).
200. YU, T. F., BALIS, M. E., KRENITSKY, T. A., DANCIS, J., SILVERS, D. N., ELION, G. B., GUTMAN, A. B.: Rarity of X-linked Partial Hypoxanthine-Guanine Phosphoribosyltransferase Deficiency in a Large Gouty Population. Ann. intern. Med. **76**, 255 (1972).
201. YU, T. F., GUTMAN, A. B.: Study of the Paradoxical Effects of Salicylate in Low, Intermediate, and High Dosage on the Renal Mechanisms for Excretion of Urate in Man. J. clin. Invest. **38**, 1298 (1959).
202. YU, T. F., GUTMAN, A. B.: Uric Acid Nephrolithiasis in Gout; Predisposing Factors. Ann. intern. Med. **67**, 1133 (1967).
203. ZALOKAR, J., LELLOUCH, J., CLAUDE, J. R., KUNTZ, D.: Serum Uric Acid in 23923 Men and Gout in a Subsample of 4257 Men in France. J. chron. Dis. **25**, 305 (1972).
204. ZALOKAR, J., LELLOUCH, J., CLAUDE, J. R., KUNTZ, D.: Epidemiology of Serum Uric Acid and Gout in Frenchmen. J. chron. Dis. **27**, 59 (1974).
205. ZÖLLNER, N.: The Treatment of Gout. Germ. med. Mth. **2**, 253 (1957).

III. Ätiologie und Pathogenese der Hyperuricämie

1. The Etiology and Pathogenesis of Gout

By

J. B. WYNGAARDEN and W. N. KELLEY

With 20 Figures

Gout is a clinical disorder which chiefly affects the joints and produces a characteristic type of acute and chronic arthritis, related to the presence of crystals of sodium urate. The cardinal biochemical feature is hyperuricemia. In *primary gout* hyperuricemia is attributable to an inborn error of metabolism. In *secondary gout*, hyperuricemia occurs as a complication of an acquired disorder or of the use of certain drugs. Both primary and secondary gout are markedly heterogeneous conditions. A classification of gout is presented in Table 1.

Primary and secondary gout evolve through similar stages of asymptomatic hyperuricemia, recurrent acute gouty arthritis or renal lithiasis, and chronic tophaceous gout. This chapter deals with the etiology and pathogenesis of hyperuricemia and gout. Major emphasis will be placed upon the genetic and biochemical bases of primary gout.

Definition and Significance of Hyperuricemia

The definition of hyperuricemia favored by the authors is one based upon the limited solubility of sodium urate in extracellular body fluids. Since sodium is the most abundant cation of extracellular fluid, uric acid exists primarily as monosodium urate. The solubility product of sodium urate in aqueous solution is 4.9×10^{-5} M. At a sodium concentration of 0.13 M, plasma water is saturated with urate at 6.4 mg per 100 ml (PETERS and VAN SLYKE, 1946). Additional urate may be bound to nondiffusible elements of plasma.

Early claims of substantial binding of urate to plasma protein molecules (ADLERSBERG et al., 1942) were not confirmed by various studies based on ultrafiltration (YU and GUTMAN, 1953a) and electrophoresis (VILLA et al., 1958). Utilizing more sensitive techniques of gel filtration and immunoelectrophoresis, ALVSAKER (1965a, 1965b, 1966) demonstrated reversible interactions between urate and four macromolecular components in human plasma. These components were identified as albumin, low density α-lipoprotein, α_2-macroglobulins, and an α_1-α_2-globulin. KLINENBERG and KIPPEN (1970) found substantial binding of urate to albumin *in vitro* utilizing the technique of equilibrium dialysis. Additionally, KATZ and EHRLICH (1968) have identified a serum acid mucopolysaccharide component migrating in the region of α- and β-globulins which increases urate solubility.

The importance of urate binding to plasma proteins *in vivo* is still controversial (SKEIKH and MOLLER, 1968). ALVSAKER (1966) found that 25 to 30 percent of urate was bound to plasma proteins at room temperature. However, others have found 20 to 26 percent of urate in plasma bound at 4° C, but only 5 percent or less at temperatures above 20° C (WYNGAARDEN, 1955a, SKEIKH and MOLLER, 1968; KLINENBERG and KIPPEN, 1970). Additionally, BLUESTONE and coworkers (1969

Table 1. Classification of hyperuricemia and gout

Type	Metabolic	Inheritance
Primary		Polygenic
Normal excretion (75 to 80% of primary gout)	Overproduction of uric acid and/or underexcretion of uric acid (specific defects undefined; some reported to have reduced levels of an α_1–α_2 urate-binding globulin in plasma)	Autosomal dominant forms (? glutathione reductase variants; ? $\alpha_1\alpha_2$ globulin deficiencies)
Overexcretion (20 to 25% of primary gout)	Overproduction of uric acid (specific defects undefined; excessive hepatic xanthine oxidase activity reported in some; superactive variants of glutathione reductase reported in some)	
Associated with specific enzyme defects		
Glucose-6-phosphatase: deficiency or absence	Overproduction plus underexcretion of uric acid; glycogen storage disease, Type 1 (von Giercke)	Autosomal recessive
PP-ribose-P synthetase variants; increased activity	Overproduction of PP-ribose-P and of uric acid	X-linked (?)
Hypoxanthine-guanine phosphoribosyltransferase: deficiency, partial or "virtually complete" (Lesch-Nyhan syndrome)	Overproduction of uric acid; increased purine biosynthesis *de novo* driven by surplus PP-ribose-P	X-linked
Secondary		
Associated with increased nucleic acid turnover	Overproduction of uric acid	
Associated with decreased renal excretion of uric acid	Reduced renal functional mass. Inhibited tubular secretion of uric acid. Enhanced tubular reabsorption of uric acid	

and 1970) reported that several drugs, including salicylates, phenylbutazone, sulfinpyrazone, and probenecid, reduce urate binding to plasma macromolecules *in vitro*.

On the basis of a provisional estimate of an average binding of 10 percent of plasma urate at 37° *in vivo* (POSTLETHWAITE et al., 1973a) we suggest that extracellular fluids are supersaturated with sodium urate at concentration values above 7.0 mg per 100 ml. The potentiality for precipitation of urate crystals therefore exists whenever true plasma urate values exceed this limit.

The physiochemical definition of hyperuricemia is amply validated by experience. With the FOLIN method (1933) only 2 percent of 1190 determinations of serum urate values in 234 gouty patients in three laboratories were below 6.0 mg per 100 ml (JACOBSON, 1937; TALBOTT and COOMBS, 1938; GOLDTHWAIT et al., 1958). Ninety-four percent of 177 serum analyses in 21 gouty patients exceeded 7.0 mg per 100 ml (JACOBSON, 1937).

Statistical definitions of hyperuricemia encounter theoretical difficulties on several scores. These include (1.) asymmetry of urate distributions with skewness toward high values (HAUGE and HARVALD, 1955; MIKKELSON et al., 1965; HALL et al., 1967); (2.) bimodality of some frequency histograms (LAWRENCE, 1960; DECKER et al., 1962; COBB, 1963; BURCH et al., 1966), e.g. of Filipino males living in Northwestern North America (DECKER et al., 1962); (3.) positive correlations of serum urate values with "factors of plenty" (ACHESON and CHAN, 1969); and (4.) racial differences, e.g. mean values of 7.06 mg per 100 ml among adult male Maori of New Zealand (PRIOR et al., 1966).

Potential Pathophysiologic Mechanisms of Hyperuricemia

In theory, hyperuricemia could result from increased absorption of precursor purines or from increased plasma protein binding, increased production, decreased excretion, or decreased destruction of uric acid, or from combinations of these abnormalities.

A purine-free diet results in an average reduction of the serum urate level of 1 to 1.2 mg per 100 ml in gouty subjects (GUTMAN and YU, 1952; SEEGMILLER et al., 1961) but, with rare exceptions (RIESELBACH et al., 1970), does not correct hyperuricemia. Ingestion of 4 g yeast RNA per day for 4 days results in comparable elevations of serum urate levels in nongouty (NUGENT and TYLER, 1959; SEEGMILLER et al., 1962) and gouty subjects (YU et al., 1962). Therefore, hyperuricemia does not appear to be attributable to abnormal absorption of precursor purines.

Such uricolysis as occurs in man (WYNGAARDEN and STETTEN, 1953) can be accounted for almost entirely by the action of intestinal flora upon uric acid entering the gastrointestinal tract in gastric, biliary, pancreatic, and intestinal secretions (SORENSEN, 1959; SORENSEN, 1960). There is no evidence that extrarenal disposal of uric acid is diminished in gout. On the contrary, in hyperuricemia the fraction of urate disposal accounted for by extrarenal routes is increased, and in patients with high-grade renal disease it may constitute the major component of urate disposal (SORENSEN, 1962).

There is considerable evidence that both increased production of uric acid and reduced renal excretion of uric acid play important roles in the pathogenesis of hyperuricemia in primary gout. This evidence will be considered in detail below.

Genetics

Familial Incidence of Gout

Gout has been recognized as a familial disorder since antiquity. GALEN ascribed gout to "debauchery, intemperance and an hereditary trait." A familial incidence of gout of 38 to 81 percent has been reported by English observers (COHEN, 1955). In the United States the familial incidence reported has generally ranged from 6 to 18 percent (ROSENBERG, 1941; NEEL, 1947), but figures up to 75 percent (TALBOTT, 1955) have been obtained after persistent questioning.

Asymptomatic Hyperuricemia in Families of Gouty Patients

FOLIN and LYMAN first recorded asymptomatic hyperuricemia in a man in whose family gout occurred in 1913. In the first extensive study, by TALBOTT in 1940, 25 percent of 136 asymptomatic blood relatives of 27 gouty persons had hyperuricemia. In five studies reviewed by SMYTH (1957) about 25 percent of first-

Table 2. Hyperuricemia in relatives of gouty patients

Number of gouty patients	Number of relatives	Number of gouty relatives	Number of hyperuricemic relatives	Percent hyperuricemic	References
27	136	3	34	25	
19	87	3	21	24	Wyngaarden
44	136	0	16	11	and Kelley
3	29	11	21	72	(1972)
32	261	16	71	27	

Source: Smyth (1957).

degree relatives of gouty subjects were hyperuricemic. Twenty percent of the hyperuricemic relatives had gout (Table 2).

Hypothesis of an Autosomal Dominant Gene

The first studies of familial hyperuricemia assigned the defect to an autosomal dominant gene whose penetrance was low. Smyth et al. (1948) found that a frequency diagram of serum urate values among relatives of gouty patients was bimodal for both males and females, with nadirs of 6.0 and 5.0 mg per 100 ml, respectively. Using these critical levels, they classified 10 of 48 male relatives and 11 of 39 female relatives as hyperuricemic. The distribution of hyperuricemic individuals in 19 pedigrees conformed quite closely with segregation of a dominant autosomal gene for hyperuricemia. In this mode of inheritance, the ratio of hyperuricemic to normal postpubertal offspring should be 1:1 when only one parent is hyperuricemic. Among sons of such matings six of 13 above age 16 were hyperuricemic. Among daughters of the same matings, two of six above 16 years were hyperuricemic.

Stecher et al. (1949) published a frequency distribution of serum urate values of 137 relatives of gouty persons (excluding spouses) which was shifted toward high values in comparison with a similar plot of 1024 determinations on individuals from the general hospital population. This distribution was also suggestively bimodal, the nadir being 6.0 to 6.4 mg per 100 ml, and 23 of 147 determinations of 137 relatives fell above this range. Among relatives, they observed hyperuricemia in 15 to 21 percent of mothers, brothers, sisters, and sons, but in none of the 45 daughters of index cases. These workers also concluded that hyperuricemia was an autosomal dominant trait.

When this conclusion was put to the numerical test for male offspring, a correction being applied for small family size, the expected number of hyperuricemic individuals was 31. Actually 26 were found among 51 men. These figures were regarded as showing satisfactory conformity with the expected 1:1 ratio. Since 26 hyperuricemic sons were observed where 31 were expected, penetrance was estimated at about 84 percent in heterozygote males. Since there were only 8 hyperuricemic females as against with 54 hyperuricemic males, despite nearly equal sex distribution of the 203 individuals in the study, penetrance was estimated to be about one-seventh as high in women as in men, or about 14 percent. Since no hyperuricemic daughters of gouty patients were found, no critical analysis could be applied to female offspring. Both groups of investigators excluded sex-linked inheritance on the basis of male-to-male transmission patterns. Recessive inheritance was excluded by Stecher et al. (1949) on the basis of a probability analysis. In neither of these studies was a rigorous statistical analysis performed to exclude a unimodal distribution with skewness toward high values.

Hypothesis of Multifactorial Inheritance

The hypothesis of an autosomal dominant gene for hyperuricemia was questioned by HAUGE and HARVALD (1955) in their study of 261 relatives of 32 gouty subjects. Plots of serum uric acid values in both controls and relatives fitted unimodal distributions. No clear separation could be made between normal and abnormal uric acid values, although mean values for both male and female relatives of gouty patients were higher than mean values of their respective control groups. Data on male sibs conformed satisfactorily to the sum of two normal distributions, but those on female relatives did not. The writers therefore excluded inheritance due to a single autosomal dominant gene and concluded that insofar as the higher uric acid values observed in these sibs were genetically determined, multifactorial inheritance was responsible.

In 1954, NEEL and associates restudied 271 members of 19 gouty families first studied 18 years earlier by SMYTH et al. (1948). The new results showed significant skewing to the right, and evidence for bimodality was less convincing than earlier. The hypothesis of multifactorial inheritance was regarded as at least as tenable as the "one gene-hyperuricemia" hypothesis.

Hyperuricemia in Population Studies

A study of 2000 Blackfoot and Pima Indians showed an association of hyperuricemia with obesity and surface area, but in addition there were strong hereditary determinants of serum urate levels, which appeared to be polygenic. Transmission patterns suggested that some of the genes were autosomal dominants and others possibly sex-linked dominants (BURCH et al., 1966). The studies of MIKKELSEN et al. (1965 and 1967) of 6000 residents of Tecumseh, Michigan, and of HALL et al. (1967) of 5000 residents of Framingham, Massachusetts also favored multifactorial inheritance. Frequency histograms showed skewness toward high values without evidence of bimodality.

By contrast, population studies conducted by LAWRENCE (1960) in England, and by COBB (1963) and associates (DUNN et al., 1963) in groups of Pittsburgh executives and medical students, by DECKER et al. (1962) in Filipino males living in Northwestern North America, and by BURCH et al. (1966) in the Chamarros and Carolinians of the Mariana Islands all showed bimodal distributions of serum uric acid values.

When all available data are considered, they suggest a possible synthesis of views. In the species at large, serum uric acid concentrations are controlled by multiple genes. The probability of selecting out an apparently dominant genetic factor increases when the basis of selection is racial, when the group is an isolate, or when the study concerns several generations of families in which gout occurs, as in the studies of SMYTH et al. (1948) and STECHER et al. (1949). Evidence for polygenic control will be more prominent when the population is heterogeneous or when only sibs of gouty subjects are studied, as in the investigations of HAUGE and HARVALD (1955).

It is doubtful whether additional population studies will contribute much more to our understanding of hereditary mechanisms. Further progress in understanding the heredity of hyperuricemia will require a definition of the precise biochemical mechanism of hyperuricemia in each isolate or family, and study of

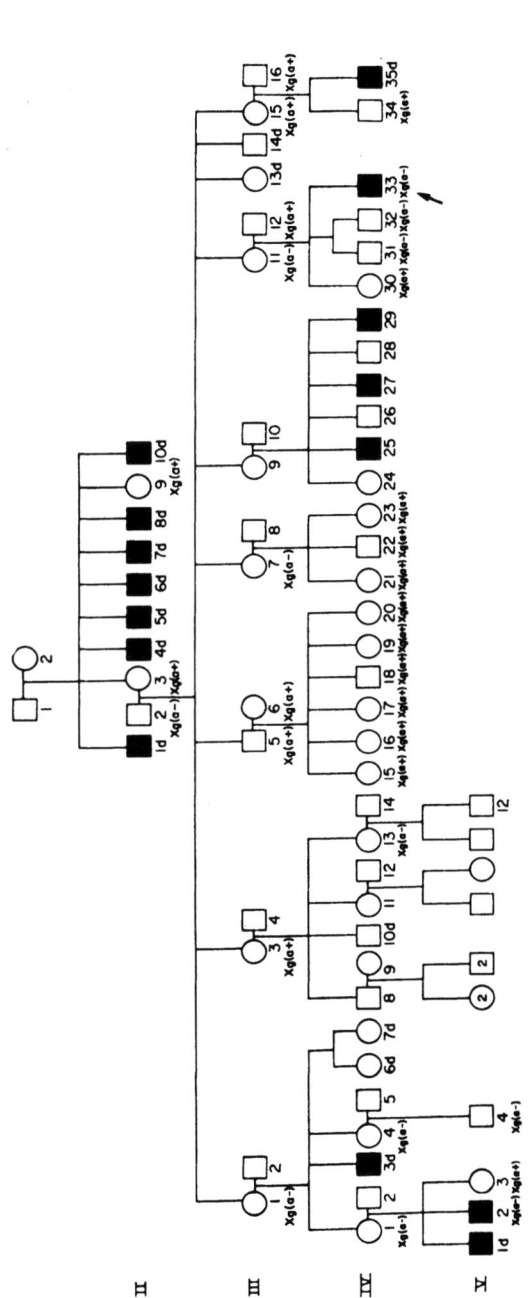

Fig. 1. Pedigree of family showing cases of Lesch-Nyhan syndrome (solid symbols). Note maternal transmission to male offspring only. (From NYHAN, 1968)

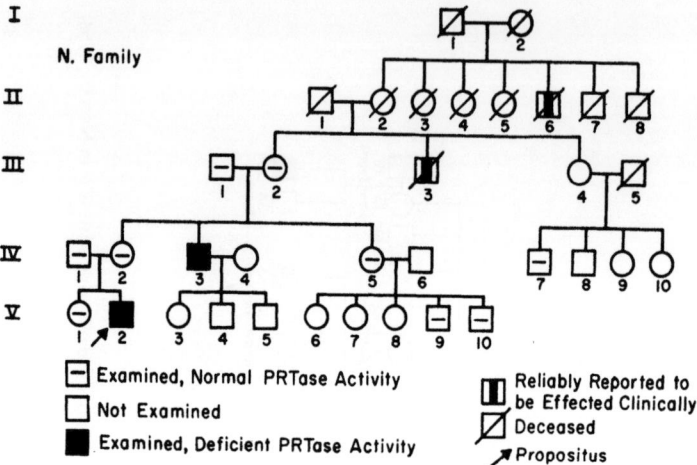

Fig. 2. Pedigree of a family with partial PRT deficiency, gout, and spinocerebellar ataxia. (Reproduced from KELLEY et al., 1969, with permission of Ann. Intern. Med.)

the transmission of that trait. The mechanisms of inheritance of known rare subtypes or primary gout will be discussed below.

Genetic Control of Uric Acid Excretion

In a study of uric acid excretion in 37 patients with primary gout and 96 of their first-degree relatives, SCOTT and POLLARD (1970) found a graded correlation between clearance values of patients and relatives, closer in the case of male than of female relatives. These observations suggest that insofar as familial correlations in the control of renal handling of urate are of genetic origin, they are also multifactorial.

X-linked Hyperuricemia

Complete and Partial Deficiencies of Hypoxanthine-Guanine Phosphoribosyltransferase (PRT)

Hypoxanthine-guanine phosphoribosyltransferase deficiency is an X-linked condition, clinically manifest in fully expressed form only in the hemizygous male. A representative pedigree of "virtually complete" deficiency (Lesch-Nyhan syndrome) is shown in Fig. 1, and one of partial deficiency in Fig. 2. Examples of complete (LESCH and NYHAN, 1964) or partial (GREENE and SEEGMILLER, 1969) deficiencies among half-brothers are known. In both instances the half-brothers were related through their mothers. No examples of male-to-male transmission of PRT deficiency have been identified (LESCH and NYHAN, 1964; KELLEY et al., 1969).

Heterozygous subjects may be mildly hyperuricemic or hyperuricaciduric, may show abnormalities of kinetics of uric acid synthesis or turnover, and may show values of erythrocyte PRT activity intermediate between normal values and values in deficient subjects (KELLEY et al., 1969; EMMERSON and WYNGAARDEN, 1969). However, in most obligate heterozygotes, especially those who are mothers of children with virtually complete PRT deficiency, erythrocyte PRT activity values are normal (KELLEY et al., 1969; KOGUT et al., 1970; SPERLING et al., 1970) and the mutant enzyme is absent (McDONALD and KELLEY, 1972). A selective growth or survival advantage of PRT-competent erythrocytes in competition with high grade PRT-deficient cells appears to be a likely explanation, for the mature erythrocyte cannot synthesize purine ribonucleotides *de novo*. An alternative explanation is that there is selective inactivation of the X chromosome which codes for the mutant PRT enzyme in erythropoietic cells.

Subjects who are heterozygous for PRT deficiency are mosaics: their fibroblasts grown in tissue culture show two populations of cells, one capable, the other incapable of incorporating hypoxanthine into nucleotides and nucleic acids (ROSENBLOOM et al., 1967a). These results are consistent with LYON's hypothesis (1961) of early random irreversible inactivation of one of the X chromosomes in cells of female subjects. When fibroblasts in tissue culture are allowed to grow to confluence the majority of cells may appear normal in their ability to utilize hypoxanthine or guanine. This phenomenon may reflect metabolic cooperation, a process by which some product of a competent cell is transferred to an incompetent cell (SUBAK-SHARPE et al., 1966; FRIEDMAN et al., 1968; SUBAK-SHARPE, 1969). In this instance, the transfer apparently involves a nucleotide or one of its products synthesized in the PRT-competent cell with which the deficient cell is in contact (COX et al., 1970).

A mouse fibroblast line deficient in PRT activity has been successfully transformed with competent mouse DNA by SZYBALSKA and SZYBALSKI (1962).

Hyperuricemia in Autosomally Inherited Conditions

Glucose 6-Phosphatase Deficiency

There are many examples of this disorder among sibs, both male and female, whose parents are clinically normal. In addition, several patients affected with Type I glycogen storage disease (both male and female) have had phenotypically normal children (VAN CREVALD, 1961; SIDBURY, 1965; ALEPA et al., 1967). Studies on intestinal glucose-6-phosphatase activity in patients with type I glycogen storage disease and their families support autosomal recessive inheritance (WILLIAMS et al., 1963; FIELD et al., 1965; FIELD and DRASH, 1967). FIELD and DRASH (1967), who studied the parents of five children with type I glycogen storage disease, found that all of them had lowered intestinal glucose-6-phosphatase activity. In one family the maternal grandfather and one of his brothers had lowered intestinal glucose-6-phosphatase, while another brother and the maternal grandmother had normal values.

Glutathione Reductase Variants

During a survey by LONG (1967) of 1473 Negro male outpatients in search of variants of erythrocyte glucose-6-phosphate dehydrogenase, an electrophoretically fast variant of glutathione reductase was detected. In a subgroup of 196 consecutive samples there was no association between common G-6-PD variants and the glutathione reductase variant. The gene frequency of the reductase variant was 0.133 and of the usual form of the enzyme it was 0.867. A subsequent study of 125 presumably healthy Negroes, 79 males and 46 females selected at random from the population, showed a gene frequency of 0.132 for the glutathione reductase variant, almost identical with that of the hospital outpatient population. Studies of nine Negro families (LONG, 1967) were consistent with an autosomal mode of inheritance of the enzyme variant. The striking frequency of

Table 3. Frequency of glutathione reductase phenotypes in general negro population and in negro males with gout or other medical illnesses

GSSG-R phenotype	General Negro population, percent	Negro male patients	
		Gout	Other illnesses
S	75.16	5	150
FS	23.06	15	40
F	1.78	8	6

Source: LONG (1967).

the fast variant among 28 gouty patients (1.9 percent of the 1473 subjects), the predicted random distribution of the trait, and the findings in the last 196 general medical patients of the G-6-PD study (all Negro males), are shown in Table 3.

In a subsequent study by LONG (1970) of 522 Negro volunteers, 10 phenotypes of glutathione reductase were detected by acrylamide-gel electrophoresis of plasma. These were judged to be products of five alleles at the same autosomal locus. Gene frequencies were 0.2644 for type 1, 0.6322 for type 2, 0.0086 for type 4, 0.0431 for type 5, and 0.0517 for type 6. Mean plasma urate levels were higher in those who were heterozygous or homozygous for type 1 and type 6 variants than in those homozygous for the usual form of the enzyme, type 2 (type 2, 5.17 mg per 100 ml; type 1, 7.24 mg per 100 ml; type 6, 6.48 mg per 100 ml). Red cells with type 1 or 6 isoenzyme show greater glutathione reductase activity and less activation by FAD than those with type 2 or 5.

Adenine Phosphoribosyltransferase (A-PRT) Deficiency

Four families with partial A-PRT deficiency are known. In one, values about 20 percent of normal were found in four members of three generations. Transmission of the trait from father to two daughters but not to a third established the autosomal location of the gene for A-PRT (KELLEY et al., 1968a; HENDERSON et al., 1969). The propositus of this pedigree was hyperlipoproteinemic. None of these A-PRT-deficient subjects was hyperuricemic.

In the second family, A-PRT deficiency was more severe. The propositus had activity values of 8 percent of normal in erythrocytes and was hyperuricemic. The family study disclosed discordance of the two traits, with examples of all four possible combinations of findings (Fig. 3) (KELLEY et al., 1970a).

It is likely that a complete or high-grade deficiency of A-PRT would require a double dose of abnormal allele and be inherited as an autosomal recessive condition. Two such patient have now been identified.

Deficiency of an α_1-α_2 Urate Binding Globulin

ALVSAKER (1966) described a reduced capacity of plasma from seven gouty patients to bind urate, which he attributed to a specific reduction in a plasma component which migrates as an α_1-α_2-globulin. This deficiency appeared to be inherited in an autosomal manner and the patients exhibiting reduced levels were heterozygous for this defect (ALVSAKER, 1968). KLINENBERG and KIPPEN (1970) described reduced binding of urate to plasma proteins in three patients with severe tophaceous gout, although plasma from seventeen other gouty subjects including three with tophi exhibited a normal urate binding capacity.

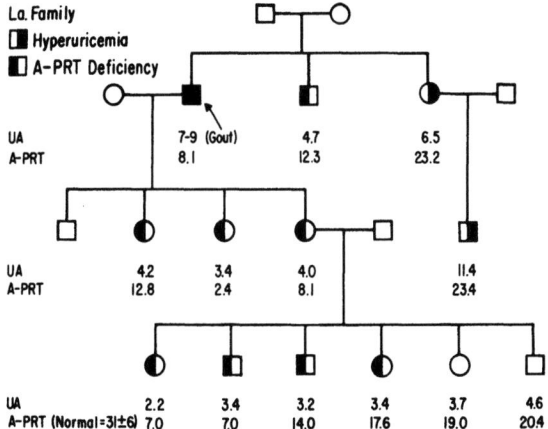

Fig. 3. Pedigree of a family with partial adenine phosphoribosyltransferase (A-PRT) deficiency and hyperuricemia. Note lack of concordance of the two traits

Idiopathic Uric Acid Nephrolithiasis

This condition has been described among Israeli subjects with normal serum and urinary uric acid values. The defect appears to be one leading to undue acidity of the urine (FRANK et al., 1960; BARZEL et al., 1964). It is reported to be a disorder distinct from gout and inherited as an autosomal dominant condition.

Subtypes of Uncertain Genetic Patterns

PP-ribose-P Synthetase Variants

Qualitatively different defects of this enzyme, leading to a marked increase in the rate of synthesis of PP-ribose-P and of uric acid have been described in two families, in each case in two brothers (SPERLING et al., 1972; BECKER et al., 1972; BECKER et al., 1973). In one family, PP-ribose-P synthesis and plasma urate values were normal in a third (nongouty) brother, three sons of one subject, both parents, and one maternal aunt. This family pattern is consistent with X-linked recessive inheritance (SPERLING et al., 1972a). Studies of the purified enzyme in this and other families will be required to establish that this is the basic genetic defect.

Hyperuricemia and Hyperlipoproteinemia

The common denominator with reference to hyperuricemia is probably the presence of hypertriglyceridemia in each of these types of hyperlipoproteinemia. A rank-order correlation between serum urate and triglyceride values has been described (BERKOWITZ, 1964). The mode of inheritance of the familial forms of these hyperlipoproteinemias is not yet certain. A distinction between primary and secondary hyperlipoproteinemia is essential when gout is also present. Type IV hyperlipoproteinemia sometimes coexists with partial PRT deficiency (KELLEY et al., 1969) or glucose-6-phosphatase deficiency (HOWELL et al., 1962a). Hypertriglyceridemia has been reported in 75 to 84 percent of patients with idiopathic primary gout (BERKOWITZ, 1964; FELDMAN and WALLACE, 1964; BERKOWITZ, 1966a; BENEDEK, 1967; BARLOW, 1968) and hyperuricemia in 82 percent of patients with hypertriglyceridemia (BERKOWITZ, 1964).

Biochemistry of Purine Compounds

Biosynthesis of the Purine Ring

In 1943 BARNES and SCHOENHEIMER fed ammonium citrate containing ^{15}N to pigeons and rats and demonstrated that the purines of internal organs and the uric acid of the avian excreta contained appreciable ^{15}N in the ring structure and substituent amino groups. Following these early studies, the use of labeled substrates in bacterial, avian, and mammalian systems soon defined the origin of the individual atoms of the purine ring (Fig. 4). Glycine contributes carbon atoms 4 and 5, and nitrogen atom 7 (SHEMIN and RITTENBERG, 1947; BUCHANAN et al., 1948; KARLSON and BARKER, 1949). Carbon atoms 2 and 8 come from formate

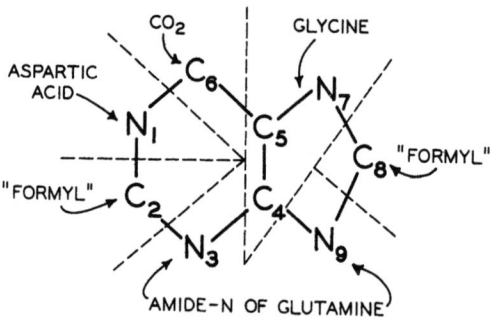

Fig. 4. Origins of the atoms of the purine ring.

(SONNE et al., 1948; KARLSON and BARKER, 1949), carbon atom 6 comes from CO_2 (BUCHANAN et al., 1948; HEINRICH and WILSON, 1950), nitrogen atoms 3 and 9 come from the amide-N of glutamine (SONNE et al., 1956; LEVENBERG et al., 1956; GOLDTHWAIT et al., 1956), and nitrogen atom 1 comes from aspartic acid (LEVENBERG et al., 1956).

A key intermediate in the synthesis of purines is 5-phosphoribosyl-1-pyrophosphate (PP-ribose-P). This high-energy compound is involved in purine synthesis in two types of reactions; in one it is a substrate, together with L-glutamine, in the first specific reaction of purine synthesis *de novo* (HARTMAN and BUCHANAN, 1958a); in the other it participates with purine bases in the direct synthesis of purine ribonucleotides by a condensation reaction with liberation of inorganic pyrophosphate (FLAKS et al., 1957a; LUKENS and HERRINGTON, 1957a). PP-ribose-P is formed by transfer of the terminal pyrophosphate group of ATP to carbon-1 of ribose-5-phosphate (KORNBERG et al., 1955; REMY et al., 1955).

$$\text{Ribose-5-phosphate} + \text{ATP} \xrightarrow{Mg^{2+}} \text{PP-ribose-P} + \text{AMP} \tag{1}$$

In this reaction, inorganic phosphate is an allosteric activator of the synthetase (FOX and KELLEY, 1971a) which is subject to regulation by a number of ribonucleotides in a mechanism termed "heterogeneous metabolic pool inhibition" (FOX and KELLEY, 1972a).

The first specific step of purine synthesis *de novo* is that in which 5β-phosphoribosyl-1-amine is generated. There may be two reactions for synthesis of phosphoribosylamine. In the better studied of the two (GOLDTHWAIT et al., 1956; HARTMAN, BUCHANAN, 1958a), the pyrophosphate group of PP-ribose-P is dis-

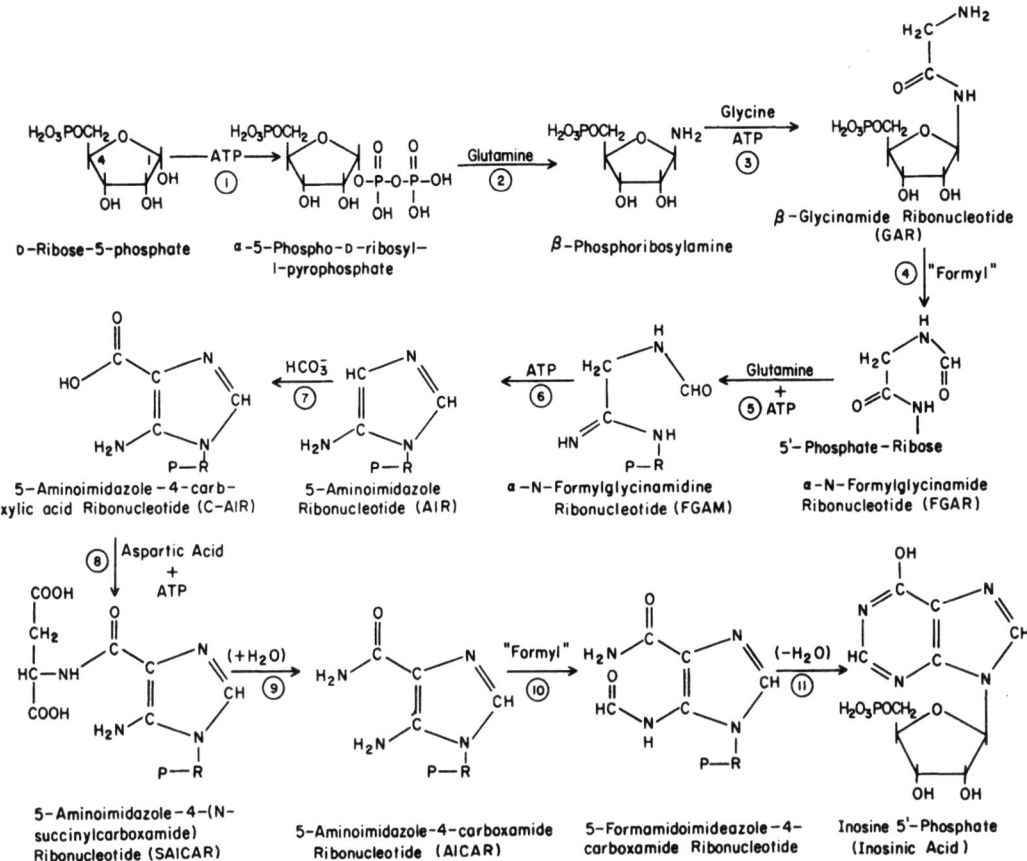

Fig. 5. Biosynthesis of the purine ring. The encircled numbers in this figure and in Fig. 6 refer to numbered reactions in the text

placed by the amide group of glutamine, and there is an inversion of the substituents to yield the β linkage characteristic of the glycosidic bond of all known ribonucleotides (HARTMAN and BUCHANAN, 1958a) (Fig. 5).

$$\alpha\text{-PP-ribose-P} + \text{glutamine} + H_2O \xrightarrow{Mg^{2+}} \beta\text{-phosphoribosylamine} + \text{glutamine acid} + PP \quad (2a)$$

This reaction is irreversible, and it thus becomes potentially important in the control of purine synthesis. The enzyme catalyzing this reaction, glutamine phosphoribosylpyrophosphate amidotransferase, is the site of a synergistic feedback control by adenine and guanine ribonucleotides (WYNGAARDEN and ASHTON, 1959a; HOLMES et al., 1973a). The regulation of purine biosynthesis will be discussed more fully below.

An alternative pathway for the synthesis of phosphoribosylamine by a direct reaction of ammonia with ribose-5-phosphate was described in bacterial extracts by NIERLICH and MAGASANIK (1961).

$$\text{Ribose 5-P} + NH_3 + ATP \xrightarrow{Mg^{2+}} \beta\text{-phosphoribosylamine} + ADP + P_i \quad (2b)$$

Because it has been shown to occur nonenzymatically at high ammonium chloride concentrations its biological significance has been doubted. Nevertheless, suggestive evidence for such a pathway was provided by LE GAL et al. (1967) in bacteria, by WAYGOOD and KAPOOR (1962) in plants, by HERCOVICS and JOHNSTONE (1964) in Ehrlich ascites cells, and by REEM (1968, 1972) in pigeon liver and human splenic extracts. Indirect evidence also points toward participation of NH_3 in synthesis of phosphoribosylamine in man *in vivo* (SPERLING et al., 1973). By contrast, WESTBY and GOTS (1969) have described bacterial mutants which lack any activity of glutamine PP-ribose-P amidotransferase (*pur F* mutants), and show complete dependence upon exogenous purines for growth, yet have normal assay values for ribose 5-P aminotransferase in extracts *in vitro* (WESTBY and GOTS, 1969). A final verdict on the importance of a second pathway for the formation of phosphoribosylamine is not yet possible.

The stepwise synthesis of the purine ring is shown in Fig. 5. Phosphoribosylamine reacts with glycine to yield glycinamide ribonucleotide, the first intermediate in which one finds the fundamental components of a nucleotide, namely the combination of base, sugar, and phosphoric acid. ATP is involved in this condensation as an energy source (GOLDTHWAIT et al., 1956; HARTMAN et al., 1956; HARTMAN and BUCHANAN, 1958b). Nucleotides of adenine and guanine show no inhibitory effects upon the enzyme catalyzing this reaction (NIERLICH and MAGASANIK, 1965a).

$$\text{Phosphoribosylamine} + \text{glycine} + \text{ATP} \xrightarrow{Mg^{2+}} \text{glycinamide ribonucleotide} + \text{ADP} + P_i \quad (3)$$

Glycinamide ribonucleotide receives a one-carbon "formyl" unit from an active folic acid derivative (GOLDTHWAIT et al., 1956; HARTMAN et al., 1956), N^5, N^{10}-methenyl tetrahydrofolic acid (THFA) (WARREN and BUCHANAN, 1957a; WARREN and BUCHANAN, 1957b).

$$\text{Glycinamide ribonucleotide} + N^5, N^{10}\text{-methenyl-THFA} + H_2O \rightarrow \alpha\text{-N-formylglycinamide ribonucleotide (FGAR)} + \text{THFA} + H^+. \quad (4)$$

The formyl derivative then receives the amide group of glutamine to form the corresponding amidine compound (MELNICK and BUCHANAN, 1957; MIZOBUCHI and BUCHANAN, 1968), following which ring closure generates the five-membered imidazole ring (LEVENBERG and BUCHANAN, 1957). Each of these reactions requires ATP as an energy source.

$$\text{FGAR} + \text{glutamine} + \text{ATP} + H_2O \xrightarrow{Mg^{2+}} \alpha\text{-formylglycinamidine ribonucleotide (FGAM)} + \text{glutamic acid} + \text{ADP} + P_i; \quad (5)$$

$$\text{FGAM} + \text{ATP} \xrightarrow{Mg^{2+}K^+} \text{5-aminoimidazole ribonucleotide} + \text{ADP} + P_i. \quad (6)$$

5-Aminoimidazole ribonucleotide (AIR) now receives a carboxyl group at C-4 by a CO_2-fixation reaction which requires a high concentration of bicarbonate (LUKENS and BUCHANAN, 1957b). The carboxyl serves as a point for condensation of this intermediate with aspartic acid through an amide linkage involving another ATP as the source of energy (LUKENS and BUCHANAN, 1957b). Hydrolysis of the intermediate yields 5-aminoimidazole-4-carboxamide ribonucleotide, a compound lacking only carbon atom 2 of a complete purine ribonucleotide.

$$\text{AIR} + CO_2 \rightarrow \text{5-aminoimidazole-4-carboxylic acid ribonucleotide (C-AIR)}; \quad (7)$$

$$\text{C-AIR} + \text{aspartic acid} + \text{ATP} \xrightarrow{Mg^{2+}} \text{5-aminoimidazole-4-N-succinocarboxamide ribonucleotide (SAICAR)} + \text{ADP} + P_i; \quad (8)$$

$$\text{SAICAR} \rightarrow \text{fumaric acid} + \text{5-aminoimidazole-4-carboxamide ribonucleotide (AICAR)}. \quad (9)$$

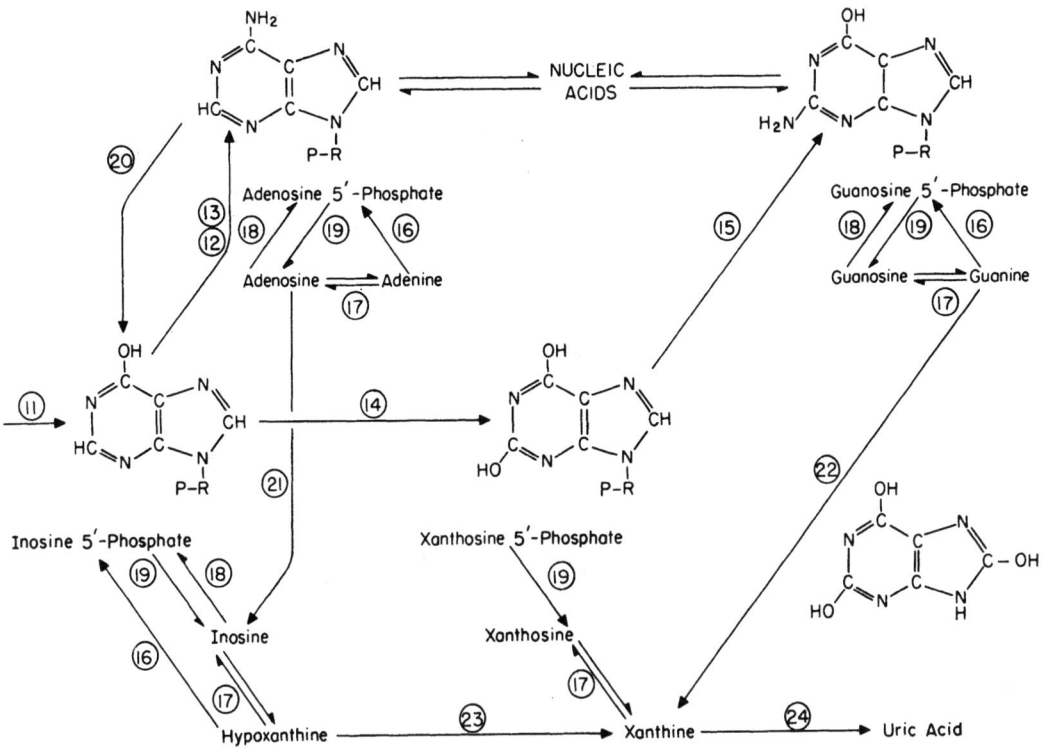

Fig. 6. Biosynthesis of purine ribonucleotides, ribonucleosides, and bases

AIC-ribonucleotide receives a second formyl group from a tetrahydrofolic acid derivative (FLAKS et al., 1957b; FLAKS et al., 1957c), and ring closure completes the biosynthesis of the purine structure by forming inosine-5′-monophosphate (IMP) (FLAKS et al., 1957c).

$$\text{AICAR} + \text{N}^{10}\text{-formyl-THFA} \xrightarrow{\text{K}^+} \text{5-formamidoimidazole-4-carboxamide ribonucleotide} + \text{THFA}; \tag{10}$$

$$\text{5-formamidoimidazole-4-carboxamide ribonucleotide} \rightarrow \text{IMP} + \text{H}_2\text{O}. \tag{11}$$

Biosynthesis of Other Nucleotides

IMP may be considered the parent purine compound. It is an intermediate in the formation of adenosine-5′-monophosphate (AMP) and guanosine-5′-monophosphate (GMP), the purine nucleotide components of nucleic acids (Fig. 6). The conversion of IMP to AMP (ABRAMS and BENTLEY, 1955) occurs in two steps. There is an initial condensation of IMP with aspartic acid to form adenylosuccinic acid (AMP-S) (CARTER and COHEN, 1956; JOKLIK, 1957). Energy for this reaction is derived from guanosine triphosphate (LIEBERMAN, 1956). This reaction is inhibited by AMP (WYNGAARDEN and GREENLAND, 1963). Cleavage of AMP-S yields AMP and fumaric acid. The latter reaction is freely reversible (LIEBERMAN, 1956). This reaction is analogous to cleavage of SAICAR (Reaction 9) and is probably catalyzed by the same enzyme, adenylosuccinase. Mutant strains of several microorganisms which lack the ability to catalyze one reaction cannot catalyze the other.

$$\text{IMP} + \text{L-aspartic acid} + \text{GTP} \xrightarrow{Mg^{2+}} \text{AMP-S} + \text{GDP} + P_i; \qquad (12)$$

$$\text{AMP-S} \rightarrow \text{AMP} + \text{fumaric acid}. \qquad (13)$$

Conversion of IMP to GMP also occurs in two steps. There is first an irreversible oxidation of IMP to xanthosine-5'-monophosphate (XMP), with nicotinamide adenine dinucleotide (NAD) as hydrogen acceptor (MAGASANIK et al., 1957; LAGERKVIST, 1958a). This reaction is inhibited by GMP (MAGER and MAGASANIK, 1960). The second reaction involves amination of XMP at the 2 position, and the specific donor is the amide group of glutamine (LAGERKVIST, 1958b). The second step requires ATP. These reactions proceed according to the following overall schemes:

$$\text{IMP} + \text{NAD}^+ + \text{H}_2\text{O} \xrightarrow{K^+} \text{XMP} + \text{NADH} + \text{H}^+; \qquad (14)$$

$$\text{XMP} + \text{glutamine} + \text{ATP} \xrightarrow{Mg^{2+}} \text{GMP} + \text{glutamic acid} + \text{AMP} + P_i. \qquad (15)$$

The combined influences of "forward" control, based on the availability of GTP and ATP, each of which is concerned with the synthesis of the other nucleotide, and of feedback inhibition, by which AMP and GMP each controls its own biosynthesis, may regulate the production of these ribonucleotides. In addition, AMP may be converted to IMP by adenylic deaminase and thus potentially serve as a source of guanyl ribonucleotides. Adenylic deaminase is stimulated by ATP and strongly inhibited by GTP (SETLOW et al., 1966). GMP may be deaminated to IMP. This reaction is strongly inhibited by ATP (MAGER and MAGASANIK, 1960). These various reactions and their controls may serve to provide the cell with the proper balance of adenyl and guanyl ribonucleotides, and also allow for replenishment of one from the other when necessary.

Salvage Pathways

Two general mechanisms exist for synthesis of ribonucleotides from purine bases or ribonucleosides which result from catabolism of endogenous ribonucleotides, from ingestion of purine-containing foods, or from administration of purine compounds. These involve phosphoribosyltransferase reactions in which free bases condense with PP-ribose-P to form ribonucleotides in one step, or phosphorylase reactions in which free bases react with ribose-1-phosphate to form ribonucleosides, some of which may then be converted to ribonucleotides by operation of kinase reactions.

The phosphoribosyltransferase reaction has the following general form:

$$\text{Base} + \text{PP-ribose-P} \rightarrow \text{base-ribose-phosphate} + PP_i. \qquad (16)$$

This reaction is responsible for the conversion of purines (FLAKS et al., 1957a; LUKENS and HERRINGTON, 1957b), pyrimidines (LIEBERMAN et al., 1955), nicotinamide (PREISS and HANDLER, 1957), and certain other nitrogenous bases to their respective ribonucleotides. Two different mammalian purine phosphoribosyltransferases (formerly termed ribonucleotide pyrophosphorylases) have been identified, one (A-PRT) acting upon AIC and adenine (FLAKS et al., 1957a; HORI and HENDERSON, 1966), the other (HG-PRT) acting upon hypoxanthine and guanine (LUKENS and HERRINGTON, 1957a; HENDERSON et al., 1968a). A-PRT will also accept adenine analogues such as 2,6-diaminopurine and 8-azadenine. HG-PRT (or simply PRT) will catalyze the conversion of xanthine to XMP, but at only about 0.3 percent of the rate of the reaction will hypoxanthine or guanine (KELLEY et al., 1967a). PRT will also catalyze the conversion of 6-thiopurine (LUKENS and HERRINGTON, 1957a), 6-thioguanine, 8-azaguanine, allopurinol (MCCOLLISTER et al., 1964), and oxipurinol to their respective ribonucleotides. These enzymes have been studied in beef liver (FLAKS et al., 1957a; LUKENS and HERRINGTON, 1957a), ascites cells (HORI and HENDERSON, 1966), and human erythrocytes (PREISS and HANDLER, 1957; HENDERSON et al., 1968a; CRAFT et al., 1970). In man, PRT activity is widely distributed and is especially rich in brain, where activity is greatest in basal ganglia (KELLEY et al., 1969). Activity is low in muscle and bone marrow (KELLEY et al., 1969). The K_{eq} of both phosphoribosyltransferases is far toward the ribonucleotide; a value of 290 has been estimated for A-PRT (HORI and HENDERSON, 1966). Both phosphoribosyltransferases are inhibited by purine ribonucleoside monophosphates. Adenine phosphoribosyltransferase is inhibited by AMP (HORI and HENDERSON, 1966). Hypoxanthine-guanine phosphoribosyltransferase is inhibited by IMP and GMP whether the substrate is hypoxanthine or guanine (HENDERSON et al., 1968a). The inhibitions are formally competitive against PP-ribose-P, and appear to involve product inhibition at the substrate site (HENDERSON et al., 1968a).

The two-step pathway has the following general form:

$$\text{Base} + \text{ribose-1-phosphate} \to \text{base-ribose} + P_i \tag{17}$$

$$\text{Base-ribose} + \text{ATP} \to \text{base-ribose-phosphate} + \text{ADP} \tag{18}$$

Purine nucleoside phosphorylase is widely distributed in mammalian tissue and active with guanine, hypoxanthine, and, to a lesser extent, with xanthine, but not with adenine (FRIEDKIN and KALCKAR, 1961; KRENITSKY et al., 1968). In the case of hypoxanthine, the equilibrium point is far toward the ribonucleoside. The phosphorylase has been extensively studied in human erythrocytes (KRENITSKY et al., 1968; SANDBERG et al., 1955).

Present indications are that the phosphoribosyltransferases are responsible for a much more extensive recycling of purine bases back into nucleotide pools than was initially appreciated. Studies in subjects who lack activity of HG-PRT, and of their cells in culture, indicate that recycling of hypoxanthine and guanine via the nucleoside phosphorylase-nucleoside kinase route is not very active. Kinases capable of phosphorylating inosine or guanosine have been described in animal tissues (PIERRE and LE PAGE, 1968), and labeled inosine is incorporated into adenine and guanine nucleotides in liver of both normal and PRT-deficient subjects (WADA et al., 1968). These kinases appear to be absent in human fibroblasts (FRIEDMAN et al., 1969). Normally the action of purine nucleoside phosphorylase upon inosine or guanosine is probably largely degradative. The situation with adenosine is quite different. Adenosine kinase is an active enzyme with an extensive distribution in mammalian tissues (CAPUTTO, 1951; KORNBERG and PRICER, 1951). For example, adenosine is readily converted to acid-soluble nucleotides by dog heart muscle (GOLDTHWAITE, 1957).

By either of these salvage pathways only one high-energy bond, in the form of PP-ribose-P or ATP, is expended in the resynthesis of a ribonucleotide, whereas synthesis of AMP or GMP *de novo* from glutamine and PP-ribose-P requires the expenditure of a minimum of six high-energy bonds.

Economy of Purine Biosynthesis in the Mammal

Purine biosynthesis *de novo* is especially active in liver. All enzymes of purine biosynthesis, nucleotide interconversion, degradation, and base salvage are found in the soluble portion of the cell, except for uricase which when present is particulate, and is found in lysosomes. Uricase is not present in birds, higher apes, or man. There is evidence that the enzymes of purine biosynthesis *de novo* are not in free solution, circulating within the cytosol at random, but rather that they exist in a macromolecular aggregate of molecular weight well in excess of 1 million daltons capable of conducting the complete synthesis of inosinic acid (WYNGAARDEN et al., 1969a). Nonhepatic tissues other than placenta appear capable of only limited synthesis of purines *de novo*. The mature human erythrocyte actively synthesizes PP-ribose-P, and purine ribonucleotides from free bases via phosphoribosyltransferase reactions, but it cannot synthesize phosphoribosylamine (WYNGAARDEN et al., 1958a). Therefore, it is incapable of purine synthesis *de novo*. Circulating leukocytes contain assayable PP-ribose-P amidotransferase activity (HOLMES et al., 1973b).

Data of LAJTHA and VANE (1958) suggest that some nonhepatic tissues, for example bone marrow, are dependent upon an advanced purine precursor originating in liver for their source of nucleic and purine bases. HENDERSON and LE PAGE (1959) suggested that erythrocytes may transport an auxiliary supply of purines. LERNER and LOWY (1973) have assigned this function to adenosine synthesized in the liver and delivered to distant tissues by the erythrocytes. The critical role of phosphoribosyltransferase pathways in nonhepatic tissues is thus clear. In the presence of a limited capacity for purine synthesis *de novo*, and partial dependence upon purine imports, recovery of purine bases generated by catabolic reactions becomes a function of major importance to the cell. Because of the restricted distribution in man of catabolic enzymes capable of acting upon free purines, those bases generated in nonhepatic or nonintestinal tissue are largely protected from catabolism and available for recycling, unless lost from the cell and transported to the liver.

Nucleic Acid Catabolism

Enzymatic hydrolysis of polynucleotide chains of nucleic acid occurs through the action of various nucleases (HEPPEL and RABINOWITZ, 1958). The major products released by ribonuclease a and b and by deoxyribonuclease I and II are oligonucleotides. The oligonucleotides are further cleaved by phosphodiesterases to yield 5'- and 3'-mononucleotides.

The mononucleotides are split by group-specific nucleoside-5-phosphatases (HEPPEL and HILMOE, 1951), as well as by nonspecific phosphatases (SCHMIDT, 1955), to yield the corresponding purine or pyrimidine nucleoside and orthophosphate. The purine nucleoside is then split by purine nucleoside phosphorylase (FREIDKIN and KALCKAR, 1961) to yield a free purine base and ribose-1-phosphate, or deoxyribose-1-phosphate.

$$\text{Purine mononucleotide} \rightarrow \text{purine nucleoside} + P_i; \tag{19}$$

$$\text{Base-ribose} + P_i \rightarrow \text{base} + \text{ribose-1-phosphate} \tag{17}$$

In addition to these general reactions, AMP and adenosine are acted upon by specific deaminating enzymes. AMP is converted to IMP by adenylic deaminase

(Reaction 20, Fig. 6) (NIKIFORUK and COLOWICK, 1956) and adenosine to inosine by adenosine deaminase (Reaction 21, Fig. 6) (KALCKAR, 1947).

A number of purine bases other than adenine and guanine occur as minor constituents of nucleic acids. The mononucleotides derived from certain bacterial and bacteriophage DNAs contain small quantities of 6-methylaminopurine (DUNN and SMITH, 1958). Ribosomal and transfer RNAs of bacterial and mammalian cells contain small amounts of hypoxanthine, as well as of several methylated purine bases, including 1-methylguanine, N^2-methylguanine, N^2-dimethylguanine, 7-methylguanine, 2-methyladenine, N^6-methyladenine, N^6-dimethyladenine, 1-methyladenine, and 1-methylhypoxanthine (BOREK and SRINIVASAN, 1966). tRNAs contain approximately four times as many methyl groups as rRNAs. The 16 S species of bacterial ribosomal RNA contains approximately 20 percent more methyl groups than the 23 S species. Methylations occur at the polynucleotide level (GOLD and HURWITZ, 1964; HURWITZ et al., 1965) and a number of different methylating enzymes have been identified which will methylate specific purine sites in DNA (GOLD and HURWITZ, 1964), rRNA (HURWITZ et al., 1965), or methyl-deficient tRNA (BOREK and SRINIVASAN, 1966). In all known instances the methyl donor is S-adenosyl-methionine. Most of the methylated bases listed above have been identified in human urine in small quantities.

Catabolism of Ingested Nucleoproteins

Nucleic acids of dietary nucleoproteins are liberated in the intestinal canal by the action of proteolytic enzymes. Nucleic acids are degraded to nucleotides by nucleases and phosphodiesterases secreted by the pancreas. The nucleotides are chiefly hydrolyzed to nucleosides by various nucleotidases and phosphatases, and the nucleosides are either absorbed intact, or cleaved phosphorolytically to the free base. The small intestinal mucosa of man is rich in nucleoside phosphorylase and xanthine oxidase, and ingested nucleoprotein purines may potentially be converted to uric acid in the gastrointestinal mucosa. The uric acid may be further catabolized by intestinal bacteria or may be absorbed. From experiments in which human subjects ingested ^{15}N-labeled nucleic acid (WILSON et al., 1954), it appeared that the purine moieties were converted to uric acid largely by direct routes without prior incorporation into body nucleic acids. However, small quantities of dietary nucleosides and even nucleotides may be utilized directly for synthesis of nucleic acids (ROLL et al., 1949).

Formation of Uric Acid

The free purine bases that result from nucleoside cleavage are adenine, guanine, hypoxanthine, and xanthine. Since purine nucleoside phosphorylase acts most readily upon inosine and guanosine (FRIEDKIN and KALCKAR, 1961; HUENEKENS et al., 1956), the major bases generated are very probably hypoxanthine and guanine. In bacteria, free adenine is deaminated (SCHMIDT, 1955), but mammalian tissues lack adenase so that adenine does not give rise directly to hypoxanthine. If it is not recovered to its nucleotide, it may be excreted. Normal human subjects excrete 1—2 mg of adenine per day in urine (WEISSMANN et al., 1957a). By contrast, the other purine bases are readily converted to uric acid. Guanine is deaminated to xanthine by guanase (Reaction 22, Fig. 6). Hypoxanthine is oxidized to xanthine by xanthine oxidase (Reaction 23), and then further oxidized to uric acid by the same enzyme (Reaction 24) (BERGMANN and DIKSTEIN, 1956). Thus, whereas adenine, hypoxanthine, and guanine arise exclusively from cleavage of the corresponding nucleoside, xanthine has at least three direct precursors, namely, xanthosine (or deoxyxanthosine), hypoxanthine, and guanine.

In man, xanthine oxidase is found in high activity only in liver and small intestinal mucosa (ENGELMAN et al., 1964; WATTS et al., 1965). Traces of activity are found in heart and skeletal muscle, kidney and spleen, and none is present in leukocytes, erythrocytes, stratum corneum, or fibroblasts in tissue culture (WATTS et al., 1965). The enzyme is a flavoprotein containing iron and molybdenum, capable of oxidizing a wide variety of purines, aldehydes, and pteridines. In the rat (ROWE and WYNGAARDEN, 1966) and certain other species, xanthine oxidase is an inducible enzyme, its activity in liver depending on protein intake, and perhaps other factors.

Because of the restricted distribution of xanthine oxidase and its great activity in liver, uric acid synthesis appears largely to be a hepatic process in man. Presumably purine degradation products of other tissues are transported to the liver for further oxidation. Plasma contains small quantities of xanthine and hypoxanthine, together amounting to about 0.1 to 0.3 mg per 100 ml (SEGAL and WYNGAARDEN, 1955; JORGENSEN and POULSEN, 1955), but no other uric acid precursors have been detected in normal plasma in significant quantity, with the possible exception of IMP following anoxic muscle injury (HOFFMAN et al., 1951).

Uric Acid Ribonucleoside

Since the discovery of uric acid ribonucleoside in beef erythrocytes (DAVIS et al., 1922) and liver (FALCONER and GULLAND, 1939), the possibility has been entertained that this nucleoside is an intermediate of an alternative pathway of uric acid synthesis. Its existence in human erythrocytes has been claimed (NEWTON and DAVIS, 1922) and denied (OVERGAARD-HANSEN and NIELSON, 1957; FORREST et al., 1961). Although FALCONER and GULLAND (1939) originally concluded that the beef compound was a 9-N-ribosyl derivative, more recent spectral studies (BIRKOFER et al., 1963) indicate that the ribosyl group is attached to the N-3 position of uric acid (FORREST et al., 1961). This structure has been confirmed by synthesis (BIRKOFER et al., 1963; LOHRMAN et al., 1964). The ribonucleoside is cleaved to uric acid and ribose-1-phosphate by a specific phosphorylase found in several species and purified extensively from dog small intestinal mucosa (LASTER and BLAIR, 1963). It is now known that the ribonucleoside is formed by the action of phosphatase or 5'-nucleotidase upon uric acid ribonucleotide ((3-N-ribosyluric acid)-5'-phosphate), which is formed by a direct condensation of uric acid and PP-ribose-P (HATFIELD and FORREST, 1962; HATFIELD and WYNGAARDEN, 1964b). Therefore, the pathway does not result in net synthesis of uric acid. Small amounts of the ribonucleotide exist in beef erythrocytes (HATFIELD et al., 1963).

The enzyme catalyzing synthesis of the ribonucleotide has been purified over 5000-fold from beef erythrocytes. It also catalyzes reaction with xanthine, uracil, orotic acid, and thymine (HATFIELD and WYNGAARDEN, 1964a, 1964b). With xanthine and uric acid the products are both 3-N-ribosephosphate derivatives (HATFIELD et al., 1963). The K_m values for the pyrimidine substrates are lower than those for uric acid or xanthine. For this reason the enzyme is considered to be a 2, 4-diketo pyrimidine phosphoribosyltransferase with overlapping activity toward 2, 6-diketo purines with unsubstituted nitrogen atoms. Competition experiments indicate that the enzyme is identical with orotate phosphoribosyltransferase (BEARDMORE and KELLEY, 1971). In addition, a phosphoribosyltransferase derived from Lactobacillus plantarus forms a 9-N-ribose-phosphate derivative of uric acid (HATFIELD et al., 1964c), but it is not known whether such a compound is synthesized in mammalian tissues.

Regulation of Purine Biosynthesis De Novo

Rate-limiting Step

A number of arguments collectively suggest that the rate of formation of 5-phosphoribosyl-1-amine, is limiting for the entire sequence: (1.) Phosphoribosylamine is the first specific purine precursor, and no branching of the succeeding pathway occurs prior to synthesis of inosinic acid. (2.) No intermediates of the *de-novo* pathway accumulate unless a genetic or chemical block of a reaction is introduced, e.g. in bacteria (GOTS and GOLDSTEIN, 1959) or in tissue culture of surviving mammalian cells (BROCKMAN and ANDERSON, 1963; BROCKMAN and CHUMLEY, 1965). (3.) The activities of PP-ribose-P synthetase (FOX and KELLEY, 1971a), of glutamine PP-ribose-P amidotransferase (CASKEY et al., 1964; WYNGAARDEN, 1972), and of ribose-5-P aminotransferase (REEM, 1968) are all regulated by purine ribonucleotides, but that of GAR-synthetase is not (NIERLICH and MAGASANIK, 1965a), and no functional inhibition is observed in the portion of the sequence from GAR to IMP (WYNGAARDEN et al., 1958a). Although inhibition of the amidation of FGAR to FGAM by AMP and GMP can be demonstrated with the isolated enzyme, the required concentrations of inhibitor ribonucleotides are unphysiologically high (HOWARD and APPEL, 1968). (4.) Bacterial purine auxotrophs grown on limiting concentrations of purines show derepression of synthesis of the first amidotransferase as well as of five other enzymes concerned with purine synthesis *de novo* (NIERLICH and MAGASANIK, 1963; MOMOSE et al., 1966). (5.) Measures which raise intracellular concentrations of PP-ribose-P accelerate purine biosynthesis; measures which lower PP-ribose-P concentrations reduce the rate of purine biosynthesis (HENDERSON and KHOO, 1965a; KELLEY et al., 1970b). (6.) The availability of glutamine can be rate limiting for purine synthesis under certain circumstances (RAIVIO and SEEGMILLER, 1971).

The regulation of the rate of formation of phosphoribosylamine may therefore be the single most important factor in the control of purine synthesis *de novo*. The chief and perhaps sole functional reaction for its synthesis is the glutamine PP-ribose-P amidotransferase reaction (see reaction 2a, above). The major factors determining the rate of this reaction are the concentrations of substrates, the intrinsic activity of the enzyme catalyzing it, and the effects of inhibitors or activators upon it.

Substrates

5-phosphoribosyl-1-pyrophosphate

Only a small fraction of pentose phosphate is converted to PP-ribose-P (KATZ and ROGNSTAD, 1967). PP-ribose-P synthetase from bacteria (SWITZER, 1967), Ehrlich ascites tumor cells (WONG and MURRAY, 1969) or human erythrocytes (FOX and KELLEY, 1971a) is inhibited by a large number of purine and pyrimidine nucleoside mono-, di-, and triphosphates. The smallest native form of the human enzyme has a molecular weight of 60000 and is composed of two subunits of equal molecular weight. However, the active form of the enzyme *in vivo* appears to be a polymer of this native form ranging in molecular weight from 240000 to over 1000000 (FOX and KELLEY, 1971a). It is found in virtually all tissues with highest activity in testes. Nucleotide inhibition is noncompetitive and cumulative (SWITZER, 1967; WONG and MURRAY, 1969; Fox and KELLEY, 1972). This mechanism conforms with the concept of "heterogeneous metabolic pool inhibition (FOX and KELLEY, 1972).

ATKINSON and FALLS (1967 and 1968) postulate that the activity of biosynthetic reaction activity is controlled by the "energy charge" of the cell, as well as by cumulative feedback inhibition.

$$\text{"Energy charge"} = \frac{\text{ATP} + 1/2\,\text{ADP}}{\text{ATP} + \text{ADP} + \text{AMP}}$$

This concept predicts that the synthesis of PP-ribose-P will be inhibited by nucleoside diphosphates and monophosphates, irrespective of specific feedback effects. Observations in bacteria (SWITZER, 1967) and mammalian cells (WONG and MURRAY, 1969; FOX and KELLEY, 1971a) support the concept. The experiments of KLUNGSOYR et al. (1968) suggest an interaction between energy charge modulation and cumulative product inhibition in control of activity of bacterial PP-ribose-P synthetase.

Normal levels of PP-ribose-P range from 1 to 5×10^{-6} M erythrocytes; and perhaps as high as 1.3×10^{-5} M in fibroblasts in tissue culture (FOX and KELLEY, 1971b). These values are 1 to 10 percent the Michaelis constant for PP-ribose-P of the human amidotransferase (HOLMES et al., 1973a; WOOD and SEEGMILLER, 1973), which is 4.7×10^{-4} M.

Methylene blue raises the intracellular concentration of PP-ribose-P in Ehrlich ascites cells *in vitro* (HENDERSON and KHOO, 1965a), in human fibroblasts in tissue culture (GREENE and SEEGMILLER, 1969), and in human erythrocytes *in vitro* (KELLEY et al., 1970b), presumably by accelerating the regeneration of NADP in the oxidative pathway of glucose metabolism and thereby stimulating the rate of production of ribose-5-phosphate. Purine biosynthesis *de novo* is enhanced. PP-ribose-P synthesis is also stimulated *in vitro* by glucose, fructose and mannose (HENDERSON and KHOO, 1965a; GREENE and SEEGMILLER, 1969). Intracellular PP-ribose-P concentrations may be reduced by stimulating PP-ribose-P consumption with allopurinol (Fox et al., 1970), orotic acid (KELLEY et al., 1970c), adenine (GREENE and SEEGMILLER, 1969), or 2,6-diaminopurine (GREENE and SEEGMILLER, 1969). Such measures reduce the rate of purine biosynthesis *de novo* in normal cells (KELLEY et al., 1970b). PP-ribose-P concentration values are elevated in cells with deficient hypoxanthine-guanine phosphoribosyltransferase activity (ROSENBLOOM et al., 1968), as well as in cells with overactive variant forms of PP-ribose-P synthetase (SPERLING et al., 1972a; BECKER et al., 1973). Fibroblasts from subjects with either of these enzyme abnormalities synthesize purines at an excessive rate. The sum total of the observations cited above underscore the critical role that rates of generation, and steady-state levels, of PP-ribose-P exert upon the rate of purine biosynthesis *de novo*.

L-*Glutamine*

This compound is often regarded as a storage form of ammonia-N:

α-Ketoglutarate + NH_3 + NADH + H^+ → L-glutamate + H_2O + NAD^+

L-Glutamate + NH_3 + ATP → L-glutamine + H_2O + P_i + ADP.

The reversible fixation of ammonia by α-ketoglutarate is catalyzed by glutamic acid dehydrogenase, an enzyme subject to complex regulation by purine ribonucleotides and certain steroids. FRIEDEN (1963) has discussed the possibility that the inhibition of glutamic acid dehydrogenase, which catalyzes a reaction usually operating to convert glutamic acid to α-ketoglutaric acid, may indirectly influence the rate of glutamine synthesis and thereby that of purine synthesis.

The reaction of L-glutamate, NH_3, and ATP is catalyzed by glutamine synthetase, an enzyme found in high activity in liver (SPECK, 1949), cerebral cortex (SELLINGER and VERSTER, 1962), and rat kidney (RECTOR and ORLOFF, 1959), but apparently absent from dog kidney (KREBS, 1935; RECTOR and ORLOFF, 1959). Glutamine synthetase of E. coli is a decameric enzyme which requires adenylylation by ATP for conversion from inactive to active state (KINGDON et al., 1967). The active enzyme is subject to cumulative endproduct inhibition; each of eight end products of pathways entered by glutamine contributes a fractional inhibition of residual enzyme activity; all eight end products are required in saturating concentrations for complete inhibition. These include glycine, alanine, histidine, tryptophan, glucosamine-6-phosphate, carbamylphosphate, and CTP, as well as AMP, an end product of the purine biosynthetic pathway (SHAPIRO and STADTMAN, 1970). The enzyme from sheep brain has similar properties but is an octomer (PAMILJANS et al., 1962).

Normal human fibroblasts grown in a glutamine-free medium for 1 or 2 days show a roughly linear increase in purine synthesis with increasing glutamine concentrations, the maximal stimulation being five to tenfold (RAIVIO and SEEGMILLER, 1971). The K_m of glutamine in the PP-ribose-P amidotransferase reaction is 0.5 mM with rat liver enzyme (CASKEY et al., 1964), 0.7 to 1.1 mM with pigeon liver enzyme (WYNGAARDEN and ASHTON, 1959a; CASKEY et al., 1964; ROWE and WYNGAARDEN, 1968), and 1.6 mM with human placental (HOLMES et al., 1973a) or lymphoblast enzyme (WOOD and SEEGMILLER, 1973). Liver, brain and kidney of all species studied are rich in glutamine (WAELSCH, 1951). Glutamine concentration values in rat liver cell water range from 3 to 7 mM (KENNAN, 1962; BERGMEYER, 1970). These values are sufficiently high to suggest that the amidotransferase may be nearly saturated with respect to glutamine under normal conditions, at least in the rat. If this is the case, changes in the concentration of glutamine would not be associated with a concomitant change in the rate of PRPP amidotransferase or purine biosynthesis *de novo*.

The plasma levels of glutamine in both normal and gouty men are about 0.7 mM (SEGAL and WYNGAARDEN, 1955). L-glutamine of plasma is the immediate precursor or perhaps 80 percent of urinary ammonia (OWEN and ROBINSON, 1963; PITTS, 1964). Two glutaminases are present in the kidney and liver (ERRERA, 1949a; ERRERA and GREENSTEIN, 1949b). One, designated as glutaminase I, is activated (or stabilized) by phosphate (KREBS, 1935; SAYRE and ROBERTS, 1958) and splits off the amide nitrogen of glutamine to form glutamic acid and ammonia. Its pH optimum is 8; it is found in the mitochondria. The other, designated as glutaminase II, is in reality a glutamine-transaminase-ω-deamidase system and is activated by α-keto acids. Alpha-ketoglutaramide is the hypothetical direct precursor of ammonia (MEISTER, 1957). The pH optimum of this enzyme is about 9, and it is found in the soluble fraction of the cell.

Glutamine Phosphoribosylpyrophosphate Amidotransferase

The enzyme has been studied in bacteria (NIERLICH and MAGASANIK, 1965b), yeast (NAGY, 1970), pigeon, chicken, and rat liver (CASKEY et al., 1964; ROWE and WYNGAARDEN, 1968; ROWE et al., 1970), Ehrlich ascites cells (HENDERSON and KHOO, 1965b), mouse adenocarcinoma 755 cells (HILL and BENNETT, 1969), human placenta (HOLMES et al., 1973a), and human lymphoblasts in culture (WOOD and SEEGMILLER, 1973). The avian enzyme has a molecular weight of about 200000 and on dilution dissociates into molecules of about 100000 daltons. In the presence of reducing agents these molecules further dissociate into electrophoretically identical subunits of 50000 molecular weight. The enzyme is activated by PP-ribose-P and Mg^{++}, which are required for the subsequent binding of glutamine. The avian enzyme contains 12 atoms of nonheme iron per 200000 molecular weight. The human placental enzyme has a molecular weight of 133000 in the presence of PP-ribose-P, and of 270000 in the presence of ribonucleotides (see below).

End-Product Inhibition

The avian enzyme is inhibited by purine-5'-ribonucleotides, but not by ribonucleosides, or bases (WYNGAARDEN and ASHTON, 1959a). The K_i values for various ribonucleotide inhibitors range from 10^{-5} to 10^{-3} M. The enzyme may be desensitized to its inhibitors without loss of catalytic activity. The enzyme has two inhibitor-binding sites, one for 6-aminopurine and one for 6-hydroxypurine ribonucleotides, and both sites appear to be distinct from either substrate site. Some of the iron atoms are concerned with inhibitor binding, while others appear to be involved in maintaining the dimer and tetramer structure (ROWE and WYNGAARDEN, 1968). Sigmoidal kinetics are observed with variations of PP-ribose-P concentrations in the presence of ribonucleotide inhibitors (ROWE et al., 1970). Furthermore, the inhibitory effects of AMP and GMP acting in concert are synergistic. With the human enzyme, ribonucleotide inhibitors convert the active form of the enzyme (133000 mol. wt.) to an inactive form (270000 mol. wt.) (HOLMES et al., 1973c, in press). These results define a special type of end-product control of purine biosynthesis, which is maximal when the two types of negative effectors are present in optimal concentration and ratio, and reversible by excess PP-ribose-P (WYNGAARDEN, 1972; HOLMES et al., 1973a; HOLMES et al., 1973c). The synergistic nature of the inhibition permits a more effective curtailment of the first reaction when both types of inhibitor are present in abundance, but allows for a more moderate control when only one kind is in excess (Fig. 7).

Production of Uric Acid in Gout

Chemical Balance

In theory, the rate of purine synthesis may be assessed from the difference between intake and excretion in the dynamic steady state. In practice this approach fails because urinary uric acid represents a variable fraction of total purine turnover, and there are no convenient methods for measurement of extrarenal excretion of urate. Purine intake may be reduced to less than 3 mg purine-N per day by severe dietary restriction. The average urinary uric acid excretion value is then a minimal estimate of purine production. The normal urinary uric acid excretion under standard conditions of activity and dietary intake ranges from 278 to 558 per day (mean 418 ± 70 mg) (GUTMAN and YU, 1957), or from 264 to 588 mg per day (mean 426 ± 81 mg) (SEEGMILLER et al., 1961) in the male. The frequency histograms show skewness toward high values without evidence for bimodality.

Urinary uric acid values in males with primary gout extend from 150 mg per day or less to 1500 mg per day or more. Low values are found in patients with overt renal damage. From 21 to 28 percent of subjects with primary gout consis-

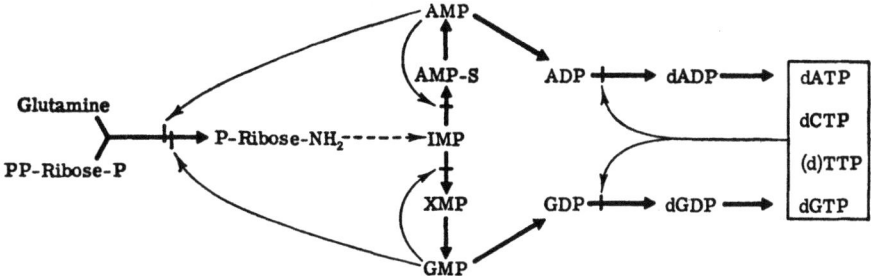

Fig. 7. Summary of feedback controls operating upon reactions of purine synthesis and utilization. (Reproduced from WYNGAARDEN, 1965, with permission of Academic, New York)

tently excrete quantities of urate exceeding the (mean +2 s.d.) value (GUTMAN and YU, 1957; SEEGMILLER et al., 1961). Such patients have arbitrarily been classified as overexcretors of uric acid. The theoretical possibility that increased urinary excretion is secondary to decreased extrarenal disposal of urate has been excluded by normal urinary recoveries of injected labeled uric acid in the majority of overexcretor patients (GUTMAN and YU, 1957). Therefore, sustained overexcretion of uric acid is evidence for excessive synthesis of purines *de novo*. However, normal urinary excretion of uric acid does not exclude overproduction of uric acid in gouty subjects, for in the hyperuricemic subject with reduced renal urate excretion, the disposal of urate by extrarenal processes may be much increased, in extreme examples accounting for over 80 percent of the urate turnover (SEEGMILLER et al., 1961).

In the past two decades the mechanism and rates of uric acid production have been under intensive study by means of two general types of biochemical techniques: (1.) The turnover study, emplying principles of isotope dilution; and (2.) precursor administration, with evaluation of the rate and extent of conversion of the substance administered into uric acid. More recently, studies in gout have been amplified by direct enzyme assays in human tissue and by the use of cell culture techniques.

The Miscible Pool of Uric Acid and its Turnover

The isotope dilution technique for measurement of the miscible pool of uric acid and the rate of its turnover was introduced by BENEDICT et al. (BENEDICT et al., 1949). Isotopic uric acid is injected intravenously and permitted to mix intimately with uric acid in the body. Urinary uric acid is isolated serially for several days, and the isotope concentration of each sample is determined. Values are plotted on semilogarithmic coordinates, and the theoretical concentration of isotope in the body at the moment of mixing (I_o) is obtained by extrapolation of the linear portion of the decay curve to zero time (Fig. 8). The miscible pool of uric acid is defined as the quantity of uric acid in the body of the recipient by which the injected uric acid is promptly diluted. The quantity of uric acid present in the miscible pool (A) can be calculated from knowledge of the amount of uric acid injected (a), of the concentration of isotope in it (I_i), and of the concentration of isotope in the uric acid of the body at the moment of mixing (I_o):

$$A = a\left(\frac{I_i}{I_o} - 1\right).$$

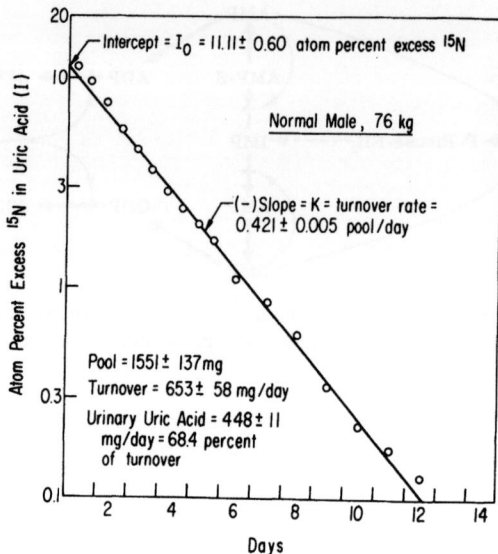

Fig. 8. Determination of miscible pool of uric acid and its turnover. The line has been fit by least squares analysis of points of days 2—10 inclusive. Points of day 1 are frequently high because of excretion of infused ^{15}N-uric acid before mixing is complete. Late points (e.g. days 11, 12) often trend upward from the linear plot, possibly because of recycling of labeled urate from compartments in slow equilibrium with the major miscible pool

After mixing has occurred, a further progressive decline in the concentration of isotope in uric acid occurs because of the continuous dilution of the labeled uric acid pool by newly synthesized nonisotopic uric acid molecules. From the rate of decline in isotope concentration (K), the rate of addition of unlabeled uric acid (KA) can be calculated (BENEDICT et al., 1949). In the normal subject, this addition can be presumed to represent newly synthesized uric acid. The majority of studies have employed the original technique of determining the isotope concentration of uric acid isolated from urine. SORENSEN (1959; 1962) has injected ^{14}C-labeled uric acid intravenously and has calculated the specific activity of uric acid from the radioactivity value and uric acid content of a volume of serum, on the reasonable assumption that (in man) all ^{14}C in serum is in the form of uric acid.

In about 25 normal male subjects (WYNGAARDEN and KELLEY, 1972b), the rapidly miscible pool was an average of 1200 mg uric acid, with values ranging from 866 to 1587 mg. In three normal females, the pool ranged from 541 to 687 mg (WYNGAARDEN and KELLEY, 1972b). These values confirmed earlier analytic values of GUDZENT (1928).

From the rate of decline in concentration of ^{15}N or ^{14}C in urinary uric acid, it was calculated that 45 to 85 percent of the uric acid of the miscible pool was normally replaced each day by newly formed, nonisotopic molecules. The turnover of uric acid averaged 695 mg per day, with values ranging from 513 to 1108 mg per day. In each case, the quantity of uric acid entering the pool exceeded the amount in urine by 100 to 260 mg per day (SORENSEN, 1959; BENEDICT et al., 1949). The significance of this surplus will be discussed below.

In gouty subjects, the miscible pool is generally enlarged to 2000 to 4000 mg in patients without tophi (WYNGAARDEN and KELLEY, 1972b) and may reach 18000 to 31000 mg in patients with severe tophaceous disease (BENEDICT et al., 1950). Even so, the value the miscible pool may represent only a small fraction of the total urate in the body, for only the peripheral layers of tophi are readily exchangeable with urate in solution in body fluids (BENEDICT et al., 1950). In one patient, the amount of uric acid in the tophaceous compartment participating in a slow exchange with soluble uric acid was estimated by SORENSEN (1962) to be 300 times larger than the rapidly miscible pool.

Because of the possibility of exchange of labeled urate of the miscible pool with unlabeled urate of the solid phase, the turnover technique may not provide a reliable measure of the rate of synthesis of urate in subjects with tophaceous gout. Nevertheless, the value for turnover of urate agrees very well with that obtained by another calculation for rate of synthesis (SEEGMILLER et al., 1961; KELLEY et al., 1969), viz.,

$$\frac{\text{Basal urinary uric acid, mg per day}}{\text{Urinary recovery of injected isotopic uric acid, fraction of administered dose}}$$

In gouty patients whose miscible pool is within, or just above, the normal range it is sometimes possible to calculate that all the urate measured in the miscible pool is in solution. In two patients meeting these criteria, SORENSEN (1959) found excessive turnover of uric acid. However, in five other patients meeting these criteria, SEEGMILLER et al. (1961) found a normal turnover of uric acid, and these five patients also showed normal incorporations of isotopic glycine into uric acid (see below).

Incorporation of Labeled Precursors into Uric Acid

The rate of generation of uric acid has been studied in both normal and gouty subjects by observing the rate at which isotope appears in uric acid when a labeled precursor is administered. Studies of this type have been performed with glycine-^{15}N, glycine-1-^{14}C, glycine-2-^{14}C, ammonium-^{15}N, formate-^{14}C, 4-aminoimidazole-5-carboxamide-4-^{13}C and 4-^{14}C, hypoxanthine-8-^{14}C, and adenine-8-^{14}C and 8-^{13}C.

Incorporation of Labeled Glycine into Urinary Uric Acid

A large number of studies of incorporation of labeled glycine into urinary uric acid have been performed since the technique was introduced by BENEDICT and associates in 1952 (BENEDICT et al., 1952; BENEDICT et al., 1953). The discussion below is based on studies of incorporation of glycine-1-^{14}C, glycine-U-^{14}C, and glycine-^{15}N under standardized experimental conditions. The few studies in which glycine-2-^{14}C was administered orally (GUTMAN et al., 1958), or in which glycine-^{15}N was given in small amounts (BISHOP et al., 1955) will be omitted, since they are not strictly comparable.

After the subject has been prepared with a very-low-purine diet for about 5 days, labeled glycine is given orally with a light breakfast (BENEDICT et al., 1952), or injected intravenously (SORENSEN, 1962). The labeled glycine will be diluted with glycine of dietary origin and by glycine of various intracellular and extracellular pools. Variations in the amount of diluting unlabeled glycine and in the size and turnover of the hepatic glycine pool could influence the specific activity of uric acid, quite apart from differences in the rates of purine synthesis. Efforts to assess the significance of such factors as explanations for abnormal enrichment of urate in gout, by measurements of enrichment of other products of glycine metab-

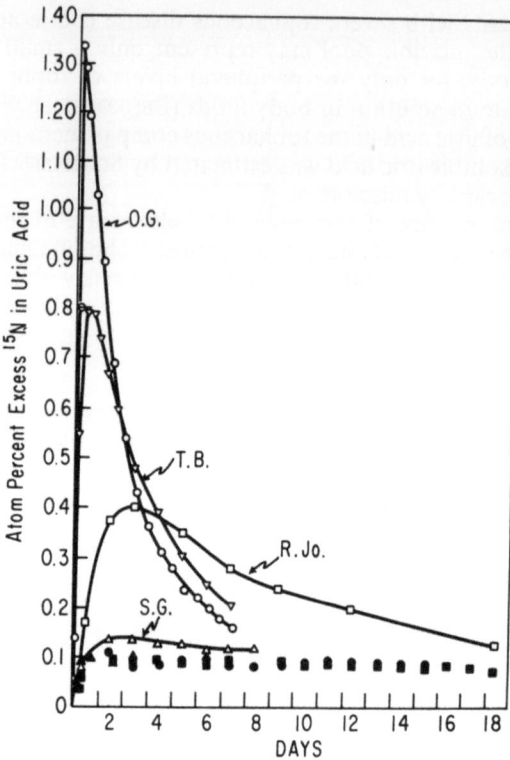

Fig. 9. Incorporation of (1-^{14}C)-glycine into urinary uric acid in 3 control subjects (solid symbols), one patient with idiopathic gout and mild overexcretion (S.G.), one patient with high-grade but partial PRT deficiency (R.Jo.), and two patients with variant forms of PP-Ribose-P synthetase (T.B., O.G.). From SPERLING et al., 1973

olism, such as hippurate (SEEGMILLER et al., 1961; SPERLING et al., 1973) or creatinine (GUTMAN and YU, 1963a), have been reassuring, and have not disclosed evidence of abnormal labeling or turnover kinetics of glycine in gout.

Glycine-1-^{14}C is given in tracer doses of a few milligrams, whereas doses of 0.1 g per kg are required with ^{15}N-glycine. This quantity of ^{15}N-glycine is approximately equal to the free glycine pool in man, which is 80 to 90 mg per kg (GUTMAN et al., 1958; WATTS and CRAWHALL, 1959). Since glycine enters the purine sequence beyond the rate-limiting step of purine synthesis, one would anticipate that approximately one-half as much isotope would be incorporated into uric acid when such a glycine load is given as when a tracer dose is given. Average incorporation values for ^{14}C and ^{15}N in control and gouty subjects (WYNGAARDEN, 1966) as well as a direct appraisal of this question in four control subjects given glycine-1-^{14}C with and without carrier glycine (GUTMAN et al., 1958) confirm this prediction.

The studies of BENEDICT et al. (1952, 1953) established that the incorporation of glycine-^{15}N into urinary uric acid was excessive in gouty subjects with abnormally large excretions of urate but normal or only slightly elevated in subjects with normal excretion values (Fig. 9). Subsequent studies with glycine-^{15}N or glycine-1-^{14}C have extended these observations. Figure 10 summarizes the majority of published incorporation values observed in studies in which glycine-

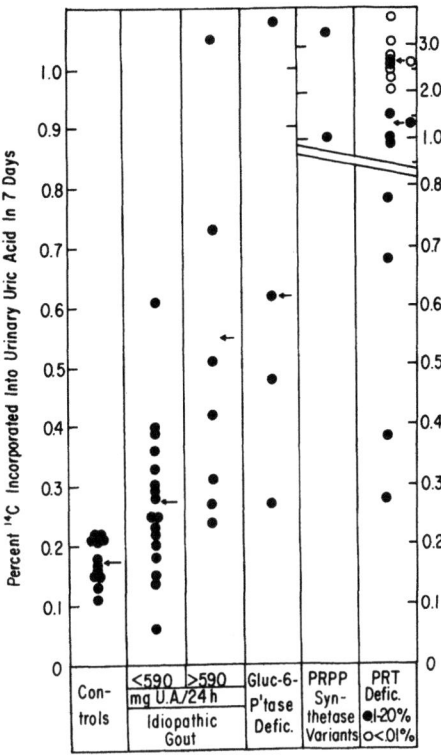

Fig. 10. Summary of incorporations of glycine-1-^{14}C and glycine U-^{14}C into urinary uric acid. Values represent data from published studies (SPERLING et al., 1972; BECKER et al., 1972; WYNGAARDEN and KELLEY, 1972) in which glycine was administered to subjects on purine-restricted diets

1-^{14}C or U-^{14}C was administered. Those in which glycine-^{15}N were employed have been summarized elsewhere (WYNGAARDEN, 1966). In gouty subjects with uric acid excretions of less than 590 mg per day, the cumulative incorporation of ^{14}C is excessive in one-half to two-thirds of the cases. In subjects with excretions of more than 590 mg per day, incorporation is invariably excessive, often exceeding normal values by several fold.

Incorporation of Labeled Glycine into Total Body Uric Acid

Newly synthesized isotopic urate will be diluted within an expanded miscible pool of unlabeled urate in gouty subjects. In addition, as renal function deteriorates, the fraction of the urate turnover excreted in urine each day may decline, and that excreted into the gastrointestinal tract may increase. Several of the gouty subjects of Fig. 10 with apparently normal incorporation values had extensive tophaceous deposits and impaired renal function. These factors could mask over-incorporation. SEEGMILLER and co-workers (1961) measured the fraction of intravenously injected uric acid (labeled with a different isotope) that was not recovered in the urine during the experiment. In two of five gouty subjects whose glycine-^{14}C incorporation values were normal, excessive incorporation was revealed when appropriate corrections were made for extrarenal disposal.

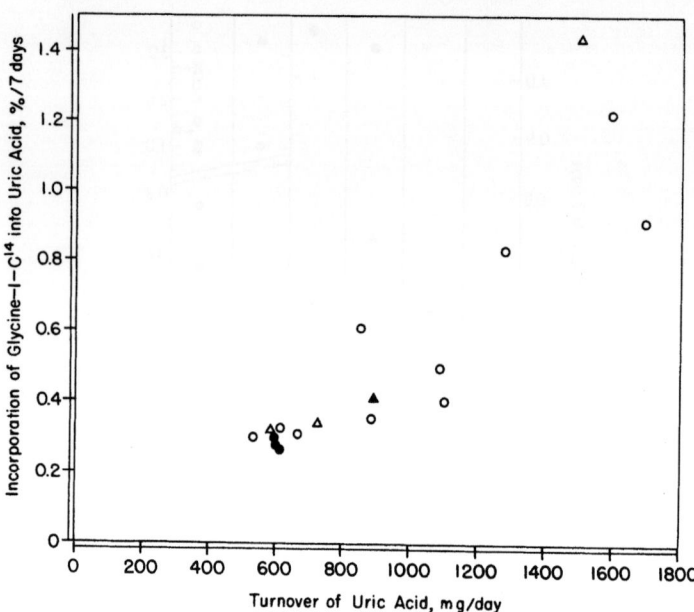

Fig. 11. Comparison of incorporation of glycine-1-^{14}C into uric acid and turnover of uric acid. The incorporation values have been corrected for extrarenal disposal. (Replotted from SEEGMILLER et al., 1961)

Glycine incorporation values are indices rather than definitive measurements of rates of purine production. There is no independent quantitative method for assessing purine production that is reliable under all circumstances. The 24-h urinary uric acid values generally represent about two-thirds of the turnover in normal man but may represent a much smaller fraction in gouty subjects (SORENSEN, 1955; NUGENT and TYLER, 1959; SEEGMILLER et al., 1961). The turnover of uric acid, as determined by isotope dilution, may not be a measure of production in subjects in whom solid urate contributes to the dilution process. Turnover measurements may overestimate uric acid production in gouty subjects just as excretion measurements may underestimate production.

Figure 11 compares incorporation values of glycine-^{14}C into uric acid (corrected for extrarenal disposal) with turnover of uric acid-^{15}N. Although a positive correlation clearly exists, an appreciable scatter of values is apparent. The imprecision of glycine incorporation as a measure of purine production in the range of uric acid turnover of 500 to 1200 mg per day, in which the turnovers of the majority of gouty subjects fall, is clear. Taken together, the glycine incorporation studies suggest that subjects with primary gout show a spectrum of rates of production of uric acid ranging from values within the normal range to elevated values four or five times the normal, or, in the case of patients with phosphoribosyltransferase deficiency or other rare types of flamboyant overproduction, perhaps twenty times the norm.

Incorporation of Ammonium-^{15}N into Urinary Uric Acid

When ^{15}N-labeled ammonium chloride was administered to control and gouty subjects, excessive incorporation (uncorrected for extrarenal loss) occurred only in the overexcretor group (GUTMAN et al., 1962a).

Incorporation of Formate-^{14}C into Urinary Uric Acid

The incorporation of formate-^{14}C into urinary uric acid is excessive in gouty patients with excessive excretion values of uric acid and is normal in patients with normal urinary excretion values (SPILMAN, 1954; SPILMAN, personal communication; VILLA et al., 1958). Erratic results bearing no relationship to urinary urate values have been reported in patients in whom experimental conditions were not standardized (BUCHANAN and ROLLINS, 1961).

Incorporation of Glycine, 5-Aminoimidazole-4-Carboxamide, Hypoxanthine or Adenine into Urinary Uric Acid and Purine Bases

In both nongouty and gouty subjects, 5-aminoimidazole-4-carboxamide (AIC) (SEEGMILLER et al., 1955; SEEGMILLER et al., 1957) and adenine (SEEGMILLER et al., 1968) are rapidly converted to uric acid. The pathways of utilization involve initial conversion to ribonucleotide forms (FLAKS et al., 1957a) (Reaction 16). SEEGMILLER et al., found that approximately 20 percent of AIC-^{13}C administered was excreted in urine as uric acid in 14 days in normal man (1955). There was a biphasic incorporation, consisting of a prompt and extensive conversion of ingested AIC-^{13}C into uric acid, followed by a slower, less direct conversion process. In all of five gouty subjects studied (SEEGMILLER et al., 1957), incorporation of AIC into uric acid was somewhat greater than normal irrespective of urinary urate excretion. The degree of abnormality was magnified when appropriate corrections were made for dilution factors within the urate pool and for uricolysis on the basis of simultaneous studies with uric acid-^{14}C.

In a similar study with adenine-8-^{13}C, SEEGMILLER et al. (1968) found a prompt incorporation of ^{13}C into urinary uric acid, with maximal labeling on the first or second day and a first-order decline in isotope abundance thereafter. Three gouty subjects, who were known overproducers of uric acid and overincorporators of glycine-^{15}N, incorporated twice as much ^{13}C into urate as two controls.

When AIC or adenine was administered together with glycine-^{15}N a marked and comparable suppression of incorporation of ^{15}N into urinary uric acid was observed in normal and gouty subjects (SEEGMILLER et al., 1955; SEEGMILLER et al., 1968). This probably resulted from the activation of feedback inhibition of purine synthesis by nucleotides derived from AIC or adenine, rather than from the diversion of PP-ribose-P from the pathway of purine synthesis *de novo*, for reasons discussed below.

Further indications of the complexity of pathways between IMP and uric acid came from studies of the incorporation of labeled glycine or labeled purine bases into urinary purine bases in nongouty and gouty subjects (WYNGAARDEN, 1957; WYNGAARDEN et al., 1958b; WYNGAARDEN et al., 1959b). Following the administration of glycine-1-^{14}C, there was a prompt and striking labeling of urinary hypoxanthine, indicative of the operation of an IMP cleavage pathway. Early labeling of adenine and 7-methylguanine suggested that other nucleotides were also subject to cleavage shortly after formation. Early labeling of 7-methylguanine, now known to be a constituent of DNA, and soluble and ribosomal RNAs (BOREK and SRINIVASON, 1966) was particularly impressive in gouty subjects (WYNGAARDEN et al., 1958b). Labeled hypoxanthine administered intravenously was promptly converted to uric acid. Labeled adenine in tracer dose was only slowly and sparingly converted to uric acid (WYNGAARDEN et al., 1959b), in contrast to larger doses which were converted to uric acid more promptly (SEEGMILLER et al., 1968). Labeled AIC gave rise to extensive labeling of all urinary

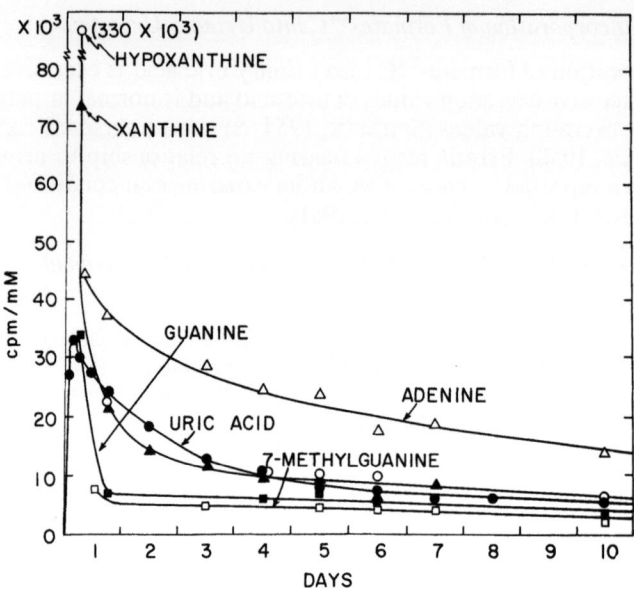

Fig. 12. Specific activity values of urinary purines in a patient with chronic myelogenous leukemia following the intravenous administration of AIC-4-^{14}C. (From WYNGAARDEN, 1957, with permission of Metabolism)

purine bases, in particular hypoxanthine and xanthine (WYNGAARDEN et al., 1959b). (Fig. 12) These findings strengthen the concept that IMP cleavage contributes to the rapid synthesis of uric acid in normal and gouty man. The findings that urinary 7-methylguanine is labeled promptly in gouty subjects and that excretion of 5-ribosyluracil (pseudo-uridine) (an important constituent of soluble and ribosomal RNA) (DUNN and SMITH, 1958; CANTONI et al., 1962) may be increased in gouty subjects (ADLER and GUTMAN, 1962; WEISSMANN et al., 1962) suggest that certain species of RNA may turn over sufficiently rapidly to contribute to hyperuricemia in certain patients.

Overproduction of Uric Acid in Gout

All the tracer studies discussed thus far involve the isolation of uric acid from urine and the determination of its isotopic enrichment following the administration of labeled uric acid or some labeled precursor of uric acid. These studies have demonstrated overproduction of uric acid in a substantial percentage of gouty subjects, but have not disclosed the mechanism.

Present concepts of control of purine synthesis de novo suggest three general categories of abnormalities which may potentially lead to overproduction of uric acid (WYNGAARDEN, 1969b). These are (1.) metabolic defects, remote or proximate, which increase the substrate levels of L-glutamine or phosphoribosylpyrophosphate; (2.) defects which increase the amount or intrinsic activity of the first enzyme of the pathway of purine synthesis; or (3.) defects which reduce the concentrations of one or more negative effectors (nucleotide inhibitors) of the first enzyme.

Studies of mechanisms of hyperuricemia in the three subtypes of primary gout associated with well-documented specific enzymatic defects will be presented first.

In each of these the driving force of excessive purine biosynthesis *de novo* is postulated to be a surplus of the substrate PP-ribose-P. Data on the pathogenesis of hyperuricemia in idiopathic gout will be presented next. Finally, selected examples of mechanisms of hyperuricemia in secondary gout will be discussed.

Gout Associated with Specific Enzymatic Defects

Glucose-6-Phosphatase Deficiency in Gout

Patients with glycogen storage disease Type I (glucose-6-phosphatase deficiency) have hyperuricemia from infancy, and may develop gouty arthritis by the end of the first decade of life, sometimes of disabling severity (JEUNE et al., 1957; HOWELL, 1963; HOLLING, 1963; FINE et al., 1966; VON-HOYNINGEN-HEUNE, 1966; KELLEY et al., 1968b). Chronic tophaceous gout and gouty nephropathy may account for a major portion of the morbidity in these patients as they become adults. Over 40 cases of glycogen storage disease and gout have been recorded (SEEGMILLER, 1969).

Hyperuricemia in glycogen storage disease Type I is often in the range of 10 to 16 mg per 100 ml plasma (HOWELL et al., 1962a; KELLEY et al., 1968b). Two and perhaps three distinct pathophysiologic mechanisms contribute to the hyperuricemia of this disorder. They are reduced excretion of uric acid because of the presence of marked hyperlacticacidemia and ketonemia; increased production of uric acid *de novo*, possibly a consequence of increased synthesis of phosphoribosylpyrophosphate; and perhaps increased binding of urate in plasma by lipoproteins which are present in increased amounts.

Patients with glucose-6-phosphatase deficiency are unable to produce free glucose from phosphorylated carbohydrates. Recurrent hypoglycemia acts as a stimulus both to glycogenolysis and gluconeogenesis. One consequence is hyperlacticacidemia (JEANDET and LESTRADET, 1961; HOWELL et al., 1962a; ALEPA et al., 1962). Blood lactate levels may be 50 mg per 100 ml or more (normal 5 to 18 mg per 100 ml). Recurrent hypoglycemia also results in ketonemia and elevated blood levels of β-hydroxybutyrate (HOWELL et al., 1962a). Both lactate and β-hydroxybutyrate suppress tubular urate secretion (YU et al., 1957; SHAPIRO, 1964). Renal clearances of uric acid are low in Type I glycogen storage disease (HOWELL et al., 1962a).

The hyperuricemia of Type I glycogen storage disease is also associated with excessive uric acid production. Urinary excretion values are high when expressed in terms of body weight (KELLEY et al., 1968b). The urinary uric acid/creatinine ratio may be >0.75 (KAUFMAN et al., 1968). By tracer methods, both the turnover of the urate pool (ALEPA et al., 1967; KELLEY et al., 1968b) and glycine-1-^{14}C incorporation into urinary urate (ALEPA et al., 1967; JAKOVCIC and SORENSEN, 1967; KELLEY et al., 1968b) may be excessive (Table 4). The pattern of increased purine production is that of accelerated biosynthesis *de novo*. This finding has theoretically been attributed to the overproduction of phosphoribosylpyrophosphate (HOWELL, 1963; KELLEY et al., 1968b). The intracellular surfeit of carbohydrate intermediates that cannot be released as free glucose may lead to an excessive production of phosphorylated ribose compounds, including PP-ribose-P. The active operation of the oxidative pathway of glucose-6-phosphate catabolism has been demonstrated in liver in this disease (HOWELL et al., 1962a). However, neither an elevated synthesis of PP-ribose-P, nor elevated intracellular levels of this compound, have yet been documented. GREENE and SEEGMILLER (1969) found normal levels of PP-ribose-P in erythrocytes and cultured fibroblasts

Table 4. Turnover and synthesis of uric acid in glycogen storage disease, Type I

Subject	Sex	Age yr.	Serum urate mg/100 ml	Pool size mg	Turnover rate pool/day	Turnover uric acid mg/day	Excretion uric acid mg/day	Turnover excreted %	Recovery of isotope in urinary uric acid in 7 days. Administered uric acid %	Recovery of isotope in urinary uric acid in 7 days. Administered glycine Uncorrected %	Recovery of isotope in urinary uric acid in 7 days. Administered glycine Corrected %
Normal control subjects[a]	6M 2F	26 (19—38)	4.3 (2.9—5.5)	978 (541—1,290)	0.62 (0.46—0.80)	590 (431—729)	429 (357—536)	73 (65—82)	73 (63—82)	0.24 (0.16—0.29)	0.32 (0.27—0.37)
Patients with Type I glycogen storage disease	M[a]	14	10.9	1,380	0.85	1,176	528	45	54	1.09	2.02
	M[a]	17	16.4	2,843	0.48	1,365	569	42	39	0.61	1.56
	F[a]	19	14.7	1,917	0.61	1,175	343	29	35	0.48	1.37
	M[b]	34	15.0	1,920	0.42	807	362	45	42	0.26	0.62
	M[c]	18	17.0	2,251	0.39	884	318	36	32	0.11	0.34

[a] Ref. KELLEY et al. (1968).
[b] Ref. LONG (1967).
[c] Ref. JAKOVCIC and SORENSEN (1967).

in two patients with this disorder. This result was perhaps to be expected, since these tissues do not contain glucose-6-phosphatase activity even in normal subjects. The critical organ for study will be the liver.

The hyperlipoproteinemia of glycogen storage disease may include elevations of triglycerides, phospholipids, and cholesterol (HOWELL et al., 1962a). Lipoprotein electrophoresis discloses a Type IV pattern. The possibility that lipoproteins may bind urate in this and other disorders requires further study.

Hypoxanthine-Guanine Phosphoribosyltransferase Deficiency in Gout

SEEGMILLER et al. (1967) discovered a deficiency of hypoxanthine-guanine phosphoribosyltransferase (PRT) in certain patients with flamboyant overproduction of uric acid. A virtually complete deficiency of this enzyme activity is associated with a childhood syndrome of choreoathetoses, spasticity, mental retardation, and bizarre compulsive self-mutilation, known as the Lesch-Nyhan syndrome (LESCH and NYHAN, 1964). There is prodigious overproduction and overexcretion of uric acid, and renal stones and secondary renal damage are common. In a few patients, severe gouty arthritis has occurred.

Among adult patients with marked overproduction of uric acid, a portion has been found to have a high-grade, but partial, deficiency of PRT activity (KELLEY et al., 1967b). Six affected individuals, three of them in one family, were found among 110 gouty patients admitted for special study at the Clinical Center of the National Institutes of Health over a 14-year period. A total of 18 patients were described in a general review of the topic written in September, 1968 (KELLEY et al., 1969). SPERLING et al. (1970) found only one subject with a partial deficiency of PRT activity among 52 adult male gouty overproducers of urate. In 1972 YU et al. estimated that PRT deficiency accounted for about 1.6 percent of cases of primary gout. All patients with PRT deficiency are males, and the disorder is X-linked. The Lesch-Nyhan syndrome and adult PRT deficiency are sufficiently distinct entities to warrant a full description apart from brief inclusion here. Accordingly, they are considered in extenso in Chapter IX.

Presenting symptoms in patients with partial PRT deficiency may be typical acute gouty arthritis, renal stones, crystalluria, or neurological dysfunction. Gouty arthritis usually presents in the second or third decade. Three quarters of all known patients have formed renal stones, half of them before the age of 10. In 20 percent of patients there have been neurological manifestations, including mental retardation, mild spastic quadriplegia, dysarthria, cerebellar ataxia, and seizure. These suggest that there may be a relationship to the debilitating disease found in patients with complete PRT deficiency. Neurological findings have occurred in patients with 0.5 percent or less of normal PRT activity in erythrocyte lysates with guanine as substrate (EMMERSON and WYNGAARDEN, 1969). As little as 1 percent of normal enzyme activity in hemolysates is associated with no discernible neurological involvement (KOGUT et al., 1970). A few patients have had a mild macrocytic anemia (KELLEY et al., 1969).

Gouty subjects with PRT deficiency tend to have serum urate values above 10 mg per 100 ml. Urinary uric acid excretion is elevated unless renal failure is present, often being well above 1000 mg per day (Fig. 13). Patient TS of Fig. 13, whose uric acid excretion falls within the normal range, had a glomerular filtration rate of only 10 ml per min. Turnover studies of Patient TS disclosed a urate production of 1693 mg per day, only 34 percent of which was disposed of in the urine. The elevated excretion of uric acid in PRT-deficient subjects is reflected in a uric acid/creatinine ratio above 0.75 (normal, 0.15 to 0.75) (KAUFMAN et al., 1968).

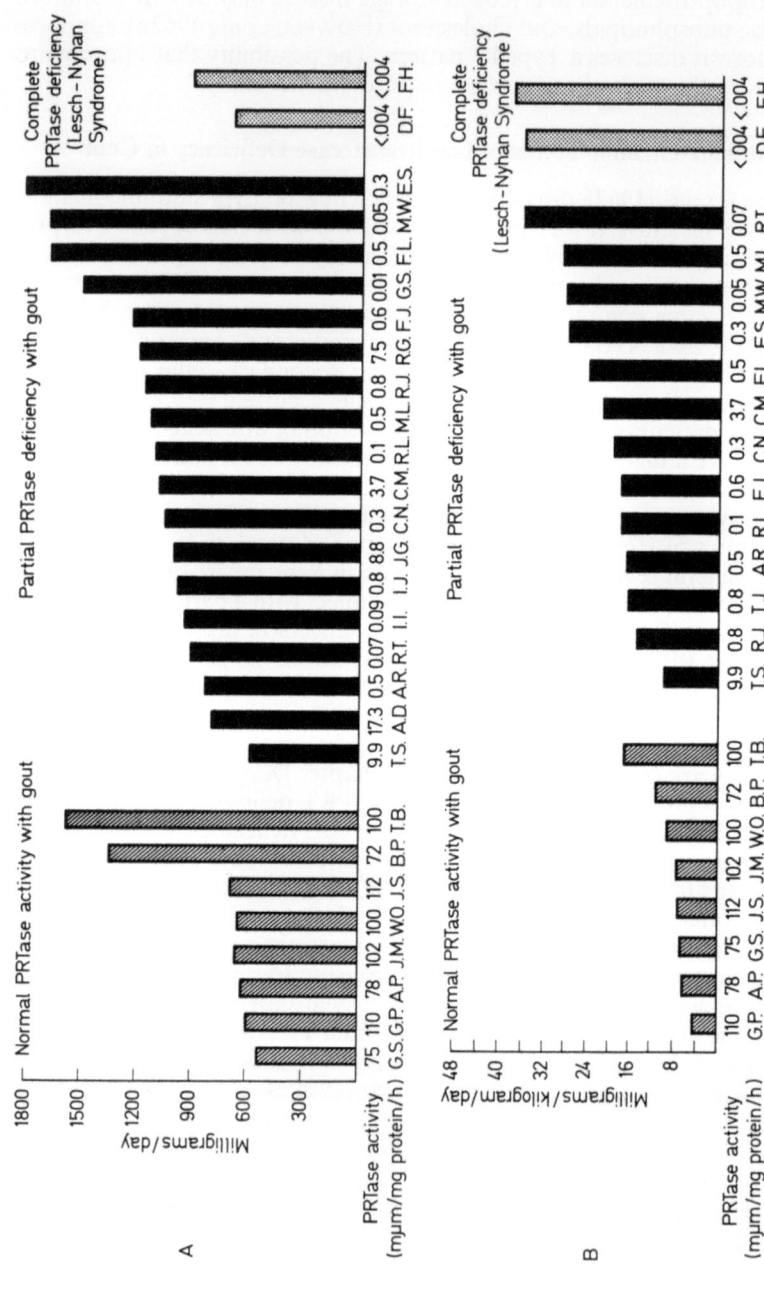

Fig. 13. Daily uric acid excretions in Patients producing excessive quantities of uric acid. Comparison of patients with normal, partially deficient, and "virtually completely" deficient hypoxanthine-guanine phosphoribosyltransferase (PRT) activity. A. Excretion values in mg/day (upper limit of normal is 590 mg per day). B. Excretion values in mg/kg/day (upper limit of normal is 6 to 7 mg/kg/day). Source: KELLEY et al., 1969

Table 5. Specific activity of phosphoribosyltransferases in erythrocytes in hyperuricemic subjects

Subject	Number	PRT activity, nmoles/mg protein/h (mean ± s.d.)		
		Hypoxanthine	Guanine	Adenine
Normal controls	32	103 ± 18	103 ± 21	31.1 ± 6.0
Gout				
Normal uric acid production	6	99 ± 13	106 ± 10	31.2 ± 6.9
Excessive uric acid production				
Normal PRT activity	10	103 ± 18	104 ± 22	30.4 ± 5.3
Partial deficiency	24	0.03—34	0.009—17.3	26—74
Lesch-Nyhan syndrome	9	< 0.01	< 0.004	39—94

Source: KELLEY et al., (1969), except that data of KOGUT et al. (1970), EMMERSON and WYNGAARDEN (1969), SPERLING et al. (1970), and YU et al. (1972) on patients with partial PRT deficiency have been added, with corrections for differences in control values. Activity with hypoxanthine and guanine was reduced in parallel in patients with partial PRT deficiency, except in the L. family reported by KELLEY et al., in which activity with hypoxanthine as substrate was 20 times higher than with guanine.

In most patients with gout and normal PRT activity, the values are within the normal range.

Turnover studies with labeled uric acid disclosed enlarged urate pools and increased urate turnovers in all five patients in one study (KELLEY et al., 1969). Glycine-1-^{14}C incorporation into urinary uric acid is excessive, particularly after correction for extrarenal disposal. Values in five patients ranged from 0.88 to 3.94 percent of administered glycine in 7 days. These values are somewhat lower than are sometimes found in patients with complete PRT deficiency (4.3 to 6.1 percent) but very much higher than in normal subjects (0.1 to 0.3 percent). There is an overlap with values found in gouty overproducers with normal PRT activity (0.4 to 3.3 percent). In patients with PRT deficiency given glycine-1-^{14}C, the peak specific activity values in urinary uric acid occur earlier than in normal individuals. These results indicate that excessive purine production in these patients is the result of increased purine synthesis *de novo*, rather than an increased turnover of nucleic acids.

Activity values in dialyzed hemolysates have ranged from 0.01 to 30 percent of normal, with guanine as substrate (lowest activity detectable = 0.004 percent of normal) (Table 5). The amount of activity with either hypoxanthine or guanine varies widely from one family to another, but is about the same among members of the same family. Further evidence of heterogeneity among the mutant enzymes was obtained in studies of heat stability and electrophoretic migration of the protein. In one family, the mutant enzyme was less stable than normal; in another, it was more stable; and in a third, it exhibited normal thermolability (KELLEY et al., 1969). BENKE has recently reported an especially instructive patient with hyperuricemia and excessive production of uric acid due to a partial deficiency of PRT. The mutant form of the enzyme from this patient had an altered Km with a normal Vmax so that the enzyme initially appeared to be normal *in vitro* although it clearly functioned with reduced activity *in vivo* (SORENSEN and BENKE, 1967; BENKE and HERRICK, 1972; BENKE and HERRICK, personal communication).

Leukocytes and fibroblasts of patients with partial PRT deficiency also show low activity values, indicating that this deficiency is not confined to a single cell type.

Other Enzyme Abnormalities

An increase in the activity of the closely related enzyme, A-PRT, has been a consistent observation in hemolysates of patients with complete PRT deficiency (SEEGMILLER et al., 1967), and has also been observed in about half all patients with partial deficiency (KELLEY et al., 1969; EMMERSON and WYNGAARDEN, 1969; SPERLING et al., 1970) (see Table 5). A-PRT activity values are normal in fibroblasts of PRT-deficient patients (KELLEY 1971a). The elevated activity values of A-PRT in erythrocytes have been attributed to stabilization of the enzyme by the very high concentrations of phosphoribosylpyrophosphate in the erythrocytes of PRT-deficient subjects (GREENE et al., 1970). In addition, there is increased activity of inosinic acid dehydrogenase (IMP-DH), orotate phosphoribosyltransferase (OPRT) and orotidylic decarboxylase (ODC) in circulating erythrocytes from patients with Lesch-Nyhan syndrome (PEHLKE et al., 1972; BEARDMORE et al., 1973). The mechanisms responsible for this effect remains unclear.

Purine Metabolism in Heterozygotes

All mothers of PRT-deficient patients are obligate heterozygotes, except in the case of new mutations. In most instances heterozygotes have been clinically normal, without hyperuricemia or hyperuricaciduria (KELLEY et al., 1969; EMMERSON and WYNGAARDEN, 1969; KOGUT et al., 1970). However, three of nine heterozygotes studied by KELLEY et al. (1969) and two of three studied by EMMERSON and WYNGAARDEN (1969) were hyperuricemic. Only one of nine heterozygotes in the first series and one of three in the second showed lowered PRT activity values, intermediate between those of hemizygotes and normal controls in erythrocytes. Elevated urinary uric acid, enlarged urate pools, increased urate turnover, and enhanced glycine incorporation into urinary urate have been reported in several obligate heterozygotes (KELLEY et al., 1969; EMMERSON and WYNGAARDEN, 1969).

The fibroblasts of heterozygotes are mosaics, consisting of some cells with normal activity and some with no activity (ROSENBLOOM et al., 1967a). The proportion varies from 60 percent to virtually 100 percent of normal cells, depending on the degree of cell contact in cultures. Demonstration of PRT-deficient cells may be enhanced by the use of selective growth conditions, in which an antimetabolite is employed to kill PRT-competent cells. At the present time, this is probably the simplest relatively dependable method available for the identification of heterozygotes (MIGEON, 1970; FELIX and DE MARS, 1971). The two cell populations have also been separated by cloning techniques (MIGEON et al., 1968). Assay of hair follicles provides a promising new approach to the detection of heterozygotes for this enzyme defect (GARTLER et al., 1971).

Relationship of PRT Deficiency to Accelerated Purine Biosynthesis

According to concepts developed above, accelerated purine biosynthesis de novo in PRT deficiency must be a consequence of an alteration of the control of the activity of glutamine-phosphoribosylpyrophosphate amidotransferase, involving changes in concentrations of nucleotide regulators, or of substrates, or changes in the activity or properties of the enzyme itself.

The only information on nucleotide levels in PRT-deficient cells is that total adenyl and guanyl nucleotide concentrations are normal in cultured fibroblasts from Lesch-Nyhan patients (ROSENBLOOM et al., 1968). No analyses in erythrocytes or basal ganglia, where PRT activity is normally 5 to 10 times greater than in fibroblasts (KELLEY and MEADE, 1971b), are available.

Table 6. PP-Ribose-P concentration values in human erythrocytes

Subjects	Numbers	PP-Ribose-P Contents, in nmoles/ml	Synthesis, in nmoles of GMP/ml per 45 min, glucose present	References
Controls[a]	28	2.6 ± 0.7[b]	—	Fox et al. (1970)
	12	4.4 ± 1.8	—	Fox and Kelley (1971)
	10	3.1 ± 0.5	—	Greene and Seegmiller (1969)
	9	6.1 ± 3.1	—	Sperling, et al. (1972a)
	30	—	35.7 ± 8.4[c]	Sperling, et al. (1971; 1972a)
	10	3.0 ± 0.3	32.0 ± 5.3	Meyskens, et al. (1971)
Specific Subtypes of Gout				
Glycogen storage disease, Type I	2	2.2 ± 2.4	—	Greene and Seegmiller (1969)
PRT partial deficiency (hemizygote)	3	4.6 ± 1.3	—	Greene and Seegmiller (1969)
Lesch-Nyhan (hemizygote)	7	38.8 ± 4.0	—	Greene and Seegmiller (1969)
Lesch-Nyhan (hemizygote)	3	35.3 (21—50)	—	Fox and Kelley (1971)
Lesch-Nyhan (heterozygote)	3	4.2 (1.5—6.5)	—	Fox and Kelley (1971)
PP-Ribose-P synthetase variants	2	13.1, 17.3	—	Sperling et al. (1972a)
PP-Ribose-P synthetase variant	1		94.3	Sperling et al. (1971; 1972a)
Idiopathic Gout or Asymptomatic Hyperuricemia				
Normal 24-hours urinary uric acid excretion	28	2.6 ± 0.7[b]	—	Fox et al. (1970)
	14	2.7 ± 0.5	—	Greene and Seegmiller (1969)
	17[d]	2.8 ± 0.4	34.7 ± 6.1	Meyskens et al (1971)
Urinary excretion > 800 mg per 24 hours	51	—	52.4 ± 15.6[c]	Sperling et al. (1971; 1972a)

[a] Experimental values should be compared with control values from the same paper.
[b] These control and gouty subjects had similar values of PP-Ribose-P. Mean ± s.d. refer to data on all 56 subjects (Fox et al., 1970).
[c] P value of difference < 0.001 (Sperling et al., 1971).
[d] Eleven of 17 patients studied while on allopurinol (Meyskens et al., 1971), which lowers PP-Ribose-P concentrations (Fox et al., 1970). Also synthesis was measured as nmoles of IMP/ml/h, glucose present.

The concentration of PP-ribose-P is significantly elevated in both fibroblasts and erythrocytes from patients with complete or partial PRT deficiency (ROSENBLOOM et al., 1968; GREENE and SEEGMILLER, 1969; FOX and KELLEY, 1971b). Representative values are shown in Table 6. These elevations reflect a reduced consumption of PP-ribose-P in the deficient PRT reaction. These values are sufficiently high for modest reductions induced by orotic acid or adenine through consumption of PP-ribose-P in other phosphoribosyltransferase reactions not to suppress purine biosynthesis *de novo in vitro* as they do in normal cells (KELLEY et al., 1970c).

The activity and properties of glutamine PP-ribose-P amidotransferase have been approached indirectly. The rate of synthesis of formylglycinamide ribonucleotide is accelerated in fibroblasts from PRT-deficient subjects, but this may be a reflection of the elevated levels of substrate PP-ribose-P. Such fibroblasts appear to be at least normally susceptible to the inhibition of purine biosynthesis by derivatives of adenine or 6-methylmercaptopurine ribonucleoside, an adenosine analogue (ROSENBLOOM et al., 1968). All available data implicate excess PP-ribose-P as the driving force of accelerated purine biosynthesis *de novo* in PRT deficient subjects. In addition, PP-ribose-P amidotransferase activity is normal in leukocytes from subjects with the Lesch-Nyhan syndrome (HOLMES et al., unpublished observation).

Increased PP-Ribose-P Synthetase Activity in Gout

SPERLING et al. (1971) conducted studies of incorporation of hypoxanthine, guanine and adenine into nucleotides in gouty subjects with urinary uric acid excretion values of 800 mg per day or more, and found significantly elevated mean incorporation values for all three purine bases. Assay values of PRT and APRT were normal. The common denominator of increased base incorporation was therefore suspected of being elevated PP-ribose-P levels in the erythrocytes of these subjects. Detailed studies (SPERLING et al., 1972b) of one patient selected because of unusually rapid rates of incorporation of bases into nucleotides and exceptionally high urinary urate excretion values, 2400 mg per day, disclosed increased rates of PP-ribose-P synthesis in erythrocytes *in vitro*. One brother, who also suffered from recurrent gout and uric acid lithiasis, showed similarly increased rates of PP-ribose-P synthesis, but a normal brother, three sons, both parents and one maternal aunt were found to have normal synthesis rates for PP-ribose-P in hemolysates.

The erythrocytes of the index case were found to contain excessive PP-ribose-P synthetase activity at low phosphate concentrations (Fig. 14). Experiments employing mixtures of hemolysates from this subject or a normal control, with dialyzed hemolysate from the other, did not result in alteration of normal activity. Thus the enhanced PP-ribose-P generation reflects an abnormality of the enzyme proper and is not one of its environment (SPERLING et al., 1972a).

BECKER and associates (1972, 1973) subsequently found a related but different variant of PP-ribose-P synthetase in two overproducers, gouty brothers previously shown to exhibit increased concentrations of PP-ribose-P in erythrocytes and fibroblasts. PP-ribose-P synthetase activity elevated to 2.5 to 3 times the control values in dialyzed hemolysates at all concentrations of inorganic phosphate. Although the increased activity resided in the enzyme itself, studies of heat stability, kinetic constants, and purine nucleotide feedback inhibition did not provide evidence for a structural alteration of the enzyme.

The prevalence of variants of PP-ribose-P synthetase among overproducer gouty subjects is unknown. The indirect indications that increased erythrocyte

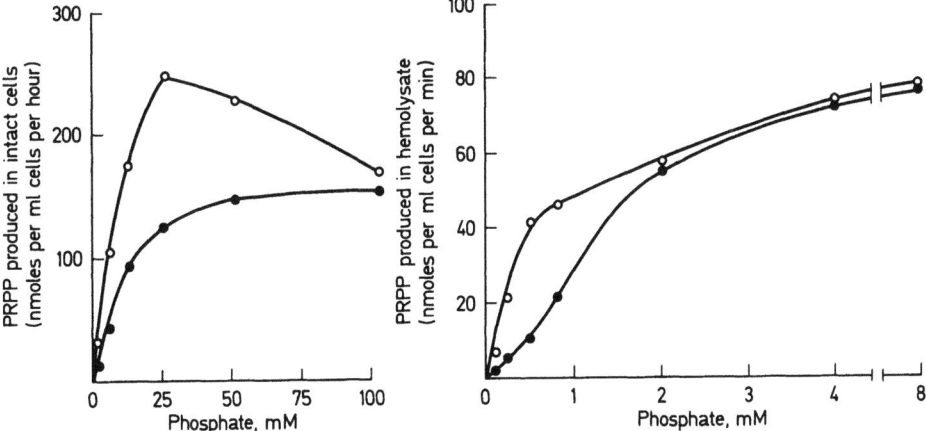

Fig. 14. Effect of inorganic phosphate concentration in incubation buffer on rate of PP-ribose-P generation in erythrocytes (left) and hemolysates (right) in a normal subject (●) and in a gouty patient (○). (Reproduced from SPERLING et al. (1972a) with permission of Flammarion Medicine — Sciences, Paris)

PP-ribose-P concentrations are common among gouty overproducers who are not PRT-deficient (SPERLING et al., 1971) suggests that this defect may not be rare. However, further studies will be necessary to determine whether the increased activity of PP-ribose-P synthetase is the basic genetic defect or merely a secondary phenomenon.

Primary Gout

The specific subtypes of primary gout discussed above account for no more than 3 or 4 percent of the total. Furthermore, all three subtypes are components of the "overexcretor" group, which itself accounts for only 20 to 25 percent of cases of primary gout. Among flamboyant overexcretors, there are a number of well-studied patients in whom glucose-6-phosphatase deficiency, PRT deficiency, and PP-ribose-P synthetase variants have been carefully excluded. Some of these present indirect or direct evidence of excessive concentration values of PP-ribose-P in erythrocytes or in fibroblasts in culture. Clearly additional defects leading to overproduction of PP-ribose-P, or underconsumption of PP-ribose-P in another competing reaction remain to be discovered.

The majority of patients with primary gout are not high-grade overexcretors. Their 24-hrs uric acid excretion values fall just above, or within, the broad normal range. Mean excretion values are higher than mean values in control subjects. Values for turnover of the miscible pool of urate and for incorporation of labeled glycine into urate tend to be higher than normal, though an appreciable percentage of both fall within the normal range. As a group, they show statistically significant increases of glycine incorporation into urate (WYNGAARDEN, 1960a), although perhaps one-fourth of individual values fall within the normal range even after correction for extrarenal disposal (WYNGAARDEN and KELLEY, 1972b; WYNGAARDEN, 1966). These data point toward mild overproduction of purines as a factor in the pathogenesis of hyperuricemia in at least the majority of members of this group, even in many with normal urinary urate excretion values.

The basis of purine overproduction in this group is obscure. The data currently available will be considered in some detail.

The Role of L-Glutamine in Gout

Amino Acids and Urinary Ammonia Production in Gout

Plasma glutamine values are normal in gout, and range from 7 to 10 mg per 100 ml or 0.5 to 0.7 mM (SEGAL and WYNGAARDEN, 1955; KAPLAN et al., 1965; YU et al., 1969; PAGLIARA and GOODMAN, 1969). Concentration values of total amino acids in plasma, exclusive of proline and aspartic acid, are about 2.7 mM in both nongouty (WYNGAARDEN, 1960a; YU et al., 1969) and gouty subjects (KAPLAN et al., 1965; YU et al., 1969; PAGLIARA and GOODMAN, 1969). Reported elevations of individual plasma amino acid values in gout largely disappear when protein intakes are standardized in the two groups (YU et al., 1969). An exception is glutamic acid, which remains higher than in controls (YU et al., 1969; PAGLIARA and GOODMAN, 1969) even after casein loading of both groups (PAGLIARA and GOODMAN, 1969). Values in gouty subjects average 68 or 72 µM, compared with 45 or 51 µM in controls (YU et al., 1969; PAGLIARA and GOODMAN, 1969). Plasma glycine values are distinctly lower in gouty subjects than in controls and serine values slightly so (YU et al., 1969).

Renal clearances of several amino acids are less in gouty subjects than in control (YU et al., 1969; KAPLAN et al., 1969). Deficits of some degree persist for glutamine, serine, and threonine even after protein restriction. The most conspicuous deficit in the gouty subjects is in the urinary excretion and clearance of glutamine. Following glutamine loading, plasma glutamine levels rise and fall indistinguishably in gouty and control subjects, but the difference in glutamine excretion and clearance persist (YU et al., 1969).

GUTMAN and YU (1963a) have reported that when glycine-^{15}N is administered, the first-day and cumulative ammonium-^{15}N values are less in gouty normal and overexcretor subjects than in control subjects with equivalently acid urines. In three subjects in each category, the average cumulative values in 7 days were 3.38 percent of administered ^{15}N in controls, 2.54 percent in gouty normal excretors, and 1.61 percent in gouty overexcretors. The enrichment values were the same in all groups: 2.61 to 2.72 atom percent excess ^{15}N. The deficit was attributed to a decrease in the quantity of ammonia produced in the gouty subjects. The ammonium/creatinine ratios were found to average 0.27 ± 0.09 in 77 gouty subjects as compared to 0.41 ± 0.10 in 17 nongouty subjects with comparable urinary pH values. In 83 gouty subjects with a urinary pH 5.7 the mean net deficit in the elimination of ammonia was 8 µeg per min in comparison with 46 nongouty controls excreting urine of the same pH. YU et al. (1965) have suggested that the increased tubular reabsorption of glutamine, and reduced urinary excretion of ammonia in primary gout (overexcretors and normoexcretors alike) are related in some way (see Glutaminase Hypothesis below).

By contrast, PLANTE et al. (1968) noted that the apparent defect in ammonium excretion in gouty subjects was not present in patients on a low-purine diet, but they did not reexamine the same patients on normal- or high-purine diets. METCALFE-GIBSON et al. (1965) found no abnormally low values of ammonium excretion in hyperuricemic subjects with creatinine clearance values above 65 ml per min. A low ammonium/titratable acidity ratio has been a well-known consequence of renal disease since the studies of HENDERSON and PALMER (1915). Tubular ammonia production also declines with age (HILTON et al., 1955). In gouty patients the earliest recognizable renal changes, as observed by both light and electron microscopy, involve the tubules (GONICK et al., 1965). Thus, even a normal glomerular filtration rate in gouty subjects may not exclude an acquired deficit in tubular function. Furthermore, values of ammonia production in gouty subjects show extensive overlap with normal values, even though mean values are different (GUTMAN and YU, 1965). The relationship of the deficit in urinary excretion of ammonium to uric acid production and hyperuricemia in gouty subjects remains conjectural.

Intramolecular Distribution of ^{14}C or ^{15}N in Urinary Uric Acid

Glycine-1-^{14}C serves as a specific label of C-4 of the purine ring. No significant recycling of isotope from the degradation products of glycine into other carbon atoms of uric acid is detected in normal (GUTMAN et al., 1958; HOWELL et al., 1961) or gouty subjects (GUTMAN et al., 1958). When glycine-1-^{14}C, α-^{15}N is administered, the ^{15}N/^{14}C ratio in urinary uric acid is significantly above 1.0 in both nongouty and gouty subjects, indicating a greater incorporation of ^{15}N than can be attributed to the entry of the intact glycine molecule into the eventual purine structure (GUTMAN et al., 1958; HOWELL et al., 1961).

When the urate molecule was degraded into fractions representing N-7 and N-(1+3+9), the latter fraction was found to contain 23 to 34 percent of the total ^{15}N on day 1 in normal subjects, and from 34 to 50 percent on day 1 in six gouty subjects (SHEMIN and RITTENBERG, 1947; HOWELL et al., 1961; GUTMAN et al., 1962a). These studies indicated that amino nitrogen derived from glycine was incorporated into the N-1 of purines via aspartic acid and into N-3 and N-9 by way of the amide-N of glutamine in both nongouty and gouty subjects (Fig. 4).

Hypothesis of Abnormal Glutamine Metabolism in Primary Gout

Further dissection of the urate molecule by GUTMAN and YU (1963a) disclosed that the increase in the percentage of ^{15}N in the N-(1+3+9) fraction in gouty subjects was accounted for by higher percentage of ^{15}N in N-(3+9) in gouty subjects than in their control subjects. The preferential increase of labeling of N-(3+9) and the reduced excretion of ammonia in these gouty subjects (see above) suggested to GUTMAN and YU (1963a) that there was a diversion of the amide nitrogen of glutamine from ammonia production into purine synthesis de novo in gout.

The Glutaminase Hypothesis: On the basis of these findings a block of glutaminase I was proposed (GUTMAN and YU, 1963a; GUTMAN and YU, 1963b). This hypothesis, as originally stated, has now been disproved by the finding of normal activities of phosphate-activated glutaminase (glutaminase I), pyruvate-activated glutaminase (glutaminase II), and nonactivated glutaminase in renal biopsy tissue from four gouty subjects by POLLAK and MATTENHEIMER (1965). In rebuttal, YU and GUTMAN (1965) have called attention to the scatter of enzyme assay results on tissue obtained by biopsy and have cited the need for a functional assay of glutaminase I *in vivo*, by measurement of transrenal glutamine differences at various urinary pH values in nongouty and gouty subjects.

The Glutamic Acid Dehydrogenase Hypothesis: The reaction catalyzed by glutamic acid dehydrogenase appears to operate chiefly in the direction of α-ketoglutaric acid. The observation by YU et al. (1969) and PAGLIARA and GOODMAN (1969) that plasma levels of glutamic acid are elevated in gout, together with those of GUTMAN and YU on ^{15}N distribution in N-(3+9), are viewed by PAGLIARA and GOODMAN (1969) as supporting a suggestion first made by FRIEDEN (1963) that faulty control or reduced activity of glutamic acid dehydrogenase could result in diversion of glutamic acid toward glutamine and purine biosynthesis.

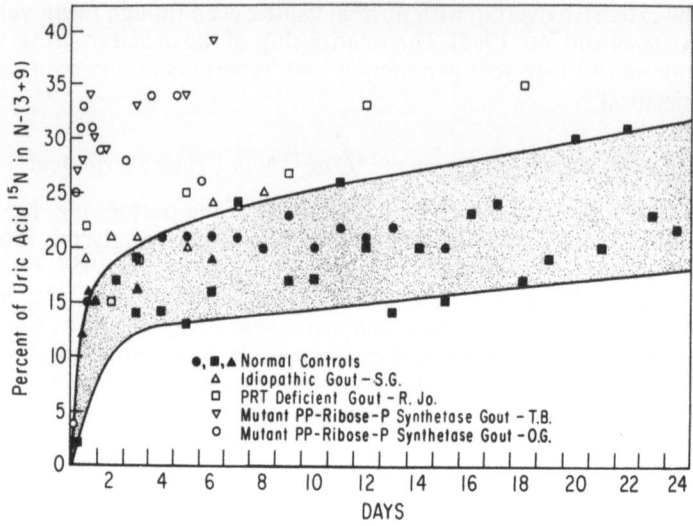

Fig. 15. Intramolecular distribution of ^{15}N in uric acid, expressed as the percentage of total ^{15}N found in N-(3+9). The shaded area includes essentially all values on the control subjects. (Reproduced from SPERLING et al., 1973, with permission of Journal of Clinical Investigation

The Kinetic Hypothesis

In the original paper (GUTMAN and YU, 1963a) in which a defect of glutamine metabolism in primary gout was proposed, the preferential labeling of N-(3+9) was provisionally attributed to "glutamine amide nitrogen containing an unduly high concentration of N^{15}." We have reexamined this proposition in four gouty subjects, three of whom had specific metabolic defects in which the driving force of excessive purine biosynthesis was known to be surplus PP-ribose-P. One patient was a mild overproducer with "idiopathic gout"; one was a marked overproducer with high-grade but "partial" PRT deficiency; two were extraordinary overproducers with superactive PP-ribose-P synthetases, though of different variant types (see Fig. 9). Following administration of ^{15}N-glycine, disproportionately high labeling of N-(3+9) was observed, most marked in the most flamboyant overproducers (Fig. 15). Thus the primary observation of GUTMAN and YU (1963a) was confirmed (SPERLING et al., 1973).

The precursor glycine pool was sampled by periodic administration of benzoic acid and isolation of urinary hippuric acid. Similarly, the precursor glutamine pool was sampled by means of periodic administration of phenylacetic acid and isolation of the amide-N of urinary phenylacetylglutamine. The enrichments and turnover kinetics of hippurate and phenylacetylglutamine were entirely normal in the gouty subjects. Thus the increased labeling of N-7 and of N-(3+9) in gout cannot be attributed to abnormal enrichments of precursor pools, and instead appears to represent the utilization of increased fractions of precursor glycine and glutamine pools for purine biosynthesis per unit of time.

A computer model simulating the kinetics of the relevant reactions was constructed, utilizing as input data the observed enrichments of hippurate and phenylacetylglutamine. The relationships of the enrichments of glutamine-amide-N to glycine-N with time are such that accelerations in the rates of purine biosynthesis, based on increasing concentrations of PP-ribose-P, resulted in progressive

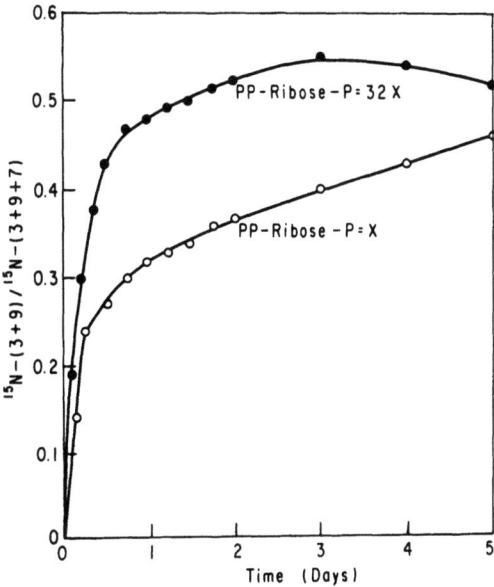

Fig. 16. Enrichment values of ^{15}N-(3+9)/^{15}N-(3+9+7) predicted by simulation model at two levels of PP-ribose-P. Compare with values in Fig. 16, and note that the simulation model omits ^{15}N-1 values from the denominator

increases in the theoretical ratio ^{15}N-(3+9)/^{15}N-(3+9+7) in uric acid during the first few hours following labeling of the glycine pool (Fig. 16). Thus the increased fractional labeling of N-3 and N-9 of uric acid in gouty overproducers fed ^{15}N-glycine appears to be a kinetic phenomenon related to the relative time-courses of enrichment of precursor glycine and glutamine pools, and the rates of transfer of ^{15}N from these pools to specific N atoms of the purine ring, and not necessarily to a specific metabolic defect of glutamate or glutamine in gout (SPERLING et al., 1973).

The Role of Phosphoribosylpyrophosphate in Gout

Phosphoribosylpyrophosphate Turnover in Gout

The rate of turnover of PP-ribose-P has been assessed in control and gouty subjects by determination of the specific activity of the ribose moiety of PP-ribose-P following the administration of labeled glucose (JONES et al., 1962). Net flux of carbon is from glucose-6-phosphate to ribose-5-phosphate via the oxidative limb of the hexose monophosphate shunt (KATZ and ROGNSTAD, 1967). Normally, only a small fraction, perhaps one sixth, of ribose-5-phosphate is converted to PP-ribose-P (KATZ and ROGNSTAD, 1967). However, measures which increase the production of ribose-5-P may be reflected in an increased synthesis of PP-ribose-P and of purines (see above). An increase in turnover of PP-ribose-P from ribose-5-P should be reflected in an increase in the specific activity of PP-ribose-P, provided that the pool of PP-ribose-P does not expand by a factor as large as the increase in PP-ribose-P production. "Aliquots" of the PP-ribose-P pool can be obtained by the administration of imidazoleacetic acid and the isola-

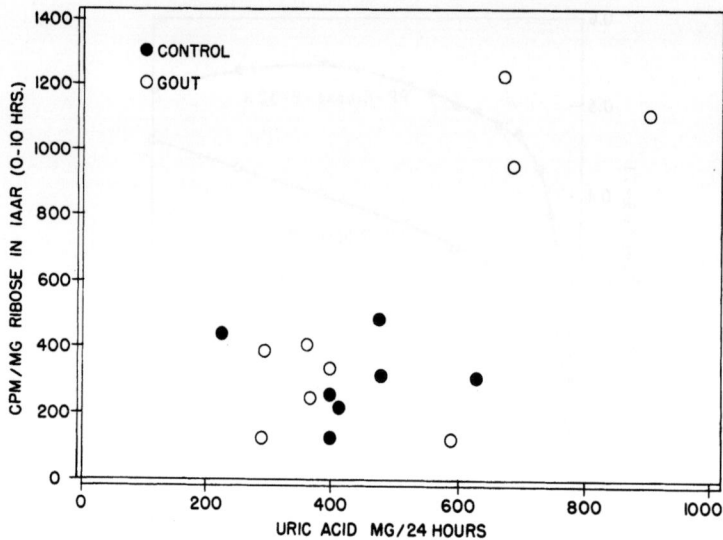

Fig. 17. Specific activity of the ribose moiety of imidazoleacetic acid ribonucleoside in control and gouty subjects. Values obtained during the 10-hr period after administration of imidazoleacetic acid and glucose-U-^{14}C are plotted against uric acid excretion values. (Reproduced from JONES et al., 1962, with permission of Journal of Clinical Investigation

tion of its ribonucleoside derivative from the urine (HIATT, 1957). The reactions occur in liver (CROWLEY, 1964) and are as follows:

$$\text{Imidazoleacetic acid} + \text{ATP} + \text{PP-ribose-P} \rightarrow \text{IAA-ribose-P} + \text{ADP} + \text{PP}_i + \text{P}_i$$
$$\text{IAA-ribose-P} \rightarrow \text{IAA-ribose} + \text{P}_i$$

This study has been performed on seven control and nine gouty subjects, including three overexcretors of uric acid (JONES et al., 1962). Specific activity values in the ribose moiety of IAA-ribonucleoside isolated from the 0- to 10-h urine samples are shown in Fig. 17. Values in gouty subjects who excreted more than 600 mg uric acid per day are clearly excessive. Those of subjects who excreted normal amounts are indistinguishable from controls. The results indicate an increase in turnover of PP-ribose-P in these gouty overexcretors. The underlying metabolic defect is unknown, except that erythrocyte PRT activity was normal in the only one in whom it was assayed. The results in the gouty normoexcretor do not rigorously exclude an increase in turnover of PP-ribose-P, for an enhancement of rate of synthesis of PP-ribose-P could take place from labeled glucose and unlabeled precursors equally, such that the specific activity of PP-ribose-P would remain unchanged, or conversely enhanced enrichment could be obscured by dilution within an enlarged PP-ribose-P pool.

Phosphoribosylpyrophosphate Concentrations in Gout

Concentration values of PP-ribose-P are normal in the erythrocytes and cultured fibroblasts of gouty subjects with normal 24-hrs urinary uric acid values (GREENE and SEEGMILLER, 1969; FOX and KELLEY, 1971b). They are elevated in patients who are deficient in PRT activity in whom there is a gross underutilization of PP-ribose-P in purine salvage (GREENE and SEEGMILLER, 1969; FOX and

KELLEY, 1971b). The elevated PP-ribose-P levels lead to marked stimulation of purine synthesis *de novo*, even though the maximal rates of synthesis of PP-ribose-P are not increased in PRT-deficient cells (ROSENBLOOM et al., 1968). Mean erythrocyte levels of PP-ribose-P are also elevated in some gouty overexcretors of uric acid with normal PRT activity (HERSHKO, 1968; SPERLING et al., 1971). In 51 gouty patients with urinary uric acid values of 800 mg per day or greater, SPERLING et al., found a mean increase of erythrocyte PP-ribose-P concentration values of 35 percent ($p = <0.001$) (1971) (see Table 6). In one of these patients with a marked elevation of PP-ribose-P concentration, SPERLING et al. (1972a) subsequently demonstrated a superactive variant form of PP-ribose-P synthetase, as discussed above. It is probable that this defect will be identified in others of this group in the future.

Glutathione Reductase Variants and Gout

A rank order association of hyperuricemia with increased enzymatic activity of a series of variant glutathione reductases has been hypothetically attributed by LONG (1970) to an increased rate of operation of the hexose monophosphate shunt, and of synthesis of ribose-5-phosphate and PP-ribose-P. Twenty-three of twenty-eight Negro patients with gout were found to have the glutathione reductase variant. The fast variant is 28 percent more active than the normal enzyme and is associated with a mean serum urate level of 7.24 mg per 100 ml, and often with gout (Table 3) (LONG, 1967). Elevated activity of erythrocyte glutathione reductase has also been observed in a group of Caucasians with untreated primary gout (LONG, 1962).

These findings have not yet been confirmed in another laboratory. It is well known that activity of glutathione reductase is increased in certain disease states, e.g. diabetes mellitus, and by certain vitamins, e.g. nicotinamide (BREWER, 1969) and riboflavin (BEUTLER, 1969). LONG's findings and hypothesis warrant further investigation.

Role of Abnormal Properties of Glutamine-PP-ribose-P Amidotransferase

When 5-aminoimidazole-4-carboxamide (AIC) (SEEGMILLER et al., 1955), adenine (SEEGMILLER et al., 1968), azathioprine (KELLEY et al., 1967c), or allopurinol (RUNDLES et al., 1963) are administered to nongouty subjects there is suppression of purine synthesis *de novo*. Comparable suppression is found in normal excretor and overexcretor gouty subjects, provided the patient has the enzymatic mechanism for converting the analogue to ribonucleotide form. Patients who are PRT-deficient do not respond to these agents with suppression in purine production (KELLEY et al., 1967c; SEEGMILLER et al., 1968; KELLEY et al., 1969). They do respond normally to adenine (SEEGMILLER et al., 1968), which is converted to adenylic acid by A-PRT, and (in tissue culture) to 6-methylmercaptopurine ribonucleoside (ROSENBLOOM et al., 1968), which is converted to its ribonucleotide by adenosine kinase (CALDWELL et al., 1966; ALLAN et al., 1966) and then behaves as an analogue of inosinic acid (BROCKMAN, 1969). Thus in these gouty subjects, including those who are PRT-deficient, it appears that both the 6-amino and 6-hydroxyribonucleotide control sites of the amidotransferase are intact. This has now been demonstrated directly in leukocyte extracts (HOLMES et al., 1973, in press).

HENDERSON and associates (1968b) found that purine biosynthesis *de novo* in fibroblasts cultured from two patients with extraordinary overexcretion and overproduction of uric acid and normal PRT activity appeared to be abnormally resistant to feedback inhibition by both 6-amino and 6-hydroxypurine compounds. They initially suggested that these patients had a mutation which had altered the regulatory properties of glutamine-PP-ribose-P amidotransferase. Such a potential defect has ample precedent in bacterial, yeast, and Ehrlich ascites tumor cell mutants (WYNGAARDEN, 1972). However, PP-ribose-P levels were above normal in fibroblasts (HENDERSON et al.,1968b), a result unanticipated on the basis of altered feedback properties of the amidotransferase. Both patients were subsequently found to have superactive variants of PP-ribose-P synthetase (BECKER et al.,1972). The increased intracellular content of PP-ribose-P could explain the observed resistance to purine ribonucleotides (HOLMES et al.,1973b).

Role of Inhibitor Ribonucleotides in Gout

Excessive purine biosynthesis could result from reduced concentrations of feedback inhibitors of glutamine PP-ribose-P amidotransferase. In normally growing or neoplastic cells, presumably it is the removal of nucleotides into nucleic acids and other products which reduces the inhibitory contraints upon the amidotransferase and allows synthesis of purines *de novo* proceed. Abnormally rapid degradation of nucleotides might have the same effect. The latter mechanism may operate in specific hyperuricemic patients. In one overproducer gouty subject studied by SEEGMILLER et al., the rate constant for turnover of labeled adenine was twice that of two other gouty subjects and two controls (1968). In addition, fibroblasts cultured from one showed a twenty-fold increase in the rate of deamination of adenylic acid to inosinic acid (HENDERSON et al., 1968b), which was thought possibly to correlate with an abnormally rapid rate of breakdown of azathioprine to uric acid in this patient *in vivo* (KELLEY et al., 1967c).

Patients with PRT deficiency cannot convert hypoxanthine and guanine to ribonucleotides. They show extraordinary acceleration of purine synthesis *de novo*. One potential explanation is an inability to maintain normal intracellular concentrations of nucleotides, resulting in relaxed feedback inhibition. However, in fibroblasts in culture the total concentrations of adenyl and guanyl ribonucleotides fall within normal limits (ROSENBLOOM et al.,1968).

The synergistic nature of feedback control of the amidotransferase by adenyl and guanyl nucleotides suggests that relaxation of control could result from a nonoptimal ratio of 6-amino and 6-hydroxyribonucleotides. WEISSMANN and GUTMAN (1957b) suggested a nucleotide imbalance in explanation of the increased excretion of 7-methyl-8-hydroxyguanine and decreased excretion of 6-succinoaminopurine in acute gout. Gouty patients given glycine-1-^{14}C show enhanced labeling of urinary 7-methylguanine, but not of urinary adenine (WYNGAARDEN et al., 1958b). Although these observations are intriguing, no conclusions can be drawn at the present time.

Xanthine Oxidase Activity in Gout

CARCASSI et al. (1969) have reported elevated values of xanthine oxidase activity in liver biopsy specimens obtained from eight overexcretor gouty subjects. Mean values were four times greater than in controls. It is not known whether the increase in xanthine oxidase activity is primary, or secondary to another metabolic lesion. PRT and PP-ribose-P synthetase activities were not assayed in these subjects, nor have xanthine oxidase assays been published from patients with secondary hyperuricemia, e.g. associated with polycythemia vera. Xanthine oxidase is an inducible enzyme in mammalian tissue (ROWE and WYNGAARDEN, 1966). Nevertheless, increased xanthine oxidase activity should augment the rate of conversion of hypoxanthine and xanthine to uric acid, and reduce their reconversion to ribonucleotides in the PRT reaction, at least in liver. It is possible that a shift in the balance of competition for hypoxanthine results in a reduction of intracellular nucleotide levels, with the relaxation of end-product inhibition of glutamine PP-ribose-P amidotransferase.

Renal Mechanisms of Uric Acid Excretion in Gout

The renal handling of urate in control and gouty subjects is discussed in detail in another chapter. The authors' views will be briefly summarized here.

According to present concepts the renal excretion of uric acid in man is regulated by a three component system: glomerular filtration, tubular reabsorption, and tubular secretion (GUTMAN and YU, 1961). It is usually assumed that virtually all urate in the plasma is freely filterable at the glomerulus (YU and GUTMAN, 1953a). However, there is evidence that some urate is bound to plasma proteins *in vivo* (POSTLETHWAITE et al., 1973a) as well as *in vitro* (ALVSAKER, 1966; 1965a; ALVSAKER, 1965b; ALVSAKER, 1966). Therefore, the assumption that urate is freely filterable at the glomerulus must be a guarded one. Indeed, the possibility exists that the bound fraction of plasma urate may be decreased (ALVSAKER, 1966; SEELINGER and VERSTER, 1962) or increased (ADLERSBERG et al., 1942; BERKOWITZ et al., 1964; BERKOWITZ, 1966) in certain gouty subjects, and that variations in binding affect filtration of urate.

The $C_{urate}C_{inulin}$ ratio tends to be lower in gouty subjects than in normal controls at any specified serum urate level (MUGLER et al., 1956; SALA et al., 1956; GUTMAN and YU, 1957; NUGENT and TYLER, 1959; SEEGMILLER et al., 1962; HOUPT and AGRYZLO, 1964). This ratio increases in gouty subjects as the plasma urate level is raised, as it does in normal controls, but higher plasma urate values are required in gouty than in normal subjects to achieve a given clearance ratio (Fig. 18) (NUGENT et al., 1964; WYNGAARDEN, 1965).

When data are plotted as rates of uric acid excretion at various serum urate levels, it appears that the curve of excretion rates has the same form in gouty subjects as in nongouty control, and that the capacity of the excretory mechanism for uric acid is not reduced in gout (Fig. 19). However, the excretion curve is shifted such that gouty subjects require serum values 2 or 3 mg per 100 ml higher than controls in order to achieve equivalent uric acid excretion rates. The sharp augmentation of rate of urate excretion occurs at approximately 13 mg per 100 ml rather than at 9 or 10 mg per 100 ml as in normal man.

The data plotted in Fig. 19 are from control and gouty subjects with normal renal mass, i.e. all subjects have a glomerular filtration rate of 100 ml per min or greater. The displacement of the curve in gouty subjects is not a consequence of sustained hyperuricemia, for in leukemic subjects the rates of uric acid excretion are generally normal or increased in relation to the titration curve in nongouty subjects (NUGENT et al., 1962; RIESELBACH et al., 1964). In most gouty normal excretors, there was a blunted augmentation of urate secretion in the range of plasma urate values from 7 to 13 mg per 100 ml in comparison with controls, as one would predict from an inspection of Fig. 19.

According to interpretations of the pyrazinamide test that limit its effect to suppression of urate secretion, a normal fraction of filtered urate escapes reabsorption in both normal producers and overproducers, at both basal and increased filtered urate loads (GUTMAN et al., 1969; RIESELBACH et al., 1970). The augmented excretion of uric acid at high plasma urate levels is attributed to increased tubular secretion of urate in gouty subjects, as in normal men, since it

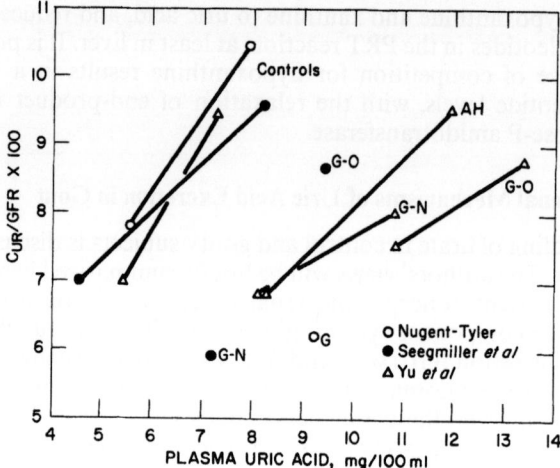

Fig. 18. Renal clearance of uric acid in nongouty and gouty subjects, plotted against plasma urate concentrations. In the pairs of points connected by lines, the right-hand member represents the value observed after the serum urate concentration was raised by feeding of RNA. G = gouty subject; AH = asymptomatic hyperuricemic; N = normal excretor; O = overexcretor. (Data of NUGENT and TYLER, 1959; SEEGMILLER et al., 1962; YU et al., 1962. Reproduced from WYNGAARDEN, 1965, with permission of Academic, New York)

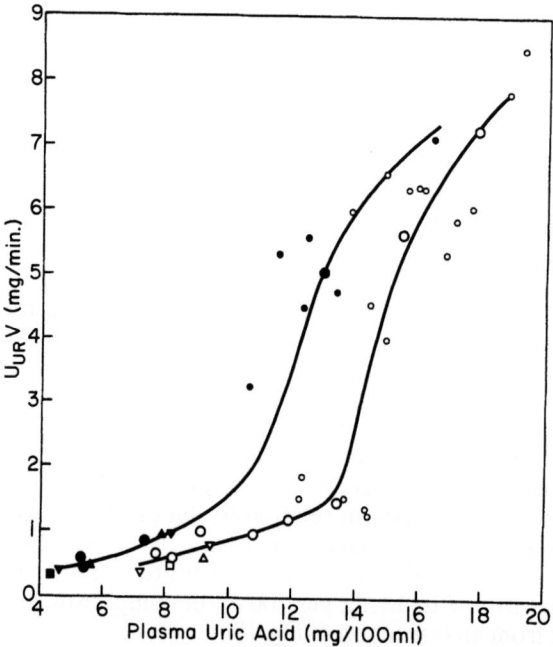

Fig. 19. Rate of uric acid excretion at various plasma urate levels in nongouty (solid symbols) and gouty (open symbols) subjects. Large symbols represent mean values; small symbols represent individual data of a few mean values selected to illustrate the degree of scatter within groups. Studies were conducted under basal conditions, after RNA feeding, and after infusions of lithium urate. (▲, △, NUGENT and TYLER, 1959; ▼, ▽, SEEGMILLER et al., 1962; ●, ○, YU et al., 1962. Reproduced from WYNGAARDEN, 1965, with permission of Academic, New York)

can be almost totally inhibited by pyrazinamide in both groups (RIESELBACH et al., 1970).

RIESELBACH and associates (1970), again utilizing the PZA suppression test, have postulated diminished renal urate secretion per nephron as the basis for hyperuricemia in patients with primary gout without demonstrable overproduction of uric acid. This study is subject to the limitations of the "PZA suppression test" (HOLMES et al., 1972). In addition, the data on "tubular secretory response" to elevated plasma urate concentrations in their study show considerable overlap of individual values, including one overproducer wholly without and one normal producer wholly within the normal range of secretory response. These observations, together with others showing low C_{urate}/C_{inulin} ratios in relation to plasma urate concentrations in certain overproducers (GUTMAN and YU, 1957; SEEGMILLER et al., 1962), suggest that it may not be appropriate to separate patients with idiopathic primary gout so sharply into primary renal gout or primary metabolic gout (SORENSEN, 1962, 1963, 1969) on the basis of mean responses. Admittedly, there are a few well-studied families in whom hyperuricemia and gout appear to be caused by an inherited renal abnormality (DUNCAN and DIXON, 1960; ROSENBLOOM et al., 1967b), and saturnine gout appears to occur on a renal basis (EMMERSON, 1965; BELL and SORENSEN, 1969), but many subjects with primary gout qualify as simultaneous overproducers and underexcretors (WYNGAARDEN, 1960b). Overproducers with partial or complete PRT deficiency are not included in this group, for they have no demonstrable impairment of renal handling of urate apart from the effects of acquired renal disease and reduced functional mass (SEEGMILLER, 1962; KELLEY, 1969).

The explanation of the shift of the velocity substrate curve of the tubular secretion of uric acid toward higher plasma urate values in a large fraction of patients with gout is unknown. It does not appear that this finding can be attributed to hemodynamic changes. Tubular blood flow may be reduced in gout but not enough to explain these findings (GUTMAN and YU, 1957). There is an active transport system for uric acid in erythrocytes (LASSEN, 1961), but little is known about the mechanism of transfer of urate from renal cells into the tubular lumen.

The reduced fractional clearance of urate in primary idiopathic gout is not a congenital component of the latent gouty condition, but rather one which becomes manifest at puberty in the male at risk, at least in our limited observations. The renal abnormality as measured could be explained by 1) an increase in plasma urate binding and an overestimation of filtered urate, e.g. in association with hyperlipidemia (see below), leading to an erroneous interpretation of abnormal tubular handling of urate in gout; 2) an increase in tubular reabsorption of filtered or secreted urate beyond that found in control subjects, or 3) an abnormally low rate of tubular secretion of urate at any given plasma urate level. Data obtained with the pyrazinamide suppression test favor the third hypothesis, but this interpretation assumes an exclusive effect of pyrazinamide upon tubular secretion, plus no reabsorption beyond the sites of secretion—assumptions that have been questioned (HOLMES et al., 1972). In the chimpanzee a second action of pyrazinamide in enhancing uric acid reabsorption has been proposed (FANELLI et al., 1970; FANELLI et al., 1971). In man there is evidence that tubular uric acid reabsorption and tubular sodium reabsorption may be closely related (HOLMES et al., 1972). The possibility that the hyperuricemia and the frequent hypertension of primary gout are related through a common mechanism involving urate and sodium reabsorption has been mentioned (HOLMES et al., 1972). The reduced fractional clearance of urate may be transiently corrected to normal in some gouty subjects by the administration of glycopyrrolate, an anticholinergic agent

(POSTLETHWAITE et al., 1973b). This substance does not affect creatinine or inulin clearance, nor does it alter plasma binding of urate, and hence these changes cannot be attributed to a change in the filtered load of urate. These data argue against the first hypothesis above, but are compatible with the second or third possibilities.

Ethanol

In his classic review on gout published in 1863, A.B. GARROD wrote: "There is no truth in medicine better established than the fact that the use of fermented liquors is the most powerful of all the predisposing causes of gout; nay, so powerful that it may be a question whether gout would ever have been known to mankind had such beverages not been indulged in."

The centuries old belief that the acute gouty paroxysm may be associated with overindulgence in drink has at long last acquired a physiologic explanation. Hyperuricemia is common in inebriated subjects (LIEBER and DAVIDSON, 1962a), and infusions of ethanol result in hyperuricemia (LIEBER et al., 1962b). As ethanol is metabolized by alcohol dehydrogenase, NAD is reduced, and this may account in part for the excessive conversion of pyruvate to lactate. The levels of hyperlacticacidemia achieved (LIEBER et al., 1962b) are adequate to suppress renal excretion of uric acid and to induce hyperuricemia (YU et al., 1957), thus increasing the probability of crystal formation.

Several epidemiologic studies have reported a correlation between serum urate levels and habitual alcohol intake (SAKER et al., 1967; EVANS et al., 1968). Furthermore, MACLACHLAN and RODNAN (1967) have observed that the combination of ethanol ingestion and fasting may have an additive or a synergistic effect on uric acid metabolism. The daily ingestion of alcohol in significant but tolerated amounts, e.g. 100 ml per 24 h, may be associated with hyperuricemia and increased urinary excretion of uric acid, both of which may return toward or to normal during protracted periods (days) of abstinence and normal diet. These cycles are not explained by reduced urinary clearance of uric acid. An effect upon purine synthesis has been postulated (MACLACHLAN and RODNAN, 1967).

Excretion of Purine Bases in Gout

Normal urine contains about 30 mg per day of purines other than uric acid. These include xanthine, hypoxanthine, 1-methylhypoxanthine, guanine, 1-methylguanine, 7-methylguanine. ^{2}N-methylguanine, 7-methyl-8-hydroxyguanine, adenine and 6-succinoaminopurine (WEISSMANN et al., 1957a; WYNGAARDEN et al.,

Table 7. Urinary excretion of purine bases in normal subjects, mg/day

Purine base	Range	Mean
Hypoxanthine	5.9—13.2	9.7
Xanthine	5.1— 8.6	6.1
Adenine	1.1— 1.7	1.4
Guanine	0.2— 0.6	0.4
1-Methylhypoxanthine	0.2— 0.7	0.4
6-Succinoaminopurine	0.8— 1.5	1.2
1 + 7-Methylguanine	5.5— 7.8	6.5
N^2-Methylguanine	0.4— 0.6	0.5
7-Methyl-8-hydroxyguanine	1.1— 2.0	1.6

Source: WEISSMANN et al. (1957), and WEISSMANN and GUTMAN (1957).

1958b; WEISSMANN and GUTMAN, 1957b; WEISSMANN et al., 1957c). Their normal excretion values are given in Table 7. The origins of adenine, guanine, hypoxanthine, xanthine, and of the methylated adenines and guanines have been discussed. Succinoadenine is the aglycone of adenylosuccinic acid (CARTER and COHEN, 1956), the intermediate in the conversion of IMP to AMP. 7-methyl-8-hydroxyguanine arises from 7-methylguanine by the action of human xanthine oxidase (SKUPP and AYVAZIAN, 1969). Bovine milk xanthine oxidase will not catalyze this reaction (WYNGAARDEN et al., 1958b).

The quantities of these bases found in the urine of gouty subjects do not differ significantly from those of normal subjects (WEISSMANN and GUTMAN, 1957b; GUTMAN et al., 1956).

Extrarenal Disposal of Uric Acid in Gout

Uricolysis in Normal Man

Urinary recoveries of injected uric acid are incomplete in normal subjects. Fifty years ago FOLIN et al. (1924) and KOEHLER (1924) reported recoveries that ranged from 28 to 91 percent and averaged about 50 percent. Recoveries ranging from 55 to 95 percent of uric acid-^{15}N or uric acid-2-^{14}C have been reported (GEREN et al., 1950; SORENSEN, 1959, 1960). The average of 14 studies with uric acid-^{15}N was 75.6 percent.

Studies of the turnover of uric acid in normal man have uniformly shown that the quantity of uric acid synthesized per day is greater than the quantity appearing in the urine. In studies with uric acid-^{15}N (WYNGAARDEN, 1955b; SEEGMILLER et al., 1961) or uric acid-^{14}C (SORENSEN, 1960; SEEGMILLER et al., 1961), the fraction of the turnover appearing in urine is essentially the same as the fraction of injected uric acid recovered in urine. Thus a significant quantity of uric acid is disposed of by entrarenal routes.

When a relatively large quantity of uric acid-1, 3-^{15}N was administered intravenously to a normal subject (WYNGAARDEN and STETTEN, 1953; BUZARD et al., 1955), about 25 percent of the isotope was found in urinary allantoin, urea, and ammonia and fecal nitrogen. In studies with uric acid-2-^{14}C, a comparable percentage of administered isotope was recovered in respiratory CO_2, urinary urea, allantoin and allantoic acid, and feces (SORENSEN, 1959). In patients with biliary catheters given uric acid-^{15}N, labeled products were recovered in bile. These results suggested that uricolysis occurred in the intestinal tract.

Sites of Uricolysis

When labeled uric acid was administered orally to normal subjects, only 9 to 11 percent was absorbed and excreted unchanged in urine (BISHOP et al., 1951; SORENSEN, 1959). With uric acid-^{15}N, 47 percent of the ^{15}N was recovered in urinary urea in 3 days (BISHOP et al., 1951). With uric acid-2-^{14}C, only 2.4 percent appeared in urea, but 55 percent of the ^{14}C was excreted as respiratory CO_2 (SORENSEN, 1959). An additional 16.3 percent was recovered in feces, 83 to 91 percent of this amount being found within the intestinal bacteria themselves.

Next, the degradation of intravenously administered uric acid was studied in a normal subject before and after an effective bacteriostasis was achieved with sulfonamide, streptomycin, and neomycin (SORENSEN, 1959). The quantity of ^{14}C recovered in degradation products was reduced from 22.5 to 3.0 percent during drug treatment (Table 8). Many intestinal organisms have the capacity to destroy uric acid (WYNGAARDEN and STETTEN, 1953).

Table 8. Recovery of intravenously administered uric acid-2-^{14}C in excretory products (5 to 10 days) before and after establishment of effective bacteriostasis of the intestinal tract

Excretory product	Recovery of ^{14}C percent of dose	
	Before bacteriostasis	During bacteriostasis
Urinary uric acid	69.0 (10 days)	55.7 (5 days)
Urinary allantoin	2.1	1.8
Urinary allantoic acid	0.2	
Urinary urea	2.2	0.7
Expired carbon dioxide	10.9	0.5
Fecal products	7.1	0.0
Total recovery in degradation products	22.5	3.0

Source: SORENSEN (1960).

SORENSEN (1959) estimated that 100 mg of uric acid or more enters the alimentary tract in saliva, gastric juice, and bile. An equal quantity may enter in pancreatic and intestinal juices. These quantities of uric acid are larger than previously estimated (LUCKE, 1932; KURTI, 1932) and adequate to account for the degradation of one-third of the uric acid normally turned over each day.

A trivial amount of uricolysis may occur within the tissues of man, amounting at most to 2 to 4 percent of the uric acid turnover (WYNGAARDEN, 1960a). Verdoperoxidase (CANELLAKIS et al., 1955) and cytochrome-cytochrome oxidase (GRIFFITH, 1952) can destroy uric acid in vitro at physiologic pH. Leukocytes (BIEN and ZUCKER, 1955; VILLA et al., 1958) of normal subjects will destroy uric acid during prolonged incubations. This activity resides primarily in myeloid cells (RATTI, 1958), which contain verdoperoxidase (AGNER, 1958). Uric acid crystals are degraded by leukocytes with the release of CO_2 from the 6 position (HOWELL and SEEGMILLER, 1962b). The mechanism of the peroxidative reaction appears to be a two-electron-one-proton oxidation, which yields allantoin and CO_2 as the initial products (HOWELL and WYNGAARDEN, 1960). The products of the peroxidative destruction of uric acid in phosphate buffer are chiefly allantoin and urea (CANELLAKIS et al., 1955).

Uricolysis in Gout

Decreased uricolysis has been proposed as a cause of hyperuricemia in gout (FOLIN et al., 1924; VILLA et al., 1958). However, urinary recoveries of injected uric acid (KOEHLER, 1924; FOLIN et al., 1924; SORENSEN, 1959; SKUPP and AYVAZIAN, 1969) are lower, on the average, than those found in nongouty subjects. In gouty subjects, the fraction of the daily turnover of uric acid recovered in urine is also smaller than in normal subjects. Extrarenal disposal of uric acid and uricolysis of ^{14}C-uric acid are enhanced in hyperuricemic subjects (POLLYCOVE et al., 1957; SORENSEN, 1959). Thus, no evidence exists to implicate failure of tissue or intestinal uricolysis in the hyperuricemia of gout. On the contrary, enhanced enteral uricolysis is a compensatory factor in gout, tending to lessen hyperuricemia and constituting the major process of disposal of uric acid in some patients with severe renal insufficiency (SORENSEN, 1962, 1963; KELLEY et al., 1969).

Dietary Factors in Primary Gout

Finally, there may be a relationship with caloric intake, obesity, protein and alcohol consumption, and gout in the genetically predisposed individual. During World Wars I und II acute gout was uncommon in Europe. When protein again became plentiful, the prevalence returned to prewar levels (ZOLLNER, 1960; BROCHNER-MORTENSEN, 1963). In Japan, where mean per capita protein intake has doubled in the past 25 years, gout has become a common disease of the middle-aged male. On the average, the patient with primary gout is overweight and drinks too much.

Epidemiological studies find associations of hyperuricemia and gout with ponderal index (EVANS et al., 1968) and alcohol ingestion (SAKER et al., 1967; EVANS et al., 1968). Uric acid production may be augmented when alcohol is consumed regularly (MACLACHLAN and RODNAN, 1967). Purine biosynthesis de novo is also greater on a high protein than on a isocaloric low protein diet (BIEN et al., 1953).

Epidemiological studies find associations of hyperuricemia and gout with ponderal index (EVANS et al., 1968) and alcohol ingestion (SAKER et al., 1967; EVANS et al., 1968). Uric acid production may be augmented when alcohol is consumed regularly (MACLACHLAN and RODNAN, 1967). Purine biosynthesis de novo is also greater on a high protein than on a isocaloric low protein diet (BIEN et al., 1953).

EMMERSON (personal communication) found in one carefully studied patient that slow weight reduction and abstinence from alcohol resulted in disappearance of all clinical and metabolic evidence for gout. Acute attacks ceased. The elevated values of serum urate concentration, of the miscible urate pool and its rate of turnover, of the rate and extent of incorporation of labeled glycine into urinary urate, of 24-h uric acid excretion, and of serum triglycerides, and the reduced fractional urinary uric acid clearance values all returned to normal. Thus both the mild overproduction and the underexcretion of urate which existed simultaneously in this subject proved to be reversible with dietary management alone. These basic observations have been duplicated, though without isotope studies, by HEYDEN (personal communication, 1972). In a recent study of fifteen obese subjects a reduction of 4 to 22 kg in weight was associated with a modest decrease in the plasma urate (mean decrease of 0.8 mg/100 ml) in twelve of the subjects with no consistant change in the urinary uric acid (NICHOLLS and SCOTT, 1972).

These studies indicate a very complex interrelationship between genetic predisposition and exogenous influences in certain patients with primary gout, and render the prospect of identification of a single precisely localized metabolic lesion in these and similar gouty subjects unlikely. It seems more probable that there are subtle departures from normal in various metabolic control mechanisms under the stress of caloric excess and ethanolism.

Secondary Hyperuricemia and Gout

A few decades ago it was widely held that all gout was hereditary (BAUER and KLEMPERER, 1947). The coexistence of gout and of polycythemia vera, for example, was viewed as chance concurrence. Additional observations have altered these views. It is now recognized that the potential for development of gout exists in all hyperuricemic subjects.

In one large American series, 13.2 percent of hospitalized males were hyperuricemic, and in 70 percent of this group hyperuricemia was attributable to a specific nongenetic cause (PAULUS et al., 1970). Gouty arthritis occurs relatively frequently in patients with polycythemia vera, myeloid metaplasia, or chronic lead intoxication, in whom hyperuricemia is usually quite severe and long standing. Gout is also becoming more common in patients taking certain drugs, the thiazide diuretics being quantitatively the most important of these. By contrast, gouty arthritis appears to be unusual in patients with hyperuricemia due to renal failure. In general, secondary hyperuricemia is caused by either increased turnover of nucleic acid purines or impaired renal excretion of uric acid. Thus in secondary gout, as in primary gout, hyperuricemia appears to have a dual pathogenesis. The differentiation of secondary metabolic gout from secondary renal gout (SORENSEN, 1962) is often valid, although these categories are not mutually exclusive.

Hematologic Disorders

Hyperuricemia and secondary gout occur in lymphoproliferative and myeloproliferative disorders (GUTMAN; 1953; HICKLING, 1953; TALBOTT, 1959; YU, 1965), multiple myeloma (BRONSKY and BERNSTEIN, 1954), secondary polycythemia (YU et al., 1953b; SOMMERVILLE, 1961), certain hemoglobinopathies, thalassemia, and pernicious anemia. All of these conditions are associated with chronically increased marrow activity.

In one large series of patients with leukemia, myeloid metaplasia, polycythemia vera, and multiple myeloma, hyperuricemia was noted in 66 percent of 113 male patients and 69 percent of 73 female patients, although only 10 patients had a history of gouty arthritis (LYNCH, 1962). Gout occurred most commonly in patients with myeloid metaplasia (6 of 22 patients). In other series, gout has occurred in a mean of 6 percent of patients with polycythemia vera; 84 percent of the gouty patients have been males. Hyperuricemia probably occurs with increased frequency in all types of leukemia, with the possible exception of chronic lymphocytic leukemia, and in general the degree of hyperuricemia is correlated with bone marrow proliferation (LYNCH, 1962). The serum urate concentration tends to be higher in these patients than in patients with primary hyperuricemia (GUTMAN, 1953; LYNCH, 1962).

SANDBERG et al. (1956) found increased uric acid excretion in acute leukemias and in all chronic leukemias, except the lymphocytic variety. In 15 patients with acute leukemia and in 2 patients with chronic myelocytic leukemia, RIESELBACH et al. (1964) found uric acid excretion rates from 0.92 to 10.3 mg per min per $1.73 M^2$ compared with a mean control value of 0.71 ± 0.22 mg per min per $1.73 M^2$. GUTMAN and YU (1962b) found a mean urinary uric acid excretion value of 634 mg per 24 hrs in 27 cases of secondary gout complicating hematologic disorders, compared to a mean value of 497 mg per 24 hrs in a control group. The fractional urate clearance, $C_{uric\ acid}/GFR$, is generally normal or increased (NUGENT et al., 1962; RIESELBACH et al., 1964). These patients show normal or low values of hypoxanthine, xanthine, and 1+7-methylguanines, and normal or high values of adenine, guanine, 7-methyl-8-hydroxyguanine, pseudouridine, and succinoadenine in the urine (YU et al., 1956). In addition, increases of urinary inosine and guanosine and of certain other purine and pyrimidine compounds have been noted in leukemic subjects (ADAMS et al., 1958).

The miscible pool of uric acid and its turnover are increased in patients with myelogenous leukemia or polycythemia vera (BISHOP et al., 1951). Incorporation of glycine-^{15}N (LASTER and MULLER, 1953; WEISSMANN et al., 1957a), glycine-1-^{14}C, and 5-aminoimidazole-4-carboxamide-4-^{14}C (WYNGAARDEN, 1957; WYNGAARDEN et al., 1959b) into urinary purine bases and uric acid show striking labeling of the bases during the first day followed by secondary maxima in bases and uric acid between 7 and 12 days (Fig. 20). Cumulative incorporation of isotope into uric acid is approximately normal during the first few days but greatly exceeds the normal after 1 to 2 weeks (WYNGAARDEN et al., 1959b). All these data

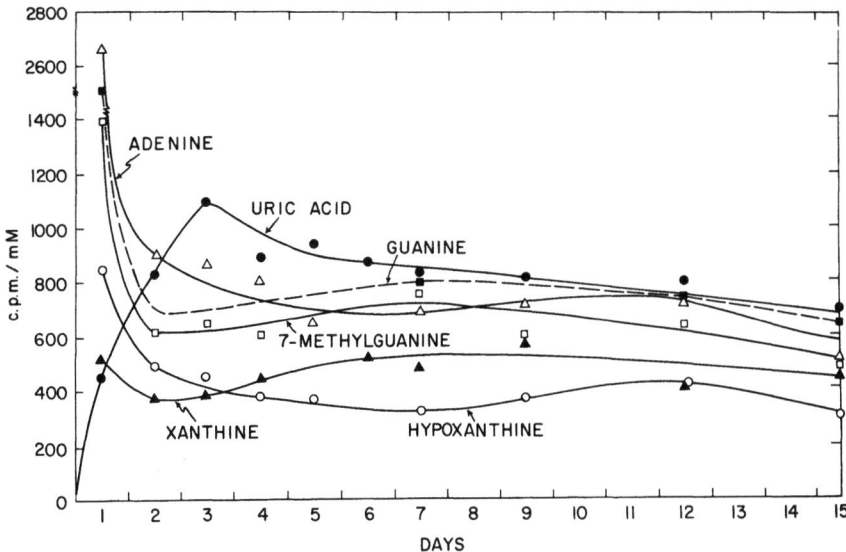

Fig. 20. Specific activity values of urinary purines in a patient with myeloid metaplasia, following the oral administration of glycine-1-^{14}C. (From WYNGAARDEN, 1957, with permission of Metabolism)

indicate an exaggerated turnover of nucleic acid purines as the cause of hyperuricemia in these subjects.

Hyperuricemia has been described in 11 of 12 males and 5 of 8 females with infectious mononucleosis (COWDRY, 1966). The increase in plasma urate values was maximal within the first 2 weeks of the disease and tended to parallel the presence of abnormal lymphocytosis.

In sickle cell disease, 6 of 13 patients were found to have a serum urate concentration greater than 6.0 mg per 100 ml (GOLD et al., 1968). Two patients had a history strongly suggestive of gouty arthritis. One patient with SS disease and gout showed both overproduction of uric acid and diminished excretion due to diminished nephron mass (BALL and SORENSEN, 1970). Hyperuricemia has also been described in about one-third of patients with SC disease but gout has occurred infrequently (RIVER et al., 1961). Gout may also complicate β-thalassemia and other chronic hemolytic anemias (MARCH et al., 1952; PAIK et al., 1970).

Drug-induced Hyperuricemia

This has become an important category in clinical medicine. Only one example will be discussed.

Diuretics

In a study of hyperuricemic men admitted to an American Veterans Administration Hospital, diuretics were considered the causative factor in 20 percent (PAULUS et al., 1970). Of new cases of gout diagnosed in Framingham, Massachusetts, over a 14-year period (mean age 58 years) 50 percent developed in subjects taking thiazides or ethacrynic acid (HEALY and HALL, 1970). The mean urate level for this group prior to diuretic therapy was 5.8 mg per 100 ml, which was higher than the mean of 5.1 mg per 100 ml for all men in this population sample. Hyperuricemia has been noted in up to 75 percent of patients treated with diuretics (DE

MARTINI et al., 1962), but it may not be appropriate to place the sole responsibility for induction of hyperuricemia or of gout upon the drug.

There are several mechanisms by which potent diuretic agents may produce hyperuricemia (WYNGAARDEN, 1970). The work of STEELE and OPPENHEIMER (1969a; 1969b) suggests that a prerequisite is sufficient salt and water loss to produce volume contraction. Following administration of furosemide or ethacrynic acid, tubular reabsorption of filtered urate is increased. In addition, inhibition of tubular secretion of urate seems likely. Neither effect appears to represent a direct action of the diuretic agent upon tubular transport of urate, for urate excretion values remain near control values when volume depletion is prevented by replacement of urinary salt and water losses with intravenous saline. Replacement studies also led SUKI et al. (1967) to postulate that thiazide-induced hyperuricemia was a byproduct of extracellular fluid volume contraction. These observations suggest that any diuretic sufficiently effective to produce volume contraction may produce hyperuricemia. Acetazolamide (AYVAZIAN and AYVAZIAN, 1961) and chlorthalidone (BRYANT et al., 1962) are also in this class.

Secondary extrarenal influences upon the kidney may be responsible for the hyperuricemia. Volume contraction leads to a generalized increase in solute reabsorption, perhaps mediated by changes in oncotic pressure (RECTOR et al., 1967; CLAPP et al., 1969; CANNON et al., 1970). In addition, furosemide induces hyperlacticacidemia sufficient to suppress tubular secretion of urate (SCHIRMEISTER et al., 1969). This is also true for diazoxide, a nondiuretic thiazide which promotes muscle glycolysis and leads to hyperlacticacidemia (SCHULTZ et al., 1966). Thiazide-induced hyperuricemia is corrected by KCl or NH_4Cl, apparently in part by causing a uricosuria and in part by causing a redistribution of urate among body compartments (ZWEIFLER and THOMPSON, 1965). Neither organomercurials nor xanthine diuretics appear to have been studied in detail in man with respect to hyperuricemia (BEYER and BAER, 1961). It is doubtful whether xanthine diuretics are sufficiently potent by themselves to produce volume contraction and hyperuricemia. The methyl xanthines are not biotransformed into uric acid.

Saturnine Gout

There is an association of gout with chronic lead poisoning, which has been attributed to the nephritis of plumbism (LUDWIG, 1957). A relatively high incidence of this type of gout still exists in Queensland, Australia (EMMERSON, 1963), and in France (RICHET et al., 1964), where patients were exposed to leaded paint in childhood. When compared to primary gout, patients with lead gout (EMMERSON, 1968) have a higher incidence of renal disease prior to the first episode of arthritis, females are more frequently affected, the arthritis is milder, the mean age of onset is younger, there is a lower incidence of renal calculi, hyperlipidemia is not observed (EMMERSON, personal communication, 1972), and patients are less likely to have a family history of gout (EMMERSON, 1968). In the United States saturnine gout is most often related to consumption of illicitly distilled (moonshine) alcohol with an appreciable lead content. In a study at a southern Veterans Administration hospital, 37 of 43 consecutive cases of gout were associated with chronic lead intoxication (BALL and SORENSEN, 1969).

In Spain 70 of 450 patients with gouty arthritis had a history of direct and prolonged contact with leaded gasoline (RAPADO, 1969). The hyperuricemia in chronic lead intoxication is due to decreased uric acid excretion (BALL and SORENSEN, 1969; EMMERSON, 1965). The pyrazinamide suppression test suggests that it is predominantly attributable to enhanced reabsorption (EMMERSON, 1965).

References

ABRAMS, R., BENTLEY, M.: Transformation of inosinic acid to adenylic and guanylic acids in a soluble enzyme system. J. Amer. chem. Soc. **77**, 4179 (1955).

ACHESON, R. M., CHAN, Y. K.: The prediction of serum uric acid in a general population. J. chron. Dis. **21**, 543 (1969).

ADAMS, W. S., SKOOG, W. A., DAVIS, F. W.: An investigation of purine and pyrimidine excretion in normal and leukemic subjects utilizing ion exchange column and paper chromatographic techniques. J. clin. Invest. **37**, 875 (1958).

ADLER, M., GUTMAN, A. B.: Uridine isomers (5-ribosyl-uracil) in human urine. Science **130**, 862 (1962).

ADLERSBERG, D., GRISHMAN, E., SOBOTKA, H.: Uric acid partition in gout and hepatic disease. Arch. intern. Med. **70**, 101 (1942).

AGNER, K.: Crystalline myeloperoxidase. Acta chem. scand. **12**, 89 (1958).

ALEPA, F. P., HOWELL, R. R., SEEGMILLER, J. E.: The occurrence of glycogen storage disease with tophaceous gout. Arthrit. and Rheum. **5**, 634 (1962).

ALEPA, F. P., HOWELL, R. R., KLINENBERG, J. R., SEEGMILLER, J. E.: Relationships between glycogen storage disease and tophaceous gout. Amer. J. Med. **42**, 58 (1967).

ALLAN, P. W., SCHNEBLI, H. P., BENNETT, L. L., JR.: Conversion of 6-mercaptopurine and 6-mercaptopurine ribonucleoside to 6-methylmercaptopurine ribonucleotide in human epidermoid carcinoma No. 2 cells in culture. Biochim. biophys. acta (Amst.) **114**, 647 (1966).

ALVSAKER, J. O.: Uric acid in human plasma. III. Investigations on the interaction between the urate ion and human albumin. Scand. J. clin. Lab. Invest. **17**, 467 (1965a).

ALVSAKER, J. O.: Uric acid in human plasma. IV. Investigations on the interactions between urate and macromolecular fraction in plasma from healthy individuals and patients with diseases associated with hyperuricemia. Scand. J. clin. Lab. Invest. **17**, 476 (1965b).

ALVSAKER, J. O.: Uric acid in human plasma. V. Isolation and identification of plasma proteins interacting with urate. Scand. J. clin. Lab. Invest. **18**, 227 (1966).

ALVSAKER, J. O.: Genetic studies in primary gout: Investigations on the plasma levels of the urate-binding α_1-α_2 globulin in individuals from two gouty kindreds. J. clin. Invest. **47**, 1254 (1968).

ATKINSON, D. E., FALL, L.: Adenosine triphosphate conservation in biosynthetic regulation: *Escherichia coli* phosphoribosylpyrophosphate synthetase. J. biol. Chem. **242**, 3241 (1967).

ATKINSON, D. E.: The energy charge of the adenylate pool as a regulatory parameter: Interaction with feedback modifiers. Biochemistry **7**, 4030 (1968).

AYVAZIAN, J. H., AYVAZIAN, L. F.: A study of the hyperuricemia induced by hydrochlorothiazide and acetazolamide separately and in combination. J. clin. Invest. **40**, 1961 (1961).

BALL, G. V., SORENSEN, L. B.: Pathogenesis of hyperuricemia in saturnine gout. New Engl. J. Med. **280**, 1199 (1969).

BALL, G. V., SORENSEN, L. B.: The pathogenesis of hyperuricemia and gout in sickle cell anemia. Arthrit. and Rheum. **13**, 846 (1970).

BARLOW, K. A.: Hyperlipidemia in primary gout. Metabolism **17**, 289 (1968).

BARNES, F. F., SCHOENHEIMER, R.: On biological synthesis of purines and pyrimidines. J. biol. Chem. **151**, 123 (1943).

BARZEL, U. S., SPERLING, O., FRANK, M., DE VRIES, A.: Renal ammonium excretion and urinary pH in idiopathic uric acid lithiasis. J. Urol. (Baltimore) **92**, 1 (1964).

BAUER, W., KLEMPERER, F.: Gout. In: Diseases of Metabolism (Ed. G. G. DUNCAN), 2nd ed. Philadelphia: Saunders 1947.

BEARDMORE, T. D., KELLEY, W. N.: Studies on the mechanism of allopurinol-induced inhibition of pyrimidine metabolism. Clin. Res. **19**, 27 (1971).

BEARDMORE, T. D., MEADE, J. C., KELLEY, W. N.: Increased activity of two enzymes of pyrimidine biosynthesis *de novo* in erythrocytes from patients with the Lesch-Nyhan syndrome. J. Lab. clin. Med. **81**, 43 (1973).

BECKER, M. A., MEYER, L. J., WOOD, A. W., SEEGMILLER, J. E.: Gout associated with increased PRPP synthetase activity. Arthrit. and Rheum. **15**, 430 (1972).

BECKER, M. A., MEYER, L. J., SEEGMILLER, J. E.: Gout with purine overproduction resulting from increased PRPP synthetase activity. Clin. Res. **21**, 217 (1973).

BENEDEK, T. G.: Correlations of serum uric acid and lipid concentrations in normal, gouty, and atherosclerotic men. Ann. intern. Med. **66**, 851 (1967).

BENEDICT, J. D., FORSHAM, P. H., STETTEN, DE W., JR.: The metabolism of uric acid in the normal and gouty human studied with the aid of isotopic uric acid. J. biol. Chem. **181**, 183 (1949).
BENEDICT, J. D., FORSHAM, P. H., ROCHE, M., SOLOWAY, S., STETTEN, DE W., JR.: The effect of salicylates and adrenocorticotropic hormone upon the miscible pool of uric acid in gout. J. clin. Invest. **29**, 1104 (1950).
BENEDICT, J. D., ROCHE, M., YU, T.-F., BIEN, E. J., GUTMAN, A. B., STETTEN, DE W., JR.: Incorporation of glycine nitrogen into uric acid in normal and gouty man. Metabolism **1**, 3 (1952).
BENEDICT, J. D., YU, T.-F., BIEN, E. J., GUTMAN, A. B., STETTEN, DE W., JR.: A further study of the utilization of dietary glycine nitrogen for uric acid synthesis in gout. J. clin. Invest. **32**, 775 (1953).
BENKE, P. J., HERRICK, N.: Azaguanine resistance as a manifestation of a new form of metabolic overproduction of uric acid. Amer. J. Med. **52**, 547 (1972).
BENKE, P. J., HERRICK, N.: Personal communication.
BERGMANN, F., DIKSTEIN, S.: Studies on uric acid and related compounds. III. Observations on the specificity of mammalian xanthine oxidase. J. biol. Chem. **223**, 765 (1956).
BERGMEYER, H. U.: Methods of Enzymatic Analysis, Book II, p. 2206. New York: Academic Press 1970.
BERKOWITZ, D.: Blood lipid and uric acid interrelationships. J. Amer. med. Ass. **190**, 856 (1964).
BERKOWITZ, D.: Gout, hyperlipidemia and diabetes interrelationships. J. Amer. med. Ass. **197**, 117 (1966).
BEUTLER, E.: Effect of flavin compounds on glutathione reductase activity: *In vivo* and *in vitro* studies. J. clin. Invest. **48**, 1957 (1969).
BEYER, K. H., BAER, J. E.: Physiological basis for the action of newer diuretic agents. Pharmacol. Rev. **13**, 517 (1961).
BIEN, E. J., YU, T.-F., BENEDICT, J. D., GUTMAN, A. B., STETTEN, D., JR.: The relation of dietary nitrogen consumption to the rate of uric acid synthesis in normal and gouty man. J. clin. Invest. **32**, 778 (1953).
BIEN, E. J., ZUCKER, H.: Uricolysis in normal and gouty individuals. Ann. rheum. Dis. **14**, 409 (1955).
BIRKOFER, L., RITTER, A., KUHLTHAN, H. P.: Uric acid-3-ribofuranoside and uric acid-3-glucopyranoside. Angew. Chem. (Eng.) **2**, 155 (1963).
BISHOP, C., GARNER, W., TALBOTT, J. H.: Pool size turnover rate, and rapidity of equilibration of injected isotopic uric acid in normal and pathological subjects. J. clin. Invest. **30**, 879 (1951).
BISHOP, C., RAND, R., TALBOTT, J. H.: Rate of conversion of isotopic glycine to uric acid in the normal and gouty humans and how this is affected by vitamin E and folic acid. Metabolism **4**, 174 (1955).
BLUESTONE, R., KIPPEN, I., KLINENBERG, J. R.: Effect of drugs on urate binding to plasma proteins. Brit. Med. J. **1969 IV**, 590.
BLUESTONE, R., KIPPEN, I., KLINENBERG, J. R., WHITEHOUSE, M. W.: Effect of some uricosuric and anti-inflammatory drugs on the binding of uric acid to human serum albumin *in vitro*. J. Lab. clin. Med. **76**, 85 (1970).
BOREK, E., SRINIVASAN, P. R.: The methylation of nucleic acids. Ann. Rev. Biochem. **35**, 275 (1966).
BREWER, G. J.: 6-phosphogluconate dehydrogenase and glutathione reductase. In: Biochemical Methods in Red Cell Genetics (Ed. J. J. YUNIS), p. 139. New York: Academic Press 1969.
BROCHNER-MORTENSEN, K.: Review of diagnostic criteria and known etiological factors in gout. In: Epidemiology of Chronic Rheumatism, Vol. 1, p. 140. Philadelphia: Davis 1963.
BROCKMAN, R. W.: Metabolism and mechanisms of action of purine analogues. In: Exploitable Molecular Mechanisms and Neoplasia, p. 435. Baltimore: Williams & Wilkins 1969.
BROCKMAN, R. W., ANDERSON, E. P.: Biochemistry of cancer (metabolic aspects). Ann. Rev. Biochem. **32**, 463 (1963).
BROCKMAN, R. W., CHUMLEY, S. W.: Inhibition of formylglycinamide ribonucleotide synthesis in neoplastic cells by purines and analogs. Biochim. biophys. Acta (Amst.) **95**, 365 (1965).
BRONSKY, D., BERNSTEIN, A.: Acute gout secondary to multiple myeloma, a case report. Ann. intern. Med. **41**, 820 (1954).
BRYANT, J. M., YU, T.-F., BERGER, L., SCHVARTZ, N., TOROSDAG, S., FLETCHER, L., JR., FERTIG, H., SCHWARTZ, M. S., QUAN, R. B. F.: Hyperuricemia induced by administration of chlorthalidone and other sulfonamide diuretics. Amer. J. Med. **33**, 408 (1962).
BUCHANAN, D. L., ROLLINS, J. M.: Lack of correlation between gout and the incorporation of isotopic formate into uric acid. Yale J. Biol. Med. **34**, 31 (1961).
BUCHANAN, J. M., SONNE, J. C., DELLUVA, A. M.: Biologic precursors of uric acid. II. The role of lactate, glycine, and carbon dioxide as precursors of the carbon chain and nitrogen atom 7 of uric acid. J. biol. Chem. **173**, 81 (1948).

BURCH, T. A., O'BRIEN, W. M., NEED, R., KURLAND, L. T.: Hyperuricemia and gout in Mariana Islands. Ann. Rheum. Dis. **25**, 144 (1966).
BUZARD, J., BISHOP, C., TALBOTT, J., II.: The fate of uric acid in the normal and gouty human. J. chron. Dis. **2**, 42 (1955).
CALDWELL, I. C., HENDERSON, J. F., PATERSON, A. R. P.: The enzymic formation of 6-(methylmercapto) purine ribonucleoside 5-phosphate. Canad. J. Biochem. **44**, 229 (1966).
CANELLAKIS, E. S., TUTTLE, A. L., COHEN, P. P.: A comparative study of the end products of uric acid oxidation by peroxidases. J. biol. Chem. **213**, 397 (1955).
CANNON, P. J., SVAHN, D. S., DEMARTINI, F. E.: The influence of hypertonic saline infusions upon the fractional reabsorption of urate and other ions in normal and hypertensive man. Circulation **41**, 97 (1970).
CANTONI, G. L., GELBOIN, H. V., LUBORSKY, S. W., RICHARDS, H. H., SINGER, M. F.: Studies on soluble ribonucleic acid of rabbit liver. III. Preparation and properties of rabbit-liver soluble RNA. Biochim. biophys. Acta (Amst.) **61**, 354 (1962).
CAPUTTO, R.: The enzymatic synthesis of adenylic acid: Adenosinekinase. J. biol. Chem. **189**, 801 (1951).
CARCASSI, A., MARCOLONGO, R., JR., MARINELLO, E., RIARIO-SFORZA, G., BOGGIANO, C.: Liver xanthine oxidase in gouty patients. Arthrit. and Rheum. **12**, 17 (1969).
CARTER, C. E., COHEN, C. H.: The preparation and properties of adenylosuccinase and adenylosuccinic acid. J. biol. Chem. **222**, 17 (1956).
CARTER, C. E., POTTER, J. L.: Distribution and properties of uric acid riboside. Fed. Proc. **11**, 195 (1952).
CASKEY, C. T., ASHTON, D. M., WYNGAARDEN, J. B.: The enzymology of feedback inhibition of glutamine phosphoribosylpyrophosphate amidotransferase by purine ribonucleotides. J. biol. Chem. **239**, 2570 (1964).
CLAPP, J. R., NAKAJIMA, K., NOTTEBOHM, G. A., ROBINSON, R. R.: Volume-mediated regulation of furosemide. Clin. Res. **17**, 426 (1969).
COBB, S.: Hyperuricemia in executives. In: The Epidemiology of Chronic Rheumatism, Vol. 1, p. 182. Philadelphia: Davis 1963.
COHEN, H.: Gout. In: Textbook of the Rheumatic Diseases (Ed. W. S. C. COPEMAN), p. 361. Edinburgh: Livingston 1955.
COWDREY, S. C.: Hyperuricemia in infectious mononucleosis. J. Amer. med. Ass. **196**, 319 (1966).
COX, R. P., KRAUSS, M. R., BALIS, M. E., DANCIS, J.: Evidence for transfer of enzyme product as the basis of metabolic cooperation between tissue culture fibroblasts of Lesch-Nyhan disease and normal cells. Proc. nat. Acad. Sci. (Wash.) **67**, 1573 (1970).
CRAFT, J. A., DEAN, B. M., WATTS, R. W. E., WESTWICK, W. J.: Studies on human erythrocyte IMP: Pyrophosphate phosphoribosyl transferase. Europ. J. Biochem. **15**, 367 (1970).
CROWLEY, G. M.: The enzymatic synthesis of 5'-phosphoribosylimidazoleacetic acid. J. biol. Chem. **239**, 2593 (1964).
DAVIS, A. R., NEWTON, E. B., BENEDICT, S. R.: The combined uric acid in beef blood. J. biol. Chem. **54**, 595 (1922).
DECKER, J. L., LANE, J. J., JR., REYNOLDS, W. E.: Hyperuricemia in a Filipino population. Arthrit. and Rheum. **5**, 144 (1962).
DEMARTINI, F. E., WHEATON, E. A., HEALEY, L. A., LARAGH, J. H.: Effect of chlorothiazide on the renal excretion of uric acid. Amer. J. Med. **32**, 572 (1962).
DE VRIES, A., FRANK, M., ATSMON, A.: Inherited uric acid lithiasis. Amer. J. Med. **33**, 880 (1962).
DUNCAN, H., DIXON, A. ST. J.: Gout, familial hyperuricemia, and renal disease. Quart. J. Med. **29**, 127 (1960).
DUNN, J. P., BROOKS, G. W., MAUSNER, J., RODNAN, G. P., COBB, S.: Social class gradient of serum uric acid levels in man. J. Amer. med. Ass. **185**, 431 (1963).
DUNN, D. B., SMITH, J. D.: The occurrence of 6-methylaminopurine in deoxyribonucleic acids. Biochem. J. **68**, 627 (1958).
EMMERSON, B. T.: Chronic lead nephropathy: The diagnostic use of calcium EDTA and the association with gout. Aust. Ann. Med. **12**, 310 (1963).
EMMERSON, B. T.: The renal excretion of urate in chronic lead nephropathy. Aust. Ann. Med. **14**, 295 (1965).
EMMERSON, B. T.: The clinical differentiation of lead gout from primary gout. Arthr. and Rheum. **11**, 623 (1968).
EMMERSON, B. T.: Personal communication (1972).

EMMERSON, B. T.: Personal communication.
EMMERSON, B. T., WYNGAARDEN, J. B.: Purine metabolism in heterozygous carriers of hypoxanthine guanine phosphoribosyltransferase deficiency. Science 166, 1533 (1969).
ENGELMAN, K., WATTS, R. W. E., KLINENBERG, J. R., SJOERDSMA, A., SEEGMILLER, J. E.: Clinical, physiological and biochemical studies of a patient with xanthinuria and pheochromocytoma. Amer. J. Med. 37, 839 (1964).
ERRERA, M.: Liver glutaminases. J. biol. Chem. 187, 483 (1949a).
ERRERA, M., GREENSTEIN, J. P.: Phosphate-activated glutaminase in kidney and other tissues. J. biol. Chem. 187, 495 (1949b).
EVANS, J. G., PRIOR, I. A. M., HARVEY, H. P. B.: Relation of serum uric acid to body bulk, haemoglobin, and alcohol intake in two South Pacific Polynesian populations. Ann. Rheum. Dis. 27, 319 (1968).
FALCONER, R., GULLAND, J. M.: The constitution of purine nucleosides. VIII. Uric acid riboside. J. Chem. Soc. (Org.) 1939 (1939).
FANELLI, G. M., JR., BOHN, D. L., REILLY, S. S.: Functional characteristics of renal urate transport in the Cebus Monkey. Amer. J. Physiol. 218, 627 (1970).
FANELLI, G. M., JR., BOHN, D. L., STAFFORD, S. S.: Renal urate transport in the chimpanzee. Amer. J. Physiol. 220, 613 (1971).
FELDMAN, E. B., WALLACE, S. L.: Hypertriglyceridemia in gout. Circulation 29, 508 (1964).
FELIX, J. S., DE MARS, R.: Detection of femal heterozygous for the Lesch-Nyhan mutation by 8-azaguanine resistant growth of cultured fibroblasts. J. Lab. clin. Med. 77, 596 (1971).
FIELD, J. B., DRASH, A. L.: Studies in glycogen storage disease. II. Heterogeneity in the inheritance of glycogen storage disease. Trans. Assoc. Amer. Phycns. 80, 284 (1967).
FIELD, J. B., EPSTEIN, S., EGAN, T.: Studies in glycogen storage disease. I. Intestinal glucose-6-phosphatase activity in patients with von Gierke's disease and their parents. J. clin. Invest. 44, 1240 (1965).
FINE, R. N., STRAUSS, J., DONNELL, G. N.: Hyperuricemia in glycogen storage disease Type I. Amer. J. Dis. Child. 112, 572 (1966).
FLAKS, J. G., ERWIN, M. J., BUCHANAN, J. M.: Biosynthesis of the purines. XVI. The synthesis of adenosine 5'-phosphate and 5'-amino-4-imidazolecarboxamide ribotide by a nucleotide pyrophosphorylase. J. biol. Chem. 228, 201 (1957a).
FLAKS, J. G., ERWIN, M. J., BUCHANAN, J. M.: Biosynthesis of the purines. XVIII. 5-amino-1-ribosyl-4-imidazolecarboxamide 5'-phosphate transformylase and inosinicase. J. biol. Chem. 229, 603 (1957c).
FLAKS, J. G., WARREN, L., BUCHANAN, J. M.: Biosynthesis of the purines. XVII. Further studies of the inosinic acid transformylase system. J. biol. Chem. 228, 215 (1957b).
FOLIN, O.: Standardized methods for determination of uric acid in unlaked blood and urine. J. biol. Chem. 101, 111 (1933).
FOLIN, O., BERGLUND, H., DERICK, C.: The uric acid problem: An experimental study on animals and man, including gouty subjects. J. biol. Chem. 60, 361 (1924).
FOLIN, O., LYMAN, H.: On the influence of phenylquinolin carbonic acid (Atophan) on uric acid elimination. J. Pharmacol. exp. Ther. 4, 539 (1913).
FORREST, H. S., HATFIELD, D., LAGOWSKI, J. M.: Uric acid riboside. Part I. Isolation and reinvestigation of the structure. J. Chem. Soc. (Org.) 1961, 963.
FOX, I. H., KELLEY, W. N.: Human phosphoribosylpyrophosphate synthetase: Distribution, purification and properties. J. biol. Chem. 246, 5739 (1971a).
FOX, I. H., KELLEY, W. N.: Phosphoribosylpyrophosphate in man: Biochemical and clinical significance. Ann. intern. Med. 74, 424 (1971b).
FOX, I. H., KELLEY, W. N.: Human phosphoribosylpyrophosphate synthetase: Kinetic mechanism and end-product inhibition. J. biol. Chem. 247, 2126 (1972).
FOX, I. H., WYNGAARDEN, J. B., KELLEY, W. N.: Depletion of erythrocyte phosphoribosylpyrophosphate in man, a newly observed effect of allopurinol. New Engl. J. Med. 283, 1177 (1970).
FRANK, M., DE VRIES, A., ATSMON, A., KOCHWA, S.: Urinary pH, ammonia and calcium excretion in renal uric acid stone patients. Israel med. J. 12, 299 (1960).
FRENCH, J. G., DODGE, H. J., KJELSBERG, M. O., MIKKELSEN, W. M., SCHULL, W. J.: A study of familial aggregation of serum uric acid levels in the population of Tecumseh, Michigan. Amer. J. Epidem. 86, 214 (1967).
FRIEDEN, C.: Glutamate dehydrogenase. V. The relation of enzyme structure to the catalytic function. J. biol. Chem. 238, 3286 (1963).

FRIEDKIN, M., KALCKAR, H.: Nucleoside phosphorylases. In: The Enzymes (Eds. P. D. BOYER, H. LARDY, K. MYRBACK), Vol. 5, p. 237. New York: Academic Press 1961.
FRIEDMAN, T., SEEGMILLER, J. E., SUBAK-SHARPE, J. H.: Metabolic cooperation between genetically marked human fibroblasts in tissue culture. Nature **220**, 272 (1968).
FRIEDMAN, T., SEEGMILLER, J. E., SUBAK-SHARPE, J. H.: Evidence against the existence of guanosine and inosine kinases in human fibroblasts in tissue culture. Exp. Cell Res. **56**, 425 (1969).
FUJIMOTO, W. Y., SEEGMILLER, J. R.: Hypoxanthine-guanine phosphoribosyltransferase deficiency: Activity in normal, mutant and heterozygote-cultured human skin fibroblasts. Proc. nat. Acad. Sci. (Wash.) **65**, 577 (1970).
GARROD, A. B.: The Nature and Treatment of Gout and Rheumatic Gout, p. 251. London: Walton and Maberly 1863.
GARTLER, S. M., SCOTT, R. C., GOLDSTEIN, J. L., CAMPBELL, B., SPARKES, R.: The Lesch-Nyhan syndrome: Rapid detection of heterozygotes by the rise of hair follicles. Science **172**, 572 (1971).
GEREN, W., BENDICH, A., BODANSKY, O., BROWN, G. B.: Fate of uric acid in man. J. biol. Chem. **183**, 21 (1950).
GOLD, M., HURWITZ, J.: The enzymatic methylation of ribonucleic acid and deoxyribonucleic acid. V. Purification and properties of the deoxyribonucleic acid methylating activity of *Escherichia coli*. J. biol. Chem. **239**, 3858 (1964).
GOLD, M. S., WILLIAMS, J. C., SPIVACK, M., GUANN, V.: Sickle cell anemia and hyperuricemia. J. Amer. med. Ass. JAMA **206**, 1572 (1968).
GOLDTHWAITE, D. A.: Mechanisms of synthesis of purine nucleotides in heart muscle extracts. J. clin. Invest. **36**, 1572 (1957).
GOLDTHWAIT, D. A., PEABODY, R. A., GREENBERG, G. R.: On the mechanism of synthesis of glycinamideribotide and its formyl derivative. J. biol. Chem. **221**, 569 (1956).
GOLDTHWAITE, J. C., BUTLER, C. F., STILLMAN, J. S.: The diagnosis of gout: Significance of an elevated serum uric acid value. New Engl. J. Med. **259**, 1095 (1958).
GONICK, H. C., RUBINI, M. E., GLEASON, I. O., SOMMERS, S. C.: The renal lesion in gout. Ann. intern. Med. **62**, 667 (1965).
GOTS, J. S., GOLDSTEIN, J.: Specific action of adenine as a feedback inhibitor of purine biosynthesis. Science **130**, 622 (1959).
GREENE, M. L., BOYLES, J. R., SEEGMILLER, J. E.: Substrate stabilization: Genetically controlled reciprocal relationship of two human enzymes. Science **167**, 887 (1970).
GREENE, M. L., SEEGMILLER, J. E.: Elevated erythrocyte phosphoribosylpyrophosphate in X-linked uric aciduria: Importance of PRPP concentration in the regulation of human purine biosynthesis. J. clin. Invest. **48**, 32a (1969).
GRIFFITHS, M.: Oxidation of uric acid catalyzed by copper and by the cytochrome-cytochrome oxidase system. J. biol. Chem. **197**, 399 (1952).
GUDZENT, F.: Gicht und Rheumatismus. Berlin: Springer 1928.
GUTMAN, A. B.: Primary and secondary gout. Ann. intern. Med. **39**, 1062 (1953).
GUTMAN, A. B., YU, T.-F., WEISSMANN, B.: The concept of secondary gout: Relation to purine metabolism in polycythemia and myeloid metaplasia. Trans. Ass. Amer. Phycns **69**, 229 (1956).
GUTMAN, A. B., YU, T.-F.: Renal function in gout with a commentary on the renal regulation of urate excretion, and the role of the kidney in the pathogenesis of gout. Amer. J. Med. **23**, 600 (1957).
GUTMAN, A. B., YU, T.-F.: Gout, a derangement of purine metabolism. Advances intern. Med. **5**, 27 (1952).
GUTMAN, A. B., YU, T.-F.: A three-component system for regulation of renal excretion of uric acid in man. Trans. Ass. Amer. Phycns **74**, 353 (1961).
GUTMAN, A. B., YU, T.-F.: Secondary gout. Ann. intern. Med. **55**, 675 (1962b).
GUTMAN, A. B., YU, T.-F.: An abnormality of glutamine metabolism in primary gout. Amer. J. Med. **35**, 820 (1963a).
GUTMAN, A. B., YU, T.-F.: On the nature of the inborn metabolic error(s) of primary gout. Trans. Ass. Amer. Phycns **76**, 141 (1963b).
GUTMAN, A. B., YU, T.-F.: Urinary ammonium excretion in primary gout. J. clin. Invest. **44**, 1474 (1965).
GUTMAN, A. B., YU, T.-F., ADLER, M., JAVITT, N. B.: Intramolecular distribution of uric acid-N^{15} after administration of glycine-N^{15} and ammonium N^{15} chloride to gouty and nongouty subjects. J. clin. Invest. **41**, 623 (1962a).

GUTMAN, A. B., YU, T.-F., BERGER, L.: Renal function in gout. III. Estimation of tubular secretion and reabsorption of uric acid by use of pyrazinamide (pyrazinoic acid). Amer. J. Med. **45**, 575 (1969).
GUTMAN, A. B., YU, T.-F., BLACK, H., YALOW, R. S., BERSON, S. A.: Incorporation of glycine 1-C^{14}, glycine 2-C^{14} and glycine-N^{15} into uric acid in normal and gouty subjects. Amer. J. Med. **25**, 917 (1958).
HALL, A. P., BARRY, P. E., DAWBER, T. R., MC NAMARA, P. M.: Epidemiology of gout and hyperuricemia: A long-term population study. Amer. J. Med. **42**, 27 (1967).
HARTMAN, S. C., BUCHANAN, J. M.: Biosynthesis of the purines. XXI. 5-phosphoribosylpyrophosphate amidotransferase. J. biol. Chem. **233**, 451 (1958a).
HARTMAN, S. C., BUCHANAN, J. M.: Biosynthesis of the purines. XXII. 2-amino-N-ribosylacetamide-5'-phosphate kinosynthetase. J. biol. Chem. **233**, 456 (1958b).
HARTMAN, S. C., LEVENBERG, B., BUCHANAN, J. M.: Biosynthesis of the purines. XI. Structure, enzymatic synthesis, and metabolism of glycinamide ribotide and (a-N-formyl)-glycinamide ribotide. J. biol. Chem. **221**, 1057 (1956).
HATFIELD, D., FORREST, H. S.: Biosynthesis of 3-ribosyluric acid (uric acid riboside). Biochim. biophys. Acta (Amst.) **62**, 185 (1962).
HATFIELD, D., GREENLAND, R. A., STEWART, H. L., WYNGAARDEN, J. B.: Biosynthesis of a new uric acid ribonucleotide. Biochim. biophys. Acta (Amst.) **91**, 163 (1964c).
HATFIELD, D., RINEHART, R. R., FORREST, H. S.: 3-ribosyluric acid. Part II. Isolation of the corresponding nucleotide from beef blood. J. Chem. Soc. 889 (1963).
HATFIELD, D., WYNGAARDEN, J. B.: 3-ribosylpurines. I. Synthesis of (3-ribosyluric acid) 5'-phosphate and (3-ribosylxanthine) 5'-phosphate by a pyrimidine ribonucleotide pyrophosphorylase of beef erythrocytes. J. biol. Chem. **239**, 2580 (1964a).
HATFIELD, D., WYNGAARDEN, J. B.: 3-ribosylpurines. II. Studies on (3-ribosylxanthine)5'-phosphate and on ribonucleotide derivatives of certain uracil analogues. J. biol. Chem. **239**, 2587 (1964b).
HAUGE, M., HARVALD, B.: Heredity in gout and hyperuricemia. Acta med. scand. **152**, 247 (1955).
HEALY, L. A., HALL, A. P.: The epidemiology of hyperuricemia. Bull. rheum. Dis. **20**, 600 (1970).
HEINRICH, M. R., WILSON, D. W.: Biosynthesis of nucleic acid components studied with C^{14}. I. Purines and pyrimidines in the rat. J. biol. Chem. **186**, 447 (1950).
HENDERSON, J. F., BROX, L. W., KELLEY, W. N., ROSENBLOOM, F. M., SEEGMILLER, J. E.: Kinetic studies of hypoxanthine-guanine phosphoribosyltransferase. J. biol. Chem. **243**, 2514 (1968a).
HENDERSON, J. F., KELLEY, W. N., ROSENBLOOM, F. M., SEEGMILLER, J. E.: Inheritance of purine phosphoribosyltransferases in man. Amer. J. hum. Genet. **21**, 61 (1969).
HENDERSON, J. F., KHOO, M. K. Y.: Synthesis of 5-phosphoribosyl-1-pyrophosphate from glucose in Ehrlich ascites tumor cells *in vitro*. J. biol. Chem. **240**, 2349 (1965a).
HENDERSON, J. F., KHOO, M. K. Y.: On the mechanism of feedback inhibition of purine biosynthesis *de novo* in Ehrlich ascites tumor cells *in vitro*. J. biol. Chem. **240**, 3104 (1965b).
HENDERSON, J. F., LE PAGE, G. A.: Utilization of host purines by transplanted tumors. Cancer Res. **19**, 67 (1959).
HENDERSON, L. J., PALMER, W. W.: On the several factors of acid excretion in nephritis. J. biol. Chem. **21**, 37 (1915).
HENDERSON, J. F., ROSENBLOOM, F. M., KELLEY, W. N., SEEGMILLER, J. E.: Variations in purine metabolism of cultured skin fibroblasts from patients with gout. J. clin. Invest. **47**, 1511 (1968b).
HEPPEL, L. A., HILMOE, R. J.: Purification and properties of 5-nucleotidase. J. biol. Chem. **188**, 665 (1951).
HEPPEL, L. A., RABINOWITZ, J. C.: Enzymology of nucleic acids, purines, and pyrimidines. Ann. Rev. Biochem. **27**, 613 (1958).
HERSCOVICS, A., JOHNSTONE, R. M.: ^{14}C-formate utilization in cell-free extracts of Ehrlich ascites cells. Biochim. biophys. Acta (Amst.) **93**, 251 (1964).
HERSHKO, A., HERSHKO, C., MAGER, J.: Increased formation of 5-phosphoribosyl-1-pyrophosphate in red blood cells of some gouty patients. Israel med. J. **4**, 939 (1968).
HEYDEN, S.: Personal communication (1972).
HIATT, H. H.: Studies of ribose metabolism. II. A method for the study of ribose synthesis *in vivo*. J. biol. Chem. **229**, 725 (1957).
HICKLING, R. A.: Gout, leukemia, and polycythaemia. Lancet **1953 I**, 57.
HILL, D. L., BENNETT, L. L., JR.: Purification and properties of 5-phosphoribosylpyrophosphate amidotransferase from adenocarcinoma 755 cells. Biochemistry **8**, 122 (1969).

HILTON, J. G., GOODBODY, M. F., JR., KRUESI, O. R.: The effect of prolonged administration of ammonium chloride on the blood acid-base equilibrium of geriatric subjects. J. Amer. Geriat. Soc. 3, 697 (1955).
HOFFMAN, G. T., ROTTINO, A., ALBAUM, H. G.: Levels of nucleotide in the blood during shock. Science 114, 188 (1951).
HOLLING, H. E.: Gout and glycogen storage disease. Ann. intern. Med. 58, 654 (1963).
HOLMES, E. W., KELLEY, W. N., WYNGAARDEN, J. B.: The kidney and uric acid excretion in man. Kidney Internat. 2, 115 (1972).
HOLMES, E. W., MC DONALD, J. A., MC CORD, J. M., WYNGAARDEN, J. B., KELLEY, W. N.: Human glutamine phosphoribosylpyrophosphate amidotransferase: Kinetic and regulatory properties. J. biol. Chem. 248, 144 (1973a).
HOLMES, E. W., JR., WYNGAARDEN, J. B., KELLEY, W. N.: The regulation of PRPP amidotransferase in man. Clin. Res. (abstract) 1973, in press.
HOLMES, E. W., JR., WYNGAARDEN, J. B., KELLEY, W. N.: Human glutamine phosphoribosylpyrophosphate amidotransferase: Two molecular forms interconvertible by purine ribonucleotides and phosphoribosylpyrophosphate. J. biol. Chem. 248, 6035 (1973).
HOLMES, E. W., JR., WYNGAARDEN, J. B., KELLEY, W. N.: Unpublished observation.
HORI, M., HENDERSON, J. F.: Kinetic studies of adenine phosphoribosyltransferase. J. biol. Chem. 241, 3404 (1966).
HOUPT, J. B., OGRYZLO, M. A.: Persistence of impaired uric acid excretion in gout during reduced synthesis with allopurinol. Arthrit. and Rheum. 7, 316 (1964).
HOWARD, W. J., APPEL, S. H.: Control of purine biosynthesis: FGAR amidotransferase. Clin. Res. 16, 344 (1968).
HOWELL, R. R., WYNGAARDEN, J. B.: On the mechanism of peroxidation of uric acids by hemoproteins. J. biol. Chem. 225, 3544 (1960).
HOWELL, R. R., SPEAS, M., WYNGAARDEN, J. B.: A quantitative study of recycling of isotope from glycine-1-C^{14}, N^{15} into various subunits of the uric acid molecule in a normal subject. J. clin. Invest. 40, 2076 (1961).
HOWELL, R. R., ASHTON, D. M., WYNGAARDEN, J. B.: Glucose-6-phosphatase deficiency glycogen storage disease: Studies on the interrelationships of carbohydrate, lipid, and purine abnormalities. Pediatrics 29, 553 (1962a).
HOWELL, R. R., SEEGMILLER, J. E.: Uricolysis by human leukocytes. Nature 196, 482 (1962b).
HOWELL, R. R.: The interrelationship of glycogen storage disease and gout. Arthrit. and Rheum. 8, 780 (1965).
HUENNEKENS, F. M., NURK, E., GABRIO, B. W.: Erythrocyte metabolism. I. Purine nucleoside phosphorylase. J. biol. Chem. 221, 971 (1956).
HURWITZ, J., ANDERS, M., GOLD, M., SMITH, I.: The enzymatic methylation of ribonucleic acid and deoxyribonucleic acid. VII. The methylation of ribosomal ribonucleic acid. J. biol. Chem. 240, 1256 (1965).
JACOBSON, B. M.: The uric acid in the serum of gouty and non-gouty individuals: Its determination by Folin's recent method and its significance in the diagnosis of gout. Ann. intern. Med. 11, 1277 (1937).
JAKOVCIC, S., SORENSEN, L. B.: Studies of uric acid metabolism in glycogen storage disease associated with gouty arthritis. Arthrit. and Rheum. 10, 129 (1967).
JEANDET, J., LESTRADET, H.: L'hyperlactacidemie cause probable de l'hyperuricemie dans la glycogenose hepatique. Rev. franc. Étud. clin. biol. 6, 71 (1961).
JEUNE, M., CHARRAT, A., BERTRAND, J.: Polycorie hepatique, hyperuricemic et goutte. Arch. franc. Pédiat. 14, 897 (1957).
JOKLIK, W. K.: Adenine succinic acid and adenylsuccinic acid from mammalian liver: Isolation and identification. Biochem. J. 66, 333 (1957).
JONES, O. W., JR., ASHTON, D. M., WYNGAARDEN, J. B.: Accelerated turnover of phosphoribosylpyrophosphate, a purine nucleotide precursor, in certain gouty subjects. J. clin. Invest. 41, 1805 (1962).
JORGENSEN, S., POULSEN, H. E.: Enzymic determination of hypoxanthine and xanthine in human plasma and urine. Acta Pharmacol. (Kbh.) 11, 223 (1955).
KALCKAR, H. M.: Differential spectrophotometry of purine compounds by means of specific enzymes. III. Studies of the enzymes of purine metabolism. J. biol. Chem. 167, 461 (1947).
KAPLAN, D., BERNSTEIN, D., WALLACE, S. L., HALBERSTAM, D.: Serum and urinary amino acids in normouricemic and hyperuricemic subjects. Ann. intern. Med. 62, 658 (1965).

KAPLAN, D., DIAMOND, H., WALLACE, S. L., HALBERSTAM, D.: Amino acid excretion in primary hyperuricaemia. Ann. rheum. Dis. **28**, 180 (1969).

KAPOOR, M., WAYGOOD, E.: Initial steps of purine biosynthesis in wheat germ. Biochem. biophys. Res. Commun. **9**, 7 (1962).

KARLSON, J. L., BARKER, H. A.: Biosynthesis of uric acid labeled with radioactive carbon. J. biol. Chem. **177**, 597 (1949).

KATZ, W. A., EHRLICH, G. E.: The solubility of monosodium urate in serum and connective tissue fractions. Arthrit. and Rheum. **11**, 492 (1968).

KATZ, J., ROGNSTAD, R.: The labeling of pentose phosphate from glucose-^{14}C and estimation of the rates of transaldolase, transketolase, the contribution of the pentose cycle, and ribosephosphate synthesis. Biochemistry **6**, 2227 (1967).

KAUFMAN, J. M., GREENE, M. L., SEEGMILLER, J. E.: Urine uric acid to creatinine ratio: A screening test for inherited disorders of purine metabolism. J. Pediat. **73**, 583 (1968).

KELLEY, W. N., ROSENBLOOM, F. M., HENDERSON, J. F., SEEGMILLER, J. E.: Xanthine phosphoribosyltransferase in man: Relationship to hypoxanthine-guanine phosphoribosyltransferase. Biochem. biophys. Res. Commun. **28**, 345 (1967a).

KELLEY, W. N.: Studies on the adenine phosphoribosyltransferase enzyme in human fibroblasts lacking hypoxanthine-guanine phosphoribosyltransferase. J. Lab. clin. Med. **77**, 33 (1971a).

KELLEY, W. N., FOX, I. H., WYNGAARDEN, J. B.: Further evaluation of adenine phosphoribosyltransferase deficiency in man: Occurrence in a patient with gout. Clin. Res. **18**, 53 (1970a).

KELLEY, W. N., FOX, I. H., WYNGAARDEN, J. B.: Essential role of phosphoribosylpyrophosphate (PRPP) in regulation of purine biosynthesis in cultured human fibroblasts. Clin. Res. **18**, 457 (1970b).

KELLEY, W. N., FOX, I. H., WYNGAARDEN, J. B.: Regulation of purine biosynthesis in cultured human cells. I. Effects of orotic acid. Biochim. biophys. Acta (Amst.) **215**, 512 (1970c).

KELLEY, W. N., GREENE, M. L., ROSENBLOOM, F. M., HENDERSON, J. F., SEEGMILLER, J. E.: Hypoxanthine-guanine phosphoribosyltransferase deficiency in gout. Ann. intern. Med. **70**, 155 (1969).

KELLEY, W. N., MEADE, J. C.: Studies on hypoxanthine-guanine phosphoribosyltransferase in fibroblasts from patients with the Lesch-Nyhan syndrome: Evidence for genetic heterogeneity. J. biol. Chem. **246**, 2953 (1971b).

KELLEY, W. N., LEVY, R. I., ROSENBLOOM, F. M., HENDERSON, J. F., SEEGMILLER, J. E.: Adenine phosphoribosyltransferase deficiency: A previously undescribed genetic defect in man. J. clin. Invest. **47**, 2281 (1968a).

KELLEY, W. N., ROSENBLOOM, F. M., HENDERSON, J. F., SEEGMILLER, J. E.: A specific enzyme defect in gout associated with overproduction of uric acid. Proc. nat. Acad. Sci. (Wash.) **57**, 1735 (1967b).

KELLEY, W. N., ROSENBLOOM, F. M., SEEGMILLER, J. E.: The effect of azathioprine (Imuran) on purine synthesis in clinical disorders of purine metabolism. J. clin. Invest. **46**, 1518 (1967c).

KELLEY, W. N., ROSENBLOOM, F. M., SEEGMILLER, J. E., HOWELL, R. R.: Excessive production of uric acid in Type I glycogen storage disease. J. Pediat. **72**, 488 (1968b).

KENNAN, A. L.: Glutamine synthesis in rats with diabetic acidosis. Endocrinology **71**, 203 (1962).

KINGDON, H. S., SHAPIRO, B. M., STADTMAN, E. R.: Regulation of glutamine synthetase. VIII. ATP: glutamine synthetase adenyltransferase, an enzyme that catalyzes alterations in the regulatory properties of glutamine synthetase. Proc. nat. Acad. Sci. (Wash.) **58**, 1703 (1967).

KLINENBERG, J. R., GOLDFINGER, S. E., SEEGMILLER, J. E.: The effectivness of the xanthine oxidase inhibitor allopurinol in the treatment of gout. Ann. intern. Med. **62**, 639 (1965).

KLINENBERG, J. R., KIPPEN, I.: The binding of urate to plasma proteins determined by means of equilibrium dialysis. J. Lab. clin. Med. **75**, 503 (1970).

KLUNGSOYR, L., HAGEMAN, J. H., FALL, L., ATKINSON, D. E.: Interaction between energy charge and product feedback in the regulation of biosynthetic enzymes. Aspartokinase, phosphoribosyladenosine triphosphate synthetase, and phosphoribosylpyrophosphate synthetase. Biochemistry **7**, 4035 (1968).

KOEHLER, A. E.: Uric acid excretion. J. biol. Chem. **60**, 621 (1924).

KOGUT, M. D., DONNELL, G. N., NYHAN, W. L., SWEETMAN, L.: Disorder of purine metabolism due to partial deficiency of hypoxanthine-guanine phosphoribosyltransferase: A study of a family. Amer. J. Med. **48**, 148 (1970).

KORNBERG, A., LIEBERMAN, I., SIMMS, E. S.: Enzymatic synthesis and properties of 5-phosphoribosylpyrophosphate. J. biol. Chem. **215**, 389 (1955).

KORNBERG, A., PRICER, W. E., JR.: Enzymatic phosphorylation of adenosine and 2,6-diaminopurine riboside. J. biol. Chem. **193**, 481 (1951).

KREBS, H. A.: Metabolism of amino-acids. IV. The synthesis of glutamine from glutamic acid and ammonia, and the enzymic hydrolysis of glutamine in animal tissues. Biochem. J. **29**, 1951 (1935).

KRENITSKY, T. A., ELION, G. B., HENDERSON, A. M., HITCHINGS, G. H.: Inhibition of human purine nucleoside phosphorylase: Studies with intact erythrocytes and the purified enzyme. J. biol. Chem. **243**, 2876 (1968).

KURTI, L.: Untersuchungen über den Harnsäurestoffwechsel bei Nierenkranken. Z. klin. Med. **122**, 585 (1932).

LAGERKVIST, U.: Biosynthesis of guanosine 5'-phosphate. I. Xanthosine 5'-phosphate as an intermediate. J. biol. Chem. **233**, 138 (1958a).

LAGERKVIST, U.: Biosynthesis of guanosine 5'-phosphate. II. Amination of xanthosine 5'-phosphate by purified enzymes from pigeon liver. J. biol. Chem. **233**, 143 (1958b).

LAJTHA, L. G., VANE, J. R.: Dependence of bone marrow cells on the liver for purine supply. Nature **182**, 191 (1958).

LASSEN, U. K.: Kinetics of uric acid transport in human erythrocytes. Biochim. biophys. Acta (Amst.) **53**, 557 (1961).

LASTER, L., BLAIR, A.: An intestinal phosphorylase for uric acid ribonucleoside. J. biol. Chem. **238**, 3348 (1963).

LASTER, L., MULLER, A. F.: Uric acid production in a case of myeloid metaplasia associated with gouty arthritis, studied with N^{15}-labeled glycine. Amer. J. Med. **15**, 857 (1953).

LAWRENCE, J. S.: Heritable disorders of connective tissue. Proc. roy. Soc. Med. **53**, 522 (1960).

LE GAL, M.-L., LE GAL, Y., ROCHE, J., HEDEGAARD, J.: Purine biosynthesis: Enzymatic formation of ribosylamine-5-phosphate from ribose-5-phosphate and ammonia. Biochem. biophys. Res. Commun. **27**, 618 (1967).

LERNER, M. H., LOWY, B. A.: The formation of adenosine in rabbit liver and its possible role as a direct precursor of erythrocyte adenine nucleotides. J. biol. Chem. **249**, 959 (1974).

LESCH, M., NYHAN, W. L.: A familial disorder of uric acid metabolism and central nervous function. Amer. J. Med. **36**, 561 (1964).

LEVENBERG, B., BUCHANAN, J. M.: Biosynthesis of the purines. XII. Structure, enzymatic synthesis, and metabolism of 5-aminoimidazole ribotide. J. biol. Chem. **224**, 1005 (1957).

LEVENBERG, B., HARTMAN, S. C., BUCHANAN, J. M.: Biosynthesis of the purines. X. Further studies in vitro on the metabolic origin of nitrogen atoms 1 and 3 of the purine ring. J. biol. Chem. **220**, 379 (1956).

LIEBER, C. S., DAVIDSON, C. S.: Some metabolic effects of ethyl alcohol. Amer. J. Med. **33**, 319 (1962a).

LIEBER, C. S., JONES, D. P., LOSOWSKY, M. S., DAVIDSON, C. S.: Interrelation of uric acid and ethanol metabolism in man. J. clin. Invest. **41**, 1863 (1962b).

LIEBERMAN, I.: Enzymatic synthesis of adenosine 5'-phosphate from inosine 5'-phosphate. J. biol. Chem. **223**, 327 (1956).

LIEBERMAN, I., KORNBERG, A., SIMMS, E. S.: Enzymatic synthesis of pyrimidine nucleotides: Orotidine-5'-phosphate and uridine-5'-phosphate. J. biol. Chem. **215**, 403 (1955).

LOHRMAN, R., LAGOWSKI, J. M., FORREST, H. S.: 3-ribosyluric acid. Part III. Unambiguous synthesis of 3-ribosyluric acid and related compounds. J. Chem. Soc. (Org.) **1964**, 451.

LONG, W. K.: Red blood cell glutathione reductase in gout. Science **138**, 991 (1962).

LONG, W. K.: Glutathione reductase in red blood cells: Variant associated with gout. Science **155**, 712 (1967).

LONG, W. K.: Association between glutathionereductase variants and plasma uric acid concentration in a Negro population. Program abstracts. Amer. Soc. Human Genetics, October 1970, p. 14a.

LOWRY, B. A., WILLIAMS, M. K., LONDON, I. M.: Enzymatic deficiencies of purine nuclyotide synthesis in the human erythrocyte. J. biol. Chem. **237**, 1622 (1962).

LUCKE, H.: Das Harnsäureproblem und seine klinische Bedeutung. Ergebn. Inn. Med. Kinderheilk. **44**, 499 (1932).

LUDWIG, G. D.: Saturnine gout: A secondary type of gout. Arch. intern. Med. **100**, 802 (1957).

LUKENS, L. N., HERRINGTON, K. A.: Enzymic formation of 6-mercaptopurine ribotide. Biochim. biophys. Acta (Amst.) **24**, 432 (1957a).

LUKENS, L. N., BUCHANAN, J. B.: Further intermediates in the biosynthesis of inosinic acid de novo. J. Amer. chem. Soc. **79**, 1511 (1957b).

LYNCH, E. C.: Uric acid metabolism in proliferative diseases of the marrow. Arch. intern. Med. **109**, 639 (1962).

LYON, M. F.: Gene action in the X-chromosome of the mouse. Nature **190**, 372 (1961).

MAC LACHLAN, M. J., RODNAN, G. P.: Effects of food, fast and alcohol on serum uric acid and acute attacks of gout. Amer. J. Med. **42**, 38 (1967).

Magasanik, B., Moyed, H. S., Gehring, L. B.: Enzymes essential for the biosynthesis of nucleic acid guanine: Inosine 5'-phosphate dehydrogenase of Aerobacter aerogenes. J. biol. Chem. **226**, 379 (1957).

Mager, J., Hershko, A., Zeitlin-Beck, R., Shoshami, T., Razin, A.: Turnover of purine nucleotides in rabbit erythrocytes. I. Studies *in vivo*. Biochim. biophys. Acta (Amst.) **149**, 50 (1967).

Mager, J., Magasanik, B.: Guanosine 5'-phosphate reductase and its role in the interconversion of purine nucleotides. J. biol. Chem. **235**, 1474 (1960).

March, H. W., Schlyen, S. M., Schwartz, S. E.: Mediterranean hemopathic syndromes (Cooley's anemia) in adults. Amer. J. Med. **13**, 46 (1952).

Mc Collister, R. J., Gilbert, W. R., Jr., Ashton, D. M., Wyngaarden, J. B.: Pseudofeedback inhibition of purine synthesis by 6-mercaptopurine ribonucleotide and other purine analogues. J. biol. Chem. **239**, 1560 (1964).

Mc Donald, J. A., Kelley, W. N.: Lesch-Nyhan syndrome: Absence of the mutant enzyme in erythrocytes of a heterozygote for both normal and mutant hypoxanthine-guanine phosphoribosyltransferase. Biochem. Genet. **6**, 21 (1972).

Meister, A.: Biochemistry of the Amino Acids. New York: Academic Press 1957.

Melnick, I., Buchanan, J. M.: Biosynthesis of the purines. XIV. Conversion of (a-N-formyl)-glycinamide ribotide to (a-N-formyl)-glycinamidine ribotide; purification and requirements of the enzyme system. J. biol. Chem. **225**, 157 (1957).

Metcalfe-Gibson, A., Mc Callum, F. M., Morrison, R. B. I., Wrong, O.: Urinary excretion of hydrogen ion in patients with uric acid calculi. Clin. Sci. **28**, 325 (1965).

Meyskens, F. L., Williams, H. E.: Concentration of phosphoribosylpyrophosphate in erythrocytes from normal, hyperuricemic, and gouty subjects. Metabolism **20**, 737 (1971).

Migeon, B. R.: X-linked hypoxanthine-guanine phosphoribosyl transferase deficiency: Detection of heterozygotes by selective medium. Biochem. Genet. **4**, 377 (1970).

Migeon, B. R., Der Kaloustian, V. M., Nyhan, W. L., Young, W. J., Childs, B.: X-linked HGPRTase deficiency: Heterozygote has two clonal populations. Science **160**, 425 (1968).

Mikkelsen, W. M., Dodge, H. J., Valkenburg, H.: The distribution of serum uric acid values in a population unselected as to gout or hyperuricemia: Tecumseh, Michigan 1959—1960. Amer. J. Med. **39**, 242 (1965).

Mizobuchi, K., Buchanan, J. M.: Biosynthesis of the purines: Purification and properties of formylglycinamide ribonucleotide amidotransferase from chicken liver. J. biol. Chem. **243**, 4842 (1968).

Momose, H., Nishikawa, H., Shus, L.: Regulation of purine nucleotide synthesis in *Bacillus subtilis*. J. biol. Chem. **59**, 325 (1966).

Mugler, A., Pernet, A., Friedrich, S.: Le pouvoir d'epuration du rein pour l'acide urique chez l'hyperuricemique d'apres l'etude de 400 clearances. In: Contemporary Rheumatology (Ed. J. Goslings, H. van Swaay), p. 574. Amsterdam: Elsevier 1956.

Nagy, M.: Regulation of the biosynthesis of purine nucleotides in Schizosaccharomyces pombe. I. Properties of the phosphoribosylpyrophosphate glutamine amidotransferase of the wild strain and of a mutant desensitized towards feedback modifiers. Biochim. biophys. Acta (Amst.) **198**, 471 (1970).

Neel, J. V.: The clinical detection of the genetic carriers of inherited disease. Medicine (Baltimore) **26**, 115 (1947).

Neel, J. V., Rakic, M. T., Davidson, R. I., Valkenburg, H. A., Mikkelsen, W. M.: Studies on hyperuricemia. II. A reconsideration of the distribution of serum uric acid values in the families of Smyth, Cotterman, and Freyberg. Amer. J. hum. Genet. **17**, 14 (1965).

Newton, E. B., Davis, A. R.: Combined uric acid in human, horse, sheep, pig, dog, and chicken blood. J. biol. Chem. **54**, 603 (1922).

Nicholls, A., Scott, J. T.: Effect of weight loss on plasma and urinary levels of uric acid. Lancet **1972 II**, 1223.

Nierlich, D. P., Magasanik, B.: Alternative first steps of purine biosynthesis. J. biol. Chem. **236**, 32 (1961).

Nierlich, D. P., Magasanik, B.: Control by repression of purine biosynthetic enzymes in aerogenes. Fed. Proc. **22**, 476 (1963).

Nierlich, D. P., Magasanik, B.: Phosphoribosylglycinamide synthetase of Aerobacter aerogenes. J. biol. Chem. **240**, 366 (1965 a).

Nierlich, D. P., Magasanik, B.: Regulation of purine ribonucleotide synthesis by end product inhibition. J. biol. Chem. **240**, 358 (1965 b).

Nikiforuk, G., Colowick, S. P.: The purification and properties of 5-adenylic acid deaminase from muscle. J. biol. Chem. **219**, 119 (1956).

NUGENT, C. A., MAC DIARMID, W. D., TYLER, F. H.: Renal excretion of uric acid in leukemia and gout. Arch. intern. Med. **109**, 54 (1962).

NUGENT, C. A., MAC DIARMID, W. D., TYLER, F. H.: Renal excretion of urate in patients with gout. Arch. intern. Med. **113**, 165 (1964).

NUGENT, C. A., TYLER, F. H.: The renal excretion of uric acid in patients with gout and in nongouty subjects. J. clin. Invest. **38**, 1890 (1959).

OVERGAARD-HANSEN, K., NIELSEN, A. T.: Does human blood contain uric acid riboside? Scand. J. clin. Lab. Invest. **9**, 194 (1957).

OWEN, E. E., ROBINSON, R. R.: Amino acid extraction and ammonia metabolism by the human kidney during the prolonged administration of ammonium chloride. J. clin. Invest. **42**, 263 (1963).

PAGLIARA, A. S., GOODMAN, A. D.: Elevation of plasma glutamate in gout, its possible role in the pathogenesis of hyperuricemia. New Engl. J. Med. **281**, 767 (1969).

PAIK, C. H., ALAVI, I., DUNEA, G., WEINER, L.: Thalassemia and gouty arthritis. J. Amer. med. Ass. **213**, 296 (1970).

PAMILJANS, V., KRISHNASWAMY, P. R., DUMVILLE, G., MEISTER, A.: Studies on the mechanism of glutamine synthesis; isolation and properties of the enzyme from sheep brain. Biochemistry **1**, 153 (1962).

PAULUS, H. E., COUTTS, A., CALABRO, J. J., KLINENBERG, J. R.: Clinical significance of hyperuricemia in routinely screened hospitalized men. J. Amer. med. Ass. **211**, 277 (1970).

PEHLKE, D. M., MC DONALD, J. A., HOLMES, E. W., KELLEY, W. N.: Inosinic acid dehydrogenase activity in the Lesch-Nyhan syndrome. J. clin. Invest. **51**, 1398 (1972).

PETERS, J. P., VAN SLYKE, K. K.: Quantitative Clinical Chemistry, 2nd ed., Vol. 1, p. 937. Baltimore: Williams & Wilkins 1946.

PIERRE, K. J., LE PAGE, G. A.: Formation of inosine-5'-monophosphate by a kinase in cell-free extracts of Ehrlich ascites cells *in vitro*. Proc. Soc. exp. Biol. (N. Y.) **127**, 432 (1968).

PITTS, R. F.: Renal production and excretion of ammonia. Amer. J. Med. **36**, 720 (1964).

PLANTE, G. E., DURIVAGE, J., LEMIEUX, G.: Renal excretion of hydrogen in primary gout. Metabolism **17**, 377 (1968).

POLLAK, V. E., MATTENHEIMER, H.: Glutaminase activity in the kidney in gout. J. lab. Clin. Med. **66**, 564 (1965).

POLLYCOVE, M., TOLBERT, B. M., LAWRENCE, J. H., HARMAN, D.: Uric acid metabolism: The oxidation of uric acid in normal subjects and patients with gout, polycythemia and leukemia. Clin. Res. Proc. **5**, 38 (1957).

POSTLETHWAITE, A. E., GUTMAN, R. A., KELLEY, W. N.: Salicylate-mediated increase in uric acid removal during hemodialysis: Evidence for urate binding *in vivo*. Clin. Res. **21**, 68 (1973a).

POSTLETHWAITE, A. E., RAMSDELL, C. M., KELLEY, W. N.: Uricosuric effect of an anticholinergic agent in hyperuricemic subjects. Arthrit. and Rheum. **16**, 127 (1973b).

PREISS, J., HANDLER, P.: Enzymatic synthesis of nicotinamide mononucleotide. J. biol. Chem. **222**, 759 (1957).

PRIOR, I. A. M., ROSE, B. S., HARVEY, H. P. B., DAVIDSON, F.: Hyperuricaemia, gout, and diabetic abnormality in Polynesian people. Lancet **1966 I**, 333.

RAIVIO, K. O., SEEGMILLER, J. E.: Role of glutamine in purine synthesis and interconversion. Clin. Res. **19**, 161 (1971).

RAPADO, A.: Gout and saturnism. New Engl. J. Med. **281**, 851 (1969).

RATTI, G.: Sull esistenza di una attivita, uricolitica nell'uomo. Reumatismo **10** suppl. 2, 33 (1958).

RECTOR, F. C., JR., ORLOFF, J.: The effect of the administration of sodium bicarbonate and ammonium chloride on the excretion of ammonia. The absence of alterations in the activity of renal ammonia-producing enzymes in the dog. J. clin. Invest. **38**, 366 (1959).

RECTOR, F. C., JR., SELLMAN, J. C., MARTINEZ-MALDONADO, M., SELDIN, D. W.: The mechanism of suppression of proximal tubular reabsorption by saline infusions. J. clin. Invest. **46**, 47 (1967).

REEM, G. H.: Enzymatic synthesis of 5'-phosphoribosylamine from ribose-5-phosphate and ammonia, alternative first step in purine biosynthesis. J. biol. Chem. **243**, 5695 (1968).

REEM, G. H.: *De novo* purine biosynthesis by two pathways in BURKITT lymphoma cells and in human spleen. J. clin. Invest. **51**, 1058 (1972).

REMY, C. N., REMY, W. T., BUCHANAN, J. M.: Biosynthesis of the purines. VIII. Enzymatic synthesis and utilization of 5-phosphoribosylpyrophosphate. J. biol. Chem. **217**, 885 (1955).

RICHET, G., ALBAHARY, C., ARDAILLOU, R., SULTAN, C., MOREL-MAROGER, A.: Le rein du saturnisme chronique. Rev. franc. Étud. clin. biol. **9**, 188 (1964).

RIESELBACH, R. E., BENTZEL, C. J., COTLOVE, E., FREI, E., III., FREIREICH, E. J.: Uric acid excretion and renal function in the acute hyperuricemia of leukemia: Pathogenesis and therapy of uric acid nephropathy. Amer. J. Med. **37**, 872 (1964).

RIESELBACH, R. E., SORENSEN, L. B., SHELP, W. D., STEELE, T. H.: Diminished renal urate secretion per nephron as a basis for primary gout. Ann. intern. Med. **73**, 359 (1970).
RIVER, G. L., ROBBINS, A. A., SCHWARTZ, S. O.: S-C hemoglobin: A clinical study. Blood **18**, 385 (1961).
ROLL, P. M., BROWN, G. B., DE CARLO, F. J., SCHULTZ, A. S.: The metabolism of yeast nucleic acid in the rat. J. biol. Chem. **180**, 333 (1949).
ROSENBERG, E. F.: Gout and male hermaphroditism: Report of a case. Ann. rheum. Dis. **2**, 273 (1941).
ROSENBLOOM, F. M., HENDERSON, J. F., CALDWELL, I. C., KELLEY, W. N., SEEGMILLER, J. E.: Biochemical bases of accelerated purine biosynthesis de novo in human fibroblasts lacking hypoxanthine-guanine phosphoribosyltransferase. J. biol. Chem. **243**, 1166 (1968).
ROSENBLOOM, F. M., KELLEY, W. N., CARR, A. A., SEEGMILLER, J. E.: Familial nephropathy and gout in a kindred. Clin. Res. **15**, 270 (1967b).
ROSENBLOOM, F. M., KELLEY, W. N., HENDERSON, J. F., SEEGMILLER, J. E.: Lyon hypothesis and x-linked diseases. Lancet **1967 a II**, 305.
ROWE, P. B., COLEMAN, M. D., WYNGAARDEN, J. B.: Glutamine phosphoribosylpyrophosphate amidotransferase: Catalytic and conformational heterogeneity of the pigeon liver enzyme. Biochemistry **9**, 1498 (1970).
ROWE, P. B., WYNGAARDEN, J. B.: The mechanism of dietary alteration in rat hepatic xanthine oxidase levels. J. biol. Chem. **241**, 5571 (1966).
ROWE, P. B., WYNGAARDEN, J. B.: Glutamine phosphoribosylpyrophosphate amidotransferase: Purification, substructure, amino acid composition and absorption spectra. J. biol. Chem. **243**, 6373 (1968).
RUNDLES, R. W., WYNGAARDEN, J. B., HITCHINGS, G. H., ELION, G. B., SILBERMAN, H. R.: Effects of a xanthine oxidase inhibitor on thiopurine metabolism, hyperuricemia and gout. Trans. Ass. Amer. Phycns **76**, 126 (1963).
SAKER, B. M., TOFLER, O. B., BURVILL, M. J., REILLY, K. A.: Alcohol consumption and gout. Med. J. Aust. **1**, 1212 (1967).
SALA, G., BALLABIO, C. B., AMIRA, A., RATTI, G., CIRLA, E.: Renal mechanism for urate excretion in normal and gouty subjects. In: Contemporary Rheumatology Ed. J. GOSLINGS, H. VAN SWAAY), p. 581. Amsterdam: Elsevier 1956.
SANDBERG, A. A., CARTWRIGHT, G. E., WINTROBE, M. D.: Studies on leukemia. I. Uric acid excretion. Blood **11**, 154 (1956).
SANDBERG, A. A., LEE, G. R., CARTWRIGHT, G. E., WINTROBE, M. D.: Purine nucleoside phosphorylase activity of blood. I. Erythrocytes. J. clin. Invest. **12**, 1823 (1955).
SAYRE, F. W., ROBERTS, E.: Preparation and some properties of a phosphate-activated glutaminase from kidneys. J. biol. Chem. **233**, 1128 (1958).
SCHIRMEISTER, J., MAN, N. K., HALLAUER, W.: Study on renal and extrarenal factors involved in the hyperuricemia induced by furosemide. In: Progress in Nephrology (Ed. G. PETERS, F. ROCH-RAMEL), p. 59. Berlin-Heidelberg-New York: Springer 1969.
SCHMIDT, G.: Nucleases and enzymes attacking nucleic acid components. In: The Nucleic Acids (Ed. E. CHARGAFF, J. N. DAVIDSON), Vol. 1. New York: Academic Press 1955.
SCHULTZ, G., GESAFT, G., LOSERT, W., SITT, R.: Biochemische Grundlagen der Diazoxide-Hyperglykämie. Naunyn-Schmiedebergs Arch. Pharmak. exp. Path. **255**, 372 (1966).
SCOTT, J. T., POLLARD, A. C.: Uric acid excretion in relatives of patients with gout. Ann. rheum. Dis. **29**, 397 (1970).
SEEGMILLER, J. E.: Diseases of purine and pyrimidine metabolism. In: Duncan's Diseases of Metabolism (Ed. P. K. BONDY), p. 516. Philadelphia: Saunders 1969.
SEEGMILLER, J. E., GRAYZEL, A. I., HOWELL, R. R., PLATO, C.: The renal excretion of uric acid in gout. J. clin. Invest. **41**, 1094 (1962).
SEEGMILLER, J. E., GRAYZEL, A. I., LASTER, L., LIDDLE, L.: Uric acid production in gout. J. clin. Invest. **40**, 1304 (1961).
SEEGMILLER, J. E., KLINENBERG, J. R., MILLER, J., WATTS, R. W. E.: Suppression of glycine-N^{15} incorporation into urinary uric acid by adenine-8-C^{13} in normal and gouty subjects. J. clin. Invest. **47**, 1193 (1968).
SEEGMILLER, J. E., LASTER, L., STETTEN, D., JR.: Incorporation of 4-amino-5-imidazolecarboxamide-4-C^{13} into uric acid in the normal human. J. biol. Chem. **216**, 653 (1955).
SEEGMILLER, J. E., LASTER, L., STETTEN, D., JR.: Uric acid formation in patients with gout: The incorporation of 4-amino-5-imidazolecarboxamide-C^{13} into uric acid. Ninth Int. Congr. Rheum. Dis., Toronto, Canada, June 23—28, 1957, Vol. 2, p. 207.
SEEGMILLER, J. E., ROSENBLOOM, F. M., KELLEY, W. N.: An enzyme defect associated with a sex-linked human neurological disorder and excessive purine synthesis. Science **155**, 1682 (1967).

SEGAL, S., WYNGAARDEN, J. B.: Plasma glutamine and oxypurine content in patients with gout. Proc. Soc. exp. Biol. (N.Y.) **88**, 342 (1955).

SELLINGER, O. Z., VERSTER, F. DE B.: Glutamine synthetase of rat cerebral cortex: Intracellular distribution and structural latency. J. biol. Chem. **237**, 2836 (1962).

SETLOW, B., BURGER, R., LOWENSTEIN, J. M.: Adenylate deaminase. I. The effects of adenosine and guanosine triphosphate on activity and the organ distribution of the regulated enzyme. J. biol. Chem. **241**, 1244 (1966).

SHAPIRO, J. R., KLINENBERG, J. R., PECK, W., GOLDFINGER, S. E., SEEGMILLER, J. E.: Hyperuricemia associated with obesity and intensified by caloric restriction. Arthrit. and Rheum. **7**, 343 (1964).

SHAPIRO, B. M., STADTMAN, E. R.: The regulation of glutamine synthesis in microorganisms. Ann. Rev. Microbiol. **24**, 501 (1970).

SHEMIN, D., RITTENBERG, D.: On the utilization of glycine for uric acid synthesis in man. J. biol. Chem. **167**, 875 (1947).

SIDBURY, J. B.: The genetics of the glycogen storage diseases. Progr. Med. Genet. **4**, 32 (1965).

SKEIKH, M. I., MOLLER, J. V.: Binding of urate to proteins of human and rabbit plasma. Biochim. biophys. Acta (Amst.) **158**, 456 (1968).

SKUPP, S., AYVAZIAN, J. H.: Oxidation of 7-methylguanine by human xanthine oxidase. J. Lab. clin. Med. **73**, 909 (1969).

SMYTH, C. J.: Hereditary factors in gout: A review of recent literature. Metabolism **6**, 218 (1957).

SMYTH, C. J., COTTERMAN, C. W., FREYBERG, R. H.: The genetics of gout and hyperuricemia: An analysis of nineteen families. J. clin. Invest. **27**, 749 (1948).

SOMMERVILLE, J.: Gout in cyanotic congenital heart disease. Brit. Heart J. **23**, 31 (1961).

SONNE, J. C., BUCHANAN, J. M., DELLUVA, A. M.: Biological precursors of uric acid. I. The role of lactate, acetate and formate in synthesis of the ureido groups of uric acid. J. biol. Chem. **173**, 69 (1948).

SONNE, J. C., LIN, I., BUCHANAN, J. M.: Biosynthesis of the purines. IX. Precursors of the nitrogen atoms of the purine ring. J. biol. Chem. **220**, 369 (1956).

SORENSEN, L. B.: Degradation of uric acid in man. Metabolism **8**, 687 (1959).

SORENSEN, L. B.: The elimination of uric acid in man studied by means of C^{14}-labeled uric acid. Scand. J. clin. Lab. Invest. **12**, suppl. 54 (1960).

SORENSEN, L. B.: The pathogenesis of gout. Arch. intern. Med. **109**, 379 (1962).

SORENSEN, L. B.: Current concepts of gout and its treatment. Med. Clin. N. Amer. **47**, 169 (1963).

SORENSEN, L. B.: Hyperuricemia and gout. Advanc. intern. Med. **15**, 177 (1969).

SORENSEN, L. B., BENKE, P. J.: Biochemical evidence for a distinct type of primary gout. Nature **213**, 1122 (1967).

SPECK, J. F.: The synthesis of glutamine in pigeon liver dispersions. J. biol. Chem. **179**, 1387 (1949).

SPERLING, O., BOER, P., PERSKY-BROSH, S., KANAREK, E., DE VRIES, A.: Altered kinetic property of erythrocyte phosphoribosylpyrophosphate synthetase in excessive purine production. Europ. J. Clin. Biol. Res. **17**, 703 (1972a).

SPERLING, O., EILAM, G., PERSKY-BROSH, S., DE VRIES, A.: Accelerated erythrocyte 5-phosphoribosyl-1-pyrophosphate synthesis. A familial abnormality associated with excessive uric acid production and gout. Biochem. Med. **6**, 310 (1972b).

SPERLING, O., FRANK, M., OPHIR, R., LIBERMAN, U. A., ADAM, A., DE VRIES, A.: Partial deficiency of hypoxanthine-guanine phosphoribosyltransferase associated with gout and uric acid lithiasis. Rev. Europ. Etud. Clin. Biol. **15**, 942 (1970).

SPERLING, O., OPHIR, R., DE VRIES, A.: Purine base incorporation into erythrocyte nucleotides and erythrocyte phosphoribosyltransferase activity in primary gout. Rev. Europ. Etud. Clin. Biol. **16**, 147 (1971).

SPERLING, O., WYNGAARDEN, J. B., STARMER, C. F.: The kinetics of intramolecular distribution of ^{15}N in uric acid following administration of ^{15}N-glycine: A reappraisal of the significance of preferential labeling of N-(3+9) of uric acid in primary gout. J. clin. Invest. **52**, 2468 (1973).

SPILMAN, E. L.: Uric acid synthesis in the nongouty and gouty human. Fed. Proc. **13**, 302 (1954).

SPILMAN, E. L.: Personal communication.

STECHER, R. M., HERSH, A. H., SOLOMON, W. M.: The heredity of gout and its relationship to familial hyperuricemia. Ann. intern. Med. **31**, 595 (1949).

STEELE, T. H.: Evidence for altered renal urate reabsorption during changes in volume of the extracellular fluid. J. lab. Clin. Med. **74**, 288 (1969a).

STEELE, T. H., OPPENHEIMER, S.: Factors affecting urate excretion following diuretic administration in man. Amer. J. Med. **47**, 564 (1969b).

SUBAK-SHARPE, J. H., BURK, R. R., PITTS, J. D.: Metabolic cooperation by cell to cell transfer between genetically different mammalian cells in tissue culture. Heredity **21**, 342 (1966).

SUBAK-SHARPE, H., BURK, R. R., PITTS, J. D.: Metabolic co-operation between biochemically marked mammalian cells in tissue culture. J. Cell Sci. **4**, 353 (1969).

SUKI, W. N., HULL, A. R., RECTOR, F. C., JR., SELDIN, D. W.: Mechanism of the effect of thiazide diuretics on calcium and uric acid. J. clin. Invest. **46**, 1121 (1967).

SWENDSEID, M. E., TUTTLE, S. G., FIGUEROA, W. S., MULCARE, D., CLARK, A. J., MASSEY, F. J.: Plasma amino acid levels in men fed diets differing in protein content. Some observations with valine deficient diets. J. Nutr. **88**, 239 (1966).

SWITZER, R. L.: End-product inhibition of phosphoribosylpyrophosphate synthetase. Fed. Proc. **26**, 560 (1967).

SZYBALSKA, E. H., SZYBALSKI, W.: Genetics of human cell lines. IV. DNA-mediated heritable transformation of a biochemical trait. Proc. nat. Acad. Sci. (Wash.) **48**, 2026 (1962).

TALBOTT, J. H.: Serum urate in relatives of gouty patients. J. clin. Invest. **27**, 749 (1940).

TALBOTT, J. H.: Gout. J. chron. Dis. **1**, 338 (1955).

TALBOTT, J. H.: Gout and blood dycrasias. Medicine (Baltimore) **38**, 173 (1959).

TALBOTT, J. H., COOMBS, F. S.: Metabolic studies on patients with gout. J. Amer. med. Ass. **110**, 1977 (1938).

VAN CREVELD, S.: Clinical course of glycogen storage disease. Chemical Weekblad **57**, 445 (1961).

VILLA, L., ROBECCHI, A., BALLABIO, C. B.: Physiopathology, clinical manifestations, and treatment of gout, Part I. Ann. rheum. Dis. **17**, 9 (1958).

VON HOYNINGEN-HUENE, C. B. G.: Gout and glycogen storage disease in preadolescent brothers. Arch. intern. Med. **118**, 471 (1966).

WADA, Y., ARAKAWA, T., KOIZUMI, K.: Lesch-Nyhan syndrome: Autopsy findings and *in vitro* study of incorporation of ^{14}C-8-inosine into uric acid, guanosine-monophosphate and adenosine-monophosphate in the liver. Tohoku J. exp. Med. **95**, 253 (1968).

WAELSCH, H.: Glutamic acid and cerebral function. Advances Protein Chem. **6**, 299 (1951).

WARREN, L., BUCHANAN, J. M.: Biosynthesis of the purines. XIX. 2-amino-N-ribosylacetamide-5'-phosphate (glycinamide ribotide) transformylase. J. biol. Chem. **229**, 613 (1957a).

WARREN, L., FLAKS, J. G., BUCHANAN, J. M.: Biosynthesis of the purines. XX. Integration of enzymatic transformylation reactions. J. biol. Chem. **229**, 627 (1957b).

WATTS, R. W. E., CRAWHALL, J. C.: The first glycine metabolic pool in man. Biochem. J. **73**, 277 (1959).

WATTS, R. W. E., WATTS, J. E. M., SEEGMILLER, J. E.: Xanthine oxidase activity in human tissues and its inhibition by allopurinol (4-hydroxypyrazolo (3, 4-d) pyrimidine). J. Lab. clin. Med. **66**, 688 (1965).

WEISSMANN, B., BROMBERG, P. A., GUTMAN, A. B.: The purine bases of human urine. II. Semiquantitative estimation and isotope incorporation. J. biol. Chem. **224**, 423 (1957a).

WEISSMANN, B., BROMBERG, P. A., GUTMAN, A. B.: The purine bases of human urine. I. Separation and identification. J. biol. Chem. **224**, 407 (1957c).

WEISSMANN, B., GUTMAN, A. B.: The identification of 6-succinoaminopurine and of 8-hydroxy-7-methylguanine as normal human urinary constituents. J. biol. Chem. **229**, 239 (1957b).

WEISSMANN, S., EISEN, A. Z., KAREN, M.: Pseudouridine metabolism. II. Urinary excretion in gout, psoriasis, leukemia, heterozygous orotic aciduria. J. Lab. clin. Med. **59**, 852 (1962).

WESTBY, C. A., GOTS, J. S.: Genetic blocks and unique features in the biosynthesis of 5-phosphoribosyl-N-formylglycinamide in *Salmonella typhimurium*. J. biol. Chem. **244**, 2095 (1969).

WILLIAMS, H. E., JOHNSON, P. L., FENSTER, L. F., LASTER, L., FIELD, J. B.: Intestinal glucose-6-phosphatase in control subjects and relatives of a patient with glycogen storage disease. Metabolism **12**, 235 (1963).

WILSON, D., BEYER, A., BISHOP, C., TALBOTT, J. H.: Urinary uric acid excretion after the ingestion of isotopic yeast nucleic acid in the normal and gouty human. J. biol. Chem. **209**, 227 (1954).

WONG, P. C. L., MURRAY, A. W.: 5-phosphoribosyl pyrophosphate synthetase from Ehrlich ascites tumor cells. Biochemistry (Wash.) **8**, 1608 (1969).

WOOD, A. W., SEEGMILLER, J. E.: Properties of 5-phosphoribosyl-1-pyrophosphate amidotransferase from human lymphoblasts. J. biol. Chem. **248**, 138 (1973).

WYNGAARDEN, J. B.: Uric acid. In: The Cyclopedia of Medicine, Surgery, Specialties (Ed. G. M. PIERSOL), p. 341. Philadelphia: Davis 1955a.

WYNGAARDEN, J. B.: The effect of phenylbutazone on uric acid metabolism in two normal subjects. J. clin. Invest. **34**, 256 (1955b).

WYNGAARDEN, J. B.: Intermediary purine metabolism and the metabolic defects of gout. Metabolism **6**, 244 (1957).
WYNGAARDEN, J. B.: Gout. In: The Metabolic Basis of Inherited Disease, 1st Ed. (Ed. J. B. STANBURY, J. B. WYNGAARDEN, D. S. FREDRICKSON), p. 679. New York: McGraw-Hill 1960a.
WYNGAARDEN, J. B.: On the dual etiology of hyperuricemia in primary gout. Arthrit. and Rheum. **3**, 414 (1960b).
WYNGAARDEN, J. B.: Gout. Advances Metab. Dis. **2**, 2 (1965).
WYNGAARDEN, J. B.: Gout. In: The Metabolic Basis of Inherited Disease, 2nd Ed. (Ed. J. B. STANBURY, J. B. WYNGAARDEN, D. S. FREDRICKSON), p. 667. New York: McGraw-Hill 1966.
WYNGAARDEN, J. B.: Pathophysiology of hyperuricemia in primary gout. Trans. Amer. Clin. Climat. Ass. **81**, 161 (1969b).
WYNGAARDEN, J. B.: Diuretics and hyperuricemia. New Engl. J. Med. **283**, 1170 (1970).
WYNGAARDEN, J. B.: Glutamine phosphoribosylpyrophosphate amidotransferase. In: Current Topics in Cellular Regulation (Ed. B. HORECKER, E. STADTMAN), Vol. V, p. 135. New York: Academic Press 1972a.
WYNGAARDEN, J. B., APPEL, S. H., ROWE, P. B.: Control of biosynthetic pathways by regulatory enzymes. In: Exploitable Molecular Mechanisms and Neoplasia, p. 415. Baltimore: Williams & Wilkins 1969a.
WYNGAARDEN, J. B., ASHTON, D. M.: The regulation of activity of phosphoribosylpyrophosphate amidotransferase by purine ribonucleotides: A potential feedback control of purine biosynthesis. J. biol. Chem. **234**, 1492 (1959a).
WYNGAARDEN, J. B., BLAIR, A. E., HILLEY, L.: On the mechanism of overproduction of uric acid in patients with primary gout. J. clin. Invest. **37**, 579 (1958b).
WYNGAARDEN, J. B., GREENLAND, R. A.: The inhibition of succinoadenylate kinosynthetase of *Escherichia coli* by adenosine and guanosine 5'-monophosphates. J. biol. Chem. **238**, 1054 (1963).
WYNGAARDEN, J. B., KELLEY, W. N.: Gout. In: The Metabolic Basis of Inherited Disease, 3rd Ed. (Eds. J. B. STANBURY, J. B. WYNGAARDEN, D. S. FREDERICKSON), p. 889. New York: Mc Graw-Hill 1972b.
WYNGAARDEN, J. B., SEEGMILLER, J. E., LASTER, I., BLAIR, A. E.: The utilization of hypoxanthine, adenine and 4-amino-5-imidazolecarboxamide for uric acid synthesis in man. Metabolism **8**, 455 (1959b).
WYNGAARDEN, J. B., SILBERMAN, H. R., SADLER, J. H.: Feedback mechanisms influencing purine ribotide synthesis. Ann. N.Y. Acad. Sci. **75**, 45 (1958a).
WYNGAARDEN, J. B., STETTEN, D., JR.: Uricolysis in normal man. J. biol. Chem. **203**, 9 (1953).
YU, T.-F.: Secondary gout associated with myeloproliferative diseases. Arthrit. and Rheum. **8**, 765 (1965).
YU, T.-F., ADLER, M., BOBROW, E., GUTMAN, A. B.: Plasma and urinary amino acids in primary gout, with special reference to glutamine. J. clin. Invest. **48**, 885 (1969).
YU, T.-F., BALIS, M. E., KRENITSKY, T. A., DANCIS, J., SILVERS, D. N., ELION, G. B., GUTMAN, A. B.: Rarity of X-linked partial hypoxanthine-guanine phosphoribosyltransferase deficiency in a large gouty population. Ann. intern. Med. **76**, 255 (1972).
YU, T.-F., BERGER, L., GUTMAN, A. B.: Renal function in gout. II. Effect of uric acid loading on renal excretion of uric acid. Amer. J. Med. **33**, 829 (1962).
YU, T.-F., GUTMAN, A. B.: Ultrafilterability of plasma urate in man. Proc. Soc. exp. Biol. (N.Y.) **84**, 21 (1953a).
YU, T.-F., SIROTA, J. H., BERGER, L., HALPERN, M., GUTMAN, A. B.: Effect of sodium lactate infusion on urate clearance in man. Proc. Soc. exp. Biol. (N.Y.) **96**, 809 (1957).
YU, T.-F., WASSERMAN, L. R., BENEDICT, J. D., BIEN, E. J., GUTMAN, A. B., STETTEN, D., JR.: A simultaneous study of glycine-N^{15} incorporation into uric acid and heme, and of Fe utilization in a case of gout associated with polycythemia secondary to congenital heart disease. Amer. J. Med. **15**, 845 (1953b).
YU, T.-F., WEISSMANN, B., SHARNEY, L., KUPFER, S., GUTMAN, A. B.: On the biosynthesis of uric acid from glycine-N^{15} in primary and secondary polycythemia. Amer. J. Med. **21**, 901 (1956).
ZOLLNER, N.: Moderne Gichtprobleme Atiologie, Pathogenese. Klin. Ergbn. inn. Med. Kinderheilk. **14**, 321 (1960).
ZWEIFLER, A. J., THOMPSON, G. R.: Correction of thiazide hyperuricemia by potassium chloride and ammonium chloride. Arthrit. and Rheum. **8**, 1134 (1965).

2. Spezielle Probleme
a) Genetik der Gicht

Von

W. KAISER

Die primäre Gicht wird heute ganz allgemein als eine Erbkrankheit angesehen. Familiär gehäuftes Auftreten der Gicht ist seit langer Zeit bekannt und auf Grund verschiedener epidemiologischer und familiärer Untersuchungen bewiesen.

HIPPOKRATES (460—357 v. Chr.), der bereits ein gutes klinisches Bild der Gicht beschrieb, beobachtete damals schon ein vermehrtes familiäres Auftreten mit gleichzeitiger Bevorzugung des männlichen Geschlechts (HIPPOKRATES, 1821). Auch GALEN (129—201 n. Chr.) wies in seinen Kommentaren über die Gicht auf deren erbliche Komponente hin (NEUWIRTH, 1943). GARROD fand 1876 sogar familiäres Auftreten in ca. 80% seiner Gichtpatienten und ordnete auch 1909 die Gicht unter die angeborenen Stoffwechselkrankheiten ein (GARROD, 1909). Bei Blutsverwandten von Patienten mit manifester Gicht tritt diese Purinstoffwechselstörung eindeutig häufiger auf. In den älteren Statistiken liegen die Werte für die davon betroffenen Familienmitglieder (mit etwa 40—80%) sicher zu hoch, denn diese Familienuntersuchungen wurden meist an ausgesuchtem Krankengut und kleinen Kollektiven durchgeführt. Die größte Schwierigkeit in den älteren Untersuchungen zur Genetik der Gicht lag jedoch darin, daß allein die Gichtarthritis bzw. die manifeste Gicht als der genetische Marker bei der Vererbung zur Verfügung stand. Damit konnte kein schlüssiges Vererbungsmuster erhalten werden, denn läßt man — wie es in diesen älteren Untersuchungen geschah — die asymptomatischen Hyperuricämiker als latente Gichtpatienten außer Betracht, so mußte die Vererbung bei der Gicht für eine stark unregelmäßige Dominanz sprechen.

Nachdem GARROD (1909) bei der Gicht eine Hyperuricämie nachweisen konnte, war erstmals einer der entscheidenden Faktoren für die Pathogenese der Gicht entdeckt. Damit war die Hyperuricämie also als eine der Voraussetzungen zur Entwicklung der Gicht erkannt und konnte seitdem erst als einer der wesentlichen genetischen Marker für den Vererbungsmodus bei der Gicht verwendet werden. Mit der Entwicklung von Methoden zur Bestimmung der Serumharnsäure waren dann auch erst die weiteren Voraussetzungen geschaffen zur genaueren Untersuchung der Häufigkeit und Vererbung der Hyperuricämie und Gicht. Als erster berichtete 1940 TALBOTT, daß bei asymptomatischen Verwandten von Gichtpatienten in vermehrtem Maße erhöhte Serumharnsäurewerte festgestellt werden können. Auch andere Familienuntersuchungen danach zeigten das gleiche Ergebnis, nämlich das häufigere Vorkommen einer asymptomatischen Hyperuricämie und einer Gicht unter den Blutsverwandten von Gichtpatienten. Im Vergleich mit der Gesamtbevölkerung zeigte sich das Risiko zur Entwicklung einer Gicht in der Verwandtschaft eines Patienten mit dieser Krankheit also absolut höher.

Als Werte für das Vorkommen von Gicht bei Verwandten von Gichtpatienten werden Zahlen zwischen 6—18% angegeben (BABUCKE, 1970; BARELLO et al., 1967; NEEL, 1947; ROSENBERG, 1941; SMYTH, 1946). Die Zahlenangaben für Personen mit einer Hyperuricämie in der klinisch gesunden, nahen Verwandtschaft von Gichtpatienten (meist als familiäre Hyperuricämie bezeichnet) lagen bei den kollektiven Untersuchungen einer Gichtpopulation bei 12—25% (RAKIC et al., 1964; SMYTH, 1957).

Personen mit einer Hyperuricämie sind also, obwohl sie keine Gichtsymptome aufweisen, latente Träger des pathogenen Erbfaktors. Die Hyperuricämie kann somit als latente Anlage bzw. asymptomatische Gicht, die Gicht als mehr oder weniger direkte klinische und pathologische Konsequenz dieser biochemischen Störung betrachtet werden.

Die ersten systematischeren Untersuchungen zur Frage des Vererbungsmodus der Gicht bzw. der Hyperuricämie wurden von SMYTH et al. (SMYTH u. FREIBERG, 1942; SMYTH et al., 1948; SMYTH, 1957) sowie STECHER et al. (1949) an allerdings relativ kleinen Kollektiven durchgeführt. Die Interpretation ihrer Ergebnisse führte zu der Annahme, daß die Hyperuricämie durch ein einziges Gen determiniert sei. Die Penetranz in beiden Geschlechtern sollte danach verschiedene Grade aufweisen, d. h. die Expressivität würde beim weiblichen Geschlecht geringer sein. Die Vererbung wurde damals in erster Linie auf die Wirkung eines einzelnen dominanten Erbfaktors mit niedriger Penetranz zurückgeführt. Allerdings schien bei einigen der untersuchten Familien die Vererbung eher autosomal recessiv zu sein. Für diese Theorie sprach eine mehr bimodale Verteilung der Serumharnsäurespiegel. Der Defekt wurde also bei dieser einige Jahre vorherrschenden Ansicht auf ein einziges Gen zurückgeführt.

Von den späteren, etwas detaillierteren Untersuchungen ist insbesondere die von HAUGE und HARVALD (1952) von Bedeutung. Bei Vergleich der Werte für den Serumharnsäurespiegel von Blutsverwandten seiner Gichtpatienten mit jenen aus einer ähnlich zusammengesetzten Kontrollgruppe waren die Werte bei den Gichtfamilien wiederum signifikant höher, die Verteilung der Werte bei diesen Familien jedoch zeigte eine normale Verteilungskurve und kein Muster, wie es nach einfachen Mendelschen Gesetzen zu erwarten gewesen wäre. Diese Untersuchungen ergaben somit keinen Anhalt für das Vorliegen eines autosomal dominanten Erbgangs, sondern ließen eher an kumulative Einflüsse bzw. das Ergebnis additiver Effekte mehrerer Gene denken. Auch bei einer Nachuntersuchung der Familien, die SMYTH et al. (1948) als Grundlage ihrer Studien gedient hatten, zeigte sich, daß die Theorie von der Entstehung der Hyperuricämie infolge eines einzelnen Gendefekts nicht zu beweisen, sondern eine Vererbung auf Grund multipler genetischer Faktoren ebenso wahrscheinlich sei (RAKICZ et al., 1964). Auch SCOTT und POLLARD (1970), die bei Verwandten ersten Grades von Gichtpatienten die Harnsäureclearance untersuchten, fanden eine gewisse Korrelation (bei männlichen Verwandten deutlicher) zwischen den Werten der Harnsäureclearance bei ihren Gichtpatienten und den Mittelwerten der Verwandten. Sie interpretierten ihre Ergebnisse als Hinweis dafür, daß das Konzept der multifaktoriellen Einflüsse, die den Harnsäurespiegel im Blut regulieren, auch für die renale Harnsäureexkretion gültig sein müsse.

Die neueren Untersuchungen zum Vererbungsmodus der Gicht sprechen dafür, daß der spezifische klinische Phänotyp Gicht bzw. der biochemische Phänotyp Hyperuricämie von mehr als einem einzigen Genotyp produziert wird. Es ist also für diesen Stoffwechseldefekt — wie für die meisten der bekannten „inborn errors" — eine genetische Heterogenität anzunehmen.

Eine der Schwierigkeiten in den älteren Untersuchungen bestand z.B. auch darin, die sekundäre Hyperuricämie von der primären, idiopathischen Hyperuricämie zu trennen. Nach den Untersuchungen von HALL (HALL et al., 1967) tritt die sekundäre Hyperuricämie bei der Normalbevölkerung in nicht ganz 3% der Personen auf. Von der Psoriasis z.B. ist die familiäre Beziehung bekannt, desgleichen das häufigere Auftreten von Psoriasis zusammen mit einer Hyperuricämie. Dasselbe gilt für die Glykogenspeicherkrankheit vom Typ I, bei der der Glucose-6-Phosphatase-Mangel die primäre Störung darstellt und die Hyperuricämie sekundär sowohl durch renale Retention als auch durch Harnsäureüberproduktion zustande kommt. Diese Krankheit wird autosomal recessiv vererbt. Auch bei der genetisch bedingten familiären Hyperlipoproteinämie vom Typ IV nach Fredrickson weist ein hoher Prozentsatz der Patienten eine Hyperuricämie auf. Diese sekundären Hyperuricämien mit ihrem spezifischen Vererbungsmodus müssen aber in Familienuntersuchungen über die Genetik der primären Gicht ausgeschlossen sein.

Aus den epidemiologischen Untersuchungen an auslesefreien, großen Bevölkerungsgruppen muß man für die Genetik der Gicht und der Hyperuricämie folgendes ableiten: HALL et al. (1967) fanden in ihrem großen Kollektiv eine Hyperuricämie (Serumharnsäurespiegel von 7 mg% und mehr) in 4,8%, die Werte für den männlichen Personenkreis betrugen 9,2%, diejenigen für Frauen 0,4%. Von besonderer Bedeutung für die Häufigkeit der Hyperuricämie sind das Alter und das Geschlecht. Die Hyperuricämie manifestiert sich bei männlichen Personen meist nach der Adoleszenz, beim weiblichen Geschlecht dagegen erst nach der Menopause. Hierfür gibt es noch keine ausreichende Erklärung. Kein Zweifel besteht an der signifikanten Verbindung zwischen dem Geschlecht und der Manifestation einer Gicht. Die Gicht ist bei Frauen eine seltene Erkrankung, die genetische Ursache dieser Geschlechtsverteilung ist noch nicht geklärt. Die Zahlen in den Literaturangaben liegen bei einem Anteil von 1—10% der weiblichen Personen an der Gesamtzahl der Gichtpatienten (HALL et al., 1967). Die Zahl der Personen, die sowohl eine Hyperuricämie als auch eine Gicht hat, nimmt mit dem Alter des Personenkreises zu (HALL et al., 1967; RAKIC et al., 1964). Dies kompliziert die Aufklärung der genetischen Komponenten erheblich. In den meisten Bevölkerungsstudien, bei denen als Grundlage der Studie ein genügend großes Kollektiv vorhanden war, zeigen die Werte für die Serumharnsäure eine kontinuierliche Normalverteilung. Eine kontinuierliche Variation kann aber nicht auf der Grundlage eines einzelnen Gens erklärt werden, sondern spricht wiederum für eine multifaktorielle Kontrolle der Hyperuricämie. Auch die Variabilität in der Schwere des Krankheitsbildes und dem Zeitpunkt des Beginns der Erkrankung spricht für eine multifaktorielle Kontrolle bei der Entstehung der Gicht. Die multigenetische Beeinflussung kommt auch zum Ausdruck in dem relativen Risiko zur Krankheitsentwicklung zwischen den einzelnen Familien. Bei der Vererbung auf der Grundlage eines einzelnen Gendefekts würde man keine Erklärung für das relativ höhere Risiko bei den schweren Graden der Krankheitsausprägung finden können.

Nimmt man eine Vererbung auf Grund multipler genetischer Einflüsse an, so ist es unwahrscheinlich, daß sich bei der Suche nach den der Störung zugrundeliegenden biochemischen Abnormitäten nur ein spezifischer Defekt erkennen läßt. Schon der Erbgang der Gicht läßt also erkennen, daß diese Störung auf verschiedene Gendefekte zurückgeführt werden muß.

Die Stoffwechselstörung, die klinisch als primäre oder idiopathische Gicht bezeichnet wird, wurde früher auf Grund ihrer klinischen Homogeneität pathogenetisch als ein einheitlicher Krankheitsprozeß betrachtet. Mit zunehmender Analyse dieser angeborenen Störung wurden unterschiedliche biochemische und pathophysiologische Faktoren erkennbar, die als Ursache einer Hyperuricämie anzuschuldigen sind. Inzwischen muß man die Hyperuricämie und ihre klinische Manifestation, die Gicht, als ein Kollektiv mit zahlreichen ursächlich unterschiedlichen Mechanismen, bzw. als Konsequenz verschiedener primärer Störungen betrachten und in pathogenetisch verschiedene Gruppen einteilen. Die Gicht ist demnach als ein Symptomenkomplex anzusehen, bei dem die Hyperuricämie und die nachfolgende Gichtarthritis bzw. Gichtniere als Hauptwirkung zutage tritt. Die genetische Kontrolle dieser Störung hängt damit auch von der Wirkung mehrerer Gene ab. Die Ursache der Hyperuricämie bzw. Gicht ist somit jeweils eine unterschiedliche Mutation, die zu verschiedenen Defekten in der Purinsynthese, der Purinreutilisation, dem Purinabbau und der Purinausscheidung führen kann, d.h. zu Defekten im Bereich verschiedener intrazellulärer Enzymsysteme oder zu Abnormitäten in Membran-Transportsystemen von Zellen. Es ist nicht überraschend, daß mehrere ganz unterschiedliche abnormale Gene zu einer ähnlichen klinischen Störung führen können. Der Funktionsverlust eines oder einer Serie von Enzymen in einem Stoffwechselweg oder in einer physiologischen Reaktion kann zum gleichen klinischen Endresultat führen, der Grad der genetischen Heterogenität ist im klinischen Syndrom nicht mehr zu erkennen. Aus diesem Grund ist es verständlich, daß die früheren kollektiven Untersuchungen zur Genetik der Gicht nur von begrenzter Aussagekraft sind, da zahlreiche ursächliche Mechanismen von mehreren verschiedenen genetischen Faktoren mit dem jeweils für sie zugrundeliegenden Vererbungsmodus abhängig sind.

Eine zahlenmäßig große Gruppe von Gichtpatienten weist eine verminderte Harnsäureclearance auf. Bei diesen Personen mit normaler Harnsäureproduktion ist die verminderte Harnsäureclearance vermutlich das Resultat einer verminderten Ansprechbarkeit der tubulären Sekretionsmechanismen auf das Harnsäure-Load. Bei der Passage der Harnsäure durch die verschiedenen Zellmembranen (z.B. Tubuluszellen) scheinen einige mehr oder weniger spezifische, aktive Transportsysteme mitzuwirken. Für andere Substrate sind eine Reihe von genetisch determinierten und spezifischen Defekten solcher aktiven Transportsysteme bekannt, die jeweilige molekulare Grundlage jedoch noch nicht geklärt. Am wahrscheinlichsten scheinen Defekte an einzelnen Enzymen oder „Carrierproteinen", die zur Verschlechterung der Passage durch die Membran führen. Für diese Gruppe der Gichtpatienten wäre also ein "inborn error" im renalen tubulären Transport anzunehmen. Hiermit wäre auch zu erklären, wie geringe metabolische Störungen durch übermäßige Belastungen (z.B. purinreiche Diät) in Erscheinung treten können. Auf diese Weise wäre bei bestimmten Patientengruppen und Familien ein Teil der Variationen in der Gichtmanifestation zu sehen, wenn sie weitgehend auf nichtgenetische Einflüsse, wie z.B. Umweltfaktoren zurückzuführen sind.

Die angeborenen Stoffwechselstörungen werden meist definiert als genetisch bestimmte biochemische Störungen auf der Grundlage von spezifischen kongenitalen Defekten in einem oder mehreren Schritten des Stoffwechsels. Dies können Defekte in der Struktur oder Funktion von Enzymproteinen sein. Die Möglichkeiten der Mutationen im Bereich von Enzymsystemen des Purinstoffwechsels sind vielfältig. Die strukturellen Mutationen sind durch eine Vielzahl verschiedener Mechanismen zu charakterisieren, z.B. durch verminderte Substrataffinität, verminderte Kofaktoraffinität, insensitive Reaktion auf Feedback-Hemmung u.a. Es kann sich dabei um Änderungen in Strukturgenen oder Kontroll- bzw. Regulatorgenen handeln.

Für jenen Teil der Gichtpopulation, der durch eine Überproduktion von Harnsäure charakterisiert ist, scheinen partielle Enzymdefekte wahrscheinlich.

Für die meisten Enzyme zieht eine Reduktion auf die Hälfte ihrer normalen Aktivität, wegen der vorhandenen funktionellen Reserven, keine offenkundige pathologische Konsequenz, d.h. klinische Störung nach sich. Es gibt jedoch Enzyme, gewöhnlich diejenigen, die geschwindigkeitsbestimmend für ihren Stoffwechselweg sind, die normalerweise ausreichende Aktivität, aber nur wenige funktionelle Reserven besitzen, so daß eine Verminderung der Aktivität zu pathologischen Störungen führt. Die Wirkung irgendeiner genetischen Änderung auf den zellulären Stoffwechsel und das klinische Bild hängt also von der Rolle des mutierten Enzyms und dem Ausmaß des Defekts ab.

Eindrucksvolle Beispiele hierfür liegen beim Lesch-Nyhan-Syndrom (LESCH u. NYHAN, 1964) und bei einigen Patienten mit Gicht (KELLEY et al., 1967) vor, bei denen als vermutlich letzte Ursache der Hyperuricämie ein inkompletter Mangel an Hypoxanthin-Guanin-Phosphoribosyltransferase (HG-PRT) nachzuweisen ist. Hier läßt sich die Wirkungskette von einem fehlenden, quantitativ verminderten bzw. qualitativ veränderten Enzym bis zum klinischen Syndrom überblicken. Die im Endeffekt vielgestaltige Wirkung, das klinische Bild des Lesch-Nyhan-Syndroms, ließ sich bei der schrittweisen Analyse auf einen einzigen Enzymdefekt zurückführen, dieser ist unmittelbarer Ausdruck des ihn verursachenden Gendefekts, der Mutation. Untersuchungen an verschiedenen Familien zeigten, daß dieses Syndrom eine an das X-Chromosom gebundene recessive Vererbung aufweist, das bedeutet, daß die betroffenen Jungen das mutante Gen von ihren gesunden heterozygoten Müttern erben. Das Gen für die HG-PRT ist an das X-Chromosom gebunden. Im allgemeinen liegen die Spiegel für die Enzymaktivitäten bei Heterozygoten zwischen den niedrigen Werten, die man beim abnormalen Homozygoten findet und denen einer auslesefreien Kontrollpopulation. Beim Lesch-Nyhan-Syndrom jedoch sind die Heterozygoten vollkommen gesund. ROSENBLOOM et al. (1967) konnten an Fibroblastenkulturen von weiblichen heterozygoten Überträgern zwei Zellpopulationen zeigen, wovon eine die mutierte HG-PRT-fehlende, und die andere die normale HG-PRT-aktive Allele aufwies. Dies stimmt mit den Erwartungen nach der Hypothese von LYON überein (1961), wonach im frühen embryonalen Stadium in den weiblichen somatischen Zellen entweder das von der Mutter oder das vom Vater stammende X-Chromosom inaktiviert wird. Diese Auswahl des Chromosoms ist willkürlich. Die Diagnose einer heterozygoten Trägerin für das Lesch-Nyhan-Syndrom kann an Zellkulturen erreicht werden (FUJIMOTO et al., 1971; GARTLER et al., 1971). Bei der im Augenblick noch bestehenden ungünstigen Prognostik der neurologischen Störungen des Lesch-Nyhan-Syndroms ist diese Diagnostik wichtig. Es ist so nämlich möglich, am Beginn einer Schwangerschaft, nachdem die Diagnose einer heterozygoten Trägerin für das Syndrom gestellt worden war, durch eine Amniocentese eine pränatale Diagnose und eventuell durch einen therapeutischen Abortus eines betroffenen Fetus ein Präventivprogramm zur Kontrolle des Lesch-Nyhan-Syndroms herbeizuführen (DE MARS et al., 1969; FUJIMOTO et al., 1968, 1971).

Die Patientengruppe mit stark und frühzeitig ausgeprägter Gicht, bei der von KELLEY et al. (1967) ein partieller Mangel der HG-PRT gefunden werden konnte, und bei der sie gleichfalls an das X-Chromosom gebunden vererbt wird (KELLEY et al., 1967, 1969), ist wahrscheinlich nicht durch eine ganz spezifische Mutation charakterisiert. Die Enzymbestimmungen lassen darauf schließen, daß ganz spezifische Formen des Enzymdefekts vorkommen, in einer Familie ist jedoch bei allen betroffenen Mitgliedern der gleiche spezifische Defekt nachweisbar. Physikalische und chemische Untersuchungen der Enzymproteine bei den verschiedenen Familien in dieser Gruppe sprechen für eine Heterogeneität in der primären Mutation des Strukturgens. Die verschiedenen Mutationen, die die Änderungen in der enzymatischen Aktivität verursachen, variieren in dem Ausmaß des jeweiligen Defizits und damit in der Schwere des Krankheitsbildes. Die varianten Formen des Enzymproteins scheinen durch eine Reihe von Allelen determiniert zu sein, von denen jedes eine unterschiedliche Strukturänderung hervorrufen kann. Das bedeutet, daß sogar für jene kleine Gruppe der Gichtpopulation, die biochemisch durch erhöhte Purinsynthese infolge inkompletten HG-PRT-Mangels charakterisiert ist, eine Vielzahl genetischer Faktoren zur Wirkung kommen müssen. Hinweise auf Änderungen in der Aktivität, den kinetischen Eigenschaften bzw. der Affinität für Substrate, Kofaktoren oder Inhibitoren bei der PRPP-Amidotransferase (HENDERSON et al., 1968) bei einer anderen Gruppe von Gichtpatienten lassen auf einen weiteren spezifischen, genetisch bestimmten Enzymdefekt als unmittelbaren Ausdruck eines Gendefekts schließen, der in der Folge zu einer Hyperuricämie und zur Gicht führt. Auch hier kann die partielle Änderung der Enzymaktivität durch verschiedene Strukturgen-Mutationen zustande kommen, die entweder die Primärstruktur des Proteins, die Geschwindigkeit seines Abbaus oder seiner Synthese und damit seine Konzentration in der Zelle regulieren.

Die Unterschiede in der Manifestationsausprägung, die Penetranz oder Schwere einer Gicht, variiert innerhalb einer Familie meist zusätzlich noch beträchtlich. Bei Individuen, die die genetische Zusammensetzung mit sich bringen, wird eventuell die Krankheit nicht manifest, weil andere Gene, modifizierende Gene oder ein Umgebungsfaktor notwendig sind, damit eines der Hauptgene zum Durchbruch kommt. Auch ist nicht auszuschließen, daß Genkombinationen an anderen Orten die pathologische Konsequenz einer Hyperuricämie vermindern oder akzentuieren können.

Wie für alle angeborenen Stoffwechselstörungen sind auch für die Entstehung einer Gicht und Hyperuricämie Umgebungsfaktoren von entscheidender Bedeutung, indem sie die biochemische und klinische Ausprägung der ursprünglichen Mutation modifizieren und evtl. verstärken können. Denn wenn auch die familiäre Abhängigkeit der Serumharnsäurewerte heute als allgemein gültig angesehen wird, so sind doch nicht alle familiär determinierten Faktoren genetisch bestimmt, sondern oft als Zusammenspiel zwischen genetischen und variablen Umgebungsfaktoren anzusehen. Familienuntersuchungen von FRENCH et al. (1967) zeigten eine signifikante Eltern-Kind-Korrelation der Serumharnsäurespiegel, was sowohl mit genetischen als auch Umgebungsfaktoren als Determinanten erklärt werden kann. Die Ausprägung eines Individuums bzw. einer Krankheit ist bekanntlich nicht allein davon abhängig, welche Gene und im Gefolge davon welche Muster oder Konzentrationen von Enzymen es mit sich bringt, sondern auch von der Umgebung, in der es aufwächst. Diese Frage des phänotypischen Durchbruchseffekts ist insbesondere für die Manifestation der Gicht von Bedeutung. Als Regel darf im allgemeinen gelten, daß Störungen, die phänotypisch erst spät im Leben auftreten, durch die Umgebung deutlicher beeinflußbar sind. Sicher sind solche Faktoren für das häufigere Vorkommen der Gicht in unserer jetzigen Wohlstandsgesellschaft verantwortlich. In Notzeiten gehen die Zahlen für die Gichtfälle zurück, in den älteren Beschreibungen der Krankheit galt die Gicht als typische Krankheit der Wohlhabenden. Ein immer wieder angeführtes Beispiel für den Einfluß solcher Umgebungsfaktoren ist der deutliche Anstieg der Gichtpatienten unter der Maori-Bevölkerung in Neuseeland im Gefolge ihrer Anpassung an die westliche Zivilisation (LENNANE et al., 1960; PRIOR u. ROSE, 1966; PRIOR et al., 1966). Das gleiche Zusammenspiel von genetischen und Umgebungsfaktoren bei der primären Gicht wird an dem häufigen Auftreten einer Hyperuricämie und Gicht bei der philippinischen Bevölkerung beobachtet, die auf Hawai und in den USA lebt. Diese weisen im Mittel signifikant höhere Serumharnsäurewerte auf als die rassisch identischen Filipinos, die in ihrer Heimat leben (DECKER et al., 1962). Die genetischen, metabolischen und exogenen Faktoren sind dabei nicht genau bekannt. Es wird aber angenommen, daß bei diesem Personenkreis in einem hohen Prozentsatz ein genetisch bestimmter tubulärer Defekt vorkommt, der es ihnen nicht ermöglicht, die Harnsäureausscheidung als Antwort auf das höhere Purinangebot der amerikanischen Diät entsprechend zu erhöhen. Das würde bedeuten, daß diätetische Änderungen, die durch die Umgebung bedingt sind, für das häufigere Vorkommen einer Hyperuricämie und Gicht in einer Rasse oder Familie mit einem wahrscheinlich latenten genetischen Potential verantwortlich sind. Die relative Bedeutung der genetischen gegenüber den Umwelteinflüssen zu differenzieren, wäre am besten möglich durch Untersuchungen an monozygoten und dizygoten Zwillingen bei jeweiliger Änderung der Lebensbedingungen. Das ist von BOYLE et al. (1967) zwar versucht worden, dabei ist jedoch zu beachten, daß die Umgebungseinflüsse je nach Bedeutung und Lokalisierung der bei den verschiedenen Familien unterschiedlichen primären Defekte auch verschieden stark ausfallen können.

Obwohl sich wahrscheinlich die grundlegende Störung für die Entstehung einer Hyperuricämie während der fetalen Entwicklung ereignet, tritt die Krankheit jahrelang nicht auf, d.h. das Alter ist eine weitere signifikante Variable bei der klinischen Ausprägung. Wenn auch ein großer Personenkreis eine Serumharnsäurekonzentration aufweist, die über der Löslichkeit der Harnsäure im Serum liegt, entwickeln nur etwa 25% davon klinische Gichtsymptome (KLINENBERG u. KIPPEN, 1970; KLINENBERG et al., 1973). Unterschiede im Zeitpunkt des Beginns oder im Schweregrad der Manifestation einer Gicht, bei vergleichbarer Serumharnsäurekonzentration, sind vermutlich auf eine Reihe genetisch bestimmter biochemischer und physiologischer Variationen zurückzuführen, die den Ausbruch der Krankheit modifizieren können. Als einer dieser Faktoren wird z.B. eine individuell unterschiedliche lokale Entzündungsbereitschaft auf Harnsäurekristalle diskutiert. Ein anderer Faktor, der die Manifestation der Gicht beeinflussen soll, wird in einer genetisch bedingten Einflußnahme auf das Bindungsvermögen von Urat an Plasmaproteine gesehen (ALVSAKER, 1968). Von ALVSAKER (1968) wurde bei Gichtpatienten eine signifikant reduzierte *in vitro*-Bindungskapazität für Harnsäure im Vergleich mit Kontrollpersonen gefunden. Eine solche Uratbindung an Plasmaproteine könnte nicht nur einen Einfluß auf die Uratablagerung, sondern auch auf die renale Exkretion der Harnsäure ausüben. Bei einigen Gichtfamilien soll diese genetisch bestimmte Verminderung der Uratbindung dominant vererbt werden und zwar unabhängig vom Vererbungsmuster der Hyperuricämie. Die Untersuchungen zum Uratbindungsvermögen, insbesondere in bezug auf ihre physiologische Bedeutung, sind nicht unwidersprochen geblieben (FARRELL et al., 1971). Sie wären jedoch ein anschauliches Beispiel, wie die Gichtmanifestation nach der primären genetischen Störung, die zur Hyperuricämie führt, zusätzlich durch andere genetische Einflüsse sekundär noch modifiziert werden kann.

Die Erblichkeit der Gicht bzw. der Hyperuricämie ist mit einem einfachen Vererbungsmodus (autosomal dominant, autosomal recessiv, an das X-Chromosom gebunden recessiv) nicht in Einklang zu bringen. Ein einheitlicher Vererbungsmodus ist durch die biochemische Heterogenität der Gicht nicht zu erwarten. Die Variabilität in der Ausprägung und dem Zeitpunkt des Krankheitsbeginns, die z.T. schon bekannten unterschiedlichen biochemischen und physiologischen Abnormitäten, die verschiedene Ansprechbarkeit auf Medikamente und vieles mehr sprechen gegen die Vererbung auf der Grundlage eines einzelnen Gens. Zumindest die multifaktorielle Kontrolle der Hyperuricämie spricht für die Beteiligung verschiedener Faktoren an vermutlich mehreren Genorten. Die Expressivität der klinischen Störung Gicht ist darüber hinaus das Ergebnis eines komplexen Zusammenspiels zwischen den genetischen und metabolischen Störungen und den variablen Umgebungseinflüssen. Die Ursache der mehr geschlechtsgebundenen Manifestation ist nicht bekannt, die Mutationen können z.B. an das X-Chromosom gebunden sein, hormonelle Einflüsse z.B. auf die renale Harnsäureexkretion sind nicht auszuschließen. Für die prospektiven Studien zur Genetik der Gicht wird es in erster Linie wichtig sein, den für die Hyperuricämie in der zu untersuchenden Familie verantwortlichen metabolischen Defekt zu identifizieren, damit in den zumindest in der metabolischen Störung einheitlichen Gichtgruppen der Vererbungsmodus untersucht werden kann. Dieser wird bei den verschiedenen Defekten unterschiedlich sein, darüber hinaus durch individuell verschiedenen genetischen "background" modifiziert werden. Da eine höhere Wahrscheinlichkeit für die Manifestation einer Gicht bei Verwandten von Gichtpatienten besteht, empfiehlt sich in Gichtfamilien eine systematischere Suche nach einer Hyperuricämie. Der augenblickliche Stand der Therapie der Gicht, der die Prognostik dieser Erkrankung bei rechtzeitiger Behandlung erheblich verbessert, ermuntert auch zu erweiterten Familienuntersuchungen und zur genetischen Beratung.

Literatur

ALVSAKER, J. O.: Genetic studies in primary gout. Investigations on the plasma levels or the urate-binding α_1-α_2-globulin in individuals from two gouty kindreds. J. clin. Invest. **47**, 1254 (1968).

BABUCKE, G.: Der rheumatische Formenkreis unter besonderer Berücksichtigung der Gicht. Dissertation Freiburg i. Br. 1970.

BARCELLO, P., SANS-SOLA, L., SANTAMARIA, A.: Estudio estadistico sobre 933 casos de gota. Rev. esp. Reum. **1**, 1 (1967).

BOYLE, J. A., GREIG, W. R., JASANI, M. K., DUNCAN, A., DIVER, M., BUCHANAN, W. W.: Relative roles of genetic and environmental factors in the control of serum uric acid levels in normouricaemic subjects. Ann. rheum. Dis. **26**, 234 (1967).

DECKER, J. L., LANE, J. J., JR., REYNOLDS, W. E.: Hyperuricemia in a male Filipino population. Arthr. and Rheum. **5**, 144 (1962).

DE MARS, R., SARTO, G., FELIX, J. S., BEHNKE, P.: Lesch-Nyhan mutation: Prenatal detection with amniotic fluid cells. Science **164**, 1303 (1969).

FARRELL, P. C., POPOVICH, R. P., BABB, A. L.: Binding levels of urate ions in human serum albumin and plasma. Biochim. biophys. Acta (Amst.) **243**, 49 (1971).

FRENCH, J. G., DODGE, H. J., KJELSBERG, M. O., MIKKELSEN, W. M., SCHULL, W. J.: A study of familial aggregation of serum uric acid levels in the population of Tecumseh, Michigan. 1959—1960. Amer. J. Epidem. **86**, 214 (1967).

FUJIMOTO, W. Y., SEEGMILLER, J. E., UHLENDORF, B. W., JACOBSON, C.: Biochemical diagnosis of an X-linked disease in utero. Lancet **1968 II**, 511.

FUJIMOTO, W. Y., SUBAK-SHARPE, J. H., SEEGMILLER, J. E.: HGPRTase-Deficiency: Chemical agents selective for mutant or normal fibroblasts in mixed and heterozygote cultures. Proc. nat. Acad. Sci. Wash. **68**, 1516 (1971).

GALEN IN NEUWIRTH, E.: Milestones in the diagnosis and treatment of gout. Arch. intern. Med. **72**, 377 (1943).

GARROD, A. E.: A Treatise on Gout and Rheumatic Gout (Rheumatic Arthritis), 3rd. Ed. London: Longmans, Green and Co. 1876.

GARROD, A. E.: Inborn Errors of Metabolism. London: Oxford University Press, 1909.

GARTLER, ST. M., SCOTT, R. C., GOLDSTEIN, J. L., CAMPBELL, B.: Lesch-Nyhan-Syndrom: Rapid detection of heterozygotes by use of hair follicles. Science **172**, 572 (1971).

HALL, A. P., BERRY, P. E., DAWBER, T. R., MC NAMARA, P. M.: Epidemology of gout and hyperuricemia. A long-term population study. Amer. J. Med. **42**, 27 (1967).

HAUGE, M., HARVALD, B.: Heredity in gout and hyperuricemia. Acta med. Scand. **152**, 247 (1955).

HENDERSON, J. F., KELLEY, W. N., ROSENBLOOM, F. M., SEEGMILLER, J. E.: Inheritance of purine phosphoribosyltransferases in man. Amer. J. hum. Genet. **21**, 61 (1969).
HIPPOKRATES: Opera omnia. Leipzig 1821.
KELLEY, W. N., ROSENBLOOM, F. M., HENDERSON, J. F., SEEGMILLER, I. E.: A specific enzyme defect—gout associated with overproduction of uric acid. Proc. nat. Acad. Sci. (Wash.) **57**, 1735 (1967).
KELLEY, W. N., GREENE, M. L., ROSENBLOOM, F. M., HENDERSON, J. F., SEEGMILLER, J. E.: Hypoxanthine-guanine phosphoribosyltransferase deficiency in gout. Ann. intern. Med. **70**, 155 (1969).
KLINENBERG, J. R., KIPPEN, I.: The binding of urate to plasma proteins determined by means of equilibrium dialysis. J. Lab. Clin. Med. **75**, 503 (1970).
KLINENBERG, J. R., BLUESTONE, R., SCHLOSSTEIN, L., WAISMAN, J., WHITEHOUSE, M. W.: Urate deposition disease. How is it regulated and how can it be modified? Ann. intern. Med. **78**, 99 (1973).
LENNANE, G. A., ROSE, B. S., ISDALE, I. C.: Gout in Maori. Ann. rheum. Dis. **19**, 120 (1960).
LESCH, M., NYHAN, W. L.: A familial disorder of uric acid metabolism and central nervous system function. Amer. J. Med. **36**, 561 (1964).
LYON, M. F.: Gene action in the X-chromosome of the mouse. Nature (Lond.) **190**, 372 (1961).
NEEL, J. V.: The clinical detection of the genetic carriers of inherited disease. Medicine (Baltimore) **26**, 115 (1947).
PRIOR, I. A. M., ROSE, B. S.: Uric acid, gout and public health in the South Pacific. N. Z. med. J. **65**, 295 (1966).
PRIOR, I. A. M., ROSE, B. S., HARVEY, H. P. B., DAVIDSON, F.: Hyperuricemia, gout and diabetic abnormality in Polynesian people. Lancet **1966 I**, 333.
RAKIC, M. T., VALKENBURG, H. A., DAVIDSON, R. T., ENGELS, J. P., MIKKELSEN, W. M., NEEL, J. V., DUFF, I. F.: Observations on the natural history of hyperuricemia and gout. I. An eighteen year follow-up of nineteen gouty families. Amer. J. Med. **37**, 862 (1964).
ROSENBERG, E. F.: Gout and male hermaphroditism. Report of a case. Ann. rheum. Dis. **2**, 273 (1941).
ROSENBLOOM, F. M., KELLEY, W. N., HENDERSON, J. F., SEEGMILLER, J. E.: Lyon hypothesis and X-linked disease. Lancet **1967 II**, 305.
SCOTT, J. T., POLLARD, A. C.: Uric acid excretion in the relatives of patients with gout. Ann. rheum. Dis. **29**, 397 (1970).
SMYTH, C. J., FREYBERG, R. H.: Hereditary nature of gout. Ann. intern. Med. **16**, 46 (1942).
SMYTH, C. J., COTTERMANN, C. W., FREYBERG, R. H.: The genetics of gout and hyperuricemia. An analysis of nineteen families. J. clin. Invest. **27**, 749 (1948).
SMYTH, C. J.: Hereditary factors in gout. A review of recent literature. Metabolism **6**, 218 (1957).
SMYTH, C. J.: Arthritis and allied conditions. In: A textbook of Rheumatology. (Ed. Hollander, I. L.), 899. Philadelphia: Lea and Febiger 1966.
STECHER, R. M., HERSH, A. H., SOLOMON, W. M.: The heredity of gout and its relationship to familial hyperuricemia. Ann. intern. Med. **31**, 595 (1949).
TALBOTT, J. H.: Serum urate in relatives of gouty patients. J. clin. Invest. **19**, 645 (1940).

b) Einfluß exogener Purine auf den Harnsäurestoffwechsel

Von

A. GRIEBSCH und W. KAISER

Mit 3 Abbildungen

Geschichtliches

Gicht war bei den mehr vegetarisch lebenden Ägyptern und Hindus seltener als bei Völkern mit überfeinerten Lebensgewohnheiten wie den Persern und später den reichen Griechen und Römern. Schon HIPPOKRATES kannte den Einfluß der Lebensweise und Diätetik bei diesem Leiden.

Im 19. Jahrhundert mehren sich die Hinweise auf die Rolle der Ernährung. So weist 1823 SCUDAMORE auf alimentäre Faktoren hin und erwähnt zwei Gichtkranke, die nach Eßexzessen regelmäßig Anfälle bekamen. 1896 schreibt EWART, daß Gicht „durch strenges Vermeiden animalischer Ernährung verhindert" werden kann.

Um die Jahrhundertwende wurde dann, besonders in Deutschland, der Zusammenhang zwischen exogener Zufuhr von Nahrungspurinen und dem Harnsäurestoffwechsel systematisch untersucht. BURIAN und SCHUR (1900, 1901 und 1903, dort auch weitere Literatur) prägten den Begriff der „endogenen Uratquote". Sie fanden nämlich, ebenso wie unabhängig von ihnen SIVÉN (1900), unter weitgehend purinkörperfreier Nahrung konstante Werte der Harn-Purin-N-Ausscheidung von rund 200 mg pro Tag (SIVÉN umgerechnet 188 mg pro Tag), was einer Harnsäureausscheidung von 480 bzw. 451 mg pro Tag entspricht. Sie nannten diese Größe „endogenen Harn-Purin-Wert". Aus einer Zusammenstellung von neun Versuchen der damaligen Literatur läßt sich eine durchschnittliche Harnsäureausscheidung unter purinarmer Kost von 450 mg Harnsäure pro Tag berechnen. Nach Verabfolgung von purinhaltiger Kost stieg die Harnsäureausscheidung in diesen Versuchen auf durchschnittlich 708 mg/Tag an, was einer Zunahme von 157% oder um etwas mehr als die Hälfte des Ausgangswertes entsprach. Diese Autoren stellten weiter fest, daß in ihren und sieben weiteren damaligen Beobachtungen ein Teil des mit der Nahrung zugeführten Oxypurin-N im Harn wieder ausgeschieden wurde; dieser Anteil lag im Mittel bei 53%. In einzelnen Versuchen stieg die Purin-N-Ausscheidung auf 241% oder um fast das $1\frac{1}{2}$fache des Ausgangswertes an.

Gaben diese Untersuchungen schon erste Hinweise über den Einfluß exogener Purine auf die Höhe der Harnsäureausscheidung, so zeigten spätere Beobachtungen über die Häufigkeit der Gicht in und nach dem ersten Weltkrieg (Literatur bei GRAFE, 1953) und besonders dem zweiten Weltkrieg (vgl. DRUBE und REINWEIN, 1959) in Deutschland, daß diese von den Ernährungsgewohnheiten abhängt und Gicht in Notzeiten selten, in Zeiten des Wohlstandes häufig ist.

Demgegenüber fehlte es nie an Ärzten, die den Einfluß einer Diät auf den Harnsäurestoffwechsel bezweifelten. 1854 schreibt GAIRDNER, daß Gicht „nicht einmal durch spärliche Diät gebessert werden kann". In USA war es vor allem TALBOTT, der bezüglich der Rolle exogener Eiweißzufuhr liberal dachte und 1938 bereits meinte, „daß man die Rolle streng niedriger Purindiät sehr übertrieben hat"; ähnlich äußerte sich SMYTH (1953), dem „Beweise für den Erfolg purinfreier Diät" fehlten, sowie BAUER und SINGH (1957) und andere.

Wirkung purinarmer und purinfreier Diät

Neuere Daten über die Abhängigkeit der Harnsäurespiegel von exogener Purinzufuhr lieferten GUTMAN und YÜ, die 1952 zeigen konnten, daß unter einer purinarmen Diät die Serumharnspiegel von 86% ihrer Patienten (n = 71) abfielen und zwar im Mittel um 1,2 mg/100 ml, im Extremfall um 3 mg/100 ml. Gleichzeitig ging die renale Harnsäureausscheidung um 200—300 mg zurück. 1959 ermittelten diese Autoren Spiegel von 5,11 mg/100 ml und Ausscheidungsraten von 701,6 mg/24 Std unter purinarmer Kost; allerdings wurden keine Ausgangswerte unter Normalkost angegeben.

1961 zeigten SEEGMILLER et al., daß unter sieben Tagen beinahe purinfreier Standarddiät die Serumplasmaspiegel von $5,32 \pm 0,93$ auf $4,69 \pm 0,68$ mg/100 ml $(\bar{X} \pm S)$ oder auf 88% des Ausgangswertes zurückgingen; Gichtkranke fielen von $9,45 \pm 1,88$ auf $8,44 \pm 1,92$ mg/100 ml oder auf 89% des Ausgangswertes ab.

Zu ähnlichen Zahlen kommen WASLIEN et al. (1968): Gesunde erreichen nach 3—6 Tagen purinarmer Kost (mit Eiereiweiß als Proteinquelle) Harnsäure-Spie-

Tabelle 1. Einfluß purinarmer und purinfreier Ernährung auf den Harnsäurestoffwechsel. Mittelwerte ($X \pm S$) von Harnsäure-Plasmaspiegel und -Ausscheidung bei verschiedenen Autoren unter purinarmer Standard-Diät (St.D.) (oben) und eigenen Ergebnissen unter purinfreier Formeldiät (F.D.)

Autor	Jahr	n	Diätform (Puringehalt) [Protein-Quelle]	Dauer (Tage)	Harnsäure plasma spiegel mg/100 ml	Harn ausscheidung mg/Tag
1. SEEGMILLER et al.	1961	22	St.D. (purinarm)	7	4,69 ± 0,68	nur graphisch dargestellt
2. WASLIEN et al.	1968	20	St.D. (purinarm) [Eier]	3–6	4,7 ± 0,6	392 ± 66
3. WASLIEN et al.	1970	7	St.D. (purinarm) [Kasein]	9	5,4 ± 1,0	394 ± 50
Mittelwert					4,79 ± 0,69	392,5 ± 61
4. GRIEBSCH u. ZÖLLNER	1970a	7	St.D. (18,6–32 mg Purin N [Milcheiweiß]	7	4,34 ± 0,81	593,1 ± 152
5. GRIEBSCH u. ZÖLLNER	1970b	5	F.D. (purin frei) [Magermilch]	8	3,15 ± 0,30	343,3 ± 96

gel von 4,9 (3,9—5,5) mg/100 ml; die Harnsäureausscheidung erreicht 373 (316—430) mg/24 Std. Auch hier fehlen Angaben über die Ausgangswerte unter frei gewählter Kost. 1970 gab diese Arbeitsgruppe bei 7 gesunden Männern unter 9tägiger purinarmer Diät (mit Kasein als Proteinträger) Harnsäurespiegel von 5,4 ± 1,0 mg/100 ml und Ausscheidungsraten von 394 + 50 mg/24 Std an. Auch wir (GRIEBSCH u. ZÖLLNER, 1970a) fanden unter purinarmer (Purin-N-Gehalt 18,2—32 mg/Tag) Standardkost Harnsäure-Plasmaspiegel von 4,34 ± 1,52 mg/100 ml und eine Harnsäureausscheidung von 593,1 ± 152 mg/Tag.

Faßt man die Ergebnisse der erwähnten Ernährungsversuche (überwiegend an Männern) mit purinarmen Standarddiäten zusammen, so ergeben sich ($n = 56$) folgende Daten: Harnsäureplasmaspiegel 4,73 ± 0,8 mg/100 ml, Harnsäureausscheidung 423 ± 80 mg/Tag.

Genauere Werte für diese Größen ergeben sich allerdings erst, wenn man statt weitgehend purinarmer Standarddiät eine purinfreie isocalorische Formeldiät verwendet (Abb. 1). So fanden wir (ZÖLLNER et al., 1972, und GRIEBSCH u. ZÖLLNER, 1974) an 5 Männern und 6 Frauen für die Harnsäureplasmaspiegel Werte von 3,15 ± 0,3 mg/100 ml und für die Harnsäureausscheidung solche von 343,3 ± 96 mg/Tag.

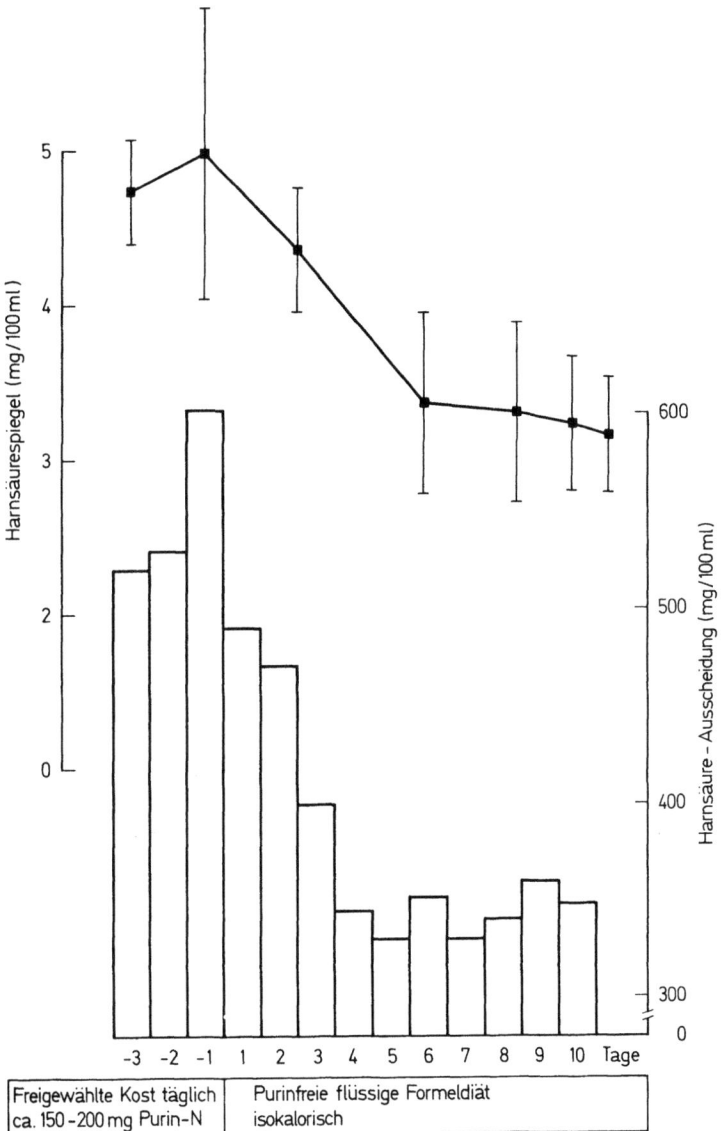

Abb. 1. Verhalten der endogenen Harnsäureproduktion (sog. endogene Uratquote): Unter völlig purinfreier flüssiger isokalorischer Formeldiät fällt die tägliche renale Harnsäureausscheidung (Säulen) von Werten zwischen 520–600 mg/Tag unter freigewählter Kost (Vorperiode -3. bis -1. Versuchstag) auf Mengen von 320–350 mg/Tag (Mittelwerte von 16 Versuchspersonen). Gleichzeitig verringern sich die Harnsäureplasmaspiegel (■ = Vierecke) von fast 5,00 auf 3,20 mg/100 ml ($n = 11$). Die senkrechten Linien geben den mittleren Fehler $\left(s_{\bar{x}} = \dfrac{s}{\sqrt{n}}\right)$ an. Modifiziert nach GRIEBSCH u. ZÖLLNER (1974)

Einfluß verschiedener exogener Purine
Auswirkungen bei Normalpersonen

Bereits in den klassischen Versuchen von NUGENT u. TYLER (1959) konnte gezeigt werden, daß die Zufuhr von exogenen Purinen in Form von Ribonukleinsäuren (RNS) die Plasma-Harnsäurespiegel deutlich anhebt. Unter einer Dosis von 4 g RNS, wie sie die meisten Autoren verwenden, steigt der Harnsäurespiegel z.B. in den Versuchen von NUGENT et al. von 4,88 mg/100 ml auf durchschnittlich 7,4 mg/100 ml. Ähnliche Daten erzielten SEEGMILLER et al. (1962), die Anstiege von 4,6 auf 8,19 mg/100 ml erreichten. WASLIEN et al. (1968) beobachteten unter der gleichen Dosis Anstiege von 4,9 auf 7,68 bzw. von 5,4 auf 8,7 mg/100 ml (1970). Wir selbst erzielten (GRIEBSCH u. ZÖLLNER, 1970a) unter Standarddiätbedingungen Spiegelanstiege von 4,5 auf 7,44 mg/100 ml und konnten eine Regression berechnen, deren Steigungsmaß +0,73 mg/100 ml Zuwachs des Harnsäurespiegels pro 1 g RNS-Zulage betrug; eine vergleichbare Anstiegsrate fanden WASLIEN et al. (1968) mit 0,65 mg/100 ml. Analog dazu betrug die Zuwachsrate für die Urinausscheidung unter RNS-Belastung +147 bzw. +152 mg/24 Std in den Versuchen von WASLIEN et al. (1968 und 1971) und 113 mg/24 Std in unseren (GRIEBSCH u. ZÖLLNER, 1970a) Versuchen unter Standarddiät. Da sich mit einer völlig purinfreien Formeldiät niedrigere Ausgangswerte erreichen lassen, werden die Anstiegsraten dadurch etwas steiler; so fanden wir (GRIEBSCH u. ZÖLLNER, 1970b) für Plasmaspiegel ein Steigungsmaß von +1,07 mg/100 ml und für die Harnsäureausscheidung ein solches von 132 mg/24 Std pro 1 g RNS-Zulage.

In weiteren Studien über die Auswirkung exogener Purine auf Spiegel und Ausscheidung der Harnsäure untersuchten wir auch andere Harnsäurevorläufer wie z.B. DNS (GRIEBSCH u. ZÖLLNER, 1970b) sowie die Mononukleotide 5'-AMP und 5'-GMP (1973); auch die purinreichen Einzeller, die reich an Eiweiß sind, wurden in ihren Auswirkungen auf den Harnsäurespiegel untersucht. Daten über die Auswirkungen der Algenarten Scenedesmus obliquus (GRIEBSCH u. ZÖLLNER, 1971), Chlorella sorokiniana (WASLIEN et al., 1970) wurden ebenso erarbeitet wie solche über bestimmte Hefearten wie Torulopsis utilis (WASLIEN et al., 1970) und andere (ABRAHAMSON et al., 1970). Einige wichtige Daten gehen aus Abb. 2 sowie aus dem Kapitel Diät hervor.

Die Rolle der exogenen Purinzufuhr für die Höhe der Harnsäureplasmaspiegel erhellt schließlich aus der Bestimmung der Normalwerte der Plasmaharnsäure in Süddeutschland, die wir (GRIEBSCH u. ZÖLLNER, 1973) mit Mittelwerten von 6,0 mg/100 ml für Männer um mehr als 1 mg/100 ml höher fanden als 10 Jahre zuvor mit der gleichen Methode (enzymatisch-spektrophotometrisch mit Uricase) im gleichen Labor am nämlichen Kollektiv (Blutspender) und die damals für Männer nur 4,86 mg/100 ml betragen hatten. Die Zunahme des Fleischverbrauchs im gleichen Zeitraum nach dem Ernährungsbericht 1972 der Deutschen Gesellschaft für Ernährung ergab nämlich eine durchschnittliche Mehrzufuhr von fast 30 g Fleischeiweiß pro Kopf der Bevölkerung und pro Tag. Der Puringehalt dieser Menge ergibt — eingesetzt in die obigen Relationen zwischen RNS und Harnsäurespiegel-Anstieg — einen theoretisch zu erwartenden Harnsäurespiegel von über 6 mg/100 ml. Auch damit ist der Einfluß der Ernährungsgewohnheiten auf die Harnsäureplasmaspiegel nachgewiesen.

Wirkung exogener Purine auf Personen mit vorbestehender Hyperurikämie

Von besonderer Bedeutung war bis Mitte der 60er Jahre die Frage, ob exogene Purine auf Normurikämiker und (familiäre) Hyperurikämiker sich gleichar-

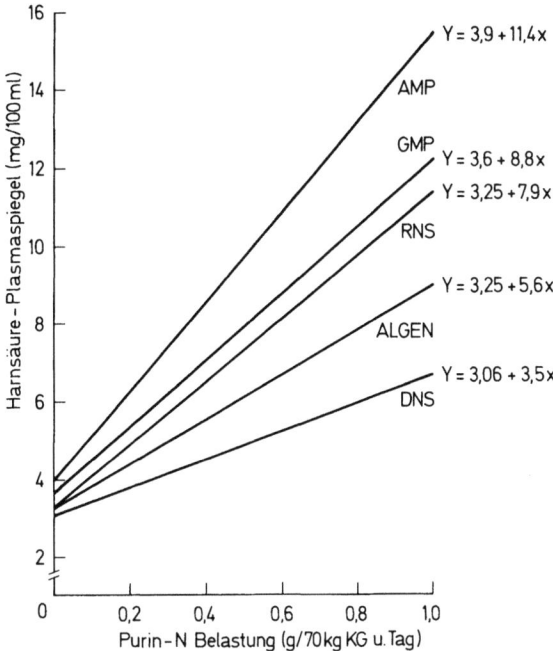

Abb. 2. Regressionen zwischen der Höhe der exogenen Purinzufuhr (Abszisse) in Form verschiedener Harnsäure-Vorläufer (berechnet in g Purin-N-Zulage pro Tag und kg KG) und dem Anstieg der Plasma-Harnsäure (P_{Hsr}: mg/100 ml, Ordinate). Man erkennt, daß hochmolekulare Purinverbindungen wie RNS, DNS und die Kombination beider, z. B. in Algen (Scenedesmus obliquus) schlechter resorbiert werden und sich weniger stark auf die Harnsäurespiegel auswirken als die Monoribonucleotide (5'-AMP und 5'-GMP). In den angegebenen Gleichungen bedeutet die erste Zahl ($\bar{x}$) den jeweiligen Ausgangswert der P_{Hsr}, die zweite Zahl das Steigungsmaß (α_{yx}). Dieses gibt an, um wieviel mg/100 ml der Plasmaspiegel (pro g Purin N-Zulage/kg KG und Tag) unter Zulage des jeweiligen Praekursors ansteigen wird (erweitert nach GRIEBSCH und ZÖLLNER, 1974)

tig auswirken. Dieses Problem war vor allem für die Erörterung der Frage erheblich, ob das Wesen der (familiären) Hyperurikämie bzw. der Gicht in einer renalen Ausscheidungsschwäche für Harnsäure liegt (THANNHAUSER, 1956, Zitat nach ZÖLLNER, 1960 u. 1969) oder ob es nach der besonders durch GUTMAN und andere vertretenen Überproduktionstheorie nicht vielmehr in einer vermehrten Synthese besteht. Im Rahmen dieser Diskussionen belasteten NUGENT et al. (1964) Gichtkranke — und im Vergleich dazu mit RNS hyperurikämisch gemachte Gesunde, die bis zu 42 Tagen diesen Harnsäurepräkursor erhalten hatten — jeweils mit einer kurzfristigen Gabe von RNS über 3 Tage. Sie konnten zeigen, daß die meisten (familiären) Hyperurikämiker bzw. Gichtpatienten weniger Harnsäure ausschieden als normourikämische Nichtgichtiker, die langfristig durch exogene Purinzufuhr hyperurikämisch gemacht worden waren. Damit war dem Einwand des Gutmanschen Arbeitskreises begegnet, die Bedingungen der akuten Purinbelastung würden diesen Unterschied nur vortäuschen.

Analog dazu konnten wir nicht nur zeigen, daß Hyperurikämiker auf eine Belastung mit z. B. RNS mit höheren Anstiegen der Harnsäureplasmaspiegel reagieren als Gesunde (GRIEBSCH u. ZÖLLNER, 1970a), sondern wir fanden bei zwei Brüdern mit Gicht in der Familie, daß die renale Harnsäureausscheidung sowohl unter purinfreier Kost wie unter Zufuhr von RNS als auch unter solcher von

DNS nur stets etwa 70—80% der Werte der Gesunden betrug (1970b). Auch dies weist — zumindest für einen Teil der Gichtpatienten — auf eine Ausscheidungsschwäche für Harnsäure hin und erklärt, warum manche (familiären) Hyperurikämiker auf die gleiche Rate exogener Purine mit höheren Harnsäurespiegeln reagieren als Gesunde.

Es ergibt sich also eine signifikante, individuell unterschiedliche Beeinflussung des Harnsäurespiegels und der renalen Harnsäureausscheidung nach exogener Zufuhr von Purinen. Den mit der Nahrung zugeführten Purinen kommt in der Ätiologie der Gicht nur die Bedeutung eines die Manifestation fördernden Faktors zu.

Einfluß der Nahrungsproteine auf den Harnsäurestoffwechsel

Da Aminosäuren direkte Präkursoren für die *de novo*-Purinbiosynthese darstellen, wäre eine Beeinflussung der Harnsäuresynthese durch den Eiweißgehalt der Nahrung theoretisch möglich. So konnte z.B. gezeigt werden, daß der Gehalt von Glutamin die Geschwindigkeit der Purinsynthese unter bestimmten Bedingungen limitieren kann (FONTENELLE u. HENDERSON, 1969).

Tatsächlich konnten BIEN et al. (1953) durch orale Zufuhr von N^{15}-markiertem Glycin an einer Normalperson und einem Gichtpatienten (Hyperexkretor) zeigen, daß die Menge des Überschusses von N^{15} im gesamten Urin-Stickstoff und in der renal ausgeschiedenen Harnsäure davon abhängt, ob die Basis-Diät wenig oder viel Eiweiß enthält. So stieg der Gehalt des Urins an Harnsäure-Stickstoff von 131 mg/Tag bei 48 g Protein auf 193 mg/Tag bei 84 g Protein/Tag oder um rund 68% des Ausgangswertes an. Eine Erhöhung der Eiweißzufuhr beschleunigt also offenbar die Harnsäuresynthese, d.h. die Purinbiosynthese stieg in einer direkten Relation zu der Gesamtstickstoffausscheidung an.

WASLIEN et al. (1968) konnten zeigen, daß zwischen einer eiweißfreien oder eiweißreichen Kost (75 g Protein/Person/Tag) signifikante Unterschiede in der Harnsäureausscheidung (354 mg/Tag bei purinfreier Kost gegenüber 392 mg/Tag bei 75 g Protein) auftreten, fanden aber bei den Plasmaspiegeln das umgekehrte Verhalten. Die höchsten Spiegel (6,0 mg/100 ml) traten nämlich bei purinfreier und die niedrigsten (4,7 mg/100 ml) bei eiweißreicher Kost auf. Für niedrigere Proteinzufuhr-Raten (22, 28 und 37 g/Tag) waren die Unterschiede zur proteinfreien Diät nicht signifikant.

1969 wiesen dann BOWERING et al. mittels flüssiger Formeldiäten an sechs Normalpersonen nach, daß unter der Gabe von 0,9, 13 und 62 g Protein-Stickstoff/Tag die Harnsäureausscheidung im Mittel 306, 388 und 1095 mg/Tag beträgt. Demgegenüber verhalten sich die Harnsäureplasmaspiegel nicht eindeutig (5,0, 5,1 und 5,3 mg/100 ml). Die Zunahme der Ausscheidung unter hoher Eiweißzufuhr konnte — nach Bestimmung des Umsatzes des "miscible pool" mittels N^{15} markierter Harnsäure — auf einen Anstieg der Umsatzrate um das Zweifache bei unveränderter Poolgröße zurückgeführt werden. Die Autoren nehmen danach an, daß die Steigerung der Harnsäureproduktion sowohl auf einer Erhöhung der Substrate für die Purin-Synthese als auch auf einem Einfluß auf die Kontrolle der Rückkoppelung des Harnsäure-Stoffwechsels beruht.

Ausmaß und Mechanismen der Resorption von Nahrungspurinen

Der größte Teil der Purine, der zu Harnsäure abgebaut wird, ist zweifellos endogenen Ursprungs (sog. endogene Uratquote). Die Fähigkeit des menschlichen Organismus zur Synthese des Purinrings ist lange bekannt. Mit Hilfe verschiedener radioaktiv markierter Verbindungen konnte die Herkunft jedes einzelnen der Kohlenstoff- und Stickstoffatome des im menschlichen Körper synthetisierten Purinrings geklärt werden (SEHMIN u. RITTENBERG, 1947; BUCHANAN et al., 1948; SONNE et al., 1948, 1956; KARLSON u. BARKER, 1949; HEINRICH u. WILSON, 1950; LEVENBERG et al., 1956; GOLDTHWAIT et al., 1956). Diese weitgehende Unabhängigkeit des Körpers von der exogenen Zufuhr ist auch Ursache für die bereits beschriebene relativ geringe Wirkung einer Ausschaltung von purinhaltigen Nahrungsmitteln auf den Serumharnsäurespiegel. Auch ist eine Reduzierung der Zufuhr auf weniger als 3 mg Purin-N/die monatelang möglich, ohne daß irgendwelche besonderen Mangelerscheinungen beim Menschen auftreten würden. Andererseits geht aus den vorangegangenen Ausführungen hervor, daß mit der Nahrung zugeführte Nucleinsäuren und Nucleinsäurebruchstücke den Serumharnsäurespiegel erhöhen, infolgedessen auch in irgendeiner Form aus dem Darm aufgenommen werden müssen.

Purine der Nahrung werden dem menschlichen Organismus zum größten Teil in Form von hochmolekularen Nucleoproteiden und Nucleinsäuren zugeführt. In geringerem Ausmaß sind in der Nahrung auch kleinere Purinkörper wie Oligonucleotide, Purinbasen und verschiedene methylierte Purinbasen enthalten (STOLL, 1973).

Proteolytische Enzyme, vor allem des Pankreas, hydrolysieren die mit der Nahrung aufgenommenen Nucleoproteine innerhalb des Dünndarms in Nucleinsäuren und Proteine. Durch Einwirkung verschiedener Nucleasen des Pankreas und der intestinalen Mucosa (Ribonucleasen a und b sowie Desoxyribonucleasen I und II) kommt es im weiteren Verlauf der Verdauung zu einer intraluminären enzymatischen Hydrolyse der Polynucleotidketten der Nucleinsäuren in Oligonucleotide.

Durch Phosphodiesterasen, vor allem der intestinalen Mucosa, werden diese Oligonucleotide — wahrscheinlich an der Zelloberfläche — zu Purin- und Pyrimidinnucleotiden hydrolysiert. Diese 5'- und 3'-Mononucleotiden können sowohl durch gruppenspezifische Nucleosid-5'-phosphatasen (HEPPEL u. HILMOE, 1951) als auch verschiedene nicht spezifische Phosphatasen (SCHMIDT, 1955) der intestinalen Mucosa bereits auf der Oberfläche oder innerhalb der Zellen sehr rasch zu den entsprechenden Purin- oder Pyrimidinnucleosiden sowie Orthophosphat gespalten werden. Die so entstandenen Nucleoside können nun als solche absorbiert werden, oder sie werden durch eine Purinnucleosid-Phosphorylase der intestinalen Mucosa intracellulär zur freien Base (Adenin, Guanin, Hypoxanthin und Xanthin) und Ribose-1-phosphat phosphorolytisch gespalten (KALCKAR, 1947a; FRIEDKIN, 1952). Diese werden anschließend intracellulär durch die Hypoxanthin-Guanin-Phosphoribosyl-Transferase (HG-PRT) oder Adenin-Phosphoribosyl-Transferase (A-PRT) in Purinbonucleotide umgewandelt.

Besondere Verhältnisse liegen bei der intracellulären enzymatischen Spaltung von AMP und Adenosin vor. Durch die Adenylsäure-Deaminase kommt es zur Bildung von IMP aus AMP (NIKIFORUK u. COLOWICK, 1956), durch die Adenosin-Deaminase von Adenosin zu Inosin (KALCKAR, 1947b). Eine Desaminierung von freiem Adenin konnte in menschlichem Gewebe nicht nachgewiesen werden, so daß Adenin nur indirekt über eine Neubildung in Adenosin oder AMP und anschließend über die Desaminierung durch spezifische Enzyme in den menschlichen Purinstoffwechsel Eingang finden kann. Geringe Mengen Adenin können normalerweise anscheinend auch resorbiert werden, da sie jedoch nicht oder nur schlecht eingebaut werden können, werden sie weitgehend renal ausgeschieden (WEISSMANN et al., 1957).

In der Mucosa des menschlichen Dünndarms kann eine hohe enzymatische Aktivität an Purinnucleosidphosphorylasen nachgewiesen werden; deren enzymatische Aktivität scheint für Inosin und Guanosin am höchsten zu sein (HEPPEL u. HILMOE, 1951; KORN u. BUCHANAN, 1955; HUENNEKENS et al., 1956). Damit kommt es bei der Verdauung von RNS intracellulär in erster Linie zur Bildung von Hypoxanthin und Guanin. Aus Guanin wird innerhalb der Dünndarmzellen durch Einwirkung des Enzyms Guanase Xanthin gebildet, Hypoxanthin wird durch Xanthin-Oxydase gleichfalls zu Xanthin oxydiert. Da beim Menschen in den Dünndarmzellen eine hohe Xanthinoxydaseaktivität nachgewiesen werden konnte, ist es sehr wahrscheinlich, daß bereits innerhalb der Mucosazellen zum größten Teil aus dem während der Verdauung der Nucleinsäuren entstandenen Xanthin Harnsäure gebildet wird. Durch diese im Dünndarmepithel lokalisierten Abbaumechanismen von exogenem Guanin, Hypoxanthin und Xanthin kommt es also bereits im Dünndarm zur direkten Harnsäurebildung. Damit wäre das Hauptresorptionsprodukt der Nucleinsäureverdauung die Harnsäure. So wären auch die Untersuchungen von WILSON et al. (1954) zu erklären, die nach oraler Verabreichung von ^{15}N-markierten Hefenucleinsäuren bei Gesunden und Gichtpatienten einen direkten Einbau von ^{15}N in Harnsäure fanden, während in den Nucleinsäuren verschiedener Gewebe kein Einbau nachgewiesen werden konnte. Auch bei Umgehung dieser im Darm lokalisierten Abbaumechanismen durch intravenöse Injektion kommt es im menschlichen Organismus anscheinend zu einer raschen Umwandlung von z.B. Hypoxanthin in Harnsäure. So fanden WYNGAARDEN et al. (1959) nach intravenöser Injektion von kleinen Dosen 8-^{14}C-Hypoxanthin einen ^{14}C-Einbau in Harnsäure von 50% der verabreichten Dosis innerhalb eines Zeitraums von 9 Tagen.

Es ist noch nicht endgültig entschieden, in welcher Form die Bruchstücke der Nucleinsäuren (Purinbasen, Nucleoside oder Nucleotide) vorwiegend oder ausschließlich die intestinalen Membranen passieren können und in die Nucleinsäuren des Körpers eingebaut werden. Auf Grund verschiedener Fütterungsversuche an Tieren ist anzunehmen, daß es auch zu einer gewissen Absorption von Nucleinsäurebruchstücken kommen kann, ehe eine Aufspaltung in die freie Base zustande gekommen ist.

Während nämlich ROLL et al. (1949) einen Einbau von ^{15}N in die Purine und Pyrimidine der Nucleinsäuren von Ratten nach Verfütterung von ^{15}N-markierter Nucleinsäure fanden, konnte in früheren Untersuchungen nach Zufuhr von ^{15}N-markiertem Guanin, Uracil und Thymin (PLENTL u. SCHOENHEIMER, 1944), Cytosin (BENDICK et al., 1949), Hypoxanthin und Xanthin (GERTLER et al., 1949) bei der Ratte kein solcher Einbau beobachtet werden. Der höhere Einbau nach oraler Gabe von Nucleinsäuren gegenüber derjenigen nach Zufuhr von freien Basen spricht deshalb auch für eine Absorption von anderen Bruchstücken. Ein Einbau von absorbierten Nucleosiden oder Nucleotiden in die Nucleinsäuren des Körpers erscheint zumindest für die Pyrimidine wahrscheinlich, denn nach Injektion von ^{15}N-markierten Pyrimidinnucleosiden oder -nucleotiden konnte ein ^{15}N-Einbau in die Nucleinsäuren der Ratten nachgewiesen werden (HAMMERSTEN et al., 1950).

Daß der Dünndarm aber zumindest eine hohe Absorptionskapazität für freie Pyrimidinbasen besitzen muß, hatten erste Untersuchungen von MENDEL u. MYERS (1910) erbracht. Diese Autoren fanden eine anscheinend komplette Absorption von Thymin, Uracil und Cytosin (in einer Dosis von 3 g) beim Kaninchen und Menschen. In Untersuchungen an isolierten Dünndarmschlingen des Hamsters und der Ratte wurde vor allem das Transportsystem für Pyrimidinbasen näher untersucht. SCHANKER u. TOCCO (1960) nahmen auf Grund solcher

Untersuchungen für den Rattendünndarm ein aktives Transportsystem für Pyrimidinbasen an, und zwar wurden Thymin, Uracil, 5-Fluorouracil und 5-Bromouracil entgegen Konzentrationsgradienten transportiert. In vivo-Untersuchungen wiesen weiter darauf hin, daß es bei intraluminärer Konzentration dieser Substanzen über 1—5 mM bei gesättigtem Transportsystem zu einer passiven Absorption durch Diffusion kam (WILSON, 1962). Dabei beanspruchten Thymin und Uracil anscheinend das gleiche Transportsystem, da der Thymintransport durch Uracil kompetitiv gehemmt werden konnte.

Bei Inkubation von isolierten Dünndarmschlingen des Hamsters mit einer Reihe von Pyrimidin-5'-Nucleotiden konnten WILSON u. WILSON (1958) sowohl Nucleoside als auch freie Basen auf der Serosaseite der Dünndarmwand, jedoch keine Nucleotide nachweisen, ein aktiver Transport entgegen einem Konzentrationsgradienten ließ sich aber nicht belegen.

Ähnliche Ergebnisse konnten zwar auch für Purinnucleotide (WILSON u. WILSON, 1962) gefunden werden, jedoch ist noch nicht sicher bekannt, ob die Purinbasen für den Transport das gleiche Transportsystem wie die Pyrimidinbasen beanspruchen. Daß Hypoxanthin den Thymintransport stark hemmt (WILSON, 1962), spricht etwas für ein gemeinsames Transportsystem; andererseits hemmen Xanthin und Harnsäure diesen Transport kaum und Adenin praktisch überhaupt nicht (SCHANKER u. TOCCO, 1962). Es scheint somit wahrscheinlich, daß einzelne Purinbasen die Zellmembran über einen mit den Pyrimidinbasen gemeinsamen Transportmechanismus passieren. Durch die innerhalb der Dünndarmzelle stattfindende rasche Metabolisierung der Purinbasen — vor allem der Oxydation durch die Xanthinoxydase bis zur Harnsäure — sind Transportstudien für die einzelnen Basen aber sehr schwierig durchzuführen.

Durch Blockierung der Oxydation von Hypoxanthin und Xanthin zu Harnsäure mit Hilfe von Allopurinol scheint es BERLIN u. HAWKINS (1968) jedoch besser möglich gewesen zu sein, den intracellulären Transport von unveränderten, d.h. intracellulär nicht metabolisierten Purinbasen in isolierten Schlingen des Dünndarms von Hamstern zu untersuchen. In diesen Untersuchungen werden Hypoxanthin, Xanthin und Harnsäure aktiv entgegen Konzentrationsgradienten in das intestinale Lumen sezerniert, und zwar war unter diesen speziellen experimentellen Bedingungen der unidirektionale transmurale Fluß von der Serosa zur Mucosa 5mal größer als der Fluß von Mucosa zu Serosa. Diese Ergebnisse sind jedoch nicht unbedingt auf die in vivo-Absorptionsverhältnisse im menschlichen Dünndarm anwendbar, denn die Absorption dürfte bei Bestehen einer normalen Blutzirkulation im Gegensatz zu den experimentellen in vitro-Bedingungen beträchtlich höher liegen.

Darüber hinaus darf man diese Ergebnisse als Hinweis dafür nehmen, daß ein Teil der aus dem Abbau von mit der Nahrung aufgenommenen Nucleinsäuren stammenden Nucleotide und Purinbasen in den Dünndarmepithelien zu Harnsäure oxydiert wird und anschließend als solche in das intestinale Lumen sezerniert werden kann. Ein Teil der mit der Nahrung zugeführten Purinkörper würde somit einer kurzen Rezirkulation unterliegen, vom Dünndarmlumen zur Zelle und von dort wieder zurück, mit dem Endergebnis einer fäkalen Harnsäureausscheidung. Bilanzmäßig liegen jedoch für die vorliegenden Beiträge von Absorption bzw. Sekretion der mit der Nahrung zugeführten Nucleinsäurebruchstücke keinerlei Angaben vor.

Bei der Bilanzierung des Beitrags zur Purinkörpersynthese aus den mit der Nahrung zugeführten Nucleinsäuren ist neben Absorption und Sekretion als ein weiterer wesentlicher Faktor die intraluminäre Zerstörung der Nucleinsäurebruchstücke durch die intestinale Bakterienflora zu beachten.

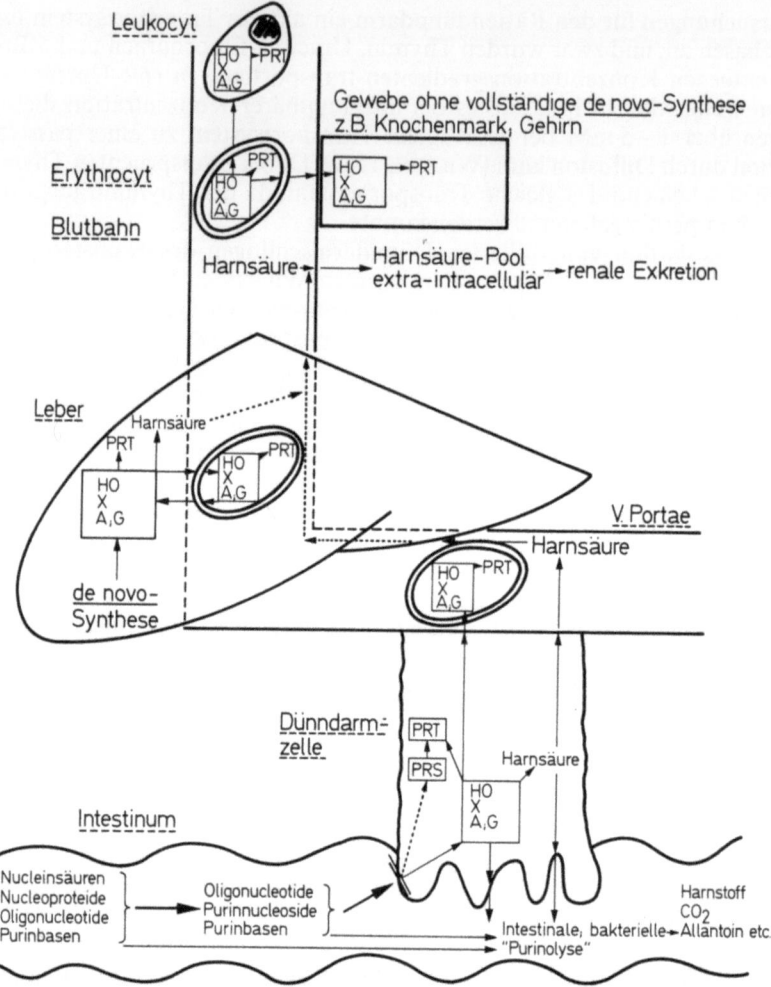

Abb. 3. Vorstellungen über Absorption, Transport und Utilisation von exogenen Purinen. HO = Hypoxanthin, X = Xanthin, A = Adenin, G = Guanin, PRS = Purinribonucleosid, PRT = Purinribonucleotid

THANNHAUSER u. DORFMÜLLER (1918) konnten z.B. an wäßrigen Lösungen von Nucleosiden (Guanosin, Adenosin und Inosin) zeigen, daß Darmbakterien des Menschen den Stickstoff derselben in Ammoniak verwandeln können und prägten den Begriff der „bakteriellen Purinolyse". Speziell in den unteren Darmabschnitten tritt die enzymatische Nucleinsäurespaltung gegenüber der bakteriellen Zersetzung zurück. Das dabei entstehende NH_3 wird resorbiert und in Harnstoff eingebaut. Damit wird zum Teil auch wieder erklärt, warum nach Zufuhr von Nahrungspurinen nur ein bestimmter Prozentsatz als Harnsäure im Urin wieder auftreten kann (10—15%) und nur 1—6% in den Faeces als unveränderte Purine, während gleichzeitig die Harnstoffausscheidung ansteigt (BRUGSCH u. SCHITTENHELM, 1912). Genauere Untersuchungen über das Ausmaß der intestinalen Urikolyse durch Darmbakterien liegen insbesondere für oral verabreichte Harnsäure vor. GEREN et al. (1950) fanden nach oraler Verabreichung von ^{15}N-Harnsäure eine Absorption und renale Exkretion in unveränderter Form von nur

9—11%, 47% des ^{15}N wurden dagegen innerhalb von 3 Tagen als Harnstoff im Urin ausgeschieden. In den Untersuchungen von SORENSEN (1959) wurde nach oraler Verabreichung von ^{14}C-Harnsäure 11,1% innerhalb von 6 Tagen als solche unverändert im Urin ausgeschieden, 13,9% des verabreichten ^{14}C fand sich in der Ausatmungsluft als CO_2 und 16,3% des ^{14}C wurde (vorwiegend innerhalb der Darmbakterien eingeschlossen) mit den Faeces ausgeschieden. Zumindest für die Harnsäure scheint also die intestinale Urikolyse quantitativ sehr bedeutend zu sein.

Die Permeabilität und die Quantität der Absorption des menschlichen Dünndarms für Harnsäure wurden von SAUNDERS u. BECK (1965) untersucht. Danach werden etwa 23% der Harnsäure aus dem Gastrointestinaltrakt absorbiert. Dieser Wert entspricht den Daten, die aus den Untersuchungen von SORENSEN (1960) berechnet werden können. Hier werden 17,4% aus dem Gastrointestinaltrakt reabsorbiert. Diese Ergebnisse sprechen für eine relative Impermeabilität der menschlichen Dünndarmmucosa für Harnsäure.

Im menschlichen Körper sind zwei Arten von Geweben vorhanden, die extracellulär angelieferte Purinbasen verwenden können: erstens solche, die sowohl einen vollständigen *de novo*-Purinstoffwechsel als auch einen Reutilisations-Stoffwechsel aufweisen und zweitens solche, denen der *de novo*-Stoffwechselweg fehlt und die dementsprechend auf die von außen an die Zelle angelieferten Purine angewiesen sind. Die ersteren verfügen über eine ausgewogene Gleichgewichtseinstellung zwischen dem *de novo*- und dem Reutilisationsstoffwechsel. Anderen Geweben des menschlichen Körpers, z.B. Knochenmark, Leukocyten, Erythrocyten und vermutlich den Gehirnzellen (LOWY u. WILLIAMS, 1960; SCOTT, 1962; SMELLIE et al., 1958; LAIJTHA u. VANE, 1958; ROSENBLOOM et al., 1967) fehlt demnach das Enzymsystem zur vollständigen *de novo*-Synthese der Purine. Da diese Zellen aber zur Aufrechterhaltung ihres Stoffwechsels Purinnukleotide brauchen, sind zumindest die Zellen des Knochenmarks und wahrscheinlich die Zellen mehrerer peripherer Gewebe auf Purinbasen angewiesen, die von außen an sie herangeführt werden. Eine dieser exogenen Quellen könnte theoretisch die intestinale Absorption von Purinbasen sein. Nachdem sich der Mensch jedoch lange Zeit ohne große Mangelerscheinungen purinfrei ernähren kann, darf die diätetische Quelle aber nicht unbedingt als essentiell angesehen werden. Nach den Untersuchungen von PRITCHARD et al. (1970) an Ratten ist vielmehr anzunehmen, daß als Organ für die Zulieferung von präformierten Purinen für andere Gewebe in erster Linie die Leber dient, für die Zulieferung von Purinbasen werden die Erythrocyten als Transportorgan angesehen (HENDERSON u. LE PAGE, 1959). Vom energetischen Standpunkt aus betrachtet erbrächte die Verwendung freier Basen z.B. aus der Diät für die Zellen große Vorteile. Zur Synthese eines Moleküls IMP über den *de novo*-Stoffwechselweg werden z.B. sechs Moleküle ATP verbraucht, während bei der Umwandlung von Hypoxanthin zu IMP nur ein Molekül ATP für die Synthese von PRPP verwendet werden muß.

Die für jede Zelle essentiellen Nucleotide können also entweder über einen *de novo*- oder "do it yourself"-Stoffwechselweg aus einfachen Metaboliten oder durch Verwendung präformierter Basen oder Nucleoside über einen Reutilisations- oder "salvage"-Stoffwechselweg gebildet werden. Die präformierten Verbindungen können dabei entweder aus diätetischen oder aus endogenen Quellen stammen.

Da ^{14}C-Adenin rasch in Nucleinsäuren eingebaut werden kann und sowohl die Aktivität als auch die Gewebsverteilung der A-PRT ausreichend ist (bei fehlender Adenin-Deaminase), wäre es denkbar, daß als signifikanter diätetischer Präkursor für die menschliche Nucleotidbildung in erster Linie Adenin in Frage kommt. Nach den Untersuchungen von PRITCHARD et al. (1970) an Ratten utilisieren die Erythrocyten jedoch eher Hypoxanthin oder Guanin. Tatsächlich nehmen Kaninchenerythrocyten *in vitro* (MAYER et al., 1967) Adenin, Guanin, Hypoxanthin und Xanthin auf und wandeln sie in Nucleotide um; die einzigen Purine jedoch, die daraus wieder freigesetzt werden, sind Hypoxanthin und Xanthin. Das würde bedeuten, daß von den vom Erythrocyten aufgenommenen Purinen für die Verwendung durch die peripheren Gewebe nur Hypoxanthin und Xanthin zur Verfügung gestellt werden. Das Transportsystem für Purine aus Organen mit einem Purinüberschuß (für die diätetischen Purine der Dünndarm, für Purine aus endogenen Quellen im wesentlichen die Leber) zu den Organen, die extracelluläre Purine benötigen, wären demnach die Erythrocyten. Als Produkte aus den verschiedenen Purinbasen würden von den Erythrocyten nur Hypoxanthin und Xanthin für die Utilisation durch die in beinahe allen menschlichen Geweben aktiven intracellulären 6-Oxypurin-Phosphoribosyltransferasen angeliefert.

Ein Teil der Unterschiede in der Höhe des Serumspiegelanstiegs für Harnsäure bei Zufuhr von exogenen Nucleinsäuren könnten evtl. ihre Erklärung haben in der unterschiedlichen Zusammensetzung der Purinbasen. So konnten z. B. CASKEY et al. (1964) zeigen, daß vor allem Nucleotide, die Adenin enthalten, eine Hemmwirkung auf das geschwindigkeitsbestimmende Enzym der Purinsynthese, die Phosphoribosyl-Glutamin-Amidotransferase, ausüben. Da die Verabreichung von ^{14}C-Adenin zu einer langsamen Umwandlung in Harnsäure führt (WYNGAARDEN et al., 1959), könnte man den Schluß ziehen, daß größere Dosen Adenin dazu verwendet werden könnten, die bei manchen Patienten mit Gicht festgestellte übermäßige *de novo*-Purinsynthese zu hemmen. Durch die geringe Umwandlung von Adenin selbst in Harnsäure würde es damit nicht zu einer direkten Harnsäureerhöhung kommen. Tatsächlich konnten SEEGMILLER et al. (1968) durch Adeninverabreichung sowohl bei Normalpersonen als auch bei Gichtpatienten eine Hemmung der *de novo*-Purinsynthese beobachten. Sie erklärten dies mit einer Rückkopplungshemmung der Purinsynthese durch die aus Adenin gebildeten Nucleotide. Trotz einer signifikant verminderten *de novo*-Synthese verringerte sich jedoch in diesen Untersuchungen die renale 24 Std-Exkretion der Harnsäure nicht, was teilweise mit einer Umwandlung des aufgenommenen Adenins in Harnsäure erklärt wurde.

Die Quantität der Resorption, die Bedeutung der Utilisation von Purinbasen, die mit der Nahrung dem Menschen zugeführt werden, kann also nur indirekt aus der Erhöhung bzw. Verminderung des Harnsäurespiegels und der renalen Harnsäureexkretion nach entsprechender Zufuhr abgeschätzt werden. Die Resorptions- bzw. Sekretionsmechanismen im Dünndarm, die Transportmechanismen im Blut bzw. die Kontrolle zur Freisetzung und Abgabe an utilisierende Zellen, sind weder im Tierexperiment noch für den Menschen geklärt. Obwohl für den Menschen keine essentielle Notwendigkeit für die Zufuhr von Purinen mit der Nahrung besteht, kommt man theoretisch — bei Erwägung der energetischen Bilanz — zu dem Schluß, daß die der Zelle aus diätetischen Quellen zugeführten präformierten Purine zu einer Energieeinsparung führen müßten, da der in allen Geweben funktionierende Reutilisationsstoffwechsel wesentlich weniger Energie benötigt als die *de novo*-Purinsynthese.

Literatur

ABRAHAMSON, L., HAMBRAEUS, L., HOFVANDER, Y., VAHLQUIST, B.: Single cell protein in clinical testing. A tolerance test in healthy adult subjects comprising biochemical, clinical and dietary evaluation. Nutr. Metabolism **13**, 186—199 (1971).

BAUER, W., SINGH, M. M.: Management of gout. New Engl. J. Med. **256**, 171—214 (1957).

BENDICK, A., GETLER, H., BROWN, G. B.: A synthesis of isotopic cytosin and a study of its metabolism in the rat. J. biol. Chem. **177**, 565—570 (1949).

BERLIN, R. D., HAWKINS, R. A.: Secretion of purines by the small intestine: general characteristics. Amer. J. Physiol. 215, 932—941 (1968).

BIEN, E. J., YÜ, T. F., BENEDICT, J. D., GUTMAN, A. B., STETTEN, D., JR.: The relation of dietary nitrogen consumption to the rate of uric acid synthesis in normal and gouty man. J. clin. Invest. 32, 778—780 (1953).

BOWERING, J., CALLOWAY, D. H., MARGEN, S., KAUFMANN, W. A.: Dietary Protein Level and Uric Acid Metabolism in Normal Man. J. Nutr. 100, 249—261 (1969).

BRUGSCH, T., SCHITTENHELM, .: Der Nuklein-Stoffwechsel. Seite 44, Jena 1910, zitiert nach THANNHAUSER und DORFMÜLLER.

BUCHANAN, J. M., SONNE, J. C., DELLUVA, A. M.: Biologic precursors of uric acid. II: The role of lactate, glycine and carbon dioxide as precursors of the carbon chain and nitrogen atom 7 of uric acid. J. biol. Chem. 173, 81—98 (1948).

BURIAN, R., SCHUR, H.: Über die Harnpurinausscheidung des Menschen. Pflügers Arch. ges. Physiol. 80, 241—343 (1900).

BURIAN, R., SCHUR, H.: Über die Stellung der Purinkörper im menschlichen Stoffwechsel. Pflügers Arch. ges. Physiol. 87, 239—354 (1901).

BURIAN, R., SCHUR, H.: Das quantitative Verhalten der menschlichen Harnpurinausscheidung. Pflügers Arch. ges. Physiol. 94, 273—336 (1903).

CASKEY, C. T., ASHTON, D. M., WYNGAARDEN, J. B.: The enzymology of feedback inhibition of glutamine phosphoribosylpyrophosphate amidotransferase by purine ribonucleosides. J. biol. Chem. 239, 2570—2579 (1964).

DRUBE, C.-H., REINWEIN, H.: Zur Klinik der Gicht, „der vergessenen Krankheit". Med. Klin. 14, 631—636 (1959).

EWART, W.: Gout and Goutiness and their Treatment. London: Baillière, Tindall & Cox 1896.

FONTENELLE, L. J., HENDERSON, J. F.: An enzymatic basis for the inability of erythrocytes to synthesize purine ribonucleotides de novo. Biochim. biophys. Acta (Amst.) 177, 175—176 (1969).

FRIEDKIN, M.: Enzymatic synthesis of desoxyxanthosine phosphorylase in mammalian tissue. J. Amer. chem. Soc. 74, 112 (1952).

GAIRDNER, W.: On Gout, Its History, Its Causes and Its Cure. 3rd ed. London: Churchill 1854.

GEREN, W., BENDICK, A., BODANSKY, O., BROWN, G. B.: Fate of uric acid in man. J. biol. Chem. 183, 21—31 (1950).

GERTLER, H., ROLL, P. M., TINKER, J. F., BROWN, G. B.: A study of the metabolism of dietary hypoxanthine and xanthine in the rat. J. biol. Chem. 178, 259—264 (1949).

GOLDTHWAIT, D. A., PEABODY, R. A., GREENBERG, G. R.: On the mechanism of synthesis of glycinamideribotide and its formyl derivative. J. biol. Chem. 221, 569—577 (1956).

GRAFE, E.: Die Gicht. Dtsch. med. Wschr. 78, 867—871 (1953).

GRIEBSCH, A., ZÖLLNER, N.: Verhalten der Harnsäurespiegel im Plasma unter dosierter Zufuhr von Nucleinsäuren. Verh. dtsch. Ges. inn. Med. 76, 849—853 (1970a).

GRIEBSCH, A., ZÖLLNER, N.: Über die dosisabhängige Wirkung oral verabreichter DNA und RNA auf Harnsäurespiegel und Harnsäureausscheidung des Gesunden und des Hyperurikämikers. Hoppe-Seylers Z. physiol. Chem. 351, 1297—1298 (1970b).

GRIEBSCH, A., ZÖLLNER, N.: Harnsäure-Plasmaspiegel und renale Harnsäureausscheidung bei Belastung mit Algen, einer purinreichen Eiweißquelle. Verh. dtsch. Ges. inn. Med. 77, 173—177 (1971).

GRIEBSCH, A., ZÖLLNER, N.: Normalwerte der Plasmaharnsäure in Süddeutschland. Vergleich mit Bestimmungen vor zehn Jahren. Z. Klin. Chem. Klin. Biochem. 11, 346—356 (1973).

GRIEBSCH, A., ZÖLLNER, N.: Effect of Ribonucleotides Given orally on Uric Acid Production in Man. Int. sympos. on purine metabolism in man, Tel Aviv, June 17—22th 1973. In: SPERLING, O., DE VRIES, A., WYNGAARDEN, J. B. (Eds.): Advanc. in Exper. Med., Vol. 41 B, pp. 443—449. New York: Plenum Press 1974.

GUTMAN, A. B., YU, T. F.: Current Principles of Management in Gout. Amer. J. Med. 13, 744—759 (1952).

GUTMAN, A. B., YU, T. F., BERGER, L.: Tubular secretion of urate in man. J. clin. Invest. 38, 1778—1781 (1959).

HAMMARSTEN, E., REICHARD, P., SALUSTE, E.: Pyrimidine nucleosides as precursors of pyrimidines in polynucleotides. J. biol. Chem. 183, 105—109 (1950).

HEINRICH, M. R., WILSON, D. W.: Biosynthesis of nucleic acid components studied with C^{14}. I. Purines and pyrimidines in the rat. J. biol. Chem. 186, 447—460 (1950).

HENDERSON, J. F., LE PAGE, G. A.: Utilization of host purines by transplanted tumors. Cancer Res. 19, 67—71 (1959).

Heppel, L. A., Hilmoe, R. J.: Purification and properties of 5-nucleosidase. J. biol. Chem. **188**, 665—676 (1951).

Hippokrates: De affect. int. lib. VII; Aphorism. VI.

Huennekens, F. M., Nurk, E., Gabrio, B. W.: Erythrocyte metabolism. I. Purine nucleoside phosphorylase. J. biol. Chem. **221**, 971—980 (1956).

Kalckar, H. M.: The enzymatic synthesis of purine ribosides. J. biol. Chem. **167**, 477 (1947a).

Kalckar, H. M.: Differential spectrophotometry of purine compounds by means of specific enzymes. III. Studies of the enzymes of purine metabolism. J. biol. Chem. **167**, 461 (1947b).

Karlson, J. L., Barker, H. A.: Biosynthesis of uric acid labeled with radioactive carbon. J. biol. Chem. **177**, 597 (1949).

Korn, E. D., Buchanan, J. M.: Biosynthesis of the purines. VI. Purification of liver nucleoside phosphorylase and demonstration of nucleoside synthesis from 4-amino-^{5}-imidazole-carboxamide, adenine, and 2,6-diaminopurine. J. biol. Chem. **217**, 183 (1955).

Laiytha, L. G., Vane, J. R.: Dependence of bone marrow cells on the liver for purine supply. Nature (London) **182**, 191—192 (1958).

Levenberg, B., Hartman, S. C., Buchanan, J. M.: Biosynthesis of the purines. X. Further studies in vitro on the metabolic origin of nitrogen atoms 1 and 3 of the purine ring. J. biol. Chem. **220**, 379 (1956).

Lowy, B. A., Williams, M. K.: The presence of a limiteal portion of the pathway de novo of purine nucleotide biosynthesis in the rabbit erythrocyte in vitro. J. biol. Chem. **235**, 2924—2927 (1960).

Mayer, J., Hershko, A., Zeitlin-Beck, R., Shoshani, T., Razin, A.: Turnover of purine nucleotides in rabbit erythrocytes. I. Studies in vivo. Biochim. biophys. Acta (Amst.) **149**, 50—58 (1967).

Mendel, L. B., Myers, V. C.: The metabolism of some pyrimidine derivatives. Amer. J. Physiol. **26**, 77—105 (1910).

Nikiforuk, G., Colowick, S. P.: The purification and properties of 5-adenylic acid deaminase from muscle. J. biol. Chem. **219** 119 (1956).

Nugent, C. A., Tyler, F. H.: The renal excretion of uric acid in patients with gout and in nongouty subjects. J. clin. Invest. **39**, 1890—1898 (1959).

Nugent, C. A., Mac Diarmid, W. D., Tyler, F. H.: Renal excretion of Urate in Patients with Gout. Arch. intern. Med. **113**, 115—121 (1964).

Plentl, A., Schoenheimer, R.: Studies in the metabolism of purines and pyrimidines by means of isotopic nitrogen. J. biol. Chem. **153**, 203—217 (1944).

Pritchard, J. B., Chavez-Peon, F., Berlin, R. D.: Purines: supply by liver to tissues. Amer. J. Physiol. **219**, 1263—1268 (1970).

Roll, P. M., Brown, G. B., Di Carlo, F. J., Schultz, A. S.: The metabolism of yeast nucleic acid in the rat. J. biol. Chem. **180**, 333—340 (1949).

Rosenbloom, F. M., Kelley, W. N., Miller, J., Henderson, J. F., Seegmiller, J. B.: Inherited disorders of purine metabolism: Correlation between central nervous system dysfunction and biochemical defects. J. Amer. med. Ass. **202**, 103—106 (1967).

Saunders, D. R., Beck, M.: Permeability of the human small intestine to uric acid. Biochim. biophys. Acta (Amst.) **102**, 618—620 (1965).

Schanker, L. S., Tocco, D. J.: Active transport of some pyrimidines across the rat intestinal epithelium. J. Pharmacol. exp. Ther. **128**, 115—121 (1960).

Schanker, L. S., Tocco, D. J.: Some characteristics of the pyrimidine transport process of the small intestine. Biochim. biophys. Acta (Amst.) **56**, 469—473 (1962).

Schmidt, G.: Nucleases and enzymes attacking nucleic acid component. In: Chargaff, Davidson, J. N. (Eds.): The Nucleic Acids, vol. 1. New York: Academic Press 1955.

Scott, J. L.: Human leucocyte metabolism in vitro. I. Incorporation of adenine-8-^{14}C and formate-^{14}C into the nucleic acid of leucemic leucocytes. J. clin. Invest. **41**, 67—79 (1962).

Scudamore, G.: A Treatise of the Nature and Course of Gout. 4th ed. London: Marlett 1823.

Seegmiller, J. E., Grayzel, A. I., Laster, L., Liddle, L.: Uric acid production in gout. J. clin. Invest. **40**, 1304—1314 (1961).

Seegmiller, J. E., Grayzel, A. I., Howell, R. R., Plato, C.: The renal excretion of uric acid in gout. J. clin. Invest. **41**, 1094—1098 (1962).

Seegmiller, J. E., Klinenberg, J. R., Miller, J., Watts, R. W. E.: Suppression of glycine-^{15}N incorporation into urinary auric acid by adenine-8-^{13}C in normal and gouty subjects. J. clin. Invest. **47**, 1193—1203 (1968).

Shemin, D., Rittenberg, D.: On the utilisation of glycine for uric acid synthesis in man. J. biol. Chem. **167**, 875 (1947).

Sivén, V. O.: Zur Kenntnis der Harnsäurebildung im menschlichen Organismus. Scand. Arch. Physiol. **11**, 134—150 (1900).
Smellie, R. M. S., Thomson, R. Y., Davidson, J. N.: The nucleic acid metabolism of animal cells in vitro. I. The incorporation of ^{14}C-formate. Biochim. biophys. Acta (Amst.) **29**, 59—74 (1958).
Smyth, C. J.: Current therapy of gout. J. Amer. med. Ass. **152**, 1106 (1953).
Sonne, J. C., Buchanan, J. M., Delluva, A. M.: Biological precursors of uric acid. I. The role of lactate, acetate and formate in synthesis of the urcido groups of uric acid. J. biol. Chem. **173**, 69 (1948).
Sonne, J. C., Lin, I., Buchanan, J. M.: Biosynthesis of the purines. IX. Precursors of the nitrogen atoms of the purine ring. J. biol. Chem. **220**, 369 (1956).
Sorensen, L. B.: Degradation of uric acid in man. Metabolism **8**, 687—703 (1959).
Sorensen, L. B.: Elimination of uric acid in man studied by means of ^{14}C-labelled uric acid. Scand. J. clin. Lab. Invest. **12**, Suppl. 54, 1—214 (1960).
Talbott, J. H., Coombs, F. S.: Concentration of serum uric acid in non-affected members of gouty families. J. clin. Invest. **17**, 508 (1938).
Thannhauser, S. J.: Über die Pathogenese der Gicht. Dtsch. med. Wschr. **81**, 492—496 (1956).
Thannhauser, S. J., Dorfmüller, G.: Experimentelle Studien über den Nuclein-Stoffwechsel. 5. Mitteilung. Über die Aufspaltung des Purinringes durch die Bakterien der menschlichen Darmflora. Hoppe-Seylers Z. physiol. Chem. **102**, 148—159 (1918).
Waslien, C. I., Calloway, D. H., Margen, S.: Uric acid Production of Men Fed Graded Amounts of Egg Protein and Yeast Nucleic Acid. Amer. J. clin. Nutr. **21**, 892—897 (1968).
Waslien, C. I., Calloway, D. H., Margen, S., Costa, F.: Uric acid levels in men fed algae and yeast as protein sources. J. Food Sci. **35**, 294—298 (1970).
Weissmann, B., Bromberg, P. A., Gutman, G. B.: The purine bases of human urine. II. Semiquantitative estimation and isotope incorporation. J. biol. Chem. **224**, 423—434 (1957).
Wilson, D., Beyer, A., Bishop, C., Talbott, J. H.: Urinary uric acid excretion after the ingestion of isotopic yeast nucleic acid in the normal and gouty human. J. biol. Chem. **209**, 227—232 (1954).
Wilson, D. W., Wilson, H. C.: Studies in vitro of the digestion and absorption of purine ribonucleotides by the intestine. J. biol. Chem. **237**, 1643—1647 (1962).
Wilson, T. H., Wilson, D. W.: Studies in vitro of digestion and absorption of pyrimidine nucleotides by the intestine. J. biol. Chem. **233**, 1544—1547 (1958).
Wilson, T. H.: Intestinal Absorption. Philadelphia: Saunders 1962.
Wyngaarden, J. B., Seegmiller, J. E., Laster, L., Blair, A. E.: Utilization of hypoxanthine, adenine and 4-amino-5-imidazole carboxamide for uric acid synthesis in man. Metabolism **8**, 455—464 (1959).
Zöllner, N.: Moderne Gichtprobleme. Ätiologie, Pathogenese, Klinik. Ergebn. inn. Med. Kinderheilk. (N. F.) **14**, 321—389 (1960).
Zöllner, N.: The renal excretion of uric acid. 5th Symp. Ges. f. Nephrol. Lausanne 1967. In: Peters, G., Roch-Ramel, S. (Eds.): Progress in Nephrology. Berlin-Heidelberg-New York: Springer 1969.
Zöllner, N., Griebsch, A., Gröbner, W.: Einfluß verschiedener Purine auf den Harnsäure-Stoffwechsel. Ernährungs-Umschau **3**, 79—82 (1972).

c) Harnsäureabbau im menschlichen Organismus

Von

W. Kaiser

Während sich in der evolutionären Entwicklung bis zu den Menschen die Stoffwechselwege des Purinaufbaus kaum änderten, traten im Abbau mehrmals aufeinander folgende Verluste an Enzymen des Purinkatabolismus auf, so daß jeweils verschiedene Endprodukte im Stoffwechsel des Stickstoffs auftreten konnten. Dies geschah vermutlich als Notwendigkeit, um in einer sich ändernden Umgebung zu überleben. Die Gründe zum Abbau der Purine vor ihrer Exkretion sind erstens die Energieeinsparung des Organismus — denn durch die weitere Oxydation zu H_2O und CO_2 wird Energie gewonnen — und zweitens die Umwandlung zu relativ leicht auszuscheidenden Endprodukten.

Die niedrigeren Lebensformen besitzen die komplette Enzymausstattung zum vollständigen Abbau der Purine. Je höher die phylogenetische Entwicklung, desto mangelhafter wird — eigentlich entgegen der Erwartung — die Fähigkeit zum Abbau. So sind die Bakterien noch mit dem vollen Enzymsystem ausgestattet (Uricase, Allantoinase, Allantoicase und Urease), so daß bei ihnen als letzte Endprodukte des Purinstoffwechsels NH_3 und CO_2 entstehen. Die Urease ging in der frühen Entwicklung der Wirbeltiere verloren, damit tritt Harnstoff als Endprodukt des Purinstoffwechsels auf. Die Amphibien waren die ersten Landtiere, und bei ihnen ist die Ausscheidung von Harnstoff als Anpassung an das Landleben anzusehen. NH_3 ist als Stickstoffendprodukt leicht in H_2O löslich, für Landtiere aber zu toxisch. Im Laufe der Evolution verwendeten deshalb verschiedene Tiergruppen auf dem Land anstatt NH_3 unterschiedliche Entgiftungsprodukte. Im Verlauf der Entwicklung der Anthropoiden ging die Uricase verloren, damit tritt die Harnsäure als Endprodukt des Purinstoffwechsels auf. Der Verlust der Uricase brachte für den Menschen die Gefahren der Hyperuricämie. Der große Vorteil der Harnsäure für Landtiere ist ihre geringe Löslichkeit, denn damit kann sie beinahe ohne Wasserverlust ausgeschieden werden. Eine geringere Wasserausscheidung mit dem Urin führt lediglich zur Kristallisation der Harnsäure und ihrer Exkretion als fester Bestandteil. Diese relative Unabhängigkeit von Wasser hat jedoch einen Nachteil, nämlich die Präcipitation der Harnsäure infolge ihrer Unlöslichkeit an unerwünschten Stellen im Organismus, z.B. in der Niere und in den Gelenken.

Lange Zeit wurde vermutet, daß die Harnsäure im menschlichen Organismus das einzige Endprodukt des Purinstoffwechsels darstellt, da weder Uricase noch eine wesentliche uricolytische Aktivität in menschlichen Geweben (ENZO, 1946; JONES, 1920; RO, 1931—32) festgestellt werden konnte. Die ersten Untersuchungen zum Ausmaß der Wiederfindung von Harnsäure im Urin nach intravenöser Injektion waren widersprüchlich. SOETBEER und IBRAHIM (1902) gaben eine vollständige Wiederfindung an, während FOLIN et al. (1924) und KOEHLER (1924) im Durchschnitt nur etwa 50% im Urin wiederfinden konnten. Die mit der Einführung der Isotopentechniken möglich gewordene bessere Quantifizierung der renalen Harnsäureausscheidung nach intravenöser Injektion ergab Wiederfindungswerte für die markierte Harnsäure (^{15}N-Harnsäure oder 2-^{14}C-Harnsäure) zwischen etwa 66 und 75% (BUZARD et al., 1952; SORENSEN, 1959, 1960; WYNGAARDEN, 1955). Diese Ergebnisse sprachen für die Beteiligung eines zusätzlichen extrarenalen Abbau- oder Ausscheidungsweges der Harnsäure. Darüber hinaus fehlte in allen Bilanzuntersuchungen die Übereinstimmung zwischen dem täglichen Harnsäure-Turnover und der täglichen renalen Harnsäureausscheidung. Die Menge der täglich synthetisierten Harnsäure übertraf die im Urin erscheinende Harnsäuremenge. Die Ergebnisse von BENEDICT et al. (1949), die nach intravenöser Injektion von 1,3-^{15}N-Harnsäure signifikante Konzentrationen von ^{15}N im Harnstoff und NH_3 des Urins fanden, wiesen erstmals darauf hin, daß ein Teil der Harnsäure einem weiteren katalytischen Abbau unterzogen sein muß. Bei quantitativer Bestimmung dieses Abbaus nach intravenöser Injektion von markierter Harnsäure (BUZARD et al., 1952; WYNGAARDEN u. STETTEN, 1953) ließen sich etwa 25% des verabreichten Isotops als Allantoin, Harnstoff und NH_3 im Urin sowie im Stickstoff der Faeces nachweisen. Nach intravenöser Injektion von 2-^{14}C-Harnsäure konnte SORENSEN (1959) im Urin einen Einbau in Harnstoff, Allantoin und Allantoinsäure sowie einen Einbau in die Faeces finden, ein Teil des Isotops erschien sogar als CO_2 in der Ausatmungsluft. Es mußte also auch bei den Menschen ein Teil der Harnsäure durch Uricase, Allantoinase, Allantoicase und Urease bis zu den einfachsten Endprodukten CO_2 und NH_3 abgebaut werden. Nach oraler Verabreichung von ^{15}N-Harnsäure fanden GEREN et al. (1950), daß nur 9—11% der verabreichten Harnsäure absorbiert und als solche unverändert im Urin ausgeschieden wurde, während 47% des ^{15}N innerhalb von 3 Tagen als Harnstoff im Urin erschien. Der hochgradige Abbau von oral verabreichter Harnsäure konnte von SORENSEN (1959) mit 2-^{14}C-Harnsäure an einer Normalperson bestätigt werden. Die Bestimmung des ^{14}C-Einbaus in die Abbauprodukte der Harnsäure ergab eine Absorption und unveränderte renale Exkretion von 11,1% innerhalb von 6 Tagen, 13,9% des verabreichten ^{14}C konnten in verschiedenen Urinbestandteilen (Allantoin und Harnstoff) nachgewiesen werden, 55% ^{14}C wurde über die Lungen als CO_2 in die Ausatmungsluft, 16,3% ^{14}C wurde über die Faeces ausgeschieden, davon 83—91% innerhalb der intestinalen Bakterien. Daraus konnte geschlossen werden, daß der Abbau von oral verabreichter Harnsäure in Zusammenhang mit ihrer Darmpassage zu bringen ist. Die intestinalen Bakterien konnten als verantwortlich für die Uricolyse, die zur Bildung von CO_2 und NH_3 über die Zwischenprodukte Allantoin, Allantoinsäure und Harnstoff führt, angesehen werden, da sie die Enzymausstattung zum kompletten Harnsäureabbau besitzen. Ein geringer Anteil der Zwischenprodukte des Abbaus wird vermutlich im Darm absorbiert und als solche im Urin ausgeschieden, während der Hauptanteil der Harnsäure zu CO_2 und NH_3 abgebaut wird. Ein Teil des entstandenen CO_2 wird von den Bakterien in ihrem Stoffwechsel weiterverwendet, der andere Teil absorbiert und über die Lungen ausgeatmet.

Zur weiteren Sicherung der Wirkung einer intestinalen Uricolyse durch Bakterien beim Menschen führte SORENSEN (1959) mit Sulfonamiden, Streptomycin und Neomycin eine weitgehende Bacteriostase im Darm einer Normalperson durch und bestimmte den Abbau intravenös verabreichter ^{14}C-Harnsäure vor und nach dieser antibiotischen Therapie. Dabei wurde bei intakter intestinaler Flora 22,5% des verabreichten ^{14}C in den verschiedenen Abbauprodukten gefunden, nach intestinaler Bacteriostase fiel der Prozentsatz auf nur 3% ab. Während also wenig Zweifel an der intestinalen Uricolyse von Harnsäure nach oraler Verabreichung bestehen konnte, war es weiterhin fraglich, ob der signifikante Harnsäureabbau nach intravenös injizierter Harnsäure allein im Intestinaltrakt oder in irgendeinem anderen Teil des Körpers stattfindet. Auch war zu klären, ob der gesamte Anteil von etwa 25—40% der Harnsäure, der täglich extrarenal beseitigt wird, durch Exkretion in den Verdauungstrakt mit nachfolgendem Abbau erklärt werden konnte. Nach den Untersuchungen von SORENSEN (1959) ist die Harnsäuremenge, die in den Intestinaltrakt ausgeschieden wird, größer als allgemein angenommen wurde. So bestimmte er die Ausscheidung von Harnsäure mit dem Speichel, dem Magensaft und der Galleflüssigkeit bei Normalpersonen auf 100 mg oder mehr. Eine ähnlich große Menge soll in der Pankreas- und Dünndarmflüssigkeit enthalten sein. Das würde bedeuten, daß etwa ein Drittel der gesamten Harnsäuremenge bei Normalpersonen auf dem extrarenalen Wege über den Darmtrakt eliminiert und abgebaut werden könnte.

Neben dieser quantitativ recht bedeutenden intestinalen Uricolyse durch Darmbakterien scheint aber noch ein Abbau von Harnsäure innerhalb des menschlichen Gewebes vorzukommen. BIEN u. ZUCKER fanden 1955 während der Inkubation von Leukozyten und Erythrozyten mit Harnsäure einen Harnsäureabbau und führten dies auf die Wirkung der in diesen Zellen nachzuweisenden Peroxydase und der Cytochrom-Oxydase der Erythrocyten zurück. Bei diesen beiden Enzymsystemen konnte nämlich *in vitro* bei physiologischem pH eine langsam stattfindende Oxydation von Harnsäure beobachtet werden (GRIFFITHS, 1952; HOWELL u. SEEGMILLER, 1962; TUTTLE u. COHEN, 1953). Die uricolytische Aktivität scheint besonders in den Zellen der myeloischen Reihe und hier in der Myeloperoxydase lokalisiert zu sein (RATTI, 1958). Der Abbau zu Allantoin und CO_2 von 6-^{14}C-Mononatriumurat durch Leukozyten war in der kristallinen Form größer als bei einer Harnsäurelösung. Nach den Untersuchungen von SORENSEN (1959) an verschiedenen post mortem entnommenen menschlichen Geweben scheint dieser Harnsäureabbau beim Menschen quantitativ jedoch minimal zu sein. WYNGAARDEN (1960) berechnete als maximale Uricolyse innerhalb menschlichen Gewebes etwa 2—4% des Harnsäure-Turnovers. Eine signifikante Korrelation zwischen dem Peroxydasegehalt und der Harnsäurekonzentration im Serum ließ sich nicht nachweisen (VORMITTAG *et al.*, 1971).

Verständlicherweise wurde nach dem Bekanntwerden dieses signifikanten extrarenalen Eliminationsmechanismus auch daran gedacht, daß eine Verminderung im Abbau der Harnsäure eine der Ursachen zur Entwicklung der Hyperuricämie sein könnte (FOLIN *et al.*, 1924; VILLA *et al.*, 1958). Auf Grund der wenigen hierzu vorliegenden Untersuchungen scheint es jedoch so zu sein, daß bei Patienten mit erhöhten Harnsäurespiegeln die extrarenale Elimination bzw. intestinale Uricolyse eher höher ist (SORENSEN, 1959). Die Wiederfindungsquote von intravenös injizierter, nicht markierter oder radioaktiv markierter Harnsäure im Urin war im Durchschnitt bei Gichtpatienten niedriger als bei Normalpersonen (FOLIN, 1924; KOEHLER, 1924; SORENSEN, 1959). Auch konnten POLLYCOVE *et al.* (1957) bei Patienten mit Hyperuricämie nach der Verabreichung von ^{14}C-Harnsäure im Vergleich zu Normalpersonen mehr $^{14}CO_2$ in der Ausatmungsluft nachweisen. Die Beobachtung von SORENSEN (1959), daß die Exkretion von Harnsäure z. B. mit dem Speichel bei Patienten mit Hyperuricämie höher ist als bei Personen mit normalen Harnsäurewerten, würde über die vermehrte Ausscheidung in den Darm auch eine vermehrte intestinale Uricolyse bei Hyperuricämie erklären können. Es ist also auf Grund dieser Befunde kaum wahrscheinlich, daß als eine der Ursachen für eine Hyperuricämie ein verminderter Harnsäureabbau anzunehmen wäre.

Literatur

BENEDICT, J. D., FORSHAM, P. H., STETTEN, DE W., JR.: The metabolism of uric acid in the normal and gouty human studied with the aid of isotopic uric acid. J. biol. Chem. **181**, 183 (1949).

BIEN, E., ZUCKER, H.: Uricolysis in normal and gouty individuals. Ann. rheum. Dis. **14**, 409 (1955).

BUZARD, J., BISHOP, C., TALBOTT, I. H.: Recovery in humans of intravenously injected isotopic uric acid. J. biol. Chem. **196**, 179 (1952).

BUZARD, J., BISHOP, C., TALBOTT, I. H.: The fate of uric acid in the normal and gouty human. J. chron. Dis. **2**, 42 (1955).

ENZO, L.: Proprietà dell' uricasi e uricolisi vel fegato umane. Boll. Soc. ital. Biol. sper. **22**, 556 (1946).

FOLIN, O., BERGLUND, H., DERICK, C.: The uric acid problem: An experimental study on animals and man, including gouty subjects. J. biol. Chem. **60**, 361 (1924).

GEREN, W., BENDICH, A., BODANSKY, O., BROWN, G. B.: Fate of uric acid in man. J. biol. Chem. **183**, 21 (1950).

GRIFFITHS, M.: Oxidation of uric acid catalyzed by copper and by the cytochrome-cytochrome oxidase system. J. biol. Chem. **197**, 399 (1952).

HOWELL, R. R., SEEGMILLER, J. E.: Uricolysis by human leukocytes. Nature (Lond.) **196**, 482 (1962).

JONES, W.: Nucleic acids. Their Chemical Properties and Physiological Conduct (Ed. 2). New York: Longmans 1920.

KOEHLER, A. E.: Uric acid excretion. J. biol. Chem. **60**, 621 (1924).

POLLYCOVE, M., TOLBERT, B. M., LAWRENCE, J. H., HARMAN, D.: Uric acid metabolism: The oxidation of uric acid in normal subjects and patients with gout, polycythemia and leukemia. Clin. Res. Proc. **5**, 38 (1957).
RATTI, G.: Sull esistenza di una attivita, uricolitica nell'uomo. Reumatismo **10**, suppl. 2, 33 (1958).
RO, K.: Über die Urikase. J. Biochem. **14**, 361 (1931—32).
SOETBEER, F., IBRAHIM, J.: Über das Schicksal eingeführter Harnsäure im menschlichen Organismus. Hoppe-Seyler's Z. physiol. Chem. **35**, 1 (1902).
SORENSEN, L. B.: Degradation of uric acid in man. Metabolism **8**, 687 (1959).
SORENSEN, L. B.: The elimination of uric acid in man studied by means of ^{14}C-labeled uric acid. Scand. J. clin. Lab. Invest. **12**, suppl. 54 (1960).
TUTTLE, A. L., COHEN, P. P.: Enzymatic oxidation of uric acid. Fed. Proc. **12**, 281 (1953).
VILLA, L., ROBECCHI, A., BALLABIO, C. B.: Physiopathology, clinical manifestations and treatment of gout. Part I. Ann. rheum. Dis. **17**, 9 (1958).
VORMITTAG, W., THUMB, N., PIETSCHMANN, H.: Peroxydasegehalt der Granulozyten des peripheren Blutes bei Arthritis urica. Z. Rheumaforsch. **30**, 119 (1971).
WYNGAARDEN, J. B.: The effect of phenylbutazone on uric acid metabolism in two normal subjects. J. clin. Invest. **34**, 256 (1955).
WYNGAARDEN, J. B.: Gout. In Metabolic Basis of Inherited Disease. (1st Ed., Ed. STANBURY, J. B., WYNGAARDEN, J. B., FREDRICKSON, D. S.), p. 679. New York: McGraw-Hill 1960.
WYNGAARDEN, J. B., STETTEN, D., JR.: Uricolysis in normal man. J. biol. Chem. **203**, 9 (1953).

d) Excretion of Uric Acid in Health and in Disease

By

L. B. SORENSEN

With 6 Figures

In normal man uric acid is excreted chiefly by way of the kidney. A smaller, but nevertheless appreciable proportion of uric acid is excreted in digestive juices into the gut. Less than one percent of all uric acid is excreted in the sweat.

Renal Excretion of Uric Acid

Normal Values for Renal Excretion of Uric Acid

The average urinary uric acid excretion in normal men on a purine-free diet is about 400 mg/24 hrs. An enzymatic spectrophotometric method revealed endogenous uric acid excretion of 401 ± 42 mg in 53 men and 321 ± 34 mg in 18 women (CRONE and LASSEN, 1956).

The renal clearance expresses the rate at which the kidneys excrete uric acid relative to the concentration of uric acid in the plasma:

$C_{ur} = U_{ur} V / P_{ur}$

where C_{ur} is ml plasma cleared of uric acid per minute, U_{ur} is mg uric acid per ml urine, V is ml urine excreted per minute, and P_{ur} is mg uric acid per ml plasma. It should be appreciated that C_{ur} is a variable parameter in the same person since $U_{ur} V$ is dependent on P_{ur} in a nonlinear fashion. In one large series, C_{ur} averaged 8.7 ± 2.5 ml per minute in normal men (GUTMAN and YU, 1957).

Isotope studies of the miscible pool of uric acid and its daily turnover have shown a fairly consistent discrepancy between the amount of uric acid calculated to be produced per day and the amount of uric acid actually found in the urine. Furthermore, only between two-thirds and three-fourths of intravenously injected

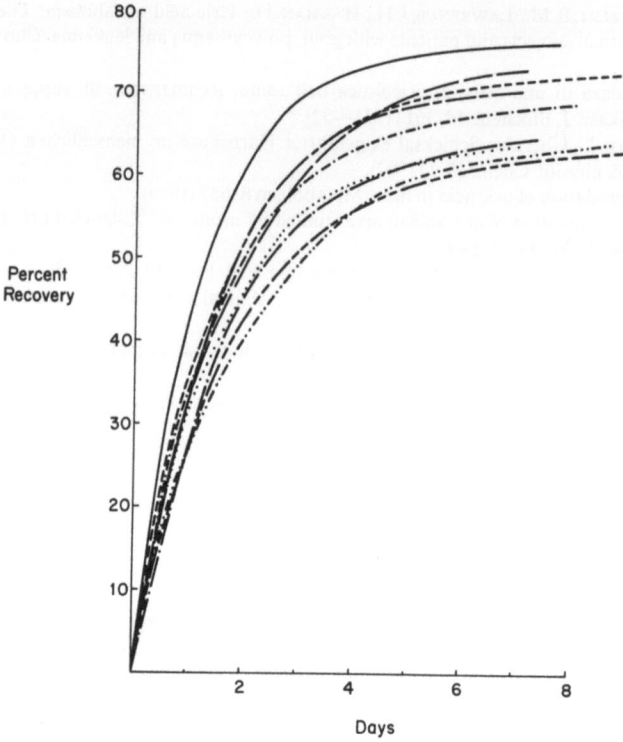

Fig. 1. Cumulative recovery from urine of ^{14}C-uric acid administered intravenously to nine nongouty subjects without overt renal disease

isotopically labeled uric acid could be recovered in the urine (Fig. 1). Nine nongouty subjects without overt renal disease excreted an average of 67.8% of injected ^{14}C-uric acid in the urine.

Normal Mechanism of Renal Excretion of Urate in Man

Until 1960 the traditional view was that uric acid is completely filtrable at the glomerulus and that all but 5 to 10% of filtered uric acid is reabsorbed in the renal tubules. With the demonstration of renal tubular secretion of urate in man (PRAETORIUS and KIRK, 1950; GUTMAN et al., 1959) this view was revised, and it is now believed that filtered urate is virtually completely reabsorbed in the proximal tubules and that the urate which appears in the final urine gains access almost entirely by a tubular secretory process. Below we shall discuss the individual parts of a "three-component mechanism" for uric acid excretion.

Filtration through the Glomeruli. Whether plasma urate is or is not completely filtrable through the glomerular membrane has been a subject of discussion for many years. A number of studies indicated that urate is freely filtrable at the glomerulus (YU and GUTMAN, 1953; LATHEM and RODNAN, 1962) while others showed evidence for protein binding of urate (MORRIS, 1958; SHINABERGER et al., 1964). Recently ALVSAKER (1966), using the techniques of gel filtration and immunoelectrophoresis, demonstrated a reversible interaction between urate and albumin, low-density β-lipoprotein, β_2-macroglobulin and α_1-α_2-globulin. Special interest has centered on the urate-binding capacity of an α_1-α_2-globulin, which was

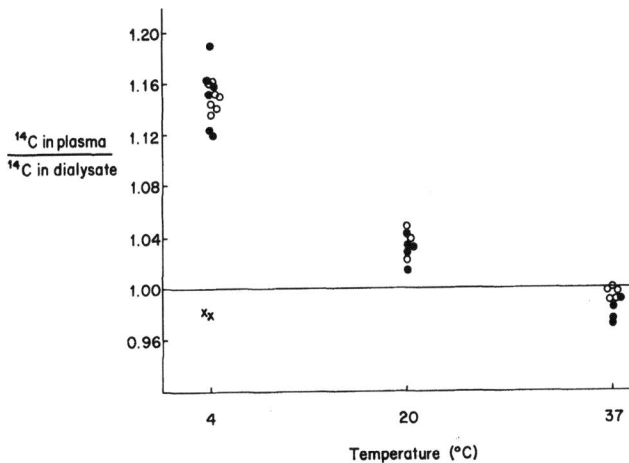

Fig. 2. Effect of temperature on urate binding to plasma proteins. The concentration of uric acid in the dialysate ranged from 2.4 to 25 mg/100 ml. Open circles, normal men; closed circles, gouty subjects; x indicates absence of binding of ^{14}C-labeled allantoin, the oxidation product of uric acid. No correction was made for possible Gibbs-Donnan effects

claimed to serve as a specific transport protein for uric acid and was found to be deficient in gouty individuals belonging to two kindreds (ALVSAKER, 1968). The existence of a specific urate binding globulin could not be confirmed in another laboratory (KLINENBERG and KIPPEN, 1970). The most recent studies (SHEIKH and MØLLER, 1968; KLINENBERG and KIPPEN, 1970) showed binding of urate to plasma proteins at 4° C. This binding, however, was markedly reduced with increasing temperature. Results obtained in our laboratory are entirely consistent with these observations. We have studied the binding of ^{14}C-urate to proteins in normal and gouty serum and plasma at different temperatures by equilibrium dialysis using plexiglass cells with a capacity of 1 ml. The effect of temperature upon binding is clearly demonstrated (Fig. 2). Plasma from normal persons and gouty subjects has similar binding characteristics. Varying the concentration of uric acid in the dialysate from 2.4 to 25 mg/100 ml did not alter the ^{14}C ratio between plasma and dialysate, indicating that absolute binding of urate is proportional to the concentration of uric acid and that within the concentration range studied a saturation limit was not reached. The marked reduction of binding at 37° C supports the view that *in vivo* binding of urate is likely to be very small and of no physiologic significance. Binding of urate to plasma proteins is therefore not a factor affecting the renal clearance of urate.

Tubular Reabsorption of Urate. Since the rate of urate excretion normally is only 8 to 10% of the amount filtered by the glomeruli, it follows that reabsorption is the predominant transfer operation within the tubules. Uric acid may be present in the urine in a lower concentration than in plasma, indicating that the tubules have reabsorbed it against a concentration gradient, a process that requires expenditure of energy. BERLINER *et al.* (1950) measured the capacity of the renal tubules to reabsorb urate in normal subjects receiving sustained infusions of urate. They found that reabsorption of urate increased with rising concentration of urate in the glomerular filtrate until a maximum was reached which was of the order of 15 mg urate per minute. At the time, it was not appreciated that the tubules also secrete urate. The figure for the reabsorptive T_m is therefore an underestimate of the true reabsorptive T_m for uric acid; it indicates the net figure, also termed the apparent reabsorptive T_m for urate. The reabsorption capacity is so extensive that under physiological conditions it is never saturated. In the normal subject, therefore, T_m per se has no regulatory influence on the concentration of plasma urate or the excretion of uric acid.

The tubular reabsorption of urate in man is presumed to be accomplished in the proximal convolution. The limited capacity of the reabsorptive process, its inhibition by potent uricosuric drugs, and studies in mongrel dogs showing that urate reabsorption is inhibited by infusion of cyanide into the renal artery (ZINS and WEINER, 1968) all indicate that reabsorption of uric acid involves active transport.

Tubular Secretion of Urate. The mechanism of tubular secretion was proposed by GUTMAN and YU (1961) to explain the paradoxical response of the kidney to salicylate, probenecid, phenylbutazone, and other uricosuric drugs. When given in low doses these drugs caused decreased uric acid excretion and urate retention, whereas high doses of the same drugs produced uricosuria (YU and GUTMAN, 1955). These findings have been explained by postulating inhibition of renal tubular secretion of urate at low doses and of tubular reabsorption with larger amounts of drugs. Evidence for tubular secretion was reported as early as 1950 by PRAETORIUS and KIRK in an apparently healthy young man with hypouricemia, whose urate clearance exceeded his inulin clearance by 46%. Further evidence for tubular secretion was presented by GUTMAN et al. (1959), who observed urate clearance up to 23% above the glomerular filtration rate in patients with reduced renal function who were given infusions of urate and mannitol and treated with large doses of sulfinpyrazone in order to suppress tubular reabsorption. Reduction of the glomerular filtration rate by previous renal disease to values of 40—80 ml/min was a prerequisite for the demonstration of urate clearance above that of inulin. Tubular secretion of urate in mammals has been demonstrated in the Dalmatian Coach Hound (YU et al., 1960) and in the rabbit (POULSEN and PRAETORIUS, 1954).

Pyrazinoic acid or pyrazinamide in a dosage of 3 g virtually abolishes urate excretion in man (YU et al., 1957a). In the Dalmatian dog the effect of these drugs was shown by the stop-flow methods to be due to almost complete suppression of tubular secretion of urate (YU et al., 1961).

The nature of the secretory mechanism of urate in man is obscure. The original hypothesis on the bidirectional transport of urate assigned the secretory component to a more distal site than that occupied by the reabsorptive component (YU and GUTMAN, 1959), as is the case with potassium. Subsequent studies suggested that the secretory flux of urate is mediated by the carrier for the organic anion system (WEINER and MUDGE, 1964). The secretion of certain organic acids, which at proper dose levels decrease urate excretion in man, was localized to the proximal tubule by stop-flow studies in the dog, e.g. salicylate, chlorothiazide and phenylbutazone. Recently, evidence has been provided which indicates that both components of the bidirectional urate transport system are limited to the proximal tubule in dogs (MUDGE et al., 1968; ZINS and WEINER, 1968). Such direct evidence is not available in man and the location of the secretory component of urate excretion to the proximal tubule is admittedly inferential. The wide interspecific variations in terms of mode of urate excretion and drug response make it hazardous to assess urate excretion in man by analogy with the results obtained from experimental animals.

Renal Mechanism for Urate Homeostasis

The human kidney has a remarkable capacity for increasing the rate of urate excretion in the presence of even a modest degree of hyperuricemia, e.g. excessive ingestion of uric acid precursors usually leads to a significant increase in urinary uric acid excretion with only a small increase in the plasma urate concentration (BRØCHNER-MORTENSEN, 1939). It has already been pointed out that change in reabsorption of urate does not serve as a regulatory mechanism until marked hyperuricemia supervenes. A priori, it would appear more reasonable if urate should share the same secretory mechanism as certain other organic acids, e.g. para-aminohippurate; this would mean that the transport of urate from renal peritubular fluid to tubular lumen would increase as substrate availability increases, until a maximum is reached where intrinsic tubular factors might become rate-limiting.

The renal mechanism for urate homeostasis has been studied by STEELE and RIESELBACH (1967a) by observing the change in urinary excretion of urate following administration of pyrazinamide. Assuming that the decrement of uric acid during pyrazinamide suppression approximates the quantity secreted by the tubules and that the residual uric acid remaining in the urine corresponds to the filtered urate that has escaped tubular reabsorption, the two components of the bidirectional transport system can be analyzed. The transport system was further characterized by relating the rate of urate secretory and reabsorptive transport to plasma urate concentration. The normal degree of variation in bidirectional urate transport in response to a wide range of plasma urate concentrations was assessed in studies at endogenously and pharmacologically elevated or depressed plasma urate levels. In these studies, the filtered load of uric acid, as well as the rates of tubular reabsorption and secretion, was expressed per unit of glomerular filtration in order to correct for a possible loss in the functioning nephron population. Since tubular secretion of urate is probably not completely suppressed by pyrazinamide, the estimates obtained with this technique represent the minimal reabsorption and secretion at a given plasma urate level. It was found that urate reabsorption remained at an average of 98% of the filtered load at all plasma levels, thereby indicating progressive augmentation of reabsorptive transport velocity with increasing filtered loads. The tubular secretion per nephron increased significantly with increasing plasma urate concentration (Fig. 3). Thus, in normal man homeostasis is attained through an alteration of the secretory rate in response to changes in the plasma urate level. Neither a reabsorptive nor a secretory T_m was reached with the plasma uric acid concentrations used in these studies. Data on the secretory rate of urate within the range of plasma urate levels studied are compatible, however, with the kinetics of an enzyme system displaying a sigmoidal velocity-substrate relationship.

The effectiveness of secretory alteration in response to an increase in plasma urate is illustrated by studies of urate secretion in the remaining kidney of transplant donors after contralateral nephrectomy. Seven to ten days after nephrectomy, urate secretion in the remaining kidney had increased 74%, whereas the fractional reabsorption remained unchanged at 98% of the filtered load (SHELP and RIESELBACH, 1968).

In the foregoing studies, the suppression of uric acid secretion by pyrazinamide was measured in short-term clearance studies not extending beyond two to three hours after oral administration of pyrazinamide. We have obtained an even greater suppression of the tubular secretion of uric acid by determining the decrement in uric acid excretion in the 12 hrs period from 3 to 15 hrs after oral intake of

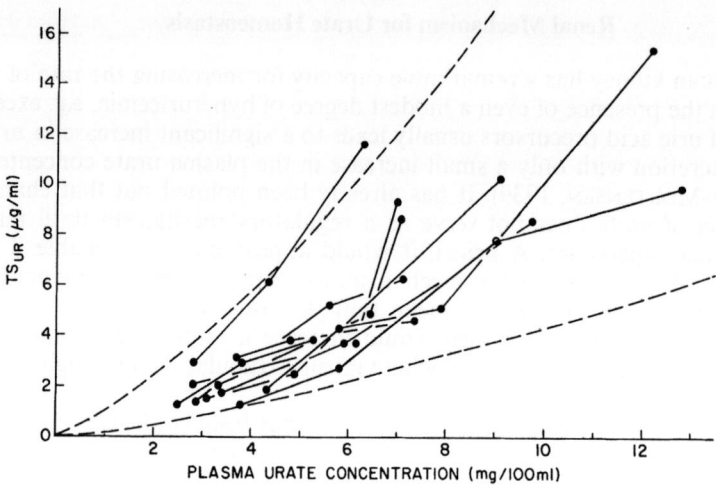

Fig. 3. Tubular secretion of urate (TS_{ur}), as a function of plasma urate concentration in normal adults, replotted by STEELE (1971) from data of STEELE and RIESELBACH (1967a). Reproduced with the permission of the author and the New England Journal of Medicine

TS_{ur} was estimated from the decrement in urate excretion produced by maximal secretory suppression with pyrazinamide, and is expressed as μg uric acid per ml glomerular filtrate. The dotted lines enclose the 95% prediction confidence limits of TS_{ur}. In every subject, increase of the plasma urate by RNA ingestion or decrease by means of allopurinol was accompanied by a change in TS_{ur} in the same direction

4 g pyrazinamide. Since the duration of the effect of a single dose of pyrazinamide is prolonged (Fig. 4), a finding also observed by YU et al. (1957a), individual variations in response, which might be due to different rates of absorption and hydrolysis of pyrazinamide, are minimized. Under these conditions, the excretion of urate fell to a mean of 11.2% (range 5.7–18.2%) of the control values (Fig. 5). Assuming that the suppression of tubular secretion of urate is complete, a mean of 99.2% (range 98.8–99.6%) of the filtered urate load was reabsorbed. Twenty-four hours after pyrazinamide intake the plasma urate had risen by an average of 2.53 mg/100 ml. The marked suppression of urinary urate implies that excreted uric acid is derived almost entirely, if not exclusively, from tubular secretion in the healthy man. Consequently, in the absence of discernible renal disease, UV_{ur} closely approximates the amount of uric acid which has been secreted. The urate excretion values factored by the creatinine or inulin clearance express secretion relative to a given population of nephrons. In the normal subject, the values for tubular secretion of urate per nephron unit have a predictable relationship to plasma urate concentration.

The urate-to-inulin clearance ratio is not always an accurate reflection of the secretory transport of urate; for example allopurinol given to gouty patients for short-term periods decreased the renal clearance of uric acid due to a disproportionate decline in tubular secretion of uric acid; conversely, the ingestion of RNA had the reverse effect (GUTMAN et al., 1969). The practice of expressing uric acid clearance as a fraction of the glomerular filtration came into being as a consequence of the filtration-partial reabsorption theory. With the demonstration that $U_{ur}V$ is derived virtually entirely from tubular secretion, parameters such as the ratio of C_{ur} to C_{in} have lost their physiologic meaning.

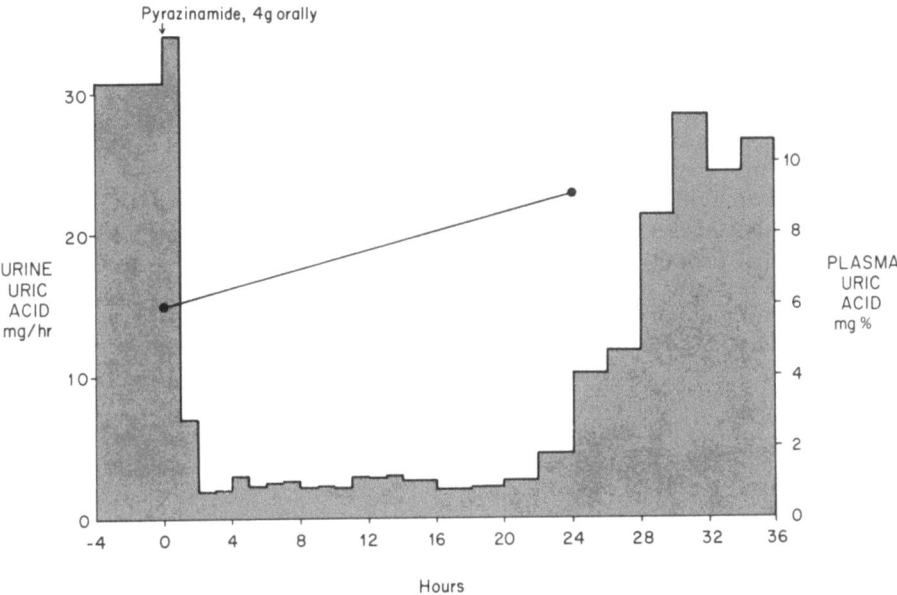

Fig. 4. Effect of a single dose of 4 g pyrazinamide on plasma and urine uric acid in a healthy man

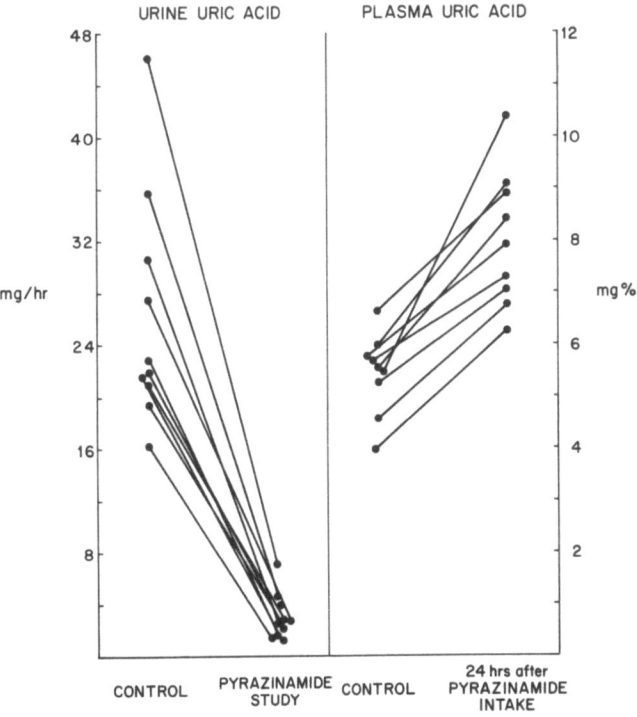

Fig. 5. Suppression of urine uric acid and rise in plasma urate after oral administration of 4 g pyrazinamide to 10 normal men

The Effect of Drugs and Intermediary Metabolites on the Renal Excretion of Uric Acid

Numerous organic acids interfere with the tubular transport system of uric acid, presumably because of competitive inhibition, i.e. the blocking effect is due to competition for an essential intermediary in the transport system. Some compounds like pyrazinoic acid only suppress uric acid excretion and do not produce uricosuria in any dose; others like salicylate exhibit a "paradoxical" action over the dosage range in common use. The potent uricosuric drug sulfinpyrazone does not cause any demonstrable retention of uric acid in any dosage. The effect of salicylate on urate excretion was studied by YU and GUTMAN (1959). They found that low concentrations of free salicylate in the tubular urine depress tubular secretion of urate. At intermediate dosage levels, there is incipient inhibition of urate reabsorption in addition to inhibition of tubular secretion, with the net result that the two effects cancel each other out. A high concentration of free salicylate in the tubular urine causes marked suppression of reabsorption as well as of secretion; since reabsorption is much more significant than secretion, the net effect is uricosuria. The uricosuric effect of salicylate was markedly enhanced by rendering the urine alkaline with sodium bicarbonate, a measure that causes a sharp increase in the urinary excretion of free salicylate. A similar paradoxical drug action was demonstrated for phenylbutazone and probenecid in a dose-dependent fashion (YU and GUTMAN, 1955). Relatively small doses of salicylate can completely counteract the uricosuric properties of probenecid and other uricosuric drugs (YU and GUTMAN, 1959). When large doses of salicylate, in the order of 5 g/day, were added to a probenecid regimen, no additive effect of the two uricosuric drugs was observed.

The use of pyrazinamide for measurement of tubular secretion and reabsorption of uric acid depends upon its capacity to suppress tubular secretion of uric acid transiently. Pyrazinamide is rapidly reabsorbed from the gastrointestinal tract and hydrolyzed in the body to pyrazinoic acid. The free acid has a more rapid and more pronounced effect on uric acid excretion than pyrazinamide, suggesting that pyrazinoic acid is the active compound (YU et al., 1957a).

Urate excretion is reduced in hyperlactic acidemia and in ketonemia, probably through inhibition of tubular secretion. Infusion of sodium lactate (YU et al., 1957b) rapidly reduces urinary uric acid excretion. Increase of plasma urate due to elevated lactic acid in arterial blood is seen in toxemia of pregnancy (HANDLER, 1960), in glycogen storage disease, Cori type I (JEUNE et al., 1957), after ingestion of sufficient ethanol to cause alcohol intoxication (LIEBER et al., 1962) and after muscular exercise (NICHOLS et al., 1951). Several cases of clinical gout have occurred in patients suffering from glycogen storage disease (ALEPA et al., 1967; JAKOVCIC and SORENSEN, 1967). MAC LACHLAN and RODNAN (1967) have shown that the combination of fasting and ingestion of large amounts of alcohol has a more profound effect on renal excretion of uric acid than either alone. Uric acid excretion is also reduced by infusion of ketone bodies (SCOTT et al., 1964; LECOCQ and MCPHAUL, 1965; GOLDFINGER et al., 1965), in ketoacidosis complicating starvation, and in uncontrolled diabetes mellitus (PADOVA and BENDERSKY, 1962), although in the last condition multiple metabolic aberrations may have opposing effects upon uric acid tubular transport. Acute gouty arthritis complicating prolonged starvation as treatment for severe obesity was observed in two nongouty subjects, who had normal uric acid prior to institution of fasting (DRENWICK et al., 1964).

A definite association between hyperuricemia and elevated serum triglycerides has been firmly established (BERKOWITZ, 1964). Hypercholesterolemia in the absence of hypertriglyceridemia was not characterized by elevated uric acid in the plasma. The mechanism whereby triglycerides cause hyperuricemia has not been definitively established, but present evidence points to a decreased renal excretion of uric acid in patients with hypertriglyceridemia.

Tubular secretion of urate can apparently be enhanced by certain compounds. Thus the uricosuria that is elicited by glycine loading is abolished by the prior administration of pyrazinamide (YU et al., 1970). Glycine-induced uricosuria is therefore assumed to be due to enhanced tubular secretion of uric acid. Similarly, the uricosuric properties of benziodarone appear to occur principally through secretory stimulation of urate, since the uricosuric effect of this drug is almost completely suppressed by pyrazinamide (GOUGOUX et al., 1970). The mechanism by which these compounds increase tubular secretion of uric acid is not clear. A stimulating effect of exogenous and endogenous substances could conceivably be related to an ability to eliminate competitive inhibitors, e.g. acylglycine derivatives which may partially occupy the organic acid secretory system under normal circumstances. Such a mechanism has been proposed to explain the stimulating effect of acetate on para-aminohippurate secretion (SCHACHTER et al., 1955).

In addition to the conventional uricosuric agents, many well known drugs whose primary use is for other purposes have marked uricosuric properties. The cholecystographic agents iopanoic acid (Telepaque) and iodipamide (Cholografin) increase the clearance of uric acid (MUDGE, 1971), and so does the urographic agent iodopyracet (BONSNES et al., 1944). Chlorprothixene, a tranquilizing agent, has a pronounced uricosuric effect (HEALEY et al., 1965).

Glycosuria increases the renal clearance of uric acid. Comparative studies on the effect of mannitol and glucose on urate excretion were made by SKEITH et al. (1967) to assess the role of the osmotic diuresis induced by concomitant glycosuria. Their data showed that glucose produced an increase in uric acid clearance per unit increase in osmolar clearance which was three times greater than that seen with mannitol. Thus, glucose has an effect on uric acid excretion in addition to its osmotic effect. Presumably, glucose diminishes tubular reabsorption of urate, since the uricosuric response by glucose also occurs after pretreatment with pyrazinamide (STEELE, 1971). Phlorizin, a glucoside which inhibits the tubular reabsorption of glucose, produces a more striking increase in urate excretion than might be expected from the degree of glycosuria, suggesting that phlorizin itself inhibits tubular reabsorption of urate (SKEITH et al., 1970).

The effect of diuretics on the excretion of uric acid has been recognized since the early clinical application of the benzothiadiazine compounds. A paradoxical action of chlorothiazide on the tubular transport of urate depending on the dose and mode of administration was reported by DEMARTINI et al. (1962). Intravenous administration of chlorothiazide caused a prompt, but transient, increase in the clearance of urate, which was distinct from its effect on electrolyte excretion; but when administered orally over a prolonged period, the drug caused urate retention and hyperuricemia. The dual action on urate transport has been interpreted as being similar to that used to explain the paradoxical effects of small and large doses of salicylate. Chlorothiazide undergoes active secretion by the organic acid system of the proximal tubule. An alternate hypothesis proposes that hyperuricemia during prolonged administration of thiazide is a consequence of extracellular fluid volume contraction, since it does not occur when volume depletion is prevented by giving salt (SUKI et al., 1967). Recently, the effects of the potent newer diuretics, ethacrynic acid and furosemide, on urate excretion were studied by STEELE and OPPENHEIMER (1969). After intravenous administration of either diuretic, there is a transient increase in uric acid excretion, followed by a marked diminution in uric acid excretion during the stage of diuretic-induced extracellular fluid volume contraction. When urinary losses were simultaneously replaced with isotonic saline solution, however, urinary uric acid excretion remained close to the control level. The immediate uricosuric response to intravenously injected furosemide or ethacrynic acid appears to be related to increased tubular secretion of uric acid, since it does not occur after pretreatment with pyrazinamide. This stimulatory effect may be mediated by redistribution of renal blood flow resulting in enhanced substrate availability at the urate secretory sites. That an acute intrarenal redistribution of blood occurs following administration of either furosemide or ethacrynic acid to dogs has been shown by BIRTCH et al. (1967). Since the decrease in uric acid excretion did not occur until after volume depletion, it seems unlikely that furosemide and ethacrynic acid inhibit tubular secretion of urate directly. Instead, it was postulated that the suppressive effects of these drugs on urate secretion during volume depletion could be mediated indirectly through generation of angiotensin, circulatory changes, or enhanced medullary lactate production during volume depletion.

Injection of angiotensin and norepinephrine to normal men in amounts sufficient to raise diastolic pressure by 20 mm Hg resulted in a marked decrease in uric acid excretion (FERRIS and GORDEN, 1968). Because of a disproportionate decrease in C_{PAH} to GFR during angiotensin infusion it was postulated that diminished renal blood flow might have limited the delivery of urate to the renal tubular sites. The changes observed in these acute experiments may be relevant to the hyperuricemia observed in many hypertensive patients (CANNON et al., 1966).

The possibility that renal urate reabsorption might be altered during changes in volume of the extracellular fluid and that such a mechanism might play a secondary role in the effect of furosemide and ethacrynic acid on urate excretion was examined by STEELE (1969) and STEELE and OPPENHEIMER (1969). After specific inhibition of the urate secretory mechanism by pretreatment with pyrazinamide, excretion of urate increased slightly during volume expansion and decreased slightly during volume contraction, suggesting that renal reabsorption of urate can be affected by changes in extracellular fluid volume. The absolute increments and decrements in urate excretion produced in this way were small, however, especially when compared to the filtered load of urate. The results may also be interpreted as reflecting changes in tubular secretion of urate effected by the factors mentioned above for ethacrynic acid and furosemide.

It has been known for a long time that uric acid excretion is dependent on urinary flow (BRØCHNER-MORTENSEN, 1937). The necessity for controlled diuresis in comparative clearance studies has been emphasized by SALA et al. (1956). Uric acid excretion is decreased at low urine volume, and rises with increasing urine output until the flow rate reaches 1.5 ml per minute. Beyond this limit there is, supposedly, no further rise in uric acid excretion. Recent preliminary studies suggest, however, that high urine flow induced by water ingestion further enhances the renal excretion of uric acid and that this increment in UV_{ur} is derived from tubular secretion (DIAMOND et al., 1971). UV_{ur} increased from 290 µg/min when V was 2.7 ml/min, to 410 µg/min when V was 6.4 ml/min; these changes could not be accounted for by alteration in GFR or by expansion of extracellular fluid volume. Increasing the urine volume to 12.1 ml/min did lead to expansion of the extracellular fluid volume. Under these conditions UV_{ur} rose to 692 µg/min and, although the postpyrazinamide urate excretion rose slightly, the increment in UV_{ur} was, for the most part, in that portion inhibited by pyrazinamide. These observations were interpreted as indicating either that increased urine flow diverts a greater portion of the renal blood flow to tubules with a greater secretory capacity for urate, or, alternatively, that a second reabsorptive site may exist distal to the secretory site inhibited by pyrazinamide, i.e., in the distal tubule or in the collecting duct where dilution of the final urine occurs; decreased reabsorption at such a site would be interpreted as increased secretion by the pyrazinamide suppression test.

The 24-hrs values for uric acid clearances are distinctly lower than those obtained in acute clearance studies. Whether the expanded extracellular fluid volume associated with the large fluid intake necessary for clearance studies diminishes tubular reabsorption of the filtered urate, as suggested by STEELE (1969), or enhances tubular secretion, as proposed by DIAMOND et al. (1971), or whether both mechanisms play a role, cannot be answered with certainty.

Urate excretion, unlike that of many other organic acids, is little affected by variation in urinary pH, indicating that nonionic diffusion plays a very minor role in tubular transport of urate.

Excretion of Uric Acid in Chronic Renal Disease

Chronic renal disease is the most common cause of hyperuricemia. There is no parallelism between plasma urate and urea nitrogen, and plasma urate may vary greatly at any level of inulin clearance. Although clinical gout as a complication to chronic renal disease has been infrequently reported (SORENSEN, 1962; RICHET et al., 1965), and the existence of true secondary renal gout has been disputed by others (BAUER and KRANE, 1964), the association of the two is more common than is generally appreciated. We have observed acute gouty arthritis in women with different types of chronic renal disease, including polycystic renal disease, retroperitoneal fibrosis, interstitial nephritis as a sequela to turpentine oil ingestion, and chronic pyelonephritis. A particularly high incidence of gout occurs in chronic lead nephropathy. EMMERSON (1963) recorded gout in 16 of 33 patients with lead nephritis. A history of prolonged ingestion of moonshine whisky, the important source of lead in the southern United States, was frequently elicited in patients with crystal-proven gout (BALL and MORGAN, 1968).

The pyrazinamide suppression technique has been applied to assess the role of residual nephrons in the maintenance of urate homeostasis in chronic renal disease (STEELE and RIESELBACH, 1967b). Such studies have shown that until severe functional loss supervenes, residual nephrons of the chronically diseased kidney retain integrity of urate reabsorptive and secretory transport. Thus the chronically diseased kidney augments urate secretion per nephron at the predicted normal rate in response to hyperuricemia. As glomerular filtration rate progressively decreases, however, the fraction of filtered urate excreted increases. With an inulin clearance of 10—15 ml per minute, the mean fractional excretion of urate was 20.8%. When the glomerular filtration rate fell below 10 ml per minute there was a striking alteration in urate transport, manifested by marked impairment in both tubular reabsorption and secretion of uric acid. In ten patients with a C_{in} of less than 10 ml per minute a mean of 45% of the filtered urate was excreted in the urine. The net effect is a sharp increase in urate excretion per nephron, which is comprised almost exclusively of filtered urate that has escaped reabsorption.

The functional integrity of the urate transport system within the residual nephrons generally seen in chronic renal disease does not apply to lead nephropathy, which affects tubular secretion more specifically (EMMERSON, 1965; BALL and SORENSEN, 1969). The markedly reduced uric acid clearance, even in the face of a modest reduction in the glomerular filtration rate, suggests a defect in tubular secretion of urate. The finding of a significant lowering of urate clearance after elevation of the plasma urate concentration by a purine load indicates an abnormal secretory response to hyperuricemia, and suggests that patients with lead-induced nephropathy may be particularly susceptible to foods high in purine content. Reduced tubular secretion of uric acid may also account for the hyperuricemia observed in some patients with chronic beryllium disease (KELLEY et al., 1969a).

The Role of the Kidney in the Pathogenesis of Primary Gout

The past 20 years have seen a polemic concerning the role of the kidney in the genesis of hyperuricemia in primary gout. The concept that hyperuricemia in primary gout is due to an abnormality in the renal excretion of urate was first proposed by GARROD (1876). It was based on the frequent incidence of albuminuria and nitrogen retention in gouty patients and on the pathologic findings in the kidney. GARROD's position was restated by THANNHAUSER (1956), who maintained that two conditions favor the incidence of hyperuricemia in man: first, the fact that most of the uric acid in the glomerular filtrate is reabsorbed in the tubules, and second, the lack of uricase in the liver, which would convert uric acid to the more soluble allantoin. These inborn stigmata predispose man to hyperuricemia. He explained the pathogenesis of gout by an increased tubular reabsorption, which aggravates the constitutionally weak ability of the human kidney to rid the body of uric acid.

During the fifties and sixties a constantly expanding amount of information on the rate of synthesis of uric acid was obtained by isotope techniques. These data, which have been reviewed by WYNGAARDEN and KELLEY (pp. 43), demonstrated unequivocally that a segment of the gouty population has overproduction of uric acid. In addition, urinary uric acid excretion determined by the enzymatic spectrophotometric method is frequently greater than normal (SEEGMILLER et al., 1961; SORENSEN, 1962; KELLEY et al., 1969b).

Behind the controversy over the role of the kidney in the pathogenesis of primary gout is the tacit assumption that all gouty subjects must carry the same metabolic defect. The debate will go on until it is recognized that hyperuricemia in primary gout is not confined to a single defect, but that multiple metabolic aberrations can cause hyperuricemia and gout. The arguments brought forward for and against altered excretion of uric acid during the past decade are reviewed below.

NUGENT and TYLER (1959) challenged earlier studies that showed no essential difference in the manner in which uric acid is excreted by subjects with gout and by normal subjects, on the grounds that these studies were performed while the normal subjects and gouty patients had markedly different plasma uric acid concentrations. To eliminate such differences, NUGENT and TYLER administered uric acid precursors orally to nongouty subjects so that their plasma urate rose to levels comparable to those found in patients with gout. Under these conditions the urate clearance and the rate of urate excretion by nongouty subjects were well above the levels observed in the gouty patients. NUGENT and TYLER concluded that abnormal renal excretion of uric acid is one important cause of hyperuricemia in some patients with gout.

These observations were further supported by the studies of two additional groups of investigators. SEEGMILLER et al. (1962) determined the urate-to-inulin clearance ratios in 7 nongouty men before and after addition of a purine load, and in 16 gouty patients who were classified by the extent of their uric acid production. In five gouty subjects who showed a normal production of uric acid, there was a diminished urate to inulin clearance ratio. LATHEM and RODNAN (1962) administered urate intravenously to gouty and nongouty subjects to study not only urate excretion at equivalent and various plasma levels, but also the dynamics of the renal tubular transport system for urate. Under conditions of intravenous urate loading, ten of eleven patients with gout showed a sluggish acceleration in uric acid excretion in response to an increase in plasma urate, indicating an impairment in uric acid excretion.

Yu et al. (1962) confirmed that normal men who had been fed RNA to raise their plasma urate to gouty levels excreted more uric acid in the urine than gouty patients, but they criticized the design of studies in which the normal group was subjected to large exogenous uric acid loads whereas the gouty group remained in a relatively steady state. They suggested that the disparity in $U_{ur}V$ is attributable to unequal conditions, when normal subjects are given a large load of uric acid and gouty subjects are not. They further showed that when gouty subjects were challenged with the same oral RNA load or with rapidly infused urate, plasma urate and urinary uric acid excretion increased and that the mean increments in these parameters were not significantly different from those observed in the normal group. In addition, GUTMAN and his associates criticized the fact that differences in renal excretion had been analyzed as a function of the filtered load.

To meet these criticisms, NUGENT et al. (1964) compared the renal excretion of urate in normal subjects who became chronically hyperuricemic by prolonged RNA ingestion with that in gouty patients during control conditions. In addition, they studied the response of these two groups to acute RNA loading. Various parameters for uric acid excretion, viz, $U_{ur}V$, C_{ur}, and C_{ur}/C_{in}, were then analyzed as functions of the plasma urate concentration which represents the physiologic variable that determines the rate of urate excretion. The figuring of urate clearance by inulin clearance was not intended to indicate the proportion of filtered urate excreted, but rather was included to correct for any loss in renal functional capacity. Regardless of the excretory parameter used for comparison of uric acid excretion, the mean values were far greater for normal subjects fed urate precursors for a long time than they were for patients with gout studied under control conditions, although some overlapping of individual values was observed. In response to an acute load of urate, the mean rate of rise in urate excretion per unit rise in plasma urate was much greater for the hyperuricemic control group than for its gouty counterpart, indicating a brisker acceleration of uric acid excretion in normal subjects.

Since the differences in urate excretion between gouty and nongouty subjects persisted when nongouty subjects were restudied after as long as 42 days on RNA feeding, it was concluded that these differences cannot be attributed to acute urate loading, but are more probably the result of impaired renal urate excretion in many patients with gout.

In support of this view are renal urate data in patients with leukemia who have increased endogenous production of uric acid (NUGENT et al., 1962). When the renal urate excretion of such patients was compared with that of patients with gout, it was found that the leukemic patients excreted much more urate per day than did the gouty patients, although their mean plasma urate concentration was lower than in patients with gout.

A reverse type of study to those reported above involved 19 gouty subjects with normal renal function, who were given allopurinol to reduce plasma urate to the normal range (HOUPT and OGRYZLO, 1964; OGRYZLO, 1965). Allopurinol apparently does not influence the renal handling of uric acid. After serum urate had been reduced to normal, the clearance of urate at 4.1 ml per min was significantly below the mean value of 7.1 ml per min in 23 nongouty men. These data indicate that the renal defect in urate excretion displayed by gouty subjects as a group persists when plasma urate is reduced to normal.

RIESELBACH et al. (1970) used the pyrazinamide suppression test to study the renal tubular transport of urate in 15 gouty patients who had been classified as either overproducers or normoproducers on the basis of uric acid turnover data. Both groups had a normal pattern of reabsorption over a wide range of filtered loads. While the tubular secretion of urate in the gouty overproducers, however, was similar to that of normals (both at elevated and at normal urate levels) diminished urate secretion was evident in the normoproducers at endogenously elevated plasma urate levels. Thus it appears that inability to accelerate urate secretion adequately provides the basis for hyperuricemia in the gouty patients with normal production rate, or, in other words, gouty normoproducers must raise their plasma urate level to provide an adequate stimulus for renal excretion of the normal daily production of urate.

Conflicting data on tubular secretion and reabsorption of uric acid measured by the use of pyrazinamide were obtained by GUTMAN et al. (1969), who maintain that it is not necessary to postulate a specific renal defect in the elimination of uric acid. On the basis of their results in 10 gouty subjects they concluded that the pattern of renal regulation of uric acid excretion in primary gout did not differ significantly from that in normal man. No turnover data were included in this report, but on the basis of a mean urinary uric acid excretion of 0.833 mg per minute at their endogenous urate level, it would appear that many of these patients produced excessive amounts of uric acid. Furthermore, tubular secretion of urate in the gouty patients averaged 0.74 mg per minute as compared to the normal mean of 0.47 mg per minute when both groups were on the same restricted diet and had similar inulin clearance.

Studies of relatively large numbers of gouty patients have, in general, shown slightly greater urinary uric acid excretion and somewhat lower uric acid clearance for gouty patients than for the controls (GUTMAN and YU, 1957; NUGENT and TYLER, 1959; LATHEM and RODNAN, 1962; HOUPT and OGRYZLO, 1964; SNAITH and SCOTT, 1971). Such studies have definite limitations, since careful scrutiny of the results reveals that the population was heterogeneous. For example, in the case of GUTMAN and YU's large series of 150 patients, who underwent detailed renal functional studies, the uric acid clearance ranged from 2.8 ml/min to 14.4 ml/min, with only modest variations in glomerular filtration rate and plasma urate level.

In conclusion, it can be said that when gouty populations are separated into overproducers and normoproducers, as they were by SEEGMILLER et al. (1962) and RIESELBACH et al. (1970), differences in the renal excretion of uric acid become readily apparent. In general, the patients who produce excessive quantities of uric acid show normal renal handling of uric acid, while gouty subjects who have normal production of uric acid have evidence of impaired renal excretion of urate. Whether the defect in urate secretion is an intrinsic tubular defect or results from a humoral inhibitor of urate secretion is not known.

Excretion of Uric Acid during Excessive Hyperuricemia in Myeloproliferative Diseases

Increased breakdown of endogenous nucleic acids is a common occurrence in leukemias, lymphomas and other neoplastic disorders, and is often aggravated by radiotherapy or chemotherapy with cytotoxic agents. If overproduction of uric acid is markedly increased and occurs suddenly, the load of uric acid filtered at the glomerular membrane may exceed the tubular capacity for reabsorption. At the same time tubular secretion of uric acid increases. Both processes lead to sharp increases in the clearance of uric acid. In one series of 26 patients with leukemia, six had urate clearance values above 30 ml/min, and in one of them C_{ur} was no less than 94 ml/min (RIESELBACH et al., 1964).

The outpouring of uric acid may assume such proportions that precipitates of uric acid are formed which may clog the lumen of the renal tubules and collecting ducts. Clinically, uric acid obstructive nephropathy is characterized by rapidly progressive acute renal failure. Prevention or prompt treatment of this complication is an essential part of effective cancer chemotherapy.

Uric acid obstructive nephropathy must be distinguished from gouty nephropathy. The latter is a consequence of chronic hyperuricemia rather than of excessive uric acid excretion. In gouty nephropathy, depositions of crystals of monosodium urate occur *de novo* in the interstitial tissue of the renal medulla, particularly in the papillary tips.

Urate Spillage in Renal Tubular Dysfunction

Some proximal tubular disorders are associated with impaired reabsorption of uric acid; these include WILSON's disease (BISHOP et al., 1954; SORENSEN and KAPPAS, 1966), FANCONI's syndrome (SIROTA et al., 1952) and cadmium intoxication (ADAMS et al., 1969). This type of defect is characterized by high uric acid clearance, which causes an abnormally low plasma urate concentration. Studies with isotopic uric acid in five patients with WILSON's disease have shown that the fraction of total urate that is eliminated through the kidney is greater than normal. Injected isotopic uric acid was almost quantitatively recovered in the urine from two of the patients. Prolonged treatment with penicillamine resulted in a reversal of the abnormalities in uric acid metabolism toward normal. Thus the plasma urate and total body pool of uric acid rose substantially, while the renal clearance and the cumulative recovery of injected uric acid in the urine diminished toward the normal range (SORENSEN and KAPPAS, 1966).

Extrarenal Elimination of Uric Acid

Excretion of Uric Acid into the Intestinal Tract

Whether uric acid is or is not catabolized in man was a subject of controversy during the first half of this century. The earlier literature on uric acid contents of digestive juices, and on the recovery of injected unlabeled or ^{15}N-labeled uric acid (either as uric acid or as degradation products) and attempts to demonstrate uricolytic activity in human tissues have been reviewed elsewhere (SORENSEN, 1960). When ^{14}C-uric acid became available, a sensitive tool was provided for an accurate assessment of the role of uricolysis in man. Reference has already been made to the fact that urinary recoveries of injected ^{14}C-uric acid are incomplete in normal subjects (Fig. 1). Thus about one-third of all uric acid is normally eliminated by extrarenal routes, and it is the fate of this portion of uric acid that is discussed in the following sections (SORENSEN, 1959; 1960; 1965).

After intravenous injection of ^{14}C-2-uric acid, a portion of the ^{14}C was found in degradation products of uric acid, viz, allantoin, allantoic acid, and urea excreted in the urine, and carbon dioxide in expired air. From 0.4 to 4.7% of injected ^{14}C-uric acid was recovered in allantoin isolated in chemically pure form from the urine of 5 individuals. Allantoic acid, which is subject to spontaneous degradation at an acid pH, was isolated by a column-chromatographic method and found to contain ^{14}C in two of five subjects who had received ^{14}C-2-uric acid intravenously. From 0.4 to 2.5% of the ^{14}C dose was recovered in urinary urea for 5—13 days after the administration of labeled uric acid. A greater amount of ^{14}C was found in carbon dioxide than in any other degradation product, indicating that carbon dioxide and ammonia are the principal uricolytic products in man. In a normal subject 11% of the injected ^{14}C was recovered in carbon dioxide of expired air over a period of 4 days.

The site of the breakdown of uric acid was next considered. The profound degradation of intravenously injected ^{14}C-uric acid together with the finding that ^{14}C was excreted in feces suggested that the gastrointestinal tract was the likely site of uricolysis in man. For example, one normal subject excreted 7.1% of the injected dose in 5 days, and a gouty patient excreted 3.8% in the stools in 4 days. The capacity of the gastrointestinal tract to degrade uric acid can be appreciated from the results of experiments dealing with orally administered ^{14}C-2-uric acid. More than 55% of the ingested ^{14}C was recovered as carbon dioxide in expired air during the first 50 hrs, while 16.3% was excreted in feces. Eleven percent of the ingested uric acid was absorbed and excreted unchanged in the urine over a period of 6 days.

Since only a trace of uric acid, if any at all, was demonstrable in feces, it may be concluded that fecal ^{14}C is present in breakdown products. Radioassay of suspensions of fecal bacteria before and after passage through a Seitz filter revealed that 83—91% of the radioactivity was retained in the filter, indicating incorporation of most of the ^{14}C into bacteria; in other words, the bacterial flora utilize carbon dioxide derived from uric acid as a result of uricolysis.

Reinvestigation of the contents of uric acid in digestive juices by means of specific enzymatic methods implied that significant amounts of uric acid gain entrance into the gastrointestinal tract. The average concentration of uric acid in mixed saliva was 3.1 mg/100 ml in 10 normal men and 1.9 mg/100 ml in 12 normal women. Saliva from a gouty patient contained 6.67 and 6.24 mg/100 ml of uric acid, corresponding to 75% of the plasma concentration. Gastric juice was found to contain small amounts of uric acid of the order of 5—10 mg per liter. The mean uric acid concentration in hepatic bile from 10 patients who had undergone cholecystectomy was 4.4 mg/100 ml. The daily excretion of uric acid in saliva, gastric juice and bile can be estimated to be about 100 mg under normal conditions. Taking into account the uric acid contained in pancreatic and intestinal juices, it is entirely within the realm of feasibility that the quantity of uric acid excreted into the gut is sufficient to account for the degradation of one third of the uric acid normally turned over each day.

The final proof of the role of the intestinal flora in uricolysis in man was established by determining the extent of degradation of intravenously administered ^{14}C-2-uric acid in a normal subject before and after effective intestinal bacteriostasis by concomitant administration of phthalylsulfathiazole, streptomycin and neomycin. The quantity of ^{14}C recovered in various degradation products was reduced from 22.5% during the control period to 3.0% during the period of intestinal bacteriostasis (Table I). Moreover, uric acid was constantly found in feces during intestinal bacteriostasis, whereas none could be demonstrated in the control experiment. A total of 930 mg uric acid was excreted in feces over a 5-day period during drug treatment. This corresponds to a daily average of 186 mg, or 26.6% of the calculated turnover. This figure is quite consistent with the recovery of 30.1% of administered ^{14}C in the feces, and indicates that essentially all of the fecal ^{14}C was present in uric acid *per se*.

Table 1. Recovery of intravenously administered ^{14}C-2-uric acid in excretory products (5 days) before and during effective intestinal bacteriostasis

Excretory product	Recovery of ^{14}C (percent of dose)	
	Before bacteriostasis	During bacteriostasis
Urinary uric acid	69.0[a]	55.7
Urinary allantoin	2.1	1.8
Urinary allantoic acid	0.2	—
Urinary urea	2.2	0.7
Expired carbon dioxide	10.9	0.5
Fecal degradation products	7.1	0.0
Total recovery in degradation products	22.5	3.0

[a] 10 days

Table 2. Uric acid turnover and recovery of intravenously administered ^{14}C-2-uric acid (6 to 11 days) in three patients with chronic renal disease

Case No.	I	II	III
Age, sex	33, ♀	57, ♀	62, ♀
Renal pathology	Chronic interstitial nephritis	Diabetic glomerulosclerosis	Chronic pyelonephritis
Renal function	C_{in}: 23 ml/min	BUN: 80 mg/100ml serum creat.: 8.0 mg/100 ml	C_{cr}: 31 ml/min
Turnover of uric acid, mg/24 h	580	424	403
Urine uric acid, mg/24 h	198	132	101
Plasma uric acid, mg/100 ml	10.36	7.20	5.81
Recovery of ^{14}C, percent of dose — Left in pool at end of study	19.02	16.31	11.31
Urinary uric acid	26.86	30.36	22.31
Urinary allantoin	1.30	1.06	0.98
Urinary urea	0.39	0.20	0.33
Expired carbon dioxide	41.97	33.36	60.86
Fecal products	11.64	9.55	10.15
Total recovery, percent	101.16	90.84	105.94

The proportion of uric acid that is broken down can be inferred from the difference between the dose of injected ^{14}C-uric acid and the quantity of ^{14}C recovered in urinary uric acid. The only situation where this relationship does not hold is in patients with tophaceous gout, for whom it has been shown that a physical exchange occurs between isotopically labeled uric acid in the miscible pool and nonlabeled uric acid deposited in tophi.

The extrarenal elimination of uric acid assumes a more significant role in clinical situations with diminished output of uric acid in the urine, either as a consequence of a decreased nephron mass or because of the presence of substances that interfere with the tubular secretion of uric acid. Marked reduction of nephrons in chronic renal disease is associated with diminished total urinary uric

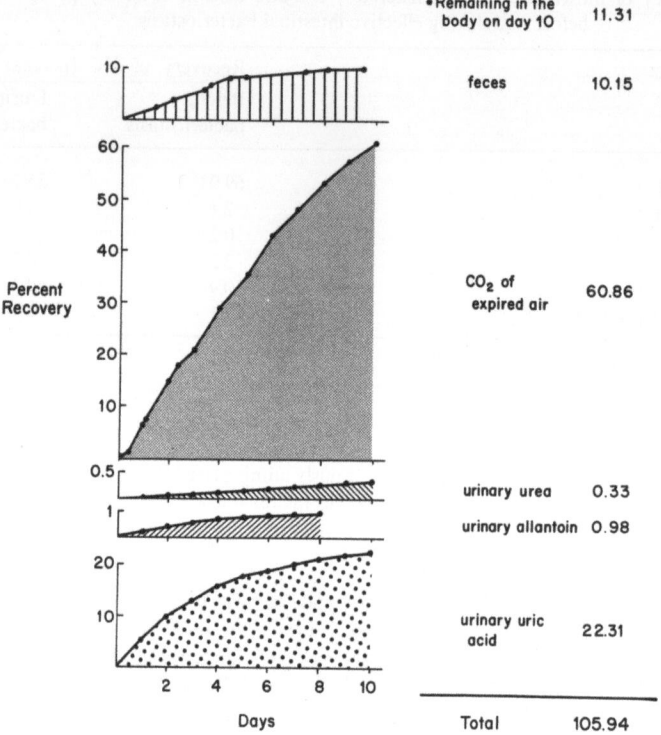

Fig. 6. Recovery of ^{14}C-2-uric acid administered intravenously to a patient with chronic renal disease

acid, even though the excretion of uric acid per nephron unit may be significantly increased. In this situation extrarenal excretion of uric acid may become the major route of elimination. To illustrate this point, we have studied the elimination of ^{14}C-2-uric acid in three patients with chronic renal disease who had low urinary uric acid excretion. The amount of ^{14}C recovered in the degradation products was 1.45, 2.06, and 3.24 times greater than that recovered in urinary uric acid (Table 2, Fig. 6).

In conclusion, then, a significant portion of uric acid is degraded in man, with carbon dioxide and ammonia as the principal uricolytic products. This breakdown is effected by the action of uricolytic enzymes of bacteria in the gut. The complete uricolytic enzyme system comprises uricase, allantoinase, allantoicase and urease. FLORKIN (1966) has pointed out that all the components of this system are present in primitive forms of life, and that as one ascends the evolutionary scale, there is successive loss of the terminal enzymes.

Excretion of Uric Acid in Sweat

Sweat contains trivial amounts of uric acid. Enzymatic spectrophotometry yielded concentrations between 0.2 and 0.4 mg/100 ml at high secretory rate (PRAETORIUS, 1950). Even if the total sweat production is estimated to be as high as one or two liters daily, the excretion through this route should not exceed 4—8 mg urate per 24 hrs, or not more than 1% of the turnover.

Uricolytic activity in human tissues

There remains the question of uricolysis within the tissues of man. It is well established that uricase is absent from human tissues. On the other hand, in the presence of peroxide, several hemoproteins, viz, cytochromoxidase, peroxidase and catalase, are capable of destroying uric acid *in vitro*. A breakdown of uric acid in human tissues has been claimed by BIEN and ZUCKER (1955), who reported that uricolysis occurs in whole blood as well as in plasma incubated with white or red blood cells. The rate of urate disappearance which they observed was so rapid that they attributed a major part of the uricolysis in man to this mechanism. On the basis of a 33% decrease in this breakdown in gouty subjects, BIEN and ZUCKER postulated that diminished uricolysis contributes to the hyperuricemia in gout. In re-examining this problem, we tested human liver, kidney, pancreas, spleen and whole blood for their ability to split off radioactive carbon dioxide from ^{14}C-6-uric acid. The amount of carbon dioxide liberated was negligible in all cases. The average value indicated a degradation of between 0.2 and 0.3% of uric acid in the substrate solution. A similar degradation, however, took place in control experiments in which tissue homogenate was replaced by Krebs-Ringer's solution. It was concluded that the trivial breakdown of uric acid in human tissues is not dependent on enzymatic action but is the result of inorganically catalyzed oxidation. The data disprove the connotation of BIEN and ZUCKER (1955) that hyperuricemia in gout is related to decreased uricolysis.

A slight breakdown does occur, however, when monosodium ^{14}C-6-urate in crystalline form is engulfed by leukocytes (HOWELL and SEEGMILLER, 1962). An analogous situation may exist in acute gouty arthritis, when microcrystals of monosodium urate are phagocytosed by leukocytes. Since the maximum rate of uricolysis *in vitro* was only 0.3 µg urate per hour per million leukocytes, any destruction by this mechanism must be small compared to intestinal uricolysis.

References

ADAMS, R. G., HARRISON, J. F., SCOTT, P.: The development of cadmium-induced proteinuria, impaired renal function, and osteomalacia in alkaline battery workers. Quart. J. Med. **38**, 425—443 (1969).

ALEPA, F. P., HOWELL, R. R., KLINENBERG, J. R., SEEGMILLER, J. E.: Relationships between glycogen storage disease and tophaceous gout. Amer. J. Med. **42**, 58—66 (1967).

ALVSAKER, J. O.: Uric acid in human plasma. V. Isolation and identification of plasma proteins interacting with urate. Scand. J. clin. Lab. Invest. **18**, 227—239 (1966).

ALVSAKER, J. O.: Genetic studies in primary gout. Investigations on the plasma levels of the urate-binding α_1-α_2-globulin in individuals from two gouty kindreds. J. clin. Invest. **47**, 1254—1261 (1968).

BALL, G. V., MORGAN, J. M.: Chronic lead ingestion and gout. Sth. med. J. (Bgham, Ala.) **61**, 21—24 (1968).

BALL, G. V., SORENSEN, L. B.: Pathogenesis of hyperuricemia in saturnine gout. New Engl. J. Med. **280**, 1199—1202 (1969).

BAUER, W., KRANE, S. M.: Gout. In: DUNCAN, G. G. (Ed.): Diseases of Metabolism, 5th ed, p. 833. Philadelphia-London: W. B. Saunders 1964.

BERKOWITZ, D.: Blood lipid and uric acid interrelationships. J. Amer. med. Ass. **190**, 856—858 (1964).

BERLINER, R. W., HILTON, J. G., YU, T. F., KENNEDY, T. J., JR.: The renal mechanism for urate excretion in man. J. clin. Invest. **29**, 396—401 (1950).

BIEN, E. J., ZUCKER, M.: Uricolysis in normal and gouty individuals. Ann. rheum. Dis. **14**, 409—411 (1955).

BIRTCH, A. G., ZAKHEIM, R. M., JONES, L. G., BARGER, A. C.: Redistribution of renal blood flow produced by furosemide and ethacrynic acid. Circulat. Res. **21**, 869—878 (1967).

BISHOP, C., ZIMDAHL, W. T., TALBOTT, J. H.: Uric acid in two patients with Wilson's disease (hepatolenticular degeneration). Proc. Soc. exp. Biol. (N.Y.) **86**, 440—441 (1954).

BONSNES, R. W., DILL, L. V., DANA, E. S.: The effect of Diodrast^{TM} on the normal uric acid clearance. J. clin. Invest. **23**, 776—782 (1944).
BRØCHNER-MORTENSEN, K.: Uric acid in blood and urine. Acta med. scand. Supplementum **84**, 1—269 (1937).
BRØCHNER-MORTENSEN, K.: On variations in the uric acid clearance after administration of purine, with special reference to the threshold problem. Acta med. scand. **99**, 525—537 (1939).
CANNON, P. J., STASON, W. B., DEMARTINI, F. E., SOMMERS, S. C., LARAGH, J. H.: Hyperuricemia in primary and renal hypertension. New Engl. J. Med. **275**, 457—464 (1966).
CRONE, C., LASSEN, U. V.: Some uric acid values in normal human subjects. Scand. J. clin. Lab. Invest. **8**, 51—54 (1956).
DEMARTINI, F. E., WHEATON, E. A., HEALEY, L. A., LARAGH, J. H.: Effect of chlorothiazide on the renal excretion of uric acid. Amer. J. Med. **32**, 572—577 (1962).
DIAMOND, H., LAZARUS, R., KAPLAN, D., HALBERSTAM, D.: Renal handling of uric acid. Evidence suggesting a fourth component. Arthrit. and Rheum. **14**, 380 (1971).
DRENICK, E. J., SWENDSEID, M. E., BLAHD, W. H., TUTTLE, S. G.: Prolonged starvation as treatment for severe obesity. J. Amer. med. Ass. **187**, 100—105 (1964).
EMMERSON, B. T.: Chronic lead nephropathy: The diagnostic use of calcium EDTA and the association with gout. Aust. Ann. Med. **12**, 310—324 (1963).
EMMERSON, B. T.: The renal excretion of urate in chronic lead nephropathy. Aust. Ann. Med. **14**, 295—303 (1965).
FERRIS, T. F., GORDEN, P.: Effect of angiotensin and norepinephrine upon urate clearance in man. Amer. J. Med. **44**, 359—365 (1968).
FLORKIN, M.: A molecular approach to phylogeny, p. 75. Amsterdam: Elsevier 1966.
GARROD, A. B.: A treatise on gout and rheumatic gout (rheumatoid arthritis), 3rd Ed., p. 272. London: Longmans, Green & Co. 1876.
GOLDFINGER, S., KLINENBERG, J. R., SEEGMILLER, J. E.: Renal retention of uric acid induced by infusion of beta-hydroxybutyrate and acetoacetate. New Engl. J. Med. **272**, 351—355 (1965).
GOUGOUX, A., MICHAUD, G., VINAY, P., LEMIEUX, G.: The uricosuric action of benziodarone in man and dog. Clin. Res. **18**, 747 (1970).
GUTMAN, A. B., YU, T. F.: Renal function in gout with a commentary on the renal regulation of urate excretion, and the role of the kidney in the pathogenesis of gout. Amer. J. Med. **23**, 600—622 (1957).
GUTMAN, A. B., YU, T. F.: A three-component system for regulation of renal excretion of uric acid in man. Trans. Ass. Amer. Phycns **74**, 353—365 (1961).
GUTMAN, A. B., YU, T. F., BERGER, L.: Tubular secretion of urate in man. J. clin. Invest. **38**, 1778—1781 (1959).
GUTMAN, A. B., YU, T. F., BERGER, L.: Renal function in gout. III. Estimation of tubular secretion and reabsorption of uric acid by use of pyrazinamide (pyrazinoic acid). Amer. J. Med. **47**, 575—592 (1969).
HANDLER, J. S.: The role of lactic acid in the reduced excretion of uric acid in toxemia of pregnancy. J. clin. Invest. **39**, 1526—1532 (1960).
HEALEY, L. A., HARRISON, M., DECKER, J. L.: Uricosuric effect of chlorprothixene. New Engl. J. Med. **272**, 526—527 (1965).
HOUPT, J. B., OGRYZLO, M. A.: Persistence of impaired uric acid excretion in gout during reduced synthesis with allopurinol. Arthrit. and Rheum. **7**, 316 (1964).
HOWELL, R. R., SEEGMILLER, J. E.: Uricolysis by human leucocytes. Nature **196**, 482—483 (1962).
JAKOVCIC, S., SORENSEN, L. B.: Studies of uric acid metabolism in glycogen storage disease associated with gouty arthritis. Arthrit. and Rheum. **10**, 129—134 (1967).
JEUNE, M., CHARRAT, A., BERTRAND, J.: Polycorihépatique, hyperuricémie et goutte. Arch. franç. Pediat. **14**, 897—909 (1957).
KELLEY, W. N., GOLDFINGER, S. E., HARDY, H. L.: Hyperuricemia in chronic beryllium disease. Ann. intern. Med. **70**, 977—983 (1969a).
KELLEY, W. N., GREENE, M. L., ROSENBLOOM, F. M., HENDERSON, J. F., SEEGMILLER, J. E.: Hypoxanthine-guanine phosphoribosyltransferase deficiency in gout. Ann. intern. Med. **70**, 155—206 (1969b).
KLINENBERG, J. R., KIPPEN, I.: The binding of urate to plasma proteins determined by means of equilibrium dialysis. J. Lab. clin. Med. **75**, 503—510 (1970).
LATHEM, W., RODNAN, G. P.: Impairment of uric acid excretion in gout. J. clin. Invest. **41**, 1955—1963 (1962).

LECOCQ, F. R., MCPHAUL, J. J., JR.: The effects of starvation, high fat diets and ketone infusions on uric acid balance. Metabolism. **14**, 186—197 (1965).

LIEBER, C. S., JONES, D. P., LOSOWSKY, M. S., DAVIDSON, C. S.: Interrelations of uric acid and ethanol metabolism in man. J. Clin. Invest. **41**, 1863—1870 (1962).

MACLACHLAN, M. J., RODNAN, G. P.: Effects of food, fast and alcohol on serum uric acid and acute attacks of gout. Amer. J. Med. **42**, 38—57 (1967).

MORRIS, J. E.: The transport of uric acid in serum. Amer. J. med. Sci. **235**, 43—49 (1958).

MUDGE, G. H.: Uricosuric action of cholecystographic agents. New Engl. J. Med. **284**, 929—933 (1971).

MUDGE, G. H., CUCCHI, J., PLATTS, M., O'CONNELL, J. M. B., BERNDT, W. O.: Renal excretion of uric acid in the dog. Amer. J. Physiol. **215**, 404—410 (1968).

NICHOLS, J., MILLER, A. T., HIATT, E. P.: Influence of muscular exercise on uric acid excretion in man. J. appl. Physiol. **3**, 501—507 (1951).

NUGENT, C. A., MACDIARMID, W. D., TYLER, F. H.: Renal excretion of uric acid in leukemia and gout. Arch. intern. Med. **109**, 540—544 (1962).

NUGENT, C. A., MACDIARMID, W. D., TYLER, F. H.: Renal excretion of urate in patients with gout. Arch. intern. Med. **113**, 115—121 (1964).

NUGENT, C. A., TYLER, F. H.: The renal excretion of uric acid in patients with gout and in nongouty subjects. J. clin. Invest. **38**, 1890—1898 (1959).

OGRYZLO, M. A.: Discussion. Arthrit. and Rheum. **8**, 680—683 (1965).

PADOVA, J., BENDERSKY, G.: Hyperuricemia in diabetic ketoacidosis. New Engl. J. Med. **267**, 530—534 (1962).

POULSEN, H., PRAETORIUS, E.: Tubular excretion of uric acid in rabbits. Acta Pharmacol. (Kbh.) **10**, 371—378 (1954).

PRAETORIUS, E.: Personal communication (1950) to H. POULSEN: Urinsyre, Xantin og Hypoxantin, p. 44. Copenhagen: J. Jørgensen 1956.

PRAETORIUS, E., KIRK, J. E.: Hypouricemia with evidence for tubular elimination of uric acid. J. Lab. clin. Med. **35**, 865—868 (1950).

RICHET, G., MIGNON, F., ARDAILLOU, R.: Goutte secondaire des néphropathies chroniques. Presse méd. **73**, 633—638 (1965).

RIESELBACH, R. E., BENTZEL, C. J., COTLOVE, E., FREI, E., FREIREICH, E. J.: Uric acid excretion and renal function in the acute hyperuricemia of leukemia: pathogenesis and therapy of uric acid nephropathy. Amer. J. Med. **37**, 872—884 (1964).

RIESELBACH, R. E., SORENSEN, L. B., SHELP, W. D., STEELE, T. H.: Diminished renal urate secretion per nephron as a basis for primary gout. Ann. intern. Med. **73**, 359—366 (1970).

SALA, G., BALLABIO, C. B., AMIRA, A., RATTI, G., CIRLA, E.: Renal mechanisms for urate excretion in normal and gouty subjects. In: Contemporary Rheumatology, Proceedings IIIrd European Rheumatology Congress, The Hague-Sceveningen, 1955, pp. 581—583. Amsterdam: Elsevier 1956.

SCHACHTER, D., MANIS, J. G., TAGGART, J. V.: Renal synthesis, degradation and active transport of aliphatic acyl amino acids. Amer. J. Physiol. **182**, 537—544 (1955).

SCOTT, J. T., MCCALLUM, F. M., HOLLOWAY, V. P.: Starvation, ketosis and uric acid excretion. Clin. Sci. **27**, 209—221 (1964).

SEEGMILLER, J. E., GRAYZEL, A. I., HOWELL, R. R., PLATO, C.: The renal excretion of uric acid in gout. J. clin. Invest. **41**, 1094—1098 (1962).

SEEGMILLER, J. E., GRAYZEL, A. I., LASTER, L., LIDDLE, L.: Uric acid production in gout. J. clin. Invest. **40**, 1304—1314 (1961).

SHEIKH, M. I., MØLLER, J. V.: Binding of urate to proteins of human and rabbit plasma. Biochim. biophys. Acta (Amst.) **158**, 456—458 (1968).

SHELP, W. D., RIESELBACH, R. E.: Increased bidirectional urate transport per nephron following unilateral nephrectomy. In: Abstracts of the American Society of Nephrology, Vol. II, p. 60 (1968).

SHINABERGER, J. H., PABICO, R. C., SHEAR, L., KNOCHEL, J. P., BARRY, K. G.: The effect of albumin on peritoneal extraction of uric acid. Evidence for *in vivo* protein binding of urate. Clin. Res. **12**, 463 (1964).

SIROTA, J. H., YU, T. F., GUTMAN, A. B.: Effect of Benemid (p-[di-n-propylsulfamyl]-benzoic acid) on urate clearance and other discrete renal functions in gouty subjects. J. clin. Invest. **31**, 692—701 (1952).

SKEITH, M. D., HEALEY, L. A., CUTLER, R. E.: Urate excretion during mannitol and glucose diuresis. J. Lab. clin. Med. **70**, 213—220 (1967).

SKEITH, M. D., HEALEY, L. A., CUTLER, R. E.: Effect of phloridzin and uric acid excretion in man. Amer. J. Physiol. **219**, 1080—1082 (1970).
SNAITH, M. L., SCOTT, J. T.: Uric acid clearance in patients with gout and normal subjects. Ann. rheumat. Dis. **30**, 285—289 (1971).
SORENSEN, L. B.: Degradation of uric acid in man. Metabolism **8**, 687—703 (1959).
SORENSEN, L. B.: The elimination of uric acid in man studied by means of ^{14}C-labeled uric acid. Scand. J. clin. Lab. Invest. **12**, Suppl. 54, 1—214 (1960).
SORENSEN, L. B.: The pathogenesis of gout. Arch. intern. Med. **109**, 379—390 (1962).
SORENSEN, L. B.: Role of the intestinal tract in the elimination of uric acid. Arthrit. and Rheum. **8**, 694—706 (1965).
SORENSEN, L. B., KAPPAS, A.: The effects of penicillamine therapy on uric acid metabolism in Wilson's disease. Trans. Ass. Amer. Phycns. **79**, 157—164 (1966).
STEELE, T. H.: Evidence for altered renal urate reabsorption during changes in volume of the extracellular fluid. J. Lab. clin. Med. **74**, 288—299 (1969).
STEELE, T.: Control of uric acid excretion. New Engl. J. Med. **284**, 1193—1196 (1971).
STEELE, T. H., OPPENHEIMER, S.: Factors affecting urate excretion following diuretic administration in man. Amer. J. Med. **47**, 564—574 (1969).
STEELE, T. H., RIESELBACH, R. E.: The renal mechanism for urate homeostasis in normal man. Amer. J. Med. **43**, 868—875 (1967a).
STEELE, T. H., RIESELBACH, R. E.: The contribution of residual nephrons within the chronically diseased kidney to urate homeostasis in man. Amer. J. Med. **43**, 876—886 (1967b).
SUKI, W. N., HULL, A. R., RECTOR, F. C., JR., SELDIN, D. W.: Mechanism of the effect of thiazide diuretics on calcium and uric acid. J. clin. Invest. **46**, 1121 (1967).
THANNHAUSER, S. J.: The pathogenesis of gout. Metabolism **5** 582—593 (1956).
WEINER, I. M., MUDGE, G. H.: Renal tubular mechanisms for excretion of organic acids and bases. Amer. J. Med. **36**, 743—762 (1964).
YU, T. F., GUTMAN, A. B.: Ultrafiltrability of plasma urate in man. Proc. Soc. exp. Biol. (N.Y.) **84**, 21—24 (1953).
YU, T. F., GUTMAN, A. B.: Paradoxical retention of uric acid by uricosuric drugs in low dosage. Proc. Soc. exp. Biol. (N.Y.) **90**, 542—547 (1955).
YU, T. F., BERGER, L., GUTMAN, A. B.: Suppression of tubular secretion of urate by pyrazinamide in the dog. Proc. Soc. exp. Biol. (N.Y.) **107**, 905—908 (1961).
YU, T. F., BERGER, L., GUTMAN, A. B.: Renal function in gout. II. Effect of uric acid loading on renal excretion of uric acid. Amer. J. Med. **33**, 829—844 (1962).
YU, T. F., BERGER, L., KUPFER, S., GUTMAN, A. B.: Tubular secretion of urate in the dog. Amer. J. Physiol. **199**, 1199—1204 (1960).
YU, T. F., BERGER, L., STONE, D. J., WOLF, J., GUTMAN, A. B.: Effect of pyrazinamide and pyrazinoic acid on urate clearance and other discrete renal functions. Proc. Soc. exp. Biol. (N.Y.) **96**, 264—267 (1957a).
YU, T. F., GUTMAN, A. B.: Study of the paradoxical effects of salicylate in low, intermediate and high dosage on the renal mechanisms for excretion of urate in man. J. clin. Invest. **38**, 1298—1315 (1959).
YU, T. F., KAUNG, C., GUTMAN, A. B.: Effect of glycine loading on plasma and urinary uric acid and amino acids in normal and gouty subjects. Amer. J. Med. **49**, 352—359 (1970).
YU, T. F., SIROTA, J. H., BERGER, L., HALPERN, M., GUTMAN, A. B.: Effect of sodium lactate infusion on urate clearance in man. Proc. Soc. exp. Biol. (N.Y.) **96**, 809—813 (1957b).
ZINS, G. R., WEINER, I. M.: Bidirectional urate transport limited to the proximal tubule in dogs. Amer. J. Physiol. **215**, 411—422 (1968).

e) Sekundäre Hyperuricämie und sekundäre Gicht

Von

N. ZÖLLNER

Mit 2 Abbildungen

Geschichtliches und Definitionen

In seinem Lehrbuch des Stoffwechsels und der Stoffwechselkrankheiten (1929) unterscheidet THANNHAUSER als erster deutlich zwischen primärer und sekundärer Gicht, wobei er die sekundäre Gicht „als Folge einer schweren, anatomisch sichtbaren Nierenerkrankung" ansieht. Dementsprechend diskutiert er die Gicht bei Schrumpfniere und entzündlichen Nierenkrankheiten, bei Bleivergiftung und bei Alkoholikern.

Die klare Definition, die THANNHAUSER für die sekundäre Gicht gab, als er sie der „primären konstitutionellen Gicht" gegenüberstellte, wurde weithin nicht zur Kenntnis genommen bzw. vergessen. Noch 1947 erklären W. BAUER und F. KLEMPERER in einem Lehrbuch, daß die Gicht immer hereditär auftritt. Das Zusammentreffen z. B. von Gicht und Polycythaemia vera wurde für zufällig angesehen, obwohl bereits 1943 BARRICK und MILLER einen Teil der Literatur über Gicht bei Blutkrankheiten zusammengestellt hatten.

Die endgültige Einführung des Begriffs „sekundäre Gicht" ist das Verdienst von GUTMAN (1953), der ihn allerdings in Ergänzung von THANNHAUSER in erster Linie für die Gicht im Gefolge von Blutkrankheiten mit vermehrtem Zellumsatz verwendete. Wir haben dann 1960 (ZÖLLNER, 1960) die Definitionen von THANNHAUSER und GUTMAN erstmals zusammengefaßt und darüber hinaus darauf hingewiesen, daß sekundäre Hyperuricämie und sekundäre Gicht nicht nur bei Krankheiten des Blutes und der Nieren, sondern auch bei anderen Krankheiten, z. B. der Glykogenose, vorkommen können.

Natürlich ist die Feststellung, daß Gicht im Gefolge anderer Leiden auftreten kann, nicht erst in diesem Jahrhundert getroffen worden; entsprechende klinische Beobachtungen sind sehr viel älter. So wurde der Zusammenhang von Blei und Gicht schon im 18. Jahrhundert erkannt, als nachgewiesen werden konnte, daß die „Kolik von Devonshire", die meistens von Gicht gefolgt war, durch Blei verursacht wurde (MUSGRAVE, zit. von THANNHAUSER, 1929). Auch GARROD und andere englische Autoren geben an, daß unter den Gichtkranken ein hoher Prozentsatz von Bleiarbeitern zu finden sei, und einen ähnlichen Bericht gibt es von einem Knappschaftsarzt, Dr. JACOB, „Über die Gicht bei den Bleiarbeitern im Oberharz" (ebenfalls zitiert nach THANNHAUSER, 1929).

Auf Grund klinischer Erfahrung konnte bereits um die Jahrhundertwende von MINKOWSKI formuliert werden, daß „das Blei offenbar diejenigen Gewebselemente zu schädigen vermag, deren Funktion gestört sein muß, wenn die Gicht entstehen soll". MINKOWSKI hat aber nicht den Schritt getan, den Begriff einer sekundären Gicht zu prägen, weil er gleichzeitig zu erkennen glaubte, daß die Einwirkung des Bleis allein für die Ausbildung der Gicht nicht ausreicht.

Obwohl heute sekundäre Erkrankungen an Gicht bei hämatopoetischen Krankheiten sehr viel häufiger sind als bei Krankheiten der Niere oder des Stoffwechsels, ist die Kenntnis des Zusammenhangs zwischen Blutkrankheiten und Gicht wesentlich jünger. Ältere Autoren hielten ein Zusammentreffen von Gicht und Leukämie für selten. So schreibt NAEGELI 1919: „Für die Auffassung des Wesens der Gicht ist diese so eminent seltene Kombination trotz der jahrelang

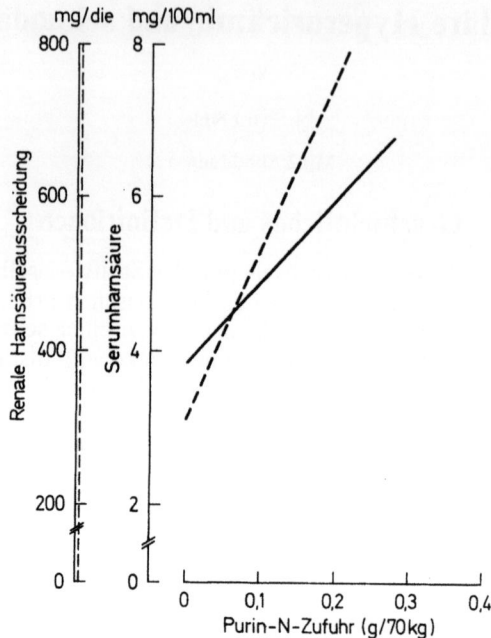

Abb. 1. Lineare Beziehung zwischen Purinzufuhr (Abszisse, im vorliegenden Fall als Ribomononucleotid [AMP]) einerseits und Serumharnsäure bzw. renaler Harnsäureausscheidung andererseits

vermehrt gebildeten Harnsäure entschieden wichtig", und FORKNER stellt 1938 fest: "The simultaneous occurrence of the two conditions is so rare that any real relationship seems doubtful." HEILMEYER (HEILMEYER u. BEGEMANN, 1951) schließt sich diesen Erfahrungen an: „Wenn trotzdem gichtische Erscheinungen bei Leukämien kaum beobachtet werden, ...". Wahrscheinlich haben die älteren Autoren die zeitlichen Beziehungen nicht deutlich genug gesehen; vom Beginn einer vermehrten Purinbelastung an dauert es im allgemeinen Jahre, bis der erste Gichtanfall auftritt, eine Erfahrung, die wir nach der Währungsreform erneut machen konnten (ZÖLLNER, 1960).

Vereinfacht kann man sagen, daß eine vermehrte Harnsäurebildung (bzw. eine verminderte Fähigkeit zur Harnsäureausscheidung) zwar innerhalb kurzer Zeit zur Hyperuricämie führt, daß von da an aber noch längere Zeit bis zur Manifestation der gichtischen Gelenkkrankheit vergeht. Die Uratnephrolithiasis ist dieser Verzögerung in sehr viel geringerem Maße unterzogen, und so ist es zu verstehen, daß bei Leukämien mit kurzem Verlauf wohl die renalen Komplikationen durch Harnsäure häufig sind, nicht aber die Gicht.

Die mathematisch eindeutigen Beziehungen zwischen Purinumsatz, Harnsäurespiegel im Plasma und Harnsäureausscheidung im Harn sind in den letzten Jahren durch die Arbeiten von ZÖLLNER et al. (1972) grundsätzlich klargestellt worden. Neuere Arbeiten mit Ribomononucleotiden (Abb. 1) erlauben es weitgehend, aus dem Plasmaspiegel bzw. der renalen Harnsäureausscheidung von Gesunden auf den Purinumsatz rückzuschließen. Bei normaler Nierenfunktion ist im klinisch interessanten Bereich der Plasmaharnsäurespiegel eine Funktion der Harnsäurebildung, vermehrte Harnsäurebildung führt obligatorisch zum Ansteigen des Harnsäurespiegels. Wirken mehrere Faktoren additiv, z.B. die derzeitige hohe alimentäre Purinbelastung der Bevölkerung und eine Leukose, so kommt es auch zu einer additiven Beeinflussung der Harnsäurespiegel.

Die Beziehung zwischen einer Einschränkung der Nierenfunktion und der Hyperuricämie ist ebenso eindeutig geklärt. Genaue zahlenmäßige Angaben sind jedoch erst teilweise möglich, weil kein Modell für eine ethisch vertretbare, reproduzierbare, graduierbare und reversible Einschränkung der Harnsäureausscheidung bei gesunden Versuchspersonen bekannt ist. Alle Rückschlüsse auf die Zusammenhänge zwischen Einschränkung der Harnsäureausscheidung und Hyperuricämie beruhen entweder auf experimentell nicht übersehbaren klinischen Beobachtungen oder auf pharmakologischen (z.B. Saluretica oder Pyrazinamid) bzw. toxikologischen Versuchen. (Berechtigterweise wird auch der umgekehrte Weg beschrieben, und eine bei gleichem stationärem Plasmaspiegel verminderte renale Harnsäureausscheidung wird als ein Beweis für eine Einschränkung der entsprechenden Funktionen in der Niere gewertet.)

Beim derzeitigen Stand der Beobachtungen und Befunde darf im Zusammenhang mit der Niere, dem wichtigsten Ausscheidungsorgan für die Harnsäure, als sicher angenommen werden, daß

chronische Nierenkrankheiten die Fähigkeit zur Harnsäureausscheidung einschränken können,

diese Einschränkung bevorzugt bei Krankheiten auftritt, die mit tubulären Insuffizienzen einhergehen (vgl. Kap. SÖRENSEN),

metabolische und pharmakologische Einflüsse die Fähigkeit zur Ausscheidung von Harnsäure isoliert (eventuell zusammen mit wenigen anderen Substanzen) beeinträchtigen können

und daß eine solche isolierte Einschränkung Ursache der familiären Gicht ist.

Die Fähigkeit zur Harnsäureausscheidung ist definiert durch die Beziehung zwischen dem Plasmaspiegel der Harnsäure und der Harnsäureausscheidung pro Zeiteinheit, sei es im akuten Versuch (WYNGAARDEN, 1965) oder im chronischen Ernährungsexperiment (ZÖLLNER u. GRIEBSCH, 1974) (Abb. 2).

Offensichtlich ist es grundsätzlich möglich, daß in der Pathogenese der sekundären Hyperuricämie und der sekundären Gicht die Einflüsse einer vermehrten Harnsäurebildung und einer verminderten Fähigkeit zur Harnsäureausscheidung zusammenwirken. Dieses Zusammenwirken kommt in der Pathogenese der sekundären Gicht auch tatsächlich vor, z.B. bei der Glykogenose. Experimentell läßt sich zeigen, daß die Hyperuricämie, welche bei reichlicher Fructosezufuhr auftritt, sowohl durch eine vermehrte Harnsäurebildung als auch durch eine Verminderung der Harnsäureausscheidung zustande kommt.

Die im Konzept klare Trennung zwischen primärer und sekundärer Gicht bzw. primärer und sekundärer Hyperuricämie ist heute nicht mehr aufrecht zu erhalten. Über das Dilemma hilft auch die neuere Unterscheidung zwischen genetischer und aquirierter Hyperuricämie nicht hinweg. Die begrifflichen Schwierigkeiten sind verschiedener Art. Sie hängen damit zusammen, daß bei genauer Betrachtung nicht alle Fälle eindeutig primär oder sekundär sind. Häufig wirken primäre, in der Regel genetische Ursachen zusammen mit Umweltfaktoren, z.B. Ernährung, anderen Krankheiten, z.B. Bleivergiftung oder sogar anderen genetisch bedingten Krankheiten, z.B. Thalassämie, bei der Ausbildung von Hyperuricämie bzw. Gicht.

In solchen Fällen kommt es nur auf den Standpunkt an, ob man den Befund der Hyperuricämie oder die festgestellte Gicht als primär oder sekundär bezeichnet. Dies gilt sogar für die klassische („primäre") Gicht, die in Notzeiten nicht vorkommt, also eindeutig ernährungsbedingt ist. Der richtige Standpunkt dürfte allerdings sein, an die Stelle des Entweder/Oder ein Sowohl als Auch zu setzen.

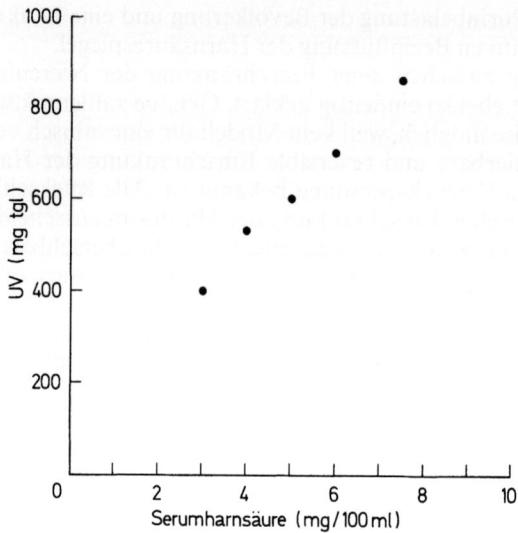

Abb. 2. Lineare Beziehung zwischen Serumharnsäure und renaler Harnsäureausscheidung ($u\,v$) im chronischen Versuch bei Gesunden

Schon DENT hat darauf hingewiesen, daß sich sehr viele genetisch bedingte Stoffwechselstörungen nur in einer passenden Umwelt manifestieren.

Gicht, d. h. an dieser Stelle die Arthritis urica, ist genau gesehen immer sekundär, nämlich die Reaktion auf die Bildung von Harnsäuremikrokristallen, die ihrerseits wiederum eine örtliche Erhöhung der Uratkonzentration über das Löslichkeitsprodukt, meist im Zusammenhang mit einer Hyperuricämie, voraussetzt. Eine sekundäre Gicht ohne sekundäre Hyperuricämie ist allerdings nicht bekannt, frühere Annahmen zum Gegenteil sind unbewiesen geblieben. Dagegen gibt es viele Fälle von sekundärer Hyperuricämie ohne das gehäufte Auftreten von Gicht; die Hyperuricämie bei Down-Syndrom ist hierfür ein Beispiel.

Für die Entstehung einer sekundären Gicht sind Höhe und Variationen einer sekundären Hyperuricämie nicht belanglos. Konstante, geringe Hyperuricämien (bis etwa 8 mg/100 ml), wie sie zur Zeit in Deutschland häufig sind, führen praktisch nie zur Auslösung einer Gicht. Bei deutlicher, chronisch konstanter Erhöhung des Harnsäurespiegels (über 9 mg/100 ml) kann man dagegen, unabhängig von ihrer Ursache, mit Gichtanfällen beinahe sicher rechnen. Die durch reichlichen Alkoholgenuß erzeugte vorübergehende Verstärkung der Hyperuricämie ist eine bekannte Ursache von Anfällen.

Letztlich sei erwähnt, daß es nicht nur eine primäre Hyperuricämie bzw. primäre Gicht gibt. Es sind mindestens zwei Defekte im Purinstoffwechsel beschrieben, die durch den Mangel einer Transferase zur Mehrproduktion von Harnsäure führen, und die häufigste Form der familiären Gicht des Erwachsenen dürfte auf einen tubulären Transportdefekt zurückzuführen sein. Schwierig wird die Zuordnung beim Glucose-6-phosphatase-Mangel (der Glykogenose I), bei welchem die Erhöhung der Harnsäurespiegel als unvermeidliche Folge des genetischen Stoffwechseldefekts angesehen werden kann; hier kann die Hyperuricämie als „primär" angesehen werden, obwohl sie „eigentlich" sekundär zu einer Störung des Kohlenhydratstoffwechsels auftritt (vgl. Tabelle 1,2). Eine nahezu vollständige Auflistung findet sich bei NEWCOMBE (1975).

Tabelle 1. Primäre Hyperuricämie mit Gicht (modifiziert nach ZÖLLNER, 1974)

Verminderte renale Harnsäureausscheidung (wahrscheinlich die Ursache der häufigsten Form, nämlich der familiären Gicht des Erwachsenen)
2. Vermehrte Harnsäurebildung
   a) Enzymdefekte
      Adenin-Phosphoribosyltransferase
         Mangel (wenige Fälle von juveniler Gicht)
      Hypoxanthin-Guanin-Phosphoribosyltransferase
         Partieller oder kompletter (Lesh-Nyhan-Syndrom) Mangel
      Glucose-6-phosphatase
         Mangel (Glykogenspeicherkrankheit I)
      Phosphoribosylpyrophosphat-Synthetase
      Glutathion-Reduktase
      Xanthin-Oxydase
         vermehrte Aktivität (?)
   b) Vermehrte Harnsäurebildung mit unbekannter Ursache

Tabelle 2. Wichtige Ursachen (und Beispiele) sekundärer Hyperuricämien mit Gicht (modifiziert nach ZÖLLNER, 1974; bei den eingeklammerten Angaben müssen wahrscheinlich für das Zustandekommen einer Gicht hereditäre Faktoren ebenfalls vorliegen)

Vermehrte Harnsäurebildung	Verminderte renale Harnsäureausscheidung
Störungen der Hämatopoese	Nierenkrankheiten
Polycythämie	vgl. Kap. SÖRENSEN, aber auch isolierte tubuläre
Osteomyelosklerose	Defekte, wie das Bartter-Syndrom
Chronische myeloische Leukämie	Hyperlactacidämien
(sekundäre Polycythämie bei Herz- und	hohe Alkoholspiegel
Lungenkrankheiten)	Glucose-6-phosphatase-Mangel
(Hämolytische Anämien)	Sarkoidose
Glucose-6-phosphatase-Mangel	Ketoacidosen
(vermehrte Zufuhr von Nahrungspurinen,	Fasten
Fettsucht)	Diabetes mellitus
	Vergiftungen
	Blei
	Arzneimittel
	Saluretica
	Pyrazinamid
	Salicylate und Probenecid in niederer Dosis

Tabelle 3. Häufigkeit (Prozent der Fälle) der verschiedenen Formen der Gicht (modifiziert nach ZÖLLNER, 1974, eigene Schätzungen sind kursiv geschrieben)

	Idiopathische	Sekundäre Gicht
Ausscheidungsdefekt	80—95	*1—2—5*
Vermehrte Harnsäurebildung	*2—5—20*	*1—3—10*

Die Tabellen auf S. 168 stellen trotz der eben diskutierten Vorbehalte die primären und die sekundären Hyperuricämien mit Gicht einander gegenüber.

Wichtige Beispiele sekundärer Hyperuricämien

Während sich die bisherigen Erörterungen vorwiegend auf die Ursachen der sekundären Gicht konzentriert haben, wird im weiteren die sekundäre Hyperuricämie diskutiert. Es wurde bereits erwähnt, daß eine ausgeprägte Hyperuricämie (mit Werten über 9 mg/100 ml) unabhängig von ihrer Genese nahezu zwangsläufig zur Gicht führt, und daß plötzliche Anstiege der interstitiellen Harnsäurekonzentration ebenfalls recht regelmäßig Gichtanfälle auslösen können.

Blutkrankheiten

Die frühen Untersuchungen über den Harnsäurestoffwechsel bei Blutkrankheiten durch SALKOWSKI, MAGNUS-LEVY (1909/10) und KRAUSS sind nur zum Teil durch Bestimmungen von Harnsäureausscheidung und Harnsäureclearance mit enzymatischer Methodik ergänzt worden. LAWRENCE (1955) gibt an, daß die Harnsäureausscheidung bei chronisch-lymphatischer Leukämie normal, bei chronisch-myeloischer und bei den akuten Leukämien dagegen auf das Zwei- bis Zweieinhalbfache erhöht sei. Dabei bestehe eine Korrelation der Harnsäureausscheidung mit der Schwere des leukämischen Prozesses, nicht aber mit der Leukocytenzahl. SANDBERG et al. (1956) sowie KRAKOFF (1957) haben die Feststellung bestätigt und durch detaillierte Angaben eindrucksvoll erläutert. Ihren Zahlen kann man entnehmen, wie stark die Harnsäurebildung vermehrt sein kann, so z. B. bei einem vierjährigen Knaben mit akuter Lymphoblastenleukämie, der täglich 2,8 g Harnsäure (165 mg/kg KG, oder das 25fache der Norm) ausschied. Die Nierensteinbildung durch Urate bei der Leukämie ist entsprechend häufig. WEISBERGER und PERSKY (1953) geben 4,76%, verglichen mit 0% bei anderen metastasierenden Malignomen und 0,07% in der allgemeinen Krankenhausbelegschaft ihrer Serie an. Einmalig ist der vorzüglich beschriebene Fall von VINING und THOMSON (1934) einer aleukämischen Leukämie (durch Autopsie gesichert) mit schwerer tophöser Gicht bei einem fünfjährigen Knaben. Erwähnenswert sind bei diesem Fall eine gewisse, nicht näher in Erfahrung zu bringende familiäre Belastung sowie die starke leukämische Veränderung der Niere, kombiniert mit weißen Uratniederschlägen.

Zusammenfassend darf man feststellen, daß Gicht bei Leukämien trotz stark erhöhter Harnsäurebildung selten ist. In den Fällen mit erhöhter Plasmaharnsäure bewirkt möglicherweise die kurze Lebensdauer (TIVEY, 1954/55), daß es nicht zur Ausbildung der Gicht kommt. Das gelegentliche Vorkommen einer Gicht bei chronisch-myeloischer Leukämie weist jedenfalls in diese Richtung.

HEILMEYER und BEGEMANN (1951) machen keine Angaben über Gicht als Komplikation der perniziösen Anämie, WILKINSON (1949) erwähnt in einem Bericht über 1600 Patienten mit perniziöser Anämie weder Gicht noch Nierensteine.

Besonders interessant ist das Studium der Zusammenhänge zwischen familiärem hämolytischen Ikterus und Gicht, da mehrere Stammbäume vorliegen. Der älteste ist 1885 von MURCHISON beschrieben, und HUTCHINSON und PANTON (1896) haben die Familiengeschichte ergänzt. Von fünf Familienmitgliedern in drei Generationen mit hämolytischem Ikterus litten drei (eines davon eine Frau) an Gicht. LESCHKE hat 1922 ebenfalls hämolytischen Ikterus bei vier Familienmitgliedern in drei Generationen beobachtet; zwei der vier Männer litten an Gicht.

DEITRICK (1940) berichtet über hämolytischen Ikterus mit Gicht bei Vater und Sohn, während OWEN und ROBERTS (1937) den Fall eines Patienten mitteilen, der mit 10 Jahren an hämolytischem Ikterus, mit 26 Jahren an Gicht erkrankte und bei dem die jung verstorbene Mutter an Gelbsucht gelitten hatte, während der Vater Gichtiker war. Von besonderem Interesse ist indes ein Stammbaum von TILESTON und GRIFFIN (1910), denn es gelang, eine der Personen des Stammbaumes in einem 25 Jahre später von FITZ (1935) beschriebenen Kranken wiederzuerkennen (gleiche Initialen des Namens O.A.S., gleiches Alter, gleiche Zahl der Geschwister gleichen Geschlechtes, gleiche Familienvorgeschichte und gleicher Lebensraum, New England), so daß der Stammbaum ergänzt werden kann. In dieser Familie ist bei zwei Mitgliedern hämolytischer Ikterus mit Gicht aufgetreten, daneben sind aber sowohl hämolytischer Ikterus ohne Gicht als auch Gicht ohne hämolytischen Ikterus vorgekommen. Damit wäre das Zusammentreffen von familiärem hämolytischen Ikterus und Gicht ein Produkt zufälliger Kreuzung. Dieser Schluß ist wahrscheinlich richtig, denn erstens ist Gicht als sporadische Komplikation des familiären hämolytischen Ikterus nicht beschrieben, zweitens zeigen die erwähnten Familien außerhalb des Tileston-Griffin-Fitz-Stammbaumes die für die primäre Gicht typische Geschlechtsverteilung (eine von vier Frauen, aber sieben von neun Männern hatten Gicht), und drittens zeigt der erwähnte Fall von OWEN und ROBERTS (1937), wie der Patient von je einem Elternteil die Blutkrankheit und die Gicht erben kann. Man kann annehmen, daß bei vorhandener Gichtanlage eine Krankheit mit dauernder vermehrter Blutneubildung infolge der vermehrten Harnsäurebildung vermehrt zur Gichtmanifestation führt. So ist es vermutlich auch zu erklären, warum die Auseinandermendelung von Gicht und hämolytischem Ikterus nicht öfter beschrieben ist.

Analoge Argumente, wie für den familiären hämolytischen Ikterus, gelten für eine Familie mit der Kombination von Thalassämie und Gicht (MARCH et al., 1952). Auch hier ist nicht anzunehmen, daß die Thalassämie Ursache der Gicht ist, sondern das Zusammentreffen ist als zufällig anzusehen, wobei wiederum der dauernden Blutregeneration bei Personen mit Gichtanlage die Rolle eines auslösenden Faktors zukommt.

Während bei den bisher besprochenen Hämoblastosen und Anämien, mit der möglichen Ausnahme der chronisch myeloischen Leukämie, eine sekundäre Gicht nicht zustande kommt, sondern höchstens eine familiäre Gicht manifestiert wird, gehört bei der Polycythaemia vera und bei den Krankheiten der Gruppe der myeloischen Metaplasie die sekundäre Gicht zu den bekannten Komplikationen.

Den ältesten Hinweis auf die Häufigkeit der Gicht bei Polycythaemia vera macht WEBER (1934), der ohne zahlenmäßige Angabe behauptet, daß Gicht eine wohlbekannte Komplikation der Polycythämie sei, die er selbst mehrmals beobachtet habe. TINNEY et al. berichteten dann 1945 aus der Mayo Clinic, daß in ihrer Serie von 168 Fällen von Polycythämie Gicht achtmal aufgetreten sei; ihre Patienten waren Männer zwischen 51 und 67 Jahren. In einer Serie von 125 Fällen aus Kopenhagener Krankenhäusern fand VIDEBAEK (1950) elf Gichtfälle (sieben von 74 Männern, vier von 51 Frauen). TALBOTT (1959) gibt zwei weitere ihm persönlich mitgeteilte Serien (LAWRENCE, BERLIN und HUFF, sowie DAMON und HOLUB) von zusammen 466 Polycythaemia vera-Kranken mit 32 Fällen sekundärer Gicht bekannt. Nimmt man noch die bei TALBOTT zitierte Serie von WASSERMAN und BASSEN (fünf Gichtiker unter 253 Polycythämiefällen) hinzu, so ergibt sich bei 1012 Fällen von Polycythämie eine Gichthäufigkeit von 5,5%. Man kann also der geistreichen Bemerkung WEBERS (1934) wohl zustimmen, daß die ältesten Beschreibungen der Polycythämie unter Berichten über Gichtiker zu finden sein mögen.

Soweit in den genannten Serien angegeben, liegt die Häufigkeit einer Nephrolithiasis bei der Polycythämie zwischen vier und elf Prozent. Mit Ausnahme der skandinavischen Untersuchung waren Männer in einem über die Geschlechtsverteilung der Polycythämie hinausgehenden Maße von der sekundären Gicht betroffen.

Im deutschen Schrifttum ist Gicht bei Polycythaemia vera in neuerer Zeit mehrfach beschrieben worden, z. B. von ACHENBACH (1955). Wir selber sind mehrfach durch Gichtanfälle auf das Vorliegen einer Polycythämie aufmerksam gemacht worden. Seit einer frühen Beschreibung durch KÖNIG und ZÖLLNER (1962) haben wir darauf verzichtet, weitere Fälle mitzuteilen; es lohnt aber bei jedem Fall von Gicht das Blutbild sorgfältig anzusehen.

REIFENSTEIN berichtete 1939 über eine Frau mit „Erythrämie, Gicht und subleukämischer Myelose", bei der im Alter von 52 Jahren eine sehr große Milz festgestellt worden war, vier Jahre später eine Gicht und noch zwei Jahre später eine Anämie. Seither sind ab und zu Berichte über myeloische Metaplasie (LASTER u. MULLER, 1953), Osteomyeloreticulose (FISCHER u. KLINGHARDT, 1958) oder Myelosklerose (HICKLING) mit Gicht publiziert; LINKE konnte bereits 1954 siebzehn Fälle zusammenstellen. LASTER und MULLERs Patient hatte mit 20 Jahren eine normale Milz (bei einer Operation gesehen), mit 60 Jahren eine palpable Milz mit normalem peripherem Blutbild, mit 61 Jahren wurde eine große Milz mit myeloischer Metaplasie entfernt. 27 Monate nach der Operation trat der erste Gichtanfall auf, bei der Autopsie fanden sich Harnsteine, im Knochenmark „myeloische Metaplasie". Der Einbau des markierten Glycins in die Harnsäure dieses Patienten erfolgte wie bei der Polycythaemia vera mit einem späten Konzentrationsmaximum.

HICKLING fand bei 30 Fällen von Osteomyelosklerose zweimal Gicht, LINMAN und BETHELL (1957) geben bei 56 Patienten mit "agnogenic myeloid metaplasia" einen Gichtanfall an. Im Gegensatz zu letzteren Autoren hat BALDINI in einer Serie von 45 Patienten sechs sichere und einen fraglichen Gichtkranken (eine Häufigkeit von 13%) und vier Fälle mit Nephrolithiasis beobachtet. Auch von BALDINIs sechs Fällen mit Gicht hatten zwei eine zuverlässige Vorgeschichte von Polycythaemia vera. (In der Linman-Bethell-Serie finden sich fünf Fälle von Polycythämie.) Von den neun Polycythämiekranken mit Gicht von TINNEY et al. (1945) wiesen wenigstens vier Milzvergrößerungen von einem für Polycythämie außergewöhnlichen Umfang auf, und auch in WEBERs (1934) Fall wurden eine beträchtlich große Milz, außerdem Myelocyten im Blut, beobachtet. Der von ACHENBACH (1955) beschriebene Polycythämiekranke mit Gicht hatte ebenfalls Myelocyten (5%) im peripheren Blut und zeigte im zellreichen Sternalmark reichlich Megakaryocyten; die sehr große Milz ergab bei der Punktion das Bild einer myeloischen Metaplasie. In zwei der von TALBOTT (1959) mitgeteilten Serien von Polycythämiekranken mit Gicht starb ein Viertel bis ein Drittel der Gichtiker an Leukämie. Es wäre deshalb zu prüfen, ob das Auftreten einer Gicht bei Polycythämie nicht der Vorbote des Auftretens leukämischer Veränderungen bzw. einer myeloischen Metaplasie der Milz sein kann.

Arzneimittel

Im Kapitel über Hyperuricämie durch therapeutische Maßnahmen wird von MERTZ die Problematik ausführlich dargestellt, so daß die heute häufige arzneimittelbedingte Hyperuricämie hier kurz abgehandelt werden kann.

Seitdem die Saluretica in die Therapie eingeführt wurden, hat die arzneimittelinduzierte Hyperuricämie stark zugenommen. Nichtsdestoweniger ist nach wie vor unklar, ob Saluretica allein ausreichen, eine deutliche Hyperuricämie hervorzurufen oder ob nur das Zusammentreffen von Salureticabehandlung mit einer Gichtanlage oder massiver Purinbelastung eine ausgeprägte Hyperuricämie hervorrufen kann.

Neben den Thiaziden haben auch Etacrynsäure, Chlorthalidon und Acetazolamid die Eigenschaft, die Harnsäureausscheidung zu verringern und Hyperuricämie hervorzurufen. Der gemeinsame Mechanismus ist unklar. Es ist unwahrscheinlich, daß die im amerikanischen Schrifttum angenommene Verringerung des extracellulären Flüssigkeitsraumes als Ursache in Frage kommt, weil dieser Effekt sich innerhalb weniger Tage ausgleichen müßte. Bemerkenswert ist dagegen die Angabe, daß die durch Thiazid induzierte Hyperuricämie durch die Gabe von KCl und NH_4Cl ausgeglichen werden kann (ZWEIFLER u. THOMPSON, 1965).

Die Angaben über die Häufigkeit des Zusammentreffens von Hyperuricämie und Gicht sind widersprüchlich. Sie schwanken zwischen Feststellungen, daß etwa ein Fünftel aller Hyperuricämiker in einer Krankenhauspopulation Thiazide erhalten hätten (wobei offen bleibt, ob Hyperuricämie oder Thiazidbehandlung zeitlich vorangehen), und der Behauptung, daß nahezu die Hälfte aller Männer, welche Gicht entwickelten, unter Salureticabehandlung standen. Mangels genau vergleichbarer Kontrollpopulationen lassen sich hier keine endgültigen Feststellungen treffen. Unsere eigenen Erfahrungen sprechen dafür, daß bei der Mehrzahl der in der ambulanten Praxis gesehenen Gichtfälle eine Salureticabehandlung keine Rolle spielt, doch fehlt auch für diese Angabe eine Kontrollpopulation. Die Wirkung des Pyrazinamids ist bereits im Kapitel III, 1 d dargestellt; die Substanz hat heute nur noch experimentelles Interesse.

Bemerkenswert ist der paradoxe Effekt vieler uricosurischer Substanzen, d. h. die Feststellung, daß z.B. Salicylate oder Probenecid in niedriger bis sehr niedriger Dosierung den Harnsäurespiegel durch eine Hemmung der tubulären Ausscheidung erhöhen. Insofern als eine große Zahl von Substanzen mit den genannten Verbindungen, aber auch mit den Dicumarinen oder dem Phenylindandion strukturell entfernte Ähnlichkeiten aufweisen (vgl. ZÖLLNER, 1960), ist in der Praxis immer damit zu rechnen, daß Arzneimittel Hyperuricämie hervorrufen. Es empfehlen sich entsprechende Auslaßversuche.

Von einigen carcinostatisch wirkenden Verbindungen wird behauptet, daß sie zu vermehrter Harnsäurebildung führen. Die entsprechenden Angaben sind schwer nachzuprüfen, weil kaum unterschieden werden kann, inwieweit die Substanz direkt in den Purinstoffwechsel eingreift und inwieweit es sich um den bekannten Effekt der Tumorbehandlung auf die Harnsäurebildung handelt. Mit einer vermehrten Harnsäurebildung und mit einer Hyperuricämie rechnet man bei einer Tumorbehandlung ohnedies.

Blei

Die Bleigicht scheint in einzelnen Ländern immer noch häufig zu sein. EMMERSON (1963) hat über eine verhältnismäßig große Incidenz dieser Gicht in Queensland berichtet, und in den Vereinigten Staaten soll vor allem der Genuß von "Moonshine"-Whisky recht häufig zur Bleivergiftung führen (BALL u. SÖRENSEN, 1969).

Sarkoidose und Berylliose

In schweren Fällen von Sarkoidose und Berylliose tritt die Hyperuricämie recht häufig auf. Besonders deutlich ist das Zusammentreffen bei Fällen mit eingeschränkter Diffusionskapazität der Lungen (für Kohlenmonoxid). Da diese Fälle in der Regel auch eine Hyperlactacidämie zeigen, wird angenommen, daß bei ihnen die Hyperuricämie renaler Genese ist und der bekannten Wirkung der Hyperlactacidämie bei hohem Alkoholspiegel (vgl. Tabelle 2 und Seite 168) entspricht.

Fasten und Diabetes

Es ist seit langem bekannt, daß absolutes Fasten zu einer Hyperuricämie mit Werten über 10,0 mg/100 ml führt und daß bei bekannter familiärer Vorbelastung dabei Gichtanfälle auftreten können. Tatsächlich tritt die Erhöhung des Harnsäurespiegels auch bereits bei Verringerungen der Nahrungszufuhr auf 600—300 kcal/Tag auf und ist ein von der Praxis längst sanktioniertes Maß für die Zuverlässigkeit der Einhaltung von Diätvorschriften.

Die klinischen Erfahrungen sprechen dafür, daß die Hyperuricämie bei der Einschränkung der Nahrungszufuhr der Ketoacidose entspricht. Diese Beobachtung wird bestätigt durch die Feststellung, daß auch die diabetische Ketoacidose mit Hyperuricämie einhergeht.

Für die Erklärung der Wirkung auf die Harnsäure stehen zwei Hypothesen zur Verfügung. Einmal wird postuliert, daß eine Verschiebung des NADH/NAD$^+$-Quotienten für die Störung des tubulären Harnsäuretransportes verantwortlich sei. Die zweite Hypothese vergleicht die Wirkung der chronischen Ketoacidose mit der der Saluretica und bezieht sie auf eine Verarmung des Elektrolytpools.

Unabhängig von der Richtigkeit der einen oder anderen Ansicht ist festzuhalten, daß vielen Stoffwechselvorgängen mit Verschiebungen im Redoxgleichgewicht (Lactat/Pyruvat, Hydroxybutyrat/Acetoacetat) oder Verringerungen des Körpergehaltes an Kalium (und/oder Natrium) eine Hyperuricämie gemeinsam ist.

Hyperparathyreoidismus

Im angelsächsischen Schrifttum (vgl. SCOTT et al., 1964) wird mehrfach festgestellt, daß beim Hyperparathyreoidismus die Hyperuricämie häufig sei. Unsere eigenen Erfahrungen können dies nicht bestätigen. Bisher hat sich auch kein Mechanismus finden lassen, welcher die Hyperuricämie beim Hyperparathyreoidismus erklären ließe, sieht man von der Niereninsuffizienz bei der Nephrocalcinose ab. Prospektive Untersuchungen sind hier notwendig, weil mit JACKSON und HARRIS (1965) anzunehmen ist, daß der Hyperparathyreoidismus auch mit der Pseudogicht einhergehen kann.

Psoriasis

Seit der Mitteilung von EISEN und SEEGMILLER (1961), daß bei ausgedehnter Psoriasis Hyperuricämie häufig sei, haben wir die Frage des Zusammenhanges zwischen Psoriasis und Hyperuricämie in der Klinik sorgfältig beobachtet. In unserem großen Krankengut konnten wir keine auffällige Häufung von Psoriasis feststellen, und viele von uns untersuchten Psoriatiker sind normouricämisch. Sollte tatsächlich eine Beziehung zwischen Psoriasis und Hyperuricämie bestehen, so muß sie als so wenig evident angesehen werden, daß zu ihrer Bestätigung Untersuchungen an einem sorgfältig ausgewählten Kontrollkollektiv unerläßlich sind.

Schlußbemerkungen

Das Gebiet der sekundären Hyperuricämie und der in ihrem Gefolge auftretenden sekundären Gicht ist eines der interessantesten Gebiete der Gichtforschung.

Die Wirkung von bekannten (und neuen) Arzneimitteln ist noch nicht ausreichend erklärt, ganz abgesehen davon, daß Arzneimittel in sorgfältig geplanten Versuchen hervorragende Modelle für genetische, aber auch anders bedingte Krankheiten, welche den Harnsäurestoffwechsel beeinflussen, liefern können.

Die genauere Beschreibung der metabolischen Voraussetzungen für Störungen der Harnsäureausscheidung (Lactacidose, Ketoacidose, Kaliumverarmung) unter sorgfältiger Berücksichtigung quantitativer Aspekte dürfte die Voraussetzung für vernünftige Untersuchungen über den Einfluß metabolischer Parameter auf die Harnsäureausscheidung liefern.

Die Geschichte der sekundären Gicht zeigt, daß klinische Beobachtungen immer noch zu neuen Feststellungen führen können, obwohl diese Feststellungen bereits Jahrzehnte früher hätten getroffen werden können.

Literatur

ACHENBACH, W.: Atypische Polycythämie. Myelosklerose und Gicht. Medizinische **1955**, 807.
BALDINI, M.: Persönl. Mitteilung.
BALL, G. V., L. B. SORENSEN: Pathogenesis of hyperuricemia in saturnine gout. New Engl. J. Med. **280**, 1199 (1969).
BARRICK, L. E., MILLER, J. R.: Gout. Quart. Bull. North. Univ. med. Sch. **17**, 133 (1943).
DEITRICK, J. E.: The association of congenital hemolytic jaundice and gout. Int. Clin. **3**, 264 (1940).
EBSTEIN, W.: Natur und Behandlung der Gicht. Wiesbaden 1822, 2. Auflage 1906.
EISEN, A. Z., SEEGMILLER, J. E.: Uric acid metabolism in psoriasis. J. clin. Invest. **40**, 1486 (1961).
EMMERSON, B. T.: Chronic lead nephropathy: The diagnostic use of calcium EDTA and the association with gout. Aust. Ann. Med. **12**, 310 (1963).
FISCHER, E., KLINGHARDT, G. W.: Osteomyeloreticulose mit Gicht. Acta haemat. (Basel) **19**, 82 (1958).
FITZ, R.: Three cases with intermittently painful joints, splenomegaly and anemia. Med. Clin. N. Amer. **18**, 1053 (1935).
FORKNER, C. E.: Leukemia and alied disorders, p. 42. New York: MacMillan 1938.
GUTMAN, A. B.: Primary and secondary gout. Ann. intern. Med. **39**, 1062 (1953).
HEILMEYER, L., BEGEMANN, H.: Handbuch der Inneren Medizin, Bd. II. Berlin-Göttingen-Heidelberg: Springer 1951.
HOLBØLL, S. A.: Untersuchungen über den Grundumsatz bei Patienten mit Leukämie und Lymphogranulomatose. Acta med. scand. **72**, 326 (1929).
HUTCHINSON, J.: On the importance of perseverance in inquiries as to the inheritance of gout. Arch. Surg. (London) **7**, 197 (1896).
JACKSON, H. JR.: Studies in nuclei metabolism — I. Adenine nucleotide in human blood. J. biol. Chem. **57**, 121 (1923).
JACKSON, W. P. U., HARRIS, F.: Gout with hyperparathyroidism: Report of a case with examination of synovial fluid. Brit. med. J. **1965 II**, 211.
KÖNIG, E., ZÖLLNER, N.: Sekundäre Gicht bei Osteomyelosklerose und bei Polycythaemia vera. Med. Klin. **57**, 1741 (1962).
KRAKOFF, I. H.: Urinary uric acid excretion in leukemia. In: The Leukemias, Etiology, Pathophysiology, Treatment, p. 407. New York: Academic Press 1957.
LASTER, L., MULLER, A. F.: Uric acid production in a case of myeloid metaplasia associated with gouty arthritis, studied with N^{15}-labeled glycine. Amer. J. Med. **15**, 857 (1953).
LAWRENCE, J. S.: Physiology and function of the white blood cells. J. Amer. med. Ass. **157**, 1212 (1955).
LESCHKE, E.: Hämolytischer Ikterus und Gicht. Med. Klin. **13**, 896 (1922).
LINMAN, J. W., BETHELL, F. H.: Agnogenic myeoloid metaplasia. Amer. J. Med. **22**, 107 (1957).
MAGNUS-LEVY, A.: Uric acid in gout. Harvey Lect. **5**, 251 (1909/1910).
MARCH, H. W., SCHLYEN, S. M., SCHWARTZ, S. E.: Mediterranean hemopathic syndromes (Cooley's anemia) in adults. Amer. J. Med. **13**, 46 (1952).
MURCHISON, C.: Clinical Lectures on Diseases of the Liver, Jaundice, and Abdominal Dropsy, 3 rd. ed. London 1885.
NAEGELI, O.: Blutkrankheiten und Blutdiagnostik. Berlin u. Leipzig 1919.

NEWCOMBE, D. S.: Inherited Biochemical Disorders and Uric Acid Metabolism. Aylesbury, Engl.: HM + M Publishers.
OWEN, T. K., ROBERTS, J. C.: Acholuric jaundice and gout. Brit. med. J. **1937 II**, 661.
REIFENSTEIN, G. H.: A case of erythremia, gout and subleukemic myelosis. Amer. J. med. Sci. **197**, 215 (1939).
SANDBERG, A. A., CARTWRIGHT, G. E., WINTROBE, M. M.: Studies on leukemia. I. Uric acid excretion. Blood **11**, 154 (1956).
SCOTT, J. T., DIXON, A. ST. J., BYWATERS, E. G. L.: Association of hyperuricemia and gout with hyperparathyreoidism. Brit. med. J. **5390**, 1070 (1964).
STANBURY, J. B., WYNGAARDEN, J. B., FREDRICKSON, D. S.: The Metabolic Basis of Inherited Diseases. New York: McGraw-Hill 1972.
TALBOTT, J. H.: Gout and blood dyscrasias. Medicine **38**, 173 (1959).
THANNHAUSER, S. J.: Lehrbuch des Stoffwechsels und der Stoffwechselkrankheiten. München: Bergmann 1929.
THANNHAUSER, S. J., CZONICZER, G.: Kennen wir Erkrankungen des Menschen, die durch eine Störung des intermediären Purinstoffwechsels verursacht werden? Dtsch. Arch. klin. Med. **135**, 224 (1921).
TILESTON, W., GRIFFIN, W. A.: Chronic family jaundice. Amer. J. med. Sci. **139**, 847 (1910).
TINNEY, W. S., POLLEY, H. F., HALL, B. E., GIFFIN, H. Z.: Polycythemia vera and gout: report of eight cases. Proc. Mayo Clin. **20**, 49 (1945).
TIVEY, H.: The natural history of untreated acute leukemia. Ann. N. Y. Acad. Sci. **60**, 322 (1954/55).
TIVEY, H.: The prognosis for survival in chronic granulocytic and lymphocytic leukemia. Amer. J. Roentgenol. **72**, 68 (1954).
VIDEBAEK, A.: Polycythaemia vera. Course and prognosis. Acta med. scand. **138**, 179 (1950).
VINING, C. W., THOMSON, J. G.: Gout and aleukaemia in a boy aged five. Arch. Dis. Childh. **9**, 277 (1934).
WEBER, F. P.: Erythraemia with migraine, gout, and intracardiac thrombosis. Lancet **1934 II**, 808.
WEISBERGER, A. S., PERSKY, L.: Renal calculi and uremia as complications of lymphoma. Amer. J. med. Sci. **225**, 669 (1953).
WILKINSON, J. F.: Megalocytic anaemias. Lancet **1949**, 249, 292, 336.
WYNGAARDEN, J. B.: Gout. Advanc. Metab. Dis. **2**, 2 (1965).
ZÖLLNER, N.: Grundlagen der Gichtforschung. Münch. med. Wschr. **116**, 865 (1974).
ZÖLLNER, N.: Moderne Gichtprobleme, Ätiologie, Pathogenese, Klinik. Ergebn. inn. Med. **14**, 321 (1960).
ZÖLLNER, N., GRIEBSCH, A.: Diet and Gout. In: Purine Metabolism in Man, vol. 41B, p. 435. New York: Plenum Press 1974.
ZÖLLNER, N., GRIEBSCH, A., GRÖBNER, W.: Einfluß verschiedener Purine auf den Harnsäurestoffwechsel. Ernährungs-Umschau **3**, 79 (1972).
ZWEIFLER, A. J., THOMPSON, G. R.: Correction of thiazide hyperuricemia by potassium chloride and ammonium chloride. Arthrit. Rheum. **8**, 1134 (1965).

IV. Pathogenese der Harnsäureablagerungen und des Gichtanfalles

Pathogenese der Harnsäureablagerungen und des Gichtanfalles

Von

P.-U. Heuckenkamp

Mit 4 Abbildungen

Pathogenese der Harnsäureablagerungen

Eigenschaften der Harnsäure

Harnsäure liegt in den Körperflüssigkeiten bei einem pH von 7,4 fast ausschließlich als monovalentes Uration vor. Diese Eigenschaft läßt sich auf den schwach sauren Charakter der Harnsäure zurückführen (pKa = 5,75). Mononatriumurat bildet den Inhalt von Tophi bei Patienten mit Gicht.

Harnsäure besitzt die Fähigkeit, im Plasma und auch in proteinfreien Flüssigkeiten übersättigte Lösungen zu bilden (SEEGMILLER et al., 1963). SEEGMILLER et al. (1963) gelang es, im Plasma Harnsäurekonzentrationen von 300 mg/100 ml innerhalb von einer Stunde bei Inkubation mit Harnsäure im Überschuß und einer Temperatur von 37° C herzustellen. Läßt man dieses Plasma weiterhin bei einer Temperatur von 37° C stehen, wobei man sorgfältig auf eine Vermeidung bakterieller Verunreinigungen zu achten hat, so fällt die Harnsäurekonzentration binnen 24 Std auf einen Spiegel von 13 mg/100 ml ab: Dieser Konzentrationsabfall erwies sich als die Folge einer Ausfällung von Mononatriumurat-monohydratkristallen (SEEGMILLER et al., 1963). Im Verlauf der Inkubation fallen dann noch weitere Uratkristalle aus, allerdings mit langsamerer Geschwindigkeit; nach 96 Std beträgt die Plasmaharnsäurekonzentration nur noch 8,5 mg/100 ml bei einem pH von 6,8.

Wird anstelle von Kohlensäure ein Krebs-Ringer-Bicarbonatpuffer der Inkubationslösung zugesetzt, so lassen sich innerhalb einer Stunde Harnsäurekonzentrationen von nur 180 mg/100 ml herstellen. Bei diesem Versuchsansatz kommt es nicht zu einer Ausfällung von Natriumuratkristallen, sondern die Lösung bleibt in übersättigter Form bestehen. Die Zugabe von Natriumuratkristallen (als Kristallisationskeim) führt zu einer Ausfällung von Natriumurat in kristalliner Form.

Im alkalischen Bereich nimmt die Löslichkeit von Natriumurat mit steigendem pH zu. Im sauren Milieu hingegen, beispielsweise in den abführenden Harnwegen, werden die Uratsalze großenteils in freie Harnsäure überführt. Daher treten Ablagerungen in den ableitenden Harnwegen gewöhnlich in Form von *Harnsäure*konkrementen auf.

Harnsäureablagerungen

Bei der Gicht werden Natriumuratkristalle in den bindegewebigen Strukturen des Körpers abgelagert. Dieses Salz entspricht chemisch Mononatriumurat-monohydrat.

Werden solche Uratkristallablagerungen sichtbar, wie beispielsweise im Knorpel von Helix und Antihelix des Ohres oder in der Umgebung von Fuß- und Fingergelenken, spricht man von Tophi. Keineswegs aber neigen allein die oberflächlichen Bindegewebsstrukturen des Körpers zur Tophusbildung: häufig werden Uratkristalle im interstitiellen Bindegewebe der Nieren abgelagert. Bei entsprechenden klinischen Befunden spricht man hierbei von einer Gichtniere.

Der zur Ausfällung von Natriumuratkristallen führende Mechanismus ist noch weitgehend ungekannt. BRØCHNER-MORTENSEN (1958) gibt eine durchschnittliche Krankheitsdauer bei Gichtikern bis zum Auftreten sichtbarer Tophi von 13,2 Jahren an. Dadurch wird verständlich, daß eine experimentelle Nachahmung einer Tophusbildung schwierig ist. Trotzdem gelang es HIS (1900), durch subcutane Injektion von Uratkristallen die Entstehung eines histologisch charakteristischen Tophus' zu beobachten.

Die Bedeutung des Natriumurates für die Tophusbildung

Die Ablagerungen von Uratkristallen im Bindegewebe bei Patienten mit Gicht ist eine direkte Konsequenz der geringen Löslichkeit dieser Substanz in biologischen Flüssigkeiten (SEEGMILLER et al., 1963). Nach diesen Autoren werden Tophi selten unterhalb eines Plasmaharnsäurespiegels von 8 mg/100 ml beobachtet. Andererseits führt eine Senkung des Plasmaharnsäurespiegels unter 7 mg/ 100 ml gewöhnlich zu einer sichtbaren Auflösung tophöser Ablagerungen (GUTMAN u. YÜ, 1957; BARTELS u. MATOSSIAN, 1959; THOMPSON et al., 1962).

Fortdauernde, erhöhte Harnsäurekonzentrationen führen zu einer Vergrößerung der Tophi mit Destruktion benachbarter Gewebsstrukturen. Ein Durchbruch nach außen führt nicht selten zu Infektionen, die sich klinisch jedoch stets von einem akuten Gichtanfall abgrenzen lassen.

Uratkristalle sind erstmals von dem Erfinder des Mikroskopes, ANTONI VAN LEEUWENHOEK (1679), gesehen worden (McCARTY, 1970a). Er war sich der chemischen Natur der aus tophösem Material gewonnenen Kristalle nicht bewußt, denn die Harnsäure wurde erst durch SCHEELE im Jahre 1776 entdeckt. BRANDENBERGER et al. (1947) wiesen mit Hilfe von Röntgenuntersuchungen nach, daß es sich bei dem im Tophus abgelagerten Material um Mononatriumurat-monohydrat handelt; diese Autoren widerlegten damit die frühere Auffassung von DE-GRACIANSKY (1938), der mit Hilfe optischer Kristallographie *Harnsäure*kristalle beobachtet haben wollte. SOKOLOFF (1957) weist jedoch darauf hin, daß von DE-GRACIANSKY (1938) möglicherweise Säuren zur Decalcifizierung der Knochen verwendet wurden, die die Uratkristalle zu Harnsäure verwandelt haben könnten. Die Befunde von BRANDENBERGER et al. (1947) sind später von HOWELL et al. (1963) bestätigt worden.

Von zentraler Bedeutung für die Tophusbildung ist die Serumharnsäurekonzentration. Konzentrationen von 400 mg/100 ml führen im physiologischen Bereich spontan zur Auskristallisierung von Mononatriumurat-monohydrat (KLINENBERG, 1969; SEEGMILLER et al., 1963). KLINENBERG (1969) hat weiterhin nachgewiesen, daß Seren von Gichtikern und Gesunden, die mit Natriumuratkristallen über zwei Stunden hinweg inkubiert wurden, zu einer Auflösung dieser Kristalle führten, wenn die ursprüngliche Serumharnsäurekonzentration unter 7 mg/ 100 ml gesenkt wurde. Höhere Konzentrationen führten hingegen zur Präcipitation von weiteren Uratkristallen.

Dieses in vitro-Modell liefert auch eine Erklärung, daß Uratkristalle bei hohen Serumharnsäurekonzentrationen abgelagert und bei niedrigeren aufgelöst werden.

Langdauernde Hyperuricämien führen unabhängig von der sie verursachenden Krankheit zur Bildung von Tophi. Uratablagerungen im Verlaufe einer Polycythaemia vera sind bekannt (ZÖLLNER, 1968). Möglicherweise kommt auch eine latente Gicht (MERRILL, 1955) durch eine zusätzliche Hyperuricämie zur Manifestation. SORENSEN (1962) vertritt die Auffassung, daß jeder Patient, der nur lange genug eine Hyperuricämie aufweist, früher oder später Gicht mit Tophusbildung und Arthritiden entwickelt. Der Grund, weshalb beispielsweise eine manifeste Gicht nur äußerst selten den Verlauf einer chronischen Niereninsuffizienz kompliziert, liegt nach Auffassung von SORENSEN (1962) und ZÖLLNER (1968) in der oft kurzen Lebenserwartung dieser erkrankten Patienten. SORENSEN (1962) berichtet über drei Patienten mit chronischer Niereninsuffizienz, bei denen ein typischer, akuter Gichtanfall beobachtet wurde.

Der Nachweis nekrotischer Bezirke im Zentrum von Tophi hat die Vermutung aufkommen lassen, daß die Urate direkt cytotoxisch wirken könnten (GIESEKING, 1969). GIESEKING (1969) machte die Beobachtung, daß es durch Kontakt des Kollagens mit Harnsäure zu einer Fibrinolyse kommt, bevor eine Ausfällung von Uratkristallen im Bindegewebe nachgewiesen werden konnte. Nach der Meinung dieses Autors könnte die Fibrinolyse möglicherweise eine direkte Folge einer durch Harnsäureüberschwemmung bedingten Wasserstoffionenkonzentration sein; die Ausfällung von Natriumuratkristallen wäre demnach ein davon unabhängiger, sekundärer Prozeß. GIESEKING (1969) konnte erstmals am Beispiel isolierter Gichttophi zeigen, daß der Transport von Urat- oder Harnsäuremolekülen durch die Capillargefäßwand hindurch erfolgt, und zwar nicht durch die Intercellularspalten des Capillarendothels, sondern transcellulär durch das Cytoplasma der Endothelzellen hindurch, ein Vorgang, der von MOORE u. RUSKA (1957) als Cytopempsis bezeichnet wurde. Die Richtung des Transportes läßt sich allerdings nur vermuten.

Untersuchungen über die äußere Form von Uratkristallen entstammen den Untersuchungen von INAGAKI u. MORIOKA (1968). Mit Hilfe übersättigter Serumharnsäurelösungen konnten die beiden Japaner zeigen, daß die Tophusbildung sich überwiegend in Form aggregierter Kristallblöcke entwickelt, die später den Kern für das sphärische Wachstum nadelartiger Kristalle bilden. INAGAKI u. MORIOKA (1968) sehen hierin Parallelen zum Kristallwachstum von Mineralien.

Die Prädilektion bestimmter Gewebe bzw. Gewebsstrukturen für Uratsalzablagerungen ist nicht völlig geklärt. Ebenso fehlen uns Kenntnisse über die Faktoren, die zur Tophusbildung führen. Auf die besondere Affinität der Knorpelgewebe, Natriumuratsalze zu binden, hat erstmals Sir WILLIAM ROBERTS (1892) in seiner berühmten "Croonian Lecture" hingewiesen. Nach seiner Meinung ist der von ihm nachgewiesene hohe Natriumgehalt dieser Gewebe verantwortlich für die Auskristallisierung von Natriumurat „im kritischen Moment". Demnach sollen Uratsalze von der Synovia in die oberflächlichen Schichten des Gelenkknorpels diffundieren und dort irgendwann auskristallisieren. Am Beispiel eines Tarsusknochens vom Schwein, der in eine übersättigte Natriumuratlösung getaucht wurde, gelang ROBERTS (1892) der Nachweis, daß innerhalb von zwei bis drei Tagen Uratsalze im Knorpel auskristallisierten: Die gelenknahen Flächen zeigten kalkig aussehende Inkrustierungen, die sich nicht durch Schaben oder Wischen entfernen ließen.

Nahezu 60 Jahre wurden keine weiteren Untersuchungen über die Bedeutung der Matrix des Bindegewebes für die Tophusentstehung durchgeführt. Lediglich BRUGSCH u. CITRON (1908) haben ebenfalls die Affinität des Knorpels, Urate in vitro zu absorbieren, erkannt. 1957 hat SOKOLOFF diese Befunde bestätigen können. Uratkristalle findet man im Knorpel, in der Synovia, in den subcutanen

Schichten der Haut und auch im Interstitium der Nieren bei Patienten mit Gicht. Darüber hinaus wurden aber auch Uratkristallablagerungen vereinzelt in der Cornea des Auges (SLANSKY u. KUWABARA, 1968), in den Augenlidern, den Nasenflügeln, im Scrotum, Penis, in der Zunge, der Epiglottis, im Kehlkopf, in der Aorta und im Herzmuskel nachgewiesen (LÖFFLER u. KOLLER, 1955). SOKOLOFF (1957) hat darauf hingewiesen, daß allen diesen Geweben eine Grundsubstanz, nämlich die der sauren Mucopolysaccharide, gemeinsam ist.

GREILING et al. (1961) versuchten mit Hilfe von Titrationsversuchen den Nachweis zu erbringen, daß das Chondroitinsulfat in seiner Eigenschaft als schwache Säure gewissermaßen als Kationenaustauscher wirkt. Demnach soll das Natriumion des Uratsalzes gegen Wasserstoff ausgetauscht werden, so daß Harnsäure gebildet wird, die weniger löslich ist und ausfällt. Harnsäure ist jedoch tatsächlich weniger löslich in destilliertem Wasser, dafür aber von größerer Löslichkeit in den Gewebsflüssigkeiten mit einem pH von 7,43 (PETERS u. VAN SLYKE, 1946). Außerdem erklärt die Hypothese von GREILING et al. (1961) nicht, warum Natriumurat- und nicht Harnsäurekristalle in den betreffenden Geweben vorgefunden werden. KATZ und SCHUBERT (1970) weisen in diesem Zusammenhang darauf hin, daß das Chondroitinsulfat nicht als freie Säure vorliegt und demnach keine freien Wasserstoffionen zur Verfügung stehen.

Zweifellos aber bestehen Zusammenhänge zwischen dem hohen Polysaccharidgehalt des Knorpels (EINBINDER u. SCHUBERT, 1950) und der Ausfällung von Uratkristallen. LAURENT (1964) konnte in diesem Zusammenhang zeigen, daß bei Inkubation von jeweils 15 mg Harnsäure mit Chondroitin-4-sulfat in steigender Konzentration (6,3—18,8 g/100 ml) die Löslichkeit der Harnsäure sich umgekehrt proportional zur Konzentration des Polysaccharids verhält. In einem weiteren Versuchsansatz gelang LAURENT (1964) auch der Nachweis, daß die Natriumsalze der Harnsäure innerhalb oder in unmittelbarer Nachbarschaft des Knorpels gebildet werden müssen. Diese Versuche geben somit eine Erklärung für die herabgesetzte Löslichkeit der Urate in bindegewebigen Strukturen.

KATZ u. SCHUBERT (1970) haben die Untersuchungen von LAURENT (1964) und GREILING et al. (1961) fortgeführt und erweitert. Im Gegensatz zu den letzteren verwendeten KATZ u. SCHUBERT (1970) anstelle des Chondroitinsulfates Proteinpolysaccharide, also die intakten Moleküle der Bindegewebsmatrix. Das aus Rindernasenknorpel herausgelöste Proteinpolysaccharid besteht aus einem Proteinanteil, der Chondroitinschwefelsäure und einem kleinen Anteil von Keratinsulfat.

Incubation von Proteinpolysacchariden in steigender Konzentration bei pH 7,4 mit Natriummonourat führt zu einer zunehmenden Konzentration gelöster Urate (Abb. 1). Die obere Löslichkeitsgrenze von Natriumurat im NaCl-Puffer (4° C) liegt bei 5,7 mg/100 ml, im Knorpelextrakt hingegen bei 25 mg/100 ml (KATZ u. SCHUBERT, 1970). Eine Erhöhung der Incubationstemperatur auf 37° C führt zu keiner Veränderung der Löslichkeit der Uratsalze in dem Proteinpolysaccharidhomogenat. Wird der Knorpelextract jedoch zuvor mit Trypsin inkubiert, so beobachtet man eine Ausfällung von Uratsalzen. KATZ u. SCHUBERT (1970) deuten demnach ihre Ergebnisse so, daß chemische Veränderungen der Bindegewebsmatrix auch in vivo eine Vorbedingung für die Uratkristallausfällung sein könnten.

Die Befunde von KATZ u. SCHUBERT (1970) stehen somit im Widerspruch zu denjenigen von LAURENT (1964). Dies ist möglicherweise darauf zurückzuführen, daß letzterer mit einem isolierten Polysaccharidextrakt gearbeitet hat, dessen Löslichkeitsbedingungen anders sind als die der unveränderten Matrix.

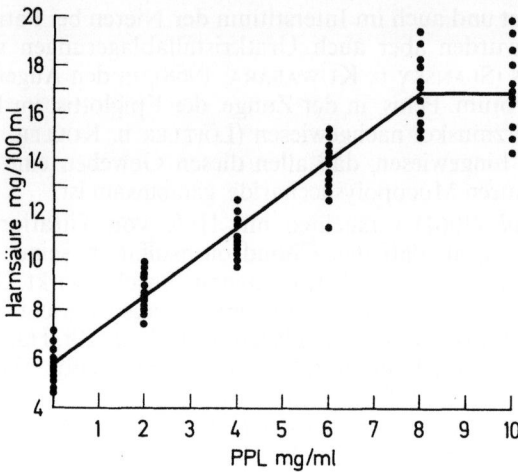

Abb. 1. Wirkung von Proteinpolysaccharid (PPL) auf die Löslichkeit von Mononatriumurat (als Harnsäure gemessen) bei einem pH von 7,4, gelöst in einem 0,021 M Kaliumpuffer, der 0,130 M NaCl enthielt. (Reproduziert aus: KATZ, W. A., SCHUBERT, M.: The interaction of monosodium urate with connective tissue components. J. clin. Invest.. **49**, 1783 (1970). Mit freundlicher Genehmigung der Herausgeber des J. clin. Invest.

Unklar bleibt jedoch, wodurch die Urate im Knorpel in Lösung gehalten werden. Es wäre denkbar, daß sich reversible (chemische und/oder physikalische) Bindungen zwischen den Uraten und dem Proteinmolekül einstellen. Es fehlen jedoch Mitteilungen über derartige Bindungsfähigkeiten im Bindegewebe.

Neuerdings wurde von ALVSAKER (1968) ein uratbindendes Protein im menschlichen Serum beschrieben. Dieses Protein, das in der α_1-α_2-Globulinfraktion des Serums zu lokalisieren ist, soll demnach in der Lage sein, 13—33% der Harnsäure im Plasma zu binden. Patienten mit Gicht haben nach Untersuchungen von ALVSAKER (1966, 1968) einen Mangel an diesem Protein. Möglicherweise besteht hierfür gar eine genetische Determination.

KLINENBERG (1968), der die Untersuchungen von ALVSAKER (1968) im wesentlichen bestätigen konnte, fand bei Gichtkranken nur die Hälfte der Uratbindung an die Plasmaproteine gegenüber Gesunden. Die von KLINENBERG (1968) und KLINENBERG u. KIPPEN (1970) verwendete Methode (Äquilibriumdialyse) ist reproduzierbar; das Protein befindet sich innerhalb einer semipermeablen Membran und wird gegen ein großes Volumen eines Uratpuffers dialysiert. Nach Einstellung eines Äquilibriums läßt sich aus der Differenz von freier Harnsäure im Puffer und der Harnsäure innerhalb der semipermeablen Membran das an Eiweiß gebundene Urat errechnen. Folgende Faktoren beeinflussen die Uratbindung an Proteine: pH, Puffermolarität, Temperatur, die Konzentration des freien Urates und die Proteinkonzentration innerhalb der Membran.

Die physiologische Bedeutung der Plasmauratbindung ist unbekannt. Eine beeinträchtigte Uratbindung in vivo könnte mit einer verminderten Uratlöslichkeit einhergehen und somit dazu beitragen, daß Harnsäure bei bestehender Hyperuricämie in Gelenken, Tophi und den Nieren abgelagert wird (KLINENBERG *et al.*, 1973). Die normale Bindungsfähigkeit liegt bei 29 µg pro Milliliter Plasma, d.h. daß 20% der im Serum nachweisbaren Harnsäure gebunden sein müßte (KLINENBERG, 1968). Nach Ansicht von KATZ u. EHRLICH (1969) scheint es sich um ein in der α- und β-Globulinfraktion wanderndes Protein zu handeln, das den Mucopolysacchariden zuzuordnen ist.

Es bedarf jedoch noch der Bestätigung dieser Befunde durch weitere Untersuchungen und einer genaueren Charakterisierung. Auch bleibt zweifelhaft, ob es sich bei diesem im Serum nachweisbaren Mucopolysaccharid um eine Substanz handelt, die identisch oder zumindest verwandt ist mit den Mucopolysacchariden des Bindegewebes. Es besteht jedoch Einigkeit darüber, daß Urate an Eiweiße gebunden werden können (McCarty, 1970b). Diese Auffassung steht im Widerspruch zu früheren Ansichten, wonach eine nennenswerte Urat-Eiweißbindung im Plasma verneint wurde (Wyngaarden, 1966).

Die Bedeutung des pH, der Glykolyse, der Temperatur und der Milchsäure für die Uratablagerungen

Knorpel und Sehnen sind vergleichsweise avasculäre Gewebe. Die Aufrechterhaltung der Energie ist sehr wahrscheinlich auf Grund der niedrigen Sauerstoffspannung in diesen Geweben nur durch die Glykolyse gewährleistet: hierbei entsteht Milchsäure. Nach Meinung von Seegmiller und Howell (1962) kommt es zu einem pH-Gradienten zwischen dem avasculären Gewebe und dem Plasma. Das saurere Milieu avasculärer Gewebe soll die Präcipitation von Natriummonourat in Knorpel und Sehnen begünstigen (Seegmiller et al., 1963). Außerdem beeinflußt das avasculäre Gewebe ungünstig den Abtransport von Milchsäure zu den sie weiter verbrennenden (oder zu Glucose synthetisierenden) Organen, was die Aufrechterhaltung eines sauren Milieus unterstützt.

Katz u. Schubert (1970) haben jedoch folgende Einwände gegen die oben ausgeführten Theorien:
1. Das Ausmaß der pH-Verschiebung ist nur sehr gering und übersteigt selten mehr als 0,5 pH-Einheiten. Selbst wenn deutlich größere pH-Verschiebungen zum sauren hin nachweisbar wären, so sollte anstelle von Natriummonourat Harnsäure zur Ausfällung gelangen.
2. Andere Gelenkerkrankungen, so etwa die primär chronische Polyarthritis, verursachen ebenfalls eine Ansäuerung der Gelenkflüssigkeit (Ropes u. Bauer, 1953; Steele u. McCarty, 1966), und dennoch kommt es bei gleichzeitig bestehender Hyperuricämie (etwa auf Grund einer Nierenerkrankung) nur äußerst selten zu Uratablagerungen und Tophusbildung.

Schon frühzeitig war aufgefallen, daß bestimmte Organregionen, die starken Temperaturschwankungen ausgesetzt sind, Prädilektionsstellen für die Tophusbildung darstellen (Garrod, 1861). Dies betrifft z.B. Helix und Antihelix der Ohren und das Großzehengrundgelenk. Loeb (1972) hat den Nachweis erbringen können, daß die Löslichkeit von Natriumurat im Plasma um einen Faktor 4 abnimmt, wenn die Temperatur von 37° C auf 10° C gesenkt wird. Loeb (1972) vertritt daher die Ansicht, daß es Körperregionen gibt, die in Hinblick auf die Temperatur, der sie ausgesetzt sind, selbst bei normalen Uratkonzentrationen chronisch *übersättigt* sind. Temperaturveränderungen könnten demnach wesentlich dazu beitragen, daß es an bestimmten Prädilektionsstellen zur Tophusbildung kommt. Genauere Daten über Temperaturunterschiede stammen aus Untersuchungen von Slansky u. Kuwabara (1968): sie fanden zwischen der Orbita und der äußeren Oberfläche der Cornea ein Temperaturgefälle von 6° C. Der Temperaturunterschied zwischen Innen- und Außenseite der Cornea beträgt 0,8° C (Slansky u. Kuwabara, 1968). Diese an sich bestechenden Theorien erklären aber nicht die Uratausfällungen im Interstitium der Nieren, die Temperaturschwankungen nur unwesentlich ausgesetzt sein dürften.

Bedeutung mechanischer Einflüsse auf die Tophusbildung

Die Bevorzugung mancher Organe und Gewebe könnte auch durch deren leichtere Verletzbarkeit erklärt werden (GARROD, 1861; FREUDWEILER, 1901). Bei 18 von 20 untersuchten Leichen ohne zu Lebzeiten nachgewiesene Hyperuricämie fand GARROD (1861) Läsionen an der Oberfläche des 1. Metatarsalköpfchens. Aber auch hierbei handelt es sich höchstens um zusätzliche Faktoren, denn FREUDWEILER (1901) fand bei künstlich nekrotisch gemachtem Knorpelgewebe keine stärkere Uratbindung in einem Inkubationsansatz als bei unversehrtem Knorpel.

Zusammenfassung

Nach den bisher vorliegenden Untersuchungen handelt es sich offensichtlich um eine Vielzahl von Faktoren, die zur Uratsalzablagerung in bestimmten Geweben beitragen. Die Löslichkeitsverhältnisse dieser Prädilektionsorgane sind vermutlich von großer Bedeutung für die Tophusentstehung. Neuerdings wird auch noch der Natriumkonzentration in diesen Geweben eine Rolle am Zustandekommen der Uratablagerungen zugemessen (KLINENBERG et al., 1973). Im physiologischen Bereich der Natriumkonzentration ist demnach die Uratlöslichkeit erheblich geringer als in natriumfreien Puffern.

Urate werden teilweise an Plasmaproteine gebunden. Ein spezifisches uratbindendes Protein konnte hingegen bisher nicht nachgewiesen werden. Ob dies aber etwas mit der Uratablagerung und Tophusentstehung zu tun hat, bleibt ungeklärt.

Die Pathogenese des akuten Gichtanfalles

Die Bedeutung der Harnsäure und ihrer Salze für die Pathogenese des akuten Gichtanfalles

Nach der Entdeckung der Harnsäure durch SCHEELE im Jahre 1776 erkannte erstmals GARROD (1861) einen Zusammenhang zwischen Harnsäure und Gicht. Etwa 30 Jahre zuvor sah DZONDI (1829) noch „skorische Reize" als die Ursache akuter Gichtanfälle an. GARROD (1861) hat in seiner Abhandlung über die Natur der Gicht erstmals die Ansicht vertreten, daß Natriumuratablagerungen in der Synovia, in Knorpel und Sehnen nicht Folge, sondern Ursache der entzündlichen Reaktion sind. Bei neun Fällen konnte GARROD jedesmal Uratsalze in den Gelenken nachweisen. Er erkannte auch, daß die Uratsalze nicht dem Knorpel aufliegen, sondern im Interstitium eingebaut sind. GARROD beschrieb auch die Bevorzugung bradytropher Gewebe für die Ablagerung von Harnsäuresalzen. Es muß heute als Verdienst dieses englischen Klinikers angesehen werden, das Vorkommen von Uratablagerungen in den Gelenken als pathognomisch für die Diagnose der Gicht erkannt zu haben. Die Ursache für die Auskristallisation von Uraten in der Gelenkflüssigkeit sah er in einer Verschiebung der „Serumalkalinität" zum neutralen pH hin.

Andererseits fiel GARROD (1861) bereits auf, daß die Entstehung des akuten Gichtanfalles nicht allein durch die Harnsäurekonzentration im Blut erklärt werden kann. Auch bleibt ungeklärt, weshalb es zu keinen akuten Gichtattacken in den uratreichen Tophi kommt. Zunächst aber wurden in Erweiterung der Garrodschen Erkenntnisse um die Jahrhundertwende wesentliche Einsichten in die Pathogenese des akuten Gichtanfalles gewonnen.

ROBERTS (1892) beschrieb Uratkristalle in Gelenkergüssen von Patienten mit Gicht. HIS (1900) und FREUDWEILER (1901) haben nach Injektion von Uratkristallen in die Bauch- und Gelenkhöhle von Kaninchen eine gichtähnliche Entzündung erzeugen können. Aber auch die Phagocytose von Uratkristallen durch Leukocyten wurde von HIS (1900) und FREUDWEILER (1901) bereits beschrieben. In der Synovia wurden histologisch Nekrosen nachgewiesen, die man auf eine Giftwirkung von Uraten zurückführte (FREUDWEILER, 1901). FREUDWEILER (1901) verglich erstmals auch verschiedene Uratsalze und Harnsäure auf deren unterschiedlich entzündungserzeugende Wirkung. Dabei zeigte sich, daß sich die Kaliumsalze der Harnsäure nach Injektion am raschesten auflösten, die Natriumsalze hingegen die längste Verweildauer besaßen. Auch bewirkten die Kaliumurate eine geringere Leukocytose. BROGSITTER (1927) vertrat die Ansicht, daß die Urate zuerst in Form eines Tophus innerhalb des Gelenkknorpels abgelagert werden, der durch zunehmende Vorwölbung, wodurch ein mechanischer Reiz entsteht, zu einer Knorpelläsion mit nachfolgender Uratfreisetzung führt. Das harnsaure Salz wirkt nach seiner Ansicht als Entzündungsreiz auf die „blutgefäßreichen, ausgiebig nervös versorgten Synovialgefäße".

Die ursprüngliche Ansicht von GARROD (1861), wonach die akute Gelenkentzündung des Gichtkranken eine Reaktion auf Natriumuratkristalle darstellt, ist später oft angezweifelt worden (HENCH, 1940; GUTMAN u. YÜ, 1952; SOKOLOFF, 1957). Durch die Anwendung neuer, zuverlässiger Methoden zur Bestimmung von Harnsäure im Serum konnte gezeigt werden, daß keine Beziehung zwischen Veränderungen der Harnsäurekonzentration im Serum und dem Auftreten akuter Gichtanfälle besteht (SEEGMILLER et al., 1963). Intravenöse Harnsäureinfusionen, die eine deutliche Hyperuricämie verursachten (26 mg-%), bewirkten weder bei Gesunden noch bei Gichtkranken einen akuten Gichtanfall (BERLINER et al., 1950).

Hyperuricämie tritt häufig infolge hämatopoetischer Krankheiten und chronischer Niereninsuffizienz auf, ohne daß es zu akuten entzündlichen Gelenkerkrankungen kommt. Das gleiche gilt für hyperuricämische Verwandte von Patienten mit Gicht (SEEGMILLER et al., 1963). Colchicin, das den akuten Gichtanfall beendet, hat jedoch keinen Einfluß auf den Serumharnsäurespiegel. Auf der anderen Seite sind Probenecid und andere, den Harnsäurespiegel senkende Präparate, ohne Wirkung im akuten Gichtanfall; im Gegenteil, unter ihrer Anwendung läßt sich oft ein akuter Anfall provozieren (SEEGMILLER et al., 1963). Schließlich berichtete SOKOLOFF (1957) über Uratablagerungen in Gelenken, die niemals von einer akuten Entzündung heimgesucht wurden; andererseits fehlen oft Uratablagerungen in solchen Gelenken, in denen sich typische Gichtattacken abgespielt haben.

Das Interesse hatte sich demnach zunächst auf Abweichungen im Purinmetabolismus während des akuten Gichtanfalles konzentriert. WEISSMANN u. GUTMAN (1957) beobachteten eine vermehrte renale Ausscheidung von 8-Hydroxy-7-methylguanin während des akuten Anfalles, wohingegen die Ausscheidung von 6-Succinoaminopurin abnahm. Nach Ansicht dieser Autoren besteht eine Störung im Gleichgewicht zwischen den Adenyl- und Guanylvorläufern der Nucleinsäuren. SEEGMILLER et al. (1963), die keinen signifikanten Unterschied in der Einbaurate von Glycin in Harnsäure während des akuten Gichtanfalles fanden, sprechen sich aber gegen pathologische Veränderungen im Purinstoffwechsel als Ursache für den akuten Anfall aus.

Wenn auch die Harnsäurekonzentration im Serum allein nicht die Entstehung des akuten Gichtanfalles erklären kann, worauf bereits GARROD (1861) hingewiesen hatte, so ist ein normaler Harnsäurespiegel während des akuten Geschehens, von BRØCHNER-MORTENSEN (1941) noch mit 10—30% angegeben, die Ausnahme. SEEGMILLER et al. (1963) weisen darauf hin, daß einige der beschriebenen Fälle von akuter Gicht bei normalem Harnsäureserumspiegel möglicherweise Beispiele für Chondrocalcinosis („Pseudogicht") darstellen. Bei dieser Krankheit werden Calciumpyrophosphatkristalle in der Synovialflüssigkeit anstelle von Uratablagerungen vorgefunden. In der Tat können durch verschiedene Kristalle, intraarticulär appliziert, typische gichtähnliche Anfälle ausgelöst werden (FAIRES u. MCCARTY, 1962; MCCARTY, 1970b; TSE u. PHELPS, 1970).

Die ersten Mitteilungen über das Vorkommen von Uratkristallen in Gelenken von Gichtkranken (GARROD, 1861; ROBERTS, 1892; FREUDWEILER, 1901) sind zunächst in Vergessenheit geraten. Erst MCCARTY u. HOLLANDER haben 1961 bei 15 von 18 Patienten mit akutem Gichtanfall Mononatriumuratkristalle in der Synovialflüssigkeit nachgewiesen und damit die ursprüngliche Beobachtung von GARROD (1861) bestätigt. Die beiden Autoren verglichen den optischen Nachweis von Uratkristallen durch polarisiertes Licht mit dem durch ein gewöhnliches Lichtmikroskop: mit der zuletzt genannten Methode gelang der Kristallnachweis nur in 11 von 18 Fällen, weswegen der ersteren Technik seither der Vorrang eingeräumt wird. Daß es sich bei den beobachteten Kristallen tatsächlich um Urate handelt, ließ sich durch Uricaseverdauung beweisen (MCCARTY u. HOLLANDER, 1961).

FAIRES und MCCARTY (1961) beobachteten in der Synovialflüssigkeit von Patienten im akuten Gichtanfall in 90% eine intraleukocytäre Natriumuratansammlung. Um zu beweisen, daß Uratkristalle einen Gichtanfall auszulösen vermögen, haben FAIRES u. MCCARTY (1961) zwei gesunden Männern und einigen Hunden Mononatriumuratkristalle (jeweils 20 mg, suspendiert in 0,9%iger NaCl) intraarticulär injiziert; 2 Std danach konnte in jedem Fall ein klassischer Gichtanfall beobachtet werden. Die anschließende Untersuchung aspirierter Gelenkflüssigkeit unter dem Polarisationsmikroskop ergab, daß die injizierten Natriumuratkristalle von Leukocyten phagocytiert waren. Dies entsprach den Befunden beim spontanen Gichtanfall (MCCARTY, 1961; SEEGMILLER et al., 1962a). Proportional zum Schweregrad der entzündlichen Symptome verhielt sich die intraleukocytäre Uratkristallansammlung, unabhängig davon, ob es sich um eine spontane Attacke oder eine durch Kristallinjektion hervorgerufene handelte (MCCARTY, 1961; SEEGMILLER et al., 1962a). SEEGMILLER et al. (1962a) haben im akuten Anfall bis zu 90% aller Uratkristalle innerhalb von Granulocyten vorgefunden. ZVAIFLER u. PEKIN (1963) haben ebenfalls über Uratphagocytose in der Gelenkflüssigkeit bei 22 von insgesamt 27 Patienten mit akuter Gicht berichtet. Die Ähnlichkeit der Entzündungsreaktion beim Hund läßt weiterhin den Schluß zu, daß es sich hierbei um keine speciesspezifische Reaktion handelt (FAIRES u. MCCARTY, 1961, 1962a, b).

SEEGMILLER et al. (1962a), die die Ergebnisse von MCCARTY u. HOLLANDER (1961) bestätigt haben, geben die erforderliche Kristallgröße für die Erzeugung einer akuten Entzündung mit einer Länge von 0,5—8,0 μ an. Hiermit ließ sich nach intraarticulärer Injektion (pH der Suspension 7,2) sowohl bei Gesunden als auch bei Gichtkranken und Patienten mit chronischer Polyarthritis nach 3—4 Std eine akute Entzündung hervorrufen (SEEGMILLER et al., 1962a). Das Ausmaß der Symptome schwankte allerdings selbst innerhalb der Gruppe von Gichtpatienten, wobei Patienten mit nichttophöser Gicht am heftigsten reagierten. Wurden statt dessen amorphe Urate (20 mg) intraarticulär gespritzt, so kam es nur selten zu einer Entzündung. Allerdings zeigte sich hierbei, daß mit zunehmendem Entzündungsvorgang größere Uratkristallmengen nachweisbar wurden (SEEGMILLER et al., 1962a), vermutlich weil ein Teil des amorphen Urates in kristalline Form überführt worden ist. SEEGMILLER et al. (1962a) sehen auch darin einen Beweis, daß die Uratsalze erst in kristalliner Form entzündungserregend wirken.

Die entzündungsauslösende Eigenschaft der Uratkristalle ist nicht auf Gelenke beschränkt, denn durch subcutane Kristallinjektion läßt sich ebenfalls eine akute Entzündung erzeugen (SEEGMILLER et al., 1962a). SEEGMILLER et al. (1962a) beschrieben in der gleichen Publikation eine akute, entzündliche Reaktion nach subcutaner und intraarticulärer Injektion von Natriumorotatkristallen, die derjenigen nach subcutaner Uratinjektion glich. Auch die Injektion von Calciumpyrophosphatdihydrat-, Calciumoxalat- und Calciumphosphatkristallen in die Gelenkhöhle von Tieren und Menschen verursachte eine akute Entzündung (FAIRES u. MCCARTY, 1962; MCCARTY, 1970b; TSE u. PHELPS, 1970). Die intraarticuläre Verabfolgung von kristallinem Diamantstaub bewirkt keine Entzündung (TSE u. PHELPS, 1970). Nach Meinung von MCCARTY (1970b) und TSE u. PHELPS (1970) ist die elektrisch-negative Oberflächenspannung, die Diamantkristalle nicht besitzen, entscheidend für die Entstehung einer „kristallinduzierten Synovitis" (MCCARTY et al., 1966; PHELPS u. MCCARTY, 1969). Die kristallinduzierte Synovitis bzw. Arthritis ist nach den Untersuchungen von MCCARTY et al. (1966) dosisabhängig, vollständig reversibel und weitgehend unabhängig von der chemischen Zusammensetzung des Kristalles.

Ausgehend von den Beobachtungen, daß Mononatriumuratkristalle in fast allen Gelenken Gichtkranker angetroffen werden (ZEVELY et al., 1956; SOKOLOFF, 1957; MCCARTY u. HOLLANDER, 1961; SEEGMILLER et al., 1962a, b) und daß darüber hinaus experimentell durch intraarticuläre Injektion von Urat- und anderen Kristallen ein dem akuten Gichtanfall in allen Einzelheiten ähnliches Geschehen ausgelöst werden konnte (FAIRES u. MCCARTY, 1961, 1962a, b; SEEGMILLER et al., 1962a; MCCARTY et al., 1966; MCCARTY, 1970a, b; TSE u. PHELPS, 1970), hat sich das Interesse auf den Entstehungsmechanismus der kristallinduzierbaren Entzündung gerichtet.

Die gegenwärtigen Vorstellungen über das Zustandekommen eines akuten Gichtanfalles gehen auf SEEGMILLER u. HOWELL (1962) zurück. Danach sind folgende Bedingungen Voraussetzung für die akute Attacke:

1. In den Geweben der Gelenke müssen Mononatriumuratkristalle, die sich aus einer hyperuricämischen Körperflüssigkeit in kristalliner Form abgesetzt haben, vorhanden sein.
2. Es entwickelt sich dann eine entzündliche Reaktion auf diese Kristalle.
3. Die zusätzliche Ausfällung weiterer Kristalle am Ort der Entzündung steigert den bereits eingeleiteten Entzündungsvorgang.

Eine Ablagerung von Uratkristallen findet nach der Vorstellung von SEEGMILLER u. HOWELL (1962) erst dann statt, wenn die Uratkonzentration in den Körperflüssigkeiten die Löslichkeitsgrenze von Natriumurat überschreitet. Nun ist die Ablagerung von Uratkristallen nicht immer eine Folgeerscheinung hyperuricämischer Zustände, wie etwa im Falle chronischer Nierenerkrankungen oder bei hyperuricämischen Verwandten von Gichtkranken. Bei der zuletzt genannten Gruppe sind es beispielsweise nur 10—15%, die klinisch an akuter Gicht erkranken (HAUGE u. HARVALD, 1955). Allerdings ist unklar, wie sich der erste Kristallkeim bildet, der dann, wie experimentell nachgewiesen wurde (SEEGMILLER et al., 1963), zur Ausfällung weiterer Kristalle führt.

Die Phagocytosetätigkeit der Granulocyten ist mit einer vermehrten glykolytischen Energieentfaltung verbunden (KARNOVSKY, 1962). Die dadurch entstehende Lactatbildung soll zu einem pH-Abfall in der Gelenkhöhle führen, wodurch es zu einem pH-Gradienten zwischen der Gelenkflüssigkeit und dem Blut kommt (SEEGMILLER et al., 1963; GOLDFINGER et al., 1965) (siehe auch: „Mechanismus der Harnsäureablagerung"). Ein erhöhter Lactatspiegel wurde von SEEGMILLER et al. (1963) im Gelenkerguß nachgewiesen. Hierdurch sollen weitere Kristalle aus der hyperuricämischen Körperflüssigkeit ausgefällt werden, was den in

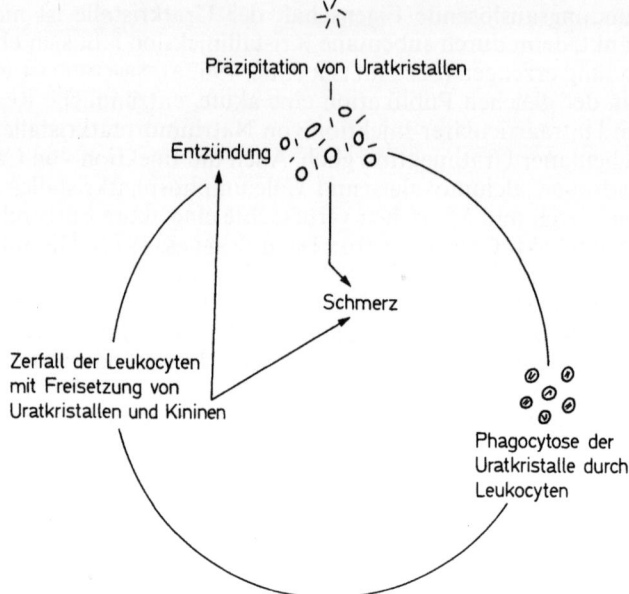

Abb. 2. Schematische Darstellung der Hypothese über die Pathogenese der akuten Gichtarthritis als einer sich selbst unterhaltenden entzündlichen Reaktion. [Modifiziert nach SEEGMILLER, J. E., HOWELL, R. R.: The old and new concepts of acute gouty arthritis. Arthr. and Rheum. 5, 616 (1962)]

Gang gebrachten Entzündungsvorgang im Gelenkspalt durch Phagocytose weiterer Urate mit erneuter Milchsäurebildung fortsetzt. SEEGMILLER u. HOWELL (1962) haben diese Theorie entwickelt und graphisch zur Darstellung gebracht (Abb. 2). Danach unterhält sich der Entzündungsprozeß von einem bestimmten Schwellenwert der Uratkristalle im Gelenk an, der allerdings nicht näher definiert ist, selbst, und schreitet weiter fort.

Dem ist aber entgegengehalten worden, daß die pH-Verschiebung nach Uratkristallinjektionen nur 0,1—0,2 pH-Einheiten über eine 4—5 stündige Meßperiode beträgt (STEELE u. MCCARTY, 1966). DUNCAN et al. (1968) haben in keinem Fall in der Gelenkflüssigkeit während eines akuten Anfalles pH-Werte, die niedriger als 7,23 waren, vorgefunden. Sie bezweifeln daher die Bedeutung der Acidose für das Zustandekommen des Gichtanfalles. Darüber hinaus haben Patienten mit chronischer Polyarthritis bei gelegentlich gleichzeitig bestehender Hyperuricämie trotz vergleichsweise niedriger intraarticulärer pH-Werte zwischen 6,8—7,2 keine Gichtanfälle und intraartikulären Uratkristalle (MCCARTY, 1970 b, c).

Wir haben es demnach mit einem Circulus vitiosus zu tun, der durch die Verabfolgung von Colchicin erfolgreich unterbrochen werden kann. Colchicin unterbindet die Phagocytosefähigkeit der Granulocyten (HOWELL u. SEEGMILLER, 1962 a, b; SEEGMILLER et al., 1962): "Colchicine destroys the appetite of the leucocyte for microcrystals" (STETTEN, 1968). MALAWISTA u. SEEGMILLER (1965) haben nachgewiesen, daß eine Vorbehandlung mit Colchicin die Phagocytose von Urat-, aber auch Orotatkristallen stark herabsetzt.

Die Bedeutung der Leukocyten und ihrer Enzyme

Die älteste Mitteilung über die Fähigkeit von Leukocyten, Uratkristalle zu phagocytieren, verdanken wir dem Dermatologen RIEHL (1897). HIS (1900) und FREUDWEILER (1901) haben diesen Befund unter Verwendung synthetischer Urate bestätigt. Aber erst 60 Jahre danach wurde dieses Phänomen von FAIRES u. MCCARTY (1961) neu entdeckt. HOWELL und SEEGMILLER (1962a, b) haben in vitro Granulocyten mit radioaktiv markierter Harnsäure bzw. Uratkristallen inkubiert und danach die Bildung von $^{14}CO_2$ aus Urat-6-^{14}C gemessen: Dabei gelang ihnen der Nachweis, daß die neutrophilen Granulocyten nur Uratkristalle, nicht aber gelöste Harnsäure phagocytieren und abbauen können. Der Abbau der intracellulär angereicherten Uratkristalle kommt durch die Enzyme Peroxydase und Verdoperoxydase zustande (HOWELL u. SEEGMILLER, 1962a). Dadurch ist eine langsame Uricolyse innerhalb der Granulocyten möglich, d.h. also, daß Harnsäure unter bestimmten Umständen auch beim Menschen nicht Endstufe des Nucleinsäureabbaus ist (CANELLAKIS *et al.*, 1955).

Die Vermutung, daß die Peroxydaseaktivität der Granulocyten von Gichtkranken möglicherweise höher als die von Gesunden sein könnte, ist durch neuere Untersuchungen von VORMITTAG *et al.* (1971) ausgeschlossen worden.

Uratkristalle lassen sich nach ZVAIFLER u. PEKIN (1963) während eines akuten Gichtanfalles nur innerhalb von Granulocyten der Gelenkhöhle nachweisen, nicht jedoch in denjenigen des zirkulierenden Blutes, obwohl nach den Ergebnissen dieser Autoren die Harnsäurekonzentration im Blut und in der Synovialflüssigkeit annähernd gleich sein soll. REEVES (1965) hat jedoch später zeigen können, daß die Harnsäurekonzentration im Serum von Patienten, in deren Gelenken Uratkristalle gefunden wurden, niedriger als in der Gelenkflüssigkeit war.

Auf alle Fälle kommt den segmentierten neutrophilen Granulocyten eine entscheidende Bedeutung für die Entzündungsvorgänge während der akuten Gichtattacke zu. Dies erhellt auch aus Versuchen an Hunden, die, nach Vorbehandlung mit Vinblastin, wodurch es zu einer ausgeprägten Leukopenie kommt, keine Entzündungszeichen nach intraarticulärer Uratkristallinjektion erkennen lassen (PHELPS u. MCCARTY, 1966). Wurden diese Tiere zu einem späteren Zeitpunkt mit normalem Blut perfundiert, so reagierten sie auf eine Uratkristallinjektion wie gesunde Hunde mit einem typischen akuten Anfall (PHELPS u. MCCARTY, 1966; MCCARTY *et al.*, 1966). Nach intramuskulärer Injektion von Antileukocytenserum läßt sich bei Hunden ebenfalls eine Leukopenie erzeugen; auch hierbei unterbleibt der Gichtanfall nach Injektion von Uratkristallen (CHANG u. GRALLA, 1968).

Leukocyten, die Uratkristalle phagocytiert haben, sollen eine erhöhte Absterbequote im Vergleich zu anderen Leukocyten besitzen (FRITZE *et al.*, 1967, SCHUMACHER u. PHELPS, 1971). Dadurch gelangen diese Kristalle erneut in die Gelenkhöhle und können wieder von anderen Granulocyten phagocytiert werden.

AYVAZIAN u. AYVAZIAN (1963) erklären die von ihnen beobachtete gesteigerte Harnsäureausscheidung bei gleichbleibender Uratkonzentration im Serum während des akuten Gichtanfalles mit einem vermehrten Harnsäurenachschub aus dem arthritischen Entzündungsgebiet durch gesteigerten Granulocytenzerfall mit Uratbildung aus den Purinkörpern der Zellkerne.

Die Inkubation synthetischer Uratkristalle mit menschlichen, segmentierten Granulocyten führt zu einer raschen Phagocytose der Kristalle. SCHUMACHER u. PHELPS (1971) konnten mit Hilfe elektronenmikroskopischer Untersuchungen zeigen, daß bereits 3 min nach Zugabe von Uratkristallen zu einer Leukocytensuspension 10% der im Inkubationsansatz vorhandenen Granulocyten Urate phagocytiert hatten.

Nach Einverleibung der Uratkristalle ins Zellinnere findet man die Kristalle von einer intakten Membran umgeben; (die Einheit „Kristall- umgebende Membran" wird Phagosom bezeichnet) (SCHUMACHER u. PHELPS, 1971). Bald darauf kommt es im Zellinneren zu einer Verbindung der Phagosomenmembran mit Lysosomen; man spricht dann von Phagolysosomen.

Innerhalb weniger Minuten nach Inkubationsbeginn läßt sich eine Degranulierung der Leukocyten beobachten (RAJAN, 1966). Dieser Vorgang ist gleichbedeutend mit einer intracellulären Freilassung der in den Lysosomen (= Granula) gespeicherten Enzyme, insbesondere saurer Hydrolasen (WEISSMANN, 1967). Dies führt zu einer Autolyse und somit zur Nekrose der Granulocyten. Bereits 8 min nach Inkubationsbeginn sind 4% der Granulocyten, die Uratkristalle phagocytiert haben, nekrotisch. Nach 2 Std ließen sich bei der Hälfte aller Granulocyten intracelluläre Kristalle nachweisen: 37% davon waren nekrotisch (SCHUMACHER u. PHELPS, 1971). SCHUMACHER u. PHELPS (1971) konnten in diesem Zusammenhang erstmals zeigen, daß sich Uratkristalle gelegentlich auch innerhalb von Mono- und Thrombocyten vorfinden. Lymphocyten sind dagegen stets frei von Uratkristallen.

Aus den Untersuchungen von SCHUMACHER u. PHELPS (1971) geht demnach hervor, daß der Phagocytosevorgang sehr rasch ist. Die Membran der Phagosomen wird zerstört, die Zellen degranulieren und lösen sich schließlich auf, wobei die Kristalle wieder frei werden (RAJAN, 1966; SCHUMACHER u. PHELPS, 1971).

Andere Autoren konnten keine Phagosomenmembran nachweisen (BLUHM et al., 1969). Nach Ansicht von SCHUMACHER u. PHELPS (1971) ist dies jedoch die Folge einer zeitlich verspäteten Beobachtung, d.h. also, daß die Membranen infolge der raschen Phagocytose bereits aufgelöst waren.

Die Auflösung der Phagosomenmembran erfolgt enzymatisch unter Mitwirkung lysosomaler Enzyme; hierzu sind zu zählen die saure Phosphatase, die β-Glucuronidase und das Lysozym (ANDREWS u. PHELPS, 1971). Während des Gichtanfalls läßt sich daher auch eine erhöhte Aktivität lysosomaler Enzyme in der Gelenkflüssigkeit nachweisen (PHELPS et al., 1966).

Mit Hilfe isolierter leukocytärer Granula konnte RAJAN (1966) deren proteolytische Aktivität (mit Hämoglobin als Substrat) direkt nachweisen. WEISSMANN et al. (1969) haben Lysate aus Granula leukocytärer Herkunft hergestellt und in die Gelenke von Kaninchen eingespritzt. Hierdurch kam es zu einer Hyperplasie und Hypertrophie synovialer Zellen mit Rundzellinfiltration in die Synovia, später auch zu Pannusbildung mit Zerstörung der normalen Knorpelstruktur. Somit sind die im Spätstadium zu beobachtenden destruktiven Gelenkveränderungen Folge der Wirkung lysosomaler Enzyme, die nach Uratphagocytose aus Granulocyten freigesetzt werden. Entscheidend für die Phagocytose ist auch die Größe der Kristalle. RAJAN (1966) beobachtete, daß nur Kristalle in der Größenordnung zwischen 0,5—8,0 µ phagocytiert werden. Diese Beobachtung bestätigt frühere Befunde von SEEGMILLER et al. (1962a).

Kristallbildung und Auslösung des Gichtanfalles

Mononatriumuratkristalle werden in praktisch allen Gelenken, die von einem akuten Gichtanfall betroffen sind, vorgefunden. Nach Meinung von BROGSITTER (1927) lösen sich auf eine noch ungeklärte Weise Uratkristalle aus dem Knorpel- oder Synovialgewebe heraus und gelangen so in die Gelenkhöhle. Dieser Mechanismus könnte auch die akuten Anfälle erklären, die während Allopurinolbehandlung trotz sehr niedriger Serumharnsäurespiegel beobachtet werden.

Ganz anders sehen DUNCAN et al. (1968) sowie RIDDLE et al. (1967) das Problem der Uratkristallentstehung. Elektronenmikroskopische Untersuchungen hatten zu der Vermutung Anlaß gegeben, daß das Cytoplasma intakter neutrophiler Granulocyten selbst der Ort der Kristallbildung sein könnte (RIDDLE et al., 1967). In Erweiterung der genannten Untersuchungen mit Hilfe ultradünner Granulocytenschnitte gelangten DUNCAN et al. (1968) zu der Vorstellung, daß sich zunächst nicht-kristalline Harnsäure in der Gelenkflüssigkeit kurz vor Beginn des Anfalles ansammelt. Danach sollen die Urate ins Cytoplasma der Neutrophilen gelangen und durch Ausscheidung des zur Lösung notwendigen Wassers konzentriert und als nadelartige Kristallstrukturen ausgefällt werden. DUNCAN et al. (1968) gelang auch der Beweis für ihre Vermutung: aus einer kristallfreien Gelenkflüssigkeit von zwei Gichtpatienten isolierte neutrophile Granulocyten, die feucht auf einem verschlossenen Objektträger gebracht und auf 4° C abgekühlt wurden, ließen innerhalb von 24—48 Std im Zellinneren eine spontane Kristallisation erkennen. (Vor Abkühlung ließen sich zuverlässig keine Kristalle erkennen.) DUNCAN et al. (1968) nehmen weiterhin an, daß im Verlaufe des Alterungsprozesses die Zellen absterben und die im Cytoplasma befindlichen Kristalle zum Austritt weiterer Granulocyten aus der Blutbahn führen.

Man sollte freilich erwarten, daß intracellulär gebildete Kristalle als Kaliumurate ausfallen, denn Kalium ist das prädominierende Kation im Zellinneren. Nach Untersuchungen von HOWELL et al. (1963) sowie FAIRES u. MCCARTY (1962) besteht aber kein Zweifel, daß es sich bei den während des Gichtanfalles auftretenden Uratkristallen um Natriumurate handelt. Auch hatte FREUDWEILER bereits 1901 nachweisen können, daß Kaliumuratkristalle sich im Gegensatz zu den Natriumsalzen der Harnsäure rasch auflösen. Inwieweit die in vitro gewonnenen Ergebnisse von RIDDLE et al. (1967) und DUNCAN et al. (1968) in vivo anwendbar sind, steht nach Ansicht von MCCARTY (1970c) noch aus.

Die Bedeutung der Kinine, des Hageman-Faktors (Faktor XII) und des Complementsystemes für die Pathogenese des akuten Gichtanfalles

Verschiedene Aspekte des entzündlichen Geschehens im akuten Gichtanfall erinnern an Eigenschaften vasoaktiver Polypeptide. Zum weiteren Verständnis der Pathogenese des Gichtanfalles ist es daher unumgänglich, kurz das wichtigste des Kininsystems zu beschreiben.

Man unterscheidet drei verschiedene Kinine: das Bradykinin, bestehend aus neun Aminosäuren, das Dekapeptid Kallidin (= Lysyl-Bradykinin) und das aus elf Aminosäuren zusammengesetzte Methionyl-Lysyl-Bradykinin. Diese Kinine besitzen die Fähigkeit, Blutgefäße zu erweitern und dadurch Blutdruckabfall und Schock zu erzeugen. Weiterhin lösen sie Schmerz aus, kontrahieren die glatte Muskulatur, steigern die Gefäßpermeabilität und ermöglichen den Gefäßaustritt von Leukocyten (HABERMANN, 1966; WEBSTER, 1966; WERLE, 1967; MELMON u. CLINE, 1967a; WILHELM, 1971).

Es versteht sich, daß in Anbetracht dieser für den Organismus sehr weitreichenden Eigenschaften die Kinine in einer inaktiven Form im Blut und anderen Körperflüssigkeiten zirkulieren. Die inaktiven Vorstufen sind die mit den α_1- bzw. α_2-Globulinen im tierischen und menschlichen Plasma zirkulierenden Kininogene (WERLE, 1955). Die Aktivierung der Kininogene zu Kininen erfolgt durch die im Blutplasma vorkommenden spezifischen Kininogenasen (Endopeptidasen), auch als Kallikreine bezeichnet. Diese Enzyme, im Organismus weit verbreitet, sind u.a. im Plasma, in verschiedenen Drüsen und auch innerhalb von Granulocyten nachgewiesen worden (MELMON u. CLINE, 1967a).

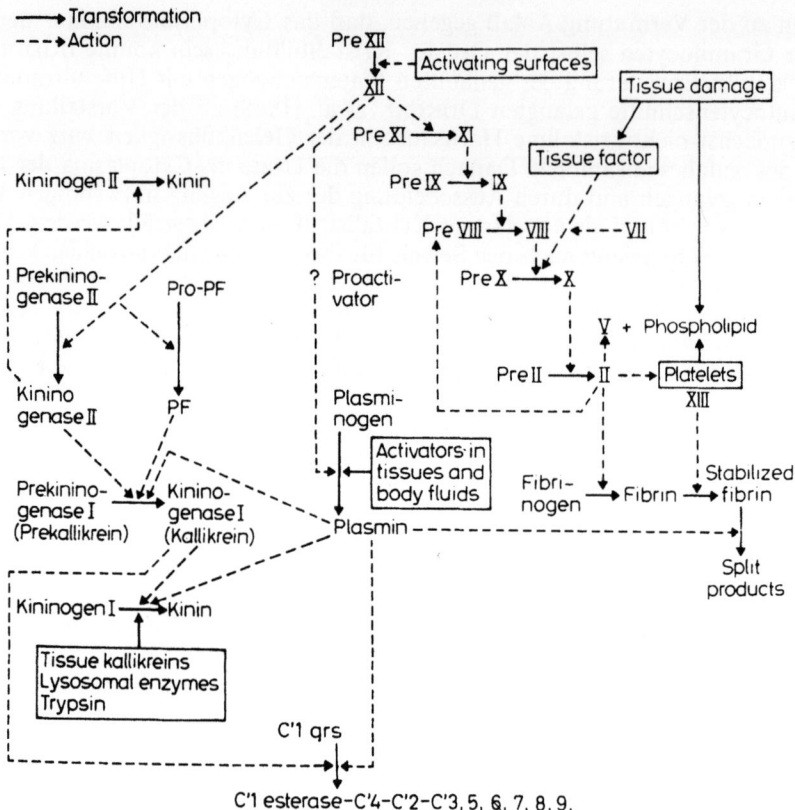

Abb. 3. Darstellung von Reaktionen, die Hageman-Faktor (Faktor XII) abhängig sind, wie das Gerinnungssystem, die Fibrinolyse, das Complementsystem und die Kininaktivierung (Reproduziert aus: EISEN, V., BRUCKNER, F. E.: Proteolysis and its inhibition in joint diseases. In: Neue Aspekte der Trasylol-Therapie. Stuttgart-New York: Schattauer 1970. Mit freundlicher Genehmigung des Autors (EISEN, V.) und des Schattauer Verlages

Auch die Kallikreine bzw. Kininogenasen müssen zunächst enzymatisch von einer inaktiven Vorstufe (Kallikreinogen bzw. Präkininogenase) in eine aktive Komponente verwandelt werden, bevor es zu einer Kininfreisetzung aus den genannten Plasmaproteinen kommt. Hierbei kommt dem Hageman-Faktor (Faktor XII des Blutgerinnungssystems) eine entscheidende Bedeutung zu (MELMON u. CLINE, 1967a). (Die Kallikreinaktivierung kann aber noch durch andere Faktoren eingeleitet werden.)

Die zentrale Bedeutung des Hageman-Faktors besteht darin, daß er drei voneinander verschiedene, aber untereinander in enger Beziehung stehende Systeme entscheidend beeinflußt, nämlich

1. die Blutgerinnung und die damit im Zusammenhang stehende Fibrinolyse,
2. das Kallikrein-Kininogen-Kininsystem und
3. das Complementsystem.

In Abb. 3 sind diese Beziehungen schematisch dargestellt.

Der Hageman-Faktor muß auch zuerst von einer inaktiven in eine aktive Form überführt werden, bevor er auf andere Systeme einwirken kann. Die Aktivierung von Faktor XII läßt sich durch Glas, Ellaginsäure (RATNOFF u. CRUM,

1964) und eine Reihe kristalliner Substanzen mit negativer Oberflächenladung, u.a. auch Uratkristalle (KELLERMEYER, 1965), auslösen. Hageman-Faktor-Aktivierung läßt sich aber auch mit Hilfe proteolytischer Enzyme, die von phagocytierenden Leukocyten freigesetzt worden sind, nachweisen (EISEN, 1969). Es ist bisher jedoch nicht gelungen, physiologischerweise vorkommende Substanzen in tierischen und menschlichen Geweben nachzuweisen, die eine Hageman-Faktor aktivierende Eigenschaft besitzen (KELLERMEYER u. BRECKENRIDGE, 1966).

Der Vollständigkeit halber muß erwähnt werden, daß es in Geweben und im Blut Inhibitoren gibt, die aktivierte Komponenten, beispielsweise Kallikrein, sehr rasch spalten. Auch die Kinine haben eine außerordentlich kurze Halbwertszeit; innerhalb von Sekunden werden sie durch Plasmakininasen (z.B. Carboxypeptidase N) gespalten und damit inaktiviert (ERDÖS, 1966). Kininasen kommen außerhalb des Plasmas u.a. auch in Granulocyten vor (MELMON u. CLINE, 1967a, b).

Kinine im akuten Gichtanfall

GOLDFINGER et al. (1964) haben erstmals den Nachweis erbringen können, daß in der Synovialflüssigkeit von Gichtpatienten während einer akuten Arthritis Kinine vorkommen; die Konzentrationen, gemessen an der Größe der Kontraktion eines isolierten Rattenuterus, lagen zwischen 0,002 und 0,1 µg/ml Gelenkflüssigkeit. Eine intraarticuläre Injektion von Bradykinin erzeugte bei Hunden eine arthritisähnliche, schmerzhafte Entzündung, die durch vorherige Einspritzung von Carboxypeptidase B, einem spezifischen, kininspaltenden Enzym, verhindert werden konnte (MELMON et al., 1967). Dabei zeigte sich eine deutliche Korrelation zwischen der Kininkonzentration und dem Ausmaß an Schmerzhaftigkeit, Schwellung und Wärme im Gelenk.

Einen 50fachen Anstieg der Kininkonzentration in den Gelenken von Gichtpatienten beobachteten GOLDFINGER et al. (1964) nach intraarticulärer Injektion gereinigter Uratkristalle. Auch hierbei stellte sich eine schmerzhafte, entzündliche Reaktion ein, die einem akuten Gichtanfall entsprach. EISEN (1966), EISEN u. VOGT (1970) und WEBSTER (1966) konnten ebenfalls den Nachweis erbringen, daß Uratkristalle in Synovialflüssigkeiten und auch im Plasma eine Kininfreisetzung induzieren. In einigen Gelenken von Patienten im akuten Gichtanfall wurden Kininkonzentrationen von mehr als 50 ng/ml gemessen (EISEN, 1966). Wie weitere Untersuchungen zeigen, lassen sich Kinine in allen entzündlichen Gelenkflüssigkeiten, unabhängig von der Ätiologie, nachweisen (MELMON et al., 1967), so beispielsweise bei Patienten mit chronischer Polyarthritis. An der Auslösung des Schmerzes beim akuten Gichtanfall sind nach Untersuchungen von SICUTERI et al. (1965) neben den Kininen auch die 5-Hydroxytryptamine beteiligt.

Kinine können also eine dem Gichtanfall ähnliche entzündliche Reaktion hervorrufen. Im Gegensatz jedoch zu dem prompten Effekt nach intraarticulärer Kinininjektion verstreichen etwa 4 Std bis zur Ausbildung einer Entzündungsreaktion, wenn anstelle von Kininen Uratkristalle injiziert werden (MELMON et al., 1967). Diesen Unterschied erklären MELMON et al. (1967) damit, daß die Uratkristalle zunächst — auf eine noch nicht geklärte Weise — einen (Zeit erfordernden) Austritt von Granulocyten aus der Blutbahn in die Gelenkflüssigkeit bewirken. Die Granulocyten führen dann zu einer Aktivierung bzw. Freisetzung von Kininen, worauf sich die typische Gelenksentzündung entwickelt.

MELMON u. CLINE (1967b) und GREENBAUM u. KIM (1967) haben in lysosomalen und extralysosomalen Strukturen von Kaninchengranulocyten Enzyme nachweisen können, die in der Lage waren, Kinine aus ihren inaktiven Vorstufen (beispielsweise aus Bradykininogen) freizusetzen. Darüberhinaus sollen die Kinine selbst in inaktiver Form innerhalb von Granulocyten vorkommen (MELMON u. CLINE, 1967a). Wurden Leukocytenpräparationen, zu 60—80% aus Granulocyten bestehend, in vitro mit menschlichem Plasma inkubiert, so stieg die Konzentration der Kinine rasch um das 2- bis 3fache an (MELMON u. CLINE, 1967b). Die Größe der bereits nach 5 min nachweisbaren Kininbildung war dabei proportional der Konzentration der Granulocyten; 2—3 Std später konnte keine Kininaktivität mehr gemessen werden.

GREENBAUM u. KIM (1967) haben die kininaktivierenden Faktoren in lysosomalen und extralysosomalen Fraktionen der neutrophilen Granulocyten lokalisieren können.

Normalerweise werden Kinine durch Kininasen oder Endopeptidasen sehr rasch zerstört (ERDÖS, 1966). Das pH-Optimum der Kininasen liegt bei 8,5 (GREENBAUM u. KIM, 1967). Das leicht saure Milieu, das man in Entzündungsbereichen antrifft, trägt nach Ansicht von LEWIS (1964, 1970) zu einer Anreicherung von Kininen bei, weil darin die Kininase gehemmt wird.

Bedeutung des Hageman-Faktors

Der Hageman-Faktor wird nach Kontakt mit Uratkristallen, deren Oberfläche elektrisch negativ geladen ist, aktiviert (KELLERMEYER u. BRECKENRIDGE, 1965). KELLERMEYER u. BRECKENRIDGE (1966) haben in weiteren Untersuchungen sowohl Hageman-Faktor (Faktor XII) als auch Plasmathromboplastinantecedent (PTA = Faktor XI) in der Gelenkflüssigkeit von Gesunden und Gichtpatienten nachweisen können. Diese beiden Faktoren sind essentiell für die Aktivierung des "intrinsic thromboplastin systeme" (GASTON, 1964).

KELLERMEYER u. BRECKENRIDGE (1966) haben nachweisen können, daß sich der Zusatz von Gelenkflüssigkeit, die vorher mit Uratkristallen inkubiert wurde, zu einem recalcifizierten Serum beschleunigend auf die Gerinnungszeit auswirkt. Nach Meinung dieser Autoren wird durch die Uratkristalle zunächst Faktor XII aktiviert, der seinerseits PTA (Faktor XI) mobilisiert. Werden die anderen Gerinnungsfaktoren hinzugefügt, so kann auf diese Weise Serum zum Gerinnen gebracht werden. Welche Bedeutung allerdings dem Hageman-Faktor und PTA normalerweise in der Gelenkflüssigkeit zukommt, ist noch unbekannt.

Werden Uratkristalle im Serum von Patienten mit hereditärem Hageman-Faktor-Mangel inkubiert, so unterbleiben sowohl die Faktor XII-abhängige PTA-Aktivierung mit anschließender Gerinnung (KELLERMEYER u. BRECKENRIDGE, 1965), als auch die kininabhängige Vasodilatation (WEBSTER u. RATNOFF, 1961). Wird Gelenkflüssigkeit gesunder Menschen nach vorheriger Inkubation mit Uratkristallen einem Serum von Patienten mit angeborenem Hageman-Faktor-Mangel zugemischt, so läßt sich bei letzterem die Gerinnung aktivieren (KELLERMEYER u. BRECKENRIDGE 1965, 1966). Es ist in diesem Zusammenhang von Interesse, daß Hühner, die physiologischerweise keinen Hageman-Faktor besitzen, nach intraarticulärer Uratkristallinjektion keine Gichtarthritis entwickeln (KELLERMEYER, 1968). In einer neuen Veröffentlichung konnte jedoch von SPILBERG (1974) der Nachweis erbracht werden, daß Hühner nach intraarticulärer Injektion von kristallinem Natriumurat (Größe 0,5—8,0 µ) in allen Fällen eine typische Arthritis entwickelten. Da es hierbei zu keiner Freisetzung von Kininen in der Gelenkflüssigkeit kommt, bezweifelt SPILBERG (1974) die Bedeutung des Kinin-Kallikreinsystems und die Mitwirkung von Hageman-Faktor für die Gichtarthritis des Huhnes.

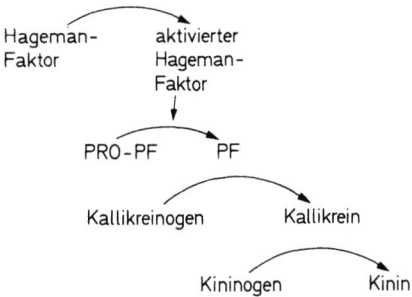

Abb. 4. Darstellung der Sequenz, die nach Aktivierung des Hageman-Faktors zur Freisetzung von Kininen führt. *PF* Permeabilitätsfaktor. [Modifiziert nach KELLERMEYER, R. W.: Inflammatory process in acute gouty arthritis. J. Lab. clin. Med. **70**, 372 (1967)]

In diesem Zusammenhang sind die Beobachtungen von DONALDSON et al. (1972) von Bedeutung, die nämlich das Vorkommen einer rheumatoiden Arthritis bei einem Patienten mit Hageman-Factor-Mangel beschrieben. Der Zweifel an der Bedeutung von Factor XII für die Entstehung einer entzündlichen Gelenksreaktion wird dadurch unterstrichen.

Da aber durch die Vermittlung des Hageman-Faktors auch noch andere Systeme als die der Gerinnung aktiviert werden können, so ist die Vermutung naheliegend, daß Uratkristalle auch die entzündliche Reaktion im Gelenk des Gichtkranken hervorrufen, so beispielsweise die Hageman-Faktor abhängige, capilläre Permeabilitätssteigerung (MARGOLIS, 1959), die Gefäßdilatation (RATNOFF u. MILES, 1964) und die Schmerzauslösung (MARGOLIS, 1958). GRAHAM et al. (1965) fanden darüber hinaus, daß aktivierter Hageman-Faktor zu einer randständigen Zusammenballung von Leukocyten im Blutgefäßsystem mit anschließendem Gefäßaustritt führt.

Vermutlich ist aber noch ein weiterer Faktor, von MILES (1964) als "permeability factor" (PF) oder, da sich diese Substanz erst nach Verdünnung des Serums mit Kochsalzlösung nachweisen läßt, als PF/dil (dil = diluted) bezeichnet, in die durch den Hageman-Faktor auslösbare Kininaktivierung zwischengeschaltet. Abbildung 4 zeigt schematisch die von KELLERMEYER (1966, 1967) entwickelte Vorstellung.

Wird Synovialflüssigkeit zuerst mit einem spezifisch gegen den Hageman-Faktor gerichteten Antikörper vorbehandelt und diese anschließend mit Faktor XII aktivierenden Substanzen wie Glas oder Uratkristallen in Berührung gebracht, dann unterbleiben alle Hageman-Faktor-abhängigen Reaktionen, insbesondere die sonst nach Uratkristallinjektion zur Ausbildung kommende Arthritis (KELLERMEYER, 1967). Auch dieser Versuchsansatz unterstreicht die Bedeutung des Hageman-Faktors an der Entzündungsentstehung. Ähnlich sind auch die Ergebnisse von EISEN (1964) zu interpretieren: Eine Aktivierung des Hageman-Faktors unterbleibt, wenn Uratkristalle oder Serum zuvor mit Hexadimethrinbromid behandelt werden. Hexadimethrinbromid lagert sich der Oberfläche von Kristallen mit negativer Oberflächenspannung an, dadurch verhindert es den Kontakt der Kristalle mit den durch sie aktivierbaren Substanzen (RATNOFF u. MILES, 1964).

All diese Untersuchungen unterstreichen die Bedeutung des Hageman-Faktors für das Zustandekommen verschiedenartiger Reaktionen. Allerdings sind Zweifel an der Mitwirkung der Kinine, die durch Hageman-Faktor aktiviert werden, für die im Gichtanfall (auf natürliche Weise oder durch Uratkristallinjektion hervorgerufen) beobachteten Veränderungen wie Chemotaxis mit Leukocytenaustritt und Permeabilitätssteigerung aufgekommen. PHELPS et al. (1966b) haben Bradykinin direkt in die Gelenkhöhle von Hunden injiziert, wodurch es unmittelbar danach zwar zu schmerzhaften Sensationen, nicht aber zu Leukocyteninfiltration und pH-Abfall kam. Weiterhin verursachte die Injektion von Uratkristallen nach vorheriger Instillation von Carboxypeptidase-B, einem kininspaltenden Enzym, trotzdem einen typischen Gichtanfall mit Leukocytenansammlung im Gelenk; die schmerzauslösende Wirkung der Kinine konnte aber mehrere Stunden nach einmaliger Carboxypeptidase-B-Behandlung unterbunden werden (PHELPS et al., 1966b). MELMON et al. (1967) halten dem zwar entgegen, daß im Hundeplasma keine größeren Kininmengen freigesetzt werden, so daß es fragwürdig bleibt, die Befunde von PHELPS et al. (1966b) auf den Menschen zu übertragen.

Einwände gegen die Rolle des Bradykinins als Entzündungsvermittler wurden auch von MILES (1964) vorgebracht, der nämlich feststellen konnte, daß der Bradykinineffekt sich nur an den Venolen abspielt und auch nicht das histologische Bild der Capillarwandschädigung verursacht, das sich im Spätstadium der Arthritis urica entwickelt. Andererseits bezweifeln JASANI et al. (1969) auf Grund des Vorkommens von Kininase in der Gelenkflüssigkeit, die freie Kinine sofort zerstören würde, die beschriebenen Kininkonzentrationen in der Gelenkhöhle. Da aber das pH-Optimum der Kininasen im alkalischen Bereich (pH 8,5) liegt (GREENBAUM u. KIM, 1967) und andererseits SEEGMILLER et al. (1963) einen pH-Abfall ins saure Milieu während des Gichtanfalles messen konnten, ist es möglich, daß die Kininasen während der akuten Entzündung ihre Wirkung nur zum Teil entfalten können.

Die leukotaktische Wirkung der Uratkristalle kann auch nicht eindeutig durch die Anwesenheit von Kininen erklärt werden. Nach Untersuchungen von PHELPS u. MCCARTY (1969) ließ sich durch Uratkristalle, die nach vorangehender intraarticulärer Injektion von Carboxypeptidase-B in die Gelenkhöhle eingebracht wurden, eine für den Gichtanfall typische Granulocyteninfiltration nachweisen. Carboxypeptidase-B zerstört aber die Kinine, so daß die Leukotaxis auf die Uratkristalle direkt zurückgeführt werden kann. Nach Untersuchungen von EISEN (1966), GREENBAUM u. KIM (1967) sowie MELMON u. CLINE (1967) stammen die von ihnen nachgewiesenen Kinine im akuten Gichtanfall aus neutrophilen Granulocyten der Gelenkhöhle. Somit werden die Kinine nicht für die leukotaktische Eigenschaft im akuten Gichtanfall verantwortlich gemacht, wohl aber für die kontinuierlich fortschreitende Entzündungsreaktion mit Schwellung, Schmerz und Wärmebildung.

Den Untersuchungen von JASANI et al. (1969) zufolge entstammen die Kinine während einer akuten Arthritis nicht den Leukocyten, sondern dem Plasma. Gegen eine entscheidende Mitwirkung der Kinine für die Pathogenese des akuten Gichtanfalles spricht sich auch MERTZ (1971) aus, der nach intravenöser Injektion von mindestens 2 mal 400000 IE Trasylol K, einem potenten Kallikreininhibitor, kein Nachlassen der Entzündungsreaktion feststellen konnte. Diese Beobachtung steht aber im Widerspruch zu den Ergebnissen von SPILBERG u. OSTERLAND (1970a, b), die nach intraartikulärer Trasylolinjektion bei Kaninchen eine bedeutend schwächere entzündliche Reaktion nach anschließender Uratkristallinjektion fanden. SPILBERG u. OSTERLAND (1970a, b) beschreiben in ihren Versuchen auch eine Hemmung der proteolytischen Aktivität lysosomaler Granulocytenenzyme, so daß nicht sicher entschieden werden kann, inwieweit das Trasylol hierbei eine antientzündliche Wirkung über das Kallikrein-Kininsystem entfaltet.

Bedeutung des Complements

Den Kininen kann nach den bisherigen Untersuchungen eine wesentliche Bedeutung am Zustandekommen der im akuten Gichtanfall beobachteten Leukotaxis nicht zuerkannt werden (GRAHAM et al., 1965). VAN ARMAN u. CARLSON (1970) vertreten die Meinung, daß die Kinine nur die erste von zwei zu unterscheidenden Phasen im akuten Gichtanfall bewirken, nämlich eine kurzdauernde Schmerzreaktion. Für die zweite, mit Leukotaxis und intraartikulärem Leukocytenaustritt einhergehende Reaktion kommt nach neueren Ergebnissen dem Complementsystem eine entscheidende Bedeutung zu: RATNOFF u. LEPOW (1963) konnten erstmals zeigen, daß C'_1-Esterase, ein proteolytisches Enzym, das durch Antigen-Antikörperkomplexe aus den drei Komponenten der ersten Complementfraktion, nämlich C'_{1q}, C'_{1r} und C'_{1s}, entsteht, in der Lage ist, Gefäßpermeabilität zu induzieren. Auch die C'_1-Esterase wird, ähnlich dem Kallikrein, von einem spezifischen Inhibitor in freier Form zerstört (RATNOFF u. LEPOW, 1963). RATNOFF u. LEPOW (1963) vermuten, daß die Permeabilitätssteigerung durch Aktivierung einer histaminartigen Substanz zustande kommt.

WARD et al. (1966) konnten mit Hilfe der isolierten Complementfraktionen C'_5 und C'_6 nach Incubation mit Immunpräcipitaten einen chemotaktischen Faktor bei Kaninchen nachweisen. Die leukotaktische Wirkung erwies sich wenigstens 10- bis 20mal so stark wie die durch Bradykinin, Kallidin oder Histamin verursachte.

DA SILVA et al. (1967) machen Anaphylatoxin, ein Spaltprodukt von C'_3, das durch Wechselwirkung zwischen C'_1, C'_4 und C'_2 entsteht, für die Permeabilitätssteigerung verantwortlich. Hierdurch könnte man sich den Gefäßaustritt von Leukocyten erklären. Auf die Bedeutung des Complements für den akuten Gichtanfall haben erstmals NAFF u. BYERS (1967) hingewiesen. Diese Autoren haben Natriumuratkristalle (3,5 mg-%) mit normalem menschlichen Serum 90 min bei 37° C incubiert und danach die $C'H_{50}$ Aktivität bestimmt. Der Aktivitätsverlust betrug hierbei 75%. Ein Complementaktivitätsverlust konnte von NAFF u. BYERS (1967) auch mit Hageman-Faktor-Mangelserum beobachtet werden, so daß dem Faktor XII keine Bedeutung für die C'-Aktivierung zuzukommen scheint. Aber auch die Uratkristallphagocytose durch neutrophile Granulocyten war 15mal so stark im C'-haltigen wie im decomplementierten (R_4-)Serum.

MCCARTY (1970c), der ebenfalls die ursprünglichen Versuche von NAFF u. BYERS (1967) bestätigen konnte, vermutet, daß es sich dabei um eine Verunreinigung der Uratkristalle mit pyrogenen Substanzen gehandelt hat. Zu ähnlichen Resultaten kommen auch SPILBERG u. OSTERLAND (1970a, b), die nach vorheriger Decomplementierung des Serums mit Cobragift, das in der Lage ist, C'_3 und C'_5 selektiv zu zerstören (BALLOW u. COCHRANE, 1969), keine Änderung der leukotaktischen Wirkung von Uratkristallen beobachten konnten. PHELPS u. MCCARTY (1969) haben die oben beschriebenen Versuche wiederholt, dabei aber die Uratkristalle auf 200° C erhitzt und somit sicher pyrogenfrei gemacht: dabei ließ sich die von NAFF u. BYERS (1967) beschriebene C'-aktivierende Wirkung der Uratkristalle nicht mehr nachweisen.

Mit Hilfe von Micropore Filtern gelang WARD (1968) der Nachweis, daß durch drei aktivierte Complementfraktionen, nämlich C'_5, C'_6 und C'_7 eine deutliche leukotaktische Wirkung entfaltet werden konnte. Diese Versuchsanordnung ist deshalb von so großer Wichtigkeit, als sie eine spezifische Wanderung von neutrophilen Granulocyten in eine Richtung ermöglicht. Danach besteht kein Zweifel, daß Faktoren des Complementsystems leukotaktisch wirksam sind. Inwieweit dies auch für den akuten Gichtanfall zutrifft, bedarf weiterer Untersuchungen.

Chemotaktische Eigenschaften der Uratkristalle

Intraarticuläre Uratkristallinjektion bewirkt einen massiven Leukocytenaustritt aus der Blutbahn in die Gelenkhöhle. PHELPS (1969a) hat mit Hilfe einer besonderen Technik [Verwendung einer Boyden-Kammer: hierbei handelt es sich um eine Plastikkammer, in der die Zahl der durch einen Millipore-Filter eindringenden Leukocyten, die einer chemotaktischen Substanz ausgesetzt sind, ermittelt werden kann (PHELPS u. STANISLAW, 1969)] den Nachweis erbracht, daß Uratkristalle nicht direkt chemotaktische Eigenschaften haben, aber eine zum Teil auf die Uratkristalle hin gerichtete Bewegung der Granulocyten induzieren. Das Ausmaß der Beweglichkeit ist aber nicht von der Kristallform abhängig, sondern verhält sich proportional zur Konzentration des gelösten Urates. Mit Uricase, Indometacin und Colchicin konnte dieser Effekt aufgehoben werden. Aus dem Überstand eines Incubationsmediums, bestehend aus Uratkristallen und Granulocyten, der nach einer bestimmten Zeit durch Zentrifugieren gewonnen wurde, konnte PHELPS (1969b) eine Substanz gewinnen, die sich auf entfernt gelegene Granulocyten chemotaktisch wirksam erwies. Eine nähere Charakterisierung dieses Faktors ist aber noch nicht erfolgt, mit Kininen oder Complementfraktionen scheint er aber nicht identisch zu sein. Es bleibt allerdings offen, inwieweit andere Zellen an der Bildung dieses chemotaktisch wirkenden Stoffes beteiligt sind, denn nach Mitteilung von PHELPS (1969b) enthielt die Granulocytensuspension stets Verunreinigungen mit Erythro-, Lympho- und Thrombocyten.

Faktoren, die einen Gichtanfall auslösen können

Frühzeitig wurde bereits die Bedeutung leiblicher Genüsse für die Auslösung akuter Gichtanfälle erkannt. Bereits GARROD (1863) hat sich ausgiebig diesen Umständen gewidmet: "there is no truth in medicine better established than the fact that the use of fermented liquors is the most powerful of all the predisposing causes of gout; nay, so powerful, that it may be a question whether gout would ever have been known to mankind had such beverages not been indulged in." GARROD machte noch Unterschiede zwischen solchen alkoholischen Getränken, die akute Attacken auslösen (beispielsweise Wein und Bier), und solchen, die dies weniger konnten (destillierte Spirituosen). Seiner Meinung nach lag der Unterschied in der Zusammensetzung der Alkoholica, wobei der Zusatz an Säuren, Tartraten und Sulfaten in Wein und Bier den Ausschlag geben soll. Diese Unterschiede haben sich inzwischen aber als unwesentlich herausgestellt. Nach Ansicht von THANNHAUSER (zitiert bei ZÖLLNER, 1957) spielen lokale Überempfindlichkeitsreaktionen eine entscheidende Rolle beim Zustandekommen des akuten Gichtanfalles. Dabei kommen seiner Meinung nach als exogene, den Gichtanfall auslösende Stoffe, bestimmte Nahrungsbestandteile, Alkohol und auch Traumata in Betracht. Allerdings geht THANNHAUSER nicht so weit wie VILLA et al. (1958), die die Bedeutung der Uratkristalle für den akuten Anfall ganz bestreiten und diesen nur auf der Basis allergischer Mechanismen erklären. Nach ZÖLLNER (1957) sind es insbesondere ketogene Kostformen (Fettmahlzeiten, Milchsäure enthaltende Produkte), die einen Anfall auslösen können.

Seit Einführung zuverlässiger Methoden zur Bestimmung der Harnsäure weiß man, daß diejenigen alimentären Einflüsse, die einen akuten Gichtanfall auszulösen vermögen, eine vorübergehende Hyperuricämie verursachen. Hinsichtlich des Alkohols wissen wir seit den Untersuchungen von LIEBER et al. (1962), daß es nach oraler Zufuhr von Alkohol (hierfür wurde Whisky verwendet) zu einem starken Lactat- und Harnsäureanstieg im Blut kommt. Da aber bereits die alleinige Infusion von Lactat ebenfalls zu einer Erhöhung der Serumharnsäure und einer verminderten Harnsäureausscheidung führt (GIBSON u. DOISY, 1923; YÜ et al., 1957; BURCH u. KURKE, 1968), vermuten LIEBER et al. (1962), daß Milchsäure auch in ihren Experimenten für die Hemmung der Harnsäureausscheidung mit sich daraus ergebender Hyperuricämie verantwortlich ist. Die Lactatproduktion nach Alkoholaufnahme hat möglicherweise zweierlei Ursachen: einmal reduziert Alkohol infolge seiner Oxydation zu Acetaldehyd NAD zu NADH; hierdurch soll vermehrt Pyruvat zu Lactat reduziert werden (LIEBER et al., 1962).

Eine andere Erklärung geben KREISBERG et al. (1971). Bei acht freiwilligen Versuchspersonen wurde der Lactatumsatz mittels Infusion von radioaktiv markierter Milchsäure bestimmt. Danach wurde diesen Versuchspersonen in stündlichen Intervallen Alkohol in Form von Whisky (30—60 ml/Std) zu trinken verabreicht, worauf es zu einem sofortigen steilen Lactatanstieg im Blut kam. Ein konstanter Spiegel wurde 120—180 min danach erreicht, obwohl auch weiterhin Alkohol in gleichen Mengen getrunken wurde. KREISBERG et al. (1971) erbrachten den Nachweis, daß die Lactatausflußrate um mehr als 50% der Einflußrate abnimmt. Darüber hinaus konnte gezeigt werden, daß sich unter Alkoholzufuhr die Inkorporation von Lactat in Glucose bereits 30 min nach Beginn des Versuches deutlich verringert und nach 120—180 min ihren tiefsten Wert erreicht. Demnach kommt die Lactatacidämie nach Alkoholkonsum nicht durch vermehrte NADH-Bereitstellung zur Lactatbildung aus Pyruvat in der Leber zustande, sondern ist die Folge einer verminderten Verwertung, wie am Beispiel der reduzierten Gluconeogenese trotz erhöhtem Lactatspiegel gezeigt werden konnte (KREISBERG et al., 1971).

MACLACHLAN u. RODAN (1967) haben in Erweiterung der oben genannten Ergebnisse Patienten mit Gicht sowohl fasten, als auch größere Alkoholmengen trinken lassen, eine Kombination, wie sie bei Trinkern häufig angetroffen wird. Auch hierbei stiegen Lactat und Harnsäure im Serum bei gleichzeitig verminderter renaler Harnsäureausscheidung stark an. Darüber hinaus kam es während einer 2—3tägigen Versuchsperiode bei acht von neun Patienten zu einem oder mehreren akuten Gichtanfällen. Die Mehrzahl der Anfälle trat während sehr rascher Veränderungen des Serumuratspiegels auf. Diese Beobachtung bestätigt auch frühere Mitteilungen von BRØCHNER-MORTENSEN (1940) und ZÖLLNER (1957), die einerseits eine vorübergehende plötzliche Erhöhung des Serumuratspiegels im Anfall nachweisen konnten, andererseits über eine vorübergehende Schwankung der Uratdeponierung im Gewebe unmittelbar vor dem Gichtanfall berichteten. Diese Untersuchungen liefern eine Erklärung für die frühzeitig beobachtete Beziehung von Alkohol und Gicht.

Ähnliche Beziehungen lassen sich aber auch noch für andere Nahrungsfaktoren nachweisen. So ist die Hyperuricämie häufig Folge von Fettsucht (MURPHY u. SHIPMAN, 1963; SHAPIRO et al., 1964), Fastenkuren, wodurch es zu vermehrter körpereigener Fett- und Eiweißverbrennung kommt (LENNOX, 1925; ADLERSBERG u. ELLENBERG, 1939; DRENICK et al., 1964; RUNCIE u. THOMPSON, 1969), und diabetischer Ketoacidose (PADOVA u. BENDERSKY, 1962). All diese metabolischen Störungen führen ebenso wie fettreiche Ernährung zu unterschiedlich ausgeprägten Ketosen.

Die Vermutung war naheliegend, daß Ketonkörper ebenfalls über eine Hemmung der renalen Harnsäureausscheidung eine Hyperuricämie verursachen (HARDING et al., 1925; HARDING et al., 1927; QUICK, 1932; MORGANO u. ALCOZER, 1949; MURPHY u. SHIPMAN, 1963; SCOTT et al., 1964; LECOCQ u. MCPHAUL, 1964). Den direkten Beweis dafür lieferten die Versuche von GOLDFINGER et al. (1965), die mittels direkter Infusion von β-Hydroxybutter- und Acetessigsäure bei freiwilligen Versuchspersonen eine deutliche Abnahme der Harnsäure-Inulin-Clearancerate bei gleichzeitigem Serumharnsäureanstieg nachweisen konnten. So war also der Nachweis erbracht, daß die Anhäufung saurer Intermediärprodukte hemmend auf die Harnsäureausscheidung wirkt.

Hyperlactatacidämie ist auch Folge von Fructoseaufnahme (BERGSTRÖM et al., 1969). Letztere führt ebenfalls zu einem Anstieg von Harnsäure im Serum (PERHEENTUPA u. RAIVIO, 1967; SAHEBJAMI u. SCALETTAR, 1971). Allerdings kommen für die durch Fructose induzierte Hyperuricämie, die abhängig von der zugeführten Dosis ist (HEUCKENKAMP u. ZÖLLNER, 1971), noch andere Faktoren in Betracht, die auf die erhöhte Fructosephosphorylierung und die damit im Zusammenhang stehende gesteigerte Abbaurate von Leberadeninnucleotiden zurückzuführen sind (MÄENPÄÄ et al., 1968; WOODS et al., 1970; HEUCKENKAMP et al., 1971).

Derartig akute Erhöhungen des Serumharnsäurespiegels treten auch im Verlaufe von Transfusionen, Röntgenbestrahlungen, bei Patienten mit Leukämien und Carcinomen, in der Operationsnachperiode sowie bei Pneumonien im Lösungsstadium auf, und können einen Gichtanfall auslösen (ZÖLLNER, 1957).

Was auch immer die einen Gichtanfall provozierenden Faktoren sein mögen, so unterliegt es nach ZÖLLNER (1960) keinem Zweifel, daß der Serumharnsäurespiegel unter Verwendung spezifischer Untersuchungsmethoden im akuten Anfall stets erhöht ist. Voraussetzung dafür ist allerdings, daß die Patienten zuvor nicht mit Phenylbutazon, Salicylaten, Cortison bzw. seinen Derivaten, ACTH oder uricosurisch wirkenden Substanzen behandelt wurden.

Die Bedeutung von ACTH und Steroiden für die Pathogenese des akuten Gichtanfalles

Es ist eine bekannte Tatsache, daß akute Gichtanfälle durch unspezifische Streßsituationen ausgelöst werden können. Hierzu sind Infektionen, Traumata, Operationen, Unterkühlungen, Röntgenbestrahlungen und viele andere Stimuli zu rechnen. Streßsituationen gehen bekanntlich mit einer vermehrten Nebennierenrindenaktivität einher. Es war daher naheliegend, zu untersuchen, ob sich Gichtanfälle bei Gichtkranken und Gesunden nach Injektion von ACTH auslösen lassen würden.

ROBINSON et al. (1948) beobachteten bei einem Gichtpatienten, der neun Monate beschwerdefrei war, nach intramuskulärer Injektion von 50 mg ACTH über einen Zeitraum von 5 Tagen einen leichten Gichtanfall drei Tage nach Beendigung der letzten ACTH-Injektion. Die zeitliche Spanne zwischen Absetzen des Medikamentes und Auftreten der klinischen Symptome ist nach Ansicht von ROBINSON et al. (1948) auf eine vollständige Unterdrückung der Nebennierenrindenaktivität zurückzuführen. ROBINSON et al. (1949) fanden bei Gichtikern eine verminderte 17-Ketosteroidausscheidung, ein Befund, der allerdings nicht konstant ist (BUTT u. MARSON, 1952). HELMAN (1949) konnte bei vier Gichtpatienten die Beobachtungen von ROBINSON et al. (1948) bei fast identischer Versuchsanordnung bestätigen. Gesunde Versuchspersonen hingegen reagierten nicht mit einer Arthritis zu irgendeinem Zeitpunkt während oder nach Absetzen der ACTH-Behandlung. Es sei aber noch bemerkt, daß ACTH nicht nur in der Lage ist, einen akuten Anfall zu provozieren, sondern einen solchen auch weitgehend zu kupieren (LÖFFLER u. KOLLER, 1955).

Die Bedeutung der Steroide für die Genese des akuten Gichtanfalles ist neuerdings wieder von CASEY et al. (1968) und SCHILLING et al. (1969) diskutiert worden. Diese Autoren wiesen eine periphere Störung des Stoffwechsels von Dehydroepiandrosteron nach, und zwar zeigte sich eine Erhöhung des Ätiocholanolon im Plasma während eines akuten fieberhaften Schubes. Die fiebererzeugende Eigenschaft von Ätiocholanolon für den Menschen ist erwiesen (KAPPAS et al., 1957). Möglicherweise findet hierin auch die starke Bevorzugung des männlichen Geschlechtes für die Gicht eine Erklärung.

Molekulare Grundlagen des akuten Gichtanfalles

An der Beteiligung segmentierter Granulocyten, gefäßaktiver Peptide und der Freisetzung intraleukocytärer Enzyme nach Uratkristallphagocytose besteht kein Zweifel. Neuere Erkenntnisse geben bereits annähernd Aufschluß über die Vorgänge im akuten Gichtanfall auf molekularer Ebene. Hierüber soll abschließend berichtet werden.

Ausgangspunkt für die Wirkung von Uratkristallen auf die segmentierten Granulocyten sind die Untersuchungen von WALLINGFORD u. MCCARTY (1971), die zeigen konnten, daß Siliciumdioxydkristalle zu einer Hämolyse von Erythrocyten führen und, nachdem sie dann von Makrophagen phagocytiert wurden, eine Ruptur der Phagolysosomen induzieren. Diese Wirkung läßt sich durch starke Wasserstoffakzeptoren, wie z.B. Polyvinylpyridin-N-oxyd (PVPNO) verhindern. Zwischen PVPNO und den Siliciumdioxydkristallen bilden sich Wasserstoffbrücken.

MCCARTY (1973) konnte erst kürzlich zeigen, daß auch Uratkristalle Erythrocyten hämolysieren: 10 mg Urat/ml Erythrocytensuspension bewirken innerhalb von 14 Std eine sechsmal größere Hämolyse als Erythrocyten in einem uratfreien Kontrollansatz. Diese hämolytische, d.h. also membranolytische Wirkung der Uratkristalle läßt sich ebenfalls durch PVPNO blockieren. Auch normales Plasma übt eine erhebliche Hemmwirkung auf den membranolytischen Effekt der Uratkristalle aus (MCCARTY, 1973). Die Hemmwirkung von Plasma und PVPNO unterbleibt jedoch, wenn letztere Substanzen von Erythrocyten und Uratkristallen durch eine Dialysemembran getrennt werden. Somit sind also nicht in Lösung befindliche Ionen, sondern der direkte Kontakt der Inhibitoren mit dem Zielobjekt verantwortlich für die beobachtete Hemmwirkung. Diese Beobachtung liefert die Grundlage für die sich anschließenden Beobachtungen und Überlegungen.

Mononatriumuratkristalle (und auch Siliciumdioxydkristalle) sind polymerisierte schwache Säuren (pKa 10^{-10}). Auf ihrer Oberfläche befinden sich positiv geladene Wasserstoffatome. Diese können eine Verbindung eingehen mit Molekülen negativer Oberflächenladung. Negativ geladene Oberflächen lassen sich bei Proteinen, Phospholipiden von Zellmembranen und auch bei anionischen Polymeren wie PVPNO nachweisen (MCCARTY, 1973). Kommt es zu einer Verbindung negativ und positiv geladener Oberflächen, so übt die Wasserstoffbindung, die zwar pro Mol sehr gering ist (2—10 kcal/Mol), tausender solcher elektrischen Felder eine starke Oberflächenspannung aus.

Nach den Vorstellungen von MCCARTY (1973) spielt sich im akuten Gichtanfall folgendes ab:

Uratkristalle, von einer Proteinhülle umgeben, werden von Granulocyten phagocytiert. Im Zellinneren befindet sich nun das Phagosom. Anschließend kommt es zur Fusion von Lysosomen mit Phagosomen, wobei das Phagolysosom entsteht. Die Enzyme der Lysosomen, die bei der Fusion freiwerden, verdauen die die Uratkristalle umgebende Proteinhülle. Zwischen den Uratkristallen und der Phagolysosomenmembran kommt es infolge der entgegengesetzten elektrischen

Ladung zu einer Oberflächenbindung. Da die Uratkristalle sich nicht biegen lassen, muß es die Phagolysosomenmembran tun. Dabei entstehen Risse in der Membran, durch die die intraphagolysosomalen Enzyme lysosomaler Herkunft ins Cytoplasma übertreten und die Autolyse der Zelle bewirken. Anschließend treten durch Defekte in der Zellmembran hydrolytische Enzyme aus der Zelle heraus und sind dann, wie von PHELPS et al. (1966) nachgewiesen werden konnte, in der Gelenkflüssigkeit nachweisbar. Mit dem Zelltod gelangen letzten Endes auch die Kristalle wieder in die Gelenkflüssigkeit, und der Circulus vitiosus ist vollständig.

WEISSMANN et al. (1972) haben die Untersuchungen von WALLINGFORD u. PHELPS (1971) dahingehend erweitert, daß sie isolierte Fraktionen von Kaninchenleberzellen, die sowohl Mitochondrien als auch Lysosomen enthielten, mit Uratkristallen reagieren ließen. Weiterhin wurden isolierte menschliche Lysosomen granulocytärer Herkunft und künstliche Lipidmembranen (Liposomen), deren chemische Zusammensetzung bekannt ist, mit Uratkristallen zur Reaktion gebracht. Aus diesen Untersuchungen geht folgendes hervor:

Uratkristalle verursachen eine dosisabhängige Freisetzung lysosomaler, nicht jedoch mitochondrialer Enzyme. Während einer 60 minütigen Inkubation nimmt der Enzymanstieg in einem Ansatz mit 20 mg Uratkristallen/ml um das Doppelte gegenüber der Kontrolle zu. Isolierte menschliche Granulocyten bewirken nach Kontakt mit Uratkristallen (40 mg/ml) einen Anstieg lysosomaler Enzyme von 40%.

Das Ausbleiben einer Enzymfreisetzung aus den Mitochondrien, die sich von den Lysosomen durch eine an Cholesterin arme Membran unterscheiden, gab zu der Vermutung Anlaß, daß der Cholesteringehalt ausschlaggebend ist für die Wirkung der Uratkristalle an entsprechenden Membranen. WEISSMANN et al. (1972) haben daraufhin Untersuchungen mit künstlichen Lipidmembranen (Liposomen), in die Anionen (CrO^{2-}) ("marker anion") eingebracht wurden, durchgeführt. Nach Kontakt mit Uratkristallen verdoppelte sich der Anionenaustritt gegenüber der Kontrolle, wenn zuvor Cholesterin in die Membranen inkorporiert wurde. Ohne Cholesterin unterblieb die Freisetzung von CrO_4^{2-}.

Diese Untersuchungen erlauben den Schluß, daß der Cholesteringehalt entscheidend wichtig für den Kontakt der Kristalle mit der Membran und somit auf die Enzymfreisetzung ist.

Werden zudem die Liposomen mit Spuren von 17-β-Oestradiol (weibliche Liposomen) bzw. Testosteron (männliche Liposomen) versehen, so kommt es ebenfalls zu einem unterschiedlich großen Austritt von „Erkennungsanionen" nach Inkubation mit Uratkristallen. Mit weiblichen Liposomen nimmt die Konzentration der Ionen um 70%, mit männlichen um 100% gegenüber Kontrollversuchen zu. MCCARTY (1973) weist in diesem Zusammenhang jedoch darauf hin, daß die oben genannten Versuche noch keine eindeutige Antwort auf die Frage nach der Geschlechtsbevorzugung des Mannes für die Gicht geben. Zum einen haben Männer höhere Serumharnsäurespiegel als Frauen, was sie von daher schon für die Gicht prädisponieren läßt. Dann überwiegen bei Männern Stoffwechselanomalien mit primärer Überproduktion von Harnsäure. Schließlich deutet auch die zunehmende Häufung sekundärer Gicht bei Frauen (30%) (MCCARTY, 1973) darauf hin, daß das geringe Vorkommen von primärer Gicht bei letzteren genetisch determiniert ist und nicht hormonell durch Membranen erklärt zu werden braucht.

Die Kenntnis über die Eigenschaften natürlicher Membranen ist augenblicklich noch so unvollständig, daß man noch nicht von einem präzisen molekularen Mechanismus des Gichtanfalles sprechen kann.

Literatur

ADLERSBERG, D., ELLENBERG, M.: Effect of carbohydrate and fat in diet on uric acid excretion. J. biol. Chem. **128**, 379—385 (1939).

ALVSAKER, J. O.: Uric acid in human plasma. V. Isolation and identification of plasma proteins interacting with urate. Scand. J. clin. Lab. Invest. **18**, 227—239 (1966).

ALVSAKER, J. O.: Genetic studies in primary gout. Investigations on the plasma levels of the urate-binding alpha 1-alpha 2-globulin in individuals from two gouty kindreds. J. clin. Invest. **47**, 1254—1261 (1968).

ANDREWS, R., PHELPS, P.: Release of lysosomal enzymes from polymorphonuclear leucocytes (PMN) after phagocytosis of monosodium urate (MSU) and calcium pyrophosphate dihydrate (CPPD) crystals: effect of colchicine and indomethacine. Arthr. and Rheum. **14**, 368 (1971).

AYVAZIAN, J. H., AYVAZIAN, L. F.: Changes in serum and urinary uric acid with the development of symptomatic gout. J. clin. Invest. **42**, 1835—1839 (1963).

BALLOW, M., COCHRANE, C. G.: Two anticomplementary factors in cobra venom: hemolysis of guinea pig erythrocytes by one of them. J. Immunol. **103**, 944—952 (1969).

BARTELS, E. C., MATOSSIAN, G. S.: Gout: six year follow-up on probenecid therapy. Arthr. and Rheum. **2**, 193—202 (1959).

BERGSTRÖM, J., HULTMAN, E., ROCH-NORLUND, A. E.: Lactic acid accumulation in connection with fructose infusion. Acta med. scand. **184**, 359—364 (1968).

BERLINER, R. W., HILTON, J. G., YÜ, T. F., KENNEDY, T. J.: The renal mechanism for urate excretion in man. J. clin. Invest. **29**, 396—401 (1950).

BLUHM, G. B., RIDDLE, J. M., BARNHARDT, M. I.: Ultrathin study of exudative leucocytes provoked by acicular urate crystals. Arthr. and Rheum. **12**, 657—658 (1969).

BRANDENBERGER, E., DE QUERVAIN, F., SCHINZ, H. R.: Röntgenografische und mikroskopisch-kristalloptische Untersuchungen an Harnsteinen. Helv. med. Acta **14**, 195—211 (1947).

BRØCHNER-MORTENSEN, K.: The uric acid content in blood and urine in health and disease. Medicine (Baltimore) **19**, 161—229 (1940).

BRØCHNER-MORTENSEN, K.: 100 gouty patients. Acta med. scand. **106**, 81—107 (1941).

BRØCHNER-MORTENSEN, K.: Gout. Heberden Oration. Ann. rheum. Dis. **17**, 1—8 (1958).

BROGSITTER, A. M.: Histopathologie der Gelenk-Gicht. Leipzig: F. C. W. Vogel 1927.

BRUGSCH, T., CITRON, J.: Über die Absorption der Harnsäure durch Knorpel. Z. exp. Path. Ther. **5**, 401—405 (1908).

BURCH, R. E., KURKE, N.: The effect of lactate infusion on serum uric acid. Proc. Soc. exp. Biol. (N.Y.) **127**, 17—20 (1968).

BUTT, W. R., MARSON, F. G. W.: 17-Ketosteroid excretion in gout. Brit. med. J. **1952 II**, 1023—1024.

CANELLAKIS, E. S., TUTTLE, A. L., COHEN, P. P.: A comparative study of the end-products of uric acid oxidation by peroxidases. J. biol. Chem. **213**, 397—404 (1955).

CASEY, J. H., HOFFMAN, M. M., SOLOMON, S.: The excretion of urinary dehydroepiandrosterone in gout. Arthr. and Rheum. **11**, 444—451 (1968).

CHANG, Y. H., GRALLA, E. J.: Suppression of urate crystal-induced canine joint inflammation by heterologous anti-polymorphonuclear leukocyte serum. Arthr. and Rheum. **11**, 145—150 (1968).

DA SILVA, W. D., EISELE, J. W., LEPOW, I. H.: Complement as a mediator of inflammation. III. Purification of the activity with anaphylatoxin properties generated by interaction of the first four components of complement and its identification as a cleavage product of C'3. J. exp. Med. **126**, 1027—1048 (1967).

DE GRACIANSKY, R.: Recherches sur l'acide urique dans la goutte. Paris: Thesis 1938.

DONALDSON, V. H., GLUECK, H. I., FLEMING, T.: Rheumatoid arthritis in a patient with Hageman trait. New Engl. J. Med. **286**, 528—530 (1972).

DRENICK, E. J., SWENSEID, M. E., BLAHD, W. H., TUTTLE, S. G.: Prolonged starvation as treatment for severe obesity. J. Amer. med. Ass. **187**, 100—105 (1964).

DUNCAN, H., BLUHM, G. B., RIDDLE, J. M., BARNHART, M. I.: Synovial urate crystals in acute gouty arthritis. A study of their origin and significance. Clin. orthop. **59**, 277—285 (1968).

DZONDI, K. H.: Was ist Rheumatismus und Gicht, und wie kann man sich dagegen schützen und am schnellsten davon befreien? Halle: C. A. Schwetschke 1829.

EINBINDER, J., SCHUBERT, M.: Separation of chondroitin sulfate from cartilage. J. biol. Chem. **185**, 725—730 (1950).

Eisen, V.: Effect of hexadimethrine bromide on plasma kinin formation, hydrolysis of p-tosyl-L-arginine methyl ester and fibrinolysis. Brit. J. Pharmacol. 22, 87—103 (1964).

Eisen, V.: Urates and kinin formation in synovial fluid. Proc. roy. Soc. Med. 59, 302—305 (1966).

Eisen, V.: Kinin formation in human diseases. In: The scientific basis of medicine, p. 146. University of London: Athlone Press 1969.

Eisen, V., Bruckner, F. E.: Proteolysis and its inhibition in joint diseases. In: Neue Aspekte der Trasylol Therapie, S. 3—12. Stuttgart-New York: Schattauer 1970.

Eisen, V., Vogt, W.: Plasma kininogenases and their activators. In: Handbuch der exp. Pharmakologie, Bd. 25: Bradykinin, Kallidin and Kallikrein, p. 82—130. Berlin-Heidelberg-New York: Springer 1970.

Erdös, E. G.: Hypotensive peptides: bradykinin, kallidin and eledoisin. Adv. Pharmacol. 4, 1—90 (1966).

Faires, J. S., McCarty, D. J.: Acute arthritis in man and dog produced by intrasynovial injection of sodium urate crystals. Clin. Res. 9, 329 (1961).

Faires, J. S., McCarty, D. J.: Acute arthritis in man and dog after intrasynovial injection of sodium urate crystals. Lancet 1962 II, 682—684 (1962a).

Faires, J. S., McCarty, D. J.: Acute synovitis in normal joints of man and dog produced by injections of microcrystalline sodium urate, calcium oxalate and corticosteroid esters. Arthr. Rheumat. 5, 295 (1962b).

Freudweiler, M.: Experimentelle Untersuchungen über die Entstehung der Gichtknoten. Dtsch. Arch. klin. Med. 69, 155—205 (1901).

Fritze, E., Kallweit, C., Müller, H. O.: Die Uratphagozytose der Granulozyten und ihre Beeinflussung durch Colchicin. Zugleich ein methodischer Beitrag zur Bestimmung ihrer Phagozytoseaktivität in vitro. Z. Rheumaforsch. 26, 44—56 (1967).

Garrod, A. B.: Die Natur und Behandlung der Gicht und der rheumatischen Gicht. Würzburg: J. M. Richter 1861.

Garrod, A. B.: The nature and treatment of gout and rheumatic gout. London: Walton & Maberly 1863.

Gaston, L. W.: The blood-clotting factors. New Engl. J. Med. 270, 236—242 (1964).

Gibson, H. V., Doisy, E. A.: Note on effect of some organic acids upon uric acid excretion of man. J. biol. Chem. 55, 605—610 (1923).

Gieseking, R.: Feinstrukturelle Befunde am Gichtknoten. Verh. dtsch. Ges. Path. 53, 356—363 (1969).

Goldfinger, S., Melmon, K. L., Webster, M. E., Sjoerdsma, A., Seegmiller, J. E.: The presence of a kinin-peptide in inflammatory synovial effusions. Arthr. and Rheum. 7, 311—312 (1964).

Goldfinger, S. E., Howell, R. R., Seegmiller, J. E.: Suppression of metabolic accompaniments of phagocytosis by colchicine. Arthr. and Rheum. 8, 1112—1122 (1965).

Goldfinger, S. E., Klinenberg, J. R., Seegmiller, J. E.: Renal retention of uric acid induced by infusion of beta-hydroxybutyrate and acetoacetate. New Engl. J. Med. 272, 351—355 (1965).

Graham, R. C., Ebert, R. H., Ratnoff, O. D., Moses, J. M.: Pathogenesis of inflammation. II. In vivo observations of the inflammatory effects of activated Hageman factor and bradykinin. J. exp. Med. 121, 807—817 (1965).

Greenbaum, L. M., Kim, K. S.: Kinin-forming and kininase activities of rabbit polymorphonuclear leucocytes. Brit. J. Pharmacol. 29, 238—247 (1967).

Greiling, H., Herbertz, T., Schuler, B., Stuhlsatz, H. W.: Biochemische Untersuchungen über die Ursache der Harnsäureablagerung im Bindegewebe der Gicht. Z. Rheumaforsch. 21, 50—55 (1962).

Gutman, A. B., Yü, T. F.: Gout, a derangement of purine metabolism. Advanc. intern. Med. 5, 227—302 (1952).

Gutman, A. B., Yü, T. F.: Protracted uricosuric therapy in tophaceous gout. Lancet 1957 II, 1258—1260.

Habermann, E.: Das Kininsystem — pathophysiologische Bedeutung und therapeutische Konsequenzen. Internist. (Berl.) 7, 364—369 (1966).

Harding, V. J., Allin, K. D., Eagles, B. A., Van Wyck, H. B.: Effect of high fat diets on content of uric acid in blood. J. biol. Chem. 63, 37—53 (1925).

Harding, V. J., Allin, K. D., Eagles, B. A.: Influence of fat and carbohydrate diets upon level of blood uric acid. J. biol. Chem. 74, 631—643 (1927).

Hauge, M., Harvald, B.: Heredity in gout and hyperuricemia. Acta med. scand. 152, 247—257 (1955).

Hellman, L.: Production of acute gouty arthritis by adrenocorticotropin. Science **109**, 280—281 (1949).

Hench, P. S.: Gout and gouty arthritis. In: Modern medical therapy in general practice, Vol. 3, p. 3359. Baltimore: Williams and Willkins 1940.

Heuckenkamp, P.-U., Zöllner, N.: Fructose-induced hyperuricaemia. Lancet **1971 I**, 808—809.

Heuckenkamp, P.-U., Schill, K., Zöllner, N.: Zum Mechanismus des Serumharnsäureanstiegs unter konstanter Fructoseinfusion beim Menschen. Verh. dtsch. Ges. inn. Med. **77**, 177—180 (1971).

His, W.: Schicksal und Wirkungen des sauren harnsauren Natrons in Bauch- und Gelenkhöhle des Kaninchens. Dtsch. Arch. klin. Med. **67**, 81—108 (1900).

Howell, R. R., Eanes, E. D., Seegmiller, J. E.: X-Ray diffraction studies of the tophaceous deposits in gout. Arthr. and Rheum. **6**, 97—103 (1963).

Howell, R. R., Seegmiller, J. E.: A mechanism of action of colchicine. Arthr. and Rheum. **5**, 303 (1962a).

Howell, R. R., Seegmiller, J. E.: Uricolysis by human leucocytes. Nature **196**, 482—483 (1962b).

Inagaki, K., Morioka, S.: Development of urate crystals in tophus. Yokohama med. Bull. **19**, 103—108 (1968).

Jasani, M. K., Katori, M., Lewis, G. P.: Intracellular enzymes and kinin enzymes in synovial fluid in joint diseases. Origin and relation to disease category. Ann. rheum. Dis. **28**, 497—511 (1969).

Kappas, A., Hellman, L., Fukushima, D. K., Gallagher, T. F.: The pyrogenic effect of etiocholanolone. J. clin. Endocr. **17**, 451—453 (1957).

Karnovsky, M. L.: Metabolic basis of phagocytic activity. Phys. Rev. **42**, 143—168 (1962).

Katz, W. A., Ehrlich, G. E.: The solubility of monosodium urate in serum and connective tissue fractions. Arthr. and Rheum. **11**, 492 (1968).

Katz, W. A., Ehrlich, G. E.: Deposition of urate crystals in man. Ann. rheum. Dis. **28**, 327 (1969).

Katz, W. A., Schubert, M.: The interaction of monosodium urate with connective tissue components. J. clin. Invest. **49**, 1783—1789 (1970).

Kellermeyer, R. W.: Activation of Hageman factor by sodium urate crystals. Arthr. and Rheum. **8**, 741—743 (1965).

Kellermeyer, R. W.: Inflammatory process in acute gouty arthritis. III. Vascular permeability-enhancing activity in normal human synovial fluid; induction by Hageman factor activators; and inhibition by Hageman factor antiserum. J. Lab. clin. Med. **70**, 372—383 (1967).

Kellermeyer, R. W.: Mechanism of inflammation in acute gouty arthritis: Activation of permeability factor activity in synovial fluid by urate crystals. Proc. Cent. Soc. Clin. Res. **39**, 42—43 (1966).

Kellermeyer, R. W.: Hageman Factor and acute gouty arthritis. Arthr. and Rheum. **11**, 452—459 (1968).

Kellermeyer, R. W., Breckenridge, R. T.: The inflammatory process in acute gouty arthritis. I. Activation of Hageman factor by sodium urate crystals. J. Lab. clin. Med. **65**, 307—315 (1965).

Kellermeyer, R. W., Breckenridge, R. T.: The inflammatory process in acute gouty arthritis. II. The presence of Hageman factor and plasma thromboplastin antecedent in synovial fluid. J. Lab. clin. Med. **67**, 455—460 (1966).

Klinenberg, J. R.: Binding of urate to plasma proteins determined by the method of equilibrium dialysis. Arthr. and Rheum. **11**, 828—829 (1968).

Klinenberg, J. R.: Current concepts of hyperuricemia and gout. Calif. Med. **110**, 231—243 (1969).

Klinenberg, J. R., Bluestone, R., Schlosstein, L., Waisman, J., Whitehouse, M. W.: Urate deposition disease. Ann. intern. Med. **78**, 99—111 (1973).

Kreisberg, R. A., Owen, W. C., Siegal, A. M.: Ethanolinduced hyperlacticacidemia: inhibition of lactate utilization. J. clin. Invest. **50**, 166—174 (1971).

Laurent, T. C.: Solubility of sodium urate in the presence of chondroitin-4-sulphate. Nature **202**, 1334 (1964).

Lecocq, F. R., McPhaul, J. J.: The effects of starvation, high fat diets and ketone infusions on uric acid balance. Clin. Res. **12**, 274 (1964).

Lennox, W. G.: Study of retention of uric acid during fasting. J. biol. Chem. **66**, 521—572 (1925).

Lewis, G. P.: Plasma kinins and other vasoactive compounds in acute inflammation. Ann. N.Y. Acad. Sci. **116**, 847—854 (1964).

Lewis, G. P.: Kinins in inflammation and tissue injury. In: Handbuch der experimentellen Pharmakologie, Bd. **25**: Bradykinin, Kallidin and Kallikrein, p. 516—530. Berlin-Heidelberg-New York: Springer 1970.

LIEBER, C. S., JONES, D. P., LOSOWSKY, M. S., DAVIDSON, C. S.: Interrelation of uric acid and ethanol metabolism in man. J. clin. Invest. **41**, 1863—1870 (1962).
LOEB, J. N.: The influence of temperature on the solubility of monosodium urate. Arthr. and Rheum. **15**, 189—192 (1972).
LÖFFLER, W., KOLLER, F.: Die Gicht. In: Handbuch der inneren Medizin, 4. Aufl., 7. Bd., 2. Teil: Stoffwechsel-Krankheiten. Berlin-Heidelberg-New York: Springer 1955.
MACLACHLAN, M. J., RODNAN, G. P.: Effects of food, fast and alcohol on serum uric acid and acute attacks of gout. Amer. J. Med. **42**, 38—57 (1967).
MÄENPÄÄ, P. H., RAIVIO, K. O., KEKOMÄKI, M. P.: Liver adenine nucleotides: fructose-induced depletion and its effect on protein synthesis. Science **161**, 1253—1254 (1968).
MARGOLIS, J.: Activation of plasma by contact with glass: evidence for a common reaction which releases plasma kinin and initiates coagulation. J. Physiol. (Lond.) **144**, 1—22 (1958).
MARGOLIS, J.: Hageman factor and capillary permeability. Austral. J. exp. Biol. **37**, 239—244 (1959).
MALAWISTA, S. E., SEEGMILLER, J. E.: The effect of pretreatment with colchicine on the inflammatory response to microcrystalline urate. A model for gouty inflammation. Ann. intern. Med. **62**, 648—657 (1965).
MCCARTY, D. J.: Phagocytosis of urate crystals in gouty synovial fluid. Amer. J. med. Sci. **243**, 288—295 (1962).
MCCARTY, D. J.: A historical note: Leeuwenhoek's description of crystals from a gouty tophus. Arthr. and Rheum. **13**, 414—418 (1970a).
MCCARTY, D. J.: Crystal-induced inflammation of the joints. Ann. Rev. Med. **21**, 357—366 (1970b).
MCCARTY, D. J.: Pathogenesis and treatment of the acute attack of gout. Clin. Orthop. **71**, 28—39 (1970c).
MCCARTY, D. J.: Mechanisms of the crystal deposition diseases—gout and pseudogout. Ann. intern. Med. **78**, 767—771 (1973).
MCCARTY, D. J., HOLLANDER, J. L.: Identification of urate crystals in gouty synovial fluid. Ann. intern. Med. **54**, 452—460 (1961).
MCCARTY, D. J., PHELPS, P., PYENSON, J.: Crystal-induced inflammation in canine joints. I. An experimental model with quantification of the host response. J. exp. Med. **124**, 99—114 (1966).
MELMON, K. L., CLINE, M. J.: Kinins. Amer. J. Med. **43**, 153—160 (1967).
MELMON, K. L., CLINE, M. J.: Interaction of plasma kinins and granulocytes. Nature **213**, 90 (1967).
MELMON, K. L., WEBSTER, M. E., GOLDFINGER, S. E., SEEGMILLER, J. E.: The presence of a kinin in inflammatory synovial effusion from arthritides of varying etiologies. Arthr. and Rheum. **10**, 13—20 (1967).
MERRILL, J. P.: The treatment of renal failure. New York-London: Grune and Stratton 1955.
MERTZ, D. P.: Gicht und Hyperuricämie. Arch. klin. Med. **212**, 143—190 (1966).
MERTZ, D. P.: Gicht. Stuttgart: Thieme 1971.
MILES, A. A.: Large molecular substances as mediators of the inflammatory reaction. Ann. N.Y. Acad. Sci. **116**, 855—865 (1964).
MOORE, D. H., RUSKA, H.: The fine structure of capillaries and small arteries. J. biophys. biochem. Cytol. **3**, 457—461 (1957).
MORGANO, G., ALCOZER, G.: Correlazioni fra il ricambio dell' acido urico e il ricambio dei corpi chetonici. I. Comportamento dell' uricemia e dell' uricuria dopo carico di acido betaidrossibutirrico in soggetti sani ed eucrinici in condizioni basali e dopo apporto glucidico. Arch. E. Maragliano Pat. Clin. **4**, 1125—1140 (1949).
MURPHY, R., SHIPMAN, K. H.: Hyperuricemia during total fasting: renal factors. Arch. intern. Med. **112**, 954—959 (1963).
NAFF, G. B., BYERS, P. H.: Possible implication of complement in acute gout. J. clin. Invest. **46**, 1099 (1967).
PADOVA, J., BENDERSKY, G.: Hyperuricemia in diabetic ketoacidosis. New Engl. J. Med. **267**, 530—534 (1962).
PERHEENTUPA, J., RAIVIO, K.: Fructose-induced hyperuricaemia. Lancet **1967 II**, 528—531.
PETERS, J. P., VAN SLYKE, D. D.: Quantitative clinical chemistry, 2nd Ed. Baltimore: Williams & Wilkins 1946.
PHELPS, P., MCCARTY, D. J.: Crystal-induced inflammation in canine joints. II. Importance of polymorphonuclear leukocytes. J. exp. Med. **124**, 115—125 (1966a).
PHELPS, P., PROCKOP, D. J., MCCARTY, D. J.: Crystal induced inflammation in canine joints. III. Evidence against bradykinin as a mediator of inflammation. J. Lab. clin. Med. **68**, 433—444 (1966b).

PHELPS, P.: Polymorphonuclear leukocyte motility in vitro. II. Stimulatory effect of monosodium urate crystals and urate in solution; partial inhibition by colchicine and indomethacin. Arthr. and Rheum. 12, 189—196 (1969a).

PHELPS, P.: Polymorphonuclear leukocyte motility in vitro. III. Possible release of a chemotactic substance after phagocytosis of urate crystals by polymorphonuclear leucocytes. Arthr. and Rheum. 12, 197—204 (1969b).

PHELPS, P., MCCARTY, D. J.: Crystal-induced arthritis. Postgrad. med. 45, 87—93 (1969).

PHELPS, P., STANISLAW, D.: Polymorphonuclear leukocyte motility in vitro. I. Effect of pH, temperature, ethyl alcohol and caffeine, using a modified Boyden chamber technique. Arthr. and Rheum. 12, 181—188 (1969).

QUICK, A. J.: Relationship between chemical structure and physiological response. III. Factors influencing excretion of uric acid. J. biol. Chem. 98, 157—169 (1932).

RAJAN, K. T.: Lysosomes and gout. Nature 210, 959 (1966).

RATNOFF, O. D., CRUM, J. D.: Activation of Hageman factor by solutions of ellagic acid. J. Lab. clin. Med. 63, 359—377 (1964).

RATNOFF, O. D., LEPOW, I. H.: Complement as a mediator of inflammation. Enhancement of vascular permeability by purified human C'1 esterase. J. exp. Med. 118, 681—697 (1963).

RATNOFF, O. D., MILES, A. A.: The induction of permeability-increasing activity in human plasma by activated Hageman factor. Brit. J. exp. Path. 45, 328—345 (1964).

REEVES, B.: Significance of joint fluid uric acid levels in gout. Ann. rheum. Dis. 24, 569—571 (1965).

RIDDLE, J. M., BLUHM, G. B., BARNHART, M. I.: Ultrastructural study of leucocytes and urates in gouty arthritis. Ann. rheum. Dis. 26, 389—401 (1967).

RIEHL, G.: Zur Anatomie der Gicht. Wien. klin. Wschr. 10, 761—763 (1897).

ROBERTS, W.: The Croonian Lectures on the chemistry and therapeutics of uric acid gravel and gout. Lecture IV. Chemistry of uratic precipitation. Brit. med. J. 1892 II, 61—65.

ROBINSON, W. D., CONN, J. W., BLOCH, W. D., LOUIS, L. H.: Role of the adrenal cortex in urate metabolism and in gout. J. Lab. clin. Med. 33, 1473—1474 (1948).

ROBINSON, W. D., CONN, J. W., BLOCK, W. D., LOUIS, L. H., KATZ, J.: Role of the anterior pituitary and adrenal cortex in urate metabolism and in gout. Ann. Rheum. Dis. 8, 312—313 (1949).

ROPES, M. W., BAUER, W.: Synovial fluid changes in joint disease. Cambridge: Harvard University Press 1953.

RUNCIE, J., THOMSON, T. J.: Total fasting, hyperuricaemia and gout. Postgrad. med. J. 45, 251—253 (1969).

SAHEBJAMI, H., SCALETTAR, R.: Effects of fructose infusion on lactate and uric acid metabolism. Lancet 1971 I, 366—369.

SCHEELE, K. W.: Examen chemicum calculi urinarii. Leipzig: Opuscula II (1776).

SCHILLING, F., OERTEL, G. W., TREIBER, L.: Periodisches Fieber und Ätiocholanolon-Fieber bei chronischen rheumatischen Leiden. Z. Rheumaforsch. 28, 117—125 (1969).

SCHUMACHER, H. R., PHELPS, P.: Sequential changes in human polymorphonuclear leucocytes after urate crystal phagocytosis. An electron microscopic study. Arthr. and Rheum. 14, 513—526 (1971).

SCOTT, J. T., MCCALLUM, F. M., HOLLOWAY, V.: Starvation, ketosis, and uric acid excretion. Ann. Rheum. Dis. 23, 83—84 (1964).

SEEGMILLER, J. E., HOWELL, R. R.: The old and new concepts of acute gouty arthritis. Arthr. and Rheum. 5, 616—623 (1962).

SEEGMILLER, J. E., HOWELL, R. R., MALAWISTA, S. E.: The inflammatory reaction to sodium urate. Its possible relationship to the genesis of acute gouty arthritis. J. Amer. med. Ass. 180, 469—475 (1962a).

SEEGMILLER, J. E., HOWELL, R. R., MALAWISTA, S. E.: A mechanism of action of colchicine in acute gouty arthritis. J. clin. Invest. 41, 1399 (1962b).

SEEGMILLER, J. E., LASTER, L., HOWELL, R. R.: Biochemistry of uric acid and its relation to gout. New Engl. J. Med. 268, 712—716, 764—773, 821—827 (1963).

SHAPIRO, J. R., KLINENBERG, J. R., PECK, W. E., GOLDFINGER, S. E., SEEGMILLER, J. E.: Hyperuricemia associated with obesity and intensified by caloric restriction. Arthr. and Rheum. 7, 343 (1964).

SICUTERI, F., FANCIULLACCI, M., FRANCHI, G., DEL BIANCO, P. L.: Serotonin—bradykinin potentiation on the pain receptors in man. Life Sci. 4, 309—316 (1965).

SLANSKY, H. H., KUWABARA, T.: Intranuclear urate crystals in corneal epithelium. Arch. Ophthal. 80, 338—344 (1968).

SOKOLOFF, L.: The pathology of gout. Metabolism 6, 230—243 (1957).

Sorensen, L. B.: The pathogenesis of gout. Arch. intern. Med. **109**, 379—390 (1962).
Spilberg, I.: Urate crystal arthritis in animals lacking Hageman factor. Arthr. and Rheum. **17**, 143—148 (1974).
Spilberg, I., Osterland, C. K.: Anti-inflammatory effect of Trasylol in acute experimental arthritis induced by urate crystals. In: Neue Aspekte der Trasylol Therapie, p. 23—26. Stuttgart-New York: Schattauer 1970a.
Spilberg, I., Osterland, C. K.: Anti-inflammatory effect of the trypsin-kallikrein inhibitor in acute arthritis induced by urate crystals in rabbits. J. Lab. clin. Med. **76**, 472—479 (1970b).
Steele, A. D., McCarty, D. J.: An experimental model of acute inflammation in man. Arthr. and Rheum. **9**, 430—442 (1966).
Stetten, D., jr.: Basic sciences in medicine: the example of gout. New Engl. J. Med. **278**, 1333—1336 (1968).
Thompson, G. R., Duff, J. F., Robinson, W. D., Mikkelsen, W. M., Galindez, H.: Long term uricosuric therapy in gout. Arthr. and Rheum. **5**, 384—396 (1962).
Tse, R. L., Phelps, P.: Polymorphonuclear leukocyte motility in vitro. V. Release of chemotactic activity following phagocytosis of calcium pyrophosphate crystals, diamond dust, and urate crystals. J. Lab. clin. Med. **76**, 403—415 (1970).
Van Arman, C. G., Carlson, R. P.: The two distinct phases of inflammatory response in the dog's knee joint. In: Bradykinin and related Kinins. Cardiovascular, Biochemical, and Neural Actions, p. 525—535. New York-London: Plenum Press 1970.
Villa, L., Bobecchi, A., Ballabio, C. B.: Physiopathology, clinical manifestations, and treatment of gout. Part I. Physiopathology and pathogenesis. Ann. rheum. Dis. **17**, 9—15 (1958).
Vormittag, W., Thumb, N., Pietschmann, H.: Peroxydasegehalt der Granulozyten des peripheren Blutes bei Arthritis urica. Z. Rheumaforsch. **30**, 119—124 (1971).
Wallingford, W. R., McCarty, D. J.: Differential membranolytic effects of microcrystalline sodium urate and calcium pyrophosphate dihydrate. J. exp. Med. **133**, 100—112 (1971).
Ward, P. A., Cochrane, C. G., Müller-Eberhard, H. J.: Further studies on the chemotactic factor of complement and its formation in vivo. Immunology **11**, 141—153 (1966).
Ward, P.: Chemotaxis of polymorphonuclear leukocytes. Biochem. Pharmacol. Suppl. **17**, 99—105 (1968).
Webster, M. E., Ratnoff, O. D.: Role of Hageman factor in the activation of vasodilator activity in human plasma. Nature **192**, 180 (1961).
Webster, M. E.: The kallikrein-kininogen-kinin system. Arthr. and Rheum. **9**, 473—482 (1966).
Weissmann, B., Gutman, A. B.: The identification of 6-succinoamino purine and of 8-hydroxy-7-methyl guanine as normal human urinary constituents. J. biol. Chem. **229**, 239—250 (1957).
Weissmann, G.: The role of lysosomes in inflammation and disease. Ann. Rev. Med. **18**, 97—112 (1967).
Weissmann, G., Spilberg, I., Krakauer, K.: Arthritis induced in rabbits by lysates of granulocyte lysosomes. Arthr. and Rheum. **12**, 103—116 (1969).
Weissmann, G., Rita, G. A.: Molecular basis of gouty inflammation: interaction of monosodium urate crystals with lysosomes and liposomes. Nature New Biology **240**, 167—172 (1972).
Werle, E.: In: Polypeptides which stimulate plain muscle. Edinburgh-London: Livingstone 1955.
Werle, E.: Plasmakinine. Dtsch. med. Wschr. **92**, 1573—1580 (1967).
Wilhelm, D. L.: Kinins in human disease. Ann. Rev. Med. **22**, 63—84 (1971).
Woods, H. F., Eggleston, L. V., Krebs, H. A.: The cause of hepatic accumulation of fructose 1-phosphate on fructose loading. Biochem. J. **119**, 501—510 (1970).
Wyngaarden, J. B.: In: Gout. The metabolic basis of inherited disease, p. 667—728. New York: McGraw-Hill 1966.
Yü, T. F., Sirota, J. H., Berger, L., Halpern, M., Gutman, A. B.: Effect of sodium lactate infusion on urate clearance in man. Proc. Soc. exp. Biol. (N.Y.) **96**, 809—813 (1957).
Zevely, H. A., French, A. J., Mikkelsen, W. M., Duff, I. F.: Synovial specimens obtained by knee joint punch biopsy. Amer. J. Med. **20**, 510—519 (1956).
Zöllner, N.: Nucleinstoffwechsel. In: Thannhauser's Lehrbuch des Stoffwechsels und der Stoffwechselkrankheiten, 2. Aufl. Stuttgart: Thieme 1957.
Zöllner, N.: Gicht. Internist (Berl.) **1**, 333—345 (1960).
Zvaifler, N. J., Pekin, T. J.: Significance of urate crystals in synovial fluids. Arch. intern. Med. **111**, 99—102 (1963).

V. Die pathologische Anatomie der Gicht

Die pathologische Anatomie der Gicht

Von

E. UEHLINGER

Mit 21 Abbildungen

Eine vorzügliche Darstellung der Morphologie der Gicht verdanken wir F. LANG im Handbuch der speziellen pathologischen Anatomie und Histologie, Band IX/3, S. 309—339, Berlin: Springer 1937.

Alle geweblichen Prozesse lassen sich bei Gicht auf eine wiederholte Hyperuricämie zurückführen. Die Hyperuricämie zwingt den Organismus, den Harnsäurespiegel des Serums so rasch als möglich auf den Normalwert abzusenken 1. durch Erhöhung der renalen Harnsäureausscheidung, 2. durch Einlagerung von Natriumurat in die Gelenke, Sehnen, Sehnenscheiden, Schleimbeutel und in die Haut. Die damit verbundenen Gewebsschäden bestimmen das morphologische Bild der Gicht: die Gelenkgicht und die Gichtniere.

Die Gelenkgicht

Im Beginn der Gelenkgicht steht die vermehrte Harnsäureausscheidung in die Gelenkflüssigkeit. Der Harnsäuregehalt der Gelenkflüssigkeit kann im Gichtanfall ungemein hohe Werte erreichen. In einer zweiten Phase wird die Harnsäure sowohl vom Gelenkknorpel wie von der Gelenkkapsel aufgenommen und als amorphes Natriumurat ausgefällt. Anschließend wird das amorphe Natriumurat teils extracellulär, teils intracellulär in optisch einachsige Kristallnadeln umgeprägt. Sowohl in der amorphen, wie in der kristallinen Form wirkt das Natriumurat ungemein entzündungserregend, während dem in Wasser gelösten Natriummonourat keine entzündungserregende Wirkung zukommt.

Bevorzugte Lokalisation sind das *Großzehengrundgelenk* und das *Kniegelenk*. Die Befallsrate variiert je nach Auswertung nur der klinischen Erscheinungen, der Röntgen- oder der Sektionsbefunde. Bei der Zusammenstellung der Sektionsbefunde ist zu berücksichtigen, daß die Schulter- und Wirbelsäulengelenke nur selten systematisch kontrolliert werden. Unter Berücksichtigung dieser Einschränkung ist die *Verteilung der Gelenkgicht* auf Grund der Auswertung von 32 Obduktionen des Path. Institutes der Universität Zürich in den Jahren 1960—1969 in absteigender Häufigkeit folgende:

Großzehengrundgelenk	27
Kniegelenk	23
Fingergelenk	6
Fußwurzelgelenke	6
Sprunggelenke	6
Hüftgelenk	4
Ellbogengelenk	4
Acromio-Claviculargelenk	2
Handwurzelgelenke	1

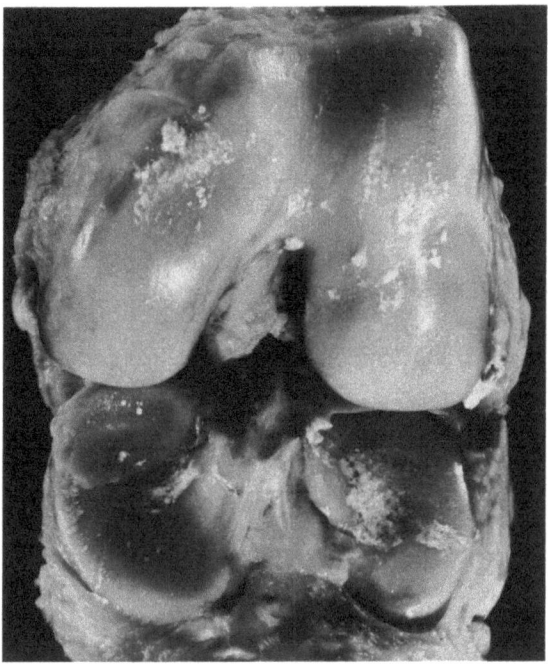

Abb. 1. Leichte Uratgicht des Kniegelenks. Gelenkknorpel mit schneeweißen Uratspritzern. Mann, 56 Jahre. (SN 2301/60. Path. Inst. Zürich)

Die Bevorzugung der großen Gelenke einerseits, der kleinen Finger- und Zehengelenke andererseits findet sich in allen Statistiken. Die Zahl der gleichzeitig befallenen Gelenke ist begrenzt. Die Auswertung des Züricher Obduktionsgutes ergibt folgende Werte:

Befall eines einzigen Gelenkes	5
Befall von 2 Gelenken	14
Befall von 3 Gelenken	7
Befall von 4 Gelenken	4
Befall von 5 Gelenken	1
Befall von 6 Gelenken	1

Führend ist die Zweierkombination und in dieser der gleichzeitige Befall von Großzehengrundgelenk und Kniegelenk.

In bezug auf *seltene Lokalisationen* der Arthritis urica sei auf folgende Arbeiten verwiesen: *Arthritis urica der Wirbelsäule*: HALL u. SELIN, MICHAEL et al.; *Arthritis urica der Sacro-iliacal-Gelenke*: ALARCÒN-SEGOVIA et al., LAMBETH et al., MALAWISTA, S. E., et al.; *Arthritis urica des Schultergelenkes*: PIGUET; *Gicht der Patella*: PELOQUIN u. GRAHAM.

Die *Form des Gelenkbefalls* wird bestimmt durch die Oberflächenrelation Gelenkknorpel/Gelenkkapsel. Je größer der Gelenkkapselanteil, um so mehr bestimmt die Uratspeicherung in der Gelenkkapsel Form und Verlauf der Gelenkgicht. Überwiegt die Knorpelfläche, so gestalten die Urateinlagerung in den Gelenkknorpel und die Knorpelschleifschäden die Gelenkzerstörung. Entsprechend sind zu unterscheiden eine vorwiegend chondrale und eine vorwiegend synoviale Form der Gelenkgicht.

Die vorwiegend *chondrale Form* der Gelenkgicht zeigen die *Knie- und Sprunggelenke*, wie auch die Handwurzel- und Fußwurzelgelenke. Die Harnsäureinsuda-

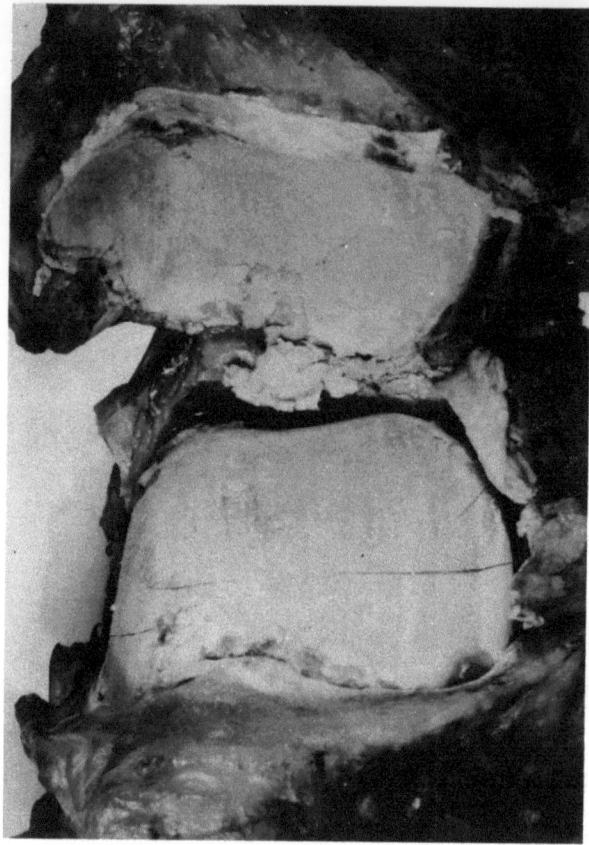

Abb. 2. Schwere Uratgicht des proximalen Sprunggelenkes. Schneeweiße Uratinsudation der Gelenkknorpel. Mann, 75 Jahre (SN 447/59. Path. Inst. Zürich)

tion des Gelenkknorpels wird durch den hohen Natriumgehalt des Gelenkknorpels, der denjenigen des Blutes um das 8fache übertrifft, und den hohen Wassergehalt der oberflächlichen Knorpelschichten maßgebend gefördert (LANG). Durch die Insudation mit Harnsäure wird der Knorpel kreideweiß und verliert seinen Glanz. Je nach der Dauer und Schwere der Hyperuricämie variiert der Knorpelbefund zwischen wenigen mattweißen Uratspritzern (Abb. 1) und einer gleichmäßigen schneeweißen Insudation der ganzen Knorpelgleitfläche (Abb. 2). Weißer Gelenkknorpel, flammend gerötete Gelenkkapsel und goldgelbes paraartikuläres Fettgewebe ergeben zusammen ein ungemein farbenfrohes Bild, welches für die fortgeschrittene Gelenkgicht so kennzeichnend ist. Die Insudation des Gelenkknorpels mit Harnsäure erreicht eine Schichttiefe von 1 mm. Sie macht den Knorpel hart und spröde. Die unmittelbaren Folgen sind *Knorpelschleifschäden* in Form von Splitterungen, Usuren und Schleifrillen (Abb. 3 u. 4). Die Schleifdefekte öffnen der Harnsäure den Zugang zu den tieferen Knorpelschichten, die schließlich ebenfalls in den mechanischen Abnützungsprozeß einbezogen werden. Die Endstadien der chondralen Gelenkgicht haben viel Ähnlichkeit mit der deformierenden Arthrose.

Die Uratspeicherung im Gelenkknorpel ist oft umfangreicher als der klinisch manifeste Gelenkbefall. So beschreiben TALBOTT und TERPLAN einen Fall von

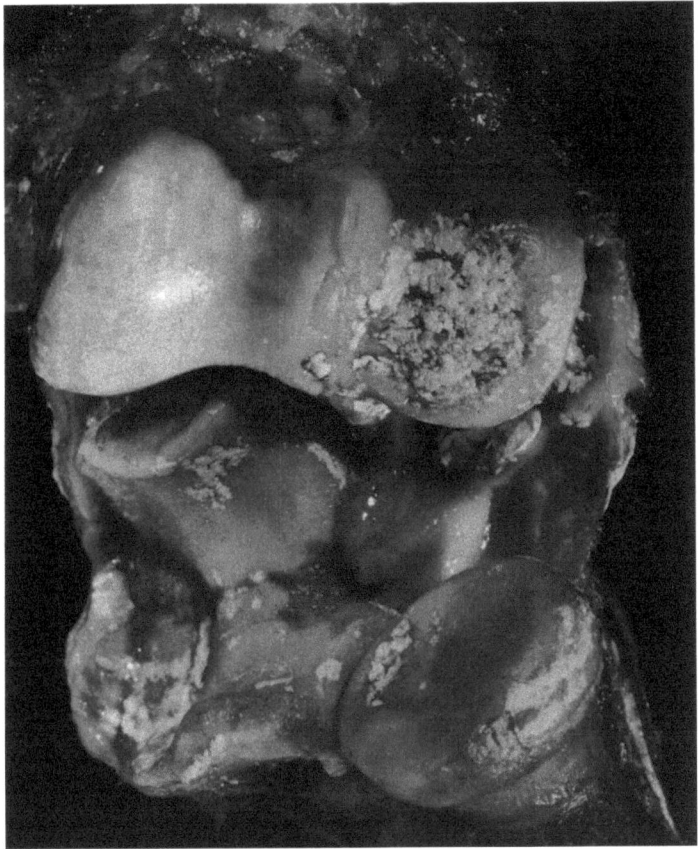

Abb. 3. Uratgicht des Ellbogengelenkes. Exulceration des uratimprägnierten radialen Humeruscondylus. Mann, 68 Jahre. (SN 2240/65. Path. Inst. Zürich)

schwerster Uratinkrustation beider Kniegelenke, ohne daß der Patient je Schmerzen in seinen Kniegelenken verspürt hatte.

Die *synoviale Form* der Gelenkgicht ist die Gicht der *Zehen- und Fingergelenke* mit verhältnismäßig großen Kapselanteilen (Abb. 5, 6 u. 13). Der Anstieg der Harnsäurekonzentration in der Gelenkflüssigkeit hat zunächst eine unspezifische Synovitis zur Folge mit arterieller Hyperämie, Schwellung der Histiocyten, Fibrocyten und Deckmesothelien und einer zottigen Proliferation der inneren Kapselschichten. Diese Frühsynovitis erleichtert den Übertritt der Harnsäure aus der Gelenkflüssigkeit in das Kapselgewebe, wo sie als amorphes Natriumurat ausgefällt wird. Die Umformung zum *Gichttophus* wird eingeleitet durch die Transformation des amorphen Natriumurates in Kristallnadeln. Durch Zusammenschluß der Kristalle zu Rosetten wird die örtliche Konzentration der Urate gesteigert. Zugleich wird das kristalline Urat zum *Fremdkörper*. Die Kristalldrusen werden durch einen Wall von ein- und mehrkernigen Histiocyten eingefaßt und gegen die Umgebung abgeschirmt (Abb. 7). Mit jedem Gichtanfall nimmt die Zahl der kristallinen Uratdrusen zu. Ältere Kristalldepots wirken bei Nachschüben als Abscheidungszentren (LANG). Gichttophus reiht sich an Tophus zu Ketten und Knoten. Die Konglomerate erreichen Kirsch- und Kastaniengröße und können

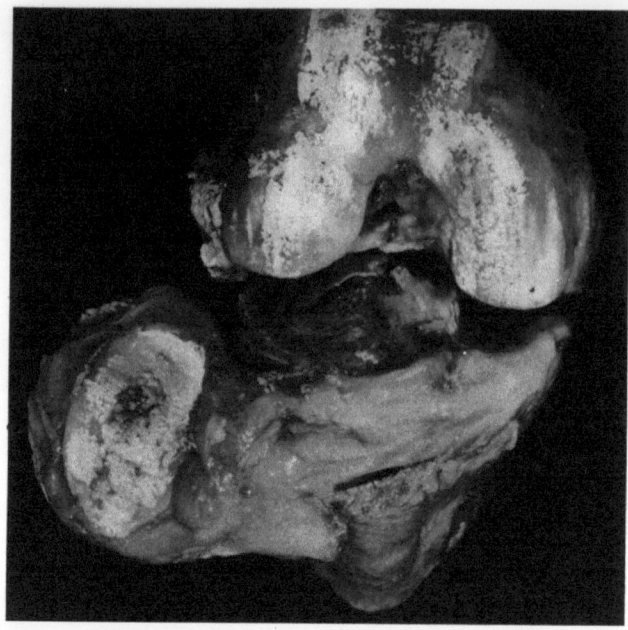

Abb. 4. Uratgicht des Kniegelenks. Femurcondylen und Patella mit Schliffurchen in den uratimprägnierten Gelenkknorpeln. Mann, 64 Jahre. (SN 889/68. Path. Inst. Zürich)

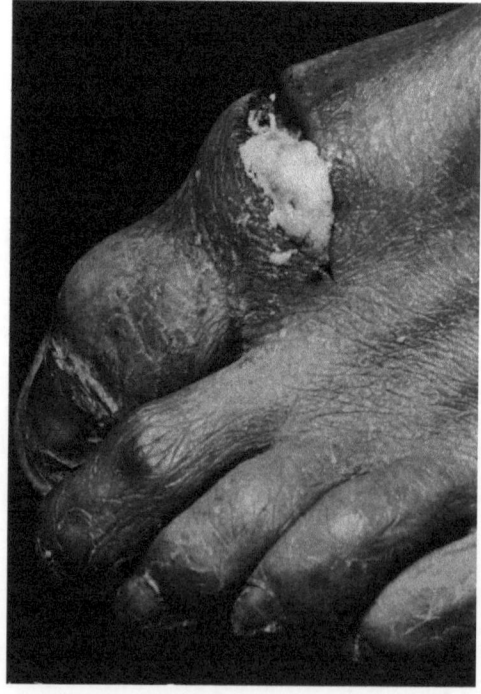

Abb. 5. Großzehengicht. Schneeweißer Uratbrei aus dem angeschnittenen Großzehengrundgelenk herausquellend. Mann, 75 Jahre. (SN 447/59. Path. Inst. Zürich)

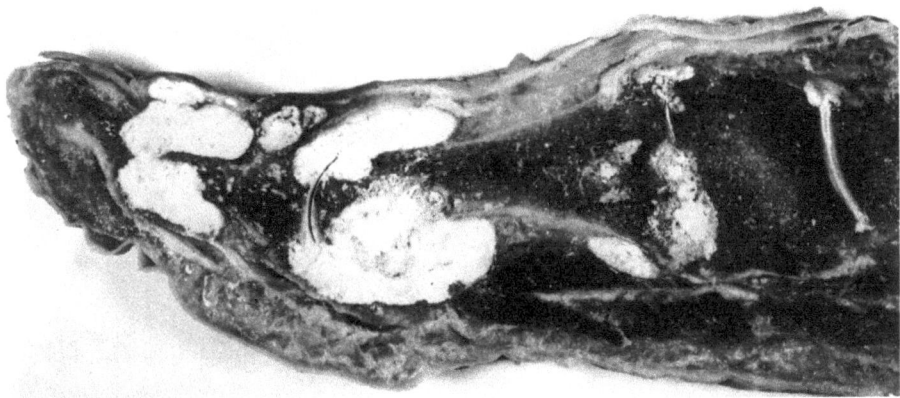

Abb. 6. Uratgicht. Längsschnitt durch Großzehe. Destruktion des Metatarso-phalangeal- und des Interphalangealgelenkes durch Urattophi. Mann, 75 Jahre. (SN 447/59. Path. Inst. Zürich)

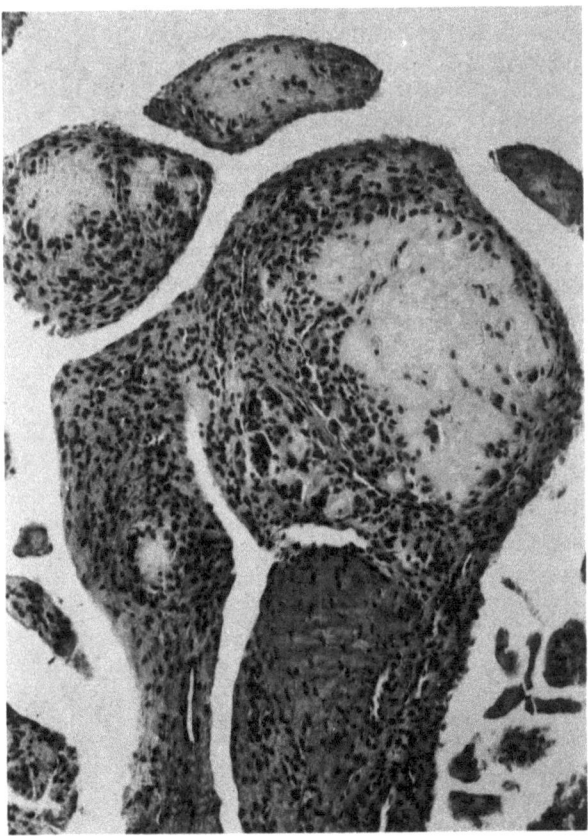

Abb. 7. Gelenkgicht. Synovitis villosa urica mit charakteristischem Gichttophus. Excisat aus einem Interphalangealgelenk. Vergr. 100:1. Frau, 65 Jahre. (MB 3968/68. Path. Inst. Zürich)

an Zehen und Fingern als bucklige Kapselverdickungen durch die Haut durchgetastet werden (Abb. 13).

Die Gichttophi neigen zur sekundären Verkalkung, ebenso die Uratdepots in Gelenkknorpeln und Menisken (DODDS u. STEINBACH).

In einer letzten Phase werden auch die *Phalangen* in den gichtischen Entzündungs- und Destruktionsprozeß einbezogen. Die subchondralen Spongiosazerstörungen stehen in engster Beziehung zum anatomischen Aufbau der Interphalangeal- und Metacarpophalangealgelenke. Auf dem Sagittalschnitt bildet die Gelenkkapsel zu beiden Seiten der Phalangenköpfchen Taschen. Diese sind auf der Ulnar- und Dorsalseite tiefer ausgebuchtet als auf der Radial- und Volarseite. Die Taschentiefe erreicht bis 3 mm. Die der Phalange zugewandte Taschenwand ist mit dem Periost verschmolzen und vermittelt den Zugang zur metaphysären Corticalis. Die paraossären Kapseltaschen sind die eigentlichen Träger der Zerstörung der ossären Gelenkkonstituenten. Die Gichttophi in diesen Taschen reizen das Periost. Ihre ein- und mehrkernigen Phagocyten werden zu Osteoclasten umgeschult und lösen die Corticalis im Haftgebiet der Kapseltaschen auf. Durch die Corticalislücken dringen Harnsäure wie Gichttophi in die subchondralen Markräume ein. Epi- und metaphysäre Spongiosa werden rücksichtslos den vordringenden Gichttophi geopfert. Der Gelenkknorpel wird besonders in den Randabschnitten unterminiert, die epiphysäre Spongiosa, als Träger des Gelenkknorpels, zerstört. Der Gelenkknorpel wird nun von zwei Seiten, sowohl vom Gelenkraum aus durch Harnsäureinsudation, wie von der Unterseite durch Gichttophi angegriffen. Dieser Zweifrontenkrieg vollendet in kürzester Zeit die vollständige Gelenkzerstörung mit Zerstückelung und Kantenabbrüchen des Gelenkknorpels. Besonders markant kommt die Gelenkdestruktion im Mazerationspräparat zum Ausdruck. Abb. 12a zeigt einen destruktiven Gichttophus im Metatarsophalangealgelenk I mit tiefer Usur in der Grundphanlanx (Abb. 8—12, 12a).

Die Zerstörung des subchondralen Spongiosagerüstes führt zu einer Gelenklockerung und, je nach Muskelzug, zur Hyperflexion, Hyperextension, Subluxation und Luxation (Abb. 13).

Der Einbruch der Gicht in die subchondrale Spongiosa ist im *Röntgenbild* genau erkennbar und verfolgbar. Kennzeichnend für die synoviale Form der Gichtarthritis ist die tief ausgeschnittene, an den Gelenkknorpel anschließende Corticalis-Usur, die Bildung ausgestanzter Lochdefekte in der subchondralen Spongiosa, die fortschreitende Abtrennung der Phalangenepiphysen von den Metaphysen. Die Konturen der ossären Restbestände gleichen einer Hellebarde (DIHLMANN).

Das Röntgenbild der rheumatischen Arthritis der kleinen Finger- und Zehengelenke unterscheidet sich vom Röntgenbild der Gichtarthritis dadurch, daß die Corticalisusuren nicht so tief greifen, daß die ausgestanzten Lochdefekte fehlen, und durch die schwere Begleitosteoporose.

Das Bestehen einer gelenkunabhängigen primären ossären Gicht ist umstritten. Es handelt sich um Tophi in Phalangen, Metacarpalia, Metatarsalia, Hand- und Fußwurzelknochen, die auf Schnitt keine Beziehungen zu Nachbargelenken aufweisen und im Röntgenbilde zu Lochdefekten führen. JAFFE scheint gegen die Anerkennung gelenksunabhängiger Knochenmarkstophi keine Bedenken zu haben. Ich persönlich habe aber doch Bedenken, denn entsprechende Befunde kann man nur im Rahmen einer schweren Gelenkgicht erheben, und auf Stufenschnitten haben sich nach meiner Erfahrung stets noch Gelenkbeziehungen nachweisen lassen.

Unter dem Titel: «le syndrom de Tietze goutteux. Goutte aigue des cartilage» beschreibt MUGLER, A. eine Gichtverlaufsform, bei der die Schmerzhaftigkeit der Knorpelabschnitte der ersten drei Rippen das Krankheitsbild beherrscht.

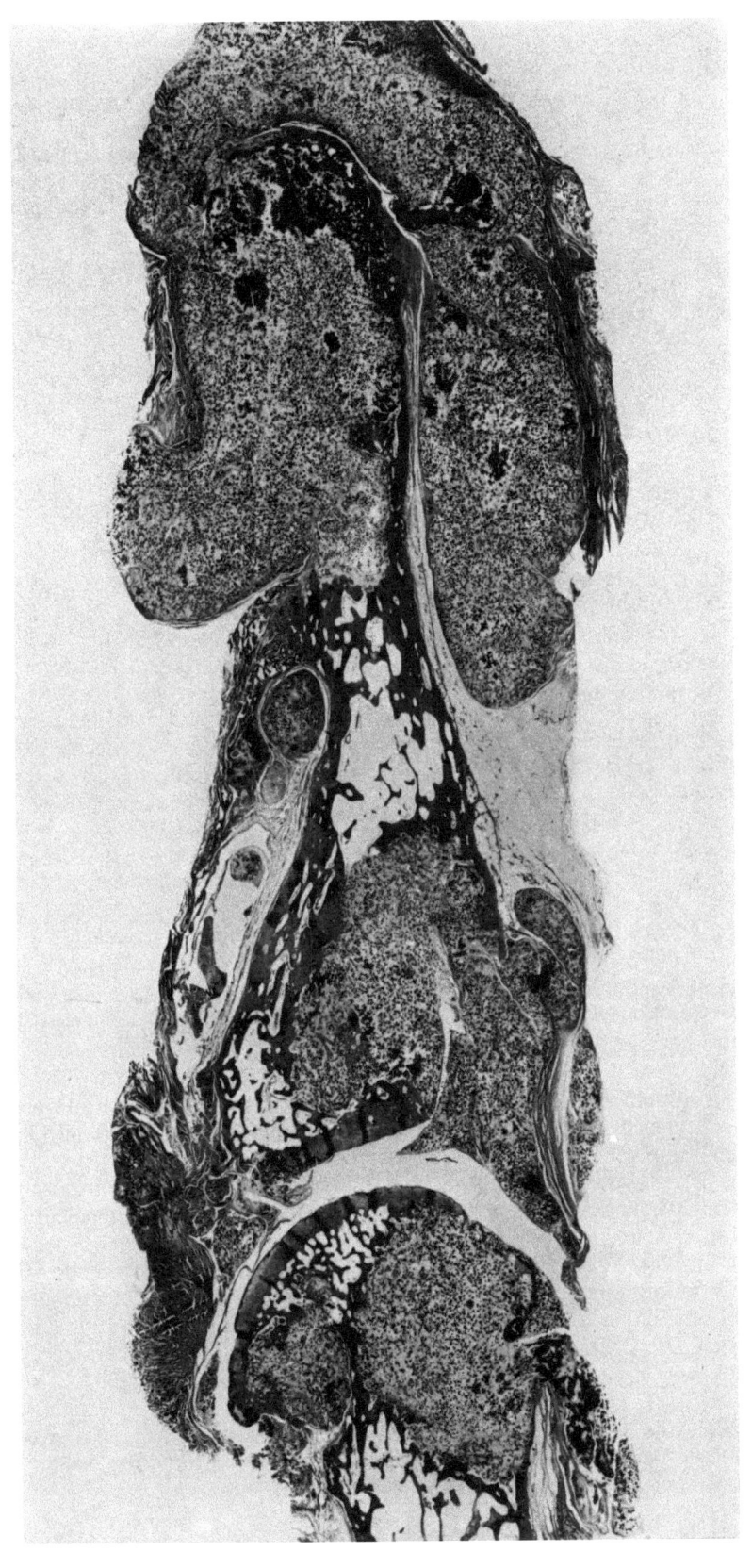

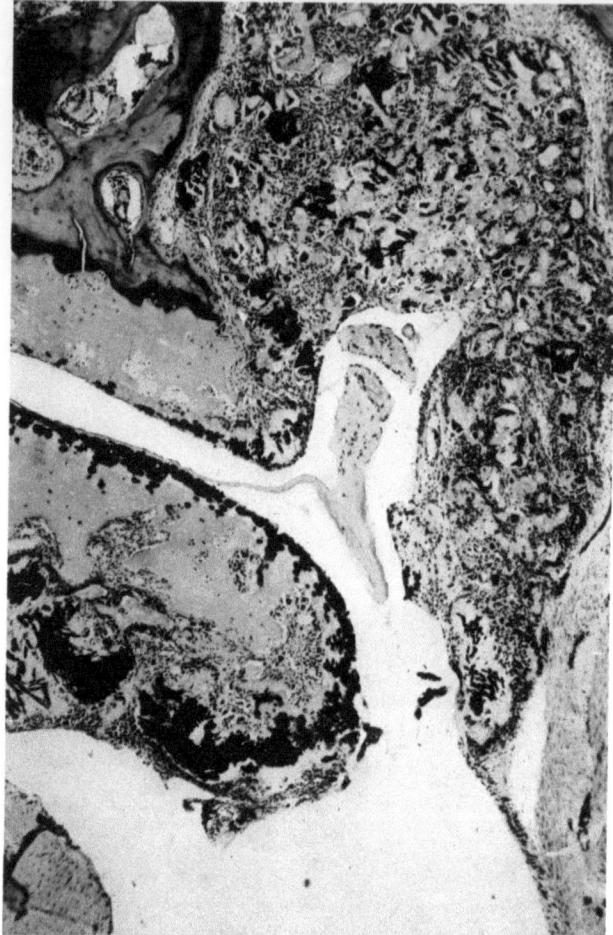

Abb. 9. Interphalangealgelenk mit Uratgicht. Uratinsudation der Knorpelgleitfläche und Unterminierung des Gelenkknorpels im ossären Haftgebiet der Gelenkkapsel durch Urattophi. Übersicht. Vergr. 30:1. Mann, 67 Jahre. (SN 1143/59. Path. Inst. Zürich)

MUGLER gibt an, daß die Schmerzen wahrscheinlich auf eine Urat-Einlagerung in die knorpeligen Rippenabschnitte zurückzuführen seien. Anatomische Untersuchungen liegen aber nicht vor.

Die *Sehnengicht* ist gekennzeichnet durch einen kettenartigen Zusammenschluß miliarer kristalliner Gichttophi zwischen den kollagenen Fibrillenbündeln (Abb. 14).

Die *Gicht der Schleimbeutel* ist eine der Gelenkgicht parallel gehende Speicherung von amorphem und kristallinem Natriumurat in einem Schleimbeutel. Der Binnenraum füllt sich mit einem kreideweißen Uratbrei. Die Wandung der Bursa dehnt sich. Die Urate werden von einem Wall aus ein- und mehrkernigen Histio-

Abb. 8. Destruktive Uratgicht. Längsschnitt durch Finger. Breiter Einbruch der Uratgranulome in die Mittelphalanx. Abtrennung des Köpfchens der Grundphalanx von der Metaphyse. Mann, 67 Jahre. (SN 1143/59. Path. Inst. Zürich)

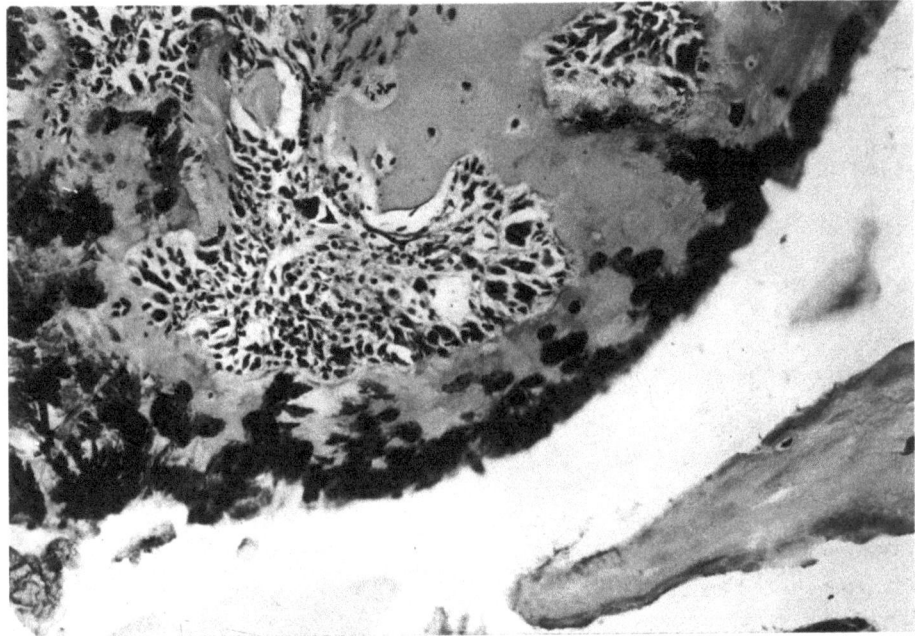

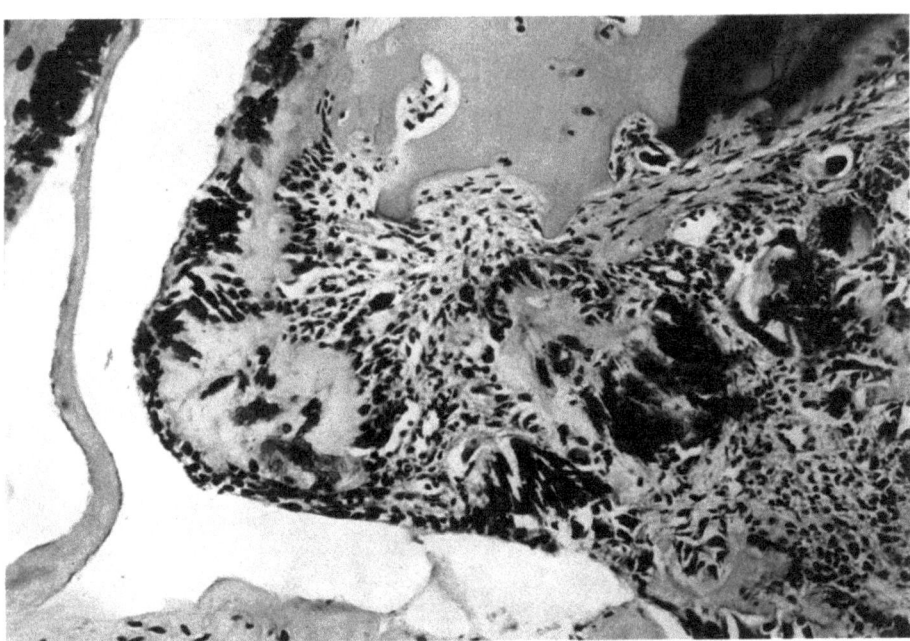

Abb. 10. Interphalangealgelenk mit Uratgicht. Uratinsudation der Knorpelgleitfläche und Unterminierung des Gelenkknorpels im ossären Haftgebiet der Gelenkkapsel mit Urattophi. a) Übersicht. Vergr. 30:1. b) u. c) Detailbilder. Vergr. 125:1. Mann, 67 Jahre. (SN 1143/59, Path. Inst. Zürich)

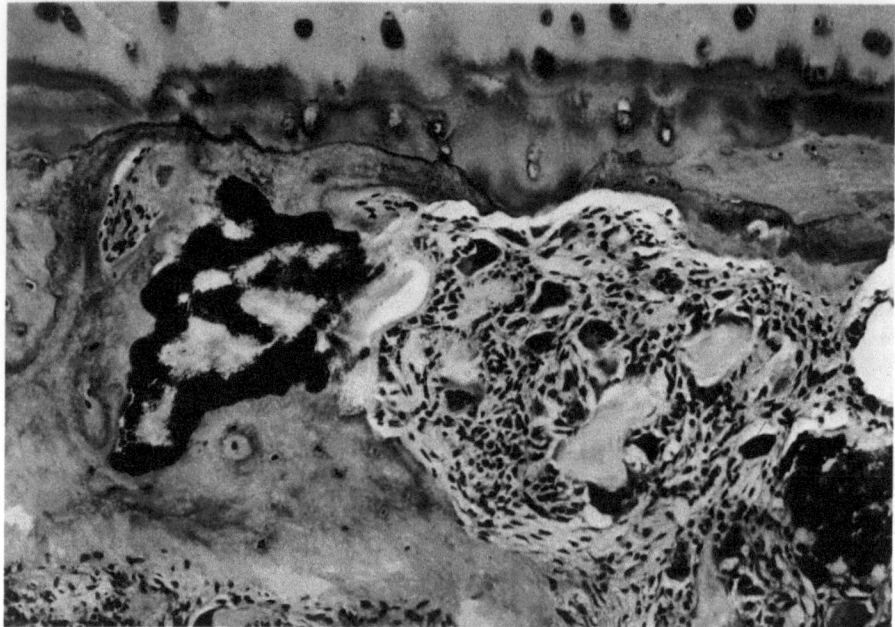

Abb. 11. Interphalangealgelenk mit Uratgicht. Destruktion der subchondralen Spongiosa durch Gichttophi (Urate schwarz). Vergr. 125:1. Mann, 67 Jahre. (SN 1143/59. Path. Inst. Zürich)

cyten eingekreist. Die Füllmasse kann bis Kastaniengröße erreichen. Bevorzugte Lokalisation sind die Bursa olecrani und die Bursa praepatellaris (Abb. 15, 16).

Trotz der intermittierenden Hyperuricämie sind *Uratablagerungen in den Gefäßen* ungemein selten. TRAUT et al. beschreiben bei 2 Gichtpatienten kristalline Uratablagerungen in Arterien, Herzklappen und Herzmuskel.

Die Gichtniere

Unter der Bezeichnung Gichtniere werden alle bei der Gicht zu beobachtenden Nierenveränderungen zusammengefaßt: Uratsteine, interstitielle Nephritis, glomeruläre und vasculäre Nephropathie. Die einzige Gicht-spezifische Nierenschädigung sind Uratniederschläge und Uratgranulome (TALBOTT u. TERPLAN). Reine Formen sind selten, Kombinationen häufig. Sie bilden einen integrierenden Bestandteil der Gicht. Sie sind oft schicksalbestimmend. Häufigste Todesursachen bei Gicht sind Urämie, Herzversagen und Hirnblutung bei renaler Hypertonie.

Zwischen der Schwere der Gelenkgicht und der Schwere des Nierenschadens, wie er im Begriff der Gichtniere zusammengefaßt ist, besteht kein Parallelismus (TALBOTT u. TERPLAN).

a) *Uratsteine und Urattophi*

Jede Erhöhung des Harnsäurespiegels im Serum hat einen vermehrten Übertritt von Harnsäure in den Primärharn zur Folge. Die tubuläre Wasserrückresorption führt zur Konzentrationssteigerung der im Primärharn gelösten Salze und schließlich zur körnigen Ausfällung des Natriumurates in den Sammelröhren

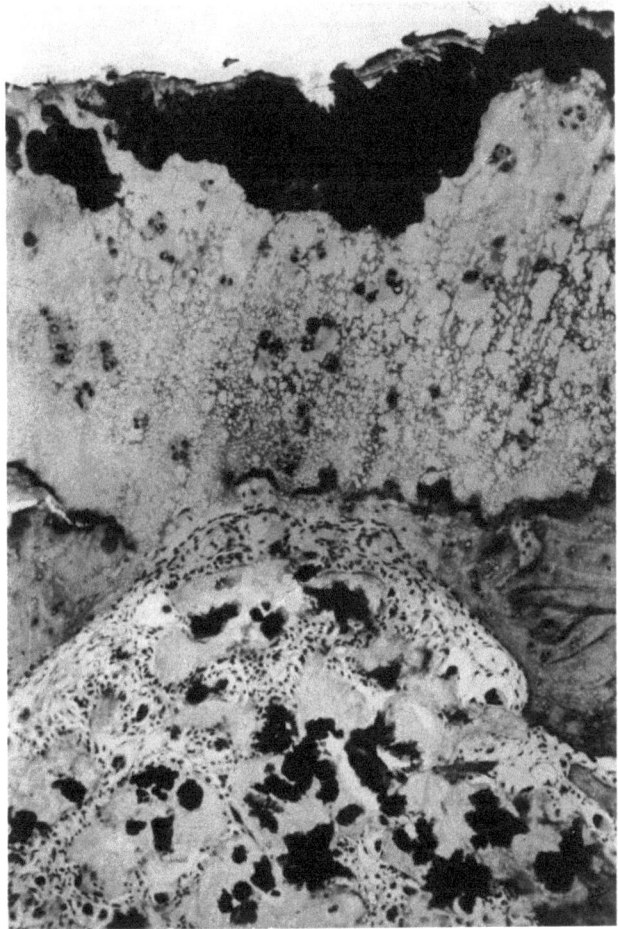

Abb. 12. Interphalangealgelenk mit Uratgicht. Gleichzeitige Arrosion des Gelenkknorpels durch Uratinsudation der Gleitfläche (schwarz) und durch Urattophi in der subchondralen Spongiosa. Vergr. 75:1. Mann, 67 Jahre. (SN 1143/59. Path. Inst. Zürich)

und/oder Nierenbecken. Die Häufigkeit von Uratsteinen bei Gicht schätzt ZOLLINGER auf 10—25%.

Die intracanaliculäre Ausfällung von Natriumuraten führt zur Bildung von *Marktophi*. ZOLLINGER fand sie in 13 von insgesamt 22 Gichtfällen. Sie sind für Gicht pathognomisch. Sie liegen vorwiegend im cortico-medullären Grenzgebiet und bilden kreideweiße Stippchen mit Strichrichtung gegen die Papillenspitze (Abb. 17). Entstehen und Vergehen der Marktophi verläuft nach ZOLLINGER in 3 Phasen. Die erste Phase umfaßt die Ausfällung von amorphem Natriumurat in den Sammelröhren. Durch Blockade der Lichtung wird der Harn im zugeordneten Nephron aufgestaut und die Kanälchen ausgeweitet (lokale Nephrohydrose). In der zweiten Phase werden die Urate vom Epithel der Sammelröhren aufgenommen und intracellulär in nadelförmige Kristalle umgeprägt. Die Kristalle schließen sich zu einer Kristallrosette. Die anliegenden Tubulusepithelien sterben ab und werden durch ein- und mehrkernige Histiocyten ersetzt, welche die Kri-

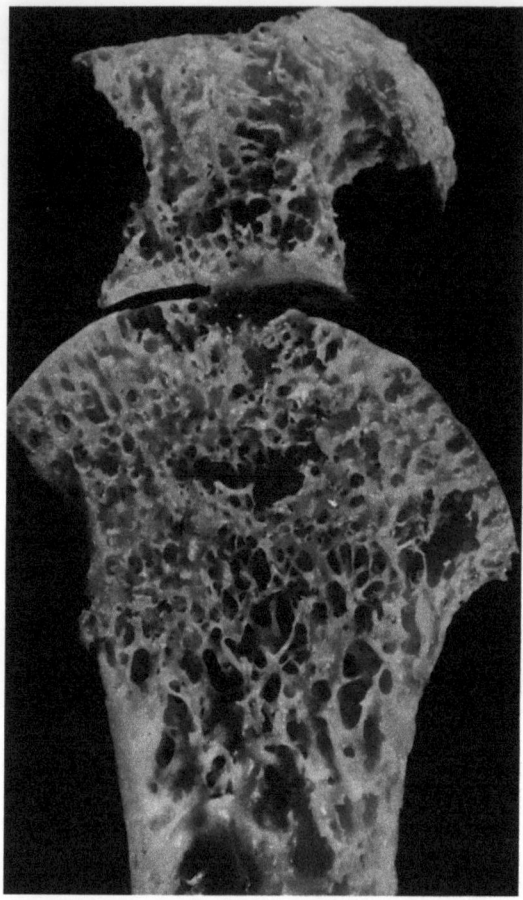

Abb. 12a. Schwere Arthritis urica des Großzehengrundgelenkes. Tiefgreifende Usur der Grundphalanx. Mazerationspräparat. E. Kaspar, 67 Jahre. (MB 9305/47 Path. Inst. Zürich)

stalldruse einkreisen (Abb. 18). In der dritten und letzten Entwicklungsphase werden die kristallinen Urate wieder aufgelöst. Der Histiocytenwall kollabiert. Der Tophus vernarbt. Das zugeordnete Nephron geht zugrunde.

b) *Interstitielle Nephritis*

Uratsteine im Nierenbecken begünstigen bakterielle Infektionen der ableitenden Harnwege; die Marktophi vermitteln einen unmittelbaren Kontakt zwischen Harn und Zwischengewebe. Beide Vorgänge begünstigen die Entwicklung einer *interstitiellen Nephritis*. Sie ist bei Gicht ungemein häufig, aber für Gicht nicht pathognomonisch. Zur Entwicklung einer interstitiellen Nephritis kann es aber auch ohne Steine und ohne Tophi kommen. Die Pathogenese dieser Form der interstitiellen Nephritis ist nicht abgeklärt. Die Folgen der interstitiellen Nephritis sind ein fortschreitender Parenchymuntergang, der maßgebend zur letalen Niereninsuffizienz beitragen kann.

c) *Glomeruläre Nephropathie*

Sie steht in engster Beziehung zu der mit der Gicht verknüpften Störung des intermediären Eiweiß-Stoffwechsels. Zusätzlich zur Harnsäure dürften noch an-

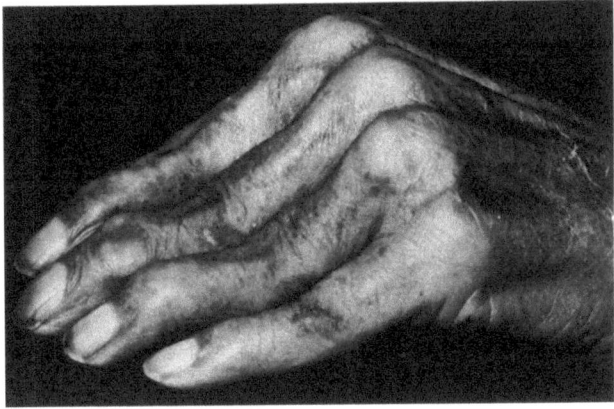

Abb. 13. Gichthand mit Hyperextension im proximalen und Tophi im distalen Interphalangealgelenk. Mann, 75 Jahre. (SN 447/59. Path. Inst. Zürich)

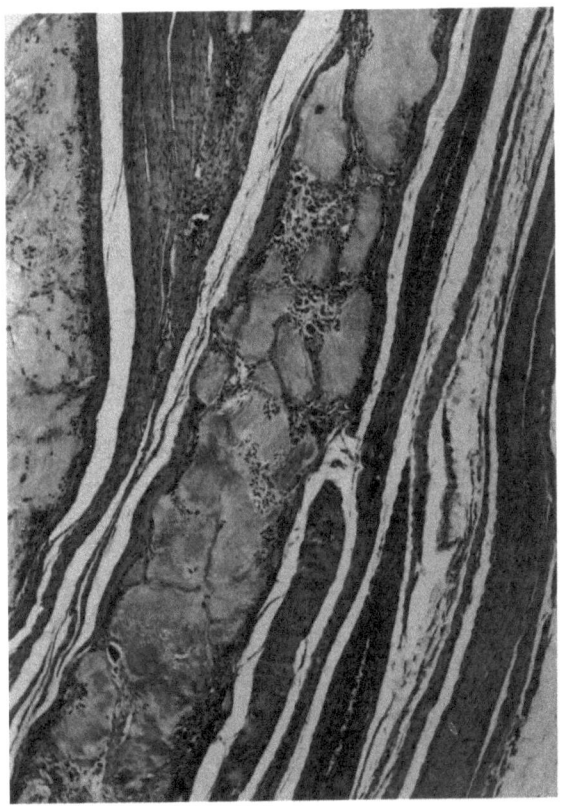

Abb. 14. Sehnengicht. Zwischen den kollagenen Fibrillenbündeln bandförmige Agglomeration von Gichttophi. Vergr. 50:1, Mann, 73 Jahre. (SN 81/58. Path. Inst. Zürich)

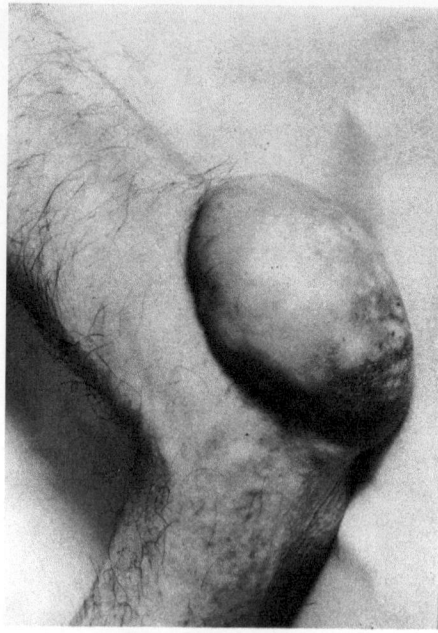

Abb. 15. Kastaniengroßer Gichttophus über dem Olecranon. Mann, 80 Jahre. (SN 147/60. Path. Inst. Zürich)

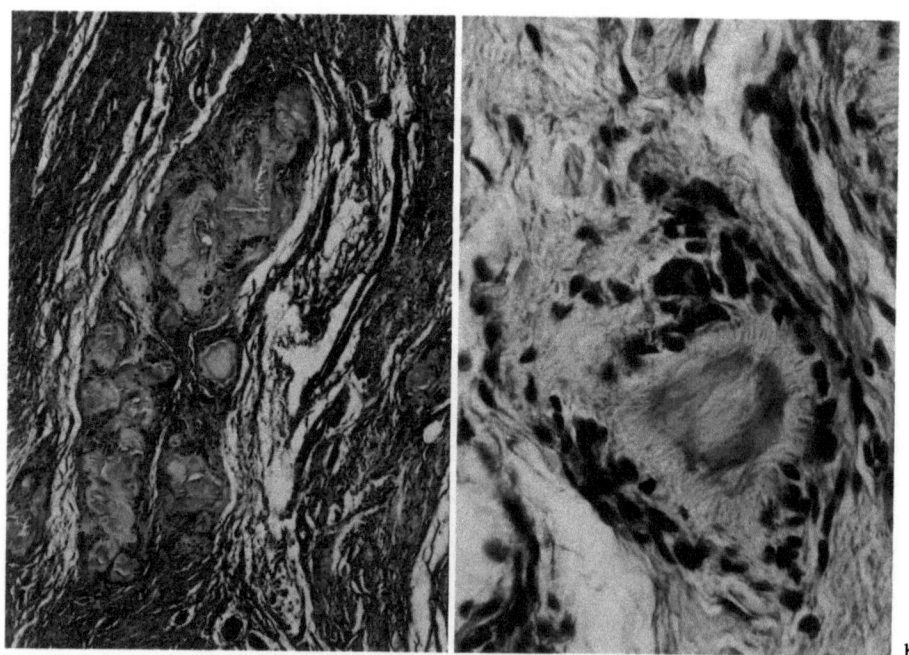

Abb. 16. Bursitis urica. Agglomeration von Gichttophi. a) Übersicht. Vergr. 150:1. b) Ausschnitt. Vergr. 400:1. Mann, 52 Jahre. (MB 2522/63. Path. Inst. Zürich)

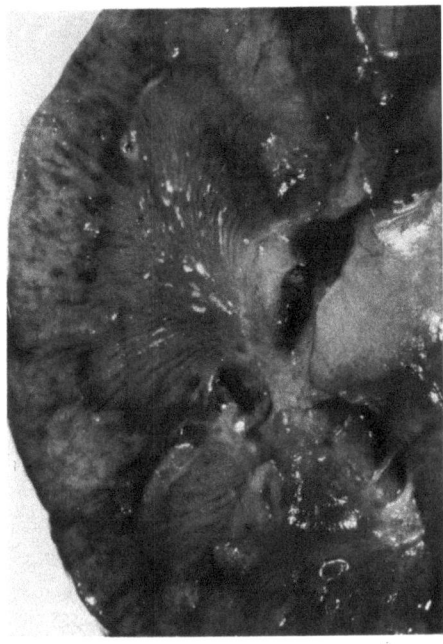

Abb. 17. Gichtniere. Markpyramiden mit radiären Uratspritzern. Mann, 59 Jahre. (SN 2474/68. Path. Inst. Zürich)

dere reguläre und irreguläre Zwischenprodukte gebildet und renal ausgeschieden werden (beispielsweise Lipoproteine). Die damit verbundene Überlastung der glomerulären Filter hat eine Schädigung der Basalmembranen der Glomerulumschlingen zur Folge. Sie zeigt sich morphologisch in einer Verstärkung des Mesangiums durch kollagene Fibrillen (Mesangiumsklerose), in einer Anlagerung von Eiweiß an die Basalmembranen der Glomerulumschlingen (Glomerulumsklerose) und einer Wandhyalinose der Arteriolen. Beide Prozesse zusammen, die Mesangiumsklerose und die Glomerulosklerose bezeichnet man als glomeruläre Nephropathie (Abb. 20). Die Rückwirkungen auf die Nierenfunktion bestehen in einer leichten Proteinurie und einer Erschwerung der renalen Harnsäureausscheidung (LICHTENSTEIN).

Die gichtische glomeruläre Nephropathie ist ungemein häufig. ZOLLINGER macht darüber folgende Angaben: Auf 22 Obduktionen von Gichtpatienten fand sich 21mal eine glomeruläre Nephropathie, davon schwer 4mal, mittelschwer 14mal, angedeutet 3mal. Nur bei einem einzigen Patienten wurde sie vermißt.

d) *Vasculäre Nephropathie*

Zwischen der glomerulären Nephropathie und der vasculären Nephropathie bestehen fließende Übergänge. Das führende klinische Symptom der vasculären Nephropathie ist die *Hypertonie*, der führende anatomische Befund die *vasculäre Schrumpfniere*.

Die Glomerulosklerose ist die Vorstufe der Schlingenhyalinose. Die fortschreitende Imprägnation der Glomerulumschlingen mit Hyalin führt schließlich zum Schlingenverschluß und zum glomerulären Totalschaden. Gleichzeitig erfahren auch die Wandungen der präglomerulären Arteriolen eine zunehmende Hyalinisierung. Eine zunehmende Hyalinisierung der Glomerula und Arteriolen hat schwere Rückwirkungen auf das *Nierenparenchym* und den *Blutdruck* zur Folge.

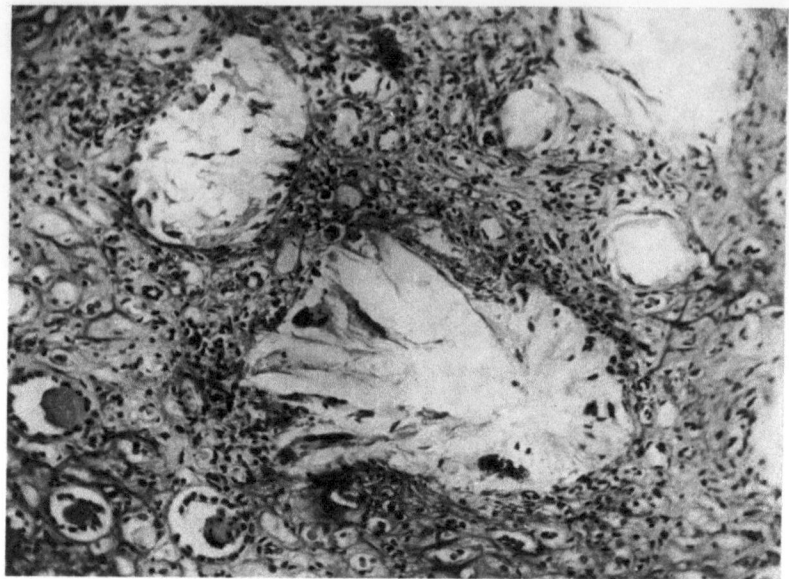

Abb. 18. Gichtniere mit kleinem Gichttophus im Marklager. Kristallbüschel aus Uraten umschlossen von ein- und mehrkernigen Histiocyten. Vergr. 150:1. (SN 1357/42. Path. Inst. Zürich)

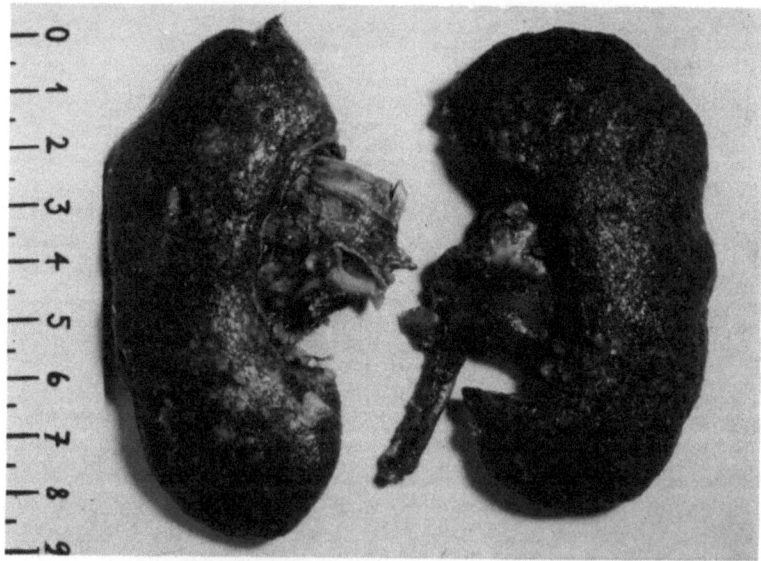

Abb. 19. Arteriolosklerotische Schrumpfnieren bei hypertoner Gicht. BD 200/100 mm Hg. Nierengewicht 85 g. Mann, 52 Jahre. (SN 1266/50. Path. Inst. Zürich)

Die funktionelle Ausschaltung eines Glomerulums zieht zwangsläufig den Untergang des zugeordneten tubulären Systems nach sich. An seine Stelle treten radiäre Narbenstränge und lymphocytäre Infiltrate. Die Nieren schrumpfen. Die Oberfläche granuliert. Die Gewichtsverluste betragen 20—30 g und erreichen ausnahmsweise 50% des Normalgewichtes. Der Endzustand entspricht der *roten* (benignen) *Granularatrophie*.

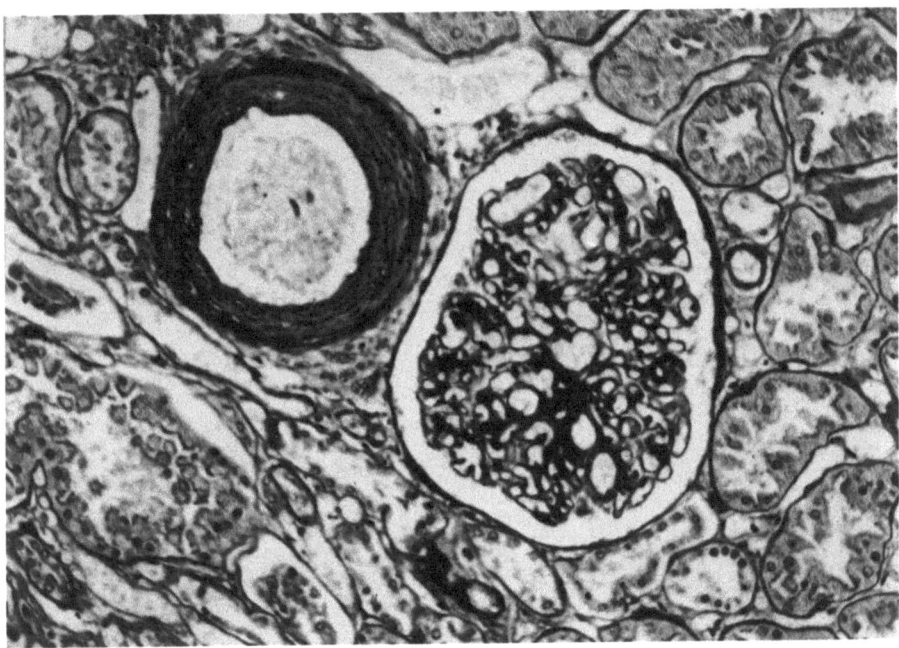

Abb. 20. Hypertonie-Gicht. Gichtniere mit Mesangiumsklerose und Mediahypertrophie einer muskulären Arterie. Vergr. 160:1. Mann, 83 Jahre. (SN 1860/70. Path. Inst. Zürich)

Glomerulumhyalinose und Sklerose der präglomerulären Arteriolen erhöhen maßgebend die renalen Durchströmungswiderstände. Zunächst versucht der Organismus durch Erhöhung des Blutdruckes und durch eine Hyperplasie der muskulären Mittelschicht der mittelgroßen Nierenarterien die Strömungswiderstände zu überwinden (Abb. 21). Je höher der Blutdruck, um so stärker die Eiweißinsudation der Glomerulumschlingen wie der Arteriolen. Zusätzlich zur quantitativen Störung des Harnsäureumsatzes wirkt sich die kompensatorische Erhöhung des Blutdruckes als wichtiger Förderungsfaktor der vasculären Nierenschäden aus. Höchste Blutdruckwerte führen schließlich zur *Arteriolonekrose* und letalen Niereninsuffizienz.

Es ist das Verdienst von FAHR, auf die engen Beziehungen zwischen gichtiger Glomerulumnephrose-Glomerulumhyalinose, benigner roter arteriolosklerotischer und maligner blasser arteriolonekrotischer Nephrosklerose und Hypertonie hingewiesen zu haben. Nach FAHR ist die Gichtniere ein Musterbeispiel des Überganges einer benignen Nephrosklerose mit dem klinischen Äquivalent des roten Hochdruckes in die maligne arteriolonekrotische Schrumpfniere mit dem klinischen Äquivalent des blassen Hochdruckes und der letalen Niereninsuffizienz. Über den zeitlichen Vortritt der Prozesse — Gichtniere oder Hypertonie — nimmt FAHR nicht eindeutig Stellung. Im Gegensatz dazu spricht sich ZOLLINGER sehr eindeutig für das Primat des gichtischen Nierenschadens aus. Er schreibt: „An der renalen Natur der Hypertonie bei Gicht kann wohl kaum gezweifelt werden."

Zum Schluß seien die vasculären Vorgänge in der Gichtniere in ihrer natürlichen Zeitfolge nochmals kurz zusammengefaßt: Glomerulo- und Mesangiumsklerose — glomeruläre Hyalinose ohne Nierenschrumpfung — benigne rote arteriolosklerotische Schrumpfniere mit Hypertonie und ohne Niereninsuffizienz

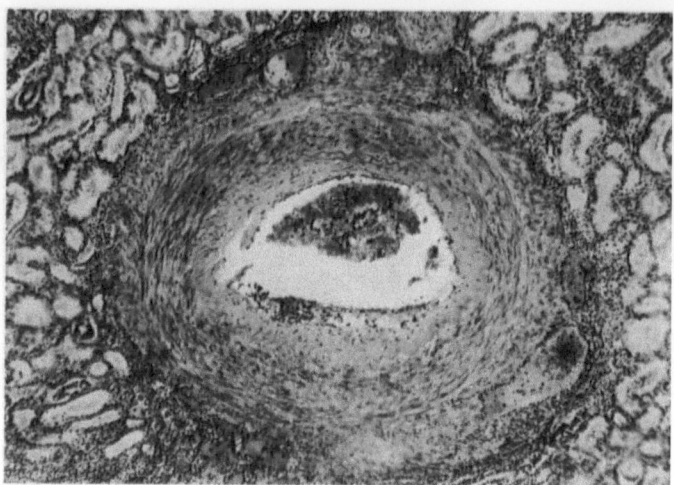

Abb. 21. Hypertone Gicht. Muskuläre Nierenarterie mit Hyperplasie der Media und Intimafibrose. Vergr. 65:1. Mann, 65 Jahre.

— maligne weiße arteriolonekrotische Schrumpfniere mit Hypertonie und Niereninsuffizienz. Auf jeder Stufe kann der vasculäre Nierenprozeß zum Stillstand kommen. Jede Stufe ist aber zugleich die anatomische Vorbereitung, gewissermaßen der Aufmarsch zur nächsten Schadensstufe. Das Endstadium der malignen Nephrosklerose, wie es von FAHR gezeichnet worden ist, wird nur selten erreicht. In seinem Beobachtungsgut von 22 Gichtpatienten fand ZOLLINGER eine schwere Arteriosklerose 16mal, eine Arteriolosklerose 13mal, eine maligne Nephrosklerose nur 1mal. In meinem Beobachtungsgut von 32 Gichtpatienten fand sich eine benigne Arteriolosklerose der Niere und *arteriolosklerotische* Schrumpfniere 20mal, eine maligne arteriolonekrotische Schrumpfniere 3mal. Die Zahlen stimmen gut überein.

Gicht und assoziierte Krankheiten

a) Von besonderem Interesse sind *Kombinationen der Gicht mit anderen Skeletkrankheiten und intermediären Stoffwechselstörungen*. Kombinationen mit einer *Ostitis deformans Paget* finden sich wohl in jedem größeren Beobachtungsgut (PAGET, TALBOTT, TRAUT et al., UEHLINGER). GOODMAN u. ERAGAN beobachteten bei einer 66 Jahre alten Negerin mit Polyarthritis urica, Hypertonie und Myxödem eine *Hyperostosis frontalis interna*. Diese Kombination ist zweifellos sehr selten, doch dürften zwischen den einzelnen Krankheitsbildern keine inneren Beziehungen bestehen.

b) HUNDER et al. beschreiben die Kombination eines *Femurkopfinfarktes* mit einer Gicht. Der 34 Jahre alte Patient erkrankte 3 Jahre nach einer posttraumatischen Femurkopfnekrose an einer charakteristischen, polyartikulären Gicht. Die histologische Untersuchung des resezierten Femurkopfes bestätigte die Diagnose einer avasculären Nekrose im cranialen Kopfquadranten. Darüber hinaus waren aber Schenkelhals, Femurkopfknorpel und Hüftgelenkskapsel mit Harnsäurekristallen dicht durchsetzt. Ist der Knocheninfarkt nur das Vorspiel für die spätere Gelenkgicht oder bestehen keine pathogenetischen Beziehungen? Die Frage kann vorläufig nicht beantwortet werden. Immerhin ist bemerkenswert, daß in Frankreich die Kombination Femurkopfnekrose und Gicht nicht allzu selten beobachtet wird (MAUVOISIN) und unter 101 Patienten der Mayoklinik der Jahre 1960/63 mit Femurkopfnekrose 4 eine Gicht hatten. Vielleicht bildet der chronische Alkoholismus die unsichere Brücke zwischen avasculärer Kopfnekrose und Gicht.

c) Gicht und assoziierte Störungen des intermediären Stoffwechsels: Zwischen Gicht und *Diabetes mellitus* besteht eine Syntropie. Nach MARTIN besteht bei 20% der Patienten mit Polyarthritis urica zugleich ein Diabetes mellitus und in weiteren 35% eine pathologische Zuckerbelastungskurve. Beiden Krankheiten gemeinsam ist die Tendenz zur Hypertonie und zum familiären Vorkommen. Die Diabetesniere mit Glomerulosklerose Kimmelstiel und Arteriolosklerose hat morphologisch viel Ähnlichkeit mit der gichtischen Glomerulonephrose und Gicht-Arteriolosklerose. Beide Krankheiten bilden gewissermaßen eine Schicksalsgemeinschaft. Es sei hier auf die Arbeiten von BARTELS et al., ISCHMAEL et al. und MARTIN verwiesen.

d) In der Syntropie zwischen *primärem Hyperparathyreoidismus*, Hyperuricämie und Uratgicht kommt dem Hyperparathyreoidismus das Primat zu. Auf Grund der Analyse von 11 Fällen kommen SCOTT et al. zum Ergebnis, daß es naheliege, in diesen Fällen eine ganz besondere Form der hyperparathyreoiden Nierenschädigung anzunehmen (Nephrocalcinose) mit fast selektiver Behinderung der Harnsäureausscheidung.

e) Kombinationsfälle von *Uratgicht* und *primärer chronischer rheumatischer Polyarthritis* kommen vor, sind aber selten. Sie sind wegen der Überlagerung und Verflechtung der Gelenkerscheinungen schwierig diagnostisch zu sichern. Eine einschlägige Beobachtung verdanken wir OWEN et al.:

Der 64jährige Patient hatte während der letzten 15 Jahre wiederholt klassische Gichtanfälle des Großzehengrundgelenkes, später auch der Zeigefinger-Interphalangeal-Gelenke. Im Laufe der Zeit entwickelte sich eine chronische deformierende Polyarthritis mit zunehmender symmetrischer Gelenkversteifung und periartikulären Rheumaknoten. Die Diagnose Uratgicht ergibt sich aus dem typischen Befall der Großzehengrundgelenke, dem Nachweis von Uratkristallen im Gelenkpunktat des Zeigefingers und dem erhöhten Harnsäurespiegel im Serum bis zu Werten von bis 13,2 mg-%. Die Diagnose primäre chronische Polyarthritis ergibt sich aus dem charakteristischen Gelenkbefall, den gelenknahen Usuren an den Phalangen der Finger, aus den periarticulären Rheumaknoten und der rheumapositiven Serologie. Die Polyarthritis spricht auf Colchicin gut an, nicht aber auf Aspirin. Absetzen des Colchicins führt zu einem Rückfall der Polyarthritis.

f) KAPLAN u. KLATSKIN haben 4 Fälle, BUNIM et al. einen weiteren Fall des gleichzeitigen Vorkommens von *Hyperurikämie*, miliarer *Lebersarkoidose* und *Psoriasis* beobachtet. Nach einer Zusammenstellung von KAPLAN und KLATSKIN hatten von 105 Patienten mit Psoriasis 4 gleichzeitig eine Gicht und von 103 Patienten mit Gicht 3 gleichzeitig eine Psoriasis. Die eigenartige Kombination weist auf innere Zusammenhänge, ohne daß darüber schon präzise Vorstellungen bestehen. In diesem Zusammenhang sei noch darauf hingewiesen, daß der erste gesicherte Fall von Sarkoidose, der 1877 von HUTCHINSON beschrieben worden ist, gleichzeitig eine Gicht hatte.

Literatur

ALARCÓN-SEGOVIA, D., CENTINA, J. A., DÍAZ-JOUANEN, E.: Sacroiliac joints in primary gout. Amer. J. Roentgenol. **118**, 438—443 (1973).
BARTELS, E. C., BALODIMUS, M. C., CORN, L. R.: Association of gout and diabetes mellitus. Med. Clin. N. Amer. **44**, 433—438 (1960).
BAUER, R.: „Osteomyelitis urica". Fortschr. Röntgenstr. **108**, 266 (1968).
BERNHEIM, C., OTT, H., ZAHND, G., MARTIN, E.: Goutte et diabète. Schweiz. med. Wschr. **98**, 33—41 (1968).

BROGSITTER, AD. M.: Histopathologie der Gelenkgicht. Dtsch. Arch. klin. Med. **153**, 257—326 (1926).
BROWN, J., MALLORY, G. K.: Renal changes in gout. N. England J. Med. **243**, 325—329 (1950).
BUNIM, J. J., MCEWEB, C.: Tophus of the mitral valve in gout. Arch. Path., Chicago, **29**, 700—704 (1940).
BUNIM, J. J., KIMBERG, D. V., THOMAS, L. B., VAN SCOTT, E. J., KLATSKIN, G.: The syndrom of sarcoidosis, Psoriasis and Gout. Comb. clin. Staff Conf. at the NJH Ann. int. Med. **57**, 1018—1040 (1962).
Combined Staff Clinic: Uric acid metabolism and gout. Amer. J. Med. **9**, 799—817 (1950).
DIHLMANN, W., FERNHOLZ, H. J.: Gibt es charakteristische Röntgenbefunde bei der Gicht? Dtsch. med. Wschr. **94**, 1909—1911 (1969).
DODDS, W. J., STEINBACH, H. L.: Gout associated with calcification of cartilage. N. England J. Med. **275**, 745—749 (1966).
FAHR, TH.: Gichtniere. Handbuch der speziellen pathologischen Anatomie und Histologie. Band VI/1, S. 430—434. Berlin: Springer Verlag 1925.
FASSBENDER, H. G.: Zur Pathologie der Gicht. Therapiewoche **22**, 105—108 (1972).
FINEBERG, S. K., ALTSCHUL, A.: The nephropathy of gout. Ann. Intern. Med. **44**, 1182—1194 (1956).
GOODMAN, D. H., ERAGAN, A.: Gout, myxedema, and hyperostosis frontalis interna. Report of a case in negro woman. J. Amer. med. Ass. **173**, 1734—1735 (1960).
GREENBAUM, D., ROSS, J. H., STEINBERG, V. L.: Renal biopsy in gout. Brit. med. J. **1961 I**, 1502—1504.
GÜNTHER, R.: Ein Beitrag zur Kenntnis der Arthritis urica. Zbl. allg. Path. Anat. **95**, 1—8 (1956).
GUTMAN, A. B., YU, T. F.: Current principles of management of gout. Amer. J. Med. **13**, 744—759 (1952).
HALL, M. C., SELIN, G.: Spinal involvement in gout. A case report with autopsy. J. Bone Jt Surg., Am. Ed. **42**, 341—343 (1961).
HARTLEIB, J.: Über einen ungewöhnlichen Fall von Gicht bei einem 18 jährigen Mann. Zbl. allg. Path. Anat. **92**, 198—203 (1954).
HEMMATI, A., VOGEL, W.: Schwere Knochendestruktionen bei Gicht-Arthritis. Chirurg **40**, 285—287 (1969).
HUNDER, G. G., WORTHINGTON, J. W., BICKEL, W. H.: Avascular necrosis in a patient with gout. J. Amer. med. Ass. **203**, 47—49 (1968).
HUTCHINSON, I.: Illustrations of clinical Surgery, pag. 42. London 1877.
ISHMAEL, W. K., OWENS, J. N., PAYNE, R. W., HONICK, M. D.: Diabetes mellitus in patients with gouty arthritis. J. Amer. med. Ass. **190**, 396—398 (1964).
JACKSON, W. P. U., HARRIS, F.: Gout with hyperparathyroidism: Report of a case with examination of synovial fluid. Brit. med. J. **1965 II**, 211.
JAFFE, H. L.: Gout in Metabolic, degenerative, and inflammatory diseases of bones and joints. pp. 479—505. Philadelphia: Lea and Febiger 1972.
KAPLAN, L., KLATSKIN, G.: The syndrome of sarcoidosis, Psoriasis and Gout. Yale J. Biol. Med. **32**, 335 (1960).
KATZ, J. L., WEINER, H., GUTMANN, A., YU, T.: Hyperuricemia, gout and the executive suite. J. Amer. med. Ass. **224**, 1251—1257 (1973).
KOLLER, F., ZOLLINGER, H. U.: Gichtische Glomerulosklerose. Schweiz. med. Wschr. **75**, 97—105 (1945).
LAMBETH, J. T., BURNS-COX, C. J., MACLEAN, R.: Sacroiliac gout associated with hemoglobin E and hypersplenism. Radiology, **95**, 413—415 (1970).
LANG, F. J.: Gelenkgicht (Arthritis urica). Handb. d. spez. patholog. Anatomie u. Histologie Band IX/3, S. 309—341. Berlin: Springer Verlag 1937.
LICHTENSTEIN, 1., SCOTT, H. W., LEVIN, M. H.: Pathologic changes in gout: Survey of eleven necropsied cases. Amer. J. Path. **32**, 871—887 (1956).
LITTEN, M.: Ein Fall von schwerer Gicht mit Amyloiddegeneration. Virchows Arch. path. Anat. **66**, 129—139 (1876).
NEGRI, L., TADDEI, L.: Rara osservazione di grave cotta articolare viscerale con particola re riguardo al quadro radiologico, anatomo-patologico ed istichimico. Arch. De Vecchi Anat. pat., Firenze, **45**, 47—109 (1965).
MALAWISTA, S. E., SEEGMILLER, J. E., HATHAWAY, B. E., SOKOLOFF, L.: Sacroiliac gout. J. Amer. med. Ass. **194**, 954—956 (1965).
MARTEL, W.: The overhanging margin of bone: a roentgenologic manifestation of gout. Radiology **91**, 755—756 (1968).
MAUVOISIN, F., BERNARD, J., GÉMAIN, J.: Aspects tomographiques des hanches chez un goûtteux. Rev. Rhumat. **22**, 336—337 (1955).

MAUVOISIN, F., BERNARD, J.: A propos de la nécrose aseptique de la tête fémorale chez l'adulte. Progr. Med. Paris **83**, 183—184 (1955).

MUGLER, A.: Le syndrom de Tietze goutteux. Goutte aiguë des cartilage. Rev. rhum. **26**, 113—122 (1959).

MUNCK, A.: Die Niere bei der Gicht. Beitr. path. Anat., Jena, **133**, 409—429 (1966).

OWEN, D. S., TOONE, E., IRBY, R.: Coexistente Rheumatoid arthritis and chronic tophaceous gout. Am. J. med. Ass. **197**, 953—956 (1966).

PELOQUIN, L. A., GRAHAM, J. H.: Gout of the patella: report of a case. New England J. Med. **253**, 979—980 (1955).

PHILIPS, R. W.: Reversal of renal insufficiency in gout: Report of a case treated with probenecid (Benemid). Arch. int. Med. **66**, 823 (1955).

PIQUET, B.: Une localisation rare de la goutte (ostéo-arthropathie uratique glénoïdienne). Rev. Rhum. **31**, 506—508 (1964).

POMMER, G.: Mikroskopische Untersuchungen über Gelenkgicht. Jena: Gustav Fischer 1929.

PRUNIER, PH.: Complications rénales de la goutte. Press méd., Paris, **75**, 139—141 (1967).

REUBI, F., VORBURGER, C.: Die Gichtniere. Münch. med. Wschr. **104**, 2152—2155 (1962).

ROSENBERG, E. F., ARENS, R. A.: Gout: Clinical, pathologic and roentgenographic observations. Radiology **49**, 169—177 (1947).

ROSENQUIST, R. C., SMALL, C. S., DEEB, P. H.: Unusual manifestations of gout. Arch. Path. (Chicago) **68**, 1—10 (1959).

SCOTT, J. T., DIXON, A. ST. J., BYWATERS, E. G. L.: Association of hyperuricemia and gout with hyperparathyroidism. Brit. med. J. **1964, I**, 1070—1073.

SEEGMILLER, J. E., HOWELL, R. R., MALAWISTA, S. E.: The inflammatory reaction to sodium urate. Its possible relationship to the genesis of acute gouty arthritis. J. Amer. med. Ass. **180**, 469—475 (1962).

SHERMAN, M. S.: Pathologic changes in gouty arthritis. Arch. Path. (Chicago) **42**, 557—563 (1946).

SIMON, L.: Ein Fall einer durch Gicht verursachten schweren Knochenzerstörung. Fortschr. Röntgenstr. **96**, 835 (1962).

SPILBERG, I.: Current concepts of the mechanism of acute inflammation in gouty arthritis. Arthr. and Rheum. **18**, 129—134 (1975).

TALBOTT, J. H.: Gout. New York: Grune & Stratton 1957.

TALBOTT, J.-H., TERPLAN, K. L.: The kidney in gout. Medecine **39**, 405—468 (1960).

VI. Klinik, Diagnose und Differentialdiagnose der Gicht

1. Klinische Wertigkeit der Hyperuricämie Beziehung zu anderen Krankheiten

Von

G. WOLFRAM

Die Bedeutung der Hyperuricämie für die Manifestation einer Gicht ist unbestritten. Mit zunehmender Höhe des Harnsäurespiegels steigt die Wahrscheinlichkeit klinischer Komplikationen. Die Rolle der Hyperuricämie als Risikofaktor in diesem Sinne ist durch epidemiologische Untersuchungen an einer ausreichend großen Zahl von Personen genau bekannt.

In neuerer Zeit werden unter dem Begriff der „Uricopathie" den Störungen des Purinstoffwechsels weittragende pathologische Wirkungen auf den Fett- und Kohlenhydratstoffwechsel, auf die Leber und auf die Herzkranzgefäße zugesprochen. Abgesehen davon, daß das Wort „Uricopathie" „eine die Unterschiede verwischende Zusammenfassung eindeutig verschiedener Störungen des Harnsäurestoffwechsels" darstellt (ZÖLLNER, 1974), ist die Beziehung zwischen Hyperuricämie oder Gicht und Hyperlipidämien, Diabetes mellitus, Fettleber, Coronarkrankheit und Adipositas noch keineswegs geklärt. Teils fehlt die klare Unterscheidung zwischen Ursache und Wirkung, teils kennt man zwar statistisch gesicherte Beziehungen, aber nicht den Wirkungsmechanismus. Das gemeinsame Auftreten von mehreren dieser Faktoren beim gleichen Patienten erschwert die Abgrenzung von pathogenetisch bedeutsamen Merkmalen und die Wertung des einzelnen Stoffwechseldefektes in seiner Bedeutung für die vorzeitige Entstehung einer Coronarsklerose. Die Aufklärung dieser Zusammenhänge ist nicht nur von akademischem Interesse, sondern hat praktische Konsequenzen für die Therapie, z.B. der symptomlosen Hyperuricämie. In diesem Kapitel sollen die relevanten Befunde zu diesem Thema aus der Literatur referiert und ihre Wertigkeit diskutiert werden.

Hyperuricämie und Übergewicht

Es entspricht der allgemeinen klinischen Erfahrung, daß Gichtkranke heute sehr häufig Übergewicht haben. In der Literatur findet man nicht selten eine Häufigkeit des Übergewichtes bei Gicht von 50% und mehr (KUZELL et al., 1955; BRØCHNER-MORTENSEN, 1958; GAMP et al., 1965; HALL, 1965; BENEDEK, 1967; GRAHAME u. SCOTT, 1970; THIELE et al., 1971; MERTZ u. BABUCKE, 1971). Hier dürfen aber Ursache und Folgen nicht verwechselt und der Einfluß anderer Faktoren, etwa der falschen Ernährung mit gleichzeitigen Störungen des Kohlenhydrat- und Fettstoffwechsels, nicht übersehen werden. Statistisch gesicherte Ergebnisse mit vergleichbaren Parametern liegen praktisch nicht vor. Daß in einem Kollektiv von Gichtkranken nicht immer die Übergewichtigen vorherrschen müssen, zeigen frühere Untersuchungen (TALBOTT, 1967), aber auch Berichte aus jüngster Zeit (GÜNTHER et al., 1968; FRANK, 1974). Auch für Patienten mit symptomloser Hyperuricämie findet man unterschiedliche Angaben. Sie reichen von einer Häufigkeit des Übergewichtes von 49% (BABUCKE u. MERTZ, 1974) über eine geringgradige Korrelation zwischen Harnsäurespiegel und Körpergewicht (LAWEE, 1969; LANESE, 1969; PAULUS et al., 1970) bis zur kontrollierten Studie, die im Durchschnitt keinen Unterschied des Körpergewichtes von Hyperuricämikern und Personen mit normalen Harnsäurespiegeln feststellen kann (FRANK, 1974).

Anhand des großen Zahlenmaterials der epidemiologischen Studien wurde eine Beziehung zwischen dem Körpergewicht und der Höhe des Serumharnsäurespiegels in randomisiert ausgewählten Bevölkerungsgruppen nachgewiesen (DUNN et al., 1963; HALL et al., 1967; MYERS et al., 1968; KLEIN et al., 1973; ZALOKAR et al., 1974). Zum gleichen Ergebnis kamen HOLLISTER et al., (1967). Dagegen wurde bei einer Personengruppe in Schottland (ANUMONYE et al., 1969) und bei 999 Blutspendern in München (GRIEBSCH u. ZÖLLNER, 1973) zwar bei höherem Körpergewicht ein höherer Harnsäurespiegel, jedoch keine statistisch signifikante Beziehung zwischen diesen beiden Größen gefunden. KASL et al. beobachteten 219 Männer zwei Jahre lang und konnten ebenfalls keine Beziehung zwischen Harnsäurespiegel und Körpergewicht feststellen. Es ist denkbar, daß für die statistische Sicherung dieser Befunde größere Personenzahlen, wie sie bei den epidemiologischen Studien vorlagen, notwendig sind. Übergewichtige haben einen höheren Harnsäurespiegel, der bei Reduktion des Körpergewichtes absinkt (KŘIŽEK, 1966). Diese Befunde legen die Deutung nahe, daß übergewichtige Personen mehr Nahrung und damit mehr Purinkörper aufnehmen und deshalb der Harnsäurespiegel im Serum ansteigt (ZÖLLNER, 1963). Befunde, die einen veränderten Harnsäurestoffwechsel des Übergewichtigen beschreiben, stehen vorerst noch isoliert und warten auf Bestätigung (EMMERSON, 1973). Bei Untersuchungen der Beziehung zwischen Körpergewicht und Serumharnsäure führten positive und negative Ergebnisse (BURCH et al., 1966, PRIOR et al., 1966; O'BRIEN et al., 1966; HEALEY et al., 1966; EMMERSON et al., 1969) zur Hypothese, daß Unterschiede im Harnsäurestoffwechsel verschiedener Rassen bestehen. Da der Harnsäurespiegel aber von vielen Faktoren beeinflußt wird, genügt es schon, wenn ein Faktor hier und der andere dort überwiegt, um derartige Unterschiede vorzutäuschen (ACHESON, 1970).

Zusammenfassend läßt sich sagen, daß auf Grund des Zahlenmaterials der epidemiologischen Studien eine geringgradige statistische Beziehung zwischen Körpergewicht und Harnsäurespiegel in der Bevölkerung besteht. Es ergibt sich aber aus den bisher vorliegenden Daten kein ausreichender Anhalt dafür, daß Übergewicht allein die Hyperuricämie begünstigt. Erhöhte Purinzufuhr mit der Nahrung führt zu einem Anstieg des Harnsäurespiegels, beim Patienten mit einem angeborenen Defekt des Harnsäurestoffwechsels stärker als beim Gesunden (ZÖLLNER et al., 1972). Unterschiede im Puringehalt der Nahrung des Übergewichtigen und des Normgewichtigen könnten auch Unterschiede im Harnsäurespiegel erklären.

Hyperuricämie und Fettleber

Im Rahmen einer therapeutischen Studie fielen SCOTT et al. im Jahre 1966 bei Gichtpatienten pathologische Werte der Bromsulphaleinretention auf (SCOTT et al., 1966). Seit dieser Zeit sind mehrere Arbeiten erschienen, die über eine auffällige Häufung von pathologischen Befunden an der Leber von Gichtkranken berichten (SCHILLING, 1967; GRAHAME et al., 1968; KNICK et al., 1968; HENNECKE u. SÜDHOF, 1970; TREMEL u. POHL, 1971; KLEIN, 1971; SCHILLING, 1971; BABUCKE u. MERTZ, 1974). Bemerkenswert sind darunter die Befunde an jungen Patienten mit primärer Hyperuricämie (HENNINGES u. MERTZ, 1971). Die Veränderungen betreffen den Tastbefund und die Laborwerte, sie werden in den meisten Fällen als Ausdruck einer Leberverfettung interpretiert. Bei einem Teil dieser Patienten konnte diese Diagnose histologisch verifiziert werden. Nicht selten wurde dabei auch ein entzündlicher Reizzustand mit mesenchymalen Begleitreaktionen beobachtet (SCHILLING, 1967).

Bisher schlugen alle Versuche fehl, gichtspezifische Veränderungen des Lebergewebes, etwa wie bei der Gichtniere, als pathologisch anatomisches Substrat der klinischen und laborchemischen Veränderungen nachzuweisen. Der histologische Befund entspricht dem einer Fettleber (TREMEL u. POHL, 1971), wie er auch bei Diabetes, Hyperlipidämie oder Alkoholabusus beobachtet wird. Im Zusammenhang mit der Entstehung auf dem Boden einer Störung des Harnsäurestoffwechsels ist interessant, daß pathologische Leberbefunde bei Gicht und bei symptomloser Hyperuricämie gleich häufig gesehen werden (TREMEL u. POHL, 1971). Nach anderen Untersuchungen nimmt die Lebergröße nur scheinbar mit der Höhe des Harnsäurespiegels zu, denn nach Berücksichtigung der Körperfettmasse fällt diese Beziehung weg (ZALOKAR et al., 1974). Bisher gibt es keine vernünftige Hypothese, die die Genese einer Fettleber durch eine Störung im Purinstoffwechsel erklären könnte (s. MERTZ, 1973). In der Literatur wird die Leberverfettung bei Gicht deshalb häufig mit einer diabetischen Stoffwechsellage (HENNECKE u. SÜDHOF, 1970), mit einer Hyperlipidämie und Übergewicht (KNICK et al., 1968) oder mit Alkoholkonsum (GRAHAME u. SCOTT, 1968) in Verbindung gebracht. Diese Stoffwechselstörungen und Folgen der Fehlernährung sind in der Tat bei Patienten mit Gicht häufig zu beobachten (Tab. 1). Leider wurden die bisher vorliegenden Untersuchungen nicht nach einem einheitlichen Plan und einheitlichen Definitionen, z.B. des Übergewichtes, aufgebaut, so daß sie nur sehr bedingt vergleichbar sind, auf keinen Fall jedoch gemeinsam ausgewertet werden können. Dies wäre aber notwendig, um bei einer Gruppierung nach drei, vier oder mehr möglichen Ursachen noch zu sinnvollen Fallzahlen zu kommen. Diese Situation wird in der Tab. 1 deutlich. In allen Publikationen ist das Auftreten von Stoffwechselstörungen nur in Prozentwerten angegeben, die Häufung mehrerer Störungen bei einem Patienten ist daraus nicht zu entnehmen und damit auch nicht die Bedeutung dieser einzelnen Faktoren für die Entstehung der Fettleber. Außerdem wurde der objektive Nachweis einer Fettablagerung im histologischen Präparat nur in einem geringen Teil der Fälle durchgeführt. Aus diesen Gründen können zum jetzigen Zeitpunkt nur Argumente für und gegen die einzelnen Faktoren, die für die Entstehung der Fettleber bei Patienten mit Gicht verantwortlich sein könnten, angeführt werden.

Zu einer Zeit, da im Durchschnitt 8% der Calorien unserer Nahrung in Form von Alkohol zugeführt werden, ist die alkoholische Fettleber keine Seltenheit. Nur in wenigen Publikationen über die Gicht sind jedoch Angaben über den Anteil der Patienten, die erhöhten Alkoholkonsum zugegeben haben, enthalten. Die Prozentzahlen reichen von 6,5—33% (PAULUS et al., 1970; GRAHAME u. SCOTT, 1968). Die anderen Autoren verzichten, teils wegen der Unzuverlässigkeit derartiger Angaben, auf diese wichtige Information. Die Bedeutung des Alkohols für die Entstehung einer Fettleber bei Gichtkranken kommt dadurch zum Ausdruck, daß auch bei diesen Patienten die Bromsulphaleinretention mit der Menge des Alkoholkonsums ansteigt (GRAHAME u. SCOTT, 1968). Erhöhter Alkoholkonsum geht nicht selten mit einer Hypertriglyceridämie einher, die ebenfalls die Entstehung einer Fettleber begünstigt. Bei den primären Hyperlipidämien werden sehr oft Fetteinlagerungen in der Leber gefunden. In der Tab. 1 liegt die Häufigkeit einer Hyperlipidämie bei Gicht zwischen 21 und 87%. Die Häufigkeit einer Kombination von Hyperlipidämie und Fettleber bei Gichtkranken läßt sich aus den in der Tabelle zusammengestellten Werten leider nicht rekonstruieren. Ledig-

Tabelle 1. Die Häufigkeit von Leberbeteiligung und von Stoffwechselstörungen bei Hyperuricämie und Gicht

	Anzahl der Patienten n	Häufigkeit pathologischer Leberbefunde %	Histologischer Befunde vorhanden n	Übergewicht %	Gesamtlipid- oder Triglyceridspiegel erhöht %	latenter oder manifester Diabetes %	Alkoholabusus %
GRAHAME et al. (1968)							
a) Gicht	73	75	—	44	—	—	33
b) Hyperuricämie	16	75	—	44	—	—	19
KNICK et al. (1968)	52	83	35	83	$\bar{x}$ 260 mg%	60	—
HENNECKE u. SÜDHOF (1970)	100	86	19	56	87	20	—
TREMEL u. POHL (1971)	27	44	27	81	70	87 (n = 39)	—
KLEIN (1971)	79	40	—	—	60 (n = 25)	18	—
HENNINGS u. MERTZ (1971)	50	64	7	78	—	16	—
BABUCKE u. MERTZ (1974)	675	41	46	49	21		

lich KLEIN berichtet, daß er keine klare Beziehung zwischen Fettleber und Gesamtlipiden finden konnte; in dieser Arbeit fehlen jedoch histologische Befunde. Ein Diabetes ist ebenfalls häufig als Ursache einer Fettleber bei Gicht zu diskutieren. Unter den Gichtpatienten mit Diabetes ist der Bromsulphaleintest häufiger pathologisch als unter den Patienten ohne Diabetes (HENNECKE u. SÜDHOF, 1970). Bemerkenswert ist in diesem Zusammenhang die Häufigkeit von asymptomatischem Diabetes bei Gicht (KNICK et al., 1968), der häufig nicht bekannt ist, aber in Kombination mit Übergewicht die Entstehung einer Fettleber begünstigt. Zwischen Übergewicht und Diabetes besteht auch bei Patienten mit Gicht eine statistische Korrelation. Adipöse Gichtkranke haben häufiger einen Diabetes (33%) als untergewichtige (14%) (BERNHEIM et al., 1968). Die diabetische Fettleber ist seltener bei den jugendlichen Diabetikern als bei den übergewichtigen Erwachsenen mit Diabetes. Dabei hängt die Menge der Fettablagerungen in der Leber nicht von der Dauer und der Schwere des Diabetes, sondern vom Grad des Übergewichtes ab (BERINGER u. THALER, 1970). Auch bei Gichtkranken ist die Korrelation des Körpergewichts mit dem Grad der Leberverfettung statistisch zumindest auffällig (KNICK et al., 1968). Auf Grund dieser Befunde und des hohen Anteils der Adipösen unter den Gichtkranken (Tab. 1) muß die „Mastfettleber" als weitere Form der Fettleber bei Gichtkranken angesehen werden. Dafür sprechen auch die Korrelation zwischen Körpergewicht und Lebergröße (ZALOKAR et al., 1974), und die Tatsache, daß die Gichtkranken mit dem größten Gewicht die höchste Bromsulphaleinretention hatten, und dies auch, nachdem der Einfluß von Unterschieden im Plasmavolumen rechnerisch korrigiert worden war (GRAHAME et al., 1968).

Die Fettleber ist in vielen Fällen nicht durch einen, sondern durch eine Kombination verschiedener Faktoren verursacht. Bei Patienten mit Gicht sind in erster Linie Übergewicht, Alkohol, Hyperlipidämie und Diabetes zu nennen, die allein oder in Kombination das Risiko des Gichtkranken für Fetteinlagerungen in der Leber stark erhöhen. Gichtkranke mit Fettleber, aber ohne wenigstens einen der oben genannten, für die Entstehung der Fettleber relevanten Faktoren, sind relativ selten. Bevor nicht eine ausreichende Zahl von Gichtkranken ohne weitere Stoffwechselstörungen, Übergewicht und Alkoholabusus nach vergleichbaren Kriterien untersucht wurde oder in einer Verlaufsstudie die Veränderungen der Fettleber nach Normalisierung des Körpergewichtes bzw. nach ausreichender Behandlung der Hyperlipidämie oder des Diabetes beobachtet wurden, muß es auf Grund der vorliegenden Befunde offen bleiben, ob eine enge Beziehung zwischen Hyperuricämie oder Gicht und einer Fettleber besteht. Bisher gibt es keinen Beweis für spezifische Veränderungen an der Leber als Folge einer Störung des Purinstoffwechsels.

Hyperuricämie und Diabetes

Über die Kombination von Gicht und Diabetes bestehen auf Grund einander widersprechender Befunde seit dem vorigen Jahrhundert sehr unterschiedliche Auffassungen (BECKETT u. LEWIS, 1960). Dies wird auch in Übersichtsartikeln der letzten Jahre deutlich (MIKKELSEN, 1965; HEIDELMANN u. THIELE, 1973; MERTZ, 1973). Manche Autoren sind der Ansicht, daß beide Krankheiten sehr selten gemeinsam auftreten. So fand JOSLIN 1952 unter 1500 Diabetikern nur einen Patienten mit einer Gicht, und TALBOTT berichtete 1953 in seinem Buch über die Gicht nur von zwei Patienten mit Gicht und Diabetes. WHITEHOUSE u. CLEARY sahen nur in 1,6% von 509 Diabetikern eine Gicht. BECKETT u. LEWIS fanden 1960 bei 800 Diabetikern 19 Patienten mit Hyperuricämie, einer von diesen hatte eine

Gicht. In seiner Übersicht berichtet MIKKELSEN von einer Häufigkeit der Hyperuricämie bei Diabetes zwischen 2 und 50%, und der Gicht zwischen 0,1 und 9%. Dagegen wird die Häufigkeit einer pathologischen Glucosetoleranz oder eines Diabetes bei Gicht mit 7—74% der Patienten beschrieben (MIKKELSEN, 1965; BERNHEIM et al., 1968a u. b; MCKECHNIE, 1964; BERKOWITZ, 1966; DENIS u. LAUNAY, 1969; SCHILLING, 1972; HERMAN, 1958; KNICK et al., 1968; ISHMAEL, 1964; CAMUS, 1968; WEISS et al., 1957; TREMEL u. POHL, 1971). Nach einer neueren Untersuchung ist bei Diabetikern nicht mit einem vermehrten Auftreten von Gicht oder Hyperuricämie zu rechnen (HASSLACHER et al., 1974). Diesen Zahlen stehen Mitteilungen gegenüber, die bei Gichtkranken eine Diabeteshäufigkeit von 3% (KUZELL et al., 1955) bzw. etwa die gleiche Häufigkeit des Diabetes bei Gichtkranken und Kontrollpersonen fanden (FRANK, 1974).

Trotz dieser gelegentlich gehäuft beobachteten Kombination von Gicht und Diabetes konnte in mehreren epidemiologischen Untersuchungen keine Beziehung zwischen Harnsäure- und Blutzuckerspiegel nachgewiesen werden (HALL, 1965; HALL et al., 1967; MYERS et al., 1968; LAWEE, 1969; KLEIN et al., 1973; ZALOKAR et al., 1974; HERMAN et al., 1974). Dieses Ergebnis kann so gedeutet werden, daß zwischen der Gicht und einem manifesten, insulinpflichtigen Diabetes des normalgewichtigen Erwachsenen tatsächlich keine statistisch zu sichernde Beziehung besteht. In den epidemiologischen Untersuchungen wurden keine Provokationsteste durchgeführt, so daß ein latenter Diabetes nicht erfaßt werden konnte. Der Diabetes bei Gicht ist in den meisten Fällen nicht insulinpflichtig (WHITEHOUSE u. CLEARY, 1966; BECKETT u. LEWIS, 1960), und es gibt Untersuchungen, in denen der manifeste Diabetes bei Gichtkranken nicht häufiger als in der übrigen Bevölkerung beobachtet wurde, während eine latente diabetische Stoffwechsellage deutlich gehäuft auftrat (SCHILLING, 1972).

Über das Auftreten von Störungen des Kohlenhydratstoffwechsels bei Hyperuricämie und Gicht sind erst dann vertrauenswürdige Aussagen zu erwarten, wenn alle, die Entstehung einer diabetischen Stoffwechsellage begünstigenden Faktoren berücksichtigt werden. In erster Linie muß das Körpergewicht in Betracht gezogen werden, da Übergewicht ein sicherer diabetogener Faktor ist. Die meisten Gichtkranken, bei denen eine Störung des Kohlenhydratstoffwechsels nachzuweisen ist, sind übergewichtig (TREMEL u. POHL, 1971; KUZELL et al., 1955; KNICK et al., 1968; GAMP et al., 1965; MERTZ u. BABUCKE, 1971; WEYLAND, 1969; BARTELS et al., 1960). Für die Bedeutung der Ernährungsweise und des Übergewichtes sprechen auch die Tatsachen, daß man die höchsten Harnsäurespiegel bei den Diabetikern mit Übergewicht findet, und daß der Durchschnitt der Harnsäurewerte in der Gruppe der nicht insulinbedürftigen, meist übergewichtigen Diabetiker höher liegt als in der Gruppe der insulinpflichtigen Diabetiker (BECKETT u. LEWIS, 1960). Die Diskrepanz zwischen der Seltenheit der Gicht bei Diabetikern und der Häufigkeit des Diabetes bei Gichtkranken (WHITEHOUSE u. CLEARY, 1966) ließe sich so erklären, daß Übergewicht sicher diabetogen wirkt, mit dem Harnsäurespiegel aber wesentlich lockerer korreliert ist (s.S. 238). Deshalb entwickeln übergewichtige Hyperuricämiker im Laufe der Zeit häufiger einen Diabetes als übergewichtige Diabetiker eine Hyperuricämie oder gar eine Gicht. Mit zunehmendem Alter steigt die Häufigkeit des Diabetes an, auch bei Patienten mit Gicht. In über zwei Drittel der Patienten mit Gicht und Diabetes geht die Gicht dem Diabetes um Jahre voraus (BARTELS et al., 1960; ISHMAEL et al., 1964; PRIOR et al., 1966; WHITEHOUSE u. CLEARY, 1966; BERNHEIM et al., 1968). Bei jüngeren Patienten mit Gicht findet man seltener einen Diabetes als bei älteren (RUNGE, nach HEIDELMANN u. THIELE, 1973, S.89). Als weiterer diabetogener Faktor ist nach neueren Untersuchungen eine Insulinresistenz bei Hypertriglyceridämie anzusehen (VOGELBERG et al., 1973). BERKOWITZ fand 1966 bei Gichtpatienten mit Hyperlipämie ($n = 25$) in 74% und bei Gichtpatienten mit normalen Triglyceridspiegeln ($n = 25$) nur in 17% eine Störung des Kohlenhydratstoffwechsels.

Über die Häufigkeit des Prädiabetes bei Gichtkranken gibt es bisher keine Mitteilung. SCHILLING fand 1972 unter 200 Männern mit Gicht nur fünfmal einen behandlungsbedürftigen Diabetes, aber bei 18 Patienten (9%) waren in der Familie Diabetiker bekannt. Andere Autoren geben die familiäre Diabetesbelastung des Gichtkranken mit bis zu 40% an (BARTELS et al., 1960; BERNHEIM et al., 1968; ISHMAEL et al., 1964; MERTZ u. BABUCKE, 1971; WHITEHOUSE u. CLEARY, JR., 1966).

Bei gesunden Erwachsenen unter üblicher Ernährung besteht keine statistisch signifikante Korrelation zwischen Blutzucker, Harnsäure und Triglyceriden im Serum (DUNN u. MOSES, 1965). Für eine direkte Verbindung zwischen Kohlenhydrat- und Purinstoffwechsel beim Patienten mit Gicht und Diabetes gibt es bisher keinen Beweis. Die Hyperuricämie bei diabetischer Ketoacidose, die u. a. durch den erhöhten Spiegel von β-Hydroxybutyrat zustandekommt (GOLDFINGER et al., 1965), ist für die chronische Hyperuricämie ohne Bedeutung. Die Hyperuricämie bei Niereninsuffizienz auf dem Boden einer diabetischen Nephropathie ist im Verhältnis zur Zahl der Diabetiker als selten zu bezeichnen. Die Angaben über eine mögliche Genkopplung als Ursache der Kombination von Gicht und Diabetes konnten bisher nicht überzeugen (BECKETT u. LEWIS, 1960).

Hyperuricämie und Hyperlipidämie

Über die Beziehungen zwischen Gicht und Hyperlipidämie bestehen trotz einer Fülle von Veröffentlichungen immer noch unterschiedliche Auffassungen. Während in einigen Arbeiten von einem gehäuften Zusammentreffen von Gicht und Hypercholesterinämie berichtet wird (MARINOFF u. LEMPERT, 1962; KOHN u. PROZAN, 1959; HARRIS-JONES, 1957), finden andere Autoren in neuerer Zeit keine Korrelation zwischen Harnsäure- und Cholesterinspiegel (LANESE et al., 1969; GÜNTHER et al., 1968; PAULUS et al., 1970). In den epidemiologischen Untersuchungen von Tecumseh und Evans County ergab sich ebenfalls keine statistisch gesicherte Korrelation zwischen Cholesterin- und Harnsäurespiegel (MYERS et al., 1968; KLEIN et al., 1973). Dieser Befund wird durch die neuen Ergebnisse einer epidemiologischen Untersuchung in Frankreich von ZALOKAR et al. gestützt, die ebenfalls keine Beziehung zwischen Harnsäure- und Cholesterinspiegel, wohl aber zwischen Harnsäure- und Triglyceridspiegel feststellten (ZALOKAR et al., 1974). Bereits vorher hatten mehrere Autoren über ein gehäuftes Auftreten einer Hypertriglyceridämie und weitgehend normaler Cholesterinspiegel bei Patienten mit Hyperuricämie oder Gicht berichtet (BERKOWITZ, 1964; BERKOWITZ, 1966; BENEDEK, 1967; GÜNTHER et al., 1967; BLUESTONE et al., 1971). Andere Autoren fanden auch die Kombination Hypercholesterinämie und Hypertriglyceridämie bei Patienten mit Hyperuricämie oder Gicht (BARLOW, 1968; KNICK et al., 1968; POLITT et al., 1968; SCHILLING, 1972). Die Häufigkeit der Hypertriglyceridämie bei Gichtpatienten wird mit 6—84% angegeben. Die Häufigkeit der Hyperuricämie bei Patienten mit Hypertriglyceridämie erreicht in einer Arbeit 82% (BERKOWITZ, 1964). Die beachtliche Streuung dieser Zahlen spricht nicht gerade für ihre Zuverlässigkeit. Wesentliche Gründe dafür sind, wie in vielen ähnlichen Untersuchungen, der Mangel an einheitlichen Kriterien und Definitionen und das inhomogene Patientengut, das durch Übergewicht, Diabetes mellitus, Alkoholkonsum und andere Störfaktoren für Triglycerid- und Harnsäurespiegel belastet ist.

Geht man von Patienten mit primärer Hyperlipidämie aus, so findet man bei der familiären Hypercholesterinämie nur sehr selten eine Hyperuricämie (JENSEN et al., 1966), während bei der kohlenhydratinduzierten Hypertriglyceridämie in etwa ein Drittel der Fälle eine Hyperuricämie beobachtet wurde (STREJČEK u. KUČEROVA, 1968). FREDRICKSON nennt für die Häufigkeit der Hyperuricämie bei den verschiedenen Typen der Hyperlipoproteinämie folgende Werte: bei Typ I und II normale Häufigkeit, bei Typ III Hyperuricämie in etwa 16%, bei Typ IV und V je in etwa 40% (FREDRICKSON u. LEVY, 1972; FREDRICKSON, 1971, persönliche Mitteilung). In einer Übersicht über die Typen der Hyperlipoproteinämien bei Gicht aus fünf Arbeiten mit insgesamt 183 Patienten, von denen 101 (= 54%) eine Hyperlipoproteinämie hatten, liegt die Häufigkeit des Typ IV bei 44%, dagegen die des Typ V bei nur 3% (LANG, 1974).

Die häufige Kombination von Hyperuricämie und Hypertriglyceridämie ist auch durch Arbeiten belegt, in denen den insgesamt 206 Patienten mit Hyperuricämie oder Gicht in Hinsicht auf Alter, Größe, Gewicht und Alkoholkonsum vergleichbare Kontrollgruppen gegenübergestellt wurden. Bei den Patienten mit Gicht trat eine Hypertriglyceridämie signifikant häufiger auf als bei den Kontrollpersonen (FELDMAN u. WALLACE, 1964; DARLINGTON u. SCOTT, 1972; MIELANTS et al., 1973; FRANK, 1974; WIEDEMANN et al., 1972). Bei symptomloser Hyperuricämie war die Hypertriglyceridämie seltener als bei Gicht (FRANK, 1974) (Tab. 2).

In der neuesten Übersicht zum Problem der Fettstoffwechselstörungen bei Gicht diskutiert LANG die Häufigkeit und die möglichen Ursachen der Kombination Purinstoffwechselstörung und Hyperlipidämie ausführlich. Von den bisher in der Literatur genannten und mehr oder minder ausführlich diskutierten Hypothesen: 1. Genetischer Zusammenhang, 2. direkter metabolischer Zusammenhang und 3. indirekter Zusammenhang über Adipositas, Störung des Kohlenhydratstoffwechsels, Fettleber, Nierenfunktionsstörungen, Alkoholabusus konnte die Mehrzahl bisher nur durch einzelne Beispiele belegt werden. Für keine der Hypothesen liegen schlüssige Beweise vor (LANG, 1974).

In der Diskussion um die Pathogenese dürfen die Berichte nicht außer acht gelassen werden, die bei Gichtpatienten mit Diabetes doppelt so häufig eine Hyperlipidämie beschreiben wie bei den Patienten ohne Diabetes (BERNHEIM et al., 1968), oder andere, die bei Gichtpatienten mit Hypertriglyceridämie häufiger eine Adipositas, eine pathologische Glucosetoleranz oder eine Hypercholesterinämie finden als bei Patienten mit normalen Triglyceridwerten (HEIDELMANN u. THIELE, 1973). Diese Befunde zeigen, daß mit Sicherheit indirekte Zusammenhänge der von LANG zitierten Art bestehen. Durch Vergleiche an 40 Gichtkranken mit Hyperlipämie, 40 Gesunden mit gleichem Alter, Geschlecht und Grad des Übergewichtes und 40 Gesunden mit geringerem Körpergewicht konnte gezeigt werden, daß die Hypertriglyceridämie in diesen Fällen mit großer Wahrscheinlichkeit auf das Übergewicht und den Alkoholkonsum zurückzuführen war (GIBSON u. GRAHAME, 1974).

Die Hypothese von einer Gen-Koppelung als Ursache der häufigen Kombination von Gicht und Hypertriglyceridämie wird bisher nur durch Vermutungen gestützt (ZALOKAR et al., 1974; BERKOWITZ, 1966; FELDMAN u. WALLACE, 1964). Für ein Syndrom aus essentieller Hyperlipidämie, Hyperuricämie und Diabetes als genetisch gekoppelte schwere Stoffwechselstörung (CAMUS, 1966) gibt es bisher keinen Beweis. Ein interessanter Hinweis ergibt sich vielleicht aus Untersuchungen an eineiigen Zwillingen, wo Triglycerid- und Harnsäurespiegel viel enger gekoppelt waren als bei zweieiigen Zwillingen (JENSEN et al., 1965). Ausgedehnte Familienuntersuchungen zur Aufklärung genetischer Zusammenhänge stehen noch aus.

Tabelle 2. Triglyceridspiegel im Serum bei Gichtpatienten und vergleichbaren Kontrollpersonen

	Anzahl der Patienten n	Durchschnittsalter Jahre	Harnsäure mg/100 ml $\bar{X}$	Triglyceride mg/100 ml $\bar{X} \pm s$	Hypertriglyceridämien n	Körpergewicht	pathologische Glucosetoleranz %	Alkoholkonsum berücksichtigt
FELDMANN u. WALLACE (1964)								
Gicht	34	52	8,8 ± 1,8	142 ± 79	8	—	0	—
Kontrollen	28	50	5,0 ± 1,3	100 ± 43	1	—	—	—
DARLINGTON u. SCOTT (1972)								
Gicht	27	53,6	—	209,2 ± 175,5	8	12,06[a]	—	+
Kontrollen	27	53,2	—	99,7 ± 41,4	0	12,51[a]	—	+
WIEDEMANN et al. (1972)								
Gicht	14	50	9,4 ± 1,3	174 ± 82	5	114[b]	14	+
Kontrollen	14	49	5,8 ± 0,7	115 ± 49	1	115[b]	7	+
MIELANTS et al. (1973)								
Gicht	31	46	6,8	241	—	—	—	—
Kontrollen	31	46	4,3	96	—	—	—	—
FRANK (1974)								
Gicht	50	52,2	8,0	213 ± 89	14	125,1[c]	46	+
Kontrollen	50	52,7	5,5	138 ± 49	16	124,9[c]	42	+
Hyperuricämie ♂	50	53,9	7,8	163 ± 82	9	113,5[c]	44	+
Kontrollen	50	54,0	5,2	171 ± 86	12	113,3[c]	36	+

[a] „Gewichtsindex": $\left(\dfrac{\text{Größe (inch)}}{\sqrt[3]{\text{Gewicht (lb.)}}}\right)$.

[b] Körpergewicht in Prozent des Idealgewichts (Metropolitan Life Insurance Tabellen).
[c] Körpergewicht in Prozent der Norm (Tabellen der Society of Actuaries).

Ein direkter Zusammenhang zwischen Purin- und Lipidstoffwechsel ist theoretisch über einen erhöhten $NADP/NADPH_2$-Quotienten möglich (GREILING, 1969). Die Erhöhung dieses Quotienten, wie sie bei acidotischer Stoffwechsellage auftritt, bedeutet eine gesteigerte Synthese von Lipiden. „Eine Erhöhung der intracellulären NADP-Konzentration führt zu einer Aktivierung der Glucose-6-Phosphat-Dehydrogenase-Reaktion. Dies bedeutet aber, daß sich auch das Ausgangsprodukt der Purinsynthese, 5-Phosphoribosyl-1-pyrophosphat im verstärkten Maße bildet, was schließlich zu einer erhöhten Harnsäuresynthese führt" (GREILING, 1969). Eine Hypertriglyceridämie wurde bereits bei einem Mangel an Hypoxanthin-Guanin-Phosphoribosyl-Transferase (KELLEY et al., 1969) und bei Glucose-6-Phosphatase-Mangel (HOWELL et al., 1962) beschrieben. Beide Enzymdefekte führen zu einem erhöhten Harnsäurespiegel. Die Entstehung der Hypertriglyceridämie ist aber auch bei diesen seltenen Enzymdefekten unklar. Bei einem Vergleich von Gichtkranken mit Hypertriglyceridämie und Gichtkranken mit normalen Triglyceridspiegeln wurde festgestellt, daß die hyperlipämischen Gichtkranken nach oraler Glucosebelastung signifikant mehr Insulin ausschütteten als die Patienten mit normalen Triglyceriden oder die gesunden Kontrollpersonen (WIEDEMANN et al., 1972). Aus diesem Ergebnis wurde auf eine direkte Beziehung zwischen Gicht und Hypertriglyceridämie geschlossen. Es ist jedoch denkbar, daß der Triglyceridspiegel per se einen Einfluß auf die Insulinwirkung und damit den Anstieg des Insulinspiegels hatte (VOGELBERG et al., 1973). Bei intravenöser Harnsäurebelastung von Hyperlipämikern und Patienten mit Gicht wurde in beiden Patientengruppen eine Verminderung der Harnsäureelimination durch die Niere gefunden. Das ähnliche Verhalten der Hyperlipämiker mit und ohne Hyperuricämie wurde als eine gleiche renal tubuläre Störung gedeutet (IRMSCHER et al., 1970). Andere Untersuchungen ergaben eine Herabsetzung von Glomerulumfiltrat und Nierenplasmastrom bei Patienten mit essentieller Hyperlipämie (DITTRICH u. SANDHOFER, 1967). Weitere Ansatzpunkte für einen renalen Mechanismus sind die Hemmung der Harnsäureausscheidung durch Ketonkörper (GOLDFINGER et al., 1965) und durch Lactat (LIEBER et al., 1962). Alkoholabusus kann zur Hyperuricämie und Hypertriglyceridämie führen.

Auch Therapiestudien konnten ex iuvantibus keine Klärung eines direkten Zusammenhanges zwischen Gicht und Hyperlipidämie bringen. Arzneimittel, die den Harnsäurespiegel beeinflussen, senken den Triglyceridspiegel nicht (GÜNTHER u. KNAPP, 1970; BLUESTONE et al., 1971). Eine Behandlung der Hypertriglyceridämie mit Clofibrat beeinflußt die primäre Hyperuricämie nicht signifikant (MERTZ u. BABUCKE, 1973). Diese Substanz ist durch ihre partiell uricosurische Wirkung für diese Fragestellung nicht sehr geeignet. Eine Behandlung der Hypertriglyceridämie mit einer kohlenhydratarmen Diät führt zu keiner Änderung des Harnsäurespiegels im Serum (STRJČEK u. KUČEROVA, 1968).

Auf Grund der vorliegenden Befunde geht eine Hyperuricämie manchmal mit einer Hypertriglyceridämie einher, selten jedoch mit einer Hypercholesterinämie. Adipositas und Alkoholabusus, die Folgen der Ernährung in unserer Wohlstandsgesellschaft, tragen sicher zu den erhöhten Triglyceridwerten des Gichtkranken bei. Von den bisher aufgestellten Hypothesen über eine direkte Verbindung zwischen Purin- und Fettstoffwechsel ist noch keine bewiesen. Auf keinen Fall ist es gerechtfertigt, von einer sekundären Hyperlipidämie bei Gicht zu sprechen.

Hyperuricämie und Gicht als Risikofaktor

Über die Beziehung zwischen Hyperuricämie, mit oder ohne Gicht, und frühzeitiger Arteriosklerose gibt es nur wenige harte Daten. Erst im letzten Jahrzehnt enthalten die Publikationen über dieses Problem Ansätze zu einer brauchbaren

Versuchsanordnung wie z. B. randomisierte Patientengruppen mit vergleichbaren Kontrollgruppen, Berücksichtigung anderer Risikofaktoren, die bei Hyperuricämikern häufig zu finden sind, oder prospektive Studien zur Morbidität der Coronarkrankheit. Das größte und zuverlässigste Zahlenmaterial liegt aus den epidemiologischen Untersuchungen zur coronaren Herzkrankheit vor.

Auf einen möglichen Zusammenhang zwischen Hyperuricämie und Arteriosklerose wurde bereits früher in vielen Arbeiten hingewiesen. Die Ergebnisse waren jedoch in Abhängigkeit von der untersuchten Population recht unterschiedlich. Prinzipiell ging man entweder von Patienten mit klinisch manifester Arteriosklerose, z. B. Herzinfarkt oder peripherer obliterierender Angiopathie, oder von Patienten mit Hyperuricämie und Gicht aus. In den meisten dieser Untersuchungen gehen Hyperuricämie und Gicht häufiger mit einer Arteriosklerose einher als diese in der übrigen Bevölkerung beobachtet wird. Einige Beispiele sollen dies erläutern.

GERTLER et al. (1951) stellten ein gehäuftes Zusammentreffen von Hyperuricämie und Herzinfarkt fest. Sie fanden bei 92 Patienten, die vor dem 40. Lebensjahr einen Herzinfarkt erlitten hatten, viermal häufiger eine Hyperuricämie als in einer Vergleichsgruppe. In einer weiteren Untersuchung an 100 Patienten mit coronarer Herzkrankheit, die zehn Jahre vorher bereits untersucht worden waren, und 146 Kontrollpersonen brachte die Einbeziehung des Serumharnsäurespiegels als Hinweis auf ein Coronarrisiko zusätzlich zum Cholesterinspiegel u. a. keine Verbesserung der Korrelation zwischen den vorhandenen Risikofaktoren und dem Auftreten eines Herzinfarktes (GERTLER et al., 1959). Andere Untersucher des Harnsäurespiegels bei Infarktpatienten fanden dagegen häufig eine Hyperuricämie (KOHN u. PROZAN, 1959; EIDLITZ, 1961; LONDON u. HUMS, 1967; UPMARK u. ADNER, 1950; DREYFUS, 1960; HANSEN, 1966). BENEDEK stellte bei 32 Patienten, die einen Herzinfarkt überstanden hatten, mit im Durchschnitt 6,7 mg-% einen signifikant höheren Harnsäurespiegel fest als bei 119 Blutspendern, die einen durchschnittlichen Harnsäurespiegel von 5,5 mg-% hatten. Cholesterin- und Triglyceridspiegel lagen aber auch signifikant höher, und die Blutspender waren im Durchschnitt sieben Jahre jünger (BENEDEK, 1967). In einer anderen Untersuchung wiesen von 113 Patienten nach einem Herzinfarkt 49% Serumharnsäurewerte über 6,4 mg-% und 31% Serumharnsäurewerte über 7 mg-% auf (SUSIĆ et al., 1969). JACOBS kommt in einer neueren Publikation sogar auf eine Häufigkeit der Hyperuricämie von über 80% bei 280 Patienten mit Herzinfarkt (JACOBS, 1972). Eine Untersuchung aus dem gleichen Jahr ergab dagegen bei 142 Patienten mit Herzinfarkt in nur 20% eine Hyperuricämie, aber auch diese Häufigkeit ist im Vergleich zur übrigen Bevölkerung noch deutlich erhöht (LIEBSCHER, 1972). Einzelne Untersucher konnten dagegen keinen signifikanten Unterschied im Mittelwert der Serumharnsäurespiegel bei Patienten mit Coronarkrankheit und sonstigen Personen feststellen (SUSIĆ, 1970; MYERS et al., 1968).

Für eine positive Korrelation zwischen peripheren obliterierenden Angiopathien und Hyperuricämie bzw. Gicht gibt es ebenfalls Hinweise (EIDLITZ, 1961). Bei 112 Männern mit peripherer arterieller Verschlußkrankheit wurde nur in 9% ein Harnsäurespiegel von mehr als 7 mg-% festgestellt. Gleichzeitig traten jedoch Diabetes, Hyperlipidämie und Hypertonus deutlich gehäuft auf (WOLLENWEBER et al., 1971). In einer anderen Untersuchung an 500 unausgewählten Patienten mit Arterienverschlüssen wurde eine Hyperuricämie bei 7,3% der Personen festgestellt (HEIDELMANN, 1973).

Diese Art von Untersuchungen hat den Nachteil, daß die einzelnen Risikofaktoren nicht klar voneinander getrennt und gesondert bewertet wurden. Eine Unterscheidung wäre jedoch unbedingt erforderlich, da Hypertonie, Diabetes, Hypercholesterinämie bei Infarktpatienten häufiger vorkommen als in einer vergleichbaren Bevölkerungsgruppe (SCHETTLER, 1972). Für die gezielte Untersuchung der einzelnen Risikofaktoren ist natürlich eine ausreichend große Zahl von Personen erforderlich.

Einen interessanten Beitrag zur Frage der Bedeutung einer Hyperuricämie als Risikofaktor für die coronare Herzkrankheit leisteten Untersuchungen an Patienten mit Coronarangiographie. Bei 742 Männern und 260 Frauen, die klinisch die Indikationen für eine Coronarangiographie erfüllten, wurde nachgewiesen, daß bei Männern und Frauen keine Korrelation zwischen dem Ausmaß der angiographisch nachgewiesenen Veränderungen der Coronararterien und der Höhe des Harnsäurespiegels bestand (ALLARD u. GOULET, 1973). Dieses Ergebnis ist besonders zu bewerten, da bei den gleichen Patienten eine sehr enge Beziehung zwischen dem Befall der Coronararterien und der Höhe des Cholesterinspiegels bestand.

Abgesehen von zahlreichen Einzelbeobachtungen (z.B. FULTON, 1952) gibt es auch Berichte über die Häufigkeit von arteriosklerotischen Komplikationen bei Patienten mit symptomloser Hyperuricämie oder manifester Gicht. Bei 504 Patienten mit primärer Gicht wurde eine Vermehrung „Atherogener Indices" festgestellt. Von den 18 Patienten, die verstarben, hatten 11 einen Herzinfarkt erlitten (KUZELL et al., 1955). In einer Studie an einem allgemeinen Krankenhaus fanden sich unter 966 Patienten 85 mit einem Serumharnsäurespiegel über 7 mg-%. Von diesen Patienten hatten nur 3% eine Gicht, aber 11% eine coronare Herzkrankheit (LAWEE, 1969). In einer ähnlichen Untersuchung an 3589 unausgewählten Krankenhauspatienten hatten 183 einen deutlich erhöhten Harnsäurespiegel (>8 mg-%). Zeichen einer Coronarsklerose bestanden bei 24% der Hyperuricämiker, aber nur bei 11% der Gesamtgruppe. Eine Herzinsuffizienz lag bei 12% — im Vergleich zu 4% — vor (VAN PEENEN, 1971). In einer anderen Untersuchung hatten von 4148 Patienten eines Krankenhauses 13,2% einen Harnsäurespiegel von 7 mg-% und höher. Von 200 der Hyperuricämiker hatten 12% eine Gicht. Die Häufigkeit der Coronarkrankheit bei diesen Patienten nahm zwar mit der Höhe des Harnsäurespiegels zu, diese Beziehung war jedoch statistisch nicht signifikant (PAULUS et al., 1970). In einer sehr sorgfältig geplanten Untersuchung wurde an 50 unausgewählten Patienten mit primärer Gicht eine Coronarsklerose signifikant häufiger als bei den Kontrollpersonen gefunden. Bei 50 Patienten mit symptomloser Hyperuricämie (>7,3 mg-%) trat die Coronarsklerose nur wenig häufiger (9/7) auf als bei den Kontrollpersonen, der Unterschied war nicht signifikant. In dieser Untersuchung konnte auch gezeigt werden, daß bei Gichtpatienten mit einer Hypertriglyceridämie im Vergleich zu normolipidämischen Gichtpatienten die Coronarsklerose häufiger ist, auch dieser Unterschied war nicht signifikant (FRANK, 1974).

Wesentlich zuverlässigere Aussagen erlauben große prospektive Studien. Dort wurde eine repräsentative Gruppe der Bevölkerung über mehrere Jahre beobachtet und in regelmäßigen Abständen kontrolliert. Diese Personen boten zu Beginn der Studie keinen Hinweis auf eine Coronarkrankheit. Im Verlauf der Untersuchung ließ sich dann prüfen, ob Personen mit einem höheren Harnsäurespiegel häufiger eine Coronarsklerose entwickelten oder nicht. Bei dieser Auswertung mußten natürlich andere bekannte Risikofaktoren, wie Hypercholesterinämie oder Hypertonie, ausgeschaltet werden. Die Framingham-Studie begann mit 5127 Personen im Alter von 30—59 Jahren. Die Beobachtungsdauer erreichte 14 Jahre und mehr. Bei den 61 Männern mit einer Gicht trat die Coronarsklerose innerhalb von zehn Jahren doppelt so häufig auf wie in der gesamten untersuchten Gruppe. Nach Unterteilung aller Personen dieser Studie in mehrere Gruppen entsprechend der Höhe des Harnsäurespiegels hatten die Männer mit Werten über 7 mg-% doppelt so häufig eine Coronarsklerose wie die Männer mit Werten unter 4 mg-%. Wenn jedoch die Gichtpatienten aus der gesamten Population herausgenommen und außerdem Hypertonie und Übergewicht als zusätzliche Risikofaktoren berücksichtigt wurden, war die Beziehung zwischen Harnsäurespiegel und dem erhöhten Risiko einer Coronarkrankheit praktisch nicht mehr gegeben. Hypertonie und Hypercholesterinämie scheinen für das erhöhte Coronarrisiko des Gichtkranken nicht verantwortlich zu sein. Der Gichtkranke hat aber offensichtlich einen höheren Blutdruck und etwas höhere Cholesterinspiegel als Männer der übrigen Bevölkerung. Für den Hyperuricämiker ist ein erhöhtes Coronarrisiko durch den erhöhten Harnsäurespiegel nicht nachgewiesen (HALL et al., 1964; HALL, 1965).

Bei einer vergleichbaren Studie von Evans County, in der 2530 Personen beobachtet werden, fand man nach sieben Jahren bei Hyperuricämikern eine mäßige Zunahme der coronaren Herzkrankheit. Die Beziehung zwischen Harnsäurewerten und Coronarsklerose war jedoch statistisch nicht mehr signifikant, wenn andere Faktoren wie Hochdruck oder Übergewicht mit berücksichtigt wurden (KLEIN et al., 1973). Eine Auswertung von Daten aus der Tecumseh-Studie, in der nahezu 6000 Personen erfaßt waren, ergab, daß der Harnsäurespiegel von Personen mit Coronarkrankheit nicht signifikant höher lag als der Durchschnittswert der gesamten untersuchten Population. Es wurde daraus der Schluß gezogen, daß keine enge Beziehung zwischen der Hyperuricämie und der Entstehung der Coronarkrankheit bestehen könne (MYERS et al., 1968).

Auf Grund der Ergebnisse der epidemiologischen Studien und einzelner brauchbarer, weniger umfangreicher Untersuchungen muß man heute zu dem Schluß kommen, daß für den Gichtkranken ein erhöhtes Risiko einer Coronarkrankheit statistisch wahrscheinlich ist, für die symptomlose Hyperuricämie allein dagegen nicht. Es gibt zwar theoretische Überlegungen und experimentelle Ansätze, die über eine verkürzte Lebensdauer der Thrombocyten (JACOBS, 1972) oder eine gesteigerte Thrombocyten-Aggregation in vitro und in vivo eine Verbindung zwischen erhöhtem Harnsäurespiegel und Veränderungen der Gefäßwand herzustellen versuchen, ein Beweis dafür steht jedoch noch aus (NEWLAND, 1968; NORDÖY u. CHANDLER, 1964; GAARDER et al., 1961). Für die Sonderstellung des Gichtkranken gegenüber dem symptomlosen Hyperuricämiker bieten die epidemiologischen Studien bisher keine vernünftige Erklärung. Die symptomlose Hyperuricämie ist weniger als Risikofaktor, sondern wegen der möglichen Kombination mit anderen Stoffwechselstörungen als Risikoindikator zu bezeichnen.

Literatur

ACHESON, R. M.: Epidemiology of serum uric acid and gout: An example of the complexities of multifactorial cansation. Proced. roy. Soc. Med. **63**, 193—197 (1970).
ALLARD, C., GOULET, C.: Serum uric acid: not a discriminator of coronary heart disease in men and women. Canad. med. Ass. J. **109**, 986—988 (1973).
ANUMONYE, A., DOBSON, J. W., OPPENHEIM, S., SUTHERLAND, J. S.: Plasma uric acid concentrations among Edinburgh business executives. J. Amer. med. Ass. **208**, 1141—1148 (1969).
BABUCKE, G., MERTZ, D. P.: Häufigkeit der primären Hyperurikämie unter ambulanten Patienten. Münch. med. Wschr. **116**, 875—880 (1974).
BARLOW, K. A.: Hyperlipidemia in primary gout. Metabolism **17**, 289—299 (1968).
BARTELS, E. C., BALODIMOS, M. C., CORN, L. R.: The association of gout and diabetes mellitus. Med. Clin. N. Amer. **44**, 433—438 (1960).
BECKETT, A. G., LEWIS, J. G.: Gout and the serum uric acid in diabetes mellitus. Quart. J. Med. **29**, 443—458 (1960).
BENEDEK, T. G.: Correlations of serum uric acid and lipid concentrations in normal, gouty and atherosclerotic men. Ann. intern. Med. **66**, 851—861 (1967).

BERINGER, A., THALER, H.: Zusammenhänge zwischen Diabetes mellitus und Fettleber. Dtsch. med. Wschr. **95**, 836—838 (1970).
BERKOWITZ, D.: Blood lipid and uric acid interrelationships. J. Amer. med. Ass. **190**, 856—858 (1964).
BERKOWITZ, D.: Gout, hyperlipidemia and diabetes interrelationships. J. Amer. med. Ass. **197**, 117—120 (1966).
BERNHEIM, C.: Gotte et diabète. II. Le diabète et ses relations avec la goutte et l'hyperuricémie induites par les salidiurétiques. Schweiz. med. Wschr. **98**, 327—334 (1968).
BERNHEIM, C., OTT, H., ZAHND, G., MARTEN, E.: Goutte et diabète. I. La goutte et ses relations avec le diabète. Schweiz. med. Wschr. **98**, 33—41 (1968).
BLUESTONE, R., LEWIS, B., MERVART, I.: Hyperlipoproteinaemia in gout. Ann. rheum. Dis. **30**, 134—137 (1971).
BRØCHNER-MORTENSEN, K.: Gout. Ann. rheum. Dis. **17**, 1—8 (1958).
BURCH, T. A., O'BRIEN, W. M., NEED, R., KURLAND, L. T.: Hyperuricaemia and gout in the Mariana Islands. Ann. rheum. Dis. **25**, 114—122 (1966).
DARLINGTON, L. G., SCOTT, J. T.: Plasma lipid levels in gout. Ann. rheum. Dis. **31**, 487—489 (1972).
DITTRICH, P., SANDHOFER, F.: Partialfunktionen der Niere bei essentieller Hyperlipämie. Klin. Wschr. **45**, 690—691 (1967).
DREYFUS, F.: The role of hypouricemia in coronary heart disease. Dis. Chest. **38**, 332—337 (1960).
DUNN, J. P., BROOKS, G. W., MAUSNER, J., RODNAN, G. P., COBB, S.: Social class gradient of serum uric acid levels in males. J. Amer. med. Ass. **185**, 431—436 (1963).
DUNN, J. P., MOSES, C.: Correlation of serum lipids with uric acid and blood sugar in normal males. Metabolism **14**, 788—792 (1965).
EIDLITZ, M.: Uric acid and arteriosclerosis. Lancet **1961 II**, 1046—1047.
EMMERSON, B. T.: Alteration of urate metabolism by weight reduction. Aust. N. Z. J. Med. **3**, 410—412 (1973).
EMMERSON, B. T., DOUGLAS, W., DOHERTY, R. L., FEIGL, P.: Serum urate concentrations in the australian aboriginal. Ann. rheum. Dis. **28**, 150—158 (1969).
FELDMAN, E. B., WALLACE, S. L.: Hypertriglyceridemia in gout. Circulation **29**, 508—513 (1964).
FRANK, O.: Untersuchungen über die Häufigkeit von Störungen des Lipid- und Kohlenhydratstoffwechsels bei primärer Gicht und symptomloser Hyperurikämie. Wien. klin. Wschr. **86**, 252—256 (1974).
FREDRICKSON, D. S., LEVY, R. I.: Familial hyperlipoproteinemia. In: The metabolic basis of inherited disease, 3rd. Ed. (J. B. STANBURY, J. B. WYNGAARDEN, D. S. FREDRICKSON, Eds.). New York: McGraw Hill 1972.
FULTON, J. K.: Essential lipemia, acute gout, peripheral neuritis and myocardial disease in a negro man. Arch. intern. Med. **89**, 303—307 (1952).
GAARDER, A. M., JONSEN, J., LALAND, S., HELLEM, A. J., OWREN, P. A.: Adenosine diphosphate in red cells as a factor in the adhesiveness of human blood platelets. Nature **192**, 531—535 (1961).
GAMP, A., SCHILLING, F., MÜLLER, L., SCHACHERL, M.: Das klinische Bild der Gicht heute. Beobachtungen an 200 Kranken. Med. Klin. **60**, 129—134 (1965).
GERTLER, M. M., GARN, S. M., LEVINE, S. A.: Serum uric acid in relation to age and physique in health and in coronary artery disease. Ann. intern. Med. **34**, 1421—1431 (1951).
GERTLER, M. M., WOODBURY, M. A., GOTSCH, L. G., WHITE, P. D., RUSK, H. A.: The candidate for coronary heart disease. J. Amer. med. Ass. **170**, 149—152 (1959).
GIBSON, T., GRAHAME, R.: Gout and hyperlipidemia. In: Purin metabolism in man. Adv. exper. med. biology, Vol. 41 B, p. 499—508. New York-London: Rheum. Press 1974.
GOLDFINGER, S., KLINENBERG, J. R., SEEGMILLER, J. E.: Renal retention of uric acid induced by infusion of β-hydroxybutyrate and acetoacetate. New Engl. J. Med. **272**, 351—355 (1965).
GRAHAME, R., HASLAM, R. M., SCOTT, J. T.: Sulphobromophthalein retention in gout and asymptomatic hyperuricaemia. Ann. rheum. Dis. **27**, 19—26 (1968).
GRAHAME, R., SCOTT, J. T.: Clinical survey of 354 patients with gout. Ann. rheum. Dis. **29**, 461—468 (1970).
GREILING, H.: Zur klinischen Biochemie der Gicht. Dtsch. med. J. **20**, 336—341 (1969).
GRIEBSCH, A., ZÖLLNER, N.: Normalwerte der Plasmaharnsäure in Süddeutschland. Z. klin. Chem. **11**, 346—356 (1973).
GÜNTHER, R., HERBST, M., KNAPP, E.: Gicht und Hyperlipämie. Wien. klin. Wschr. **79**, 218—221 (1967).

GÜNTHER, R., KNAPP, E.: Der Einfluß von Allopurinol (Zyloric®) auf Harnsäure, Kreatinin, Nüchternblutzucker und Plasmalipide bei Gichtkranken. Wien. klin. Wschr. **82**, 78—82 (1970).

GÜNTHER, R., KNAPP, E., SILLER, K.: Gicht und Plasmalipidwerte. Wien. klin. Wschr. **80**, 577—581 (1968).

HALL, A. P.: Correlations among hyperuricemia, hypercholesterolemia, coronary disease and hypertension. Arthr. and Rheum. **8**, 846—852 (1965).

HALL, A. P., BARRY, P. E., DAWBER, T. R.: The relation between hyperuricemia and gouty arthritis and the risk of developing coronary heart disease. Arthr. and Rheum. **7**, 312—319 (1964).

HALL, A. P., BARRY, P. E., DAWBER, T. R., MCNAMARA, P. M.: Epidemiology of gout and hyperuricemia: a long-term population study. Amer. J. Med. **42**, 27—37 (1967).

HANSEN, O. E.: Hyperuricemia, gout and atherosclerosis. Amer. Heart J. **72**, 570—574 (1966).

HARRIS-JONES, J. N.: Hyperuricemia and essential hypercholesterolemia. Lancet **1957 I**, 857—860.

HASSLACHER, CH., WAHL, P., VOLLMAR, J.: Diabetes und Hyperurikämie. Dtsch. Med. Wschr. **99**, 2506—2510 (1974).

HEALEY, L. A., JR., CANER, J. E. Z., DECKER, J. L.: Ethnic variations in serum uric acid. Arthr. and Rheum. **9**, 288—297 (1966).

HEIDELMANN, G., THIELE, P.: Das Gichtproblem. Dresden: Steinkopff 1973.

HENNECKE, A., SÜDHOF, H.: Leberbeteiligung bei Gicht. Dtsch. med. Wschr. **95**, 59—62 (1970).

HENNINGES, D., MERTZ, D. P.: Urikopathie von Jugendlichen. Besonderheiten im klinischen Bild. Münch. med. Wschr. **113**, 458—462 (1971).

HERMAN, J. B.: Gout and diabetes. Metabolism **7**, 703—706 (1958).

HERMAN, J. B., MEDALIE, J. H., GOLDBOURT, U.: Diabetes and uric acid — a relationship investigated by the epidemiological method. In: Purin metabolism in man. Adv. exper. med. biol. Vol. 41 B. New York-London: Rheum. Press 1974.

HOLLISTER, L. E., OVERALL, J. E., SNOW, H. L.: Relationship of obesity to serum triglyceride, cholesterol and uric acid and to plasma-glucose levels. Amer. J. clin. Nutr. **20**, 777—782 (1967).

HOWELL, R. R., ASHTON, D. M., WYNGAARDEN, J. B.: Glucose-6-phosphatase deficiency glycogen storage disease: Studies on the interrelationships of carbohydrate, lipid, and purine abnormalities. Pediatrics **29**, 553—559 (1962).

IRMSCHER, K., GRIES, F. A., DIETEL, J., LÖLLGEN-HORRES, I.: Untersuchungen zur Harnsäureclearance bei primärer Hyperlipämie, Hyperlipämie-Hyperurikämiesyndrom und primärer Gicht. Verh. dtsch. Ges. inn. Med. **76**, 686—688 (1970).

ISHMAEL, W. K., OWENS, J. N., PAYNE, R. W., HONICK, M. D.: Diabetes mellitus in patients with gouty arthritis. J. Amer. med. Ass. **190**, 396—398 (1964).

JACOBS, D.: Hyperuricaemia and myocardial infarction. S. Afr. Med. J. **46**, 367—373 (1972).

JENSEN, J., BLANKENHORN, D. H., CHIN, H. P., STURGEON, P., WARE, A. G.: Serum lipids and serum uric acid in human twins. J. Lipid Res. **6**, 193—205 (1965).

JENSEN, J., BLANKENHORN, D. H., KORNERUP, V.: Blood-uric-acid levels in familial hypercholesterolaemia. Lancet **1966 I**, 298—300.

JOSLIN, E. P., ROOT, H. F., WHITE, P., MARBLE, A.: Treatment of diabetes mellitus, 9th Ed., p. 93. Philadelphia: Lea & Febiger 1952.

KASL, S. V., COBB, S., BROOKS, G. W.: Changes in serum uric acid and cholesterol levels in men undergoing job loss. J. Amer. med. Ass. **206**, 1500—1507 (1968).

KELLEY, W., N., GREEN, M. L., ROSENBLOOM, F. M., HENDERSON, J. F., SEEGMILLER, J. E.: Hypoxanthineguanine phosphoribosyl-transferase deficiency in gout. Ann. intern. Med. **70**, 155—161 (1969).

KLEIN, W. W.: Leberfunktion bei Gicht und asymptomatischer Hyperurikämie. Z. Rheumaforsch. **30**, 230—235 (1971).

KLEIN, R., KLEIN, B. E., CORNONI, J. C., MAREADY, J., CASSEL, J. C., TYROLER, H. A.: Serum uric acid. Its relationship to coronary heart disease risk factors and cardiovascular disease, Evans Country Georgia. Arch. intern. Med. **132**, 401—410 (1973).

KNICK, B.: Aktuelle Probleme der Fettleber. Dtsch. med. J. **19**, 389—396 (1968).

KNICK, B., LANGE, H. J., RITTER, U., SCHILLING, F.: Adipositas, hypertriglyceridämie, Fettleber und latenter Diabetes bei Gichtpatienten. Therapiewoche **18**, 2071—2072 (1968).

KOHN, P. M., PROZAN, G. B.: Hyperuricemia-relationship to hypercholesteremia and acute myocardial infarction. J. Amer. med. Ass. **170**, 1909—1912 (1959).

KŘIŽEK, V.: Serum uric acid in relation to body weight. Ann. rheum. Dis. **25**, 456—459 (1966).

KUZELL, W. C., SCHAFFARZICK, R. W., NANGLER, W. E., KOETS, P., MANKLE, E. A., BROWN, B., CHAMPLIN, B.: Some observations on 520 gouty patients. J. chron. Dis. **2**, 645—669 (1955).

LANESE, R. R., HRESHAM, G. E., KELLER, M. D.: Behavioral and physiological characteristics in hyperuricemia. J. Amer. med. Ass. **207**, 1878—1882 (1969).
LANG, P. D.: Fettstoffwechselstörungen bei Gicht. Münch. med. Wschr. **116**, 909—912 (1974).
LAWEE, D.: Uric acid: The clinical application of 1000 unsolicitated determinations. Canad. Med. Ass. J. **100**, 838—841 (1969).
LIEBER, C. S., JONES, D. P., LOSOWSKY, M. S., DAVIDSON, C. S.: Interrelation of uric acid and ethanol metabolism in man. J. clin. Invest. **41**, 1863—1870 (1962).
LIEBSCHER, K.: Hyperurikämie bei Herzinfarktpatienten. Z. ges. inn. Med. **27**, 492—494 (1972).
LONDON, M., HUMS, M.: Distribution patterns of uric acid in coronary heart disease. Clin. Chem. **13**, 132—141 (1967).
MARINOFF, S. G., LEMPERT, P., MANDEL, E. E.: Association of hypercholesterolemia with hyperuricemia. A review of the literature. Chicago Med. School Quart. **22**, 135—142 (1962).
McKECHNIE, J. K.: Gout, hyperuricemia and carbohydrate metabolism. S. Afr. Med. J. **38**, 182—185 (1964).
MERTZ, D. P.: Gicht, Grundlagen, Klinik und Therapie, 2. Aufl. Stuttgart: Thieme 1973.
MERTZ, D. P., BABUCKE, G.: Epidemiologie und klinisches Bild der primären Gicht. Beobachtungen zwischen 1948 und 1968. Münch. med. Wschr. **113**, 617—623 (1971).
MERTZ, D. P., BABUCKE, G.: Die Dyslipoproteinämie bei primärer Gicht. Dtsch. med. Wschr. **98**, 1457—1462 (1973).
MIELANTS, H., VEYS, E. M., DEWEERDT, A.: Gout and its relation to lipid metabolism. II Correlations between uric acid, lipid, and lipoprotein levels in gout. Ann. rheum. Dis. **32**, 506—509 (1973).
MIKKELSEN, W. M.: The possible association of hyperuricemia and/or gout with diabetes mellitus. Arthr. and Rheum. **8**, 853—859 (1965).
MYERS, A. R., EPSTEIN, F. H., DODGE, H. J., MIKKELSEN, W. M.: The relationship of serum uric acid to risk factors in coronary heart disease. Amer. J. Med. **45**, 520—528 (1968).
NEWLAND, H.: Antagonism of the antithrombotic effect of Warfarin by uric acid. Amer. J. med. Sci. **256**, 44—49 (1968).
NORDÖY, A., CHANDLER, A. B.: Platelet thrombosis induced by adenosine diphosphate in the rat. Scand. J. Haemat. **1**, 16—23 (1964).
O'BRIEN, W. M., BURCH, T. A., BUNIM, J. J.: The genetics of hyperuricemia in Blackfeet and Pima Indians. Ann. rheum. Dis. **25**, 117—123 (1966).
PAULUS, H. E., COUTTS, A., CALABRO, J. J., KLINENBERG, J. R.: Clinical significance of hyperuricemia in routinely screened hospitalized men. J. Amer. med. Ass. **211**, 277—281 (1970).
VON PEENEN, H. J.: The causes of nonazotemic hyperuricemie. Amer. J. clin. Path. **55**, 698—705 (1971).
POLLITT, J., DOBRYSZYCKA, W., CARNEY, A., KUKRAL, J. C.: Serum cholesterol, uric acid and triglyceride concentrations in patients with Buerger's disease, arteriosclerosis obliterans, venous thromboses and Raynand's disease. J. Amer. med. Ass. **204**, 530 (1968).
PRIOR, I. A. M., ROSE, B. S., HARVEY, H. P. B., DAVIDSON, F.: Hyperuricaemia, gout and diabetic abnormality in polynesian people. Lancet **1966 I**, 333—338.
SCHETTLER, G.: Risikofaktoren beim Herzinfarkt. Dtsch. med. Wschr. **97**, 533—538 (1972).
SCHILLING, F.: Gicht-Diagnose, Differentialdiagnose und Therapie. Ärztl. Fortbild. **16**, 36—47 (1967).
SCHILLING, F.: Klinik der Gicht. Therapiewoche **22**, 92—98 (1972).
SCHILLING, F.: Klinik und Therapie der Gicht und deren Abgrenzung von der Pseudogicht. In: Fettsucht-Gicht (W. Boecker, Hrsg.), S. 139—160. Stuttgart: Thieme 1971.
SCHREIBMAN, P. H., WILSON, D. E., ARKY, R. A.: Familial type IV hyperlipoproteinemia. New Engl. J. Med. **281**, 981—989 (1969).
SCOTT, J. T., HALL, A. P., GRAHAME, R.: Allopurinol in treatment of gout. Brit. med. J. **1966 II**, 321—327.
STREJČEK, J., KUČEROVÁ, L.: Idiopathic hyperlipidemia and gout. Acta rheum. scand. **14**, 95—101 (1968).
SUSIČ, D.: Serumlipid- und Harnsäurewerte von 177 Gelegenheitsblutspendern und 116 Patienten nach Myokardinfarkt. Klin. Wschr. **48**, 847—852 (1970).
SUSIČ, D., BÄUMER, A., SCHULTZ, D.: Serum-Harnsäurewerte von 113 Patienten mit Zustand nach Herzinfarkt. Z. klin. Chem. **7**, 197—198 (1969).
TALBOTT, J. H.: Gout and gouty arthritis. In: Modern Medical Monographs 7, p. 49. New York: Grune & Stratton 1953.
TALBOTT, J. H.: Gout, 3rd Ed. New York: Grune & Stratton 1967.

THIELE, P., HEIDELMANN, G., GÄRTNER, A., SCHNEIDER, V., TELLKAMP, F.: Aktuelle Gichtprobleme. Z. ges. inn. Med. **25**, 458—466 (1970).
TREMEL, R., POHL, W.: Leberbefunde bei Gicht. Med. Klin. **66**, 777—781 (1971).
UPMARK, A. E., ADNER, M. L.: Coronary infarction and gout. Acta med. scand. **139**, 1—9 (1950).
VOGELBERG, K. H., GRIES, F. A., DIETL, J.: Klinik und Behandlung der Insulinresistenz bei primärer Hyperlipoproteinämie. Dtsch. med. Wschr. **98**, 1751—1758 (1973).
WEISS, T. E., SEGARLOFF, A., MOORE, C.: Gout and diabetes. Metabolism **6**, 103—106 (1957).
WEYLAND, N.: Beobachtungen an chronischen Gichtkranken. Münch. med. Wschr. **111**, 590—591 (1969).
WHITEHOUSE, F. W., CLEARY, W. J., JR.: Diabetes mellitus in patients with gout. J. Amer. med. Ass. **197**, 73—76 (1966).
WIEDEMANN, E., ROSE, H. G., SCHWARTZ, E.: Plasma lipoproteins, glucose tolerance and insulin response in primary gout. Amer. J. Med. **53**, 299—307 (1972).
WOLLENWEBER, J., DOENECKE, P., GRETEN, H., HILD, R., NOBBE, F., SCHMIDT, F. H., WAGNER, E.: Zur Häufigkeit von Hyperlipidämie, Hyperurikämie, Diabetes mellitus, Hypertonie und Übergewicht bei arterieller Verschlußkrankheit. Dtsch. med. Wschr. **96**, 103—107 (1971).
ZALOKAR, J., LELLOUCH, J., CLAUDE, J. R., KUNTZ, D.: Epidemiology of serum uric acid and gout in Frenchmen. J. chron. Dis. **27**, 59—75 (1974).
ZÖLLNER, N.: Eine einfache Modifikation der enzymatischen Harnsäurebestimmung. Normalwerte in der deutschen Bevölkerung. Z. klin. Chem. **1**, 178—182 (1963).
ZÖLLNER, N.: Grundlagen der Gichtforschung. Münch. med. Wschr. **116**, 865—874 (1974).
ZÖLLNER, N., GRIEBSCH, A., GRÖBNER, W.: Einfluß verschiedener Purine auf den Harnsäurestoffwechsel. Ernährungs-Umschau **3**, 79—82 (1972).

2. Verlauf der Gicht
a) Gelenkgicht
aa) Der akute Gichtanfall

Von

M. Marshall und M. Schattenkirchner

Mit 6 Abbildungen

Eine auf persönlicher Erfahrung beruhende Beschreibung des akuten Gichtanfalls von Thomas Sydenham (1683) lautet folgendermaßen:

"The victim goes to bed and sleeps in good health. About two o'clock in the morning he is awakened by a severe pain in the great toe; more rarely in the heel, ankle or instep. This pain is like that of dislocation, and yet the parts feel as if cold water were poured over them. Then follow chills and shivers, and little fever. The pain, which was at first moderate, becomes more intense. With its intensity the chills and shivers increase. After a time this comes to its height, accomodating itself to the bones and ligaments of the tarsus and metatarsus. Now it is a violent stretching and tearing of the ligaments — now it is a gnawing pain, and now a pressure and tightening. So exquisite and lively meanwhile is the feeling of the part affected, that it cannot bear the weight of the bedclothes nor the jar of a person walking in the room. The night is passed in torture, sleeplessness, turning of the part affected, and perpetual change of posture."

Diese vielzitierte, klassische Beschreibung besitzt auch heute noch ihre Gültigkeit. Aus genauen Schilderungen wissen wir, daß nicht nur der Arzt Thomas Sydenham, der sich auch wissenschaftlich mit der Gicht beschäftigte, an dieser Krankheit litt; auch eine Reihe berühmter geschichtlicher Persönlichkeiten, wie z.B. Martin Luther, Herzog Christoph von Württemberg, A. von Wallenstein, Friedrich der Grosse, Horace Walpole, J.W. von Goethe und Ch. Darwin sollen an Gicht gelitten haben.

Der akute Gichtanfall ist meist die erste eindrucksvolle klinische Manifestation einer Krankheit, deren Verlauf nach Brugsch (1930) sowie Zöllner (1959) in vier Stadien eingeteilt wird:

1. asymptomatische Gichtanlage,
2. akuter Gichtanfall,
3. interkritische Gicht,
4. chronische Gicht.

Die Klinik der akuten Gicht

Bevorzugt betroffen ist der Mann mittleren Alters, nach Hall et al. (1967) sowie Grahame u. Scott (1970) etwa von der fünften Lebensdekade an (Abb. 1). Von Männern, die das 65. Lebensjahr erreichen, erleiden 2,8% einen Gichtanfall (Hall et al., 1967). Frauen werden seltener — in weniger als 10% der Fälle (Babucke u. Mertz, 1973; Grahame u. Scott, 1970) — und dann jenseits des Klimakteriums (6. Dekade) betroffen (Grahame u. Scott, 1970). Nach neueren Untersuchungen von Henninges u. Mertz (1971) und Babucke u. Mertz (1973) ist es zu einer deutlichen Vorverlagerung des Gipfels der Erstmanifestationen der

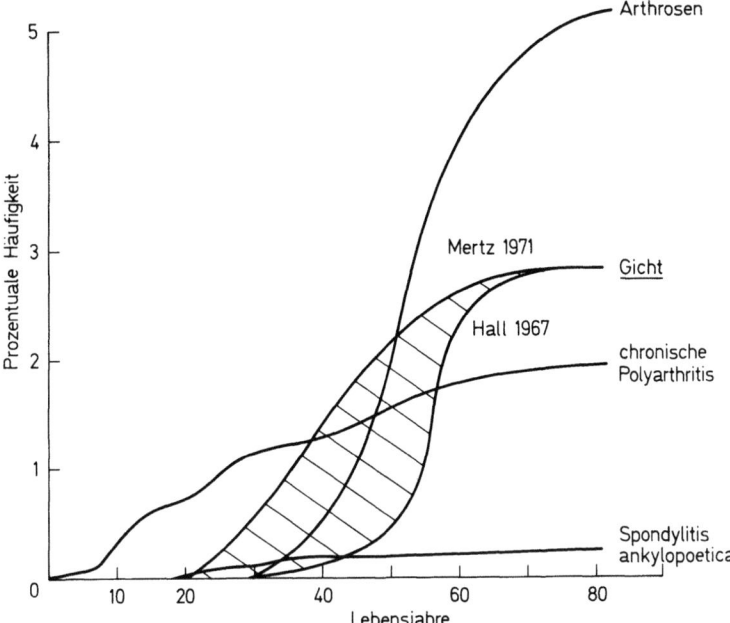

Abb. 1. Alter bei Auftreten der ersten Erscheinungen der Gicht und weiterer Gelenkkrankheiten (kumulative Häufigkeiten) in Prozenten der Gesamtbevölkerung der jeweiligen Altersstufen, bei Gicht in Prozenten der männlichen Bevölkerung (nach HALL et al., 1967; und umgerechnet nach MERTZ u. BABUCKE, 1971) (nach KORFMACHER u. ZÖLLNER, 1974)

Gicht als Gelenkerkrankung um rund zwei Jahrzehnte gegenüber früher gekommen. Dies wird auf Auswirkungen des Luxuskonsums in den hochindustrialisierten Ländern zurückgeführt.

Weiterhin besteht eine deutliche Abhängigkeit zwischen dem Lebensalter, bei dem der erste Gichtanfall auftritt, und dem Grad der Hyperuricämie insofern, als das Erkrankungsalter um so niedriger ist, je höher die Plasmaharnsäurekonzentration liegt (10 mg/100 ml entsprechend einem Alter unter 40 Jahren, 7 mg/100 ml entsprechend einem Alter über 70 Jahren) (MERTZ u. BABUCKE, 1971).

Faktoren, die für die klinische Manifestation der Gicht — bei vorhandener erblicher Disposition — von Bedeutung sind, sind Geschlecht, Alter, auch Rasse, Umweltfaktoren und Medikamente.

Auslösende Momente des Gichtanfalls

Pathogenetisch entscheidend (vgl. auch Kapitel IV) ist eine akute Änderung des Plasmaharnsäurespiegels im Sinne einer Erhöhung oder Verminderung. Diesbezüglich läßt sich folgende Einteilung treffen (in Anlehnung an ZÖLLNER, 1970):

1. Vermehrte Purinzufuhr: (Fett- und purinreiche) Festessen (Innereien, Fleischextrakt, Spinat, Erbsen, Hülsenfrüchte), Schlemmereien etc. Etwa 70% der Gichtpatienten sind lebensfrohe Pykniker (DRUBE u. REINWEIN, 1959; GARROD, 1853; LICHTWITZ u. STEINITZ, 1926). Beruflich gefährdet sind Köche, Gastwirte, Schlächter, Bierbrauer (s.u.); allerdings ist bei den heutigen nivellierten Lebens- und Eßgewohnheiten in allen zivilisierten Ländern eine berufliche ebenso wie eine soziale Disposition für Gicht nicht mehr so auffällig.

2. Verminderte Harnsäureausscheidung: Alkohol, natriuretisch wirkende Arzneimittel (Saluretica [Abb. 3], Acetazolamid, Salicylate in niedrigen Dosen, Quecksilberdiuretica), ketogene Kostformen (Fettmahlzeiten), Ketoacidose (Diabetes, Fastenkuren, Nulldiät), erhöhter Milchsäurespiegel (Glykogenose), parenterale Applikation von Penicillin. (Es handelt sich dabei um Substanzen, die direkt oder indirekt bei der tubulären Ausscheidung mit der Harnsäure konkurrieren.)

3. Vermehrte endogene Uratbildung: Zellzerfall, Pneumonie im Lösungsstadium, Röntgenbestrahlung oder Cytostaticabehandlung von Leukämien und Carcinomen, Anämien während der Regeneration, Operationsnachperiode, Bluttransfusionen (KUZELL u. GAUDIN, 1956).

4. Vermehrte Uratbildung durch Adrenalinausschüttung oder Anregung der Nebennierenrinde: Infekte, Operationen, Traumen, allergische Reaktionen, ungewohnte körperliche Anstrengungen (GUDZENT, 1928) oder allgemein physischer und psychischer Streß („Messe- oder Ausstellungsgicht").

5. Unbekannter Auslösungsmechanismus: Blei, Ergotamin, Thiamin, Insulin.

Manche Autoren beschreiben außerdem eine gewisse jahreszeitliche Rhythmik mit einem ausgesprochenen Frühjahrsgipfel und weniger ausgeprägten Herbstgipfel; nach anderen Autoren besteht diese jahreszeitliche Bevorzugung nicht (TALBOTT, 1967; ZÖLLNER, 1960).

Die Bedeutung eines Mikrotraumas als lokalisierender Faktor ist bereits länger in Diskussion (BRICOUT, 1935). In diese Richtung sprechen z. B. Beobachtungen von MUGLER (1969), daß Patienten, die Krücken benützen müssen, gehäuft Gichtanfälle an Händen und Ellbogen erleiden („aufsteigende Gicht"); weiterhin der Begriff der „Gaspedal-Gicht" nach langen Autofahrten, der Befall von Gelenken der oberen Extremität bei Lastwagenfahrern und atypische Gichtformen bei Sportlern (Knöchel und Kniegelenke bei Fußballspielern, Kniegelenke bei Skiläufern, Ellenbogen bei Tennisspielern u. a.).

Bevorzugte Lokalisationen

Akute Gichtattacken betreffen ganz bevorzugt die Gelenke: Podagra, Gonagra, Chiragra, Omagra (Abb. 2—5). Es kann aber — besonders in fortgeschritteneren Stadien der Gicht — auch ein subcutaner Tophus, eine mit Urat infiltrierte Bursa oder Sehnenscheide sich akut entzünden und extrem schmerzhaft sein.

Der eigentliche Gichtanfall betrifft synovialisausgekleidete Räume. Unter den gichtigen Bursitiden kommt die Bursitis urica olecrani besonders häufig vor. Bei gründlicher Anamneseerhebung bei Gichtpatienten erfährt man nicht selten eine Schleimbeutelentzündung am Ellenbogen vor der ersten Gelenksattacke.

Betroffen kann jedes Gelenk werden, aber bevorzugt sind die Gelenke der unteren Extremität. Diese Bevorzugung wird mit Orthostase erklärt (MUGLER, 1969); speziell beim Großzehengrundgelenk sollte aber auch die besondere mechanische Belastung beachtet werden. Es können ein oder selten auch mehrere Gelenke gleichzeitig betroffen sein, oder verschiedene Gelenke können hintereinander betroffen werden.

In etwa zwei Drittel der Fälle beginnt die Gicht mit dem Befall eines Gelenkes. In etwa 50% ist der erste Anfall im Großzehengrundgelenk lokalisiert ohne Seitenbevorzugung (die Angaben schwanken zwischen 46 und 72% [GAMP et al., 1965; BABUCKE u. MERTZ, 1973]). Der klassische Gichtanfall im Großzehengrundgelenk wird in 70 bis 95% als typisches anamnestisches Symptom angegeben.

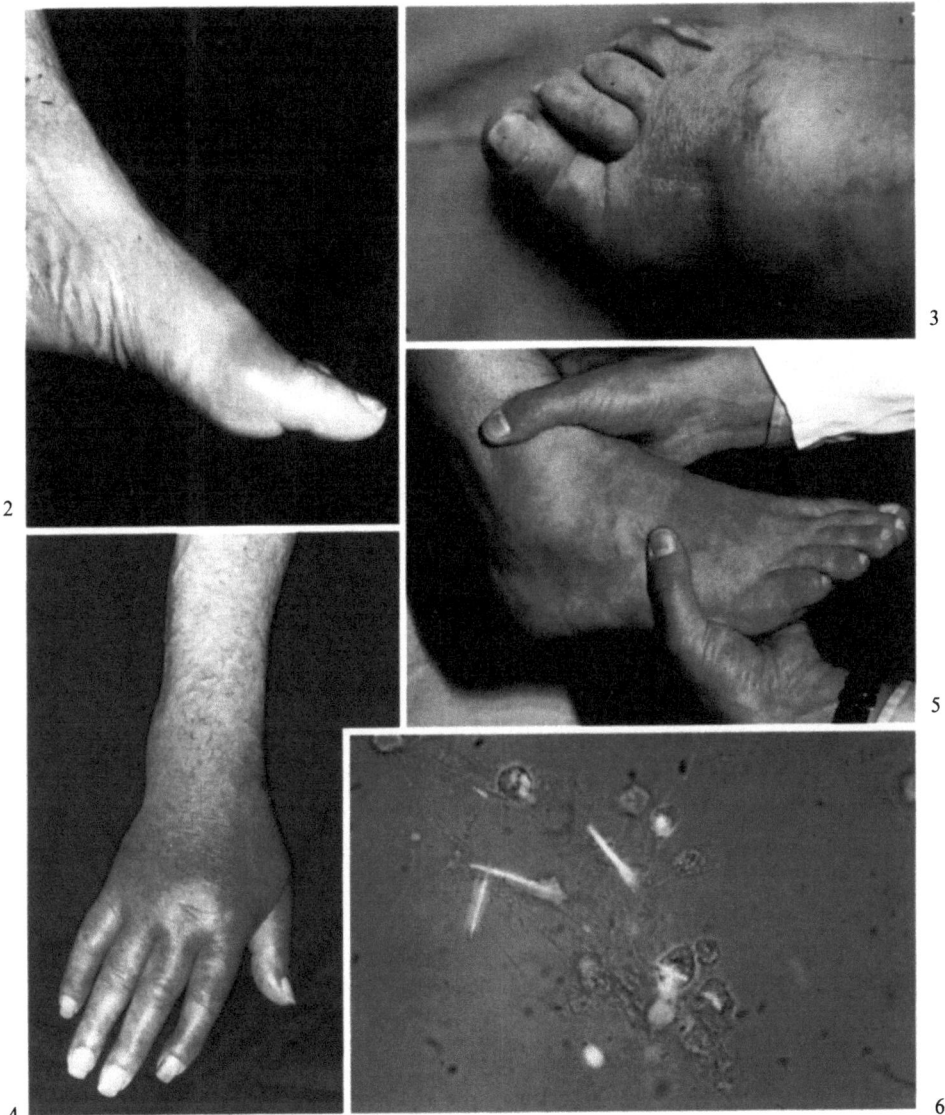

Abb. 2. Typische Podagra

Abb. 3. Podagra bei einer Frau in der Menopause unter Diureticatherapie

Abb. 4. Gichtanfall an der Hand

Abb. 5. Gichtanfall im Sprunggelenk

Abb. 6. Harnsäurekristalle — zum Teil phagocytiert — im Gelenkpunktat

Folgende Gelenke sind in absteigender Reihenfolge bevorzugt betroffen:

Tabelle 1. Reihenfolge des Gelenkbefalls bei der Gicht (Angaben in Prozent)

	Nach Schilling (1971) (n = 200)		Nach Babucke u. Mertz (1973) (n = 90; 82 Männer, 8 Frauen)		
	Erstanfall	später	gesamt	Männer	Frauen
Großzehengrundgelenk	46	74	72	74	50
Übriger Fuß	35	73	10	11	0
Kniegelenk	22	56	3,3	3,7	0
Hände	7	15	10	6,1	50
Ellbogengelenk		2	2,2	2,4	0
Schultergelenk			1,1	1,2	0
Hüftgelenk		unter 1			
Weitere Unterteilung					
Sprunggelenk			9	9.8	0
Handgelenk			6,7	6,1	12,5
Fußwurzel			4,5	4,9	0
Fingergelenk			3,3	0	40
übrige Zehengelenke			1,1	1,2	0
Daumengrundgelenk			0	0	0
Beginn monoarticulär 62 bi- bis polyarticulär 38			Erstattacke monoarticulär 85 bi- bis polyarticulär 15		

Die Reihenfolge des Gelenkbefalls stimmt auch mit Untersuchungen anderer Autoren weitestgehend überein.

Bei den Zahlen von Schilling (Tab. 1) ist zu berücksichtigen, daß es sich um ein in gewisser Weise selektioniertes Krankengut einer Rheumaklinik handelt. Bezüglich der Einteilung in monoarticulären und bi- bis polyarticulären Beginn ist anzumerken, daß sich häufig die erste Attacke an einem Gelenk abspielt und innerhalb von Tagen bis Wochen noch weitere Gelenke befallen werden können; deswegen wird diese Einteilung von Autor zu Autor differieren können.

Mitunter sind beide Großzehen gleichzeitig betroffen.

Auch wenn Babucke u. Mertz (Mertz, 1973) meinen, aus ihrem Zahlenmaterial (Tab. 1) keine nennenswerte Abweichung in der Reihenfolge des ersten Gelenkbefalls bei weiblichen gegenüber männlichen Gichtpatienten ablesen zu können, stimmen u.E. ihre Angaben gut mit Befunden von Zöllner überein (1967), wonach bei Frauen in der Menopause bevorzugt die Fingergelenke betroffen sind.

Klinische Symptomatik

Zuverlässige Vorboten sind nicht überzeugend nachgewiesen. Im individuellen Fall kann sich der Anfall aber durch mehr oder weniger unspezifische Anzeichen in Form eines Prodromalstadiums ankündigen mit vasomotorischen Störungen, Flatulenz, Obstipation, Oberbauchbeschwerden, psychischen Veränderungen wie Depressionen, Schlaflosigkeit, Nykturie, Polyurie, Palpitationen oder unklaren muskelrheumatischen Beschwerden.

Das dramatische, plötzliche Einsetzen heftigster Gelenkschmerzattacken mit intensiver entzündlicher Reaktion — häufig das Großzehengrundgelenk betreffend — ist nahezu pathognomonisch für Gicht (Abb. 2).

Der Gelenkgicht können andere Manifestationen der essentiellen Hyperuricämie vorausgehen, besonders Hypertonie (diastolische Werte über 100 mm Hg) bzw. Zeichen für Nierenschäden (Gichtniere mit Pyelonephritis und evt. Nierensteinkoliken). Aber nur in Ausnahmefällen wird die Diagnose „familiäre Hyperuricämie" vor dem ersten Gichtanfall gestellt.

Der akute Gichtanfall beginnt plötzlich oder zeigt eine Entwicklung über mehrere Stunden bis Tage. Häufig beginnt er in der Nacht und wird dann oft besonders dramatisch empfunden (manche Autoren können keine Abhängigkeit von der Tageszeit nachweisen [ZÖLLNER, 1967]); manchmal fallen die Beschwerden aber erst morgens bei Belastung des betroffenen Gelenks auf.

Lokalsymptome

Das akute Gichtgelenk gleicht einem septischen Prozeß mit den typischen Zeichen der Entzündung. Das betroffene Gelenk (meist Metatarsophalangealgelenk I) kann innerhalb weniger Stunden stark anschwellen, es wird heiß, bläulich- bis düsterrot (periarthritische Rötung) (Abb. 2—5), extrem schmerzhaft und druckempfindlich. Der Patient kann im ausgeprägten Fall weder den Druck der Bettdecke oder des Schuhs noch Erschütterungen ertragen. Das entzündliche Ödem überschreitet gewöhnlich die Gelenkgrenzen und ist ausgeprägter als bei anderen akuten Arthritiden. Es kann bei großen Gelenken mitunter eine ganz erhebliche Ausdehnung erreichen. Der Gichtschmerz ist zu einem geringen Teil durch einen Erguß in die Gelenkhöhle (denn die Synovialis ist druckempfindlich), hauptsächlich durch ein entzündliches Ödem der umgebenden Gewebe bedingt. Seltener kann es zu stärkeren, nachweisbaren Ergüssen in größeren Gelenken (Kniegelenk) kommen.

Die Haut ist gespannt und glänzend. Die oberflächlichen Venen sind erweitert, und es kommt manchmal zur Phlebitis um das entzündete Gelenk. Das glänzende, bläulichrote ("cyanotic purple") Aussehen der Haut über dem Gichtgelenk ist typisch und differentialdiagnostisch gegen eine Infektion verwertbar (in extrem seltenen Fällen kann eine Gichtarthritis mit einer infektiös-eitrigen Arthritis zusammentreffen — cave: Penicillin kann die akute Gelenkgicht verschlimmern).

Selten können Gichtanfälle auch Sehnenansätze (Ferse, Kniescheibe) und Schleimbeutel (Ellenbogen — s. o.) betreffen (SCHILLING, 1969). Nuchale oder occipitale Sehnenansatzentzündungen zeichnen sich durch akute Nackensteifigkeit aus. In Polynesien, wo die Gicht zehnmal häufiger ist als in den USA, wird die entzündliche Schwellung der Achillessehne als ein typisches Diagnosticum für Gicht angesehen (SLADE, 1967). Gicht kann sich auch in rezidivierend auftretenden Muskelschmerzen, beispielsweise in den Waden, in den Oberschenkeln und im Nacken manifestieren. Diese Schmerzen nehmen über einige Tage zu und können sich über drei bis vier Wochen hinziehen (RÜCKERT u. CHOWANETZ, 1972).

Begleitsymptome

Die systemischen Auswirkungen des akuten Gichtanfalls können denen der akuten Sepsis gleichen. Es kommt zu Störung des Allgemeinbefindens meist mit Fieber, Schüttelfrost, Tachykardie, Verdauungsstörungen, Nausea und Anorexie, Kopfschmerz, Steifheit, Polyurie und Nykturie. Fieberspitzen bis 40° C sind bei schwerem Gelenkbefall nicht selten. Manchmal besteht gleichzeitig eine Episkleritis.

Typische Laborbefunde

Im Gichtanfall haben über 98% der Patienten eine Hyperuricämie, das heißt Werte über 6,5 mg/100 ml (falls nicht eine Behandlung mit Phenylbutazon, Salicylaten oder mit uricosurischen Mitteln erfolgte). Daneben kommt es typischerweise zu Leukocytose (bis 15000/mm^3) und Akute-Phase-Reaktionen (BKS bis auf 90 mm n.W. in der ersten Stunde, α_2-Globuline und CRP stark vermehrt).

Die Synovialflüssigkeit zeichnet sich durch folgende Befunde aus: sie ist wolkig-trüb (Schrift kann nicht hindurch gelesen werden); die Farbe ist gelb bis milchig; die Viscosität ist vermindert; es finden sich keine Erythrocyten, aber eine Leukocytose bis 15000/mm^3 und mehr, überwiegend bestehend aus segmentkernigen Granulocyten (SCHILLING, 1969); Bakterien oder Kollagenfasern sind nicht nachweisbar; differentialdiagnostisch entscheidend ist die Beobachtung von Uratkristallen, zum Teil phagocytiert durch Granulocyten (Abb. 6) — am besten im polarisierten Licht in der frisch entnommenen Synovialflüssigkeit.

Die Diagnose des akuten Gichtanfalls ergibt sich somit aus Eigen- und Familienanamnese, Lokalbefund, allgemein klinischem Befund, Laborwerten mit Analyse der Synovialflüssigkeit, evtl. Röntgenbefund und gutem therapeutischen Ansprechen auf Colchicin.

Verlauf des akuten Anfalls

Die Dauer eines spontan ablaufenden Anfalls kann nicht vorausgesagt werden. Der erste Anfall kann kurzdauernd sein und innerhalb weniger Stunden ebenso schnell verschwinden, wie er aufgetreten ist, mit völliger Wiederherstellung einer normalen Gelenkfunktion. Andererseits kann ein Anfall Tage oder sogar Wochen anhalten — meist liegt die Dauer zwischen drei Tagen bis zwei Wochen. Der stark wechselnde Verlauf des akuten Gichtanfalls bezüglich Schwere und Dauer muß bei jeder Beurteilung des Erfolgs einer bestimmten Therapie berücksichtigt werden.

Unter adäquater Behandlung muß es beim akuten Gichtanfall innerhalb von 24 Std zu deutlicher Besserung und spätestens nach drei Tagen zu weitgehender Normalisierung der Funktion kommen. Bei sehr schweren Anfällen kann die völlige Wiederherstellung eine bis mehrere Wochen in Anspruch nehmen. Bestehen schwere Gelenksymptome über mehrere Wochen, kann es sich entweder um wiederholte Einzelanfälle oder um einen verzögerten Anfall handeln. Patienten mit fortgeschrittenen gichtigen Veränderungen neigen mehr zu verzögerten Verläufen der Arthritisanfälle.

Mit Abklingen der Symptome kann ein eindellbares Ödem ("pitting edema") beobachtet werden, und die Haut über der Läsion wird dünn und lose. Wenn ein akuter Anfall mehrere Tage angehalten hat, kann es zur Hautdesquamation im Bereich und in der Umgebung des betroffenen Gelenks kommen, nachdem sich die Funktion wieder normalisiert hat.

Je rascher die normale Funktion erreicht wird, um so besser ist das klinische Ergebnis. Wichtig ist der frühzeitige Gebrauch des betroffenen Gelenks nach Abklingen des Anfalls.

Weiterer Verlauf der Gelenkgicht

Nach den meisten initialen akuten Gichtattacken kommt es zur völligen subjektiven und objektiven Wiederherstellung der Gelenksfunktion.

Die meisten Attacken folgen dem klassischen Typ; allerdings sind Abweichungen vom klassischen Bild häufiger als allgemein angenommen wird (ZÖLLNER, 1970).

Die Intervalle zwischen den Attacken heißen „interkritische Phasen" ("intercritical periods"). Sie dauern unterschiedlich lange; meist wiederholen sich die Attacken innerhalb von ein bis zwei Jahren, ohne zunächst Gelenkveränderungen zu hinterlassen. Vereinzelt kann die Dauer einer interkritischen Phase acht bis zehn Jahre betragen.

Die Phasen werden fortschreitend kürzer — obwohl bei vielen Patienten die klinischen Zeichen einer chronisch tophösen Gicht fehlen. Schließlich kommt es zu Gelenksanfällen mehrmals im Jahr — oft mit einer gewissen Regelmäßigkeit (bei manchen Patienten wiederholen sich die Anfälle jeden Frühling und Herbst).

Patienten mit ausgedehnten Uratablagerungen in und um betroffene Gelenke haben bei fehlender prophylaktischer Behandlung eine höhere Anfallsfrequenz, die mit fortschreitender Zerstörung der Gelenkstrukturen wieder abnimmt.

Die Anfallsrezidive können oft bereits früher befallene Gelenke betreffen. Üblicherweise nimmt die Schwere der Gelenksymptome bei rezidivierenden Anfällen zu. Spätere Anfälle können oft mehrere Gelenke betreffen. In seltenen Fällen bleiben selbst die Wirbel-, Sternoclavicular- und Kiefergelenke nicht verschont.

Patienten, die in der fünften Dekade ihres Lebens erstmals einen Gichtanfall in milder Ausprägung erleben, erleiden in den gesamten verbleibenden Jahren im allgemeinen nur wenig Rezidive. Ein geringer Prozentsatz von Patienten zeigt eine ungewöhnlich benigne Form der Gicht mit nur einem oder einigen wenigen Anfällen insgesamt — auch ohne Therapie. (Nach Feststellungen der Framingham-Studie dürfte es sich um Anfälle bei Patienten mit nur wenig erhöhtem Plasmaharnsäurespiegel handeln. Nach eigener Erfahrung gibt es allerdings auch Patienten, die trotz deutlich erhöhter Harnsäure (9 mg/100 ml) über längere Zeit nur leichte Anfälle erleiden.)

Kurze Differentialdiagnose des Gichtanfalles

(Ausführliche Darstellung in Kapitel VI.2.a.cc)

Wenngleich akute Arthritiden bei anderen Erkrankungen kaum so akut auftreten, daß man von einem Gelenkanfall sprechen kann, und somit die anfallsartige Arthritis nahezu pathognomonisch für die Gicht ist, müssen doch bei der Diagnose der Gicht vielfach eine Reihe von anderen Krankheiten und Störungen, bei denen Mono- oder Oligoarthritiden auftreten, differentialdiagnostisch erwogen werden.

So kennen wir sehr akute Mono- oder Oligoarthritiden bei fieberhaften Infekten, zum Beispiel beim *Infekt mit Coxsackie-Viren*. Eine *Gonokokken-Arthritis* ist ebenfalls meist sehr akut und überwiegend monarticulär. Wir sehen häufig sehr akute Arthritiden der Sprunggelenke und Zehengelenke beim *M. Reiter*. Während beim M. Reiter jedoch häufig nicht nur das Großzehengrundgelenk, sondern auch andere Zehengrundgelenke befallen sind, ist ein solcher Befall fast ein Ausschlußkriterium für die Gicht, zumindest in einem frühen Stadium. Eine Urethritis wird vom Patienten meist nicht spontan angegeben. Die Conjunctivitis beim M. Reiter ist meist flüchtig und daher ein anamnestischer Befund. Die *Arthritis psoriatica* zeichnet sich ebenfalls durch akute Schübe, häufigen monarticulären Befall, bei oligoarticulärem Befall durch Asymmetrie, und häufigen Befall der Zehengelenke sowie eine ausgeprägte periarticuläre Schwellung aus. Bei der relativ hohen Morbidität sowohl der Psoriasis vulgaris als auch der Gicht ist auch ein Zusammentreffen beider Krankheiten möglich. Es ist auch bekannt, daß auf Grund des erhöhten Zellumsatzes in der Haut des Psoriasispatienten bei dieser Krankheit entsprechend der Größe der befallenen Hautfläche Hyperuricämien häufiger sind als in der Durchschnittsbevölkerung. So kann die Differentialdiagnose Arthritis psoriatica gegenüber der Gicht bzw. einer Gicht in Begleitung einer Psoriasis vulgaris gelegentlich Schwierigkeiten bereiten. Eine Hilfe bietet hierbei oft das Röntgenbild, das bei der Arthritis psoriatica schon frühzeitig typische Veränderungen zeigt.

Eine akute Sprunggelenksarthritis mit ausgeprägter periarticulärer Schwellung, häufiger beidseitig als einseitig, häufiger bei der Frau als beim Manne, finden wir nicht selten bei einer *akuten Sarkoidose.* KAPLAN (1960) hat ein promptes Ansprechen dieser Arthritis auf Colchicin beschrieben. Der Befund eines Erythema nodosum oder eine Röntgenaufnahme der Thoraxorgane klärt jedoch die Diagnose. Eine komplette internistische Durchuntersuchung empfiehlt sich jedenfalls bei jeder akuten Gelenksentzündung. Eine *chronische Polyarthritis* beginnt häufig bei Individuen jüngerer und mittlerer Altersstufen monarticulär an den unteren Extremitäten. Bei der chronischen Polyarthritis kann der Beginn akut sein, meist kommt es jedoch nicht zu einem schnellen Abklingen der Entzündungserscheinungen. Das oft allzu schnelle therapeutische Eingreifen mit Corticosteroidpräparaten kann das klinische Bild jedoch erheblich verändern. Bei der *Spondylitis ankylosans* (M. Bechterew) treten akute Mono- oder Oligoarthritiden, besonders der unteren Extremitäten in etwa einem Drittel der Patienten als Erstsymptomatik auf. Ganz selten ist ein *palindromer Rheumatismus* differentialdiagnostisch zu erwägen.

Erschwerend in der Differentialdiagnose ist die von GRIEBSCH u. ZÖLLNER (1973) festgestellte Tatsache, daß bei der Zunahme der Durchschnittswerte der Plasmaharnsäurespiegel in den letzten zehn Jahren ein Harnsäurewert im Plasma zwischen 6,5 mg-% und 8,0 mg-% die Diagnose Gicht nicht beweisen, sondern nur stützen kann. Ebenso erschwerend für die Diagnose übernommener Fälle ist oft auch der Umstand, daß heute vielfach voreilig bei allen möglichen Gelenksymptomen harnsäuresenkende Medikamente verordnet werden und somit der bei der Untersuchung gemessene Wert nicht sicher diagnostisch verwendet werden kann.

Gichtfälle, die als phlegmonöse Entzündung fehlgedeutet und chirurgisch behandelt werden oder bei Mittelfußbefall als entzündlicher Spreizfuß orthopädisch behandelt werden, stellen mit zunehmender Häufigkeit der Gicht und wachsenden Kenntnissen über diese Krankheit heute nur noch eine Seltenheit dar.

Eine akute und im eigentlichen Sinne anfallsartige Arthritis, die von einer Gichtarthritis nicht zu unterscheiden ist und deshalb *Pseudogicht* genannt wird, kann nur durch die Untersuchung des Gelenkpunktats sicher diagnostiziert bzw. ausgeschlossen werden. Man findet bei dieser Krankheit mit Hilfe des Polarisationsmikroskopes eindeutig identifizierbare rhombische Calciumpyrophosphatkristalle. Eine röntgenologische Darstellung von Kalkschatten im Kniegelenks- oder Handgelenksspalt läßt die Diagnose Pseudogicht vermuten. Über dieses Krankheitsbild wird von SCHILLING an einer anderen Stelle des Gichtbeitrages ausführlicher berichtet.

Literatur

BABUCKE, G., MERTZ, D. P.: Wandlungen in Epidemiologie und klinischem Bild der primären Gicht zwischen 1948 und 1970. Dtsch. med. Wschr. **98**, 183 (1973).

BRICOUT, C.: L'influence du traumatisme local dans le déterminisme des crises de goutte ou du rhumatisme goutteux. Congrès de la goutte et de l'acide urique. Vittel, 1935 Kongressbd., p. 242—244.

BRUGSCH, T.: Die Gicht. In: Lehrbuch der Inneren Medizin. Wien: Urban und Schwarzenberg 1930.

DRUBE, H., REINWEIN, H.: Zur Klinik der Gicht, „der vergessenen Krankheit". Med. Klin. **54**, 631 (1959).

GAMP, A., SCHILLING, F., MÜLLER, L., SCHACHERL, M.: Das klinische Bild der Gicht heute. Beobachtungen an 200 Kranken. Med. Klin. **60**, 129 (1965).
GARROD, A. B.: The nature and treatment of gout and rheumatic gout, 2. Aufl. London: Walton and Maberly 1853.
GRAHAME, R., SCOTT, J. T.: Clinical survey of 354 patients with gout. Ann. rheum. Dis. **29**, 461 (1970).
GRIEBSCH, A., ZÖLLNER, N.: Normalwerte der Plasmaharnsäure in Süddeutschland. Vergleich mit Bestimmungen vor zehn Jahren. Z. klin. Chem. **11**, 346 (1973).
GUDZENT, F.: Gicht und Rheumatismus. Berlin: Springer 1928.
HALL, A. P., BARRY, P. E., DAWBER, T. R., McNAMARA, P. M.: Epidemiology of gout and hyperuricemia. A long-term population study. Amer. J. Med. **42**, 27 (1967).
HENNINGES, D., MERTZ, D. P.: Urikopathie bei Jugendlichen. Besonderheiten im klinischen Bild. Münch. med. Wschr. **113**, 458 (1971).
KAPLAN, H.: Sarcoid arthritis with a response to colchicine. New Engl. J. Med. **263**, 778 (1960).
KORFMACHER, I., ZÖLLNER, N.: Gicht — lebenslange Behandlung unerläßlich. Dtsch. Ärztebl. **17**, 1221 (1974).
KUZELL, W. CH., GAUDIN, G. P.: Gicht. Docum. Rheumatol. Geigy, Nr. 10. Basel 1956.
LICHTWITZ, L., STEINITZ, E.: Die Gicht, in: Handbuch der inneren Medizin, 2. Aufl., Bd. IV/1. Berlin: Springer 1926.
MERTZ, D. P.: Gicht, Diabetes mellitus und Fettleber. Münch. med. Wschr. **114**, 180 (1972).
MERTZ, D. P.: Gicht. Grundlagen, Klinik und Therapie. Stuttgart: Thieme 1973.
MERTZ, D. P., BABUCKE, G.: Epidemiologie und klinisches Bild der primären Gicht. Beobachtungen zwischen 1948 und 1968. Münch. med. Wschr. **113**, 617 (1971).
MUGLER, A.: Gicht und Trauma. Münch. med. Wschr. **111**, 1615 (1969).
RÜCKERT, K.-H., CHOWANETZ, W.: Die übersehene Gicht. Münch. med. Wschr. **114**, 663 (1972).
SCHILLING, F.: Differentialdiagnose der Gicht, atypische Gicht und Pseudogicht. Therapiewoche **19**, 245 (1969).
SCHILLING, F.: Klinik und Therapie der Gicht. Vortrag VI. Bad Mergentheimer Stoffwechseltagung 1971.
SLADE, J. H.: Achilles tendon in gout. New Engl. J. Med. **277**, 160 (1967).
SYDENHAM, TH.: Opuscula omnia. Tractatus de podagra et hydrope. London 1683. (Deutsch in: Klassiker der Medizin, hrsg. von K. SUDHOFF, Leipzig: Barth 1910.
TALBOTT, J. H.: Gout, 3. Aufl. New York: Grune and Stratton 1967.
ZÖLLNER, N.: Gicht. Dtsch. med. Wschr. **84**, 920 (1959).
ZÖLLNER, N.: Moderne Gichtprobleme. Ätiologie, Pathogenese, Klinik. Ergebn. inn. Med. Kinderheilk. N. F. **14**, 321 (1960).
ZÖLLNER, N.: Diagnostische Maßnahmen bei Gicht. Dtsch. med. Wschr. **92**, 115 (1967).
ZÖLLNER, N.: Die Gicht. In: Klinik der rheumatischen Erkrankungen (Hrsg. SCHOEN, R., BÖNI, A., MIEHLKE, K.). Berlin-Heidelberg-New York: Springer 1970.

bb) Die chronische Gicht

Von

M. SCHATTENKIRCHNER und N. ZÖLLNER

Mit 6 Abbildungen

Die chronische Gicht ist gekennzeichnet durch eine ständige Beeinträchtigung der Bewegungsfunktion des betroffenen Patienten. Meist liegt eine Beteiligung mehrerer Gelenke vor. Im Stadium der chronischen Gicht sind sichtbare und tastbare Knoten (Tophi) charakteristische Befunde. Man spricht daher auch von der chronischen Knotengicht oder chronischen tophösen Gicht. Komplikationen und Begleiterkrankungen sind bei dieser klinischen Manifestationsform der Gicht häufiger und ausgeprägter als bei den anderen Erscheinungsformen dieser Krankheit. Die Definition der chronischen Gicht wird also im wesentlichen klinisch getroffen.

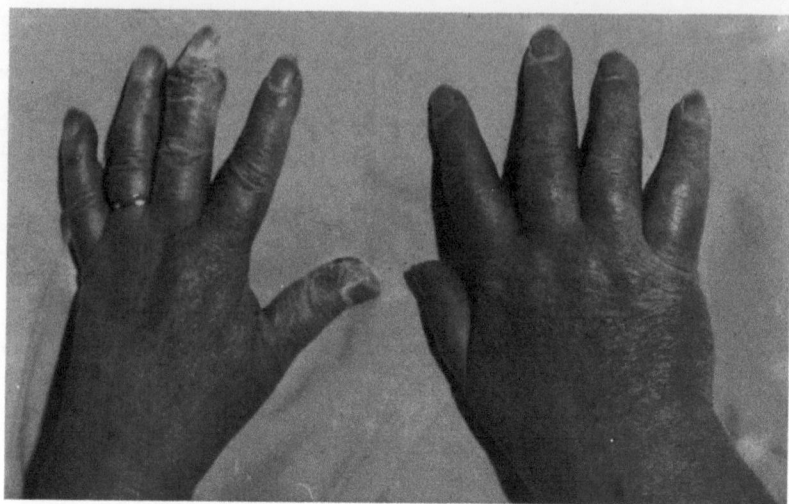

Abb. 1. 64jährige Patientin, chronische Gicht. Beginn der Krankheit sechs Jahre nach der Menopause mit 49 Jahren. Während plasmaharnsäuresenkender Therapie Abheilung exulcerierter subcutaner und paraarticulärer Tophi an der Endphalanx des linken Mittelfingers und Daumens. Plasmaharnsäure bei Aufnahme 8,4 mg-%

Entsprechend der klassischen Einteilung der Gicht in vier Stadien nach BRUGSCH (1930) sowie ZÖLLNER (1959):
1. asymptomatische Gichtanlage,
2. akuter Gichtanfall,
3. interkritische Gicht,
4. chronische polyarticuläre Gicht,

stellt die chronische Gicht das Spätstadium der Gicht dar, das meist nach jahrelangem Krankheitsverlauf erreicht wird. Nach GAMP (1965) dauert es bis zur Entwicklung einer chronischen Gicht bei der Mehrzahl der beobachteten Fälle mehr als 7 Jahre, ein Drittel der Fälle erreicht dieses Stadium jedoch schon nach fünf Jahren Krankheit.

Pathologisch-anatomisch liegt der chronischen Gicht eine Erosion des Gelenkknorpels und des subchondralen Knochens zugrunde, welche Folge einer entzündlichen Reaktion auf Uratablagerungen in diesem Bereich ist. Klinisch und röntgenologisch kommt es zu sekundären Arthrosen, z.T. mit Chondrocalcinose, welche dauernde Beschwerden verursachen. Ausgedehntere Uratablagerungen in gelenknahen Knochen werden als Knochentophi bezeichnet, die in ausgeprägten Fällen zu Gelenkdestruktionen und Gelenkdeformitäten, in Schleimbeuteln und Sehnenscheiden zu schmerzhaften Bewegungseinschränkungen führen können (Abb. 1). Tophöse Ablagerungen können auch für ein Carpal-Tunnel-Syndrom verantwortlich sein (WARD et al., 1958). Vom pathologisch-anatomischen Gesichtspunkt aus läßt sich eine Zweiteilung der klinischen Gichtmanifestation durchführen:

1. die akute Gicht, die als akute Kristall-Synovitis aufzufassen ist und keine morphologischen Veränderungen an den Gelenken aufweist,

2. die chronische Gicht mit morphologischen Veränderungen, bedingt durch tophöse Ablagerungen an den Gelenken und in den Weichteilen.

Da die morphologischen Gelenkveränderungen durch die röntgenologische Untersuchung erfaßbar sind, bietet das Röntgenbild ein wichtiges Kriterium für

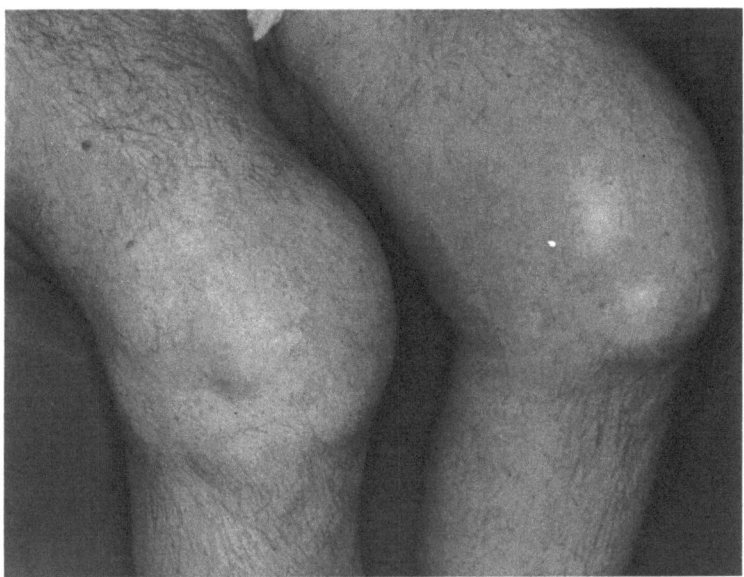

Abb. 2. Patient M. U., 50 Jahre, chronische Gicht. Knotige periarticuläre Uratablagerungen an beiden Kniegelenken, besonders auffallend in der Bursa praepatellaris links

die Diagnose chronische Gicht. Nach SCHACHERL et al. (1966) kann also die Diagnose Gicht erst im chronischen Stadium vom Röntgenologen gestellt werden. GAMP (1965) sichert die Diagnose chronische Gicht nach folgenden Punkten:
1. äußerlich sichtbare Tophi,
2. röntgenologisch nachweisbare Knochentophi,
3. klinisch manifeste Arthritis urica.

Vor Einführung wirksamer Mittel zur Behandlung der Hyperuricämie entwickelten schicksalhaft etwa 50—60% der Gichtpatienten klinisch oder röntgenologisch nachweisbare Ablagerungen von tophösem Material entsprechend Manifestationsalter, Schweregrad der Krankheit und Lebenserwartung (Committee of the Amer. Rheum. Ass., 1973). Heute ist das voll ausgeprägte Krankheitsbild, wie wir es von alten Bildern und Stichen oder von lebendigen, z.T. bitter-humorvollen Beschreibungen betroffener großer Männer her kennen, nur noch gelegentlich zu beobachten. Daß man überhaupt noch Patienten dieser Art zu sehen bekommt, ist nur darauf zurückzuführen, daß die Diagnose Gicht nicht gestellt oder diese nicht adäquat behandelt wurde. Die klinische Beschreibung nach dem heute vorhandenen Krankengut an Patienten mit chronischer Gicht ist also mehr oder weniger bestimmt durch die Beobachtung an Einzelfällen, die wir von Zeit zu Zeit einmal sehen.

Fallbeschreibung: Im Juli 1974 übernahmen wir von einer chirurgischen Abteilung einen 50jährigen Patienten, M. U., von Beruf Arbeiter in einer Speditionsfirma, der neun Wochen wegen eines großen Ulcus ventriculi, das eine fast tödliche Blutung verursacht hatte, stationär lag. Die Anamnese von Gelenkbeschwerden begann im Jahre 1964 mit akuten Arthritiden der Großzehengrundgelenke, der Mittelfußgelenke, der Sprunggelenke, der Handgelenke, der Kniegelenke und schließlich der Fingergelenke. Die Intervalle zwischen den einzelnen Gelenkattacken betrugen zunächst Monate und verkürzten sich dann auf einige Wochen. Schließlich war der Patient von ständigen Beschwerden geplagt. Die Anfälle lösten einander ab, befallene Gelenke waren nie mehr beschwerdefrei und es entwickelten sich vom Jahre 1968 an Knoten an den Kniegelenken (Abb. 2), Knoten an den Ellenbo-

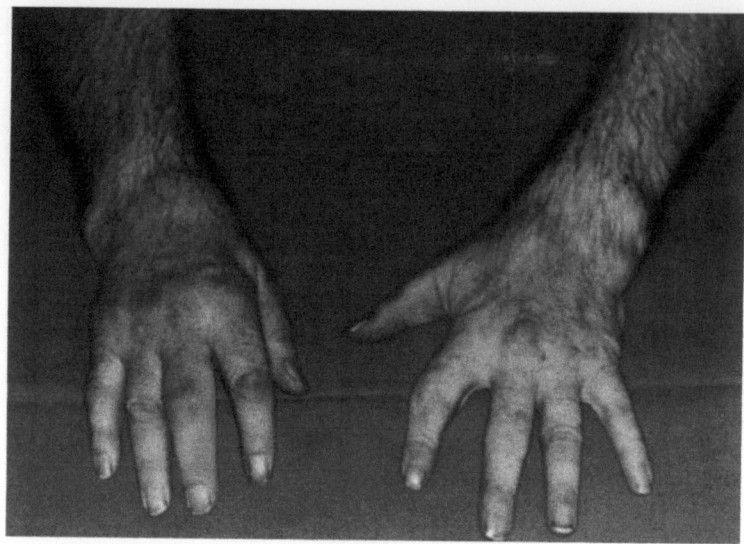

Abb. 3. Patient M. U., 50 Jahre, chronische Gichtarthritis. Multiple subcutane Tophi im Sehnen- und Gelenkbereich beider Handrücken. Ankylose des linken Zeigefingermittelgelenkes

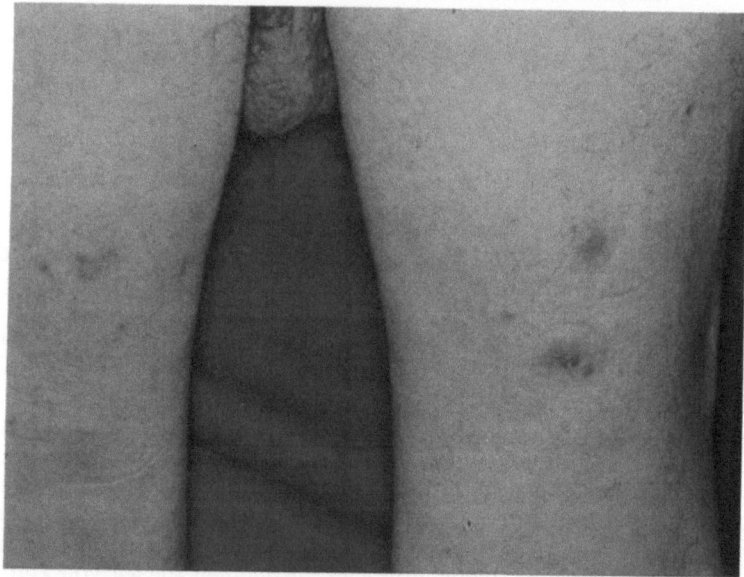

Abb. 4. Patient M. U., 50 Jahre, chronische Gicht. Hauttophi an der Dorsalseite des rechten Oberschenkels. Von andersartiger örtlicher Hautentzündung kaum zu unterscheiden

gen, die bis zu Tennisballgröße wuchsen, Knoten an den Ohrmuscheln, die der Patient gelegentlich öffnete und ausdrückte, Knoten an den Fingergelenken (Abb. 3) und in der Haut der Unterarme und Oberschenkel (Abb. 4). Der Patient lernte mit dem Mittelfinger und Daumen der rechten Hand und mit der linken Hand schreiben und konstruierte sich Hilfseinrichtungen an seinem Lieferwagen, um seinen beruflichen Verpflichtungen nachzukommen. Jedes Jahr war er wochenlang arbeitsunfähig, da er wegen entzündeter Gichtknoten und langdauernder Gichtanfälle seine Schuhe nicht anziehen konnte. Die medikamentöse Therapie bestand in intramuskulären Injektionen corticoidhaltiger Präparate. Schließlich bekam der Patient ein corticoidhaltiges orales Rheumapräparat, das er unkontrolliert in hohen Dosen einnahm, bis er wegen einer lebensbedrohlichen Magenblutung in das Krankenhaus eingeliefert werden mußte. Die Serumharnsäure betrug 10,0 mg-%. Nach Ausheilung Ulcus ventriculi wurden die Tophi über beiden Ellenbogen operativ entfernt. Die Funktionsfähigkeit war nach Wundheilung nicht mehr beeinträchtigt.

Es ist erstaunlich, wie wenig eingeschränkt trotz erheblicher Gelenkzerstörung nach dem Röntgenbild und massiver Tophi über den Gelenken und in den Sehnenscheiden die Bewegungsfunktion des betroffenen Patienten ist. Eine knöcherne Ankylose ist selten. Wir haben erstmals im beschriebenen Falle eine knöcherne Versteifung gesehen.

Die chronische Gicht ist heute das Ergebnis einer Fehldiagnose oder einer falschen Behandlung. Sie ist das Spätstadium der Gicht, das bei den modernen Möglichkeiten der Gichtbehandlung nicht mehr vorkommen darf.

Nach GRAFE (1953) soll es aber auch Gichtarthritiden geben, die von Anfang an polyarticulär und chronisch verlaufen. Es wurde der Begriff *primär-chronische Gicht* dafür geprägt. Auch MERTZ (1971) kennt diese Verlaufsform und reiht sie wie SCHILLING (1969) unter die atypischen Gichtformen ein. Nach MELLINGHOFF u. GROSS (1962) haben 20% der Gichtfälle einen primär-chronischen Verlauf. MERTZ (1971) glaubt, daß diese Zahl eher zu niedrig sei. Er weist auf SOKOLOFF (1957) hin, der feststellt, daß mit zunehmender Lebenserwartung der Gesamtbevölkerung sich auch Fälle häufen, in denen sich die Krankheit in hohem Alter manifestiert. Im höheren Lebensalter seien nach HOLLÄNDER u. SCHWARCMANN (1968) aber atypische Verlaufsformen häufiger. Ablagerungen von Harnsäure bei pathologisch-anatomischen Untersuchungen arthrotischer Gelenke, wie z.B. des Hüftgelenkes, sind bekannt, man darf aus diesem Befund jedoch nicht auf das Vorliegen einer atypischen chronischen Gichtarthritis schließen. Wir selbst halten eine primär-chronische Gicht, wenn man darunter eine von Anfang an chronisch verlaufende Gichtarthritis mit Tophusbildung versteht, für eine Seltenheit. Wir haben noch keinen solchen Fall in unserer Klinik gesehen. Auch LÖFFLER u. KOLLER (1955) erinnern sich nicht, einen solchen Fall gesehen zu haben. HILL (1951) sowie BÖNI (1965) haben bei allen ihren Fällen mit chronischer Gicht ein Vorstadium mit akuten Anfällen eruieren können. HENCH et al. (1928) fanden unter 100 Gichtpatienten 44mal ein chronisches Stadium, bei zwei dieser Fälle war die Krankheit von Anfang an chronisch verlaufen, ohne daß typische Anfälle vorgekommen wären.

GAMP (1965) hat bei 160 Fällen von Gicht nur einmal einen sicheren primär-chronischen Verlauf einer Gichtarthritis beobachtet.

Den *polyarticulären Beginn einer Gicht* sehen auch wir, jedoch nicht so häufig wie SCHILLING (1972) oder GAMP (1965). Bei diesen Fällen handelt es sich um regelrechte Gichtanfälle mit schmerzfreiem Intervall; die Anfälle dauern bei einem polyarticulären Beginn lediglich etwas länger als bei einer Monarthritis. Häufig wird eine Arthritis an einem Gelenk von einer Arthritis an einem anderen Gelenk innerhalb eines Anfalles abgelöst.

Es ist zu bedenken, daß eine primär-chronische Gichtarthritis, falls man nicht streng zu ihrer Definition klinisch und radiologisch feststellbare Tophi fordern will, im Grund eine chronische Polyarthritis ist, welche mit einem als Hyperuricämie deklarierten Harnsäurewert im Plasma einhergeht. Wir wissen aber, daß der durchschnittliche Harnsäureplasmaspiegel eines Normalkollektives beim männlichen Geschlecht in den Jahren 1962—1972 um 24% gestiegen ist (GRIEBSCH u. ZÖLLNER, 1973, dort weitere Literatur). Sicher ist auch die Morbidität der Gicht in diesem Zeitraum gestiegen; ob jedoch die Zahl atypischer Gichtformen zugenommen hat, ist bis jetzt nicht nachgewiesen. Andererseits wissen wir, daß sich hinter einer chronischen Polyarthritis ohne serologische Merkmale eine Reihe von rheumatischen Krankheiten verbergen kann, wie zum Beispiel eine rheumafaktor-negative chronische Polyarthritis (p.c.P., bzw. rheumatoide Arthritis), eine Arthritis psoriatica, eine atypische Spondylitis ankylosans mit Beteiligung peripherer Gelenke oder ein subakut verlaufender Morbus Reiter. Es ist auch zu berücksichtigen, daß die meisten sogenannten Antirheumatica einen Einfluß auf die tubuläre Harnsäuresekretion haben und so eine Hyperuricämie erzeugen können. Erhöhte Harnsäurewerte im Plasma finden sich auch bei übergewichtigen Patienten, die häufig über arthrotische Beschwerden klagen (KŘÍŽEK, 1966). Eine klare Abtrennung gegenüber einer chronischen Gichtarthritis ist in solchen Fällen zu fordern.

Der einzige nach den derzeit gültigen Kriterien gesicherte Fall eines Zusammentreffens einer chronischen Polyarthritis mit einer chronischen tophösen Gicht wurde von OWEN et al. (1966) beschrieben. Der beschriebene Patient hatte sowohl histologisch eindeutige Rheumaknoten, einen hochtitrigen Rheumafaktor im Serum, als auch chemisch und histologisch gesicherte Tophi.

Für den Beweis einer primär-chronischen Gichtarthritis halten wir das Zusammentreffen von Arthritis bzw. Polyarthritis und Hyperuricämie nicht für genügend, sondern fordern den mikroskopischen oder chemischen Nachweis von Harnsäure im Gewebe.

Diese Überlegungen über die Existenz einer primär-chronischen Gicht zeigen, daß einerseits der Anfallcharakter der Gichtarthritis, sei er beobachtet oder auch nur typisch in der Anamnese geschildert, und andererseits die Harnsäureablagerung im Gewebe — der Tophus — die beiden essentiellen Kennzeichen der Gicht sind.

Die Tophusbildung

Die Gichtknoten waren früher wegen ihrer größeren Häufigkeit das eindrucksvollste Kennzeichen der Gicht. Der englische Schriftsteller HORATIO WALPOLE (1717—1797), der an einer chronischen Gicht litt, schrieb einmal, er habe mehr „Kalksteine" als Gelenke an den Fingern, und er müsse eigentlich eine Gastwirtschaft aufmachen, denn er könne eine Zeche mit größerer Leichtigkeit und Geschwindigkeit aufkreiden als jeder andere in England. In einem anderen Brief schrieb er, daß er sich einen Chirurgen holen ließ, um sich einen erbsgroßen Kalkknoten aus dem Finger herausholen zu lassen, und er hoffe, daß die Wunde bald verheilt sei. Man glaubte also, daß es sich bei dem Inhalt des Gichtknotens um eine kalkige, kreidige Masse handle. Tophus kommt aus einem lateinischen Dialekt und bedeutet Tuff, also poröser, mürber Mineralabsatz.

Nachdem SCHEELE im Jahre 1776 Harnsäure im Urin festgestellt hatte, isolierte einige Jahre später WOLLASTON (1797) Harnsäure aus Gichtknoten. HOWELL et al. identifizierten im Jahre 1963 die abgelagerte Substanz mit Hilfe der Röntgenspektrographie eindeutig als Mononatriumurat-Monohydrat (Na-Urat·H_2O). Tophi sind demnach größere Ablagerungen von Mononatriumurat-Monohydrat im Gewebe.

Bei der histologischen Untersuchung eines kleineren Tophus erkennt man einen meist aus kristallinem Material bestehenden Kern und eine entzündliche Umgebungsreaktion. Unter den Entzündungszellen finden sich auch Fremdkörperriesenzellen (FASSBENDER, 1972). Die Größe der Tophi schwankt zwischen einem Millimeter und mehreren Zentimetern im Durchmesser.

Über den Gehalt eines Tophus an Harnsäure gibt uns eine Analyse von EBSTEIN u. SPRAGUE (1891) Auskunft. Rund 60% der Trockenmasse des Tophus ist Harnsäure. GARROD (1853) hat einen ähnlichen Wert gefunden.

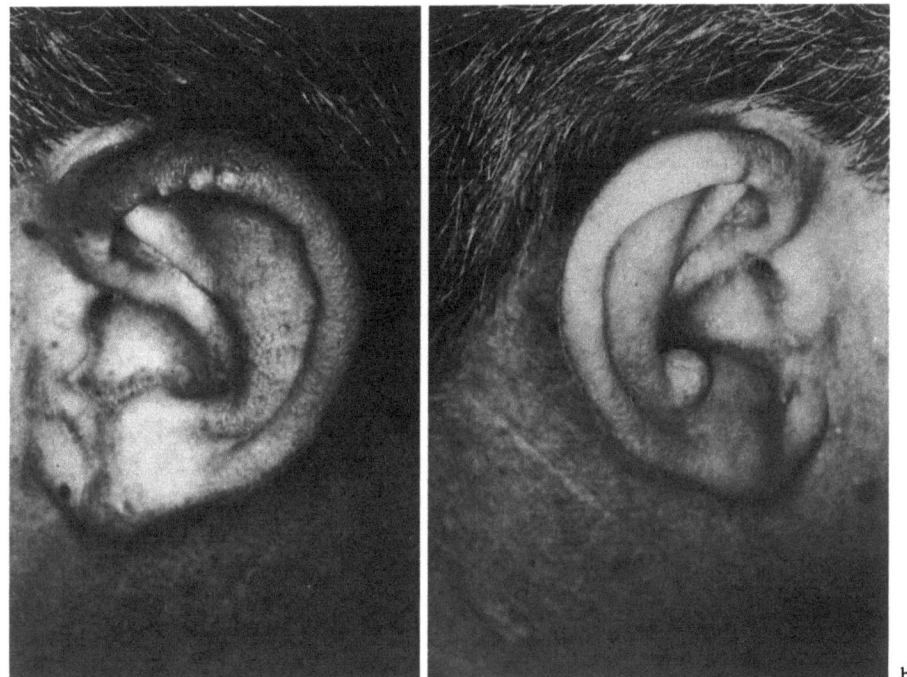

Abb. 5a u. b. 36jähriger Gichtpatient, fünf Jahre Krankheitsdauer ohne Therapie. Linke Ohrmuschel (a) mehrere reiskorngroße Tophi an typischer Stelle (Helix). Rechte Ohrmuschel (b) solitärer erbsgroßer Tophus an atypischer Stelle (Antihelix). Plasmaharnsäure bei Behandlungsbeginn 7,2 mg-%

Der Anteil der Harnsäure am Gesamtgewicht des nativen, chirurgisch entfernten Tophus liegt nach BACKMANN u. BÄUMER (1969) bei den Tophi über den Gelenken bei 11,5—16,0%, der Harnsäuregehalt von Bursawänden, zum Beispiel der Bursa olecrani, beträgt nur 2,8—4,4%. BACKMANN u. BÄUMER homogenisierten zur Bestimmung des Harnsäuregehaltes von Tophi das operativ entnommene Gewebe unter Zusatz von Lithiumcarbonat. Das Homogenat wurde durch kurzes Zentrifugieren von größeren Bindegewebspartikeln befreit. Im Überstand wurde die Harnsäure enzymatisch mit Uricase bestimmt. Das Gewicht der excidierten Tophi lag zwischen 1,5 g und 76,0 g (BACKMANN, 1972).

Tophi können klinisch diagnostiziert werden, wenn sie an typischer Stelle äußerlich sichtbar und tastbar sind, wie die pathognomonischen Gichtperlen an der Ohrmuschel (Abb. 5a u. 5b) oder die Gichtknoten über den Gelenken. Auf das Vorhandensein von Tophi im Knochen kann auf Grund einer Röntgendarstellung großer gelenknaher Cysten und größerer Usuren geschlossen werden. Die relativ kleinen Tophi in der Gelenkinnenhaut lassen sich nur histologisch diagnostizieren. Wir wissen daher nicht viel über ihre Häufigkeit und den Zeitpunkt ihres Auftretens. Durch Gelenkpunktionen läßt sich diese Frage nicht lösen. Gelenkoperationen bei Gicht werden meist nur aus anderen Gründen, wie z.B. wegen einer gleichzeitig bestehenden Meniscusläsion am Kniegelenk, durchgeführt.

Die Diagnose der äußerlich sichtbaren und tastbaren Weichteiltophi kann auch Schwierigkeiten bereiten. Die meist am Rande der Helix oder Antihelix, gelegentlich auch an anderen Stellen der Ohrmuschel liegenden Tophi sind zum

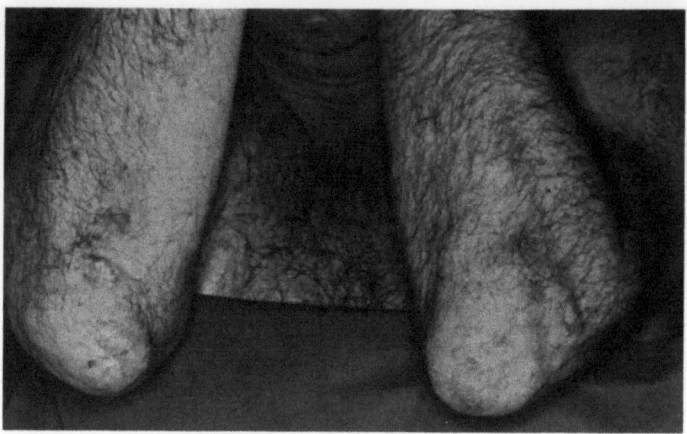

Abb. 6. 49jähriger Patient mit Arthritis urica seit acht Jahren bei Klinikaufnahme, Plasmaharnsäure 7,9 mg-%. Hühnereigroße Tophi in der Bursa olecrani beidseits. Rechts Zustand nach Abheilung einer Exulceration, durch die sich ein Teil der tophösen Masse spontan entleert hatte. Die Tophi wurden bei Beginn der Behandlung operativ entfernt

Unterschied von Knorpelmißbildungen auf ihrer Unterlage verschieblich. Tophi über den Streckseiten der Gelenke, in den Bursen, insbesondere in der Bursa olecrani (Abb. 6) sind von Rheumaknoten auseinanderzuhalten. Bezüglich der Lokalisation besteht zwischen den Gichtknoten und den Rheumaknoten in diesen Bereichen kaum ein Unterschied. Während der erbs- bis pflaumengroße Rheumaknoten am Ellenbogengelenk meist einige Zentimeter distal auf der Ulnakante liegt, liegt der Gichtknoten am Ellenbogengelenk, da es sich meist um einen Bursatophus handelt, direkt über dem Gelenk. Beide Knoten sind schmerzlos. Der Tophus ist jedoch härter, von unregelmäßiger Gestalt, oft schimmert weißlicher oder leicht gelblicher Inhalt durch die Haut hindurch, besonders wenn man sie anspannt. Der Rheumaknoten ist weich und rund.

Differentialdiagnostisch kommen auch tendinöse oder tuberöse Xanthome bei Hyperlipidämien in Frage. Heberdensche Knoten bereiten im Allgemeinen keine diagnostischen Schwierigkeiten. Selten müssen Chondrome, Ganglien, Knötchen bei der Polyvinylchloridkrankheit oder Kalkknoten bei Sklerodermie, Calcinosis universalis und Dermatomyositis von Tophi abgegrenzt werden. Im Zweifelsfalle sollte auf eine chemische oder histologische Untersuchung nicht verzichtet werden. Nach Punktion eines Knotens kann mikroskopisch ein Tophus nachgewiesen werden, wenn sich in der aspirierten Masse Natriumuratkristalle finden, wie es erstmals van LEEUWENHOEK im Jahre 1679 beschrieben hat. Mit der Murexidprobe ist die Harnsäure chemisch nachzuweisen. Häufig ist es jedoch sinnvoller, den Knoten in toto zu excidieren. Ist der Knoten für eine histologische Untersuchung bestimmt, darf er nicht wie üblich in einer Formaldehydlösung fixiert werden, in der Harnsäure löslich ist, sondern muß in 96% Alkohol fixiert werden. Im Falle eines Rheumaknotens zeigt die histologische Untersuchung ein sehr charakteristisches Bild einer zentralen fibrinoiden Nekrose umgeben von radiär angeordneten Pallisadenzellen und Granulationsgewebe mit Entzündungszellen (FASSBENDER, 1965).

Diagnose und Differentialdiagnose der ossären Tophi sind in dem Abschnitt Röntgenologie der Gicht abgehandelt.

Tabelle 1. Seltene Tophuslokalisationen. Die Autoren sind in chronologischer Reihenfolge aufgeführt

Mitralklappe	VIRCHOW (1868)
	BUNIM u. MC EWEN (1940)
Aortenklappe	COUPLAND (1873)
Verschiedene Gewebe des Auges	WEVE (1924)
	YOURISH (1953)
Nasenflügel, Augenlider, Penis, Scrotum	MINKOWSKI (1930)
Arterien	HENCH (1951)
Zunge, Epiglottis, Stimmbänder, Aryknorpel	BAUER u. KLEMPERER (1952)
	LEFKOWITZ (1965)
Myokard	TRAUT et al. (1954)
Wirbelkörper	BAUER u. SINGH (1957)
Perikard	PAULLEY et al. (1963)
Sacroiliacalgelenke	GAMP (1965)
	SCHILLING (1969)

Tophi können praktisch in allen Geweben lokalisiert sein, wie wir von Fällen excessiver Gicht wissen. Bevorzugt sind jedoch Knorpelgewebe, Sehnen- und Sehnenscheidengewebe, Schleimbeutel und Gelenkinnenhaut. Als Erklärung dafür weisen einige Autoren auf die Gefäßarmut, andere Autoren auf den hohen Gehalt an sauren Mucopolysacchariden dieser Gewebe hin.

In den Abschnitten Pathogenese der Harnsäureablagerungen und des Gichtanfalles und Pathologie der Gicht wird auf dieses Problem näher eingegangen. Tophi treten im Stratum synoviale der Gelenkinnenhaut und im Knochen unterhalb der Knorpelschicht der Gelenke auf. Sehr häufig finden sich tophöse Ablagerungen in der Bursa olecrani, in der infrapatellaren Sehne, in der Achillessehne und im subcutanen Gewebe über den Streckersehnen der Hand und über den Gelenken. Auch Tophi in der Haut sind zu beobachten (MISGELD, 1968, eigene Beobachtungen). Von den äußerlich sichtbaren Tophi sind die Tophi an der Ohrmuschel wohl die häufigste Art. Nach LÖFFLER u. KOLLER (1955) findet man sie in etwa einem Drittel aller Gichtpatienten. Seltene Lokalisationen von Tophi sind vielfach beschrieben worden, meist bei Fällen excessiver Gicht. Sie sind in Tabelle 1 zusammengestellt.

Im Muskel, in der Leber, Milz, Lunge und im Nervengewebe gibt es nach TALBOTT (1967) keine Tophi. Über die Tophusbildung in der Niere wird in einem eigenen Abschnitt über die Nierenbeteiligung bei Gicht berichtet.

Die Angaben über die Häufigkeit des Auftretens von Tophi und über die Reihenfolge der Häufigkeit an einzelnen Lokalisationen sind naturgemäß in den einzelnen klinischen Publikationen unterschiedlich. Das hängt vom beobachteten Patientengut der einzelnen Autoren ab.

Den Zeitraum zwischen Krankheitsbeginn und dem Auftreten von Tophi anzugeben, ist ebenso schwierig, da die Daten hierfür in zunehmendem Maße nur noch aus der Anamnese unbehandelter, d.h. nichtdiagnostizierter Patienten, zu entnehmen sind. Eine konsequente Therapie sowohl mit Uricosurica als auch mit Allopurinol kann entstandene Tophi zur Rückbildung bringen (YÜ u. GUTMAN, 1951; ZÖLLNER, 1970; ZÖLLNER u. SCHATTENKIRCHNER, 1967; KRÖPELIN u. MERTZ, 1972). Eine effiziente plasmaharnsäuresenkende Therapie wird auch, das darf man sicher postulieren, das Entstehen von Tophi verhindern. Folgende Tabelle zeigt die Häufigkeit von Tophi bei der Gicht nach den Angaben einzelner Autoren:

Tabelle 2. Häufigkeit von Tophi bei der Gicht aller Stadien. Die Autoren sind chronologisch aufgeführt

Autor		Zahl der Patienten	Anteil mit Tophi
Garrod	(1853)	37	47%
Strandgaard	(1899)	110	48%
Williamson	(1920)	116	57%
Hench	(1928)	100	53%
Brøchner-Mortensen	(1940)	97	34%
Mc Cracken et al.	(1948)	702 [a]	45,7%
Löffler u. Koller	(1955)	33	33–50% [b]
Bartels u. Matossian	(1957)	231	27–45% [c]
Gamp	(1965)	160	36%

[a] Aus der Literatur zusammengestellt (100 eigene Fälle).
[b] Nach 10- bzw. 20jährigem Verlauf.
[c] Nach 4- bzw. 11jährigem Verlauf.

Von der Tabelle 2 kann eine Häufigkeitsabnahme der Tophi abgelesen werden. Ob dieser Wandel mit Fortschritten in der harnsäuresenkenden Therapie in Zusammenhang gebracht werden kann, muß offen bleiben.

Betrachtet man die chronische Gichtarthritis allein, so liegt die Häufigkeit von Tophi höher als bei der Gicht aller Stadien. Die Häufigkeit der Weichteiltophi bei chronischer Gicht liegt nach Mertz u. Babucke (1971) bzw. Babucke u. Mertz (1973) bei 54%, nach Gamp (1965) bei 67%. Knochentophi finden sich nach Babucke u. Mertz (1973) in 68% der Fälle mit chronischer Gicht, nach Gamp (1965) in 80%. Beide Tophusformen werden in 21%, bzw. 10—20% gefunden.

Über den Zeitraum des Auftretens von Tophi nach dem Beginn der Gicht existieren einige Angaben in der Literatur. Selbstverständlich können nur Durchschnittswerte angeführt werden, da für das Auftreten von Tophi neben möglichen individuellen Unterschieden in der Neigung zu Harnsäureausfällungen sicher der Grad der (unbehandelten) Hyperurikämie die ausschlaggebende Rolle spielt. Es wird angenommen, daß Patienten mit Gicht, die unbehandelt einen Plasmaharnsäurespiegel, gemessen mit der enzymatischen Methode, unter 8,5 mg-% aufweisen, relativ selten zu Tophi kommen (Committee of the Amer. Rheum. Ass., 1973).

Brøchner-Mortensen (1940) stellte eine durchschnittliche Krankheitsdauer vom Krankheitsbeginn bis zum Auftreten von Weichteiltophi von 13,2 Jahren fest, von ersten Knochentophi von 11,5 Jahren. Bei kombiniertem Auftreten von Knochentophi und Weichteiltophi vergehen durchschnittlich 15,4 Jahre. Babucke u. Mertz (1973) fanden bei einem Kollektiv von Gichtpatienten durchschnittlich nach neun Jahren (2—17 Jahren) Weichteiltophi, nach 4,9 Jahren Knochentophi, das kombinierte Vorkommen nach 9,3 Jahren. Bei einem Patienten fanden Babucke u. Mertz (1973) schon beim ersten Gichtanfall einen Knochentophus an dem betroffenen Großzehengrundgelenk. Auch wir verfügen über solche Beobachtungen.

Die sich schmerzlos entwickelnden Weichteiltophi können in Ausnahmefällen schon vor dem ersten Gichtanfall entstanden sein. Garrod (1853) berichtet schon darüber. Charcot (1874) fand sogar schon 5 Jahre vor dem ersten Gichtanfall Tophi. Brugsch (in Zöllner, 1960) hat einen Fall von ausgedehnter Tophusbildung bei einem Patienten beschrieben, der nie einen Anfall hatte.

Die ersten Anregungen zur Erforschung der Gicht gingen vor 200 Jahren von der chronischen tophösen Gicht aus. Die chemische Analyse von Tophi ließ den Zusammenhang dieses Leidens mit der Harnsäure erkennen. Als WILLIAM HYDE WOLLASTON im Jahre 1797 bekanntgab, daß der Hauptbestandteil der gichtischen Konkremente (Tophi) "a neutral compound consisting of lithic acid (uric acid) ... and a mineral alkali" sei, war die Jahrhunderte alte Frage nach der materia morbi der Gicht beantwortet.

Die heutigen Kenntnisse über das Wesen der Gicht und die modernen Möglichkeiten ihrer Therapie setzen uns instande, das chronisch-tophöse Stadium dieser Krankheit aussterben zu lassen.

Literatur

BABUCKE, G., MERTZ, D. P.: Wandlungen in Epidemiologie und klinischem Bild der primären Gicht zwischen 1948 und 1970. Dtsch. med. Wschr. **96**, 183—188 (1973).
BACKMANN, L.: Chirurgische Behandlungsmöglichkeit der Gicht. Therapiewoche **22**, 140—142 (1972).
BACKMANN, L., BÄUMER, A.: Harnsäuregehalt chirurgisch entfernter Gichtknoten und gichtisch veränderter Schleimbeutel. Münch. med. Wschr. **111**, 1620—1622 (1969).
BARTELS, E. C., MATOSSIAN, G. S.: Arthr. and Rheum. **2**, 193—199 (1959); zit. n. SMYTH, CH. J.: Diagnosis and Treatment of Gout. In: Arthritis and allied conditions (HOLLANDER, J. L., Ed.), 7th Ed., p. 921—944. Philadelphia: Lea & Febiger 1966.
BAUER, W., KLEMPERER, F.: Gout, Disease of Metabolism (Ed. Duncan), 3rd Ed., Philadelphia: Saunders, W. B. 1952.
BÖNI, A.: Gelenkveränderungen bei Harnsäuregicht. In: Stoffwechsel und degenerativer Rheumatismus. Darmstadt: Steinkopff 1965.
BUNIM, J. J., McEWEN, C.: Tophus of mitral valve in gout. Arch. Path. **29**, 700—705 (1940).
BRUGSCH, T.: Die Gicht. In: Lehrbuch der Inneren Medizin. Wien: Urban und Schwarzenberg 1930.
CHARCOT, J. M.: Leçons cliniques sur les maladies de vieillards et les maladies chroniques, Paris 1874. Zit. n. LÖFFLER, W., KOLLER, F.: Die Gicht. In: Handbuch der Inneren Medizin, 4. Aufl., Bd. 7/II. Berlin-Göttingen-Heidelberg: Springer 1955.
COMMITTEE OF THE AMERICAN RHEUMATISM ASSOCIATION: Primer on the Rheumatic Diseases. Gout. Supplement to J. Amer. med. Ass. **224**, 757—766 (1973).
COUPLAND, S.: Gouty deposits on the aortic valves. Lancet **1873 I**, 447.
EBSTEIN, W., SPRAGUE, H.: Notiz betreffend die therapeutische Anwendung des Piperazins. Berl. klin. Wschr. **1891 I**, zit. n. LÖFFLER, W., KOLLER, F.: Die Gicht. In: Handbuch der Inneren Medizin, 4. Aufl., Bd. 7/II, Berlin-Göttingen-Heidelberg: Springer 1955.
FASSBENDER, H. G.: Pathologie des entzündlichen Rheumatismus. In: Rheumatismus in Forschung und Praxis (Hrsg. BELART, W.), Bd. 3: Ursachen rheumatischer Krankheiten, Bern: Huber 1965.
FASSBENDER, H. G.: Zur Pathologie der Gicht. Therapiewoche **22**, 105—108 (1972).
GAMP, A.: Gelenkveränderungen bei Harnsäuregicht. In: Stoffwechsel und degenerativer Rheumatismus (Hrsg. SCHOEN, R.). Darmstadt: Steinkopff 1965.
GARROD, A. B.: The nature and treatment of gout and rheumatic gout. London: Walton & Maberly 1853; zit. n. TALBOTT, J. H.: Die Gicht. Stuttgart: Hippokrates-Verlag 1967.
GRAFE, E.: Die Gicht. Dtsch. med. Wschr. **78**, 867—871 (1953).
GRIEBSCH, A., ZÖLLNER, N.: Normalwerte der Plasmaharnsäure in Süddeutschland. Z. klin. Chem. **11**, 346—356 (1973).
HENCH, P. S.: Gout and gouty arthritis. In: Cecil-Loeb: Textbook of medicine, 9th Ed., Philadelphia: Saunders 1951.
HOLLÄNDER, E., SCHWARCMANN, P.: Gicht im vorgeschrittenen Alter. Münch. med. Wschr. **110**, 649—653 (1968).
HOWELL, R. R., EANES, E. D., SEEGMILLER, J. E.: X-ray diffraction studies of the tophaceous deposits in gout. Arthr. and Rheum. **6**, 97—102 (1963).
KŘÍŽEK, V.: Serum uric acid in relation to body weight. Ann. rheum. Dis. **25**, 456—458 (1966).
KRÖPELIN, T., MERTZ, D. P.: Rückbildung von Gichttophi unter Langzeitbehandlung mit Allopurinol. Med. Klin. **67**, 614—618 (1972).

LEFKOWITZ, A. W.: Gouty involvement of the larynx. Report of case and review of the literature. Arthr. and Rheum. **8**, 1019—1024 (1965).
LÖFFLER, W., KOLLER, F.: Die Gicht. In: Handbuch der Inneren Medizin, 4. Aufl., Bd. 7/II. Berlin-Göttingen-Heidelberg: Springer 1955.
MELLINGHOFF, C. H., GROSS, R. H.: Erfahrungen über die Gicht, insbesondere über die urikosurische Therapie mit Anturan. Z. Rheumaforsch. **21**, 42—49 (1962).
MERTZ, D. P.: Gicht. 2. Aufl., Stuttgart: Thieme 1973.
MERTZ, D. P., BABUCKE, G.: Epidemiologie und klinisches Bild der primären Gicht, Beobachtungen zwischen 1948 und 1968. Münch. med. Wschr. **113**, 617—628 (1971).
MINKOWSKI, O.: Gicht. In: Klemperer; Neue Deutsche Klinik, Bd. IV, 1930. Zit. n. LÖFFLER, W., KOLLER, F.: Die Gicht. In: Handbuch der Inneren Medizin, 4. Aufl., Bd. 7/II. Berlin-Göttingen-Heidelberg: Springer 1955.
MISGELD, V.: Primäre Hautgicht. Eigene Beobachtungen und Beitrag zur Klinik der Gicht. Hautarzt **19**, 299—304 (1968).
OWEN, D. S., TOONE, E., IRBY, R.: Coexistent Rheumatoid Arthritis and Chronic Tophaceous Gout. J. Amer. med. Ass. **197**, 953—956 (1966).
PAULLEY, W. J., BARLOW, K. E., CUTTING, P. E. J., STEVENS, J.: Acute gouty pericarditis. Lancet **1963 I**, 21—22.
SCHACHERL, M., SCHILLING, F., GAMP, A.: Das radiologische Bild der Gicht. Radiologe **6**, 231—238 (1966).
SCHEELE, K. W.: Chemical examinations of urinary calculi. Leipzig Opuscula **2**, 73 (1776). Zit. n. TALBOTT, J. H.: Die Gicht. Stuttgart: Hippokrates-Verlag 1967.
SCHILLING, F.: Differentialdiagnose der Gicht, atypische Gicht und Pseudogicht. Therapiewoche **19**, 245—260 (1969).
SCHILLING, F.: Klinik und Therapie der Gicht und deren Abgrenzung von der Pseudogicht. In: Fettsucht-Gicht. Stuttgart: Thieme 1971.
SOKOLOFF, L.: The pathology of gout. Metabolism **6**, 230—236 (1957).
STRANDGAARD, N. J.: Gigt og urinsur diatese. Kopenhagen 1899. Zit. n. LÖFFLER, W., KOLLER, F.: Die Gicht. In: Handbuch der Inneren Medizin, 4. Aufl., Bd. 7/II. Berlin-Göttingen-Heidelberg: Springer 1955.
TALBOTT, J. H.: Die Gicht. Stuttgart: Hippokrates-Verlag 1967.
TRAUT, E. F., KNIGHT, A. A., SZANTO, P. B., PASSERELLI, E. W.: Specific vascular changes in gout. J. Amer. med. Ass. **156**, 591—594 (1954).
VIRCHOW, R.: Unusual gouty deposits. Virchow Arch. path. Anat. **44**, 137 (1868). Zit. n. TALBOTT, J. H.: Die Gicht. Stuttgart: Hippokrates-Verlag 1967.
WALPOLE, H.: Zit. n. TALBOTT, J. H.: Die Gicht. Stuttgart: Hippokrates-Verlag 1967.
WARD, L. E., BICKEL, W. H., CORBIN, K. B.: Median neuritis (carpal tunnel syndrome) caused by gouty tophi. J. Amer. med. Ass. **167**, 844—846 (1958).
WEVE, H. J. M.: Uric acid keratitis and other ocular findings in gout. Rotterdam: van Hengel 1924. Zit. n. TALBOTT, J. H.: Die Gicht. Stuttgart: Hippokrates-Verlag 1967.
WILLIAMSON, C. S.: A clinical study of 116 cases of gout. J. Amer. med. Ass. **74**, 1625 (1920). Zit. n. LÖFFLER, W., KOLLER, F.: Die Gicht. In: Handbuch der Inneren Medizin, 4. Aufl., Bd. 7/II. Berlin-Göttingen-Heidelberg: Springer 1955.
WOLLASTON, W. H.: On gouty and urinary concretions. London Phil. Trans. **87**, 386 (1797). Zit. n. Primer on the Rheumatic Diseases; Supplement to J. Amer. med. Ass. **224**, 757—766 (1973).
YOURISH, N.: Conjunctival tophi associated with gout. Arch. Ophthal. **50**, 370 (1953). Zit. n. TALBOTT, J. H.: Die Gicht. Stuttgart: Hippokrates-Verlag 1967.
YÜ, T. F., GUTMAN, A. B.: Mobilization of gouty tophi by protracted use of uricosuric agents. Amer. J. Med. **11**, 765—770 (1951).
ZÖLLNER, N.: Gicht. Dtsch. med. Wschr. **84**, 920 (1959).
ZÖLLNER, N.: Moderne Gichtprobleme, Ätiologie, Pathogenese, Klinik. Ergeb. inn. Med. Kinderheilk. **14**, 321—389 (1960).
ZÖLLNER, N.: Die Gicht. In: Klinik der rheumatischen Krankheiten (SCHOEN, R., BÖNI, A., MIEHLKE, K., Hrsg.). Berlin-Heidelberg-New York: Springer 1970.
ZÖLLNER, N., SCHATTENKIRCHNER, M.: Allopurinol in der Behandlung der Gicht und der Harnsäure-Nephrolithiasis. Dtsch. med. Wschr. **92**, 654—660 (1967).

cc) Die Differentialdiagnose der Gicht

Von

F. SCHILLING

Mit 22 Abbildungen

Außer der Niere sind es vor allem Gelenke und gelenknahe Knochen- und Bindegewebsanteile, die von den Uratablagerungen bei chronischer Hyperuricämie betroffen werden. Die primären und klinisch also überwiegend imponierenden Gichtsymptome können deshalb als Gelenk-Gicht (Arthritis urica) bezeichnet werden und erklären, warum die Gicht zu einem großen Teil ein Leiden des rheuma-klinischen Erfahrungsbereiches ist.

Die Differentialdiagnose dieses Gelenkleidens ist damit ein Teil der Rheumatologie überhaupt. Wir werden sie in der Reihenfolge unseres *Kriterienkataloges der primären Gicht* abhandeln (SCHILLING, 1969):

1. Die Hyperuricämie.
2. Der akute Anfall (im Stadium der akut rezidivierenden Gicht):
   a) articulär: Synovitis, Paraarthritis;
   b) extraarticulär: Periarthritis, Tendoperiostitis, Bursitis.
3. Die Uratablagerung (Tophus und Dauerschaden im Stadium der chronischen tophösen Gicht):
   a) articulär: chronische (destruierende) Gichtarthritis, chronische Arthritis unter dem Bild der Arthrose; paraarticulär: Knochentophus.
   b) Weichteiltophus:
   Haut-, subcutaner, Bursa-, Sehnen-Tophus

I.

Die *Hyperuricämie*, die wir für Serumharnsäurewerte oberhalb der Sättigungskonzentration für Natrium-Urat bei 6,4 mg-% (PETERS u. VAN SLYKE, 1964; GRIEBSCH u. ZÖLLNER, 1973) und damit geschlechtsunabhängig definieren (SCHILLING, 1971), ist einerseits für die Diagnose einer Gicht nahezu obligat (über 95% der Fälle). Andererseits aber ist sie epidemiologisch unter der männlichen Bevölkerung so häufig (15 bis über 30%), daß sie differentialdiagnostisch nicht einen alleinentscheidenden Stellenwert beanspruchen kann. Dabei spielt allerdings der Grad der Hyperuricämie (Durchschnittswert mehrerer Kontrollen) eine wichtige Rolle. Werte unter 8 mg-% besagen differentialdiagnostisch wenig; zwischen 9 mg-% und 10 mg-% aber sind sie hinweisend, da in diesem stark übersättigten Bereich bereits eine weit über fünfzigprozentige Wahrscheinlichkeit für eine Gichtmanifestierung besteht. Eine anhaltende Hyperuricämie über 10 mg-% schließlich bedeutet praktisch die bereits oder bald etablierte Gicht und erhärtet damit die Diagnose weitgehend.

Normouricämie sollte stets an der Diagnose Gicht zweifeln lassen. Sie ist in höchstens 5%, nach unserer Erfahrung bei knapp über 2% der Fälle vorhanden, die dann stichhaltig durch Symptome der zweiten oder dritten Kriteriengruppe als Gicht ausgewiesen sein müssen. Eine normouricämische Phase einer schon diagnostizierten Gicht sollte nicht länger als zwei Jahre hingenommen werden und muß spätestens dann zur Revision der Diagnose veranlassen.

Während noch bis in die sechziger Jahre der Nachkriegszeit hinein die Gicht häufig übersehen und zu selten diagnostiziert wurde, besteht jetzt teilweise die gegenteilige Gefahr. Unter dem Eindruck der Propagierung der Begriffe „Hyperuricämie-Syndrom" oder „Uricopathie" — Begriffsbildungen, die der Vorfeld-Diagnostik vorbehalten bleiben sollten und differenzierungspflichtig sind — wird teilweise die nosologische, an Kriterien gebundene Sauberkeit der Gicht-Diagnose vernachlässigt.

Davon bleibt unberührt, daß die Hyperuricämie als Risikofaktor (MERTZ, SCHILLING), mindestens aber als Risiko-Indiz (BÄUMER) erkannt wurde. Die Krankheit Gicht selbst ist aber weder bereits durch die Hyperuricämie konstituiert, noch ist sie gleichzusetzen mit dem Syndrom assoziierter Stoffwechselstörungen (Hyperuricämie, Hyperlipidämie, latenter Diabetes) bei Adipositas mit Fettleber und Neigung zu Gefäßsklerose und zu Arthrosen. Wir fassen dieses phänotypisch durch die Wohlstandsgesellschaft manifestierte Bild als Konstitutionspanorama auf dem Boden einer multifaktoriellen und polygenetischen Determinierung auf. Die klinische Diagnostik hat aber die Pflicht, zunächst zu differenzieren. Die Therapie wiederum muß die Gesamtheit des Symptomkomplexes berücksichtigen.

Dabei muß auch die Gefahr vermieden werden, wieder in den vorwissenschaftlichen Begriff der „Gicht" des vorigen Jahrhunderts zurückzufallen, der nicht nur alle möglichen Arthritiden, sondern auch die Heberden-Arthrose und mannigfache Erscheinungen einer sogenannten *visceralen Gicht* umfaßt hat. Die gichtige Phlebitis, die Augengicht, die akute Darmgicht sowie cerebrale Lokalisationen entstammen z.T. noch unkontrollierten Deutungen und bedürfen jedenfalls einer strengen bzw. skeptischen Überprüfung.

Nur hinzuweisen ist hier auf die *hämatologische* Differentialdiagnose der Gicht, die z.B. die konstitutionseigene Polyglobulie der primären Gicht einerseits und die Polycythaemia vera mit sekundärer Gicht andererseits betrifft, und auf die praktisch so wichtige *urologische* Differentialdiagnose der Nephropathie und des Steinleidens.

II.

Differentialdiagnose des akuten Gichtanfalls (Tab. 1)

Der akute Gichtanfall charakterisiert das erste Hauptstadium, das der akut rezidivierenden Gicht. Er ist in der Mehrzahl der Fälle monotop, in gut einem Drittel polytop, vorwiegend oligoarticulär (38%) (GAMP et al., 1965).

Wir definieren den akuten *Anfall* als örtlich begrenzten Entzündungszustand vorwiegend eines Gelenkes, der schnell (innerhalb weniger Stunden) einsetzt, von hoher Akuität und zeitlich begrenzter Aktivität ist und nach Tagen bis höchstens wenigen Wochen ad integrum ausheilt bzw. zum Ausgangszustand zurückkehrt.

Wir ordnen den Begriff des (akuten) Anfalls grundsätzlich der Gicht, den des Schubes grundsätzlich den chronischen rheumatischen Systemleiden zu und beschreiben Arthritiden dann als anfallsartig, wenn sie den Bedingungen des Anfalles entsprechen, aber nicht oder nicht sicher einer Gicht zugehören.

Der Gichtanfall spielt sich in oder an einem Gelenk oder Schleimbeutel ab, es liegt ihm eine kristallin induzierte Synovitis zugrunde. Die klassischen klinischen Zeichen der Entzündung sind alle vorhanden, insbesondere zeichnen Rötung (Paraarthritis) und deutliche Überwärmung die akute Arthritis im Gegensatz zur chronischen Gelenkentzündung aus. Eine akute Tenosynovitis urica scheint es kaum zu geben, jedenfalls haben wir in einem großen Beobachtungsgut eine solche noch nicht mit Sicherheit gesehen.

Wir unterscheiden also die *articuläre* und eine *extraarticuläre* Lokalisation, von denen die periarticulären Anfälle weniger bekannt und der Verborgenheit ihres Ausgangspunktes wegen größere diagnostische Schwierigkeiten bereiten.

Über die *Lokalisation* der Erstanfälle (a) und das Ausbreitungsmuster der Anfälle im Verlauf des akut rezidivierenden Stadiums (b) im eigenen Krankengut gibt Abb. 1 Auskunft (siehe auch Kap. Der akute Gichtanfall).

Für das Großzehengrundgelenk als Ort des ersten Gichtanfalls schwanken die Angaben zwischen 46 und 50% (GAMP et al., 1965; MERTZ u. BABUCKE, 1971) und 72 und 78% (BABUCKE u. MERTZ, 1973; DE SEZE et al., 1959).

Tabelle 1. Differentialdiagnose des akuten Gichtanfalls

A. Akute Synovitis, Arthritis und Paraarthritis
  1. Pseudogicht
  2. Akute Polyarthritis des rheumatischen Fiebers
  3. Akute und subakute Arthritis
      a) Infekte
      b) Reitersche Krankheit
      c) Episodische Synovitis (Knie) der Spondylitis ankylopoetica
  4. Psoriatische Arthritis
      „pseudo-guttöse" Form
  5. Palindromer Rheumatismus
      a) Allergische Arthritis
      b) Atypische chronische Polyarthritis
      c) Systemischer Lupus erythematodes
  6. Arthrose im Reizzustand
      Heberdenknötchen
  7. Eitrige Arthritis

B. Extraarticuläre akute Entzündungen
  1. Insertionstendopathie
      a) Mechanische Irritation
      b) Entzündliche Enthesopathie
  2. Periarthritis
      a) Periarthritis humero-scapularis
      b) Peritendinitis calcarea
  3. Bursitis (olecrani)
      a) „Rheumatoide" Bursitis
      b) Kalk-Bursitis
      c) Eitrige Bursitis
  4. Tenosynovitis
  5. a) Periostitis
      b) Phlebitis
      c) Phlegmone

Als Regeln und differentialdiagnostische Merkmale können gelten:
1. Zwei Drittel aller Fälle beginnen monoarticulär, der Rest oligoarticulär.
2. In mehr als der Hälfte der Fälle beginnt die Gicht am Großzehengrundgelenk. Die Ausbreitung erfolgt kaudo-kranial und zentripetal.
3. Gelenke der unteren Extremitäten sind etwa zehnmal häufiger der Sitz des Erstanfalls als Gelenke der oberen Extremitäten.

A. Akute Synovitis, Arthritis und Paraarthritis

Soweit bei einem synovitischen Entzündungszustand durch Punktion Exsudat zu erhalten ist, kann die *Synovia-Analyse* differentialdiagnostisch entscheidend wichtig werden (DEICHER, 1970; HÖTTL, 1970/71; DÜRRIGL u. ZERGOLLERN, 1972; THUMB, 1973; SCHILLING, 1974) (Tab. 2). Die stark entzündliche Synovialflüssigkeit ist trüb, mucinarm und zellreich. Die repräsentativen Enzyme, von denen im Routinelabor saure Phosphatase, Aldolase und Lactatdehydrogenase im allgemeinen bestimmt werden können, sind teilweise erhöht. Ihre Normalwerte entsprechen denen im Serum.

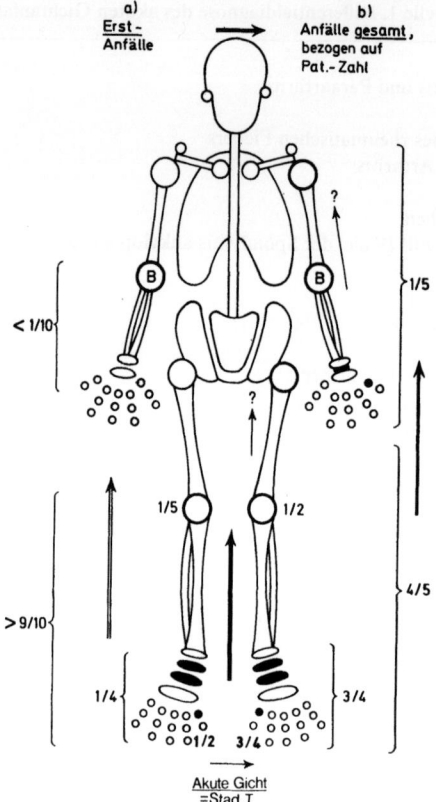

Abb. 1. Verteilung und Ausbreitung der articulären Anfälle im Stadium der akut rezidivierenden Gicht: Erstanfälle *a* und Summe der Anfälle im weiteren Verlauf *b* B = Bursitis

Lysosomale Enzymverteilungsmuster in der Synovialflüssigkeit verschiedener Gelenkerkrankungen hat GREILING 1970 untersucht; Punktatanalysen bei Arthritis urica haben HÄNTZSCHEL et al. (1972) und HÜTTL und HÜTTLOVÁ (1972) vorgelegt.

Die *mikrokristallin induzierte Synovitis* (MCCARTY u. HOLLANDER, 1961; MCCARTY, et al., 1962; FAIRES et al., 1962; SEEGMILLER et al., 1962) (vgl. Abb. 2) ist durch den Befund leukocytärer Kristallphagocytosen im Punktat ausgezeichnet, die bei mikroskopischer Betrachtung schon lichtoptisch zu erkennen sind, die Diagnose der Kristallsynovitis erlauben und bereits morphologisch deren Differentialdiagnose nahelegen (SCHILLING, 1969 und 1971). Die *Mononatriumuratkristalle* der Gicht sind stäbchen- bis nadelförmig und überragen teilweise die Peripherie des Granulocyten, der typischerweise wie von einem Pfeil durchbohrt erscheint (Abb. 3). Aber auch kleine Splitter, manchmal mehrere, kann der Zelleib enthalten. Sie müssen mit Hilfe der Mikrometerschraube als aufleuchtende anorganische Gebilde gesucht werden und können bei vorläufiger Betrachtung zunächst mit fädigen Zellstrukturen oder angelagerten Fibrinfäden verwechselt werden. Phagocytierte Knorpelsplitter oder auch früher intraarticulär injizierte Cortison-Kristalle können kaum täuschen, da sie im Gegensatz zu den Uratkristallen amorph bzw. polymorph sind.

Im frischen Gichtanfall, der zwischen 10000 und 40000 polymorphkernige Granulocyten pro mm^3 aufweist, können mehr als die Hälfte aller Zellen Kristalle enthalten, während in älteren Phasen dieser Befund durch Untergang der Freßzel-

Tabelle 2. Elementare Synovia-Analyse (Gelenkpunktat)

	nicht — wenig entzündlicher „Reizerguß"	entzündlicher Gelenk-Erguß			infektiös
		steril			
		rheumatische Arthritis	Gicht	Pseudo-Gicht	
1. Aussehen	hell	gelb — trüb			eitrig
2. Viscosität und Mucingehalt	↑	↓			
3. Zellzahl pro mm³	< 2000	6000 bis 40000	=	=	> 60000
4. Mikroskopie a) Nativ-Tropfen Ragocyten	∅	+ — + + +	0 — (+)	0 — (+)	∅
Mikrokristall- → Phagocytosen	∅	0	Na-Urat	Ca-Pyrophosphat	
b) Ausstrich Granulocyten	25%	40—70%	60 bis 90%		massenhaft
5. Chemie a) Eiweiß	< 3,0 g-%	3 bis > 5 g-%			
b) Enzyme	∅ oder niedrig	erhöht (je nach Akuität und Aktivität)			
saure Phosphatase	unter 11 mU/ml				
Aldolase	unter 3,5 mU/ml				
LDH und Isoenzyme	unter 200 mU/ml				
c) Harnsäure	dem Serumwert entsprechend				

len spärlicher wird, bis zu wenigen Prozent aller Zellen. Es muß dann u. U. länger und mit der Ölimmersion geduldig nach ihnen gesucht werden. Ein einziges sicher als Uratkristall identifiziertes Phagocytosephänomen kann bereits die zugrundeliegende Gicht beweisen. Der Phasenkontrast bringt nicht viel Vorteile. In Zweifelsfällen muß man das Polarisationsmikroskop mit Kompensator zu Rate ziehen (PHELPS et al., 1968).

Von den diagnostischen Möglichkeiten der Synoviaanalyse wird viel zu wenig Gebrauch gemacht.

Von der lichtoptischen Suche nach extracellulären Kristallen in der punktierten Synovia raten wir ab. Ohne Polarisation sind sie schwer erkennbar, als Kristalle nur zu ahnen, kaum zu differenzieren und mit Fadenkristallen zu verwechseln. — Gelöste Harnsäure kann die Synovia milchig trüben, während eine Hyperlipidämie in der Synovia keine Entsprechung findet (GREILING, 1969).

Der Mononatriumuratkristall verhält sich im Polarisationsmikroskop negativ doppelbrechend. Dies kann differentialdiagnostisch entscheidend werden, wenn Calciumpyrophosphatkristalle der zunächst zu besprechenden Chondrocalcinose zur Diskussion stehen und die morphologische Differenzierung im Stich läßt.

1. Die CPPD-mikrokristallin induzierte Synovitis (Pseudogicht) der Chondrocalcinose — Pyrophosphat-Arthropathie

Wie die Gicht ist die viel seltenere Chondrocalcinose eine Kristallablagerungskrankheit (MCCARTY, 1966; SKINNER u. COHEN, 1969). Sie hat mit jener die akute Kristallsynovitis gemeinsam und verläuft klinisch unter dem Bilde des

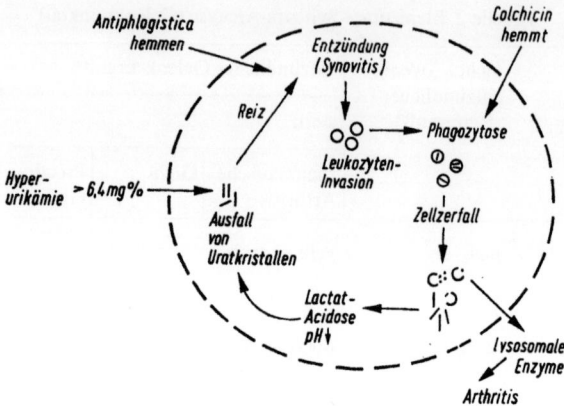

Abb. 2. Mechanismus der akuten Arthritis urica (nach SEEGMILLER u. HOWELL, 1962) als Modell der mikrokristallin induzierten Synovitis, mit den Ansätzen der antiphlogistischen bzw. antimitotischen Therapie

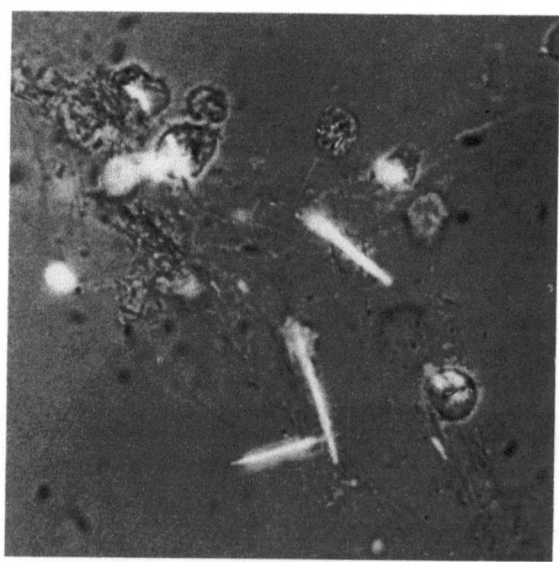

Abb. 3. Phagocytierte Mononatriumurat-Kristalle (Nadeln und Splitter) in der Synovia eines Gichtanfalls im Kniegelenk

Pseudogicht-Syndroms (MCCARTY et al., 1962). Die für diese verantwortlichen Calciumpyrophosphat-Dihydrat(CPPD)-Kristalle können den Entzündungscyclus im Gelenkinnern (Abb. 2) genauso in Gang setzen, wie die ihnen morphologisch und in der Größenordnung gleichenden Uratkristalle.

Der Dauerschaden in Knorpel- und Bindegewebe ist aber bei beiden Krankheiten verschieden, entsprechend einer anderen Stoffwechselsituation und unterschiedlichen Gewebsreaktion. Während die Uratablagerung den Knorpel zerstört, zu einer destruierenden chronischen Synovitis, subchondral sowie in bradytrophen Geweben zu tophösen Granulationen führt (FASSBENDER, 1972), lagern

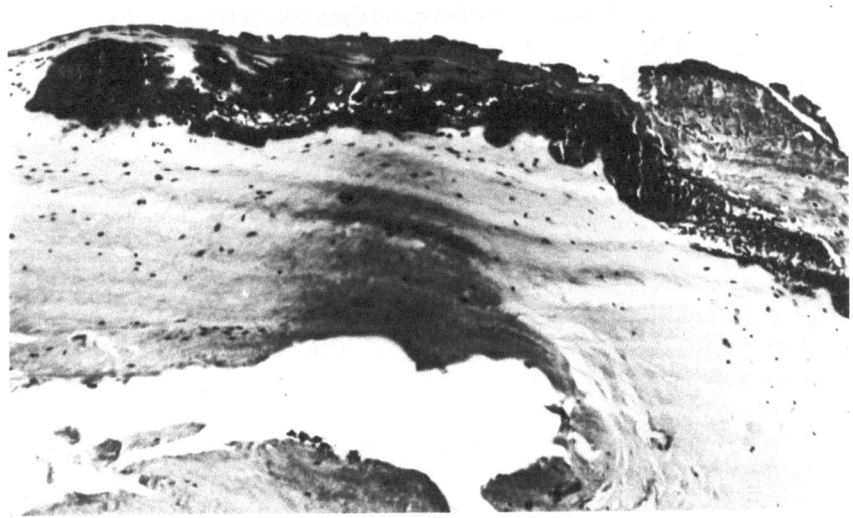

Abb. 4. Histopathologie der Chondrocalcinose (auf Kniegelenk beschränkte Form): Meniskus mit breiter oberflächlicher Kalkplatte (Calciumpyrophosphat-Inkrustation) (FASSBENDER)

sich die Calciumpyrophosphatkristalle reaktionslos in den Faserknorpel (Meniscus) oder/und in die oberflächlichen Schichten des hyalinen Gelenkknorpels ein (Abb. 4). Hier werden sie als charakteristischer feiner Kalkstreifen parallel zur Gelenkkontur röntgenologisch sichtbar (Abb. 8), durch einen schmalen, röntgenoptisch leeren Spalt von der Grenzlamelle getrennt (McCARTY u. HASKIN, 1963; TWIGG et al., 1964; ZITNAN u. SITAJ, 1963; SCHILLING, 1969). Reaktiv entstehen arthrotische Bilder. Seltener kommen aber auch destruktive Arthropathien an Knie-, Schulter-, Hand- oder/und Hüftgelenk vor (MENKES et al., 1973), die einer chronischen Polyarthritis oder auch einer Neuroarthropathie ähneln und differentialdiagnostische Schwierigkeiten bereiten können. Den Tophi entsprechende Gewebsreaktionen kennt die Chondrocalcinose nicht.

Da einerseits die Chondrocalcinose einen klinisch stummen Röntgenbefund darstellen oder als solcher auch bei anderen rheumatischen Krankheiten gefunden werden kann (MOSKOWITZ u. KATZ, 1965; DODDS u. STEINBACH, 1966; GOOD u. RAPP, 1967; BLOCH-MICHEL, 1968), andererseits aber Pseudogichtanfälle mit Nachweis von Kristallphagocytosen auch bei noch Röntgen-negativen Gelenken bzw. Fällen vorkommen, wurde eine Trennung der Begriffe Chondrocalcinose und Pseudogicht-Syndrom (CPPD-Kristallablagerungskrankheit) vorgeschlagen (SKINNER u. COHEN, 1969). Differentialdiagnostisch besonders verwirrend ist zu erfahren, daß bei gezielter Suche in 5% der Fälle einer Gicht-Serie und in 8% der Fälle einer Serie mit rheumatoider Arthritis Meniscusverkalkungen gefunden wurden (GOOD u. RAPP, 1967). Das Vorkommen solcher Verkalkungen überhaupt wird altersabhängig zwischen 0,5 und 7% (DE SEZE et al., 1969) und mit 5 auf 1619 untersuchte Personen im Alter über 44 Jahren (LAWRENCE) und mit 5,6% bei einer Untersuchung von Leichen (McCARTY et al., 1966) angegeben. Die Spannweite ist beträchtlich und für eine epidemiologische Aussage ungeeignet. Die überraschend häufige Koinzidenz von Gicht und lokalisierter Chondrocalcinose, die wir erst einmal gesehen haben, wird damit aber verständlicher.

Die der Chondrocalcinose zugrundeliegende Kollagen- oder Knorpelstoffwechselstörung ist durch laborchemische Parameter im Blutserum nicht erfaßbar, der Mineralhaushalt erscheint ungestört. Es fehlt also ein humorales Kriterium, das der Hyperurikämie als der pathophysiologischen Voraussetzung der Gicht entsprechen und dieser differentialdiagnostisch entgegengesetzt werden könnte.

Tabelle 3. Einteilung des Chondrocalcinose- bzw. Pseudogicht-Syndroms

A. Nosologisch
  I. Lokalisierte Chondrocalcinose
    1. Auf Knie und Faserknorpel beschränkt (Meniscusverkalkung)
       a) primär — doppelseitig
       b) symptomatisch (sekundär bei vorgeschädigtem Kniegelenk) — einseitig
    2. Bei Neuroarthropathien
       in arthritisch oder durch Gicht geschädigten Gelenken
  II. Polyarticuläre (systematisierte) Chondrocalcinose
    1. primär, idiopathisch, erblich
       a) familiär
       b) sporadisch
    2. sekundär, symptomatisch, metabolisch
       a) Hyperparathyreoidismus
          1. primär
          2. sekundär: chronische Niereninsuffizienz
                       Langzeit-Hämodialyse
       b) Hämochromatose
       c) Diabetes
       d) Postoperative Hypocalcämie
    3. Unter dem Bild einer destruktiven Arthropathie („Polyarthritis")
  III. Chondrocalcinose der Wirbelsäule

B. Klinisch
  1. Völlige Latenz
  2. Seltene monarthritische Anfälle
  3. Häufigere polyarthritische Anfälle
  4. Polyarthritisch chronisches Bild
  5. Wirbelsäulenbefall (röntgenologisch) — klinisch stumm

Auch ist der Purinstoffwechsel bei der Chondrocalcinose ungestört. Der noch unbekannte (Enzym-?) Defekt wird im Pyrophosphat-Stoffwechsel gesucht.

Für die Auslösung eines Pseudogicht-Anfalls könnte eine Störung des dynamischen Ionen-Gleichgewichts im Verhältnis der Serum-, Synovia- und Knorpel-Mineralien verantwortlich gemacht werden. In Analogie zum Gichtanfall bei Harnsäuresturz kommt hierfür z.B. eine postoperative Hypocalcämie in Frage (O'DUFFY, 1973).

Ältere Menschen im 6. bis zum 8. Lebensjahrzehnt erkranken häufiger, sogar das 9. ist noch befallen (ANGEVINE u. JACOX, 1973). Ein Unterschied unter den Geschlechtern ist nicht gesichert.

Wir unterscheiden entsprechend der Literatur (DE REUS, 1974) und eigener Erfahrung in 11 Fällen lokalisierte und systematisierte *Formen* bzw. Entitäten innerhalb des Syndroms der Chondrocalcinose (Tabelle 3).

Auf die Kniegelenke in Form von *Meniscus*verkalkungen beschränkte Fälle waren schon lange bekannt (WERWATH, 1928; MEYER-BORSTEL, 1931; RITTER, 1952; u.a.). Die *polyarticulär* systematisierte, teilweise familiär vorkommende Form ist zuerst in der Tschechoslowakei (ZITNAN u. SITAJ, 1958, 1960, 1963 und 1966), dann in Frankreich (RAVAULT et al., 1959 u. 1961; RUBENS-DUVAL et al., 1961; DE SEZE et al., 1961 und 1966; u.a.), in den USA (McCARTY et al., 1962; MOSKOWITZ u. KATZ, 1964 und 1967; BUNDENS et al., 1965; u.a.) und erst spät und bis vor kurzem nur vereinzelt in Deutschland beobachtet worden (SCHILLING u. SCHACHERL, 1965; ASHOFF et al., 1967; SCHILLING, 1969 und 1971; ZEIDLER et al., 1974). Als Erstbeschreibung müßte allerdings der Fall von MÜHR (1958)

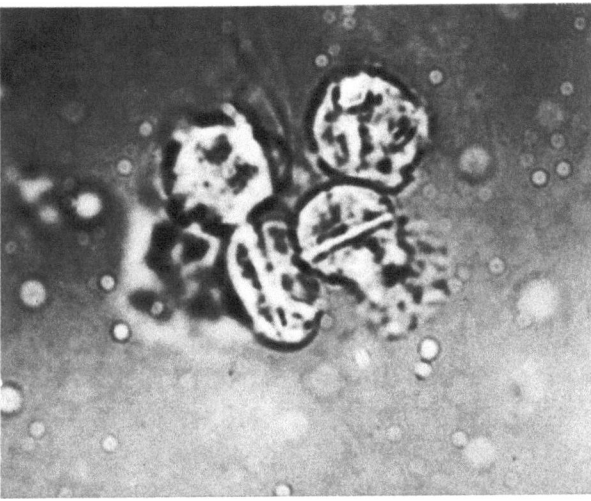

Abb. 5. Phagocytierte Calciumpyrophosphat-Kristalle (Stäbchen und Rhomboide) in der Synovia eines Pseudogichtanfalls im Kniegelenk

gelten. Sporadische Fälle wurden bislang offenbar vielfach übersehen und werden in letzter Zeit häufiger entdeckt, manchmal zufällig; einerseits wegen der nicht seltenen subjektiven Beschwerdefreiheit, andererseits wegen des heute durch Kenntnis geschärften Auges des Röntgenologen.

Prädilektionsstellen für Pseudogichtanfälle sind Knie- und Handgelenke, seltener Ellenbogen- und Fußgelenke und schließlich vereinzelt weitere kleine und große Gelenke (Abb. 10a), aber kaum das Großzehengrundgelenk. Der Anfall ist akut arthritisch mit Schwellung, Rötung, Überwärmung und Funktionsbehinderung. Den eindrucksvollsten Kniegelenkanfall mit hochschmerzhafter Akuität und flammender Paraarthritis, verkannt oder verdächtigt als Gelenkempyem, sahen wir nicht bei der Gicht, sondern mehrfach bei der Pyrophosphatsynovitis der lokalisierten Chondrocalcinose.

Die *Punktatanalyse* ergibt Befunde einer hochakuten exsudativen Synovitis mit zahlreichen Kristallphagocytosen (HÜTTL u. HÜTTLOVA, 1972). In älteren Anfallsphasen kann man auch an Entzündungszeichen verarmte Synovia mit nur vereinzelten Phagocytosen sehen. Im Gegensatz zu den Uratkristallen sind die *Calciumpyrophosphatkristalle* nicht auf die monokline Form beschränkt und sie sind polarisationsoptisch positiv doppelbrechend. Sie sind aber nicht immer so eindeutig, teilweise schwächer polarisierbar als jene; manchmal versagt diese Methode.

In den meisten Fällen liefert uns bereits die *Kristallmorphologie* mindestens Anhaltspunkte zur Erkennung der Substanz (Abb. 5): Die Stäbchen sind meist etwas gröber, dicker und stumpfer als die Urat-Nadeln, sie überragen die Zellgrenze nicht. Es kommen aber auch rhomboide Plättchen, plumpere Splitter und Körnchen vor. Gerade die Fragmente und die eher amorph erscheinenden Bröckchen entziehen sich bei Polarisation der Identifizierung, so daß wir insgesamt den Eindruck gewonnen haben, die Pyrophosphatkristalle des chondrocalcinotischen Syndroms seien chemisch gar nicht einheitlicher Natur.

Die Stäbchen zeigen beim Vergleich mit einem Gicht-Punktat im Polarisationsmikroskop ein typisches umgekehrtes Verhalten: Während der negativ dop-

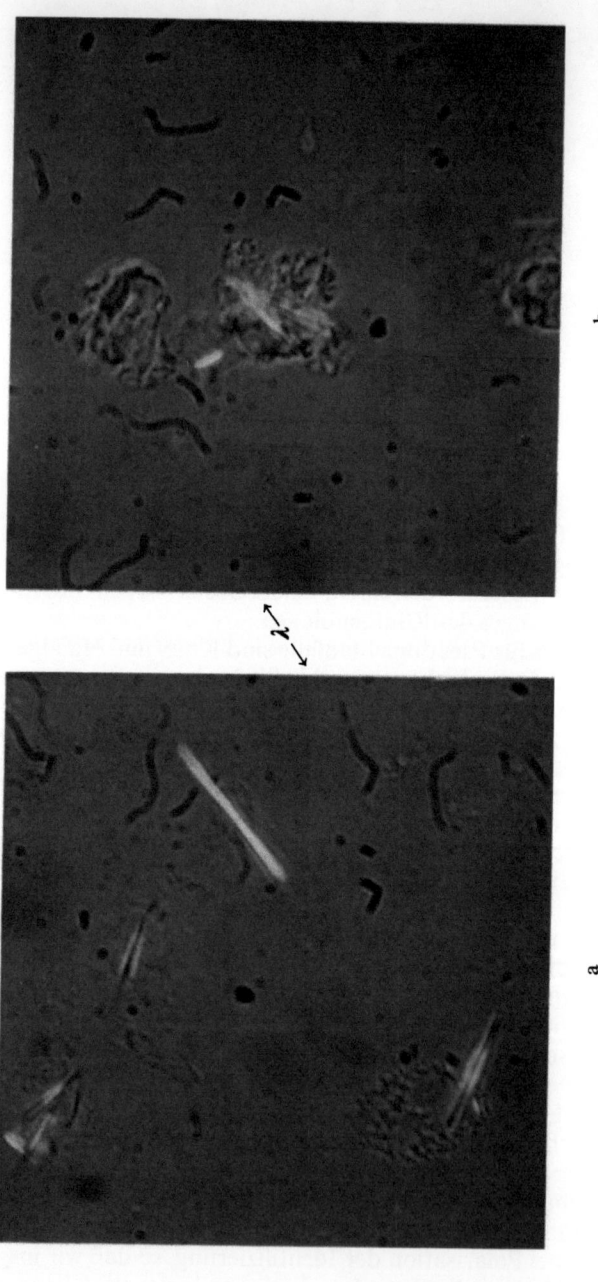

Abb. 6a u. b. Polarisationsoptisch umgekehrtes Verhalten der negativ doppelbrechenden Mononatriumurat-Kristalle (a) und der positiv doppelbrechenden Calciumpyrophosphatdihydrat-Kristalle (b) in bezug auf die Richtung der Kompensatorachse (λ)

pelbrechende Mononatriumuratkristall parallel zur Kompensatorachse gelb erscheint und beim Drehen des Gipsplättchens senkrecht zur Kompensatorachse blau wird, verhält sich der Calciumpyrophosphat-Dihydrat-Kristall umgekehrt: Mit seiner Längsachse parallel zur Kompensatorachse erscheint er blau, senkrecht wird er gelb (Abb. 6).

Für den ärztlichen Alltag mit Routinelabor ohne Polarisationsmikroskop muß als ausreichende Regel gelten: Phagocytierte Kristalle im Punktat eines Gelenkes (Kniegelenk), das im Röntgenbild Knorpelverkalkungen (Meniscusverkalkung) aufweist, bestehen mit großer Wahrscheinlichkeit aus Calciumpyrophosphat und erlauben also nicht die Diagnose Gicht.

Elektronenoptisch fanden SOLNICA et al. (1967) die Mikrokristalle innerhalb der segmentkernigen Leukocyten oder Makrophagen, und zwar die Uratkristalle in den Lysophagosomen oder umgeben von einer dicken Membran, die Calciumkristalle aber in großen Vacuolen. Elektronenmikroskopisch hat SCHUMACHER (1968) die Ultrastruktur der Synovialmembran bei Pseudogicht untersucht. Die Identifikation der Kristalle in der Synovia gelang kristallographisch (BUNDENS et al., 1965; LAGIER et al., 1966), der Kristalle im Gewebe röntgenmikroanalytisch (MOHR et al., 1974). Eine Studie über die morphologischen Veränderungen im Knorpel bei Pyrophosphat-Arthropathie stammt von BJELLE (1972).

Das anorganische Pyrophosphat im Blutplasma wurde von SILCOX und MCCARTY (1973) erhöht, von RUSSEL et al. (1970) und FALLET et al. (1972) aber normal gefunden, während diese im Gelenkpunktat ihrer Fälle eine zehnfache Erhöhung der Pyrophosphat-Konzentration bestimmen konnten. Ein somit lokalisiert wirksamer, aber genetisch determinierter Stoffwechseldefekt wird diskutiert, vielleicht ein spezifischer Phosphatase-Mangel (DYMOCK et al., 1970).

Nach eigenen Untersuchungen sind die Calcium- und anorganischen Phosphat-Werte in Blut und Urin normal, im Gelenkpunktat aber eher niedrig. Die routinemäßige Pyrophosphatbestimmung in Blut, Urin und Punktat stößt auf methodische Schwierigkeiten und ist wahrscheinlich durch schnellen Abbau des anorganischen Pyrophosphats durch die physiologischen Pyrophosphatasen stark erschwert.

Eine detaillierte lichtmikroskopische, röntgenographische und rasterelektronenmikroskopische Untersuchung mit Röntgenmikroanalyse an operativ gewonnenem Gewebsmaterial legten jüngst MOHR et al. (1974) vor. Sie kamen zu dem Schluß, daß die wahrscheinlich extracellulären Verkalkungen im Bereich der kollagenen Fasern für eine primäre Störung des Kollagens sprechen. Auch wir finden reaktionslose Kalkinkrustationen in Spalträumen des Knorpels und kristalline Einlagerungen in Stratum fibrosum und synoviale der Gelenkkapsel mit entzündlichen Reaktionen (FASSBENDER u. SCHILLING, 1973/1974) (Abb. 4).

Im Pseudogichtanfall reagieren, wie bei der echten Gicht, die systemischen Zeichen der Allgemeinentzündung teilweise besonders heftig mit: Fieber, Anstieg der Blutsenkungsgeschwindigkeit, Leukocytose, Vermehrung der akuten Phase-Proteine in der Elektrophorese.

Nach unserer Erfahrung (SCHILLING, 1971) versagt aber im Pseudogichtanfall der seit je als absolut geltende Wert des *Colchicin-Tests* als differentialdiagnostisches Unterscheidungsmerkmal, wie dies auch für die Peritendinitis calcarea und bei Hämodialyse-Patienten gesichert worden ist (MCCARTY u. GATTER, 1966; THOMPSON et al., 1968). Auch deren Anfälle sprechen auf Colchicin an. Dies entspricht an sich auch der theoretischen Erwartung. Colchicin als Mitosegift greift im synovialen Entzündungscyclus in die Phagocytose-Phase ein und unterdrückt hier den Circulus vitiosus des mikrokristallin induzierten Anfalls, ohne Rücksicht auf die chemische Natur des phagocytierten Materials. Ersatzweise oder gleichzeitig geben wir, wie im Gichtanfall (SCHILLING, 1966), Indometacin (Zäpfchen zu 100 mg im Abstand von 8 Std) oder Phenylbutazon, um antiphlogistisch in die synovitische Reaktion einzugreifen und die leukocytäre Invasion zu unterdrücken (Abb. 2).

Im rheumatologischen und orthopädischen Erfahrungsbereich ist die *lokalisierte Knie-Chondrocalcinose* am häufigsten; hier sehen wir relativ banale Fälle, meist ältere Frauen mit Kniearthrose und meist einseitiger Meniscusverkalkung, oft nach altem traumatischem oder operiertem Meniscusschaden, mit der gewöhnlichen Anamnese der Gonarthrose, aber mit vereinzelten schwersten Zuständen fieberhafter Bettlägerigkeit wegen eines sehr schmerzhaft verdickten oder wegen eines „vereiterten" Knies, das eingegipst oder antibiotisch behandelt wurde. Die Pseudogichtanfälle treten bei diesen Fällen auffallend selten auf, durch Jahre getrennt, oder sie bleiben einmalig bzw. bleiben ganz aus (klinisch stumme Fälle).

Die idiopathische Form dieser lokalisierten Knie-Chondrocalcinose, die ohne erkennbare Vorschädigung der Kniegelenke und häufiger beidseitig auftritt, ist seltener als jene symptomatische Form, zeigt keine Geschlechtsbevorzugung und ist nicht auf das höhere Alter beschränkt. Die Anfälle treten dabei häufiger auf und geraten eher in differentialdiagnostische Konkurrenz mit der Gicht.

Stets sind die lokalisierten Fälle der Chondrocalcinose am Knie auf den Faserknorpel der Menisci beschränkt (Abb. 7). Sieht man im Röntgenbild des Kniegelenks auch Verkalkungsstreifen im Bereich des Gelenkknorpels (Abb. 8), dann muß es sich um einen Fall handeln, der einer polyarticulären, also systematisierten Chondrocalcinose zugehört, und man wird mit Wahrscheinlichkeit an weiteren Prädilektionsstellen Verkalkungen finden, wenn man danach röntgenologisch sucht (Abb. 9).

Polyarticulär ausgedehnte Fälle weisen ein typisches Befallmuster auf (Abb. 10b). Dieses weicht wesentlich von dem der Gicht ab. Proximale Gelenke, besonders die stammnahen, werden von der Chondrocalcinose — ganz im Gegensatz zur Gicht — bevorzugt, und die Ausbreitung ist eher zentrifugal als — wie bei der Gicht — zentripetal. Die Hände werden von der Chondrocalcinose bald, die Füße zuletzt ergriffen. Typisch ist auch ein Verkalkungsstreifen in der Symphysis pubis (SCHILLING u. SCHACHERL, 1965).

Zur systematisierten Chondrocalcinose gehört auch ein typischer Befund an der *Wirbelsäule* mit Verkalkungen im Bereich der Bandscheiben (ZITNAN u. SITAJ, 1966; SCHILLING, 1969). Klinisch ist dieser Wirbelsäulenbefall stumm oder symptomarm, er tritt röntgenmorphologisch in Differentialdiagnose zur Spondylose oder zur Spondylitis ankylopoetica, während die Differentialdiagnose der Gicht dabei nur indirekt berührt wird. Hier sei noch erwähnt, daß diese Fälle bei der Typisierung im HLA-System das Histokompatibilitätsantigen B27 vermissen lassen, also keine entsprechende genetische Lenkung auf das Stammskelet zu erkennen geben, wie wir jedenfalls in vier eigenen Fällen feststellen konnten. In Zweifelsfällen ist damit also auch ein gewisser differentialdiagnostischer Hinweis gegenüber der typischen oder der atypischen Spondylitis ankylopoetica (z.B. der psoriatischen Spondylitis) gegeben.

Differentialdiagnostisch wichtig sind die *symptomatischen Formen* der polyarticulären Chondrocalcinose. Diese tritt dabei als Sekundärsymptom bei einem Grundleiden auf, welches auf diesem pathogenetischen Umweg durch anfallsartige Arthritiden differentialdiagnostisch überraschen kann. Es ist dies insbesondere der primäre, aber auch offenbar der sekundäre *Hyperparathyreoidismus* (ZVAIFLER et al., 1962; BYWATERS et al., 1963; VIX, 1964; RYCKEWAERT et al., 1966; JACKSON, 1965; TALON et al., 1973). Er lag zweien unserer elf Fälle von Chondrocalcinose zugrunde. Die Bestimmung mindestens des Calciumspiegels ist also bei jeder Chondrocalcinose unerläßlich und sollte in die Routine jeder differentialdiagnostischen Abklärung von nicht ganz eindeutigen akuten Arthritiden eingehen, um so auch der Abgrenzung zum Gichtanfall zu dienen.

Aufschlußreich und zum Verständnis der Pseudo-Gicht vielleicht entscheidend sind Untersuchungen über den Parathormon-Spiegel bei Chondrocalcinose von PHELPS und HAWKER (1973). Sie fanden diesen in 10 von 26 Fällen erhöht, davon viermal mit Hypercalcämie (Verdacht auf primären Hyperparathyreoidismus), dreimal mit Hypocalcämie (Verdacht auf sekundären Hyperparathyreoidismus).

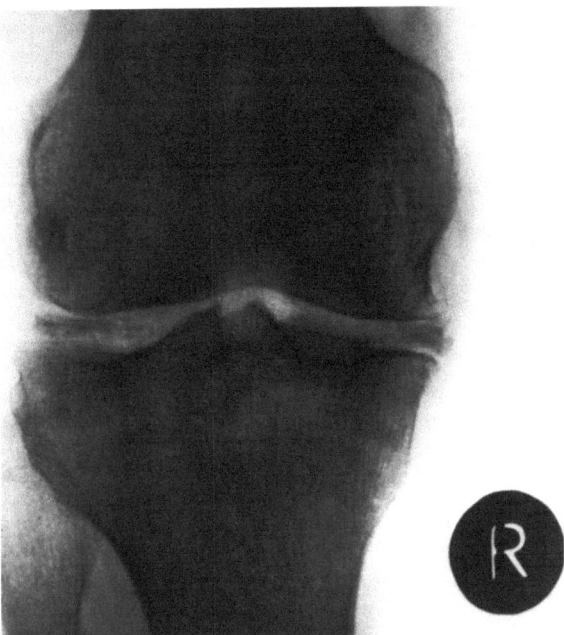

Abb. 7. Chondrocalcinose: Meniskus-Verkalkung (beider Kniegelenke) — Idiopathische Form der lokalisierten Knie-Chondrocalcinose bei einer 59jährigen Frau

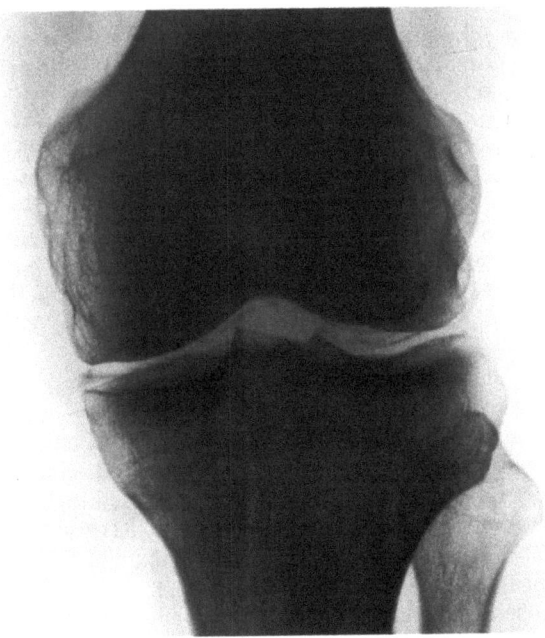

Abb. 8. Chondrocalcinose: Verkalkungen von Meniskus und hyalinem Gelenkknorpel bei systematisierter (polyarticulärer) Form — sporadischer Fall, 44jährige Frau

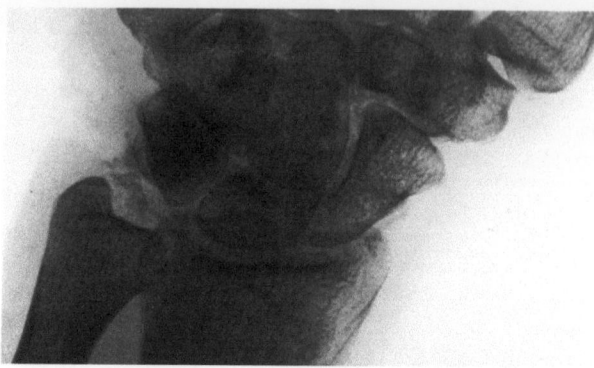

Abb. 9. Polyarticuläre Chondrocalcinose: Feinstreifige Oberflächenverkalkung von hyalinem Knorpel des proximalen Hand- und radialer Anteile des Interkarpal-Gelenks sowie unregelmäßigere Verkalkung des Discus (fibrocartilago) articularis zwischen Ulna und Carpus. — 56jährige Frau; sporadischer Fall, klinisch stumm

Beim Epithelkörper-Adenom ist die Pyrophosphat-Ausscheidung signifikant vermindert (HARTMANN, 1972). In der hypocalcämischen Phase nach Parathyreoidektomie kommen relativ häufig Pseudogicht-Anfälle vor (BILEZIKIAN et al., 1973; O'DUFFY, 1973).

Häufig aber geht der Hyperparathyreoidismus auch mit einer Hyperuricämie einher. Die dabei beschriebenen Fälle von (sekundärer) Urat-Gicht (SCOTT et al., 1964; RYCKEWAERT et al., 1966) sind verständlich, bleiben aber in ihrer Abgrenzung zur Chondrocalcinose problematisch, da sie auch mit Knorpelverkalkungen vorkommen. Immerhin aber wurden in einem solchen Falle beide Kristallformen (Urat und Pyrophosphat) in der Gelenkflüssigkeit gefunden (JACKSON, 1965).

Ein Spezialfall des sekundären Hyperparathyreoidismus ist die metabolische renale (azotämische) Osteopathie bei chronischer Niereninsuffizienz bzw. unter Langzeit-Hämodialyse (DÜRR; MALLUCHE; RITZ; ROTHENBERGER). Dabei ist die Erhöhung des Serumparathormonspiegels einerseits Folge der Hyperphosphatämie (Phosphatstau), andererseits Folge der Hypocalcämie mit peripherer Parathormon-Resistenz des Skelets bei Urämie. Abgesehen von osteomalacischen Knochenschmerzen und Erscheinungen einer Ostitis fibrosa kommt es im Rahmen der Calcium-Phosphat-Stoffwechselstörung bei Überschreiten des Ca-P-Produktes extraossal zu metastatischen Weichteilverkalkungen. Von diesen führen die (nicht-visceralen) gelenknahen Calcifikationen vorwiegend in Schleimbeuteln an Ellenbogen und Schulter sowie periarticulär in Fingern und Zehen zu tumorartig wachsenden „pseudo-tophösen" Kalkablagerungen, die — bestehend aus Hydroxylapatit-Kristallen (CONTIGUGLIA et al., 1973) — der „Kalk-Gicht" (Calcium-Phosphat-Gicht) zugehören.

Eine Arthropathie vorwiegend kleiner Gelenke mit akuten mono- oder oligoarthritischen Entzündungsreaktionen unter dem Bild einer Pseudo-Gicht kommt vor (CANER u. DECKER, 1966). Diese Form der „Pseudogicht" soll im Jahre 1970 19% der Hämodialyse-Patienten befallen haben (RITZ et al., 1973). Heute, unter wesentlich verbesserter Kontrolle der Serum-Phosphat-Spiegel, kommt eine derartige Monoarthritis kaum mehr vor (RITZ, 1974).

Die Calciumphosphat-Pseudogicht mit Pseudo-Tophi im Endstadium einer chronischen Niereninsuffizienz haben LAMOTTE et al. (1965) beschrieben. Mit diesem Ereignis kann einerseits die offenbar seltene sekundäre Harnsäure-Gicht bei chronischer Niereninsuffizienz verwechselt werden. Andererseits kann natürlich

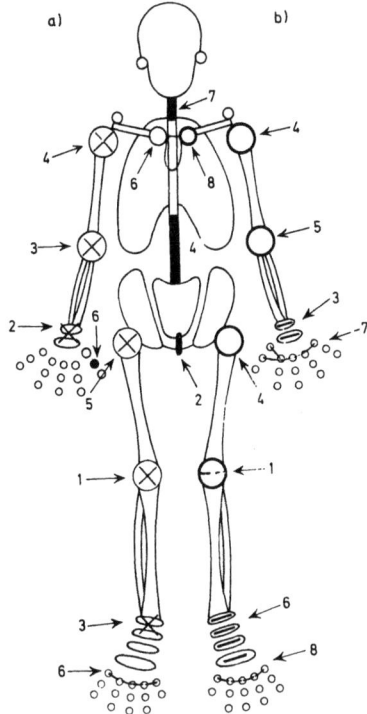

Abb. 10. Verteilung der Pseudo-Gichtanfälle *a* und der röntgenologisch erfaßten Gelenkknorpelverkalkungen *b* bei der polyarticulären Chondrocalcinose, beziffert nach der Häufigkeitsreihenfolge

die terminale Gicht-Nephropathie oder die chronische Tophus-Gicht der Dauer-Dialyse bedürfen bzw. durch diese bei sonstiger Therapie-Resistenz gebessert werden (GOLDBERG et al., 1962), was seit der Einführung von Allopurinol weniger aktuell wurde.

Die Kalkgicht ist aber im allgemeinen keine Chondrocalcinose, und ihre pseudogichtigen Erscheinungen stellen eher Periarthritiden dar (s. S. 313).

Auch die *Hämochromatose* bietet in einem Drittel der Fälle das Bild einer polyarticulären Chondrocalcinose (DE SEZE et al., 1966; ATKINS et al., 1969; DYMOCK et al., 1970; HAMILTON, 1968 und 1971). Arthritiden herrschen vor, die akute CPPD-Kristallsynovitis ist dabei häufig. Möglicherweise hemmt Eisen die Pyrophosphatase-Aktivität im Knorpel.

Schließlich gehört zu den besonderen Stoffwechselbedingungen, die eine Pyrophosphat-Kristallablagerung begünstigen oder provozieren können (metabolische Arthropathien), auch der *Diabetes* mellitus. Dieser metabolische Hintergrund einer Chondrocalcinose ist nicht selten (MCCARTY, 1969); einer unserer 11 Fälle hatte einen Diabetes.

Die Hyperuricämie spielt angesichts ihrer Häufigkeit wohl nur eine akzidentelle Rolle. Daß lokalisierte Knorpelverkalkungen aber vereinzelt auch einmal in chronisch arthritisch (rheumatoid oder durch Gicht) geschädigten Gelenken vorkommen können, wurde oben schon erwähnt.

Unspezifische *Rheumafaktor*-Titer kommen vor (BLOCH-MICHEL, 1968; MENKES et al., 1973), sollten aber im Latex-Fixationstest den Wert 1/124 und im

Waaler-Rose-Test den Wert 1/32 nicht überschreiten. Anderenfalls muß die Diagnose ernsthaft bezweifelt werden und das Vorkommen von Knorpelverkalkungen bei chronischer (rheumatoider) Polyarthritis in Erwägung gezogen werden.

Bei schweren *Arthrosen*, besonders bei einer Vorschädigung durch eine Meniscopathie oder eine Operation, aber auch bei Neuroarthropathien, z.B. bei der Tabes dorsalis (JACOBELLI *et al.*, 1973), sind es lokale metabolische Faktoren des gestörten Terrains, die zur lokalisierten Chondrocalcinose und zu Anfällen führen können.

Pseudogichtanfälle provozierend sind nicht selten *postoperative* Phasen mit Hypocalcämie, die als metabolischer Auslöser einer Kristallsynovitis durch Freisetzung von Calciumpyrophosphat aus dem Gelenkknorpel in die Gelenkflüssigkeit betrachtet werden kann (O'DUFFY, 1973).

McCARTY (1969) fand unter 200 Fällen in 37% einen Diabetes, in 27% eine Hyperuricämie und in 8,6% einen Hyperparathyreoidismus.

Die Pseudogicht stellt also einerseits die wichtigste Differentialdiagnose zur akut rezidivierenden Gicht dar und bietet andererseits in sich eine Fülle verwirrender differentialdiagnostischer Probleme. Von unseren 11 Fällen waren 2 als „akutes rheumatisches Fieber", 1 als Empyem, 3 als „Gicht", 4 als „Arthrosen" und 2 als „chronische Polyarthritis" fehldiagnostiziert worden.

2. Das rheumatische Fieber

Die akute Polyarthritis rheumatica ist eine relativ seltene Zweitkrankheit nach einem Racheninfekt mit β-hämolysierenden Streptokokken der Gruppe A (KÖTTGEN u. CALLENSEE, 1961; KÖLLE, 1969; KÖTTGEN, 1970). Das rheumatische Fieber ist längst nicht mehr auf das Kindesalter beschränkt, sondern befällt auch Erwachsene aller Altersgruppen ohne Geschlechtsbevorzugung (ANSCHÜTZ u. MENDE, 1968). Auch hat die Pathomorphose dieser einst im Sinne des „eigentlichen Rheumatismus" und von KLINGE als „Rheumatismus verus" verstandenen Krankheit eine Veränderung der arthritischen Symptomatik mit sich gebracht, die zur Quelle diagnostischer Verwechslungen wird. Bei Kindern wurde das große, erheblich exsudative, hochschmerzhafte und systematisiert polyarticuläre Krankheitsbild seltener, und auch bei Erwachsenen tauchen atypische trockene, oligoarticulär asymmetrische, sowohl flüchtige und harmlos erscheinende als auch prolongierte Formen auf. Die JONES-Kriterien mußten mehrfach modifiziert werden. Ein besonderes diagnostisches und nosologisches Problem ist der „chronische Streptokokken-Rheumatismus" (SCHATTENKIRCHNER, 1969).

Strenge Skepsis im Einzelfall wie bei der Berücksichtigung des Gestaltwandels dieser Krankheit überhaupt sei aber empfohlen. Es ist sicher, daß das rheumatische Fieber oder mindestens seine kardialen Folgen seit über 10 Jahren statistisch deutlich im Rückgang begriffen sind (ANSCHÜTZ u. WIPPERFÜRTH, 1972). Die atypische Symptomatik bietet Verkennungsmöglichkeiten in beiden Richtungen: Teils wird die Diagnose verfehlt; häufiger aber kommt es vor, daß andere akute und subakute Arthritiden und Polyarthritiden verschiedener Art dann für ein rheumatisches Fieber gehalten und als Zeuge für dessen Atypie geltend gemacht werden, wenn sie fieberhaft verlaufen und sich einer diagnostischen Einordnung zunächst entziehen.

Zu dieser Gruppe von Krankheiten gehört auch die akut rezidivierende Gicht, zumal diese bereits relativ jugendliche Menschen befällt und 10% der Anfälle mit hohem Fieber und fast stets mit mehr oder weniger ausgeprägten systemischen Entzündungszeichen einhergehen. Das entscheidende Unterscheidungskriterium, der *Antistreptolysintiter*, kann einerseits für das rheumatische Fieber nur dann verwendet werden, wenn der Titer innerhalb des frühen Krankheitsverlaufs signifikant, d. h. um mehr als eine Titerstufe ansteigt. Es bedarf also mindestens einer Kontrolluntersuchung frühestens nach 7, spätestens nach 14 Tagen.

Andererseits kann aber die Gicht einen falsch positiven „Antistreptolysintiter" bieten, dann nämlich, wenn sie mit einer Hyperlipidämie (meist Typ IV) einhergeht. Dieser diagnostische Fallstrick ist entsprechend der Häufigkeit assoziierter Fettstoffwechselstörungen bei der Gicht nicht selten gegeben und muß durch Fällung mit Dextransulfat ausgemerzt werden.

Eine sehr hohe Blutsenkungsgeschwindigkeit spricht differentialdiagnostisch für rheumatisches Fieber, jedoch keinesfalls mit entscheidendem Gewicht; denn im fieberhaften Gichtanfall kann es zu Blutsenkungsanstiegen bis über 100 mm in der ersten Stunde kommen. Die Kriterien der örtlich hohen synovitischen und paraarthritischen Akuität mit Rötung und Hitze sind allen akuten Arthritiden gemeinsam, beim rheumatischen Fieber aber selten geworden. Hilfreich ist es auch zu wissen, daß eine Monarthritis am Großzeh beim rheumatischen Fieber kaum vorkommt, sondern daß von der akuten Polyarthritis mittlere Gelenke bevorzugt werden.

Nach unserer Erfahrung werden besonders häufig Reitersche Krankheit, Pseudogicht und rheumatisches Fieber fehldiagnostisch durcheinander geworfen.

Das rheumatische Fieber bevorzugt keines der beiden Geschlechter. Seine Rezidive könnten einmal der Verkennung als akut rezidivierende Gicht Vorschub leisten.

3. Andere akute Arthritiden und subakute Polyarthritiden

a) Im Zusammenhang mit viralen oder/und bakteriellen *Infekten* verschiedener Art kommen rheumatische Erscheinungen vor, Arthralgien, flüchtige bis anfallsartige Arthritiden, vorwiegend mono- oder oligoarticular, trocken oder exsudativ, mit einer Dauer bis zu höchstens einigen Wochen und stets völlig ausheilend. Gelenkaffektionen dieser Art gehören zur Gruppe der „symptomatischen Arthritiden". Sie werden gerne als „Infektarthritis" bezeichnet; ein unscharfer Ausdruck, der auf die infektiös metastatisch-eitrige Arthritis beschränkt werden sollte. Praktisch ist dieser Begriff aber deshalb wichtig, weil er vielfach noch als Verlegenheitsdiagnose für die Vielzahl akuter Arthritiden unbekannter Ätiologie verwendet wird, worunter sich auch nicht diagnostizierte Gichtanfälle befinden.

Das Auftreten akuter synovitischer Reizzustände, die an einen Infekt geknüpft sind und von diesem im klinischen Bild mehr oder weniger beherrscht werden, ist zeitlich dem Infekt zu- oder nachgeordnet. Die parainfektiösen Zustände sind vorwiegend als toxisch („infektions-allergisch") bedingt zu verstehen, die postinfektiös nach einem Intervall auftretenden aber als immunpathologisch bedingt. Zu den letzteren gehören auch die ehemals so genannten „Rheumatoide" nach Scharlach und Ruhr, wobei wir heute das Ruhr-Rheumatoid als Abortivform des Reiter-Syndroms auffassen.

In differentialdiagnostische Konkurrenz zur akuten Gicht-Arthritis treten die akuten symptomatischen Arthritiden dann, wenn die infektiöse Grundkrankheit verborgen bleibt und die Arthritis krankheitsdominant ist. Dies kommt beim Coxsackie-Virus und bei der in Finnland häufigeren Yersinia-Infektion vor.

b) Die Diagnose der *subakuten Polyarthritis* (RAVAULT) wird nicht mehr gestellt (RAVAULT, 1964). Man kann dies bedauern, denn wir haben uns damit einer diagnostischen Kategorie begeben, die mindestens im Vorfeld der endgültigen Differentialdiagnose jenen Arthritiden eine wenigstens vorläufige Unterkunft gewähren konnte, die zwischen Akuität und Chronizität nicht so bald ihre Prozeßtendenz erkennen lassen und sehr verzögert, nach spätestens zwei Jahren ohne Dauerschaden ausheilen, ohne die Kriterien des prolongierten rheumatischen Fiebers oder die der chronischen (rheumatoiden) Polyarthritis erfüllt zu haben (BOPP, 1965).

Eine idiopathische Form subakuter Polyarthritis gibt es zweifellos. Sie ist rheuma-serologisch (Rheuma-Faktor) negativ, von durchschnittlich geringer systemischer Entzündungsaktivität, vorwiegend oligoarthritisch und heilt von selbst spurlos aus. Rezidivierende Formen („benigne rheumatoide Arthritis") können in eine chronische (rheumatoide) Arthritis übergehen und gehören damit zur Gruppe der atypischen chronischen Polyarthritis. Sicher sind auch vermeintliche Fälle des palindromen Rheumatismus und des Hydrops intermittens hierher zu zählen. Flüchtige Synovitiden der unteren Extremitäten junger Männer sind stets verdächtig auf Spondylitis ankylopoetica.

Fälle dieser Art werden besonders dann als akute Gicht verkannt, wenn sie in anfallsartigen Schüben, mono- bis oligoarticulär mit negativer Rheumaserologie und außerdem vielleicht auch noch mit Hyperuricämie verlaufen. Hier liegen tatsächlich zuweilen differentialdiagnostische Schwierigkeiten, die der Verlauf klärt, wenn nicht bereits die Beachtung einiger Schlüsselfragen die Erwägung auf eine der folgenden Diagnosen lenkt. Solche „Schlüssel" sind z.B. die anamnestische Angabe einer Urethritis oder einer Iridocyclitis, der familienanamnestische oder der verborgene Befund einer Psoriasis, ein Erythema nodosum oder eine versteckte Allergie.

Hinter subakuten Arthritiden verbergen sich also auch andere rheumatologische Entitäten: Spondylitis ankylopoetica, Reitersche Krankheit, psoriatische Arthritis und Boecksche Sarkoidose.

Es verbleibt als wahrscheinlich selbständige Entität eine meist monarticuläre „episodische Arthritis" vorwiegend des Kniegelenks, die ausheilt.

c) Die *Reitersche Krankheit*, das oculo-urethro-synoviale Syndrom (FIESSINGER-LEROY-REITER, 1916), kommt bei uns in Friedenszeiten nur sporadisch, aber nicht ganz so selten vor, wie gemeinhin angenommen wird. Die bekannte *Trias* Urethritis, Conjunctivitis und Arthritis ist nur in einem Teil der Fälle erfüllt, meist in dieser typischen Abfolge, wobei die Symptome durch ein Zeitintervall von drei bis 14 Tagen voneinander getrennt sind. Ein Viertel aller Fälle dieses Syndroms verläuft einerseits mit Hauterscheinungen als viertem Hauptsymptom, über ein Viertel der Fälle stellt andererseits aber schwer erkennbare Abortivfälle dar. Die Hälfte aller Fälle rezidiviert oder wird chronisch (chronisches Reiter-Syndrom, SCHILLING et al., 1965).

Der eitrigen *Urethritis*, die auch fehlen kann, geht bei der dysenterischen, meist epidemischen Form der Weltkriege (PARONEN, 1948), um etwa 10 Tage eine Bazillenruhr voraus. Das Reiter-Syndrom erscheint dann als Zweitkrankheit, wobei wahrscheinlich das Histokompatibilitätsantigen HLA-B 27 eine entscheidend lenkende Rolle spielt (BREWERTON et al., 1973; SCHILLING, 1974). Das Symptom Urethritis kann sich als unbedeutender Urinsedimentbefund verbergen, oder aber primär als coital übertragener Urogenitalinfekt die Krankheit einleiten: Venerische sporadische Form der Reiterschen Krankheit (CSONKA, 1964). Manchmal ist die Gonorrhoe der Einschlepp-Infekt.

Auch die *Conjunctivitis* kann als harmloser Reizzustand ablaufen, sie kann fehlen, oder aber eine schwere eitrige Sclero-Conjunctivitis darstellen, die schon beim ersten Rezidiv einen „Schichtwechsel" zur Iridocyclitis erfahren kann. Monosymptomatische Rezidive in Form einer Iritis oder seltener Scleritis werden ohne Kenntnis des Zusammenhangs nicht erkannt. Die chronische Prostatitis scheint für Rezidive und Chronizität eine Bedeutung zu besitzen.

Befallen werden ganz vorwiegend Männer. Unter mehr als 70 Fällen der eigenen Erfahrung befindet sich nur eine Frau. Allerdings verlaufen vielleicht die weiblichen Fälle so maskiert, daß sie sich der Erkennung entziehen. Jedenfalls sind geschlechtliche Ansteckung bei Partnerwechsel immer wieder eine Quelle von Rezidiven.

Diagnostisch sehr hilfreich sind, wenn vorhanden, die typischen Hautveränderungen, das *Keratoderma* blennorrhagicum vorwiegend der Fußsohlen und die Balanitis circinata parakeratotica („Reiter-Balanitis"). Beim chronischen Reiter-Syndrom wird die Verwandtschaft dieser Keratose mit der Psoriasis deutlich (WRIGHT u. REED, 1964), wobei eine dieser ähnliche Onychopathie mit subungualen Parakeratosen, krümeligen Nagelzerstörungen und rezidivierender Onycholysis manifest wird. Das chronische Reiter-Syndrom verläuft peripher unter dem Bild der atypischen chronischen Polyarthritis vom psoriatischen Typ und am Stammskelet unter dem Bild einer atypischen Spondylitis ankylopoetica. Zu diesen Verlaufsformen zählen die seltenen schwersten Fälle chronischen Siechtums, die wir im rheumatologischen Bereich kennen.

Konstantes Symptom der akuten Reiterschen Krankheit, und in der Differentialdiagnose zur akuten Gicht relevant, ist die *Arthritis*. Im Rahmen der Reiterschen Trias ist diese Arthritis diagnostisch klar einzuordnen. Aber schon beim Fehlen conjunctivaler Symptome entsteht diagnostische Unsicherheit. Arthritiden nach Urogenitalinfektionen werden gerne als „Uro-Arthritis" gekennzeichnet. Schließlich ist eine postdysenterische Arthritis oder Polyarthritis („Ruhr-Rheumatoid") im Prinzip eine monosymptomatische Reitersche Krankheit.

Die Arthritis der akuten Reiterschen Krankheit spielt sich meistens mono- oder oligarticulär an den unteren Extremitäten ab, seltener polyarticulär, diese bevorzugend. Eine auffallend häufige Lokalisation ist das Großzehengrundgelenk! Da es sich meistens um jüngere Männer handelt, liegt die Fehldiagnose Gicht nahe. Am häufigsten wird die Reitersche Krankheit als Gicht oder rheumatisches Fieber verkannt.

Das Fuß- oder das Kniegelenk sind meistens mitgegriffen. Im Kniegelenkpunktat, aber auch im Urethralabstrich, können — wenn eine günstige Färbung gelingt — die von AMOR et al. (1965) beschriebenen Einschlußkörperchen gesehen werden, die jene mit einer viralen Genese dieser Krankheit in Verbindung gebracht haben.

Nach unserer Erfahrung bevorzugt die Reitersche Krankheit, im Gegensatz zur Gicht, häufiger asthenisch konstituierte jüngere Männer als fettleibige Pykniker.

d) Die intermittierende *Hydarthrose* (Hydrops intermittens) ist selten, betrifft periodisch exsudativ und schmerzarm die Kniegelenke vorwiegend jüngerer Menschen. Die Entität ist fragwürdig, jedenfalls wird sie sicher fälschlicherweise bemüht z.B. für rezidivierende Synovitiden der frühen Spondylitis ankylopoetica und auch für Fälle akut rezidivierender Gicht. Wir kennen nur wenige Patienten, auf die diese Diagnose zutrifft: Junge Frauen mit offenbar hormonell determinierter periodischer Knieschwellung.

4. Die psoriatische Arthritis (Arthritis psoriatica, chronische Polyarthritis psoriatica; Psoriasis arthropathica)

Die Arthritis psoriatica stellt den wichtigsten Teil, jedenfalls den bedeutendsten als Entität bekannten Teil der rheumaserologisch negativen chronischen Polyarthritis dar. Wir bevorzugen den Terminus chronische Polyarthritis psoriatica, um damit den Charakter dieser im Gegensatz zur Psoriasis entzündlichen Krankheit als polyarticulär synovitischen Prozeß zu kennzeichnen. Es handelt sich um eine vom Hautleiden her geprägte Form der chronischen Polyarthritis mit einer typischen Eigenständigkeit.

Die *Häufigkeit* der Arthritis psoriatica liegt deutlich über der aus der Kombination von Schuppenflechte und chronischer Polyarthritis zu erwartenden Morbiditätsquote. Sie hat an der Gesamtzahl chronischer Polyarthritiden einen Anteil von 5%, wobei die Männer nicht absolut, aber bezogen auf ihren Anteil an allen chronischen Polyarthritiden, relativ überwiegen. Umgekehrt haben rund 5% aller Psoriatiker eine chronische Polyarthritis (HORNSTEIN, 1962). Unter Anwendung nuklearmedizinischer Untersuchungsmethoden erscheint dieser Anteil erheblich größer (EISSNER u. HAHN, 1974).

Die Arthritis psoriatica bevorzugt an der *Haut* gewisse Formen der Schuppenflechte. Neben der banalen Form der Psoriasis vulgaris sind relativ häufig die Psoriasis capitis, die Psoriasis pustulosa und die psoriatische Erythrodermie. Mit der Ausbreitung auf Handteller, Fußsohlen und Schleimhäute gewinnt sie Ähnlichkeit mit der Dermatose beim Reiter-Syndrom. Auffallend ist die Häufigkeit der psoriatischen Onychopathie, die bei der Arthritis psoriatica kaum einmal fehlt. Dabei ist der bekannte Tüpfelnagel selten, während subunguale Hyperkeratosen mit distaler Weißverfärbung, die mit einem ölig-dunkelgefärbten Streifen unregelmäßig begrenzt wird, vorherrschen (Abb. 11 und 12). Krümelnagel und Onycholysis kommen vor.

Meist ist der Hautbefall primär, die Arthritis folgt. Schübe an der Haut und an den Gelenken sind meistens nicht koinzident. In einer kleineren Zahl von Fällen erscheint die Arthritis vor der Manifestierung der Psoriasis, die im Grenzfall sogar ausbleiben kann. Wir erkennen dann die „psoriatische Konstitution" am Typ der Polyarthritis bzw. an der Morphologie der Arthritis, klinisch bzw. röntgenologisch, und sprechen von einer „Arthritis vom psoriatischen Typ" (SCHACHERL u. SCHILLING, 1967).

Gerade diese Arthritis aber hat besondere Bedeutung in der Differentialdiagnose zur Gicht.

Sowohl die Psoriasis als auch die Arthritis psoriatica sind genetisch determiniert und folgen einem bestimmten Vererbungsmodus (ANANTHAKRISHNAN et al., 1973). Die familiäre Belastung ist so bedeutend, daß familienanamnestische Hinweise auf Psoriasis in manchen Fällen zum Verständnis einer noch unklaren Arthritis führen können. — Die psoriatische Arthritis kann als eine der Organmanifestationen der Psoriasis-Krankheit aufgefaßt werden (HOLZMANN et al., 1973).

Die *klinischen Unterschiede* zwischen der chronischen (rheumatoiden) Polyarthritis und der psoriatischen Polyarthritis sind fließende, vorwiegend aber charakteristische (SCHILLING, 1969). Man findet bei der psoriatischen Arthritis einen insgesamt unruhigen Verlauf, bei häufig akutem Beginn und mit größerer Schubbereitschaft, wobei die Schübe durch hohe Akuität, getrennt durch um so vollständigere Remissionen ausgezeichnet sind, entsprechend den größeren Schwankungen der Entzündungsaktivität. Die Schübe können anfallsweisen, bei Monarthritis also pseudogichtigen Charakter annehmen, und die Remissionen können einen lang anhaltenden Stillstand der Krankheit vortäuschen, so daß diese in der Remission u. U. gar nicht erkennbar ist.

Abweichungen im Befall- und Ausbreitungsmuster kennzeichnen den psoriatischen Typ der chronischen Polyarthritis: Asymmetrischer Beginn und Asymmetrien im Verlauf; deutliche Bevorzugung der Fingerendgelenke und der Zehenzwischengelenke; Befall mehrerer Gelenke eines einzelnen Fingers oder Zehen: „Strahlbefall".

Obwohl die Arthritis psoriatica chronischen, also Prozeßcharakter hat, haben bestimmte Erscheinungsformen aber solche Akuität, daß sie als selbständige Krankheitsphasen imponieren. Dies gilt besonders für jene Sonderform der Arthritis psoriatica, die wir „*Pseudo-guttöse Arthritis bei Psoriasis inversa*" nennen (SCHILLING u. FASSBENDER, 1974). Vorwiegend bei jungen Menschen im zweiten und dritten Lebensjahrzehnt erlebt man akute Schübe, die sich klinisch charakteristischerweise unter dem Bilde plötzlich auftretender heftiger Gelenkschwellungen bemerkbar machen, mit Rötung und Schwellung an Zehen oder Fingern. Am Fuß imponiert die plumpe Schwellung mit Verfärbung und schmerzhafter Behinderung des ganzen befallenen Zehs, am Finger meistens die Rötung mit heftiger Empfindlichkeit eines Endgelenks oder aber auch eines ganzen Fingers („Wurstfinger", „Wurstzeh"). Diese akuten Arthritiden wirken in der Tat wie Gicht-Anfälle und wurden deshalb in der französischen Literatur als „pseudo-goutteuse" beschrieben (COSTE u. SOLNICA, 1966).

Bei solchen Erscheinungen achte man sorgfältig auf versteckte oder maskierte Psoriasisherde an Haut oder Schleimhäuten. Die Psoriasis inversa hat sich nicht selten vom Patienten und seiner Umgebung unbemerkt im Nabel, in der Analfalte, im und hinter dem Ohr, an der Kopfhaut oder sehr diskret und von der Reiter-Balanitis kaum unterscheidbar an der Glans penis etabliert. Besonders häufig aber und differentialdiagnostisch auf den ersten Blick hinweisend ist die typische *Onychopathie* mit subungualer Keratose, die das distale Nagelbett unregelmäßig abhebt und die im Gegensatz zur aspektiv zum Verwechseln ähnlichen Nagelmykose schneller veränderlich und auch spontan reversibel ist. Der letzteren fehlt auch der kleine ölige Streifen. In der Nachbarschaft eines plötzlich hochrot geschwollenen und sehr empfindlichen Fingerendgelenks kann diese Onychopathie die Diagnose verraten, die Topik am gleichen Finger ist aber keinesfalls obligat (Abb. 11).

In den intertriginösen Falten kann die Psoriasis inversa zum feuchten Ekzem macerieren, und die Psoriasis capitis kann als banale Schuppung verkannt werden. Das derart maskierte Bild, das man bei vorwiegend jüngeren Menschen findet, stellt nach der Pseudogicht den schwierigsten und häufigsten Fallstrick in der Differentialdiagnose zur Gicht dar.

Die *Differentialdiagnose der Fingerendgelenkarthritis* hat am häufigsten frische Heberden-Knötchen im entzündlichen Reizzustand in Betracht zu ziehen. Diese charakterisieren die Lebensphase der klimakterischen Frau, während die Psoriasis in diesem Alter sich bereits zu chronischen Dauerschäden entwickelt hat. Ein Gichtanfall am Fingerendgelenk ist selten und wird bei einer Frau kaum einmal vorkommen. Bei jüngeren Patienten ist der systemische Lupus erythematodes in Erwägung zu ziehen. Die akute entzündliche periarthritische Calcinose am Fingerendgelenk (Peritendinitis calcarea) ist täuschend ähnlich, aber ein sehr seltenes Ereignis (vgl. unten). Die chronische (rheumatoide) Polyarthritis zeitigt kaum akute Gelenkrötungen und dies schon gar nicht an den Fingerendgelenken. Die traumatische Capsulitis ist häufig. Aber auch für spontane Fingergelenkveränderungen, wie z. B. für die Heberden-Knötchen, schuldigt der Patient gerne eine Prellung an.

Häufiger als an den Fingerendgelenken ist bei der pseudoguttösen Form der Arthritis psoriatica die Manifestation an den Zehen. Hier werden tatsächlich Gichtanfälle imitiert, die aber bereits durch die Lokalisation unterscheidbar sind. An den Vorfüßen kommen echte Gichtanfälle an den Zehen II bis V nur äußerst selten vor, so daß als Regel gelten darf: Im Stadium der akut rezidivierenden Gicht gibt es die Arthritis und Paraarthritis urica praktisch nur am Großzeh, während ähnliche Zustände an den anderen Zehen auf Psoriasis sehr verdächtig sind. Panaritium und Kalkgicht müssen ausgeschlossen worden sein.

Die pseudoguttöse Arthritis psoriatica am Vorfuß überfällt den Patienten akut bis subakut, führt stets zu einer dicken, spindelförmigen bis wurstförmigen Schwellung des ganzen Zehs, der hochrot verfärbt ist mit gelegentlich livider Tönung, quälend druckempfindlich ist und beim Abrollen schmerzt. Der Zustand ist seltener flüchtig, meistens hält er wochenlang an. Er betrifft häufiger den 2. oder 5. Zeh, auch zwei Zehen gleichzeitig: „Dactylitis psoriatica" (Abb. 12).

Zugrunde liegt bereits ein morphologisch chronisches Substrat, das der Ossifizierungstendenz der psoriatischen Arthritis zugehört und die das Gelenk überschreitet. In ausgeprägten Fällen sieht man röntgenologisch die streifenförmige ossifizierende „Periostitis" an den Diaphysen der Phalangen (Abb. 13). Destruktionen treten ganz zurück.

Die Differentialdiagnose zur Gicht kann durch den Befund einer *Hyperuricämie* bei der Psoriasis erschwert werden. Hochsignifikant ist dieser Befund allerdings nicht, die statistischen Angaben darüber sind nicht einheitlich (vgl. Psoriasis-Symposium Teneriffa, 1969; YAZDI u. GAHLEN, 1969; u.a.). Mäßige Hyperuricämien bei der Psoriasis und bei der psoriatischen Arthritis kommen sicher vor; eine signifikante Überschreitung der Hyperuricämie-Morbidität der Durch-

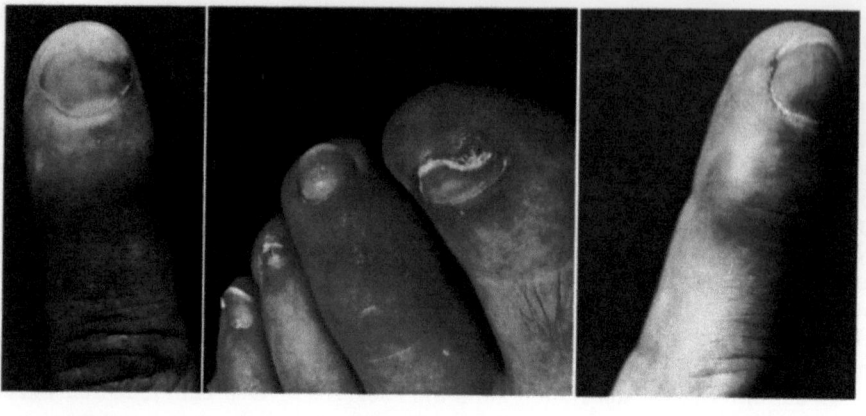

Abb. 11   Abb. 12   Abb. 14a

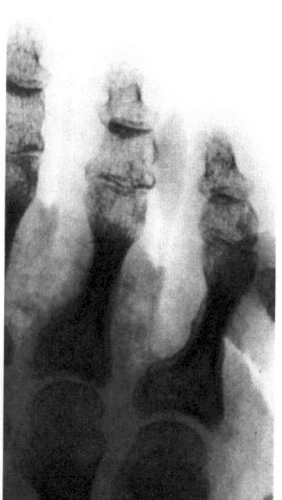

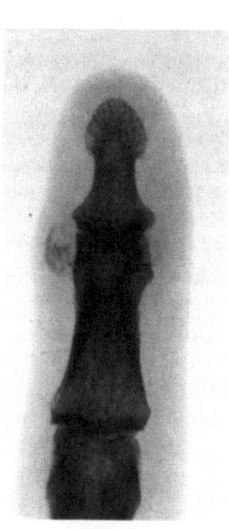

Abb. 13   Abb. 14b

Abb. 11. Psoriatische Finger-Endgelenk-Arthritis mit Rötung und Schwellung sowie mit typischer, den Nagel distal keratotisch unterminierender Onychopathia psoriatica bei einer chronischen Polyarthritis psoriatica „pseudo-guttöser" Verlaufsform mit Psoriasis inversa

Abb. 12. „Pseudo-guttöse" Form der Arthritis psoriatica: Anfallsartige Entzündung eines Zehs bei einer 24jährigen Frau mit Psoriasis nur an den Finger- und Zehennägeln. (Onychopathia und Dactylitis psoriatica)

Abb. 13. Periostal ossifizierende Proliferationen an einigen Zehen bei Psoriasis inversa mit „pseudo-guttösen" Entzündungszuständen bei einer 22jährigen Frau

Abb. 14a u. b. Periarthritischer Pseudo-Gichtanfall an einem Fingerendgelenk (a) bei Peritendinitis calcarea (b) eines 37jährigen Mannes

schnittsbevölkerung, insbesondere unter Berücksichtigung der Geschlechterunterschiede, erscheint aber nicht gesichert. Dasselbe gilt für den Zusammenhang mit der Ausdehnung der Psoriasis. Wir finden keine quantitative Proportionalität zwischen dieser und dem Harnsäurespiegel, was im Prinzip gegen den pathogenetischen Zusammenhang überhaupt spricht.

5. *Palindromer Rheumatismus*

Der von HENCH u. ROSENBERG (1944) beschriebene "palindromic rheumatism" ist ein Spezialfall innerhalb der inhomogenen Gruppe akut rezidivierender (palindromer = rekurrierender) articulärer und paraarticulärer Entzündungszustände. Die anfallsartige Attacke beginnt perakut, vorwiegend monotop und Fingergelenke bevorzugend, weist alle Zeichen der akuten Entzündung mit Schwellung auf, dauert nur Stunden bis Tage und heilt jeweils ad integrum aus. Die extraarticulären anfallsartigen Erscheinungen betreffen das periarticuläre Gewebe mit rötlicher Verfärbung der darüber liegenden Haut (Paraarthritis), Sehnenansätze, Handrücken und Ferse. Teilweise besteht Übereinstimmung mit einer akuten Enthesopathie (akute Insertionstendinitis). Milde systemische Entzündungszeichen begleiten die Attacke. Rekurrenz kann Periodik andeuten, weshalb auch Beziehungen zur „periodischen Krankheit" angenommen wurden (vgl. SCHILLING, 1969). Chronizität im Sinne eines Prozesses oder Dauerschäden werden nicht erreicht, das Röntgenbild bleibt stumm.

Die Erfahrung legt Zweifel am Vorliegen einer einheitlichen Entität nahe. Die meisten Fälle mit dieser Symptomatik stellen Grenzfälle, Vorspiele oder Frühstadien anderer rheumatologischer Krankheiten dar oder gehen über kurz oder lang in solchen auf. Wir fassen deshalb den „palindromen Rheumatismus" als Palliativ-Diagnose auf, d.h. als vorläufige, weiter differenzierungspflichtige Deskription; allerdings mit einem idiopathischen, aber kleinen „Kern", der nicht einzuordnen ist. Dieser scheint vorwiegend aus allergisch bedingten Fällen zu bestehen.

Bei der Beschreibung als palindromer Rheumatismus liegt eine als solche noch nicht erkannte akut rezidivierende Gicht mit Arthritis und Paraarthritis nahe; allerdings mit dem wesentlichen topischen Unterschied der Bevorzugung der Füße durch die Gicht. Flüchtige und rezidivierende Arthritiden einzelner Fingergelenke gehören nicht zum üblichen Bilde einer frühen Arthritis urica.

Weiterhin kann der palindrome Rheumatismus eine akute, schmerzhafte und gerötete Tenosynovitis z.B. am Handrücken bieten, was sowohl bei der Gicht als auch bei der chronischen (rheumatoiden) Polyarthritis nicht vorkommt. Vielmehr ist eine solche andernfalls auf eitrige Entzündung durch einen bakteriellen Infekt bzw. Superinfekt verdächtig, wie es z.B. bei einer langzeitig mit Cortison behandelten chronischen Polyarthritis vorkommen kann.

Unsere weiteren Fälle, die die Symptomatik des palindromen Rheumatismus erfüllten, stellen zu einem kleineren Teil sehr kaschierte Fälle von systemischem *Lupus erythematodes* dar und betrafen zwei jüngere Männer. Ein Teil gehört zur *psoriatischen* Arthritis mit latenter oder nur familiär faßbarer Psoriasis an der Haut, und ein weiterer Teil geht prozeßhaft in eine atypische *chronische Polyarthritis* über und gehört somit zum chronischen polysynovitischen Syndrom. Nie lassen diese Fälle den Rheumafaktor in einer eindeutigen Titerhöhe erkennen.

Auch die Erfahrung der Mayo-Klinik bei der Langzeitbeobachtung ihrer Fälle mit der ursprünglichen Diagnose "palindromic rheumatism" ergab schließlich die Zugehörigkeit teils zur Gicht, teils zur chronischen Polyarthritis und teils zum systemischen Lupus erythematodes (WARD u. OKIHIRO, 1959). Beim Vorliegen dieses Syndroms sollte also, abgesehen von der selbstverständlichen Harnsäurebestimmung, im Blut auch auf den Immunstatus und bei der Körperuntersuchung auf verborgene psoriatische Herde geachtet werden.

Schließlich haben wir einen jüngeren Mann beobachtet, der mit einem ähnlichen Bild zunächst auf palindromen Rheumatismus verdächtig schien, der sich dann aber als das seltene Bild der „akut rezidivierenden Peritendinitis (Periarthritis) calcarea" herausstellte (s. unten).

6. Arthrosen

Arthrosen können nur dann in der Differentialdiagnose zum akuten Gichtanfall in Erwägung gezogen werden, wenn die Sekundär-Synovitis einen besonders heftigen *Reizzustand* dieser Arthrose bewirkt: „Aktivierte Arthrose" (OTTE). Das Röntgenbild und die Punktatanalyse klären die Zugehörigkeit. Der Reizerguß einer Arthrose ist hell, mucinreich und zellarm (vgl. Tabelle 2) und im allgemeinen ohne Kristallphagocytosen. Zeigt er aber doch Merkmale stärkerer Entzündung, dann muß auch an eine pseudo-gichtige zusätzliche synovitische Reizung durch CPPD-Kristalle gedacht werden, die auf die Arthrose aufgepfropft diese komplizieren können und dann auch als Phagocytosen gefunden werden müßten.

Heftig entzündliche Reizerscheinungen können frische *Heberden-Knötchen* im Rahmen der Polyarthrose (vgl. unten) der klimakterischen Frau bieten (Abb. 18). Der doppelhöckrige Aspekt ist unverkennbar, zunächst weich cystisch und zu entzündlicher Rötung neigend. Das Heberdenknötchen kann geradezu eruptiv aufblühen, so daß die Patientin meint, sie müsse sich gestoßen haben. Später wird es derb und unempfindlich.

7. Die eitrige Arthritis (Gelenkempyem, Pyarthros)

Das infektiös vereiterte Gelenk bedarf hier nur kurzer Erwähnung. Es hat mit dem akuten Gichtanfall die örtliche und systemische Entzündungsaktivität gemeinsam. Rötung und Wärme sind beim akuten Infekt besonders stark ausgeprägt, sie können aber in ganz torpiden Fällen auch fehlen. Gleiches gilt für die akute Bursitis. Grünlich-schmutzigtrübe Synovia mit Leukocytenwerten über $60000/mm^3$ sind auf Eiter verdächtig.

Die umgekehrte Verwechslung ist häufiger. Immer wieder werden akute Gichtgelenke mit also steriler Synovitis fälschlicherweise als „vereitert" operiert.

B. Differentialdiagnose der extraarticulären Gichtanfälle

Wie die genaue Beobachtung lehrt, beginnt ein Teil der arthritischen Gichtanfälle extraarticulär als Kapselansatzentzündung, um erst von dort sozusagen ins Gelenkinnere zu gelangen und hier als Kristallsynovitis zu reagieren. Ebenso viele Gichtanfälle bleiben aber extraarticulär lokalisiert als umschrieben heftig schmerzhafte Areale oder Punkte im periarticulären straffen Bindegewebe (Periarthritis urica): Am Kapselansatz (Capsulitis), an Sehnenansätzen (Insertionstendinitis), an Retinacula (Fibrositis), in ligamentären oder periostalen Strukturen (Tendoperiostitis). Sie müssen mit dem palpierenden Finger gesucht werden und geben sich durch hohe Druckempfindlichkeit zu erkennen.

1. Insertionstendopathien

Topologisch besteht eine gewisse Übereinstimmung der extraarticulären Gichtanfälle mit den Prädilektionsstellen der *Insertionstendinosen*. Diese gehören zum Weichteilrheumatismus mit banalen Reizzuständen ohne spezifisches Substrat („Fibrositis"). Vorwiegend mechanisch-irritative und Überlastungsschäden liegen zugrunde. Mitigierte Gichtanfälle können sich hier verbergen.

Unter dem Begriff der entzündlichen *Enthesopathie* (Enthesitis) wurden Zustände zusammengefaßt (NIEPEL et al., 1966), die röntgenmorphologisch das charakteristische Bild der Tendoostitis bieten und die bestimmte chronisch entzündliche Leiden begleiten. Die Enthesitis betrifft vorwiegend jene Ansätze straff bindegewebiger Fasern am Knochen, die durch eine restierende Knorpelschicht vermittelt werden. Hier manifestiert sich bei der Spondylitis ankylopoetica, dem chronischen Reiter-Syndrom und der psoriatischen Polyarthritis bzw. Spondylitis die teilweise quälend schmerzhafte Sehnenansatzentzündung, die mit einem morphologisch charakteristischen Substrat teils destruiert, teils ossifiziert. Die Differentialdiagnose des jeweils etwas abweichend bevorzugten Befallmusters bei diesen rheumatischen Leiden wurde beschrieben (SCHILLING 1975). Bekanntester Sitz ist die Ferse („rheumatische Calcaneopathie" — DIHLMANN, 1967).

Die bradytrophen Band- und Knorpelgewebe dieser Insertionen werden offenbar auch zum Ablagerungsplatz der Uratpräcipitate bei anhaltender Hyperuricämie, die dort den Ausgangspunkt extraarticulärer Gichtanfälle darstellen. Unter ihnen bevorzugt auch die Gicht die Ferse, besonders den Achillessehnenansatz; aber nicht so häufig wie rheumatische Leiden. Weiterhin finden wir akut entzündliche Schmerzpunkte der akuten Gicht an der Spitze der Malleolen, an der Tuberositas tibiae, am Patellarrand, an den Knie-Seitenbändern, am Fibula-Köpfchen und den Humerusepicondylen; seltener am großen Rollhügel oder an den Griffelfortsätzen der Hand.

Nach unserer Erfahrung ist der periarticuläre Bindegewebsapparat des *Kniegelenks* häufigster Sitz von periarticulären Gichtanfällen (Periarthritis genus), während umschriebene Schmerzzustände an der *Ferse* zunächst entzündlich-rheumatische Ursachen ausschließen lassen müssen. Wieder ist die anfallsartige Akuität differentialdiagnostisch entscheidend, wobei am Fuß statisch-irritative Momente ins Spiel kommen und täuschen können. Ein Extremfall ist die chronisch oder akut traumatische Achillessehnenruptur, bei der immer wieder die Frage gestellt wird, ob Uratkristallinkrustationen die Zermürbung vorbereitet hätten.

Anhaltende und belastungsabhängige Insertionstendinosen an der Ferse, am Knie und am Ellenbogen haben vorwiegend orthopädische und chronisch traumatische Ursachen (Überlastungsschäden). Der Fersensporn bei der Gicht ist unspezifisch und röntgenmorphologisch vom degenerativen (tendoostotischen) Typ. Eine ossifizierend-destruierende Tendoostitis achillea oder eine manchmal fluktuierend tastbare Bursitis subachillea mit Druckusur gibt es bei der Gicht nicht, sie gehört zur Spondylitis ankylopoetica oder ihren atypischen Varianten.

Die *Epicondylitis* humeri ist allermeist eine banale Überlastungstendinose („Tennisellenbogen"), hartnäckig chronisch und von einem hier einmal etablierten Gichtanfall unterscheidbar. Dieser kann auch am Olecranon vorkommen und darf nicht mit den häufigeren Erscheinungen im Bereich des Ellenbogens (Synovitis, Bursitis) verwechselt werden. Nicht selten sind Schleimbeutel an den Reizzuständen exponierter Insertionen wie Trochanter und Malleolus beteiligt, auch im Gichtanfall.

2. Periarthritiden

a) Die *Periarthritis* (Peritendinitis) *humero-scapularis*, ohne oder mit Bursitis subdeltoidea oder subacromialis, ist nur selten als Gichtanfall diagnostizierbar. Stammnahe Gichtmanifestationen im akut rezidivierenden Stadium sind überhaupt selten und sollten mit Reserve als solche angesprochen werden. Um eine akute Periarthritis des Schultergelenks als Gichtanfall erkennen zu können, fordern wir, daß er gleichzeitig mit einem anderweitigen gesicherten Gichtanfall auftritt und somit als Teil eines polytopen Gichtanfalles verstanden werden darf.

Die akute Periarthritis humero-scapularis mit hoch entzündlicher Bursitis stellt eine Kalk-Synovitis dieses Schleimbeutels dar nach Durchbruch von Kalkmassen in denselben. Ein entsprechendes Ereignis im Sinne einer Uratkristallsynovitis in einem Schleimbeutel am Schultergelenk ist unbekannt, aber denkbar.

b) Die *Peritendinitis calcarea* (SANDSTROM, 1938) ist selten. Sie gehört zu den umschriebenen Calcinosen unbekannter Ursache („Kalk-Gicht") und stellt sich klinisch vorwiegend als Periarthritis dar. In ihrer akut rezidivierenden Form imitiert sie täuschend die akut rezidivierende Gicht. Wir nennen sie deshalb *akut rezidivierende Periarthritis (Peritendinitis) calcarea.*

Es könnte sich dabei, will man den Autoren THOMPSON et al. (1968) folgen, um ein tenosynovitisches Analogon der polyarticulären Kristallsynovitis handeln. Die gefundenen Kristalle bestehen aber aus Hydroxylapatit (McCARTY u. GATTER, 1966). Es ist auch nicht sicher, ob sich die anfallsartigen, umschrieben in Gelenknähe etablierten heftigen Entzündungszustände wirklich immer im synovialen Sehnenscheidengewebe abspielen. Bevorzugt sind die ulnare Gegend der Handgelenke (Sehne des M. flexor carpi ulnaris), Fingergelenke, Ellenbogen (radiale „Epicondylitis"), Schultern, Knie und periarticuläre oder pericapsuläre Bindegewebsanteile weiterer Gelenke. Dort gibt sich die Krankheit durch typische, meist schalenförmige, vorwiegend periarticulär angeordnete Verkalkungen zu erkennen (BUCHWALD u. SEVERIN, 1968).

Wir beobachten (SCHILLING, 1974) einen 37 jährigen Mann, der unter dieser Krankheit seit seinem zwanzigsten Lebensjahr leidet. In Abständen von einem halben bis zu mehr als einem Jahr erleidet er, leicht fiebernd, stets monoarticuläre schmerzhafte Entzündungen mit Rötung, Schwellung und Behinderung des betreffenden Gelenks, die sich innerhalb von 10 Tagen erheblich steigern, um dann schnell wieder abzuklingen. Befallen waren am häufigsten Fingermittel- und Endgelenke (Abb. 14a), seltener Handgelenke, Schulter, Knie und Ellenbogen. Am Handgelenk ging ein Anfall mit einem partiellen Carpaltunnelsyndrom einher. Das Röntgenbild zeigt inhomogene schalige bis streifenförmige Verkalkungen im pericapsulären bzw. im Bereich von Sehnengewebe, aber ohne Kontakt mit dem Knochen, also keine verknöchernde Enthesopathie darstellend (Abb. 14b). Das besondere ist die Reversibilität dieser Calcinose, die sich nach einiger Zeit auf einen kleinen Kern verdichtet. Dieser imponiert dann als harmloses Ossikel, am Fingergelenk als Bestandteil einer Arthrose. Systemische Entzündungszeichen fehlen auch im Anfall. Die weitere Besonderheit dieses Falles ist aber ein begleitendes partielles immunologisches Defektsyndrom mit IgG-Verminderung (670 mg-%) und Hypogammaglobulinämie (9 rel.-%) sowie mit dem Nachweis von Antikörpern gegen Kollagen im Antiglobulinkonsumptionstest (VORLAENDER). Das Syndrom ist in dieser Form noch nicht beschrieben worden.

Dieses polyperiarthritische Krankheitsbild mit seltenen anfallsartigen Manifestationen in Gelenknähe ist eine wahrhafte extraarticuläre Pseudo-Gicht, die als akut rezidivierende Arthritis imponiert. Seine Anfälle sprechen prompt auf Colchicin an (THOMPSON et al., 1968), dessen Spezifität damit eine weitere Einbuße erfährt (vgl. oben).

3. Bursitiden

Eine akute *Bursitis olecrani*, spontan als sackartige Schwellung am Ellenbogen bei einem Manne entstanden, mäßig schmerzhaft und stark gerötet, ist praktisch immer eine Bursitis urica, wenn ein eitriger Infekt ausgeschlossen werden kann. Sie ist die häufigste und eindrucksvollste extraarticuläre Synovitis der akut rezidivierenden Gicht, die auch anamnestisch, meist operiert, gut verwertbar ist. Sie verschwindet nach einiger Zeit wieder und hinterläßt krümelige Reste in einem schlaffen Kapselrest. Im chronischen Stadium der Gicht entstehen an derselben Stelle schmerzlose derbe Schleimbeutelverdickungen mit tophösem Inhalt, die spontan nicht mehr rückbildungsfähig sind.

Auch die *chronische (rheumatoide) Polyarthritis* kennt am gleichen Ort eine ähnliche subakut entstehende Bursitis in 5% der Fälle (GAMP u. SCHILLING, 1966). Es handelt sich um eine extraarticuläre Manifestation des polysynovitischen Syndroms. Die rheumatoide Bursitis unterscheidet sich von der gichtigen Schleimbeutelentzündung durch Blässe und Schmerzlosigkeit. Außerdem ist diese weich fluktuierende Schleimbeutelschwellung meistens noch von einem subcutanen Rheumaknoten begleitet, der distal von ihr als derber Nodus der Ellenkante aufsitzt (Abb. 19). Bei der Gicht kommt diese doppelhöckerige Silhouette nicht vor. Sie ist vielmehr typisch für die Rheumafaktor-positive chronische (rheumatoide) Polyarthritis.

Ein seltener Spezialfall der oben bereits erwähnten, durch Kalkeinbruch entstandenen akuten Schleimbeutelsynovitis am Schultergelenk ist die *pseudophlegmonöse Form der neurotrophischen Osteoarthropathie*. Diese akute *Kalk-Bursitis* stellt einen schweren Krankheitszustand mit Fieber dar und bietet ein Röntgenbild, das flockig suspendierte Kalkmassen in einem großen Schleimbeutelsack erkennen läßt (FRIED, 1970).

4. Tenosynovitis (Tendovaginitis)

Das Vorkommen einer akuten exsudativen Tenosynovitis bei der Gicht können wir nicht mit Sicherheit bestätigen. Die Tenosynovitis der polysynovitischen chronischen Polyarthritis ist blaß, schmerzlos, chronisch und neigt zu polytoper, oft symmetrischer Ausprägung. Eine akute und schmerzhafte Sehnenscheidenentzündung mit Rötung beruht meistens auf einer Vereiterung. Eine sterile flüchtige Tenosynovitis am Handrücken mit Schmerz und Rötung haben wir nur im Rahmen eines palindromen Rheumatismus erlebt. Die Peritendinitis wurde oben abgehandelt.

5. Andere extraarticuläre anfallsartige Entzündungen

Selten kommt bei der akut rezidivierenden Gicht ein Anfall am Periost, z. B. am Unterschenkel vor: *Periostitis urica*. Dieser schwere Entzündungszustand imponiert als *Phlebitis* mit flammender Hautrötung. Die fragwürdige Angabe der Literatur, bei der Gicht käme eine „Phlebitis urica" gehäuft vor, könnte in solchen Zuständen eine Quelle haben.

Der lokal pseudo-*phlegmonöse* Charakter mancher Gichtanfälle mit hohen Fieberzacken täuscht nicht selten eine Vereiterung oder gar eine Allgemeinsepsis vor, die noch heute manchen Chirurgen zum operativen Eingriff verleitet. Die Rötung der Paraarthritis urica mit Fieber gleicht örtlich und systemisch einem *Erysipel*.

III.
Differentialdiagnose der chronischen Gicht
(Tophus-Gicht) (Tab. 4)

Der Übergang des urat-speichernden Prozesses vom ersten in das zweite Hauptstadium der Gicht ist unscharf und fließend. Nach durchschnittlich 7 Jahren (zwischen 2 bis über 12 Jahre bei GAMP et al., 1965; und zwischen 4,9 und 9,3 Jahren bei BABUCKE u. MERTZ, 1973), in Grenzfällen 0 Jahren (primär chronische Form) oder nie (unter Therapie) wird die Uratablagerung (Tophus) klinisch oder röntgenologisch faßbar: articulär (A) oder weichteiltophös (B). Beide Modalitäten erscheinen ungefähr gleichzeitig, der Knochentophus meist etwas früher und einige Zeit überwiegend. Im weiteren Verlauf kombinieren sie sich zur ausgeprägten gelenkzerstörenden und knotig deformierenden Tophusgicht.

Das Stadium der chronischen Gicht zu verhindern ist die dankbare Aufgabe der Therapie, die voraussetzt, daß die Diagnose im akut rezidivierenden Stadium gestellt worden ist. Das chronische Stadium könnte und sollte also bald nicht mehr erreicht werden und damit differentialdiagnostisch gegenstandslos werden.

Tabelle 4. Differentialdiagnose der chronischen (tophösen) Gicht

A. Chronische Arthritiden
1. chronische rheumatoide Polyarthritis
2. chronische psoriatische Polyarthritis
3. periphere Arthritis bei Spondylitis ankylopoetica
4. destruktive und metabolische Arthropathien:
   Hüftkopfnekrose
   neurogene Arthropathie
   Chondrocalcinose
   Hämochromatose
5. Arthrosen
   Polyarthrose

B. Subcutane Knoten
1. Knötchen am Helix
2. Nodus rheumaticus (Rheumaknoten der c. P.)
3. tuberöse Xanthome (hypercholesterinämische Xanthomatose = „Lipoid-Gicht")
4. Pseudo-Tophi der „Kalk-Gicht"
   a) Calcinosis interstitialis und Peritendinitis calcarea
   b) Calcium-Phosphat-„Gicht" bei Niereninsuffizienz bzw.
   c) unter Dauer-Hämodialyse
5. Lipoid-Dermato-Arthritis (Reticulohistiocytose)-benigne Riesenzelltumoren
6. juxtaarticuläre fibroide Knoten der Acrodermatitis chronica atrophicans
7. Fingerknöchelpolster
8. Heberden-Knötchen

A. Die chronische Arthritis

Eine chronische Arthritis ist durch den Dauerschaden an den gelenkbildenden knorpligen oder/und knöchernen Anteilen definiert, faßbar als Deformierung und Funktionsbehinderung sowie im Röntgenbild.

Ungefähr dem Befall- und Ausbreitungsmuster der articulären Gichtanfälle (Abb. 1) folgend wird die Gicht nach durchschnittlich 7 Jahren in diesen Gelenken chronisch (Abb. 15 b). Der Dauerschaden ist am frühesten röntgenologisch nachweisbar (vgl. Kap. Röntgendiagnostik der Gicht). Das zweite Hauptstadium der Gicht ist somit auch das röntgen-positive Stadium, das der *chronischen Gicht-Arthritis* und der paraarticulären Knochentophi.

An den Füßen, insbesondere dem Großzeh wird der Röntgenbefund vor, und meist lange vor den Händen pathologisch. Es muß deshalb als Regel gelten, daß man sich bei der röntgendifferentialdiagnostischen Abklärung von Gelenkleiden nicht auf die Aufnahme der Hände beschränkt, sondern mindestens die der Vorfüße einschließen soll.

Röntgenmorphologisch sind 4 Typen des Urat-Dauerschadens am Gelenk zu unterscheiden:
1. Die ossäre (subchondrale und paraarticuläre) Destruktion mit gelenknahen Knochentophi bzw. mit Spornbildung;
2. die Urat-Synovitis mit chondro- und osteo-destruktiver Arthritis;
3. chronische Gicht-Arthritis „unter dem Bild der Arthrose" (SCHACHERL u. SCHILLING, 1966);
4. nekrotisierende Arthropathie.

Die Läsionen der ersten und der zweiten Form können sich kombinieren; die zweite Form imitiert die chronische Polyarthritis an Händen und Füßen; die dritte imitiert eine Arthrose vorwiegend am Großzehengrundgelenk, aber auch am Knie und an Fingergelenken; und die vierte Form ist als primäre Hüftkopfnekrose bekannt. Am Großzehengrundgelenk sind alle Läsionen 1 bis 3 exemplarisch zu beobachten. Zum articulären Schaden tritt nach einiger Zeit die periarticuläre Weichteilverdichtung mit typisch knotiger Weichteilkontur und schließlich mit Verkalkungstendenz hinzu.

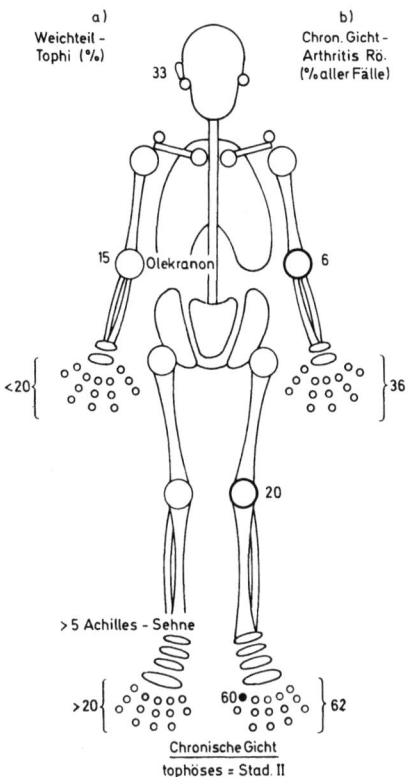

Abb. 15. Verteilung der Weichteiltophi *a* und der röntgenologisch erfaßbaren chronischen Arthritis *b* im Stadium der chronischen (tophösen) Gicht. (Die Zahlen bedeuten Prozentsatzangaben und beziehen sich auf die Gesamtzahl der Fälle in diesem Stadium)

An den kleinen Gelenken der Zehen und Finger herrschen destruktive, an den Fuß- und Mittelfuß-, Hand- und Mittelhandgelenken cystische Läsionen und an den großen Gelenken das arthrotische Bild vor. Das reparative und osteophytäre Moment ist deutlich und ist als Reaktion auf einen unterschwellig destruierenden Entzündungsreiz die Ursache für das vorwiegend arthrotische Erscheinungsbild z. B. am Großzehengrundgelenk.

Das Befallmuster bleibt zunächst caudal und peripher-distal betont (Abb. 15b), gleicht im Laufe der fortschreitenden Leidensentwicklung das Gefälle aber aus, um schließlich Hände und Füße wie größere Gelenke gleichmäßig zu verunstalten.

Während am Fuß eine typische Ausbreitungsdynamik der Zehengrundgelenkarthritis von medial (I) nach lateral (II—V) zu beobachten ist (Abb. 17b), geschieht der Befall der Fingergelenke regellos, anscheinend willkürlich und ohne bevorzugte Topik. Das betroffene Gelenk wird derb verdickt, nur selten — in synovitischen Phasen — teilweise fluktuierend, schließlich knotig-tophös aufgetrieben. Es schmerzt bei Belastung und in der entzündlichen Exacerbation. Das Gelenk wird funktionsbehindert, deformiert, destruktiv bis osteolytisch subluxiert oder versteift bzw. synostosiert. Das entstehende Bild ist aspektiv grob, bald beidseitig, aber im einzelnen meist asymmetrisch. Die tophöse Verunstaltung wird in selten gewordenen Bildern des Endstadiums dermato-dystrophisch, superinfiziert, fistelnd und mutilierend, wozu Diabetes und Angiopathie das ihre beitragen.

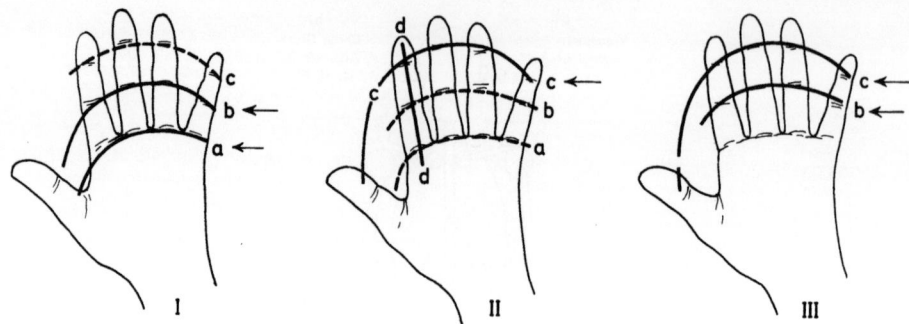

Abb. 16. „Etagen-Differentialdiagnose" der chronischen Polyarthritis (I), der psoriatischen Polyarthritis (II) und der Polyarthrose (III) an der Hand. *a* Fingergrundgelenke, *b* Fingermittelgelenke, *c* Fingerendgelenke, *d* „Strahlbefall"

Während im akut rezidivierenden Stadium der Gicht die systemischen Entzündungszeichen sich (wie der entzündliche Anfall selbst) völlig zurückbilden und in der interkritischen Phase fehlen, wird im chronischen Stadium eine dauernde leichte bis deutlicher beschleunigte Blutsenkungsgeschwindigkeit und zuweilen eine mäßige Dyproteinämie beobachtet, nicht aber Anämie oder Eisen-Erniedrigung.

Der „Rheumafaktor" kann in einem kleinen Teil der Fälle vorgefunden werden, jedenfalls in dem sehr empfindlichen Latex-Tropfentest, aber auch niedrigtitrig bei der Quantifizierung im Latex-Fixationstest. Hier mögen immunologische Sekundär-Phänomene bei anhaltender synovitischer Reizung im Spiele sein. Die bei der quantitativen Bestimmung der Immunglobuline gelegentlich gefundene IgA-Erhöhung (BALL et al., 1969) mag einer ähnlichen Erklärung zugänglich sein.

Wir finden niedrig-titrige Latexteste in 12% unserer Fälle. Der Latex-Tropfentest ist häufig positiv und quantifizierungspflichtig. Ein Latex-Fixationstest über $^1/_{120}$ und ein Waaler-Rose-Test über $^1/_{32}$ müssen aber Zweifel an der Gichtdiagnose wecken. Vierstellige Latex-Titer und dreistellige Waaler-Rose-Titer schließen sie mit wenigen Ausnahmen aus. Diese positiven Rheuma-Faktor-Titer bei einer sonst gesicherten Gicht sind als nosologisch „falsch positiv" zu bewerten. Immunpathologisch sind sie jedoch als durchaus „echt" erklärbar, etwa durch eine immunologische Reaktion mit lokaler Produktion von Antigen-Antikörperkomplexen im Milieu der Kristall-Synovitis bei etwa gegebener genetischer Prädisposition (BLOCH-MICHEL et al., 1968).

1. Die chronische (rheumatoide) Polyarthritis

Die Diagnose dieser Systemkrankheit ist die häufigste Fehlinterpretation der chronischen polyarticulären Gicht. Folgende pathogenetische und symptomatische Unterscheidungsgründe und -merkmale trennen die beiden chronischen Leiden, die sich gleichermaßen vordergründig, aber nicht ausschließlich an Gelenken abspielen, absolut differenzierungspflichtig und nosologisch prinzipiell auseinanderzuhalten sind.

a) Die rheumatoide Arthritis ist primär eine Synovitis auf wahrscheinlich immunologischer Grundlage; die der Gicht aber eine Kristall- oder eine Sekundär-Synovitis.

b) Zum Wesen der chronischen Polyarthritis gehört eine humoral faßbare systemische Entzündung, die von der Gicht erst im chronischen Stadium als Sekundärphänomen erworben wird.

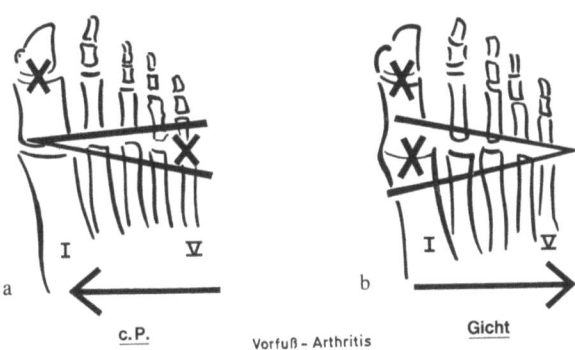

Abb. 17a u. b. Zur Differentialdiagnose des Befallmusters und der Ausbreitungsdynamik der chronischen (rheumatoiden) Polyarthritis (a) und der chronischen Gicht-Arthritis (b) am Vorfuß (vorwiegend Zehengrundgelenke und Großzehenendgelenk)

c) Den nosologischen Kern des „chronischen polyarthritischen Syndroms" bildet dessen nodöse Form, gekennzeichnet durch Rheumaknoten und signifikant-titrigen Rheumafaktor, die der Gicht im Prinzip fremd sind.

d) Die chronische Polyarthritis beginnt und breitet sich gleichermaßen an Händen und Füßen aus, schon früh mit einem möglichen Befall großer und stammnaher Gelenke, also ohne strenge distale Prävalenz oder langfristig zentripetale Ausbreitungsdynamik, wie sie der Gicht eigen sind.

e) Das Befallmuster der Hände mit regelhafter und hoher Bevorzugung der Grund- und Mittelgelenke (Abb. 16) sowie die Ausbreitungstendenz an den Vorfüßen von lateral nach medial (Beginn bei Zehengrundgelenk V bis II, meist bei III) sind typisch für die chronische Polyarthritis, in charakteristischem Gegensatz zur Gicht (Abb. 17).

f) Im Prinzip wird bald eine Symmetrie des Befallmusters erreicht, von der chronischen Polyarthritis früher und strenger als von der chronischen Gichtarthritis.

g) Die chronische (rheumatoide) Arthritis ist aspektiv durch eine weiche, z. B. spindelförmig konturierte, bei der Palpation fluktuierende Kapselschwellung ausgezeichnet, entsprechend der exsudativen Synovitis; Überwärmung fehlt oft, Rötung fast immer. Die chronische Gicht-Arthritis ist tophös und derb deformierend.

h) Röntgensymptomatisch sind die feinen Primärläsionen (Randusuren, Defekte der Grenzlamelle und der subchondralen Spongiosa-Textur) und später die paraphlogistische Ossipenie auf die chronische Polyarthritis hinweisend, die von der Gichtarthritis allerdings teilweise imitiert werden können.

i) Die Halswirbelsäule wird von der chronischen Polyarthritis in einem Drittel der Fälle mitergriffen, was der Gicht fremd ist.

k) Frauen überwiegen bei der chronischen (rheumatoiden) Polyarthritis mit zwei Dritteln; ein Konstitutionstyp wird nicht bevorzugt.

l) Die chronische Polyarthritis ist im Prinzip unheilbar.

Die chronische Gicht-Arthritis weicht also in jedem dieser Vergleichspunkte von der chronischen Polyarthritis ab. Die Beachtung des Geschlechts, anamnestisch des Verlaufsprofils und auch der Begleitkrankheiten, des Befall- und Ausbreitungsmusters, der aspektive Befund, die besonders wichtige Palpation des Gelenks, die Synovia-Analyse, die Röntgenbefunde (obwohl mit Überschneidungen), die Abwägung der Blutbefunde und schließlich die verschiedene therapeutische Ansprechbarkeit müssen vor der noch so häufigen und verhängnisvollen Verwechslung bewahren (RAVAULT et al., 1969).

Ein Fallstrick ist der manchmal „positive Rheumafaktor" bei der chronischen Gicht-Arthritis. BLOCH-MICHEL und Mitarb. (1968) haben Assoziationen „rheumatoider Symptome" bei Kristallarthritiden beschrieben.

Damit taucht die Frage nach der *Kombination von Arthritis urica und chronischer Polyarthritis* auf, oder eines „Übergangs" jener in diese. Immer wieder wurde dies als geläufig angenommen und beschrieben. Wir halten aber die meisten Fälle dieser Art für verdächtig, Fehlinterpretationen darzustellen (SCHILLING, 1971). Gicht und chronische Polyarthritis sind zunächst wesensverschiedene Krankheiten. Es gibt keine nosologischen Argumente, die für eine Syntropie verwertbar wären, und keine stichhaltige Statistik, die eine überzufällige Koinzidenz beweisen würde. Da die Gicht fast nur Männer betrifft, muß die Kombination mit einer chronischen Polyarthritis bei Frauen besonders unwahrscheinlich werden und bei Männern nach statistischer Wahrscheinlichkeit immerhin noch recht selten bleiben. In der authentischen Literatur werden gesicherte Fälle dieser Art als Einzelkasuistik veröffentlicht (ARLET u. MOLE, 1961; OWEN et al., 1966).

Die Diagnose sowohl der Gicht als auch der chronischen Polyarthritis ist an Kriterien gebunden, deren Vernachlässigung in manchen Berichten zu Konfusionen geführt hat. Besonders das chronische Stadium der Gicht kann dazu verleiten, eine polyarticuläre chronische Gichtarthritis mit einer rheumatoiden Arthritis zu verwechseln und diese als aus einer Arthritis urica hervorgegangen oder mit ihr kombiniert zu mißdeuten; dies besonders dann, wenn Knoten am Ellenbogen (Tophus oder Gicht-Bursitis, verkennbar als Rheumaknoten), eine nicht eindeutig unterscheidende Röntgensymptomatik, systemische Entzündungszeichen oder gar ein positiver Latex-Test vorliegen. Solche Fälle sind nicht so selten. Andererseits kann die chronische Polyarthritis eines Mannes mit erhöhtem Harnsäurespiegel im Blut Verwirrung stiften, was angesichts der Häufigkeit einer mittleren Hyperuricämie ebenfalls nicht selten ist, aber keinesfalls die Diagnose Gicht oder gar einer Kombinationsform rechtfertigt.

Die klare diagnostische Beachtung der Krankheitskriterien führt in den meisten Fällen zu einer eindeutigen Entscheidung. Sollte ausnahmsweise eine zweideutige Symptomatik für die Koinzidenz beider Leiden sprechen, muß jede der beiden Diagnosen für sich sicher bewiesen werden: Für die Gicht durch den Urat-Kristallnachweis im Gewebe (Tophus-Histologie oder Murexidprobe) oder in Leukocyten des Gelenkpunktates; für die chronische (rheumatoide) Polyarthritis durch den histologischen Nachweis wirklich spezifischer Strukturen (Nodus rheumaticus: Nekrose mit Histiocyten-Palisade).

2. Das Syndrom der *serologisch negativen chronischen Polyarthritis* läuft mehr als die klassische chronische (rheumatoide) Polyarthritis Gefahr, mit der chronischen Gicht-Arthritis verwechselt zu werden. Die seronegative chronische Polyarthritis ist launischer und instabiler im Verlauf als jene (MÜLLER, 1968), weniger symmetrisch und willkürlicher im Befallmuster, und kann bei einem Mann mit (zufälliger) Hyperuricämie bei fehlendem Rheumafaktor an eine chronische Gichtarthritis erinnern (vgl. RAVAULT et al., 1961).

Die *chronische Polyarthritis psoriatica* hat ein typisches Befallmuster, das sie von der chronischen „rheumatoiden" Polyarthritis, von der Polyarthrose und von der chronischen Gichtarthritis unterscheidet (Abb. 16). Es werden von der psoriatischen Arthritis einerseits die Etage der Endgelenke und andererseits die Gelenke eines einzelnen Strahls bevorzugt. Die röntgenologische Feinmorphologie ist zuweilen so typisch, daß auch ohne manifeste oder bemerkbare Psoriasis eine „Arthritis vom psoriatischen Typ" diagnostiziert und von der rheumatoiden Arthritis und von der Gicht-Arthritis abgegrenzt werden kann (SCHACHERL u. SCHILLING, 1967). Der psoriatische Wirbelsäulenbefall entspricht einer atypischen Spondylitis ankylopoetica (Spondylitis psoriatica — SCHILLING u. SCHACHERL, 1967).

Über die anfallsartigen Exacerbationen der psoriatischen Arthritis wurde oben berichtet.

Wirbelsäulenläsionen durch Uratablagerung bei der Gicht sind außerordentlich selten und sehr späte Ereignisse. Vereinzelt wurden Destruktionen beschrieben, auch eine atlantoaxiale Dislokation durch Gicht-Arthritis im Kopfgelenk.

3. Die periphere Arthritis der *Spondylitis ankylopoetica* (sog. Bechterewsche Krankheit), die diese in einem Drittel der Fälle remittierend oder chronisch werdend begleiten kann (SCHILLING, 1974), betrifft bevorzugt die Gelenke der unteren Extremitäten. Mit der Gicht kann die häufige flüchtige Synovitis des Knielenkes junger Männer mit früher Spondylitis ankylopoetica verwechselt werden.

Die *Sacroiliitis urica* ist selten, einseitig und morphologisch unterscheidbar.

Das chronische Reiter-Syndrom kann mit der chronischen Gicht nicht verwechselt werden.

4. *Destruktive Arthropathien.* — a) Die *primäre Hüftkopfnekrose* kommt bei Hyperuricämie und Gicht häufiger vor (MCCOLLUM et al., 1971). Wahrscheinlich ist hier verantwortlich oder mitverantwortlich die begleitende Hyperlipidämie (POHL, 1971). Möglicherweise sind jene Fälle der Literatur, die als Coxitis urica erschienen, auf dieser infarktähnlich nekrotisierenden Grundlage zu verstehen.

Am Hüftgelenk ist eine krankheitseigene *Coxitis urica* ein Problem (SCHULITZ, 1969). Wir neigen dazu, eine isolierte Hüftgelenkaffektion als Gicht-Symptom skeptisch zu beurteilen. Unabhängig jedenfalls von anderen gesicherten Gicht-Manifestationen sollte eine Coxarthrose oder gar eine Coxarthritis mit bzw. bei Hyperuricämie nicht ohne weiteres als „Gicht" bezeichnet werden. Selbst wenn der histologische Befund, möglicherweise sogar mit Kristallen, dafür zu sprechen scheint, ist es nosologisch immer noch problematisch, von diesem Lokalbefund ungewöhnlicher Primär-Lokalisation bereits auf die etablierte chronische Gicht schließen zu wollen.

b) Die polyarticuläre *Chondrocalcinose* in ihrer seltenen *destruktiven* Form (MENKES et al., 1973) und die *Hämochromatose* kommen differentialdiagnostisch besonders gegenüber der chronischen Polyarthritis in Frage, erinnern aber ihrer anfallsartigen Gelenkentzündungen wegen an die Gicht (s. oben).

5. *Arthrosen*

Die Arthrosen kommen im Hinblick auf die „chronische Gichtarthritis unter dem Bild der Arthrose" differentialdiagnostisch in Frage. Am Großzehengrundgelenk wird die Gicht häufig als banaler *Hallux rigidus* chronisch. Am Knie- oder am Hüftgelenk ist oft nicht zu entscheiden, ob es sich um eine Arthrose mit Hyperuricämie oder um eine dieser pathogenetisch direkt zuzuordnende Gelenkaffektion handelt. Dies kann dann nur durch den Längsschnitt des Krankheitsverlaufs und den Querschnitt aller Befunde, durch die Synovia-Analyse oder letztlich nur histologisch erwiesen werden.

Die *Polyarthrose* der Fingergelenke ist eine auf die Hände beschränkte Systemarthrose vorwiegend der klimakterischen Frau. Bei jeder dritten Frau beginnt sie um das 52. Lebensjahr, und sie ist bei Frauen zehnmal häufiger als bei Männern (STECHER, 1957). Das Befallmuster der Polyarthrose ist von dem der chronischen Polyarthritis in typischer Weise unterschieden (Abb. 16). Die chronische Polyarthritis befällt bevorzugt Fingergrund- und Mittelgelenke und verschont meistens die Endgelenke, während die Polyarthrose die Fingerendgelenke und Mittelgelenke betrifft — also ein klarer Etagenunterschied. Die Arthrose der Mittelgelenke (fälschlicherweise als „Bouchard-Arthrose" bezeichnet) tritt nur in der Hälfte der Fälle zur „Heberden-Arthrose" hinzu, im Ablauf meistens später als diese, manchmal aber auch isoliert ohne Endgelenkbeteiligung (Abb. 18a).

Unter Polyarthrose verstehen wir multiple degenerative Altersveränderungen der Fingerend- und Mittelgelenke und definieren sie als die System-Arthrose der Hand (SCHILLING, 1971). Die Analogie des Ausdrucks zur Polyarthritis erstreckt sich lediglich auf die Neigung zu einem systematisierten, bilateralen und annähernd symmetrischen Gelenkbefall. Der Polyarthrose fehlen aber eine primäre

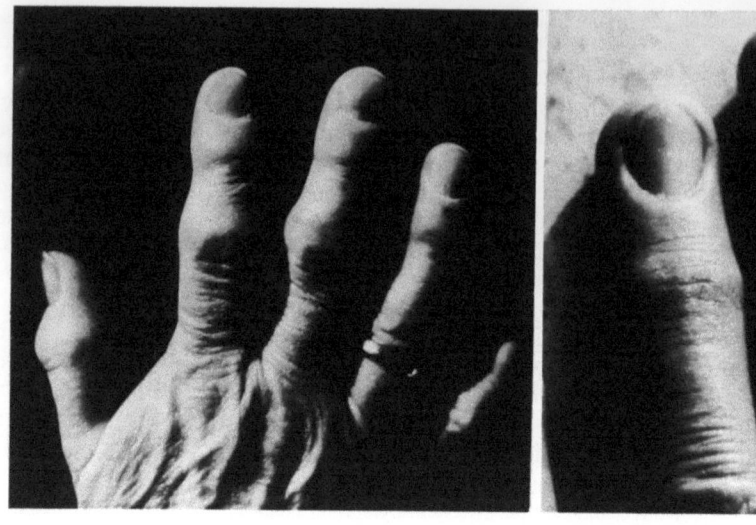

a b

Abb. 18a u. b. Polyarthrose der älteren Frau: Derbe Verdickung der Fingermittelgelenke mehr als der Endgelenke (a) (60jährige Frau); frische Heberden-Knötchen, schmerzhaft eruptiv und noch weich (b) (52jährige Frau im Klimakterium)

Lokalentzündung (Synovitis), die systemische Allgemeinentzündung und die Beziehung zu außerdigitalen Gelenkaffektionen. Unserer Polyarthrose entspricht im englischen Sprachgebrauch die „generalisierte hypertrophische Osteoarthritis" (KELLGREN u. MOORE, 1952).

Die Heberden-Knötchen beginnen bilateral dorsal an den Fingerendgelenken, manchmal entzündlich gereizt oder als mit Hyaluronsäure gefülltes paraarticuläres Cystchen (Abb. 18b) („Dorsalcyste"). Die eigentliche Endgelenkarthrose folgt mit Knorpeldegeneration, knöcherner Reaktion und Kapselmetaplasie, später auch mit Gelenkdeformierung. Die Knötchen sind dann längst hart und meistens indolent geworden und in die Fingerendgelenkarthrose als Bestandteil integriert. In dieser Form werden sie noch heute zuweilen als „Gicht-Knoten" angesprochen. Entsprechende Knoten an Mittelgelenken gibt es nicht.

Die Polyarthrose gehört zum Gicht-Begriff des vorigen Jahrhunderts. Die „Gicht" der Großmütter unserer Patienten war keine Gicht, sondern meistens die Fingergelenkarthrose der älteren Frau.

Ein besonders schwieriges differentialdiagnostisches Problem stellt die Sonderform dar, die wir *destruierende Polyarthrose* (SCHACHERL u. SCHILLING, 1967) genannt haben, im englischen Schrifttum als „erosive Osteoarthritis" bekannt (PETER et al., 1966). Zwischen 4% und 5% aller Polyarthrosen nehmen ossär destruierenden Charakter an. Die Besonderheiten dieser zerstörenden Form der Polyarthrose sind: Verschiebung der Geschlechterrelation zugunsten der Männer, Bevorzugung der Fingermittelgelenke, Beginn mit Knorpelzerstörung und cystoiden Spongiosadefekten, Entstehung einer Sekundär-Synovitis, klinisch mit entzündlichen Reizzuständen und fluktuierender Kapselschwellung, schließlich Reparationstendenz mit dem seltenen Sonderfall eines synostosierenden Durchbaus. Wir fassen die destruierende Polyarthrose als quantitative Extremform der Fingerarthrose auf, nicht aber als ein eigenes Krankheitsbild. Die Abgrenzung von der chronischen Polyarthritis gelingt durch Beachtung des Befallmusters, das bei der Arthrose die Grundgelenke ausspart, der röntgenologischen Feinmorphologie und der klinischen Umgebung.

Aufgrund ihres zunächst cystoiden Charakters wird die destruierende Polyarthrose meistens, mindestens röntgenologisch, mit der chronischen Gicht-Arthritis verwechselt. Diese befällt aber regelmäßig und ausgedehnt zuerst die Vorfüße, bevor Destruktionen an Fingergelenken erscheinen, so daß schon die routinemäßig obligate Beachtung der Vorfüße im Röntgenbild den Ausschluß der Gicht erlaubt. Eine Polyarthrose an den Zehen ist selten, und die destruierende Form gibt es an Zehengelenken überhaupt nicht.

Während im allgemeinen die Fingerendgelenke vor den Mittelgelenken arthrotisch befallen werden, ist bei der destruierenden Polyarthrose diese Reihenfolge umgekehrt häufiger zu beobachten. Beginn und Verlauf sind in einem Drittel der Fälle durch anfallsartige oder schubweise Reizzustände mit Entzündungssymptomatik ausgezeichnet. Die fast regelmäßige Verkennung als rheumatische oder Gicht-Arthritis ist dann verständlich. Im Gegensatz zur chronischen Polyarthritis fehlt eine länger als 10 min dauernde morgendliche Fingersteifigkeit, und nie kommt es zu einem deutlichen Kraftverlust beim Faustschluß. Dieser ist aber nicht selten inkomplett, da eine ausgeprägte Polyarthrose ein geringes Flexionsdefizit verursacht.

Der klinische Aspekt der befallenen Fingermittelgelenke ist durch eine derbe, manchmal spindelförmige, nicht ganz gleichmäßige oder etwas knorrige Auftreibung charakterisiert. Sie kann damit aspektiv mit einer tophösen Gelenkdeformierung Ähnlichkeit gewinnen. Die letztere ist jedoch im allgemeinen unregelmäßiger. Findet man bei der destruierenden Arthrose eine weiche und empfindliche Schwellung, eventuell mit fluktuierender Kapsel, dann liegt eine Sekundär-Synovitis vor.

Im Prinzip fehlen bei der destruierenden Polyarthrose systemische Entzündungszeichen, der Rheumafaktor und eine Hyperuricämie; die letztere stellt bei ihrer Häufigkeit als Zufallsbefund natürlich kein Ausschlußsymptom dar.

Das Bild der Polyarthrose kann durch den arthrotischen *Reparations*zustand einer chronischen Polyarthritis nachgeahmt werden, besonders dann, wenn die Fingerendgelenke beteiligt waren. Dies ist bei Jugendlichen mit juveniler chronischer (rheumatoider) Polyarthritis nicht selten, deren Fingerendgelenke bereits im 2. Lebensjahrzehnt den Aspekt von „juvenilen Heberden-Knötchen" bieten können (SCHILLING, 1974).

Ähnliches gilt für die Psoriasis, nach der in jedem Fall zu fahnden ist. Eine psoriatische Fingerendgelenkarthritis imitiert in der entzündungsfreien Intermission täuschend eine „Heberden-Arthrose", wobei die schnelle proliferative Reparationstendenz der Psoriasis-Arthritis im Spiele ist.

Über die Differentialdiagnose der Fingerendgelenkveränderungen siehe S. 296.

Die *Differentialdiagnose der Fingermittelgelenkarthrose* hat zunächst die Arthritis, seltener aber auch die Gicht zu berücksichtigen. Die degenerative Gelenkveränderung ist bei der Palpation derb, die entzündliche ist weich, fluktuierend, gleichmäßig spindelförmig aufgetrieben und mit Verlust der Hautfältchen gespannt. Subcutane Rheumaknötchen (oder als solche erscheinende kleine Exostosen) kommen an den proximalen Interphalangealgelenken selten vor. Die banalen intracutanen, verschieblichen und schmerzlosen, nicht so seltenen Fingerknöchelpolster sitzen dorsal über dem Gelenk. Sie haben mit Rheuma oder einer Gelenkaffektion nichts zu tun, sondern sind prinzipiell der Dupuytrenschen Krankheit zuzuordnen. Selten sind hier Hautknötchen einer Xanthomatosis multiplex; und extrem selten die der Lipoid-Dermato-Arthritis.

B. Subcutane Knoten

Die *Weichteiltophi* der Gicht, die chronische Hautgicht (GOTTRON u. KORTING, 1957), sind schmerzlos und sind, je nach Lokalisation (Terrain, Gewebsschicht) und Gewebsreaktion, vielgestaltig: Einerseits in der Haut (cutan, Haut-Tophi) an Fingern, Zehen, Ellenbogen und selteneren Lokalisationen flächig und kaum erhaben, weißlich bis gelblich durchschimmernd, von kreidiger, zähflüssiger oder milchiger Konsistenz, so daß pseudo-phlegmonöser Uratbrei als Eiter mißdeutet werden kann; andererseits knotig unter der Haut (subcutane Tophi) in Sehnen, Sehnenscheiden und an Sehnenansätzen, an knorpligen Strukturen, in

Schleimbeuteln und in deren Wandung und an Gelenkkapseln, sichtbar und tastbar werdend durch ihr Wachstum in Folge der Gewebsproliferationen, die terrain-abhängige histopathologisch typische Reaktionen (FASSBENDER, 1971) auf den Reiz der kristallinen Einlagerungen darstellen. Der Tophus ist spontan nicht reversibel.

Die Kristalle sind nur in alkoholfixierten Präparaten noch nachweisbar. Die Murexidprobe kann bei regressiven Veränderungen im Tophus durch Lipoidbeimengungen falsch-negativ werden.

Wir fanden bei der Auszählung von 111 Patienten mit chronischer Gicht Weichteiltophi in 51% der Fälle, davon Ohrtophi bei 33% und subcutane oder Bursa-Tophi (chronische „Bursitis" urica olecrani) am Ellenbogen bei 15% (GAMP et al., 1965). Diese Lokalisationen sind die frühesten und häufigsten (Abb. 15a).

An *Händen* und *Füßen*, wo die Weichteiltophi in Verbindung mit der chronischen tophös-destruierenden Arthritis das schon fortgeschrittene zweite Hauptstadium der Gicht anzeigen, handelt es sich vorwiegend um periarticuläre und peritendinöse Tophi. An Hand und Fingern ist das Bild knotig und regellos, periarticulär unregelmäßig konturiert und palpatorisch hart, am Handrücken von Strecksehnenknoten beherrscht. Die Differentialdiagnose gegenüber den weich synovitischen Gelenkschwellungen der Arthritis, gegenüber den kleineren parartikulären Rheumaknoten und gegenüber den derben Verdickungen der Polyarthrose hat den Konturenaspekt, die Palpation, die Symmetrie, den Etagenbefall und das Röntgenbild zu beachten (vgl. oben). Tophöse und xanthomatöse Strecksehnenknoten allerdings sind nur aus der „Umgebung", also aus dem klinischen Zusammenhang heraus zu unterscheiden.

Am Fuß ist es immer zuerst die grobe tophöse Verunstaltung des Großzehengrundgelenks, die differentialdiagnostisch praktisch ohne Konkurrenz ist. Die Differentialdiagnose an der *Ferse* aber ist in ähnlicher Weise wie der Ellenbogen reichhaltig: Hier kommen am Ansatz der Achillessehne morphologisch gleichartig tophöse wie xanthomatöse Sehnenknoten vor, und unter der Sehne die Bursitis, von der oben schon die Rede war.

1. Die tophösen perlartigen, weißlich durchschimmernden Knötchen am *Helix* der Ohrmuschel werden oft vom Patienten ausgedrückt und entleeren schmerzlos krümeliges Material. Die Chondrodermatitis nodularis chronica helicis aber ist sehr berührungsempfindlich und krustös bedeckt. Das Darwinsche Höckerchen oder Erfrierungsfolgen können mit Tophi verwechselt werden. Xanthom-Knötchen sind hier selten.

2. Am *Ellenbogen* finden sich die Tophi in der Bursa olecrani, die tumorös wächst, zunächst verschieblich bleibt, mit multi-nodulärem Tastbefund, später verbacken und verhärtet. Auf diesem besonders disponierten Terrain kommen folgende, den Tophi ähnelnde cutane und subcutane Knoten vor: Nodi rheumatici, tuberöse Xanthome und fibroide Knoten der Acrodermatitis.

Dem Tophus gegenüber sind die *Rheumaknoten*, die subcutanen Knoten der rheuma-serologisch positiven chronischen Polyarthritis mit deren pathognomonischen zentral-nekrotischen und palisadenartig histiocytär umgebenen histologischen Strukturen (FASSBENDER, 1974) am Ellenbogen die wichtigste Differentialdiagnose. Diese Knötchen sind einfach bis multipel (meist doppelhöckrig) an der Ellenkante distalwärts vom Olecranon aufgereiht und sitzen unverschieblich dem Periost auf. Der Nodus rheumaticus ist zwar auch schmerzlos, er ist aber rückbildungsfähig, er „kommt und geht". Deshalb, und weil die Knoten der chronischen Polyarthritis oft übersehen oder häufig nur tastend zu bemerken sind, wird deren Häufigkeit unterschätzt.

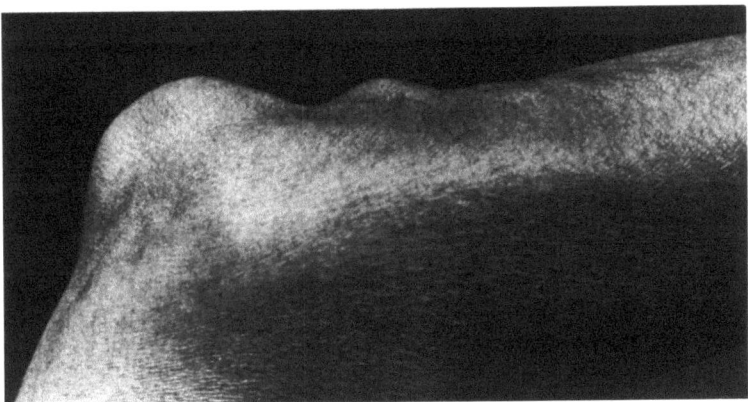

Abb. 19. Typische Silhouette am Ellenbogen bei der nodösen Form einer chronischen (rheumatoiden) Polyarthritis mit Bursitis olecrani und einem Rheumaknoten der Ellenkante

Rheuma-nodöse Einlagerungen kommen ebenso auch im Schleimbeutel des Ellenbogens vor. Die Kombination aber einer weich fluktuierenden und schmerzlosen Bursitis olecrani mit einer distal davon befindlichen knotigen Auftreibung an der Ellenkante ist typisch für die nodöse Form der chronischen (rheumatoiden) Polyarthritis und kommt bei der Gicht in dieserForm (Abb. 19) nicht vor.

3. Die „*Lipoid-Gicht*" (BÜRGER): Die tuberösen *Xanthome* der essentiellen (familiären) hypercholesterinämischen Xanthomatose haben einen Lieblingssitz ebenfalls am Ellenbogen (Abb. 20). Auch sie kommen cutan und subcutan, in Gelenknähe (periarticuläre) und an Sehnen und Sehnenscheiden (tendinöse und peritendinöse Xanthomknoten) vor. Die zugrundeliegende Stoffwechselstörung der essentiellen Hypercholesterinämie kommt häufig familiär vor (SCHILLING u. GAMP, 1957) und ist in einem Drittel der Fälle mit Hyperuricämie verbunden (ADLERSBERG et al., 1949).

Man versteht unter Xanthomen knotige Gebilde in der Haut (Schicht der Papillen) und unter der Haut an Sehnen, Gelenkkapseln, Periost, Fascien und in Gefäßwänden. Sie bestehen aus Anhäufungen der charakteristischen (aber nicht spezifischen) feinvacuolisierten Schaumzellen histiocytären Ursprungs in einem fibrös-fibroplastischen, mehr oder weniger entzündlich und großzellig durchsetzten Stroma. Bevorzugt sind die auch normalerweise im Laufe des Alterungsprozesses cholesterinophilen bradytrophen Gewebe, die auch von den Urateinlagerungen der Gicht bevorzugt werden. Die Differentialdiagnose der xanthomatösen Lipoidosen, insbesondere gegenüber dem „Rheumatismus nodosus" (vgl. oben) und gegenüber der Gicht haben wir unter ausführlicher Würdigung der Literatur eingehend dargestellt (SCHILLING u. GAMP, 1957).

Mit der echten, d.h. der Uratgicht hat die hypercholesterinämische Xanthomatose dies gemeinsam, daß sie beide eine allgemeinstoffwechselpathologische Ätiologie haben und mit Ablagerungen des repräsentativen, im Blut pathologisch vermehrten Stoffwechselproduktes (Cholesterin bzw. Harnsäure) einhergehen. Die Xanthom-Knoten bzw. die Tophi haben bezüglich der bevorzugten Lokalisation und der Neigung zur Symmetrie Ähnlichkeiten. Xanthome etablieren sich sehr selten auch am Helix auriculi, und ossäre Lipoiddepositionen in Gelenknähe mit röntgenologisch evidenten cystischen Aufhellungen kommen auch bei Sehnenxanthomen vor. Die Tophi urici sind zumindest in den Anfangsstadien weicher als Xanthome, und der Inhalt der Knoten wird in typischer Weise chemisch oder histologisch unterschieden.

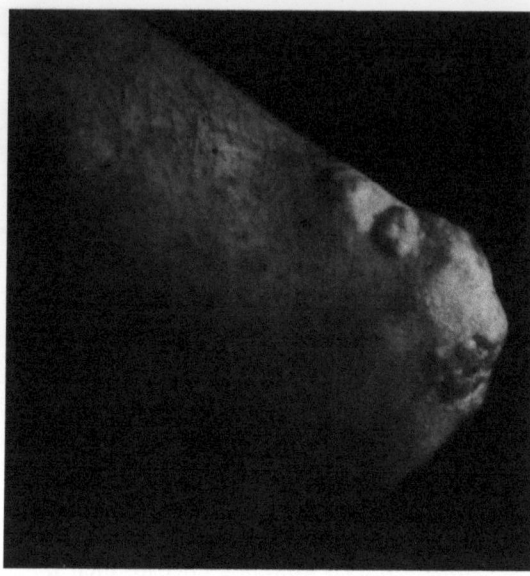

Abb. 20. Tuberöse Xanthome am Ellenbogen bei familiärer hypercholesterinämischer Xanthomatose

Besonders französische Autoren haben aber auf histologische Überschneidungen hingewiesen und sogar von einem „xanthome familiale de forme pseudo-goutteuse" (GILBERT, 1926) gesprochen. Jedenfalls muß mit der Tatsache gerechnet werden, daß ebenso wie in Rheumaknoten auch in Gichttophi sowohl Fettsubstanzen als auch cholesterinhaltige Schaumzellen vorkommen können, was als Sekundärvorgang zu verstehen ist, wenn Harnsäurekristalle als Kristallisationskern zum Ausgangspunkt scheinbar echt xanthomatöser Knötchen werden. Hinzu kommt, daß kleine Cholesterinablagerungen zwar selten aber doch verbürgt auch an den sonst der Gicht vorbehaltenen Stellen am Ohr vorkommen können; daß eine besondere Affinität der Sehnen und Sehnenscheiden sowohl für die Harnsäure- als auch für die Cholesterin-Imprägnation besteht, so daß CHAUFFARD von einer Analogie zwischen dem „tophus goutteux" und dem „tophus cholesterinique" sprach; daß röntgenologisch gleichartige Knochendefekte entstehen können; und daß Fälle gleichzeitiger Hypercholesterinämie und Hyperuricämie bekannt sind, deren Ablagerungen im Sinne ursprünglicher Harnsäureniederschläge mit Ausbildung sekundärer Cholesterindepots oder als gleichzeitiges Vorkommen beider Ereignisse gedeutet werden mußten. Es sei daran erinnert, daß wir in 45% unserer Gicht-Fälle Cholesterinwerte über 300 mg-% gefunden haben (GAMP et al., 1965).

Fälle kombinierter Lipoid- und Harnsäuregicht werden in der Literatur diskutiert (VACHTENHEIM u. SVOJITKA, 1959; OTTO, 1973).

Auf die Beziehungen zwischen *Glykogen*-Speicherkrankheit und tophöser Gicht sei hier nur hingewiesen (ALEPA et al., 1967).

4. Die „*Kalk-Gicht*": Dieses polyätiologische und polymorphe Syndrom umfaßt Weichteilverdichtungen, Verkalkungen und Ossifikationen unbekannter Ursache und bei mesenchymalen Systemerkrankungen und beansprucht zu ihrer differentialdiagnostischen Abgrenzung vorwiegend röntgenologisches Interesse (BUCHWALD u. SEVERIN, 1968). Es sind dies die Calcinosis interstitialis universalis und circumscripta, die Lipocalcinogranulomatose (pseudo-tumoröse Calcinose — TEUTSCHLAENDER) (JESSERER, 1960) und die Weichteilverkalkungen bei Kollagenosen, insbesondere der Sklerodermie und Dermatomyositis. Wir haben jenen Kalkknoten, die durch schmerzhafte Eruptionen, sogar mit Fieber und eventuell mit Ulcerationen und Sekundärinfekten vorwiegend in der Umgebung von Extremitätengelenken einhergehen können, noch die *Peritendinitis calcarea* hinzuge-

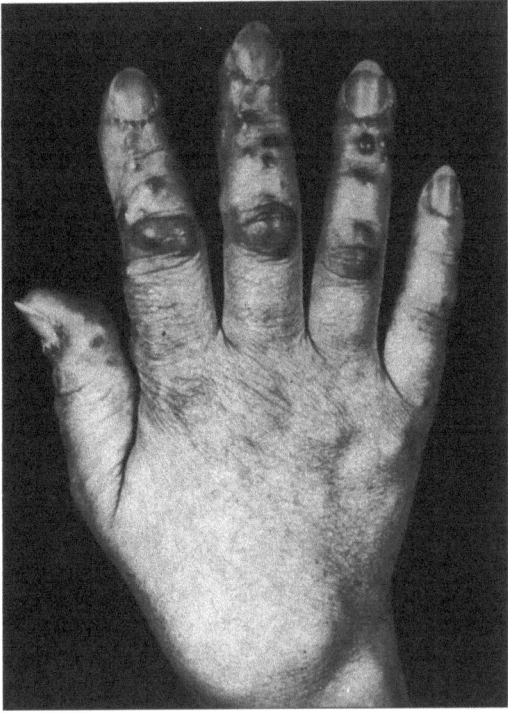

Abb. 21a. Fingergelenknahe noduläre Hauteruptionen bei Lipoid-Dermato-Arthritis; röntgenologisch mit pseudo-tophös verdichtetem Weichteilaspekt und (noch) diskreten Gelenkdestruktionen. (MEYER)

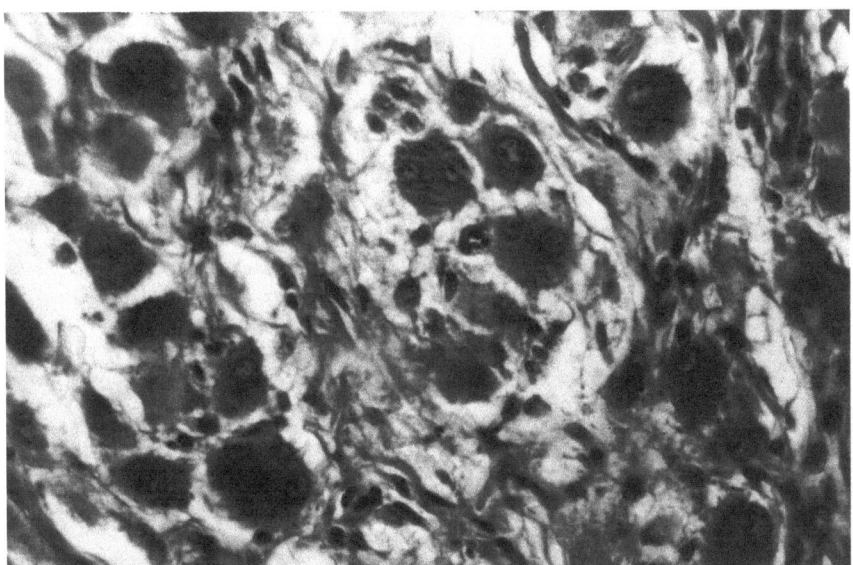

Abb. 21b. Histopathologisch zeigt ein exzidiertes Knötchen direkt unter der Epidermis tiefreichend tumorartige Ansammlungen von vielkernigen eosinophilen Riesenzellen mit Zerstörung der ortsständigen Faserstrukturen. Die Riesenzellnester lösen sich zur Subcutis hin auf und sind hier mit Fettzellen untermischt. Schaumzellen finden sich nicht. (FASSBENDER)

fügt sowie jene Pseudotophi, die bei der chronischen *Niereninsuffizienz* bzw. unter der Dauerdialyse entstehen können (RITZ *et al.*, SCHULZ u. GESSLER; — vgl. S. 289).

5. Der Rheumaknoten der chronischen (rheumatoiden) Polyarthritis kann nach cystischer Kolliquationsnekrose durch Fetteinlagerung, selten vollständig und systematisiert, eine Umwandlung in ein *Lipoid-Knötchen* erfahren (NIXON u. DURHAM, 1959).

Die *Lipoid-Dermato-Arthritis* (Reticulohistiocytosis) aber ist eine sehr seltene Haut- und Gelenkkrankheit, die durch Riesenzell-Granulome des RHS charakterisiert ist ("generalized giant cell histiocytomatosis", "multicentric reticulohistiocytosis of the skin and synovia"). Die spärliche Kasuistik ist in mancher Hinsicht uneinheitlich (vgl. BORTZ u. VINCENT, 1961; JENTZSCH, 1970). Tumorartig proliferierende histiocytäre Granulome mit mehrkernigen Riesenzellen (Riesenzell-Histiocytome) und nur fakultativ mit Schaumzellen befallen eruptiv die Haut und destruierend Gelenke und Halswirbelsäule: Cutane Knötchen mit Lieblingssitz periarticulär an den Fingern (Abb. 21a) und (nicht immer) eine in besonderer Weise synovial-proliferativ mutilierende chronische Polyarthritis (SCHWARZ u. FISH, 1960; MARTEL *et al.*, 1961) sind die Hauptsymptome dieses Syndroms. Eine Störung des intermediären Glykolipoid-Stoffwechsels soll zugrunde liegen (HORNSTEIN). Die meisten Fälle zeigen nur geringe systemische Entzündung und sind Rheumafaktor-negativ, einige aber verhalten sich ähnlich einer schweren aktiven chronischen (rheumatoiden) Polyarthritis.

Nach eigener Erfahrung ist dieses Syndrom nosologisch uneinheitlich. Dies kommt auch deutlich in der ausführlichen Publikation von JENTZSCH (1970) zum Ausdruck, deren Fall wir trotz der Bedenken der Autorin für diesem Syndrom zugehörig halten. Unter den Varianten dieser Krankheit gibt es sicher nicht nur auf die Haut beschränkte Fälle, sondern auch solche, die mit synovial-granulomatösen Destruktionen auf das Gelenksystem beschränkt sind und bleiben.

Die pseudo-tophösen Hautknötchen können auch, wie im Falle JENTZSCH, periarticuläre Verkalkungen einlagern: Lipoid-Kalkknoten.

Die dreißigjährige (mit Amyloidose kompliziert) verstorbene Patientin (JENTZSCH, 1970; mit FRANKL u. BRANDENBURG, Berlin) und eine Patientin aus Hamburg (MEYER, 1972) sind die einzigen Fälle histopathologisch belegter Lipoid-Dermatoarthritis, die ich in Deutschland gefunden habe. Die Fotografie der Hände des letzteren Falles wurde mir von Herrn Dr. Meyer dankenswerterweise zur Verfügung gestellt (Abb. 21a). Eines der digitalen cutanen Nodi haben wir (FASSBENDER, Zentrum für Rheumapathologie Mainz) feingeweblich untersucht (Abb. 21b). Häufiger sind *Riesenzelltumoren* von Finger-Sehnenscheiden.

6. Die *Acrodermatitis chronica atrophicans* (HERXHEIMER) geht in 25% der Fälle mit fibroiden Knoten in Gelenknähe („juxta-articulär") einher. Diese sind vorwiegend über den Fingergrundgelenken oder auch am Ellenbogen lokalisiert, wo sie bei Unkenntnis der zugrundeliegenden Hautkrankheit als subcutane Rheumaknoten oder auch als Tophi fehlgedeutet werden könnten. Bei der Lokalisation am Ellenbogen fehlt kaum der auf die Acrodermatitis hinweisende „Ulnar-Streifen", der selten die Form eines dermato-sklerotischen Strangs annehmen kann. Da es sich um ein Allgemeinleiden mit systemischen Entzündungszeichen (Blutsenkungsbeschleunigung und Dysproteinämie) handelt, das zuweilen sogar durch arthritische Manifestationen kompliziert sein kann (SCHILLING, 1970), ist die differentialdiagnostische Erwähnung dieses wahrscheinlich infektiös bedingten atrophisierenden Hautleidens hier am Platze.

Die chronische, entzündlich bedingte Hautatrophie schreitet zentripetal von Händen und Füßen aus fort und bevorzugt gelenknahe Hautpartien an Hand- und Fußrücken, Ellenbogen und Knien, wo zunächst Rötung, dann livide Verfärbung, z.B. streifenförmig entlang der Ulnakante, und schließlich

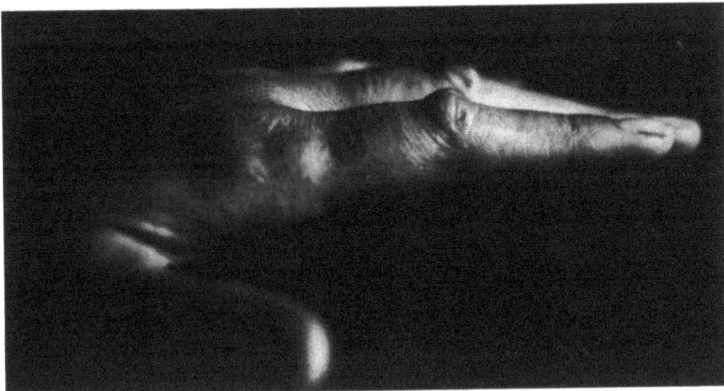

Abb. 22. Harmlose fibröse Hautknötchen über den Fingermittelgelenken: Fingerknöchelpolster

pergamentartige Verdünnung und Durchsichtigkeit vorherrschen. Hinzukommen fakultativ die fibroiden juxta-articulären Knoten. — Wir sahen bisher fünf Fälle (3 Männer) mit Acrodermatitis atrophicans, die durch eine chronische Polyarthritis kleiner und mittlerer Gelenke in den befallenen Bezirken kompliziert war, rheumaserologisch negativ, im Verlauf torpide, im Röntgenbild entweder noch stumm oder nur gering destruierend und in zwei Fällen mit knotigen Erhabenheiten der sklerosierten Haut in Ellenbogennähe.

7. Die *Fingerknöchelpolster* sind harmlose Erscheinungen einer Polyfibromatose, entsprechend der Dupuytrenschen Kontraktur, die sie oft begleiten. Es handelt sich um schmerzlose cutane Knötchen dorsal über den Fingermittelgelenken, die mit Rheuma- oder Gichtknoten verwechselt werden könnten (Abb. 22).

8. Die *Heberden-Knötchen* wurden oben schon mehrfach erwähnt. Sie haben mit Gicht nichts zu tun, sondern entsprechen dem dermatologischen Bild der „Dorsalcyste". Sie können selten einmal imitiert werden durch pseudo-tophöse Erscheinungen einer Calcinose bzw. einer Peritendinitis calcarea (vgl. oben) oder durch den arthrotischen Reparationszustand einer juvenilen oder einer psoriatischen Fingerendgelenkarthritis. Selten muß man aber auch einmal mit einem echten Urattophus an dieser Stelle rechnen, aber nur im Rahmen eines schon fortgeschrittenen tophösen Befalls der Hand.

Literatur

ADLERSBERG, D., PARETS, A. D., BOAS, E. P.: Genetics of atherosclerosis. J. Amer. med. Ass. **141**, 246 (1949).

AITKEN, R. E., KERR, J. L., LLOYD, H. M.: Primary hyperparathyroidism with osteosclerosis and calcification in articular cartilage. Amer. J. Med. **37**, 813—820 (1964).

ALEPA, F. P., HOWELL, R. R., KLINENBERG, J. R., SEEGMILLER, J.: Relationship between glycogen storage disease and tophaceous gout. Amer. J. Med. **42**, 58—66 (1967).

AMOR, F., COSTE, F., DELBARRE, F.: Sur l'origine posible du syndrome oculo-uréthro-synovial. Presse méd. **73**, 1825—1830 (1965).

ANANTHAKRISHNAN, R., ECKES, L., WALTER, H.: On the Genetics of Psoriasis An Analysis of Hellgren's Data for a Model of Multifactorial Inheritance. Arch. derm. Forsch. **247**, 53—58 (1973).

ANGEVINE, C. D., JACOS, R. F.: Pseudogout in the elderly. Arch. intern. Med. **131**, 693—696 (1973).

ANSCHÜTZ, F., MENDE, E.: Die Karditis des akuten rheumatischen Fiebers im Jugend- und Erwachsenenalter. Dtsch. med. Wschr. **93**, 7—12 (1968).

ANSCHÜTZ, F., WIPPERFÜRTH, U.: Über die Abnahme und das zunehmende Alter von rheumatischen Herzklappenfehlern. Z. Kreisl.-Forsch. **61**, 385—391 (1972).

ARLET, J., MOLE, J.: Association de goutte et de polyarthrite chronique avec ténosynovite nécrotique fistulisée. Rev. Rhumat. **1961**, 320—322.

ASSHOFF, H., BÖHM, P., SCHOEN, E., SCHÜRHOLZ, K.: Klinik der hereditären Chondrocalcinosis articularis. Dtsch. med. Wschr. **92**, 349—357 (1967).

ATKINS, C. J., MCIVOR, J., SMITH, P. M., HAMILTON, E., WILLIAMS, R.: Chondrocalcinosis and arthropathy: Studies in haemochromatosis and in idiopathic chondrocalcinosis. Quart. J. Med. **29**, 71—82 (1969).

BABUCKE, G., MERTZ, D. P.: Epidemiologie und klinisches Bild der primären Gicht. Münch. med. Wschr. **113**, 617—624 (1971).

BABUCKE, G., MERTZ, D. P.: Wandlungen in Epidemiologie und klinischem Bild der primären Gicht zwischen 1948 und 1970. Dtsch. med. Wschr. **98**, 183—188 (1973).

BALL, G. V., SCHROHENLOHER, R. E., MCBRIDE, W.: Serum immunglobulins in gout. Proc. Soc. exp. Biol. (N.Y.) **132**, 134—135 (1969).

BILEZIKIAN, J. P. et al.: Pseudogout after parathyroidectomy. Lancet **1973 I**, 445—446.

BJELLE, A. O.: Morphological study of articular cartilage in pyrophosphate arthropathy. Ann. rheum. Dis. **31**, 449—456 (1972).

BLOCH-MICHEL, H., BENOIST, M., RIPAULT, J., SIAUD, J.-R.: Arthropathies micro-cristalline associées à une maladie rhumatoide. Presse méd. **76**, 1311—1313 (1968).

BOPP, A.: Zur Differentialdiagnose der Gicht. Med. Mschr. **11**, 579—581 (1957).

BOPP, A.: Zur Differentialdiagnose subakuter rheumatischer Prozesse. Z. Rheumaforsch. **24**, 1—9 (1965).

BORTZ, A. I., VINCENT, M.: Lipid dermato-arthritis and arthritis mutilans. A. J. Med. **30**, 951—960 (1961).

BREWERTON, D. A., NICHOLLS, A., CAFFREY, M., WALTERS, D., OATES, J. K., JAMES, D. C. O.: Reiter's disease and HL-A 27. Lancet **1973** II, 996—997.

BUCHWALD, W., SEVERIN, G.: II. Röntgendiagnostik der Muskeln, Sehnen und Bänder. Pathologische Verdichtung und Aufhellung im Weichteilmantel. Sonderdruck aus Handbuch der Medizinischen Radiologie (Encyclopedia of medical radiology), Bd. VIII. Berlin-Heidelberg-New York: Springer 1968.

BUNDENS, W. D., BRIGHTIN, C. T., WEITZMAN, G.: Primary articular-cartilage calcification with arthritis (Pseudogout Syndrome). J. Bone It Surg. **47-A**, 111—122 (1965).

BYWATERS, E. G. L., DIXON, A. ST. J., SCOTT, J. T.: Joint Lesions of Hyperparathyroidism. Ann. Rheum. Dis. **22**, 171—187 (1963).

CANER, J. E. Z., DECKER, J. L.: Recurrent acute (? gouty) arthritis in chronic renal feature treated with periodic hemodialysis. Amer. J. Med. **36**, 571—582 (1964).

CONTIGUGLIA, S. R., ALFREY, A. C., MILLER, N. L., RUNNELLS, D. E., LEGEROS, R. Z.: Nature of soft tissue calcification in uremia. Kidney int. **4**, 229—235 (1973).

COSTE, F., SOLNICA, J.: Polyarthritis psoriatica. In: Rheumatismus und Bindegewebe (W. H. HAUSS, U. GERLACH, Hrsg.), S. 90—127. Darmstadt: Steinkopff 1966.

CSONKA, G.: Reiter's Syndrome. Ergebn. inn. Med. N.F. **23** (1964).

DEICHER, H.: Untersuchungsmethoden der Gelenkflüssigkeit. In: SCHOEN, R., BÖNI, A., MIEHLKE, K. „Klinik der rheumatischen Erkrankungen" Springer, Berlin-Heidelberg-New York, 1970, S. 57—64.

DELBARRE, F., BRAUN, S., SAINT-GEORGES-CHAUMET, F.: La goutte féminine. Sem. Hôp. Paris **43**, 623—664 (1967).

DIHLMANN, W.: Calcaneeopathia rheumatica (röntgenologischer Nachweis, Differentialdiagnose). Fortschr. Röntgenstr. **107**, 271—276 (1967).

DODDS, W. J., STEINBACH, H. L.: Gout associated with calcification of cartilage. New Engl. J. Med. **275**, 745—749 (1966).

DÜRR, F.: Hämodialyse und Peritonealdialyse in der Behandlung chronisch Nierenkranker. Therapiewoche **19**, 23—27 (1969).

DÜRRIGL, TH., ZERGOLLERN, V.: Praktische Bedeutung der Untersuchung der Synovialflüssigkeit. Dtsch. med. Wsch. **97**, 477—481 (1972).

DYMOCK, I. W., HAMILTON, E. B. D., LAWS, J. W., WILLIAMS, R.: Arthropathy of Haemochromatosis: Clinical and Radiological Analysis of 63 Patients with Iron Overload. Ann. Rheum. Dis. **29**, 469—476 (1970).

EISSNER, D., HAHN, K., HOLZMANN, H., HOEDE, N., SCHMIDBACH, H., WOLF, R., HÜLSE, R.: Gelenk-szintigraphische Untersuchungen bei Psoriasis-Kranken. Verh. Dtsch. Ges. Rheum. **4** (1974) (im Druck).

FAIRES, J. S., MCCARTY, J.: Acute Arthritis in man and dog after intrasynovial injection of sodium urate crystals. Lancet **1962 II**, 682—684.

FALLET, G.-H., FLEISCH, H., BISAZ, S., RUSSEL, R. G. G., BOUSSINA, I., MICHELLI, A., GABAY, R.: Etude du liquide synovial et du plasma dans la chondrocalcinose articulaire. Rev. Rhum. **39**, 189—195 (1972).

FASSBENDER, H. G., SCHILLING, F.: Chondrokalzinose — Beobachtungen an 18 Fällen (in Vorbereitung).

FASSBENDER, H. G.: Zur Pathologie der Gicht. Therapiewoche **22**, 105—108 (1972).

FASSBENDER, H. G.: Pathologie rheumatischer Erkrankungen. Berlin-Heidelberg-New York: Springer 1974.

FRIED, K.: Neurotrophische Osteoarthropathien. Fortschr. Röntgenstr. **113**, 560 (1970).

GAMP, A., SCHILLING, A.: Extraartikuläre Manifestationen der chronischen Polyarthritis am Bewegungsapparat: Sehnen-, Sehnenscheiden-, Schleimbeutelentzündung, subkutane Knoten. Z. Rheumaforsch. **25**, 42—56 (1966).

GAMP, A., SCHILLING, A., MÜLLER, L., SCHACHERL, M.: Das klinische Bild der Gicht heute. Med. Klin. **60**, 129—131 (1965).

GOLDBERG, M., CASTLEMAN, L., FRIEDMAN, I. S., WALLACE, S. L.: The artificial kidney in the treatment of chronic tophaceous gout. J. Amer. med. Ass. **182**, 870—872 (1962).

GOOD, A. E., RAPP, R.: Chondrocalcinosis of the knee with gout and rheumatoid arthritis, New Engl. J. Med. **277**, 286—290 (1967).

GOTTRON, H. A., KORTING, G. W.: Chronische Hautgicht. Arch. klin. exp. Dermat. **204**, 483—489 (1957).

GREILING, H.: Podiumsdiskussion in: Arthrosis — Arthritis — „degenerativer Rheumatismus". Verh. Dtsch. Ges. Orthop. **57**, 25—27 (1970).

GRIEBSCH, A., ZÖLLNER, N.: Normalwerte der Plasmaharnsäure in Süddeutschland. Z. klin. Chem. **11**, 348—356 (1973).

GUKELBERGER, M.: Zur Differenzierung der Gelenkpunktate. Triangel **9**, 138—147 (1970).

HAMILTON, E.: Joint disease in haemochromatosis. In: HILL, A. G. S. (Ed.): Modern Trends in Rheumatology, p. 338—347 (1971).

HÄNTZSCHEL, H., REINELT, D., OTTO, W.: Zytologische und enzymatische Untersuchungen im Gelenkpunktat zur Diagnostik der Arthritis urica. Aus: Hyperurikämie — Arthritis urica Osteoarthrosen — Osteonekrosen. Berlin: VEB Verlag Volk und Gesundheit 1972.

HARTMANN, F.: Bedeutung der Pyrophosphatausscheidung beim primären Hyperparathyreoidismus. Med. Klin. **67**, 1597—1602 (1972).

HEUER, L. J.: Entwicklung und Behandlung der renalen Osteopathie. Med. Welt (Stuttg.) **25**, 1761—1766 (1974).

HOLZMANN, H., HOEDE, N., MORSCHES, B.: Organmanifestationen der Psoriasis-Krankheit. Med. Welt (Stuttg.) (N.F.) **24**, 523—527 (1973).

HOLZMANN, H., MORSCHES, B., HOEDE, N.: Ätiopathogenese der Psoriasis-Krankheit. Med. Welt (Stuttg.) (N.F.) **24**, 429—434 (1973).

HORNSTEIN, O.: Zur nosologischen Stellung der Psoriasis arthropathica. Arch. klin. exp. Derm. **214**, 622—651 (1962).

HÜTTL, S., HÜTTLOVA, O.: Natriumuratkristalle in der Diagnostik der Arthritis urica. Beitr. Rheum. **18**, 35—39 (1972).

HÜTTL, S.: Synovial effusion I. Acta Rheumat. Balneol. Pistiniana **5** (1970).

JACKSON, W. P. U., HARRIS, F.: Gout with hyperparathyroidism: Report of case with examination of synovial fluid. Brit. med. J. **1965 II**, 211.

JACOBELLI, S., MCCARTY, D. J., SILCOX, D. C., MALL, J. C.: Calcium pyrophosphate dihydrate crystal deposition in neuropathic joints. Ann. intern. Med. **79**, 340—347 (1973).

JENTZSCH, K.: Eine besondere morphologische Verlaufsform der primär chronischen Polyarthritis (p.c.P.). Virchows Arch. Abt. A Path. Anat. **349**, 244—257 (1970).

JESSERER, H.: Calcinosis interstitialis. Med. Klin. **55**, 2229 (1960).

KELLGREN, J. H., MOORE, R.: Generalized osteoarthritis and Heberden's nodes. Brit. med. J. **1952 I**, 181.

KOHN, N. N., HUGHES, R. R., MCCARTY, D. J., FAIRES, J. S.: Significance of calcium phosphate crystals in synovial fluid of arthritic patients "pseudogout syndrome" II. Identification of crystals. Ann. intern. Med. **56**, 738—745 (1962).

KÖLLE, G.: Verlaufsformen des kindlichen Rheumatismus. Therapiewoche **19**, 240—243 (1969).

KÖTTGEN, U.: Das rheumatische Fieber. In: KSCHOEN, R., BÖNI, A., MIEHLKE, K. (Hrsg.): Klinik der rheumatischen Erkrankungen, S. 112—124. Berlin-Heidelberg-New York: Springer 1970.

KÖTTGEN, U., CALLENSSE, W.: Rheumatisches Fieber im Kindesalter. Beihefte zum Archiv für Kinderheilkunde, 45. Heft. Stuttgart: Enke 1961.

LAGIER, R., BAUD, C. A., BUCHS, M.: Crystallographic identification of calcium deposits as regards their pathological nature, with special reference to chondrocalcinosis. In: Third European Symposion on Calcified Tissues, p. 158—162. Berlin-Heidelberg-New York: Springer 1966.

LAMOTTE, M., LABROUSSE, C. L., BASSET, F.: Pseudo-goutte phosphocalcique au stade terminal d'une néphropathie chronique. Sem. Hôp. Paris 41, 511—517 (1965).

MALLUCHE, H. H.: Pathogenese und Therapie der azotämischen Osteopathie. Kassenarzt 10, 1666—1679 (1973).

MARTEL, W., ABELL, M. B., DUFF, I. F.: Cervical spine involvement in lipoid dermato-arthritis. Radiology 77, 613—617 (1961).

MATHIES, H.: Bericht über die Arbeitstagung in Teneriffa 1969 — Arthritis psoriatica. Z. Rheumaforsch. 29, 55—58 (1970).

MCCARTY, D. J.: Crystal deposition disease—calcium pyrophosphate. In: HILL, A. G. S. (Ed.): Modern Trends in Rheumatology, p. 287—302. New York: Appleton-Century-Crofts 1966.

MCCARTY, D. J., GATTER, R. A.: Recurrent acute inflammation associated with focal apatite crystal deposition. Arthr. and Rheum. 9, 804—819 (1966).

MCCARTY, D. J., HASKIN, M. E.: The roentgenographic aspects of pseudogout (articular chondrocalcinosis); an analysis of 20 cases. Amer. J. Roentgenol. 90, 1248—1257 (1963).

MCCARTY, J., HOLLANDER, J. I.: Identification of urate crystals in gouty synovial fluid. Ann. intern. Med. 54, 452—460 (1961).

MCCARTY, D. wJ., KOHN, N. N., FAIRES, J. S.: The significance of calcium phosphate crystals in the synovial fluid of arthritic patients: The "Pseudogout Syndrome". I. Clinical Aspects. Ann. intern. Med. 56, 711—737 (1962).

MCCOLLUM, D. E., MATHEWS, R. S., O'NEIL, M. T., PICKETT, P. T.: Gout, hyperuricemia and aseptic necrosis of the femoral head. In: ZINN, W. M. (Ed.): Idiopathic ischemic necrosis of the femoral head in adults, p. 133—139. Stuttgart: Thieme 1971.

MCEWEN, C.: Osteoarthritis of the fingers with ankylosis. Arthr. and Rheum. 11, 734 (1968).

MENKES, C.-J., SIMON, F., CHOURAKI, M., ECOFFET, M., AMOR, B., DELBARRE, F.: Les arthropathies destructives de la chondrocalcinose. Rev. Rhum. 40, 115—123 (1973).

MERTZ, D. P., BABUCKE, G.: Epidemiologie und klinisches Bild der primären Gicht. Beobachtungen zwischen 1948 und 1968. Münch. med. Wschr. 113, 617 (1971).

MEYER, W.: Tumoren und rheumatische Erkrankungen. Kassenarzt 12, 119—128 (1972).

MEYER-BORSTEL, H.: Meniscusverkalkungen. Chirurg 3, 424—426 (1931).

MOHR, W., HERSENER, J., WILKE, W., WEINLAND, G., BENEKE, G.: Pseudogicht (Chondrokalzinose). Z. Rheumatol. 33, 107—129 (1974).

MOSKOWITZ, R. W., KATZ, D.: Chondrocalcinosis (Pseudogout Syndrome): A family study. J. Amer. med. Ass. 188, 867—871 (1964).

MOSKOWITZ, R. W., KATZ, D.: Chondrocalcinosis coincidental to other rheumatic disease. Arch. intern. Med. 115, 680—683 (1965).

MOSKOWITZ, R. W., KATZ, D.: Chondrocalcinosis and Chondrocalsynovitis (Pseudogout Syndrome): Analysis of 24 cases. Amer. J. Med. 43, 332—334 (1967).

MÜHR, H.: Über eine generalisierte, primäre Kalkeinlagerung in die Gelenkknorpelgrenzflächen mit Demonstrierung der wahren Gelenkspalte. Fortschr. Röntgenstr. 88, 650—655 (1958).

MÜLLER, W., LANGNESS, U., PETERSEN, K. F.: Die Stellung der seronegativen chronischen Polyarthritis. Dtsch. med. Wschr. 93, 2252—2255 (1968).

NIEPEL, G. A., KOSTKA, D., KOPECKY, S., MANCA, S.: Enthesopathy, Acta rheumatologica et balneologica Pistiniana 1966, 1.

O'DUFFY, J. D.: Pseudogout Syndrome in Hospital Patients. J. Amer. med. Ass. 226, 42—44 (1973).

O'HARA, L. J., LEVIN, M.: Carpal tunnel syndrome and gout. Arch. intern. Med. 120, 180—184 (1967).

OTTO, H.: Primär chronische Polyarthritis in Kombination mit Lipoidgicht und anderen Stoffwechselstörungen. Dtsch. Gesundh.-Wes. 28, 1796—1801 (1973).

OWEN, D. S., TOONE, E., IRBY, R.: Coexistent rheumatoid arthritis and chronic tophaceous gout. J. Amer. med. Ass. 197, 953—956 (1966).

PARONEN, I.: Reiter's disease. A study of 344 cases observed in Finland. Acta med. scand. 211, suppl. 1948.

PAULLEY, J. W., BARLOW, K. E., CUTTING, P. E. J., STEVENS, J.: Acute gouty pericarditis. The Lancet, 21—22 (1963).

PETER, J. B., PEARSON, C. M., MARMOR, L.: Erosive Osteoarthritis of the hands. Arthr. and Rheum. 9, 365 (1966).

PHELPS, P., HAWKER, CH. D.: Serum parathyroid Hormone Levels in patients with calcium Pyrophosphate Crystal Deposition Disease (Chondrocalcinosis, Pseudogout). Arthr. and Rheum. **16**, 590—596 (1973).
PHELPS, P., STEELE, A. D., MCCARTY, D. J.: Compensated polarized light microscopy. Identification of crystals in synovial fluids from gout and pseudogout. J. Amer. med. Ass. **203**, 508—512 (1968).
POHL, W.: Hüftkopfnekrose bei Hyperlipämie. Z. Orthop. **109**, 873—880 (1971).
RAVAULT, P. P., BOUVIER, M.: Le rhumatisme articulaire subaigu de l'adulte. Aktuelle Rheumaprobleme (Verh. der französisch-italienisch-schweizerischen gemeinsamen wissenschaftlichen Tagung, Lausanne 1964), Zollikofer St. Gallen 1965, p. 12—22.
RAVAULT, P. P., LEJEUNE, E., MAITREPIERRE, J.: La Chondrocalcinose aeticulaire diffuse. Rev. Rhum. **27**, 1095—1102 (1959).
RAVAULT, P., LEJEUNE, E., MAITREPIERRE, J.: Aux frontières de la goutte et du rhumatisme: la polyarthrits chronique rhumatismale à forme pseudo-goutteuse. Bull. Acad. nat. Méd. (Paris) **145**, 281—287 (1961).
RAVAULT, P. P., MAITREPIERRE, J., BERTRAND, J.-N., GRABER-DUVERNAY, B.: Sur quelques difficultés de diagnostic entre goutte et polyarthrits chronique rhumatismale. Lyon Med. **221**, 7—12 (1969).
RAVAULT, P. P., VIGNON, G., LEJEUNE, E., MAITREPIERRE, J., GAUTHIER, J.: La chondrocalcinose articulaire diffuse. (A propos de 6 observations personelles). J. Méd. Lyon, **42**, 65—98 (1961).
DE REUS, H. D.: Chondrocalcinose („Pseudogicht"). Dtsch. med. Wschr. **99**, 363—365 (1974).
RITTER, U.: Zur Klinik und Röntgendiagnose der Meniscusverkalkungen. Chirurg **23**, 22—27 (1952).
RITZ, E.: Persönliche Mitteilung 1974.
RITZ, E., KREMPIEN, B., MEHLS, O., MALLUCHE, H.: Skeletal abnormalities in chronic renal insufficiency before and during maintenance hemodialysis. Kidney int. **4**, 116—127 (1973).
ROTHENBERGER, K., THOMAE, U., EBERHARD, K., KUHLMANN, H.: Kalzium-Phosphat-Stoffwechselstörungen unter Hämodialyse. Med. Welt (Stuttg.) **25**, 103—105 (1974).
RUBENS-DUVAL, A., VILLIAUMEY, J., ARISTOFF, H.: Un cas de chondrocalcinose articulaire diffuse d'allure inflammatoire. Rev. Rhum. **28**, 444—447 (1961).
RUSSEL, R. G. G., BISAZ, S., FLEISCH, H., CURREY, H. L. F., RUBINSTEIN, H. M., DIETZ, A. A., BOUSSINA, I., MICHELI, A., FALLET, G.: Inorganic pyrophosphate in plasma, urine, and synovial fluid of patients with pyrophosphate arthropathy (chondrocalcinosis or pseudogout). Lancet **1970** II, 899—906.
RYCKEWAERT, A., SOLNICA, J., LANHAM, C., DE SEZE, S.: Manifestations articulaires de l'hyperparathyroidie. Presse Med. **74**, 2599—2603 (1966).
SANDSTROM, C.: Peritendinitis calcarea. Amer. J. Roentgenol. **40**, 1—21 (1938).
SCHACHERL, M., SCHILLING, F.: Röntgenbefunde an den Gliedmaßengelenken bei Polyarthritis psoriatica. Z. Rheumaforsch. **26**, 442—450 (1967).
SCHACHERL, M., SCHILLING, F.: Die destruierende Polyarthrose. Fortschr. Röntgenstr. **113**, 551—560 (1970).
SCHACHERL, M., SCHILLING, F., GAMP, A.: Das radiologische Bild der Gicht. Radiologe **6**, 231—238 (1966).
SCHATTENKIRCHNER, M.: Der chronische Streptokokkenrheumatismus. Therapiewoche **19**, 238—239 (1969).
SCHILLING, F.: Erfahrungen mit Indometacin. Münch. med. Wschr. **107**, 2176 (1965).
SCHILLING, F.: Gicht — Diagnose, Differentialdiagnose und Therapie. Ärztl. Fortb. **16**, 36—47 (1967).
SCHILLING, F.: Röntgenmorphologische Befunde bei der Spondylitis ankylopoetica. Verh. dtsch. Ges. Rheum. **1**, 33—46 (1969).
SCHILLING, F.: Periodisches „rheumatisches Steroid-Fieber". Münch. med. Wschr. **111**, 2312—2313 (1969).
SCHILLING, F.: Differentialdiagnose der Spondylitis ankylopoetica: Spondylitis psoriatica, chronisches Reiter-Syndrom und Spondylosis hyperostotica. Therapiewoche **19**, 249—254 (1969).
SCHILLING, F.: Differentialdiagnose der Gicht, atypische Gicht und Pseudogicht. Therapiewoche **19**, 245, 260 (1969).
SCHILLING, F.: Die symptomatischen Arthritiden. Heilkunst **83**, Heft 8 (1970).
SCHILLING, F.: Klinik und Therapie der Gicht und deren Abgrenzung von der Pseudogicht. In: Fettsucht — Gicht, SCHETTLER, G., BOECKER, W., S. 139—160. Stuttgart: Thieme 1971.
SCHILLING, F.: Kombination von Arthritis urica und rheumatoider Arthritis — Alkohol und Gichtanfall. Med. Welt (Stuttg.) **22**, 1300 (1971).
SCHILLING, F.: Die Polyarthrose. Diagnostik **4**, 350—353 (1971).

SCHILLING, F.: Zur Differentialdiagnose und Anfallstherapie der Gicht und der Pseudogicht. Arzneimittel-Forsch. **21**, 1856—1857 (1971).
SCHILLING, F.: Klinik der Gicht. Therapiewoche **22**, 2, 92 (1972).
SCHILLING, F.: Die chronische Arthritis — eine Präarthrose? Z. Orthop. **112**, 555—560 (1974).
SCHILLING, F.: Diskussionsbeitrag zu „HL-A-27 beim Reiter-Syndrom". Verh. dtsch. Ges. inn. Med. **80**, 1417 (1974).
SCHILLING, F.: Spondylitis ankylopoetica — Die sogenannte Bechterewsche Krankheit und ihre Differentialdiagnose (einschließlich Spondylosis hyperostotica, Spondylitis psoriatica und chronisches Reiter-Syndrom. In: Handb. Med. Radiol. Bd. VI/2, S. 452—689. Berlin-Heidelberg-New York: Springer 1975.
SCHILLING, F.: Fibro- und Chondrocalcinose und Periarthritis calcarea — akut rezidivierende artikuläre und extraartikuläre Pseudogicht. Fortschr. Röntgenstr. (in Vorbereitung).
SCHILLING, F., FASSBENDER, H. G.: Morphologie der Arthritis psoriatica und deren „pseudoguttöse" Verlaufsform. Verh. Dtsch. Ges. Rheumat. **4**, 221—228 (1974).
SCHILLING, F., GAMP, A.: Essentielle familiäre hypercholesterinämische Xanthomatose. Acta hepat. (Hamburg) **5**, 146 (1957).
SCHILLING, F., GAMP, A., SCHACHERL, M.: Das Reiter-Syndrom und seine Beziehungen zur Spondylitis ankylopoetica. Z. Rheumaforsch. **24**, 342—353 (1965).
SCHILLING, F., SCHACHERL, M.: Chondrocalcinose (Fragekasten). Fortschr. Röntgenstr. **102**, 692—693 (1965).
SCHILLING, F., SCHACHERL, M.: Röntgenbefunde an der Wirbelsäule bei Polyarthritis psoriatica und Reiter-Dermatose: Spondylitis psoriatica. Z. Rheumaforsch. **26**, 450—459 (1967).
SCHILLING, F., SCHACHERL, M., GAMP, A., BOPP, A.: Die Beziehungen der Spondylosis hyperostotica zur Konstitution und zu Stoffwechselstörungen. Med. Klin. **60**, 165—169 (1965).
SCHULITZ, K.-P.: Zur Frage der Hüftgelenkerkrankungen bei der Gicht. Z. Orthop. **106**, 708—716 (1969).
SCHULZ, W., GESSLER, U.: Besondere Probleme der Urämiebehandlung. Inn. Med. **2**, 22—33 (1975).
SCHUMACHER, H. R.: The Synovitis of pseudogout: Electron Microscopic observations. Arthr. and Rheum. **11**, 420—435 (1968).
SCHWARZ, E., FISH, A.: Reticulohistiocytome: A rare dermatologic disease with roentgen manifestations. J. Amer. Roentgenol. **83**, 692—697.
SCOTT, J. T., DIXON, A. ST. J., BYWATERS, E. G. L.: Association of hyperuricaemia and gout with hyperparathyroidism. Brit. med. J. **1964 I**, 1070—1073.
SEEGMILLER, J. E., HOWELL, R. R.: The old and the new concepts of acute gouty arthritis. Arthr. and Rheum. **5**, 616—623 (1962).
DE SEZE, S., HUBAULT, A., KAHN, M. F.: Deux cas de chondrocalcinose articulaire diffuse simulant une polyarthrite chronique rhumatoide. Rev. Rhum. **28**, 439—444 (1961).
DE SEZE, S., RYCKEWAERT, A., HUBAULT, A., KAHN, M.-F., MITROVIC, D., SOLNICA, J.: Les chondrocalcinoses articulaires. Sem. Hôp. (Paris) **42**, 2461 (1966).
SEZE, S. DE, HUBAULT, A., MAHN, M. F., SOLNICA, J.: A propos des formes polyarthritiques de la chondrocalcinose articulaire diffuse. Discussion nosologique. Les arthropathies métaboliques. Rev. Rhum. **36**, 724—727 (1969).
SILCOX, D. G., MCCARTY, J. D.: Measurement of inorganic pyrophosphate in biological fluids. Elevated levels in some patients with osteoarthritis, pseudogout, acromegaly, and uremia. J. clin. Invest. **52**, 1863—1870 (1973).
SKINNER, M., COHEN, A. S.: Calcium pyrophosphate dihydrate crystal deposition disease. Arch. intern. Med. **123**, 636—644 (1969).
SOLNICA, J., MITROVIC, D., KAHN, M.-F.: L'intéret de la misee évidence des formations cristallines dans le liquide synovial: La différenciation morphologique et ultrastructurale des cristaux. Sem. Hôp. (Paris) **43**, 2573—2580 (1967).
STECHER, M. R.: Das Problem der Vererbung bei Gelenkerkrankungen. Documenta rheumatologica Geigy 11. Basel 1957.
TALON, J.-P., FONDIMARE, A., HOUDENT, G., DESHAYES, P.: Chondrocalcinose articulaire et hyperparathyroidisme primitif. Rhumatologie **25**, 47—52 (1973).
THOMPSON, G. R., MING TING, Y., RIGGS, G. A., FENN, M. E., DENNING, R. M.: Calcific tendinitis and soft-tissue calcification resembling gout. J. Amer. med. Ass. **203**, 464—472 (1968).
THUMB, N.: Synovialflüssigkeitsanalyse. Orthop. Prax. **2/IX**, 78—85 (1973).
TWIGG, H. L., ZWAIFLER, N. J., NELSON, CH. W.: Chondrocalcinosis. Radiology **82**, 655—659 (1964).

VACHTENHEIM, J., SVOJITKA, J.: Ein Fall kombinierter Lipoid- und Harnsäuregicht. Dtsch. Z. Verdau.-Stoffwechselkr. **19**, 239—243 (1959).

VIX, V. A.: Articular and fibrocartilage calcification in hyperparathyroidism, associated hyperuricemia. Radiology **83**, 468—471 (1964).

WARD, L. E., OKIHIRO, M. M.: II. Pan.-am. Congr. rheum. dis., Bethesda 1959. 1 Zit. nach LAMONT-HAVERS in: HOLLANDER, J. L.: Arthritis and allied conditions, p. 753 (1967).

WERWATH, K.: Abnorme Kalkablagerungen innerhalb des Kniegelenks, ein Beitrag zur Frage der primären „Meniskopathie". Fortschr. Röntgenstr. **37**, 169—171 (1928).

WRIGHT, V., REED, W. B.: The link between Reiter's syndrome and psoriatic arthritis. Ann. rheum. Dis. **23**, 12—21 (1964).

YAZDI, S., GEHLEN, W.: Häufigkeitsanalytische Untersuchung über die Serumharnsäure bei Psoriasis. Hautarzt **20**, 488—489 (1969).

ZEIDLER, H., LUSKA, G.: Das klinische und radiologische Bild der Chondrocalcinose. Verh. Dtsch. Ges. inn. Med. **80**, 1421—1423 (1974).

ZITNAN, D., SITAJ, S. et al.: Chondrocalcinosis articularis. Ann. rheum. Dis. **22**, 142—170 (1963).

ZITNAN, D., SITAJ, S.: „Chondrocalcinosis Articularis". Acta Rheumatologica Pistiniana, Piestany, Czechoslovakia 1966.

ZVAIFLER, N. J., REEFE, W. E., BLACK, R. L.: Articular manifestations in primary hyperparathyroidism, Arthr. and Rheum. **5**, 237—249 (1962).

dd) Röntgendiagnostik der Gicht

Von

M. SCHACHERL

Mit 36 Abbildungen

Wenige Wochen nach Entdeckung der X-Strahlen demonstrierte HUBER in Berlin am 9. März 1896 eine Röntgenaufnahme der Hand eines Gichtkranken (Abb. 1). HUBER traf an Hand dieser Röntgenaufnahme folgende Feststellungen:

„1. Große Gichtknoten, besonders am Daumen und Kleinfinger (a, a), weniger scharf ausgeprägt am Ring- und Mittelfinger sowie am Ulnarrande der Mittelhand. Dieselben liegen unter der Haut stets dicht an den Gelenken und scheinen mit diesen — wohl auch genetisch? — in Zusammenhang zu stehen. Da sie trotz ihrer großen Dicke einen erheblich helleren Schatten als die um das Vielfache dünneren Knochen werfen, ergibt sich, daß die Uratablagerungen für die Röntgen-Strahlen relativ durchlässig sind.

2. Hochgradige Gelenkzerstörungen mit unregelmäßigen Verdichtungen und Auswüchsen, die bis zur völligen Obliteration des Gelenkes führen können; deutlich besonders am Metacarpophalangealgelenk des ersten und fünften Fingers sowie am 1. Interphalangealgelenk des Ringfingers (b, b).

3. Damit im Zusammenhang stehende und augenscheinlich hiervon ausgehende Zerstörungen der Knochen; so ist z. B. die zweite Phalanx des Kleinfingers (c) fast völlig zerstört, der Rest — wie von dem andrängenden großen Gichtknoten — nach innen subluxiert. Interessant erscheinen besonders die Veränderungen am Nagelgliede des Ringfingers (d). Hier sieht man drei übereinander geschobene helle Kreisflächen, von dunklen Linien umsäumt. Nach allem, was bisher die Röntgen-Strahlen lehrten, kann man nur annehmen, daß es sich um blasenförmige Hohlräume handelt, welche von einer dünnen Corticalis umschlossen sind, im übrigen aber den Knochen vollkommen „aufgezehrt" haben. Wahrscheinlich sind dieselben mit den, wie oben ausgeführt, relativ durchlässigen harnsauren Salzen ausgefüllt. Ähnliche, nur nicht ebenso deutliche Hohlräume scheinen in den Knochen um das Metacarpophalangealgelenk des fünften und zweiten Fingers zu liegen.

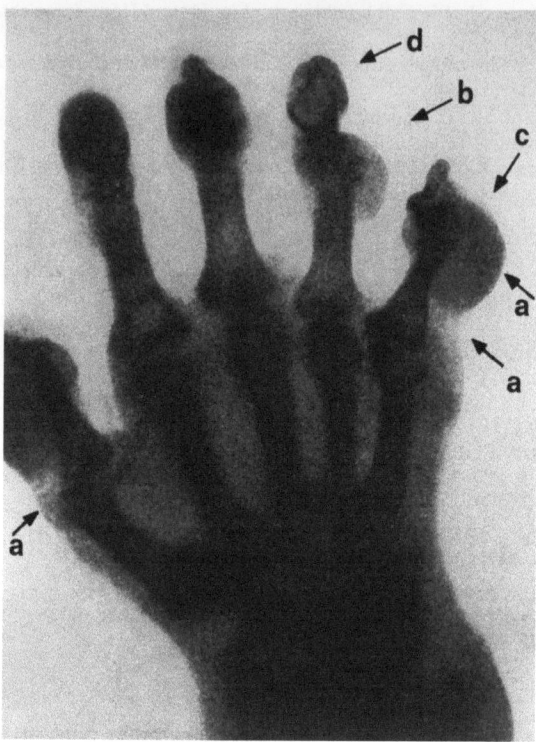

Abb. 1. Hand eines 61 jährigen Mannes, der seit 38 Jahren an Arthritis urica fast aller Gelenke leidet. (Von Huber am 9. März 1896 in der Sitzung des Vereins für Innere Medizin Berlin demonstriert)

Wenn in dem vorliegenden Fall die Durchleuchtung mit den Röntgenstrahlen für die Diagnose auch bedeutungslos war, da diese schon durch den Augenschein sicher gegeben war, so erscheint es mir doch sehr wahrscheinlich, daß dieselbe in weniger klaren Fällen auch hierfür von einigem Wert sein kann. Jedenfalls aber zeigt sie ein Bild der pathologisch-anatomischen Veränderungen, wie es bisher auf andere Weise in vivo nicht zu gewinnen war. Der Patient, selbst Arzt, hatte vordem nicht die geringste Ahnung, daß durch seine Gicht auch seine Gelenkknochen so hochgradig verändert waren."

Damit hat HUBER bereits angedeutet, daß die Radiologie für die Diagnostik der Gicht eine unterschiedliche Bedeutung besitzt, für die Beurteilung der Gicht im Einzelfalle jedoch eine grundsätzliche Bedeutung aufweist, da sie darüber informiert, ob bereits Gelenkveränderungen vorliegen oder nicht, und wenn ja, wie groß das Ausmaß der Gelenkdestruktion ist.

Die ersten speziellen Arbeiten über die Radiologie der Gicht stammen von POTAIN u. SERBANESCO (1897), STRANGEWAYS u. BURT (1905—1907), DRINBERG (1911), KÖHLER (1911), JACOBSON (1913) sowie MCCLURE u. MCCARTY (1919). STRANGEWAYS u. BURT machten bereits auf die radiologischen differentialdiagnostischen Schwierigkeiten bei der Abgrenzung der chronischen rheumatischen Polyarthritis (rheumatoiden Arthritis) von der polyartikulären Gicht aufmerksam und widerlegten die anfänglich vertretene Auffassung von POTAIN u. SERBANESCO, daß es sich bei den radiologisch dargestellten Lochdefekten um ganz spezifische Bilder handle.

In den Jahren nach dem 1. Weltkrieg sind keine größeren radiologischen Arbeiten über die Arthritis urica veröffentlicht worden, da während des Krieges und in den wirtschaftlichen Notzeiten nach dem Krieg die Gicht zu einer seltenen Krankheit wurde.

McCracken et al. sprachen 1946 von der Gicht als der „vergessenen Krankheit". Ab 1945, nach Beendigung des II. Weltkrieges, erschienen einige radiologische Arbeiten über die Gicht in Amerika (Ferguson, 1945; Rosenberg u. Arens, 1947).

In Europa setzten die Arbeiten erst 10—15 Jahre später ein, da zu diesem Zeitpunkt die Gicht auch in Europa wieder häufiger in Erscheinung trat. Drube u. Reinwein publizierten 1959 eine Arbeit mit dem Titel: „Zur Klinik der Gicht, der vergessenen Krankheit" in Anlehnung an den Titel der Arbeit von McCracken et al. In der Folgezeit erschienen dann zahlreiche radiologische Arbeiten mit z. T. größeren Fallzahlen: Brailsford (1959), Vyhnánek et al. (1960; 44 Patienten), De Sèze et al. (1960; 100 Patienten), Serre et al. (1962; 60 Patienten), Schacherl et al. (1966; 150 Patienten), Künzler (1966; 100 Patienten) sowie Dihlmann et al. (1969). 1970 konnte Schacherl über 183 Gichtpatienten berichten, die er in einem Jahr (1969) in einer Rheumaklinik radiologisch beobachten konnte.

Basisinformationen für die Röntgendiagnostik der Gicht

1. Die Gicht ist eine Stoffwechselerkrankung und besitzt ihre häufigste Manifestation an den Gelenken. Eine Übersättigung der Körperflüssigkeit mit Harnsäure ist Voraussetzung, während eine besondere Disposition der Gelenke und der Synovia die Ausfällung der Harnsäure fördert. Pommer hat die Gelenkinnenfläche als Ausgangspunkt der Harnsäureablagerungsprozesse angesehen. Kristalline Nadeln und Mikrotophi mit Fremdkörperreaktion setzen den primären Schaden, der sich durch permanente Zunahme der Harnsäureausfällungen zu einer schweren Zerstörung des Gelenkes im Verlauf mehrerer Jahre entwickelt.

2. Die Gicht ist zur Zeit keine seltene Erkrankung.

3. Die Gicht ist eine Erkrankung mit einer weitgehenden Prädominanz des männlichen Geschlechts: 95% Männer und 5% Frauen (Schilling, A.).

4. Die Gicht wird vorwiegend im 30.—60. Lebensjahr manifest.

5. Die Gicht bevorzugt mit etwa 50—60% als Erstlokalisation die Großzehengrundgelenke. Ein primärer Befall von anderen Zehengelenken und Fingergelenken ist selten.

6. Die Gicht wird in ein akut-rezidivierendes und ein chronisches Stadium unterteilt. Im akut-rezidivierenden Stadium sind radiologisch nachweisbare Gelenkveränderungen nicht zu erwarten. Dieses Stadium dauert im Durchschnitt 7 Jahre (Gamp et al.). Im beginnenden chronischen Stadium können die verschiedenen radiologischen Symptome einzeln auftreten. Im fortgeschrittenen chronischen Stadium treten meist mehrere radiologische Symptome in einer Kombination auf, die entweder ein destruktiv-arthritisches Bild oder ein arthrotisches Bild entstehen lassen.

7. Die „kleinen Gelenke" zeigen häufiger ein arthritisches Bild, während die „großen Gelenke" fast ausschließlich ein arthrotisches Bild aufweisen.

8. Prinzipiell kann jedes Gelenk befallen werden (Kuzell u. Gaudin).

9. In seltenen Fällen zeigt die Gicht ein primär polyarthritisches Bild an Händen und Füßen, das radiologisch von einer chronischen rheumatischen Polyarthritis (rheumatoiden Arthritis) nur schwer oder gar nicht abgegrenzt werden kann.

10. Das gleichzeitige Bestehen einer Gicht und einer chronischen rheumatischen Polyarthritis (rheumatoiden Arthritis) ist äußerst selten.

11. In der radiologischen Differentialdiagnose spielt die chronische rheumatische Polyarthritis (rheumatoide Arthritis) die größte Rolle. Sie beginnt nur in ganz seltenen Fällen primär und isoliert am Großzehengrundgelenk, während der Befall mehrerer Zehengrundgelenke und oft auch des Großzehenendgelenkes sowie der Finger- und Handgelenke die Regel ist.

12. Harnsäureablagerungen in den Gelenken sowie in den gelenknahen Knochenabschnitten sind in den meisten Fällen röntgenstrahlendurchlässig. Radiologisch entstehen deshalb „Knochendefekte" durch Untergang der Spongiosa. Die cystoiden Aufhellungen, die bei der chronischen rheumatischen Polyarthritis (rheumatoiden Arthritis) in etwa 50% der Fälle auftreten, haben meist einen Durchmesser unter 5 mm. Es werden aber auch gar nicht selten größere cystoide Aufhellungen gefunden, die wegen ihrer Größe dann immer verdächtig sind auf intraossale Tophusbildungen und dazu zwingen, die Harnsäure bestimmen zu lassen.

Taktische und technische Hinweise

Bei klinischem Verdacht auf eine Arthritis urica sind als Minimalprogramm beide Füße dorso-plantar zu röntgen. Bei Verdacht auf Beteiligung der Intertarsalgelenke sind Schrägaufnahmen beider Füße zusätzlich erforderlich. Wenn differentialdiagnostische Schwierigkeiten bestehen, sollten beide Hände dorso-volar ebenfalls aufgenommen werden. Für Hände und Füße sind sogenannte folienlose Filme zu bevorzugen, weil mit ihnen schärfere Aufnahmen erzielt werden können, die bei Benutzung eines Vergrößerungsglases eine Vergrößerungstechnik, wie sie von TALBOTT angegeben worden ist, überflüssig machen. Wichtig ist sodann, daß beide Füße oder Hände auf einem Röntgenfilm dargestellt werden und möglichst nur jeweils eine Exposition erfolgt, um völlig seitengleiche Bedingungen zu schaffen. Nur so ist es möglich, minimale Differenzen in der Schattendichte des Knochens zu erkennen. Weiterhin ist darauf zu achten, daß ausreichend große Filmformate benutzt werden. Für beide Hände oder Füße ist das Format 24 × 30 cm erforderlich. Die Strahlenhärte ist so zu wählen, daß nicht nur die Skeletelemente, sondern auch der Weichteilmantel zur Darstellung kommt.

Auf die Möglichkeit, durch Tomogramme exaktere Beurteilungen von pathologischen Prozessen zu erreichen, hat KERSLEY et al. hingewiesen.

Zur Beurteilung der Sesambeine des Großzehengrundgelenkes ist die Tomographie ebenfalls zweckmäßig. In manchen Fällen ist eine tangentiale Darstellung der Sesambeine zusätzlich erforderlich.

Auswertung der Röntgenaufnahmen

Da bei der Auswertung von Röntgenaufnahmen der Füße und Hände die Beurteilung zahlreicher Skeletelemente und Gelenke erforderlich ist, sollte die Befundung nach einem festgelegten Schema erfolgen, um dadurch zu einer systematischen Bildanalyse zu gelangen (SCHACHERL, 1969).

Das Befundschema sollte enthalten: eine Beurteilung
1. des Weichteilmantels,
2. der Form und Größe der Skeletelemente,
3. der Knochenkontur,
4. der Breite des radiologischen Gelenkspaltes,
5. der Knochenstruktur,
6. der Compacta,
7. der Gelenkstellung,
8. der Epiphysenentwicklung bei Jugendlichen.

Tabelle 1. Gegenüberstellung der prozentualen Beteiligung der Gelenke bei Arthritis urica mehrerer Untersucher nach Röntgenbefunden und Vergleich mit einer prozentualen Beteiligung der Gelenke nach klinischen Gesichtspunkten (die Zahlen entsprechen Prozentzahlen)

	BROCHNER-MORTENSEN: 100 Patienten 1941. Klinische Gelenkbefunde	DE SÈZE et al., 100 Pat. 1960 Radiologische Gelenkbefunde	KÜNZLER: 100 Pat., 1966. Gichtpat. der Univ. Rheumaklinik Zürich 1950–1963, Radiologische Gelenkbefunde	SCHACHERL et al.: 150 Pat., 1966. Gichtpat. der Klinik für Rheumakranke Bad Kreuznach 1950–1963. Radiologische Gelenkbefunde	SCHACHERL: 183 Pat., 1970. Gichtpat. der Klinik für Rheumakranke Bad Kreuznach im Jahre 1969. Radiologische Gelenkbefunde
Großzehgelenke	71	76	66	60	66
Zehengelenke II–V	20	31		22	8
Sprunggelenke	33	keine Angaben	49	17,3	6,5
Kniegelenke	29	keine Angaben	43	20	18,5
Hüftgelenke	1	keine Angaben	6	7,3	3
Fingergelenke	39	28 Grundgel. 20 Mittelgel. 19 Endgel.	38	24,7	15
Handgelenke	26	21	31	12	
Ellenbogengelenke	14	keine Angaben	16	6,7	2
Schultergelenke	5	keine Angaben	8	0	2,2
Sternoclaviculargelenke	1	keine Angaben	0	0	0,5
Wirbelsäule	0	keine Angaben	3	0	0
Iliosacralgel.	keine Angaben	keine Angaben	1	1,3	0

Röntgenbefunde an den einzelnen Gelenken

Die Tabelle 1 gibt einen Überblick über die Ergebnisse mehrerer Untersucher. Den Röntgenbefunden wurde eine prozentuale Aufgliederung nach klinischen Gelenkbefunden von BRØCHNER-MORTENSEN gegenübergestellt.

Die Tab. 2 bringt eine Aufgliederung der Röntgensymptome an den einzelnen Gelenken (SCHACHERL et al., 1966).

Geröntgt wurden routinemäßig die Vorfüße (140 Fälle), außerdem alle Gelenke, die Beschwerden verursachten, oder bei der klinischen Untersuchung pathologische Befunde zeigten.

Die radiologische Auswertung erfolgte nach folgenden Kriterien:
1. Osteoporose,
2. Gelenkspaltverschmälerung,
3. intraossale Tophusbildungen ohne Zerstörung der Knochenkonturen,
4. randständige intraossale Tophusbildungen mit Zerstörung der Corticalis sowie Usurierungen,
5. Osteophyten.

Tabelle 2. Aufgliederung der pathologischen Röntgenbefunde nach 5 radiologischen Symptomen an den einzelnen Gelenken (SCHACHERL et al., 1966)

	Anzahl der Patienten, bei denen Rö.-Aufnahmen der betreff. Gelenke angefertigt wurd.	Pathologische Befunde					
		Anzahl der path. Befunde	Anzahl der gefundenen Symptome				
			Osteoporose	Gelenkspaltverschmälerung	Intraossale Tophusbildungen	Usuren und durchgebrochene randständige intraossale Tophusbildungen	Osteophyten
Großzehengrundgelenke	140	90	22	44	30	41	37
Übrige Zehengelenke	140	33	12	6	9	21	3
Tarsalgelenke	80	34	2	5	12	4	27
Sprunggelenke	73	26	2	2	3	1	23
Kniegelenke	52	30	1	6	2	2	30
Hüftgelenke	39	11	0	3	5	1	8
Fingergelenke	80	37	6	13	18	14	15
Handgelenke	80	18	4	6	9	4	5
Ellenbogengelenke	17	10	0	3	3	3	10

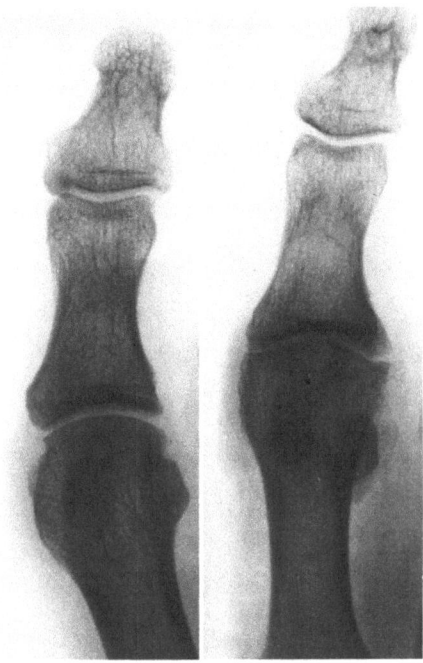

Abb. 2   Abb. 3

Abb. 2. Geringe Usurierung am Köpfchen von Metatarsale I medial und lateral bei 33jährigem Mann mit Gichtanfällen seit einem Jahr

Abb. 3. Tophusbildung im Köpfchen von Metatarsale I unterhalb des Krümmungsscheitels bei 48jährigem Mann mit Gicht seit 14 Jahren

Zehengelenke

Da sich der erste Gichtanfall in etwa 50—60% am Großzehengrundgelenk abspielt, ist dieses Gelenk besonders für die radiologische Frühdiagnose von zentraler Bedeutung.

Nach einer Lokalisationsanalyse von 183 Gichtpatienten (SCHACHERL, 1972) ergibt sich an den Vorfüßen folgende prozentuale Verteilung:

in 44% path. Befunde an Großzehengrundgelenken,
in 13% path. Befunde an Großzehengrund- und -endgelenken,
in 3% path. Befunde an Großzehenendgelenken,
in 6% path. Befunde an Großzehengelenken und anderen Zehengelenken,
in 2% path. Befunde an anderen Zehengelenken.
zusammen in 68% path. Befunde an den Zehengelenken.

Im einzelnen können folgende Röntgenbefunde an den Großzehengrundgelenken gefunden werden: Umschriebene Konturunschärfen am Köpfchen von Os metatarsale I sowie an der Basis der Grundphalanx I (Abb. 2). In diesen Abschnitten können angedeutete Aufhellungen der Knochenstruktur (intraossale Tophusbildungen) registriert werden. Eine häufig vorkommende Aufhellung im oberen inneren Quadranten des Köpfchens von Os metatarsale I ist physiologisch. In

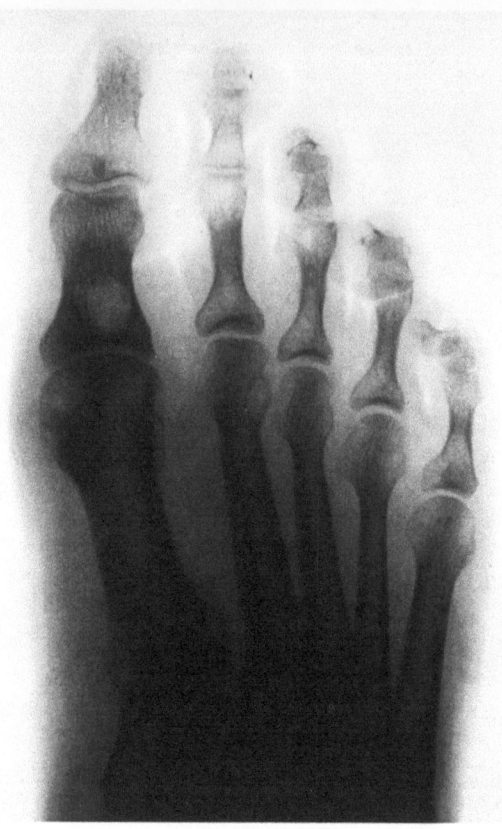

Abb. 4. Tophusbildung in der Basis der Grundphalanx I bei 42jährigem Mann mit Gicht seit 9 Jahren

anderen Fällen sieht man eine geringe Osteophytenbildung am Köpfchen von Os metatarsale I sowie an der Basis der Grundphalanx I (Abb. 3). Diese Osteophytenbildung ist abzugrenzen gegen Formvarianten des Köpfchens von Metatarsale I (SCHACHERL, 1972), die nicht als Osteophyten gedeutet werden dürfen.

In manchen Fällen erkennt man nur eine geringe Osteoporose im Bereich des Köpfchens von Os metatarsale I sowie der Basis der Grundphalanx. Im weiter fortgeschrittenen Stadium nehmen auch die einzelnen Symptome an Stärke zu, können aber immer noch allein auftreten (Abb. 4). Man beobachtet deutlichere Destruktionen der Knochenkontur am Köpfchen von Os metatarsale I sowie der Basis der Grundphalanx I. Häufiger kann man eine zentrale Usur am Scheitelpunkt des Köpfchens von Os metatarsale I beobachten, die jedoch differentialdiagnostisch von einer Osteochondrosis dissecans abgegrenzt werden muß (Abb. 5). Die Aufhellungen in der Knochenstruktur sind nun schon stärker und zeigen auch schon schärfere Ränder, jedoch keinen Sklerosierungssaum (Abb. 6). Größere Aufhellungen (mit einem Durchmesser von über 5 mm) weisen eher auf intraossale Tophusbildungen hin als Aufhellungen mit einem Durchmesser unter 5 mm. Der praktische differentialdiagnostische Wert dieser Größeneinteilung ist aber als sehr gering anzusehen.

In dem schon etwas fortgeschrittenen Stadium können auch Gelenkspaltverschmälerungen auftreten sowie kräftigere Osteophytenbildungen.

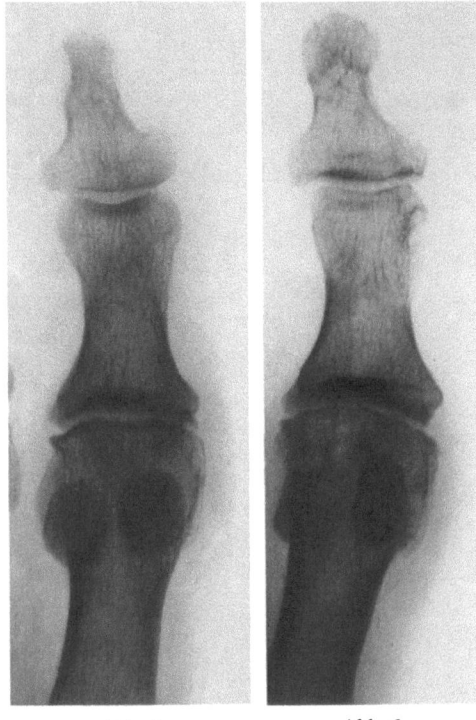

Abb. 5.   Abb. 6.

Abb. 5. Flache Usurierung in Höhe des Krümmungsscheitels des Köpfchens von Metatarsale I (zentrale Usur). 51jähriger Mann mit Gichtanfällen im Großzehengrundgelenk li. seit 2 Jahren

Abb. 6. Größere intraossale Tophusbildung im Köpfchen von Metatarsale I sowie randständig am Köpfchen der Grundphalanx mit Destruktion der Corticalis. Seit 8 Jahren bestehende Gicht bei 56jährigem Mann. Harnsäurewert 7,1 mg-%

In den noch weiter fortgeschrittenen Fällen kommt es dann zu den wie ausgestanzt wirkenden „Lochdefekten", die, wenn sie randständig liegen, den Knochenrand durchbrechen (Abb. 7). Treten solche randständigen intraossalen Tophusbildungen beiderseits am Köpfchen auf und haben sie die Knochenränder zerstört, so können Formen des Köpfchens von Os metatarsale I entstehen, die an eine Hellebarde erinnern (Abb. 8). Durch das weitere Wachstum des Tophus können stehengebliebene Knochenränder aufgebogen werden (MARTEL).

In den schweren fortgeschrittenen Fällen dominiert die intraossale Tophusbildung, die zu schweren Zerstörungen des Knochens führt (Abb. 9a u. b). In diesen schweren Fällen kann es zu Knochenzusammensinterungen kommen sowie zu Subluxationsstellungen.

Die polymorphen radiologischen Bilder lassen sich unabhängig vom Stadium im wesentlichen in drei Gruppen einteilen:

1. Vorherrschen von Usuren und intraossalen Tophusbildungen oder Usuren allein.

2. Vorherrschen von intraossalen Tophusbildungen bei erhaltener Knochenkontur.

3. Vorherrschen von Osteophytenbildungen.

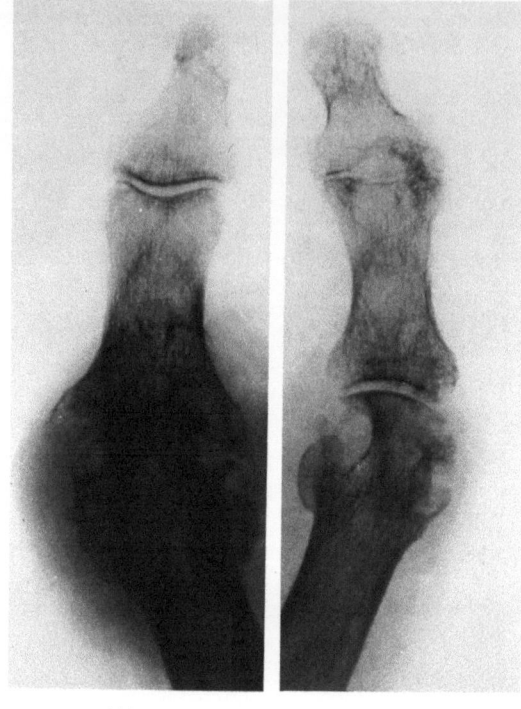

Abb. 7.   Abb. 8.

Abb. 7. Multiple intraossale Tophusbildungen, zum großen Teil randständig, mit Destruktion der Corticalis im Köpfchen von Metatarsale I sowie in der Basis der Grundphalanx. Aufgebogener Knochenrand an der Basis der Grundphalanx medial. Großer Weichteiltophus in Gelenknähe. 56jähriger Mann mit Gicht seit 10 Jahren

Abb. 8. Große intraossale Tophusbildungen medial und lateral im Köpfchen von Metatarsale I, randständig mit Zerstörung der Corticalis (Hellebarden-Bild). 63jähriger Mann mit Gicht seit 15 Jahren. Harnsäurewert 11,0 mg-%

Bei dem schon erwähnten Kollektiv von 183 Gichtkranken (SCHACHERL, 1972), von denen klinisch 44,5% dem akut rezidivierenden und 55,5% dem chronischen Stadium angehören, wurden die Röntgenaufnahmen der Vorfüße in die oben angeführten 3 Gruppen sowie eine Gruppe, die keine pathologischen Befunde zeigt, eingeteilt und nach Dauer der Erkrankung aufgeteilt. Hierbei zeigt sich, daß bei einer Dauer von 0—5 Jahren noch 44,2% keine pathologischen Prozesse erkennen lassen. Bei einer Dauer von 6—10 Jahren haben noch 37,2% keine pathologischen Veränderungen an den Vorfüßen, während bei einer Dauer der Gicht von 11—15 Jahren nur noch 5% keine pathologischen Befunde an den Vorfüßen haben.

Der Anteil an den 4 radiologischen Gruppen geht aus der Tab. 3 hervor. In selteneren Fällen kann sich eine Reflexdystrophie im Bereich der Vorfüße entwikkeln, die vermutlich durch schwere Schmerzzustände bei den Gichtanfällen ausgelöst wird. Anfangs erkennt man eine fleckige Osteoporose, die später in eine grobsträhnige Osteoporose (hypertrophe Atrophie) übergeht (DeSèze et al., Gamp).

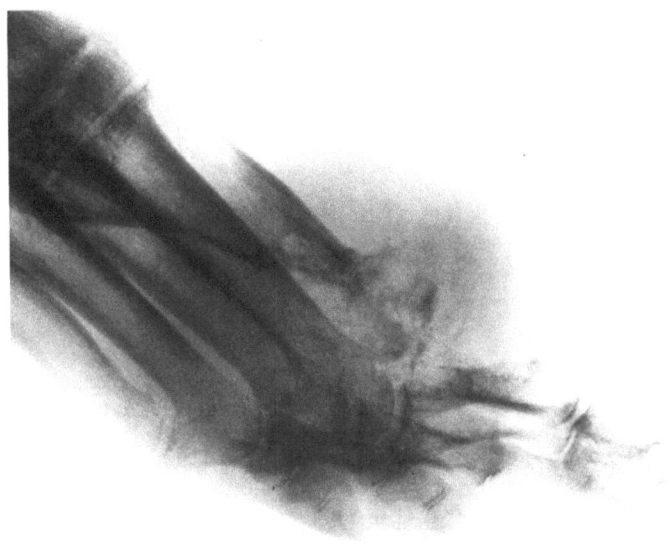

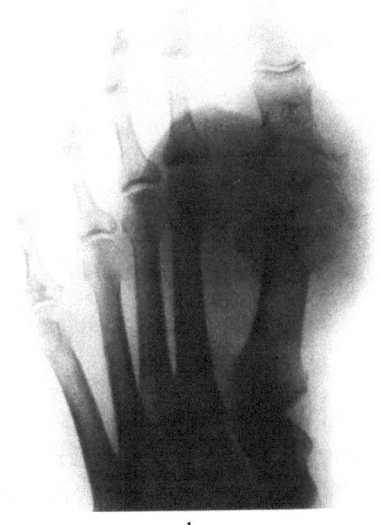

Abb. 9a u. b. Großer Weichteiltophus umlagert eine schwere destruierende Gichtarthritis des Großzehengrundgelenkes mit multiplen, nach außen aufgebrochenen Knochentophi des Köpfchens von Metatarsale I sowie der Basis der Grundphalanx. 56jähriger Mann mit Gicht seit 10 Jahren

Sesambeine der Großzehengrundgelenke

Auch im Bereich der Sesambeine des Großzehengrundgelenkes können intraossale Tophusbildungen auftreten.

Diese Sesambeine stellen phylogenetisch eine Weiterentwicklung dar, die durch den aufrechten Gang des Menschen erforderlich wurde, während die übrigen Sesambeine beim Menschen und Affen Rudimente darstellen. Beim menschli-

Tabelle 3. Aufteilung der Röntgenbefunde an den Vorfüßen nach Dauer der Gicht und nach radiologischen Symptomgruppen (die Zahlen entsprechen Prozentzahlen; SCHACHERL, 1970)

	Dauer der Gicht in Jahren			
	0–5	6–10	11–15	16 und mehr
Ohne path. Befund	44,2	37,2	5	0
Nur intraossale Tophusbildung	21,2	14,3	20	18,8
Arthritis urica	21,1	39	60	56,2
Arthritis urica unter dem Bild der Arthrose	13,5	9,5	15	25
Pathologische Befunde zusammen	55,8	62,8	95	100

chen Gang bleiben die Sesambeine unverrückt am Boden liegen und werden durch die Körperlast an den Boden noch mehr angedrückt und durch Reibung festgehalten. Sie bilden so eine unbewegliche Unterlage, gegen die der Fuß und mit ihm der ganze Körper gedreht werden kann. Der bevorzugte Befall des Großzehengrundgelenkes bei der Arthritis urica dürfte durch die besondere Druckbelastung dieses Gelenkes sowie die dadurch bedingte spezielle lokale Gefäßregulierung bedingt sein. Die Sesambeine dürften einer noch stärkeren Belastung ausgesetzt sein. Es ist deshalb nicht verwunderlich, daß in den Sesambeinen bei systematischem Suchen schon relativ früh intraossale Tophusbildungen gefunden werden. DE SÈZE u. RYCKEWAERT stellten bereits 1960 fest, daß die Sesambeine oft frühzeitig Veränderungen zeigen und mehr oder weniger vollständig zerstört werden können.

Bei gezielten Untersuchungen der Sesambeine der Großzehengrundgelenke bei Arthritis urica (SCHACHERL, 1972) durch Tomogramme und tangentiale Aufnahmen fiel auf, daß ausnahmslos das mediale Sesambein zuerst Veränderungen im Sinne von intraossalen Tophusbildungen zeigte. In 2 Fällen konnte eine vollständige Zerstörung der medialen Sesambeine nachgewiesen werden, wobei noch Knochenreste erkennbar waren, die eierschalenartig das durch die Tophusbildung stark vergrößerte Sesambein umgaben (Abb. 10a u. b).

Finger- und Handgelenke

Die Finger- und Handgelenke werden nicht so häufig befallen wie die Zehengelenke und im allgemeinen später.

Bei einer Dauer der Gicht von 0—5 Jahren wurden in dem bereits angeführten Kollektiv von 183 Gichtkranken (SCHACHERL, 1972) noch keine Beteiligung der Finger- und Handgelenke gefunden. Mit zunehmender Dauer der Gicht steigt der Prozentsatz der Mitbeteiligung von Finger- und Handgelenken kontinuierlich an (siehe Tab. 4).

Bevorzugte Lokalisationen einzelner Gelenke wie im Bereich der Füße, gibt es an den Finger- und Handgelenken nicht. Intraossale Tophusbildungen können in den Phalangen, Carpalia sowie den distalen Abschnitten von Radius und Ulna gefunden werden. Die Arthritis urica an den Händen läßt sich in den erst mäßig fortgeschrittenen Stadien nicht selten von einer chronischen rheumatischen Polyarthritis (rheumatoiden Arthritis) schwer abgrenzen (Abb. 11). In den stärker fortgeschrittenen Fällen hat die Tophusbildung in den Weichteilen und in den Knochen so stark zugenommen, daß eine differentialdiagnostische Abgrenzung leichter gelingt (Abb. 12a, b, c).

Erfahrungsgemäß werden traumatisch vorgeschädigte Gelenke von einer Arthritis urica eher befallen (MUGLER). Im Vordergrund stehen hierbei die Handge-

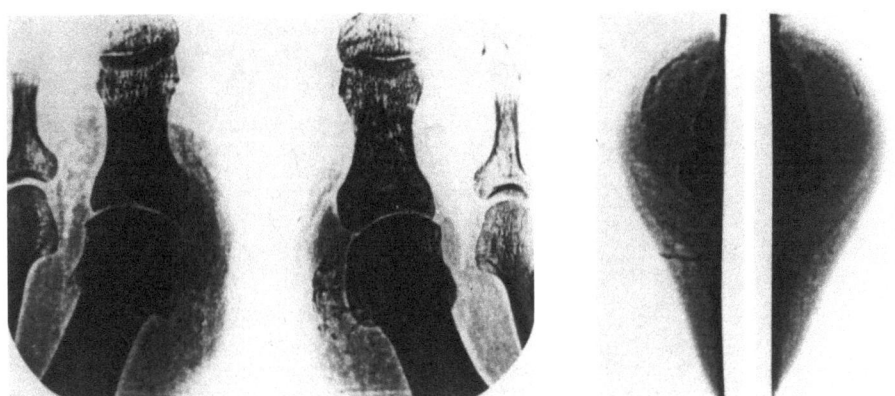

Abb. 10. (a) Intraossale Tophusbildung in den medialen Sesambeinen der Großzehengrundgelenke bds. mit deutlicher Vergrößerung der Sesambeine sowie eierschalenartigen Resten der Knochenstruktur (Harmonisierte Aufnahme) (b) Tangentiale Aufnahme der Sesambeine beiderseits (Harmonisierte Aufnahme)

lenke bei Zustand nach Radiusfraktur, Fraktur des Os naviculare sowie Schußbruchverletzungen der Handgelenke. Von 10 Patienten mit traumatischen Vorschädigungen der Handgelenke hatten 7 eindeutig auf der geschädigten Seite ihre Gichtanfälle sowie radiologisch nachweisbare arthritische Veränderungen (SCHACHERL, 1962).

Metatarsotarsalgelenke, Intertarsalgelenke und Sprunggelenke

Diese Gelenke sind häufiger befallen. Jedoch überwiegt an diesen Gelenken ein „arthrotisches Bild" mit Osteophytenbildungen. Relativ häufig werden jedoch auch intraossale Tophusbildungen in den Tarsalia und den distalen Abschnitten von Tibia und Fibula gefunden (Abb. 13). Auf seitlichen Aufnahmen des Fußes entsteht durch Osteophytenbildung und Sehnenansatzverknöcherungen das Bild des „Pied hérissé", des „struppigen" oder „borstigen" Fußes (Abb. 14), eine Bezeichnung französischer Autoren (FRANÇON u. LEROY sowie SERRE et al., 1962). Dieses Bild ist jedoch nicht spezifisch für eine Arthritis urica, wird aber häufiger gefunden, von SERRE et al. in 51%.

Auch Calcaneus-Exostosen sind keine spezifischen Zeichen für Arthritis urica. Der plantare und dorsale Fersensporn treten auch nicht häufiger auf, wie ŠTĚPÁNEK u. KŘÍŽEK durch Vergleiche mit Kontrollgruppen zeigen konnten.

Tabelle 4. Beteiligung der Finger- und Handgelenke bei Gicht, aufgegliedert nach Dauer der Gicht (SCHACHERL, 1970)

Dauer der Gicht	Zahl der Pat. mit Röntgenaufnahmen der Hände	Arthritis urica an Finger- oder Handgelenken
0–5 Jahre	58	0
6–10 Jahre	46	9 = 20%
11–15 Jahre	21	6 = 30%
16–20 Jahre	6	2 = 33%
21 u. mehr Jahre	11	4 = 36,5%

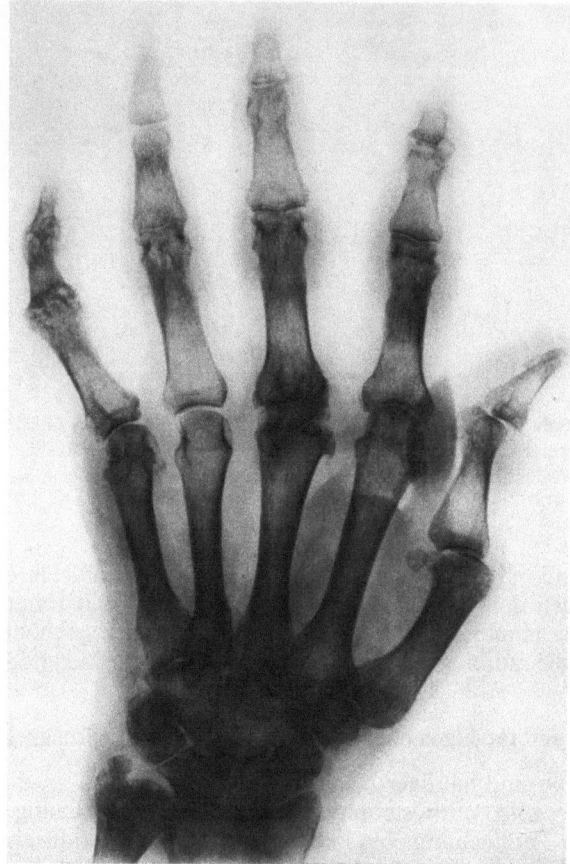

Abb. 11. Polyartikuläre, geringe bis mittelschwere Arthritis urica bei einem 43jährigen Mann mit Gicht seit 20 Jahren und einem Harnsäurewert von 12,6 mg-%

Kniegelenke

Die Kniegelenke, die nicht selten eine Mitbeteiligung zeigen, bieten radiologisch fast ausschließlich das Bild einer banalen Arthrose. Destruktive Bilder sind sehr selten und intraossale Tophusbildungen treten am Kniegelenk nicht häufig auf (Abb. 15), bereiten aber Schwierigkeiten in der Abgrenzung gegen Geröllcysten. Da die Kniearthrose wie die Coxarthrose ein sehr häufiges Krankheitsbild darstellen (nach MOHING sind 98% aller Arthrosen am Knie und Hüftgelenk lokalisiert), besteht natürlich an diesen Gelenken immer die Möglichkeit, daß eine Arthrose schon vorher bestanden hat, oder daß neben einer Arthritis urica an anderen Gelenken eine Arthrose am Kniegelenk besteht, die mit der Gicht in keinem Zusammenhang steht. Die Entscheidung, ob eine Arthritis urica am Kniegelenk vorliegt, muß in den meisten Fällen klinisch getroffen werden.

Hüftgelenke

Was für die Kniegelenke gesagt wurde, gilt auch für die Hüftgelenke. Bis vor kurzer Zeit glaubte man, daß es eine Arthritis urica des Hüftgelenkes nicht gäbe. SERRE et al. lehnten noch 1963 eine Beteiligung des Hüftgelenkes bei Arthritis

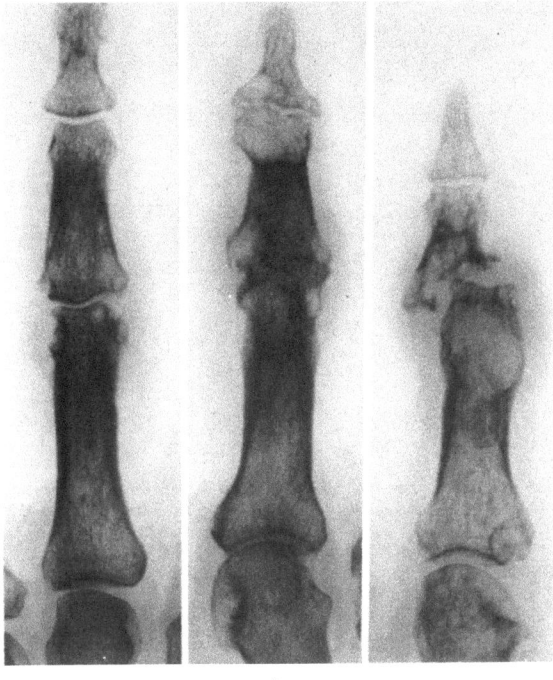

a b c

Abb. 12a—c. Arthritis urica im Bereich von Fingergelenken mit intraossalen Tophusbildungen (a) Kleine intraossale Tophusbildungen im Bereich des Köpfchens der Grundphalanx sowie der Basis der Mittelphalanx, z.T. randständig mit Destruktion der Corticalis (b) Multiple intraossale Tophusbildung im Bereich der gelenknahen Abschnitte des Fingermittel- und Endgelenkes mit Auftreibung des Köpfchens der Mittelphalanx durch intraossale Tophusbildung. 36jähriger Mann mit Gicht seit 17 Jahren (c) Schwere destruierende Arthritis urica eines Zeigefingermittelgelenkes mit Subluxationsstellung. Große intraossale Tophusbildung im Köpfchen der Grundphalanx mit deutlicher Auftreibung

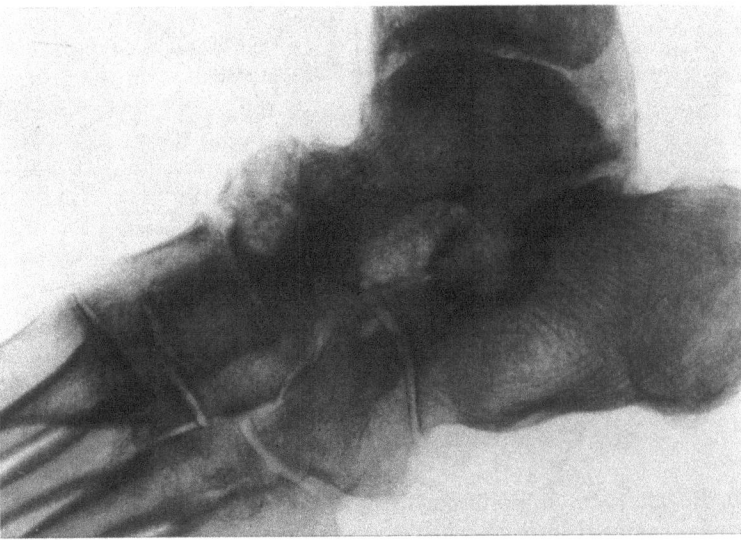

Abb. 13. Ausgedehnte intraossale Tophusbildung im Os naviculare pedis, kleine intraossale Tophusbildung im Os cuboides. 68jähriger Mann mit Gicht seit 10 Jahren

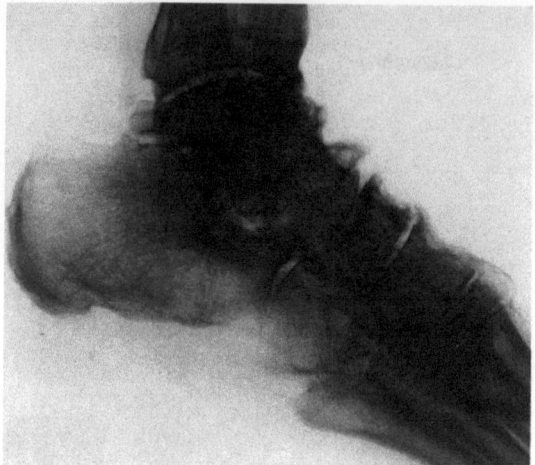

Abb. 14. Arthritis urica im Bereich des Mittelfußes mit multipler Osteophytenbildung am Talus, Os naviculare und Os cuneiforme I (Pied hérissé). Gefäßverkalkungen. 57jähriger Mann mit Gicht seit 6 Jahren

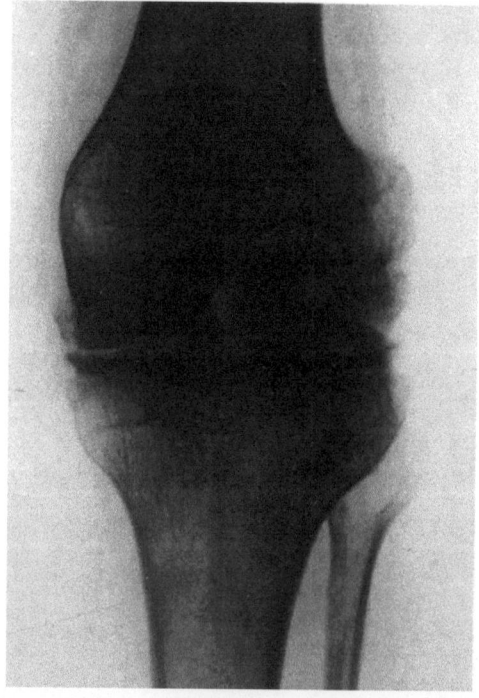

Abb. 15. Schwere Arthritis urica des li. Kniegelenkes mit Gelenkspaltverschmälerung, Usurierungen, Osteophytenbildungen sowie intraossaler Tophusbildung bei 43jährigem Mann mit Gicht seit 11 Jahren

urica ab. Im gleichen Jahr konnte jedoch WISSINGER eine Arthritis urica der Hüftgelenke diagnostizieren und histologisch durch Gelenkbiopsie sichern. HOF-MEISTER hat dann 1967 erstmals im deutschen Schrifttum eine Arthritis urica des Hüftgelenkes pathologisch-anatomisch nachgewiesen. Weitere Beobachtungen

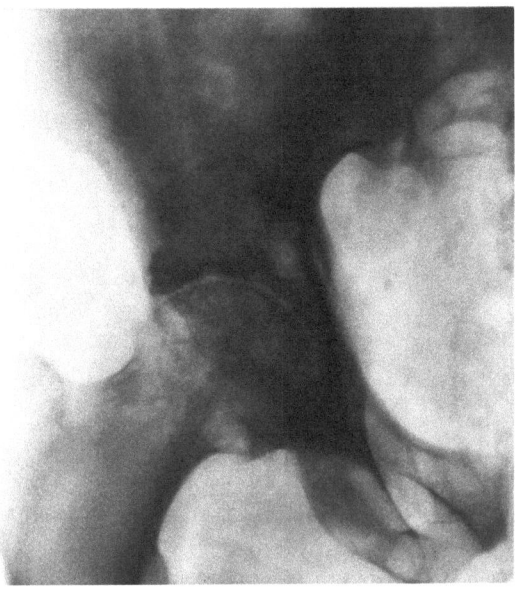

Abb. 16. Arthritis urica des re. Hüftgelenkes mit Gelenkspaltverschmälerung, Usurierungen sowie cystoiden Aufhellungen (Tophi?). 62jähriger Mann mit Gicht seit 6 Jahren

stammen von SCHULITZ (1969) und MÜLLER u. LÖHR (1969). Radiologisch ist die Diagnose einer Arthritis urica des Hüftgelenkes nicht sicher zu stellen. Das Bild ist überwiegend „arthrotisch". Eine sichere Abgrenzung von Geröllcysten, die bei Coxarthrose häufig beobachtet werden, und intraossalen Tophusbildungen ist nicht sicher möglich, wenn auch die intraossalen Tophusbildungen als differentialdiagnostisches Kriterium gegenüber den Geröllcysten keinen Sklerosesaum erkennen lassen (Abb. 16).

Ellenbogengelenke

Der Befall von Ellenbogengelenken ist nicht so selten. An diesen Gelenken herrscht ebenfalls wie an den Kniegelenken und Hüftgelenken ein arthrotisches Bild vor. In wenigen Fällen werden auch Destruktionen und intraossale Tophusbildungen gefunden (Abb. 18). Häufiger werden kräftige Sehnenansatzverknöcherungen am Olecranon beobachtet.

Schultergelenke

In vereinzelten Fällen wird eine Arthritis urica der Schultergelenke beobachtet, auch überwiegend unter einem arthrotischen Bild.

Wirbelsäule

Ein Befall der Wirbelsäule mit Harnsäureablagerungen zählt zu den Ausnahmen und wird nur in ganz schweren Fällen beobachtet. Fallbeobachtungen liegen vor von KERSLEY et al. (1950), LICHTENSTEIN et al. (1956), KOSKOFF et al. (1953), HALL u. SELIN (1960) sowie HAWKINS et al. (1965).

Beobachtet wurden Subluxationen von Wirbeln durch intraossale Tophusbildungen, Zerstörung von Intervertebralgelenken sowie Tophusbildung in Wirbelkörpern und Bandscheiben.

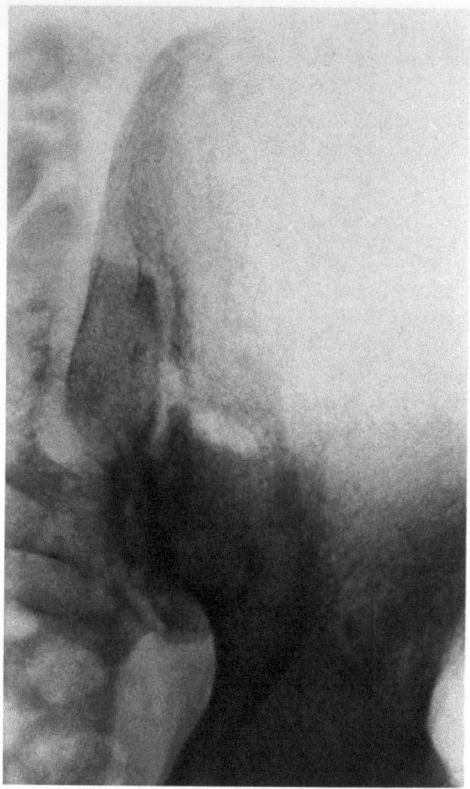

Abb. 17. Starker Verdacht auf Arthritis urica des li. Iliosacralgelenkes mit unscharfen Gelenkkonturen, kleinen cystoiden Defekten sowie subchondraler Sklerosierung. 43jähriger Mann mit Gicht seit 20 Jahren. Harnsäurewert 12,6 mg-%

Iliosacralgelenke

In schweren Fällen von Gicht können auch die Iliosacralgelenke befallen sein und zeigen intraossale Tophusbildungen, Usuren und Osteophytenbildung. MALAWISTA et al. berichten über 7 von 95 Fällen, die eine Mitbeteiligung der Iliosacralgelenke bei Gicht zeigten. Die Dauer der Gicht lag bei diesen 7 Kranken zwischen 13 und 26 Jahren. Drei Kranke hatten eine extreme periphere Arthritis urica, drei eine ausgeprägte und nur einer eine mäßige. LIPSON u. SLOCUMB berichten über einen Fall. SCHACHERL et al. (1966) sahen in 2 Fällen von 150 Gichtpatienten eine einseitige Iliosacralgelenkarthritis (Abb. 17).

Radiologische Hinweis-Symptome

Außerhalb der Gelenke können einige radiologische Symptome Hinweise auf das Bestehen einer Gicht geben:
1. breiter Thorax,
2. Gefäßverkalkungen (besonders der Arteria dorsalis pedis),
3. Verknöcherungen an Sehnenansätzen,
4. Spondylosis hyperostotica,
5. Nierensteine,
6. Engstellung des Becken- u. Kelchsystems beim i.v. Pyelogramm,
7. idiopathische Femurkopfnekrose.

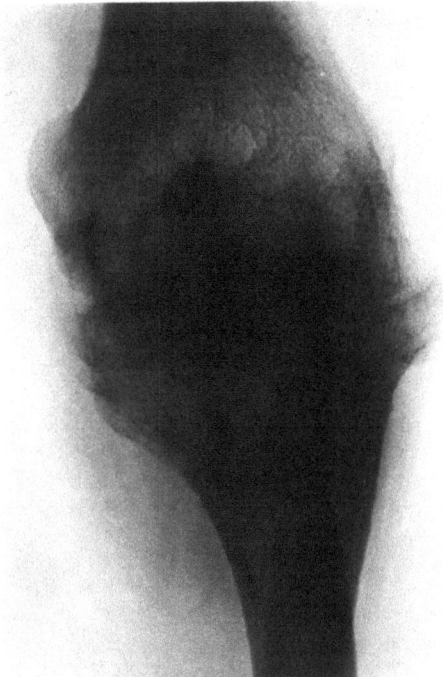

Abb. 18. Schwere Arthritis urica des li. Ellenbogengelenkes bei 57jährigem Mann mit Gicht seit 24 Jahren

Ein Teil dieser Symptome läßt sich dem Konstitutionspanorama beiordnen, das bei Gichtkranken vorwiegend angetroffen wird: Der pyknische Habitus und die Fettleibigkeit.

Diese Symptome besitzen also keinerlei Spezifität für eine Gicht, können aber an eine Gicht denken lassen.

1. Der breite Thorax

Es fällt auf, daß bei Gichtkranken der Thorax auf dem üblichen Filmformat von 36,5 × 36,5 cm seitlich häufig abgeschnitten ist, so daß ein größeres Filmformat benutzt werden muß. 60% der Thorax-Aufnahmen von Gichtkranken hatten eine Thoraxbreite von über 37 cm bei einem Focus-Film-Abstand von 1,50 m (SCHACHERL, 1972).

2. Gefäßverkalkungen

Relativ häufig sind Gefäßverkalkungen nachweisbar, besonders in der A. dorsalis pedis (DE SÈZE et al., 1960; SERRE et al., 1962).

3. Verknöcherungen an den Sehnenansätzen

Sehnenansatzverknöcherungen im Bereich des Fersenbeines, des Talus, der Patella, des Olecranon sowie des Trochanter major und minor werden beobachtet. Hierbei gibt es kein Überwiegen bei Gicht, aber ein Überwiegen bei Patienten mit Übergewicht, wie ŠTĚPÁNEK und KŘÍŽEK für den plantaren und dorsalen Fersensporn nachweisen konnten.

4. Spondylosis hyperostotica

Die vor mehr als 100 Jahren beschriebene „Zuckergußwirbelsäule" wurde 1950 von FORESTIER und ROTES-QUÉROL wieder entdeckt und als senile ankylosierende Hyperostose beschrieben. Von OTT wurde 1952 für den deutschen Sprachbereich die Bezeichnung Spondylosis hyperostotica geprägt.

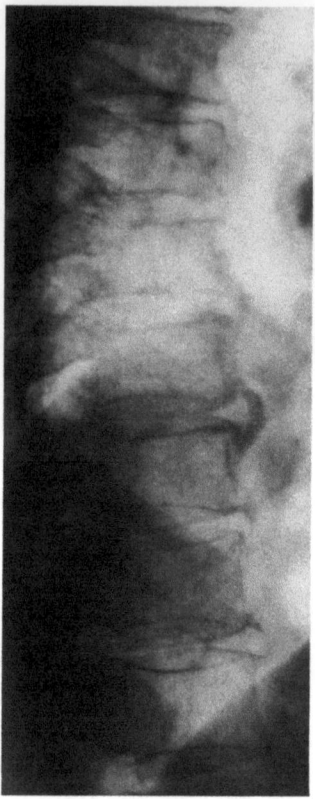

Abb. 19. Verknöcherung des vorderen Längsbandes von D8/11: Spondylosis hyperostotica bei einem 47jährigen Mann, der seit 3 Jahren an Gicht erkrankt ist. Harnsäurewert 8,0 mg-%. Kein Diabetes

Seit längerer Zeit ist bekannt, daß diese degenerative Veränderung des perivertebralen Bindegewebes mit bandförmiger Verknöcherung des Lig. longitudinale vorwiegend ventro-lateral rechts bei manifestem und latentem Diabetes gehäuft auftritt. Noch fast unbekannt aber war, daß nicht nur Störungen des Kohlenhydrathaushaltes, sondern auch die mit Hyperuricämie einhergehende Störung im Purin-Metabolismus zur Spondylosis hyperostotica neigt, worauf TEIXEIRA u. VAHIA 1956 aufmerksam gemacht haben. SCHILLING et al. fanden bei einer unausgelesenen Gruppe von 50 Gichtpatienten, bei denen systematisch die Wirbelsäule röntgenologisch untersucht worden war, 10mal eine Spondylosis hyperostotica, entsprechend einem Vorkommen von 20% (im Gegensatz zu 6% bei einer Kontrollgruppe von 350 gleichaltrigen Männern). Umgekehrt neigen Männer mit Spondylosis hyperostotica zu Hyperuricämie (30%) und zu manifester Gicht 16%. — Die Autoren glauben nicht an einen kausalen Zusammenhang, sondern sehen in Gicht und Spondylosis hyperostotica — wie in Diabetes und Spondylosis hyperostotica — einander nebengeordnete Störungen auf dem beiden gemeinsamen Boden des pyknischen Konstitutionstyps mit Adipositas (Abb. 19).

5. Nierensteine

Relevant ist sicher ein tubulärer Defekt, der bei den meisten Hyperuricämiefällen gefunden wird. Er besteht in der Produktion eines persistierend sauren

Harns. Der Urin-pH-Wert hat für die Löslichkeit der Harnsäure eine ausschlaggebende Bedeutung. Die Harnsäure liegt im Urin dieser Patienten bereits in übersättigter Lösung vor. Sie fällt im sauren Bereich aus und geht bei alkalischer Harnreaktion wieder in Lösung. Die Bildung von Harnsäurekonkrementen ist daher eine häufige Folge dieser sogenannten „Säurestarre" des Urins. Nierensteine werden in 10—25% der Fälle bei Gichtkranken gefunden. Überwiegend handelt es sich um Urat-Konkremente, die bei der Gesamtzahl von Nephrolithiasis-Fällen nur in 5—10% auftreten, so daß ein direkter Zusammenhang zwischen der Urat-Steinbildung und der Harnsäurestoffwechselstörung besteht.

6. Engstellung des Becken-Kelch-Systems beim intravenösen Pyelogramm

EBERL et al. fanden 1968 bei 22 von 35 Gichtpatienten im Ausscheidungsurogramm ein spastisch enggestelltes Hohlraumsystem. Dieser Befund ließ sich im Infusionspyelogramm reproduzieren; Nierenbecken und Nierenkelche waren kontrahiert. Der pH-Wert im Harn lag bei 25 Patienten im sauren Milieu; er schwankte zwischen 4,8 und 5,7. Von diesen Kranken zeigten 16 ein enggestelltes renales Hohlraumsystem. Von 7 Kranken, die noch kein halbes Jahr an Gicht litten, wiesen 3 bereits röntgenologische Zeichen auf. Unter den 23 Patienten, deren Gicht bereits 1—2 Jahre bekannt war, fand man 17, und unter den restlichen 5, die länger als 2 Jahre an Gicht litten, 4 mit einem positiven Röntgenbefund.

Dieses Symptom des spastisch enggestellten Beckenkelchsystems ist keinesfalls spezifisch für eine Gichtniere, kann jedoch einen wertvollen Hinweis geben.

Tabelle 5. Der bevorzugte Gelenkbefall der einzelnen Erkrankungen

Gelenke	chron. (rheum.) Polyarthritis ○	Arthritis psoriatica ●	Arthrose ◐	Arthritis urica ○
Hand				
Handgelenke	○			
Proc. styloides ulnae	○			
Daumenwurzelgelenke			◐	
Fingergrundgelenke	○			
Fingermittelgelenke	○		◐	
Fingerendgelenke		●	◐	
›Strahlbefall‹		●		
Vorfuß				
Großzehengrundgelenke				◐
Großzehenendgelenke	○			○
Zehengrundgelenke II–V	○			
Zehenmittelgelenke II–V				
Zehenendgelenke II–V		●		
›Strahlbefall‹		●		

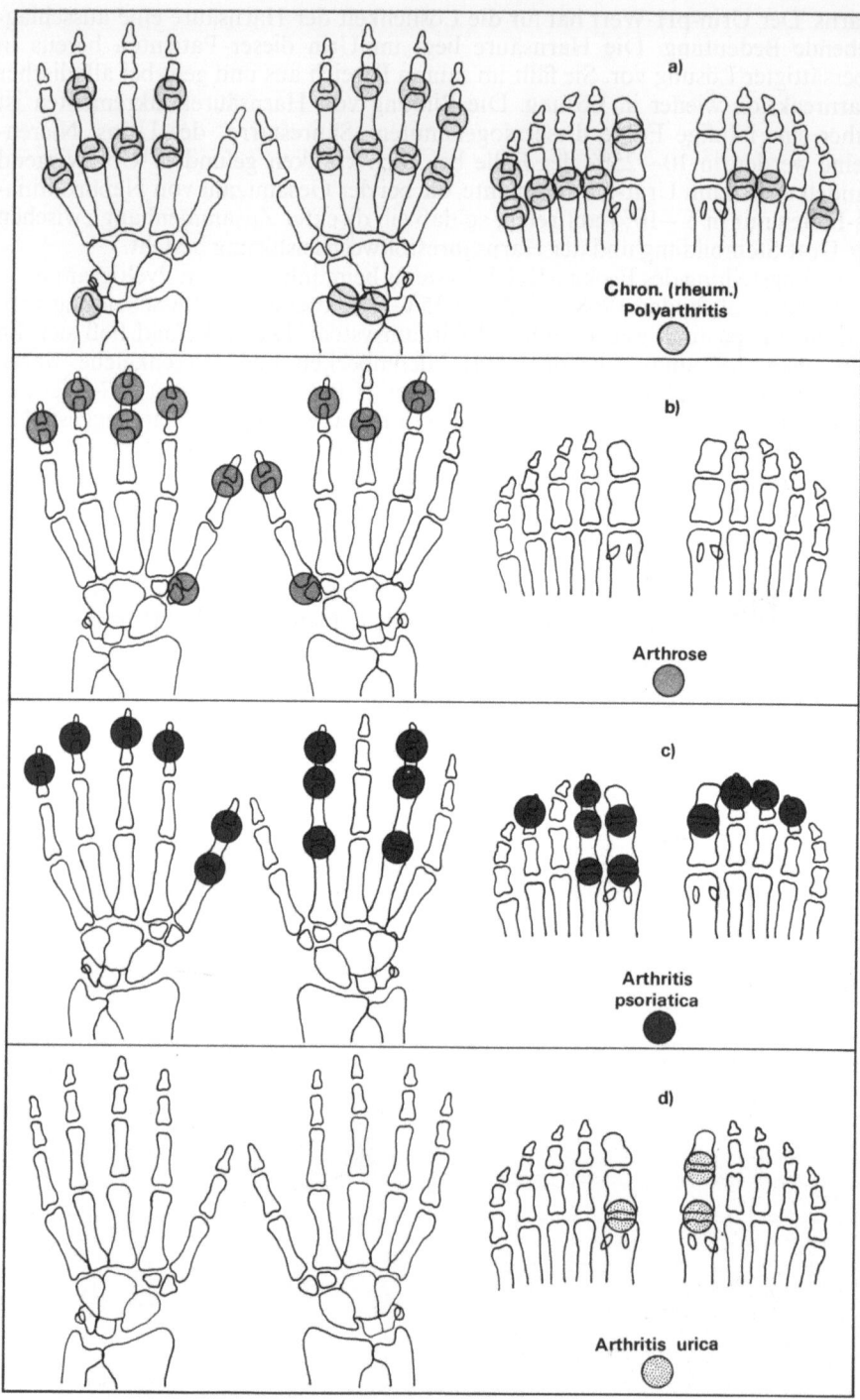

Abb. 20a—d. Typische Gelenkbefallmuster für die einzelnen Erkrankungen. (a) Chronische (rheumatische) Polyarthritis, (b) Arthrose der Fingergelenke, (c) Arthritis psoriatica, (d) Arthritis urica

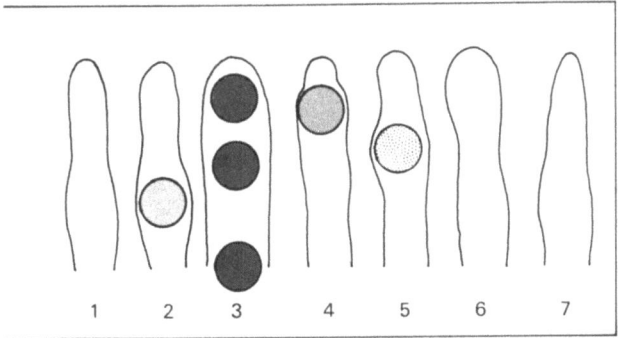

Abb. 21. Weichteilverformungen der Finger. *1* Normale Fingerform, *2* Spindelfinger bei chron. (rheum.) Polyarthritis, *3* Wurstfinger bei Arthritis psoriatica, *4* Heberden-Knoten bei Arthrose der Fingerendgelenke, *5* asymmetrische Weichteilschwellung bei Gicht (Weichteiltophus), *6* Trommelschlegelfinger bei hypertrophischer Osteoarthropathie, *7* Sklerodaktylie bei Sklerodermie

7. Idiopathische Hüftkopfnekrose

Unter den idiopathischen Hüftkopfnekrosen ist der Anteil, der durch eine Hyperuricämie hervorgerufen wird, sehr hoch. DE SÈZE et al. (1960) hatten unter 30 Femurkopfnekrosen 10 Gichtpatienten und SERRE u. SIMON (1962) sahen 5 Fälle mit Kopfnekrose bei 20 Patienten mit Hyperuricämie. Dieser Sachverhalt zwingt dazu, bei jeder Femurkopfnekrose die Harnsäure bestimmen zu lassen.

Differentialdiagnose

Besonders beim polyartikulären Erscheinungsbild muß die Gicht gegen die entzündlich-rheumatischen Erkrankungen und die Polyarthrose abgegrenzt werden. Entscheidend für die Differentialdiagnose ist häufig die Kombination von bestimmten Symptomen und Lokalisationen an bestimmten Gelenken oder Gelenketagen der Finger und Zehen. Durch die Vielzahl von Gelenken an Händen und Füßen entstehen Gelenkbefallmuster für die einzelnen Etagen.

Die Tab. 5 gibt den bevorzugten Gelenkbefall der differentialdiagnostisch wichtigsten Erkrankungen an Hand und Vorfuß wieder.

Die Abb. 20a, b, c und d geben in schematischer Form die typischen Gelenkbefallmuster für die differentialdiagnostisch wichtigsten Erkrankungen wieder.

Die Kenntnis der Weichteilverformungen der Finger erleichtert ebenfalls die differentialdiagnostischen Überlegungen (Abb. 21).

Von geradezu grundlegender Bedeutung für die Differentialdiagnose ist die Kenntnis der Geschlechtsprädominanz der einzelnen rheumatischen Erkrankungen (Abb. 22)[1].

Chronische rheumatische Polyarthritis (rheumatoide Arthritis)

Die häufig bei der chronischen rheumatischen Polyarthritis (rheumatoiden Arthritis) auftretende bandförmige Osteoporose der gelenknahen Abschnitte ist bei der Gicht äußerst selten. Cystoide Aufhellungen und Usuren treten bei beiden Erkrankungen häufig auf.

---

[1] Tabelle 5 sowie die Abb. 20a—d, 21 und 22 wurden der Arbeit SCHACHERL, M.: Radiologische Differentialdiagnose rheumatischer Erkrankungen und der Gicht an Händen und Füßen, internist. prax. **13**, 283—293 (1973), entnommen.

Chronische rheumatische Polyarthritis (rheumatoide Arthritis)

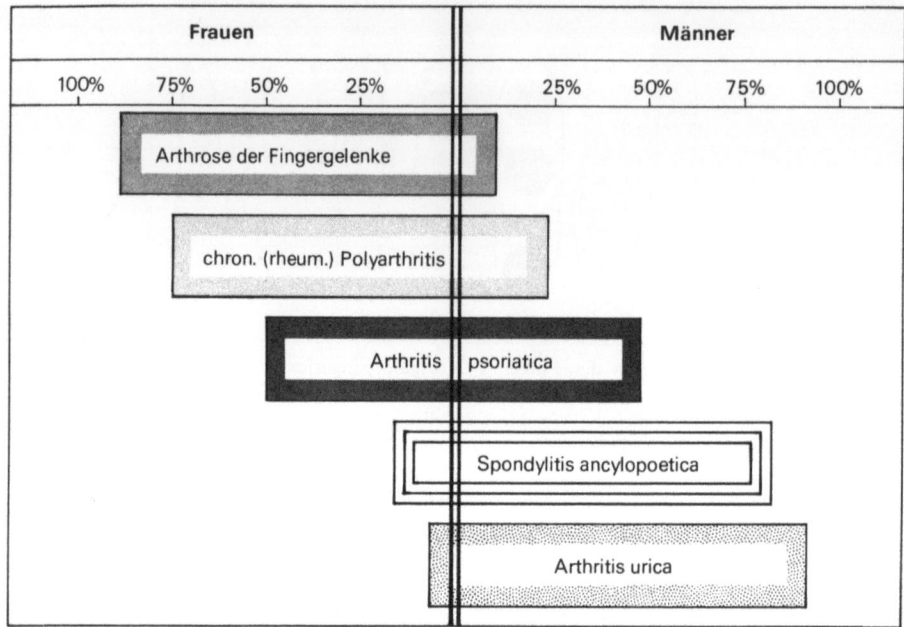

Abb. 22. Geschlechtsprädominanz für die einzelnen rheumatischen Erkrankungen

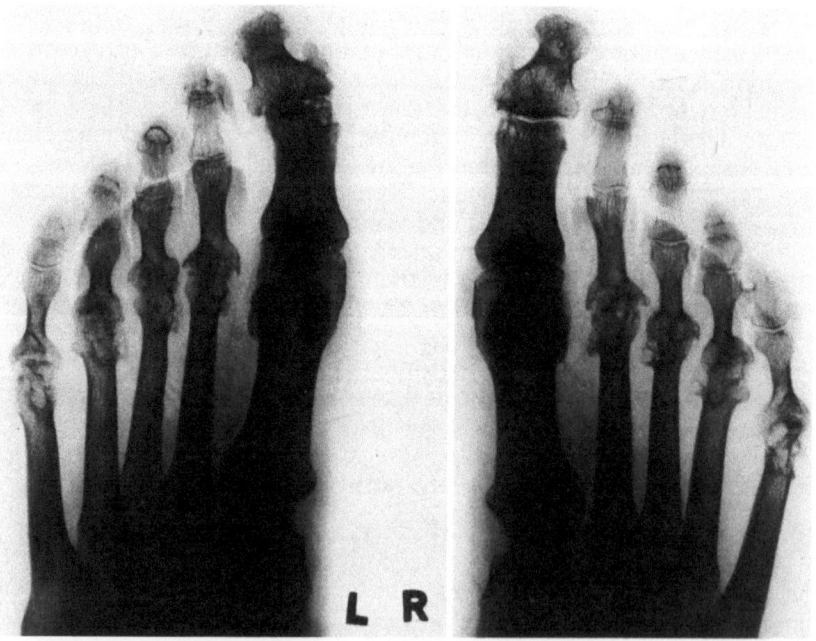

Abb. 23. Mittelschwere chronische rheumatische Polyarthritis (rheumatoide Arthritis) im Bereich der Zehengrundgelenke II—V bds. sowie des Großzehenendgelenkes bds. 65jähriger Mann mit chronischer rheumatischer Polyarthritis seit 22 Jahren

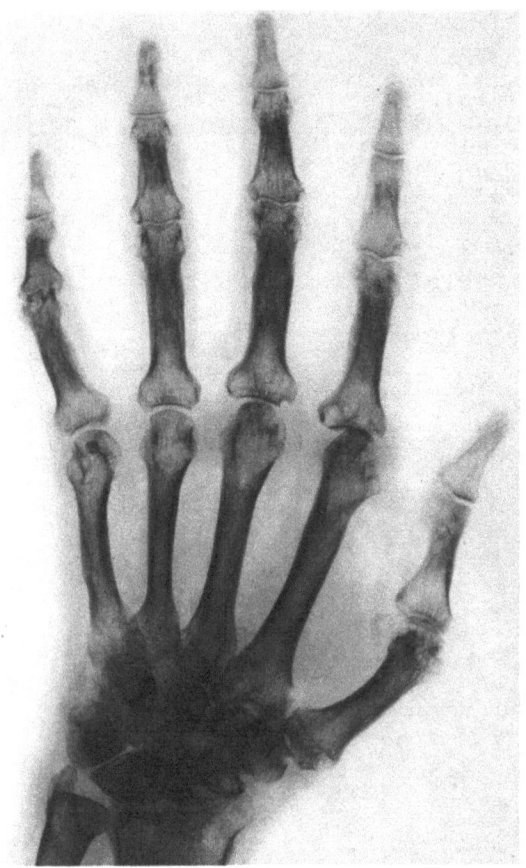 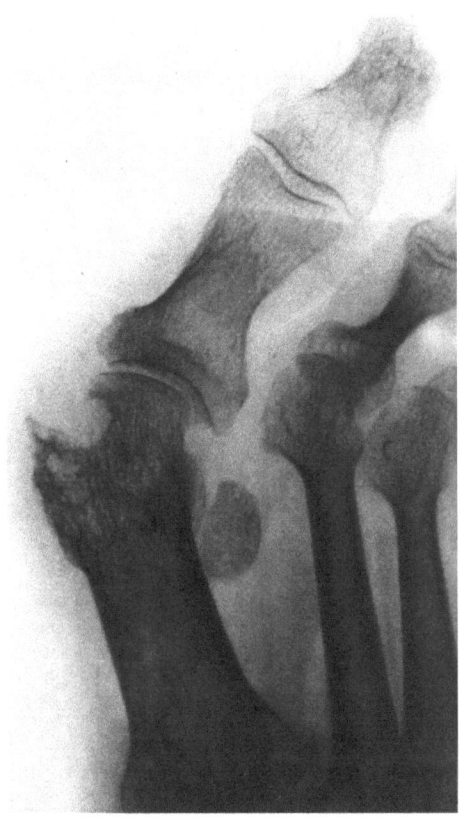

Abb. 24 Abb. 25

Abb. 24. Seit 5 Jahren bestehende chronische rheumatische Polyarthritis bei einer 52jährigen Frau

Abb. 25. Große, wie ausgestanzt wirkende Defektbildung am Köpfchen von Metatarsale I. Geringe Usurierungen an den Köpfchen von Metatarsale II und III bei 58jährigem Mann mit chronischer rheumatischer Polyarthritis seit 7 Jahren. Harnsäurewert 4,8 mg-%. Das Bild hat eine täuschende Ähnlichkeit mit einer Arthritis urica

Im Anfangsstadium der chronischen rheumatischen Polyarthritis (rheumatoiden Arthritis) sind häufig die Zehengrundgelenke V befallen, später auch die Zehengrundgelenke II—IV sowie das Großzehenendgelenk (Abb. 23). Das Großzehengrundgelenk wird meist im Anfang der Erkrankung nicht befallen, in späteren Stadien ist es häufig mitbeteiligt. Ein typisches Frühsymptom der chronischen rheumatischen Polyarthritis (rheumatoiden Arthritis) ist die Weichteilschwellung auf der Ulnaseite des Handgelenkes sowie Usurierungen am Processus styloides ulnae. Charakteristisch für die chronische rheumatische Polyarthritis (rheumatoide Arthritis) ist der Befall der Handgelenke sowie der Fingergrund- und Mittelgelenke (Abb. 24). Die Fingerendgelenke sind erst in späteren Stadien und meist bei schweren Fällen mitbeteiligt. Oft beobachtet man eine gewisse Symmetrie des Gelenkbefalles im Bereich beider Hände und Füße, während die Arthritis urica im Bereich der Fingergelenke eine ausgesprochene Asymmetrie des Gelenkbefal-

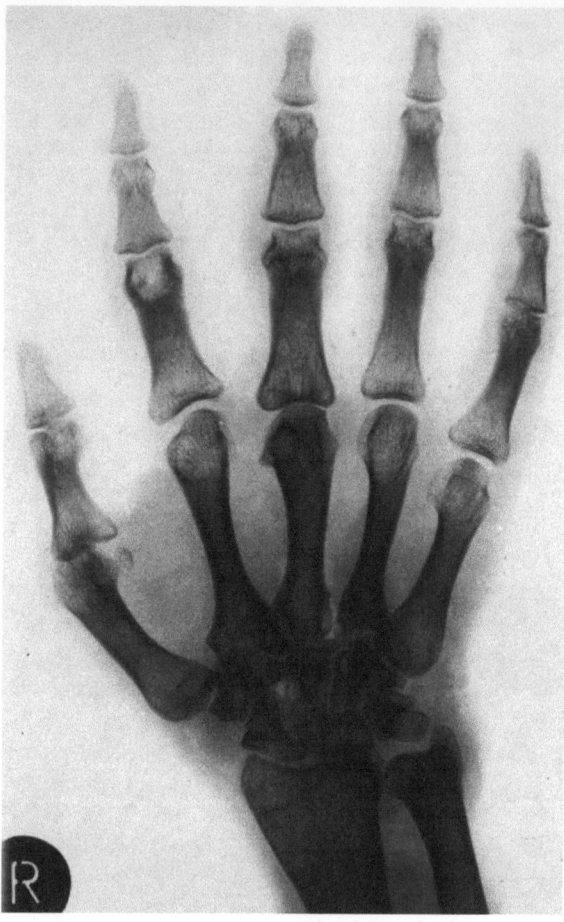

Abb. 26. Hand eines 21 jährigen Patienten mit juvenil begonnener chronischer rheumatischer Polyarthritis. Wachstumsstörungen im Bereich der Carpalia sowie von Metacarpale III re. Größere cystoide Aufhellung im Köpfchen der Grundphalanx II re.

les erkennen läßt. In fortgeschrittenen Fällen von chronischer rheumatischer Polyarthritis (rheumatoider Arthritis) entwickelt sich häufig eine partielle oder totale Carpalblockbildung, die für die Arthritis urica völlig uncharakteristisch ist (SCHACHERL, 1969).

Auch die ulnare Deviation der Finger, die pathognomonisch für die chronische rheumatische Polyarthritis (rheumatoide Arthritis) ist, wird bei Arthritis urica kaum beobachtet. Größere cystoide Aufhellungen, auch mit einem Durchmesser von mehr als 5 mm, werden bei der chronischen rheumatischen Polyarthritis (rheumatoiden Arthritis) nicht selten beobachtet. Sie bereiten dann radiologisch differentialdiagnostische Schwierigkeiten bei der Abgrenzung gegen die Arthritis urica (Abb. 25 u. 26).

Für die Differentialdiagnose weiterhin wichtig ist die Kenntnis der Geschlechtsprädominanz: Bei der chronischen rheumatischen Polyarthritis (rheumatoiden Arthritis) liegt sie mit etwa 75% bei den Frauen, während die Arthritis urica mit etwa 95% eine überwiegende Erkrankung der Männer ist.

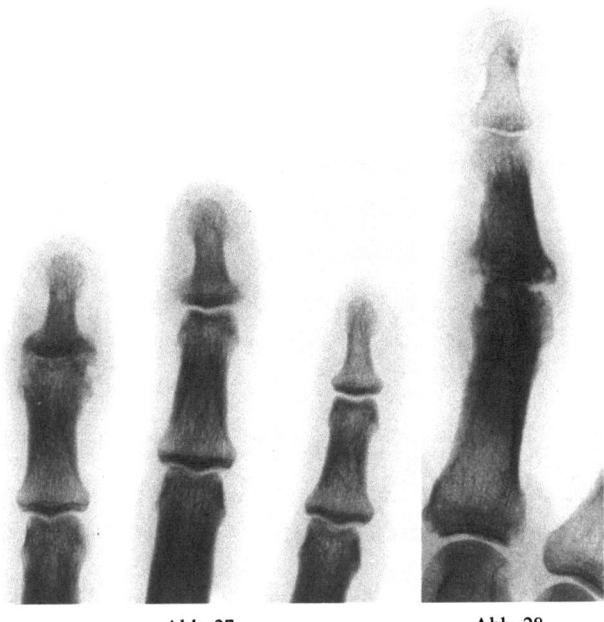

Abb. 27   Abb. 28

Abb. 27. Polyarthritis psoriatica mit ausschließlicher Fingerendgelenkbeteiligung bei einem 22jährigen Mann. Fingerendgelenk IV ohne Befund, Fingerendgelenk III zeigt eine beginnende Arthritis mit charakteristischem Knochenanbau. Fingerendgelenk II zeigt eine schon fortgeschrittene Arthritis mit stärkerer knöcherner Proliferation

Abb. 28. Arthritis psoriatica im Bereich des Fingermittelgelenkes. Typisches Nebeneinander von anbauenden und abbauenden Prozessen. Ossifizierende Periostitis unterhalb des Köpfchens der Grundphalanx

Spondylitis ancylopoetica

Bei Befall der Vorfüße ist bei Männern neben der Gicht auch an eine Spondylitis ancylopoetica (M. Bechterew) zu denken, wobei entweder ein peripheres Vorstadium vorliegen kann oder eine Spondylitis ancylopoetica mit peripherer Beteiligung. Die Spondylitis ancylopoetica ist, wie die Gicht, eine vorwiegend das männliche Geschlecht befallende Erkrankung (Männeranteil etwa 85%). Der Gelenkbefall an Händen und Füßen ist bei der Spondylitis ancylopoetica nicht so symmetrisch wie bei der chronischen rheumatischen Polyarthritis (rheumatoiden Arthritis), und häufig werden nur einzelne Gelenke befallen.

Arthritis psoriatica

Wenn eine Psoriasis vorliegt, dürfte die Stellung der Diagnose einer Arthritis psoriatica nicht schwerfallen.

Es gibt jedoch Fälle, in denen die Hautmanifestation so geringfügig ist, daß sie bei der Allgemeinuntersuchung übersehen wird (z. B. kleiner psoriatischer Herd auf der Kopfhaut unter den Haaren, psoriatischer Herd in der Ano-genitalregion oder psoriatischer Herd an den Nägeln). In seltenen Fällen besteht bereits eine Arthritis psoriatica vor der Manifestation an der Haut.

Besonders für diese Fälle ist die radiologische Diagnose wichtig sowie die Abgrenzung gegen die Gicht, da bei Psoriasis in etwa 25% eine Hyperuricämie

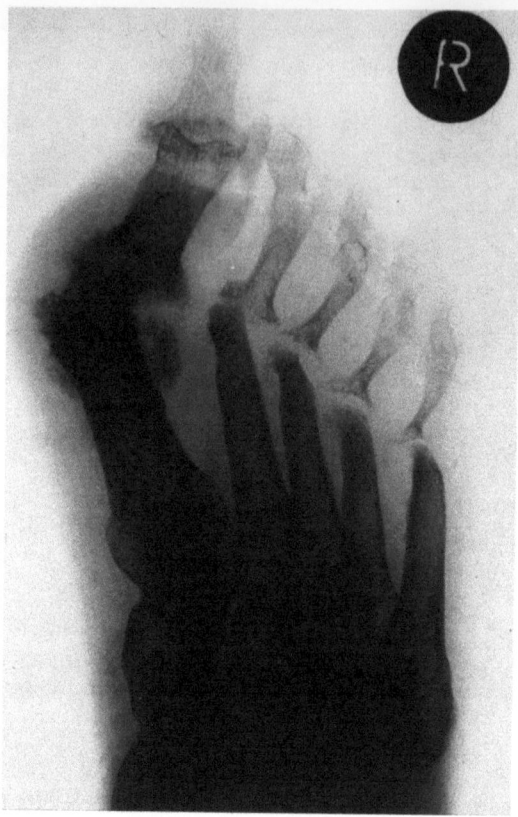

Abb. 29. Schwere Polyarthritis psoriatica mit mutilierenden Prozessen im Bereich der Zehengrundgelenke II—V (bleistiftartige Zuspitzung der Köpfchen der Metatarsalia)

besteht. Bevorzugt befallen werden bei Arthritis psoriatica die Finger- und Zehenendgelenke. Weiterhin deutet auf eine Arthritis psoriatica der sogenannte Strahlbefall hin, d.h. das Befallensein von 2 oder 3 Gelenken eines Finger- oder Zehenstrahles (SCHACHERL u. SCHILLING, 1967).

Charakteristisch ist für die Arthritis psoriatica weiterhin ein Nebeneinander von Knochendestruktion und Knochenproliferation, nicht in Form von scharf konturierten Osteophyten wie bei der Polyarthrose, sondern in Form einer unscharf begrenzten Proliferation (Abb. 27, 28). Auffällig ist weiterhin die Tendenz zu mutilierenden Prozessen, besonders im Bereich der distalen Abschnitte der Metacarpalia und Metatarsalia, die eine bleistiftartige Zuspitzung erkennen lassen (Abb. 29). Auch ein Nebeneinander von mutilierenden Prozessen sowie Synostosierungen wird nicht selten bei der Arthritis psoriatica beobachtet (Abb. 30). Eine Osteoporose der gelenknahen Abschnitte wie bei der chronischen rheumatischen Polyarthritis (rheumatoiden Arthritis) fehlt häufig. Wie die Spondylitis ancylopoetica neigt auch die Arthritis psoriatica zu fibro-ostitischen Prozessen (Abb. 31) sowie zu tendo-ostitischen Prozessen an den Sehnenansätzen (Enthesopathie nach NIEPEL et al.). Eine Geschlechtsprädominanz besteht bei der Arthritis psoriatica nicht, da auch die Psoriasis zu gleichen Teilen auf Männer und Frauen verteilt ist.

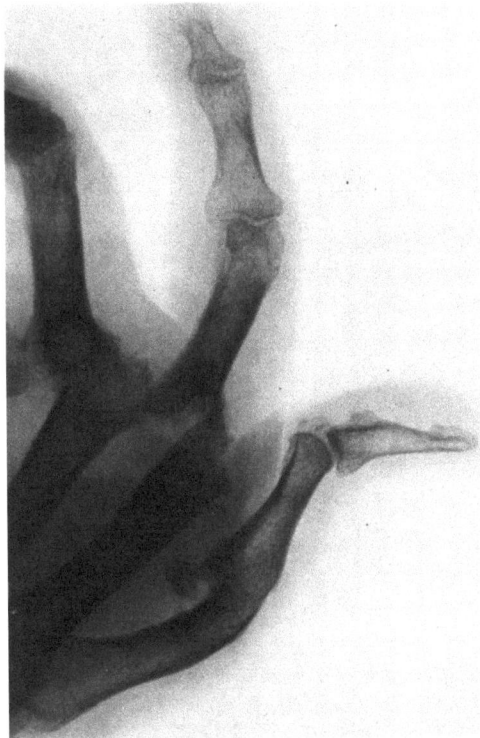

Abb. 30. Polyarthritis psoriatica. Typisches Nebeneinander von Synostosierungen und mutilierenden Prozessen. Synostosierung im Daumengrundgelenk. Schwere destruierende Arthritis mit Mutilationen im Bereich der Fingergrundgelenke II und III. Gleicher Patient wie Abb. 29

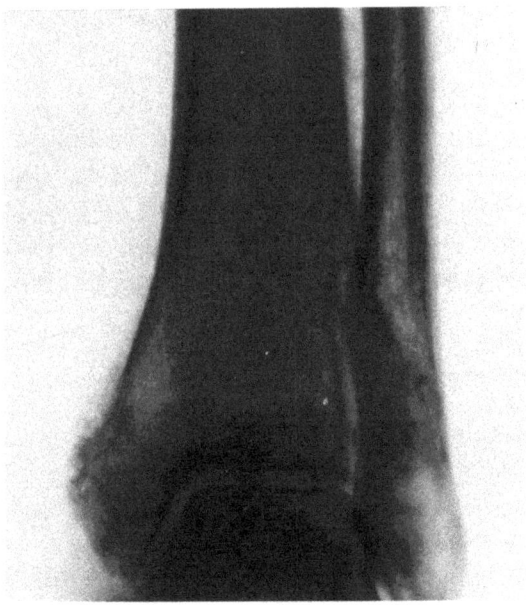

Abb. 31. Ossifizierende Periostitis am Malleolus tibialis bei einer 45jährigen Frau mit Arthritis psoriatica

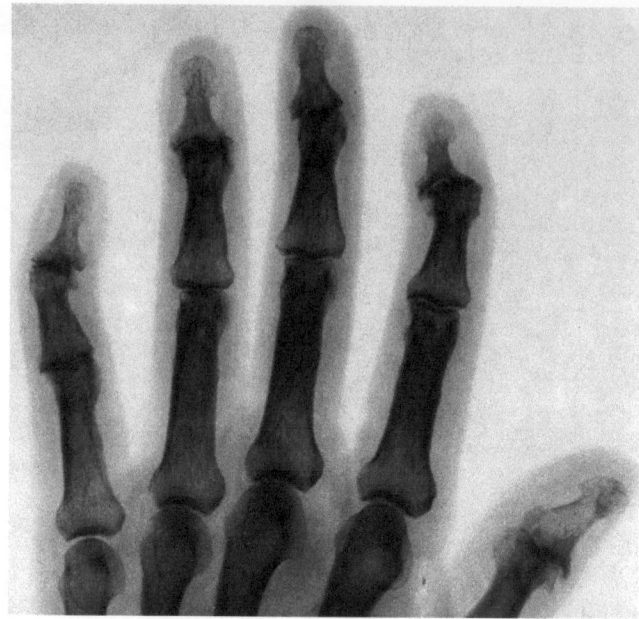

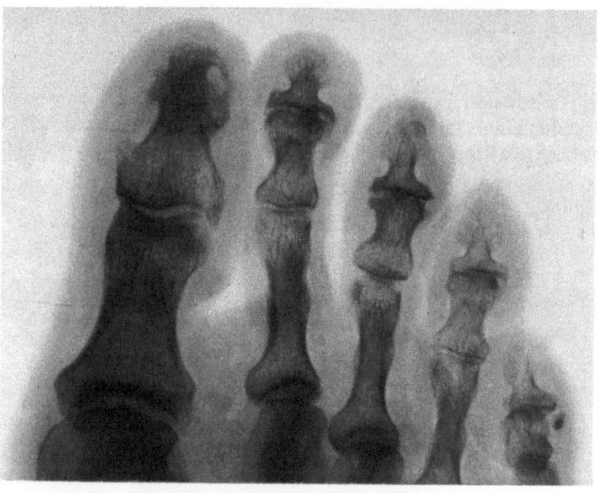

Abb. 32. (a) Typische Arthrose der Fingerendgelenke bei einem 62jährigen Mann (b) Arthrose der Zehenendgelenke II und III sowie beginnend bei IV beim gleichen Patienten

Polyarthrose und destruierende Form der Polyarthrose

Die Polyarthrose mit ihrem bevorzugten Befall der Fingerendgelenke ist unter dem klinischen Bild der Heberden-Knoten eine häufige Erkrankung. Sie läßt sich, wenn sie generalisiert auftritt, radiologisch leicht abgrenzen (Abb. 32 a, b).

Es gibt aber auch Fälle, die größere cystoide Aufhellungen in den gelenknahen Abschnitten erkennen lassen und dadurch schwer von einer Arthritis urica abgrenzbar sind (Abb. 33). Jedoch ist die Polyarthrose eine vorwiegende Erkrankung

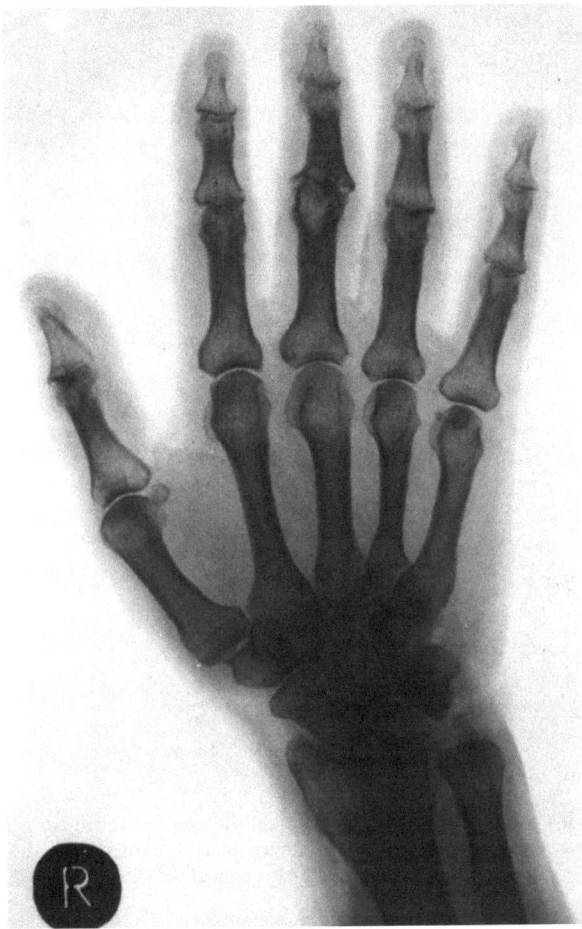

Abb. 33. Schwere Arthrose des Fingermittelgelenkes III re. bei einer 56jährigen Frau. Kleinere cystoide Aufhellungen in der Basis der Mittelphalanx. Große cystoide Aufhellung im Köpfchen der Grundphalanx

der Frauen mit einer Prädominanz von 90%, die vorwiegend in der Menopause auftritt.

Große Schwierigkeiten kann die Sonderform der Polyarthrose, die destruierende Arthrose bereiten, zumal das Vorstadium größere cystoide Aufhellungen erkennen läßt. Diese destruierende Arthrose wird häufiger im Bereich der Fingermittelgelenke, als an den Fingerendgelenken gefunden (Abb. 34a, b).

Bei der destruierenden Form der Polyarthrose sind Männer häufiger vertreten als Frauen (9,5% Männer und 3,8% Frauen). Die destruierende Form der Polyarthrose tritt insgesamt bei 4—5% der Polyarthrosen auf (SCHACHERL u. SCHILLING, 1970).

Weitere Erkrankungen, die differentialdiagnostisch eine Rolle spielen

Die besprochenen Erkrankungen des rheumatischen Formenkreises sind auf Grund ihrer relativen Häufigkeit diejenigen, die am ehesten gegen die Arthritis urica abgegrenzt werden müssen.

Weitere Erkrankungen, die differentialdiagnostisch eine Rolle spielen

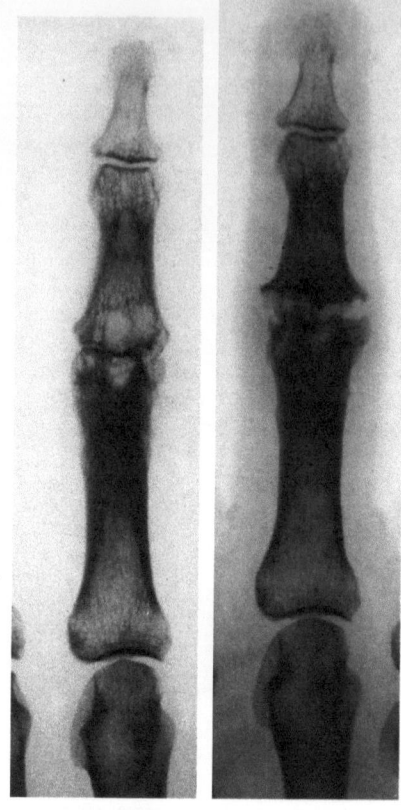

Abb. 34a u. b. Destruierende Arthrose (a) Vorstadium der destruierenden Arthrose: erhebliche Gelenkspaltverschmälerung sowie cystoide Aufhellungen in den gelenknahen Abschnitten (b) 1 Jahr später: destruierende Arthrose in diesem Gelenk

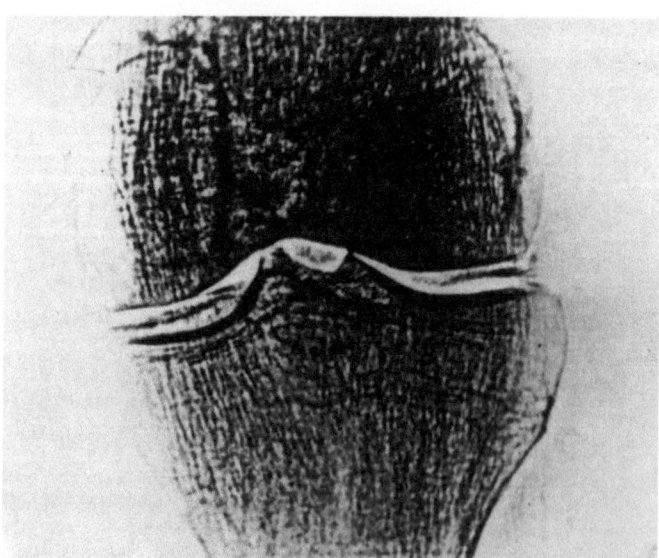

Abb. 35. Chondrocalcinosis polyarticularis: typische Meniscusverkalkungen im Kniegelenk (Harmonisierte Aufnahme)

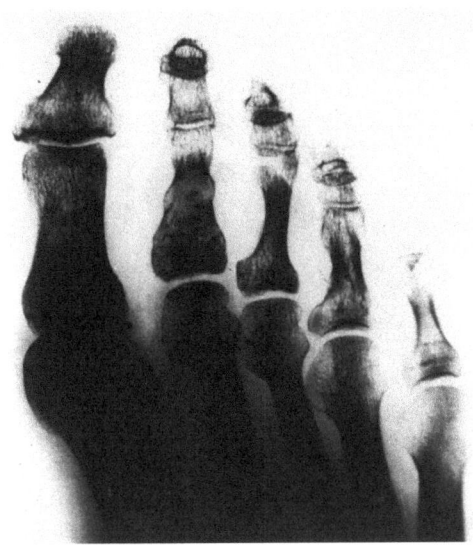

Abb. 36. Enchondrom in der Grundphalanx II mit geringer Auftreibung des Knochens

Die radiologische Diagnose der Chondrocalcinosis polyarticularis, die wegen ihrer Schmerzanfälle in den Gelenken auch Pseudogicht genannt wird, bereitet keine Schwierigkeiten, wenn die typischen Veränderungen in Form von Verkalkungen in der oberen Knorpelschicht, vorwiegend der großen Gelenke sowie Verkalkungen im Bereich der Menisci der Kniegelenke nachweisbar sind (Abb. 35).

Wegen ihrer relativen Häufigkeit seien differentialdiagnostisch noch genannt: Enchondrome, besonders in den Phalangen, die mit intraossalen Tophi verwechselt werden können (Abb. 36).

Die noch genannten Erkrankungen werden selten beobachtet und dürften radiologisch keine differentialdiagnostischen Schwierigkeiten bei der Abgrenzung gegen eine Arthritis urica bereiten:
Sarkoid-Arthritis,
Diabetische Arthropathie,
Cystoide Form der enchondralen Dysostose.

Die bakteriellen Arthritiden haben seit Entwicklung der Antibiotica radiologisch kaum noch eine differentialdiagnostische Bedeutung gegenüber der Gicht.

Literatur

BRAILSFORD, J. F.: The radiology of gout. Brit. J. Radiol. **32**, 472—478 (1959).
BRØCHNER-MORTENSEN, K.: 100 gouty patients. Acta med. scand. **106**, 81—107 (1941).
DIHLMANN, W., FERNHOLZ, H. J.: Gibt es charakteristische Röntgenbefunde bei der Gicht? Dtsch. med. Wschr. **94**, 1909—1911 (1969).
DRINBERG, E.: Die Gicht im Röntgenbilde. Diss. Berlin 1911.
DRUBE, H., REINWEIN, H.: Zur Klinik der Gicht, „der vergessenen Krankheit". Med. Klin. **54**, 631—639 (1959).
EBERL, R., PECHERSTORFER, M., ZAUNBAUER, W.: Über Veränderungen im Pyelogramm bei Gicht. Wien. med. Wschr. **118**, 1029—1030 (1968).
FERGUSON, A. B.: Gout in roentgen diagnosis of the extremities and spine. Amer. J. Roentgenol. **17**, 301 (1945).

FRANÇON, F., LEROY, J.: Le „pied hérissé" hors de la goutte. Rev. Rhum. **29**, 12—17 (1962).
GAMP, A., SCHILLING, A., MÜLLER, L., SCHACHERL, M.: Das klinische Bild der Gicht heute. Beobachtungen an 200 Kranken. Med. Klin. **60**, 129—131 (1965).
HALL, M. C., SELIN, G.: Spinal involvement in gout. A case report with autopsy. J. Bone Jt Surg. **42 A**, 341—343 (1960).
HAWKINS, C. F., ELLIS, H. A., RAWSON, A.: Malignant gout with tophaceous small intestine and megaloblastic anaemia. Ann. rheum. Dis. **24**, 224—233 (1965).
HOFMEISTER, F.: Arthritis urica der Hüftgelenke. Verh. dtsch. orthop. Ges. **1968**, 414.
HUBER: Zur Verwerthung der Röntgen-Strahlen im Gebiete der inneren Medicin. Dtsch. med. Wschr. **22**, 182—184 (1896).
JACOBSON, E.: Die Arthritis urica im Röntgenbilde. Mitt. Grenzgeb. Med. Chir. **26**, 531—552 (1913).
KERSLEY, G. D., MANDEL, L., JEFFREY, M. R.: Gout, an unusual case with softening and subluxation of the first cervical vertebra and splenomegaly. Ann. Rheum. Dis. **9**, 282—304 (1950).
KERSLEY, G. D., ROSS, F. G. M., FOWLES, S. J., JOHNSON, C.: Tomography in arthritis of the small joints. Ann. rheum. Dis. **23**, 280—287 (1964).
KÖHLER, A.: Typical alterations of the bones in gout. Arch. Roentg. Ray. **16**, 330 (1911).
KOSKOFF, Y. D., MORRIS, L. E., LUBIC, L. G.: Paraplegia as a complication of gout. J. Amer. med. Ass. **152**, 37—38 (1953).
KUZELL, W. CH., GAUDIN, G.-P.: Gicht. Documenta rheumatologica Geigy, Nr. 10. Basel 1956.
KÜNZLER, H.: Klinische Aspekte der Gichtpatienten der Universitäts-Rheumaklinik Zürich. Diss. Zürich 1966.
LICHTENSTEIN, L., SCOTT, H. W., LEVIN, M. H.: Pathologic changes in gout: survey of eleven necropsied cases. Amer. J. Path. **32**, 871—896 (1956).
LIPSON, R. L., SLOCUMB, C. H.: The progressive nature of gout with inadequate therapy. Arthr. and Rheum. **8**, 80—87 (1965).
LÖFFLER, W., KOLLER, F.: Die Gicht. In: Handbuch der inneren Medizin, 4. Auflage, Bd. VII/2, S. 435—608. Berlin-Göttingen-Heidelberg: Springer 1955.
MALAWISTA, S. E., SEEGMILLER, J. E., HATHAWAY, B. E., SOKOLOFF, L.: Sacroiliac gout. J. Amer. med. Ass. **194**, 954—956 (1965).
MARTEL, W.: The overhanging margin of bone: A roentgenologic manifestation of gout. Radiology **91**, 755—756 (1968).
MCCLURE, C. W., MCCARTY, E. D.: Roentgenographic studies in gout. Arch. intern. Med. **24**, 563 (1919).
MCCRACKEN, J. P., OWEN, P. S., PRATT, J. H.: Gout: still a forgotten disease. J. Amer. med. Ass. **131**, 367—372 (1946).
MUGLER, A.: Gicht und Trauma. Münch. med. Wschr. **111**, 1615—1619 (1969).
MÜLLER, E., LÖHR, E.: Arthritis urica des Hüftgelenkes. Fortschr. Röntgenstr. **111**, 710—711 (1969).
NIEPEL, G. A., KOSTKA, D., KOPECKÝ, S., MANCA, S.: Enthesopathy. Acta Rheumat. et Balneol. Pistiniana **1966**, 1.
POMMER, G.: Mikroskopische Untersuchung über Gelenkgicht. Jena: Fischer 1929.
POTAIN, SERBANESCO: Radiographie des extrémités chez les sujets affectés de goutte ou de rhumatisme chronique. Bull. Acad. Sci., 18. Juni 1897.
ROSENBERG, E. F., ARENS, R. A.: Gout: Clinical, pathological and roentgenographic observations. Radiology **49**, 169—177 (1947).
SCHACHERL, M.: Röntgenologische Differentialdiagnose rheumatischer Erkrankungen. Therapiewoche **19**, 307—314 (1969).
SCHACHERL, M.: Die Radiologie der Gicht. 4. Arbeitstagung der Forschungsgemeinschaft für Erkrankungen des Bewegungsapparates, Wien, 27. und 28. II. 1970. Therapiewoche **22**, 113—118 (1972).
SCHACHERL, M., SCHILLING, F.: Röntgenbefunde an den Gliedmaßengelenken bei Polyarthritis psoriatica. Z. Rheumaforsch. **26**, 442—450 (1967).
SCHACHERL, M., SCHILLING, F.: Die destruierende Polyarthrose. Fortschr. Röntgenstr. **113**, 551—560 (1970).
SCHACHERL, M., SCHILLING, F., GAMP, A.: Das radiologische Bild der Gicht. Radiologe **6**, 231—238 (1966).
SCHILLING, A.: Gicht bei der Frau. Z. Rheumaforsch. **27**, 192—198 (1968).
SCHILLING, F., SCHACHERL, M., GAMP, A., BOPP, A.: Die Beziehungen der Spondylosis hyperostotica zur Konstitution und zu Stoffwechselstörungen. Med. Klin. **60**, 165—169 (1965).

SCHULITZ, K.-P.: Zur Frage der Hüftgelenkserkrankungen bei der Gicht. Z. Orthop. **106**, 708—716 (1969).

SERRE, H., SIMON, L.: (1) L' osteonécrose primitive de la tête fémorale chez l'adulte. Rev. Rhum. **29**, 527—545 (1962).

SERRE, H., SIMON, L., GIVAUDAND, A., BENAMARA, M.: (2) La Radiographie de pied dans le diagnostic de la goutte. Ann. Radiol. **5**, 649—655 (1962).

SERRE, H., SIMON, L., CLAUSTRE, J.: A propos de l'atteinte des hanches au cours de la goutte. Rev. Rhum. **30**, 741—746 (1963).

DE SÈZE, S., RYCKEWAERT, A., LEVERNIEUX, J., MARTEAU, R.: Les lésions radiologiques de la goutte. J. Radiol. Electrol. **41**, 1—13 (1960).

DE SÈZE, S., WELFLING, J., LEQUESNE, M.: L' ostéonécrose primitive de la tête fémorale chez l'adulte. Rev. Rhum. **27**, 117—127 (1960).

ŠTĚPÁNEK, P., KŘÍŽEK, V.: Das Vorkommen des Fersensporns bei Gichtkranken. Z. Rheumaforsch. **28**, 147—152 (1969).

STRANGEWAYS, T. S. P., BURT, J. B.: A study of skiagrams from the hands of 100 cases of so called rheumatoid arthritis and chronic gout. Bull. Com. Study Special Dis. **1**, 145—164 (1905—1907).

TALBOTT, J. H., CULVER, G. J., MIZRAJI, M., CRESPO, D. I.: Roentgenographic findings: description of a magnification technic. Metabolism **6**, 277—296 (1957).

TEIXEIRA, M. A., VAHIA, M. A.: Les Spondylarthroses chez les goutteux. In: Contemporary Rheumatology, p. 595—599. Amsterdam-London-New York-Princeton: Elsevier 1956.

VYHNÁNEK, L., LAVICKA, J., BLAHOS, J.: Roentenological findings in gout: Radiol. clin. (Basel) **29**, 256—264 (1960).

WISSINGER, H. A.: Gouty Arthritis of the hip joints. J. Bone Jt Surg. **45 A**, 785—788 (1963).

b) Gichtniere

aa) Die Gichtniere

Von

N. ZÖLLNER und W. GRÖBNER

Mit 9 Abbildungen

Als Gichtniere bezeichnet man die Nierenveränderungen, die bei der Gicht und bei den ihr zugrundeliegenden Stoffwechselstörungen auftreten können. Die Häufigkeit des Zusammentreffens von Krankheiten der Niere mit der Gicht war den alten Autoren geläufig; bereits ARETAEUS von Kappadozien hat im 2. Jahrhundert nach Christus darüber berichtet. Zunächst fiel die auffällige Kombination der Gelenkkrankheit mit Steinen auf. In der zweiten Hälfte des vorigen Jahrhunderts rückten die Veränderungen am Nierenparenchym und die ersten einschlägigen chemischen Untersuchungen in den Mittelpunkt des Interesses. So berichtet DICKINSON 1861, daß er bei 250 Fällen autoptisch gesicherter schwerer Nierenkrankheiten in 7% eine Gichtanamnese festgestellt habe. Aus jener Zeit stammt auch der von TODD geprägte Ausdruck gouty kidney — Gichtniere. Unser Jahrhundert brachte zunächst vorwiegend funktionelle Untersuchungen, aus denen sich allmählich nicht nur die Mechanismen der normalen renalen Harnsäureausscheidung, sondern auch Besonderheiten bei der Gicht erschließen ließen. In den letzten Jahren hat die diagnostische Nierenpunktion Material für die anatomische Beurteilung früher Gichtnieren geliefert.

Renale Veränderungen, die anatomisch wie eine Gichtniere aussahen, aber bei Patienten zustandegekommen waren, die nie an der Gelenkgicht gelitten hatten, wurden von EBSTEIN (1906) als primäre Nierengicht bezeichnet. Der Definition dieses Begriffes verdanken wir die wichtige Anschauung, daß die Niere von der primären Stoffwechselstörung auch dann befallen sein kann, wenn keine Gelenksymptome bestehen. Soweit renale Veränderungen bei der familiären Hyperuricämie isoliert bestehen, könnten sie auch heute noch als Nierengicht bezeichnet werden, denn die Tragfähigkeit des Ebsteinschen Konzepts ist — obwohl es zweifellos auch auf einer Reihe von Fehlbeobachtungen beruhte — durch die Ergebnisse der neueren Gichtforschung bestätigt. Dennoch besteht kein Grund mehr, die von der Hyperuricämie isoliert befallene Niere — als Nierengicht — von der Niere bei Hyperuricämie mit Gelenkerscheinungen — als Gichtniere — abzutrennen.

Für das Verständnis vieler Vorgänge ist es wichtig zu unterscheiden, ob man von Uraten bzw. Urationen oder von der undissoziierten Harnsäure spricht. Häufig ist diese Unterscheidung aber nicht nötig, nicht selten auch unmöglich. Diesem Sachverhalt wird durch die Verwendung der Worte Urate bzw. freie Harnsäure Rechnung getragen, wenn eine klare Zuordnung zu harnsauren Salzen bzw. Urationen einerseits und undissoziierter Harnsäure andererseits nötig oder möglich ist. Der Begriff Harnsäure wird verwendet, wenn diese Zuordnung nicht erfolgen soll (oder kann) oder wenn ein Gemisch aus Uraten und freier Harnsäure vorliegt.

I. Pathogenese

1. Pathogenese der familiären Hyperuricämie

Die Harnsäure diffundiert frei durch den Extracellulärraum, ihr Pool beträgt etwa 1200 mg. Die Harnsäurekonzentration des Körpers stellt die Resultierende aus Zufluß und Abfluß dar. Der Zufluß erfolgt sowohl durch die endogene Neusynthese einschließlich der Reutilisation von Purinen als auch aus Nahrungspurinen. Die Ausscheidung der Harnsäure geht zu ca. 80% über die Niere, der Rest wird enteral ausgeschieden und unterliegt im Darm einer bakteriellen Zersetzung.

Die primäre Hyperuricämie resultiert entweder aus einer vermehrten Harnsäuresynthese oder aus einer Störung der renalen Harnsäureausscheidung. Gelegentlich werden beide „Defekte" kombiniert angetroffen.

Ausgangssubstanz der Harnsäuresynthese ist 5-Phosphoribosyl-1-Pyrophosphat, das mit Glutamin zum 5-Phosphoribosyl-1-Amin reagiert. Dieser Schritt ist geschwindigkeitsbestimmend für die Purinsynthese de novo und wird durch Glutamin-5-Phosphoribosyl-1-Pyrophosphat-Amidotransferase katalysiert. Über eine Reihe weiterer Zwischenstufen entsteht schließlich Inosinsäure, aus der die anderen Nucleotide, nämlich Adenyl- und Guanylsäure gebildet werden. Sie wiederum hemmen im Sinne eines Rückkopplungseffektes den ersten Schritt der Purinsynthese. Störungen in der Feedback-Regulation der Purinsynthese, eine Veränderung der Enzymaktivität der Glutamin-Phosphoribosyl-1-Pyrophosphat-Amidotransferase sowie ein Anstieg der Substratkonzentration von Glutamin oder 5-Phosphoribosyl-1-Pyrophosphat kommen als mögliche Ursachen einer vermehrten Purinsynthese de novo in Frage. Neuerdings wurden von SPERLING et al. (1972) sowie BECKER et al. (1973) in einer Gichtikerfamilie eine gesteigerte Aktivität von 5-Phosphoribosyl-1-Pyrophosphat-Synthetase, die die Bildung von 5-Phosphoribosyl-1-Pyrophosphat aus Ribose-5-Phosphat und Adenosintriphosphat katalysiert, als Ursache der Hyperuricämie beschrieben.

In den letzten Jahren wurde mit dem Lesch-Nyhan-Syndrom eine weitere Erkrankung gefunden, die mit einer vermehrten Harnsäuresynthese einhergeht. Die auffälligste biochemische Abnormalität bei diesem Syndrom ist ein Fehlen der Aktivität von Hypoxanthin-Guaninphosphoribosyltransferase, die die Um-

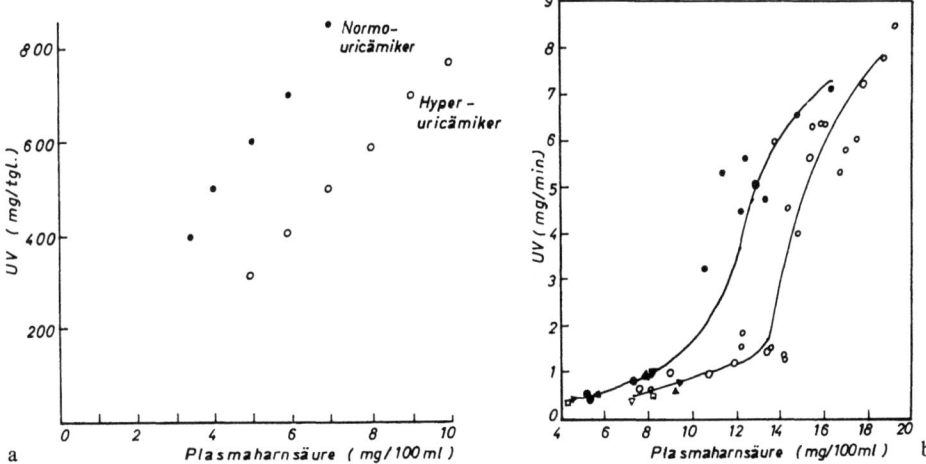

Abb. 1a. Beziehung von Plasmaharnsäure und renaler Harnsäureausscheidung während der Gabe von RNS bei Normalpersonen und Hyperuricämikern. (Nach ZÖLLNER u. GRIEBSCH, 1974)

Abb. 1b. Das Verhalten der renalen Harnsäureausscheidung bei verschiedenen Plasmaharnsäurespiegeln bei Gichtkranken (offene Symbole) und Normalpersonen (geschlossene Symbole). (Nach WYNGAARDEN, 1965)

wandlung von Hypoxanthin und Guanin zu den entsprechenden Nucleotiden katalysiert. Guanosin-5-Monophosphat sowie Inosin-5-Monophosphat sind wiederum Feedback-Inhibitoren der Purinsynthese de novo. Ein Fehlen dieses Enzyms führt somit zu einer Störung der Feedback-Regulation und damit zu einer Steigerung der Purinsynthese. Ein nur partielles Fehlen der Aktivität von Hypoxanthin-Guaninphosphoribosyltransferase wurde von KELLEY et al. (1968) bei einigen Gichtpatienten, die eine vermehrte Harnsäuresynthese zeigten, nachgewiesen.

Im Gegensatz zur vermehrten Harnsäuresynthese steht als Ursache der familiären Hyperuricämie eine Störung der renalen Harnsäureausscheidung, wie sie bei den meisten Gichtpatienten angetroffen wird. Der wesentliche Verfechter dieser auf den älteren GARROD (1876) zurückgehenden sogenannten „Ausscheidungstheorie" war THANNHAUSER, der indes bei seiner letzten zusammenfassenden Darstellung (1956) im Sinne der damals herrschenden Lehre der Nierenphysiologie als pathogenetische Mechanismen eine vermehrte Rückresorption annehmen mußte. Die Hypothese einer bei Gicht vermehrten tubulären Harnsäurerückresorption war aus allgemein-biologischen Gründen unwahrscheinlich — wie THANNHAUSER selbst wiederholt äußerte —, da alle bisher bekannten angeborenen Stoffwechselstörungen des Menschen Minusvarianten sind.

Durch die Feststellung, daß Harnsäure auch tubulär sezerniert wird, änderte sich die Situation. Aus Daten von BERLINER et al. (1950) sowie GUTMAN u. YÜ (1957) konnte wahrscheinlich gemacht werden, daß der Gichtkranke Harnsäure nicht in gleicher Weise wie der Gesunde ausscheiden kann (ZÖLLNER, 1960a). Gleichzeitig zeigten NUGENT u. TYLER (1959), daß bei gleichem Harnsäurespiegel im Plasma Gichtkranke pro Zeiteinheit weniger Harnsäure ausscheiden als Gesunde. Heute gilt es als sicher, daß bei den meisten Patienten mit Gicht eine Vermehrung der „Netto-Rückresorption" — wahrscheinlich durch Verringerung der Harnsäure-Sekretion — und somit eine Störung der Harnsäureausscheidung gefunden werden kann. Als Stoffwechseldefekt gehört die Hyperuricämie damit in die gleiche Gruppe wie die Cystinurie, bei der eine Störung des tubulären Transportes mehrerer Diaminosäuren besteht (vgl. HARRIS, 1963).

Um den festgestellten renalen Defekt zuverlässig als Ursache der Gicht ansehen zu können, bleibt nachzuweisen, daß er bereits bei der asymptomatischen Hyperuricämie, besser noch bei der Hälfte der Nachkommen Gichtkranker besteht. ZÖLLNER u. GRIEBSCH (1974) konnten in mehrwöchigen Ernährungsversuchen mittels Formeldiäten zeigen, daß nach Zulage definierter Mengen von Ribonucleinsäure oder Desoxyribonucleinsäure die Plasmaharnsäure von Hyperuricämikern stärker als die von Normalpersonen ansteigt, während sich die Zunahme der renalen Harnsäureausscheidung bei beiden Personengruppen gleich verhält. Diese Untersuchungsbefunde sprechen für eine verminderte Fähigkeit des Hyperuricämikers, Harnsäure renal auszuscheiden (Abb. 1a). Diese Ergebnisse stimmen gut mit früheren, von WYNGAARDEN (1965) zusammengefaßten Befunden überein, wobei Plasmaharnsäure und Harnsäureausscheidung bei Gichtikern und Normalpersonen verglichen werden (Abb. 1b). Eine andere Möglichkeit, die verringerte Fähigkeit zur Harnsäuresekretion festzustellen, ist die Prüfung der Ausscheidung durch andere sezernierende Epithelien. Versuche über die saliväre Ausscheidung von Harnsäure haben ergeben, daß diese mit ansteigendem Plasmaspiegel zunimmt, daß aber bei gleichem Harnsäurespiegel Gichtiker weniger Harnsäure ausscheiden als Gesunde (ZÖLLNER, 1963a, 1965a).

2. Pathogenese sekundärer Hyperuricämieformen

Die Gicht kann in eine primäre (familiäre) und in eine sekundäre Form eingeteilt werden; auch die Hyperuricämien lassen sich so einteilen. Während THANNHAUSER (1929), auf den der Begriff der sekundären Gicht zurückgeht, vorwiegend an die Harnsäureretention bei chronischen Nierenleiden dachte, rechnet man seit GUTMAN (1953) vor allem Fälle zur sekundären Gicht, bei denen eine vermehrte Harnsäureproduktion durch Krankheiten des hämatopoetischen Systems besteht. Tatsächlich ist der Bereich der sekundären Gicht damit noch nicht ausgemessen. Bei weiteren Krankheiten liegen Beschreibungen von erhöhten Plasmaharnsäurespiegeln und Gichtanfällen vor, z.B. bei der Glykogenspeicherkrankheit und — praktisch viel wichtiger — bei der Ödemtherapie mit Saluretica (vgl. ZÖLLNER, 1960a; REUTTER u. SCHAUB, 1964).

Nicht alle Fälle von Gicht oder Hyperuricämie bei Blutkrankheiten oder Insuffizienz der Niere sind ausschließlich sekundär; in manchen dieser Fälle handelt es sich um die Auslösung der angeborenen Krankheit durch die zusätzlichen Manifestationsfaktoren. An dem Vorkommen einer sekundären Gicht kann aber kein Zweifel bestehen, da anders die sehr hohe Gichtquote bei Polycythämie oder myeloischer Metaplasie nicht zu erklären wäre. Auch die Hyperuricämie bei Salureticabehandlung ist zu häufig für die Annahme, daß sie einer genetisch bedingten Voraussetzung bedürfe, und letzten Endes besteht kein Zweifel daran, daß eine Niereninsuffizienz eine Hyperuricämie hervorrufen kann.

Während die Erhöhung des Harnsäurespiegels bei organisch oder pharmakologisch bedingten Einschränkungen der Harnsäureausscheidung leicht zu verstehen ist, bedarf die Hyperuricämie des Patienten mit vermehrter Harnsäurebildung besonderer Überlegungen. Zunächst scheint es selbstverständlich, daß es bei Krankheiten mit vermehrter Zellbildung und damit vermehrtem Kernzerfall zu Hyperuricämie und Hyperuricurie kommt; aber dies ist durchaus nicht die Regel, eine mäßige Vermehrung der Harnsäureausscheidung kann mit einem normalen Plasmaspiegel einhergehen. Dennoch kommt bei diesen Krankheiten die Harnsäureurolithiasis gehäuft vor — so daß es klinisch zwei mit Neigung zur Harnsäuresteinbildung einhergehende „Syndrome" von Laboratoriumsbefunden gibt: Die Vermehrung der Plasmaharnsäure bei normaler Tagesausscheidung, Beispiel Gicht, und die Vermehrung der Harnsäureausscheidung bei normalem Plasmaharnsäurespiegel, Beispiel chronische myeloische Leukämie. Dazwischen liegen die Fälle, bei denen eine mäßige Mehrbildung von Harnsäure im Laufe der Zeit zur Ausbildung einer sekundären Gicht und Harnsäureurolithiasis führt. KÖNIG u. ZÖLLNER (1962) haben zwei Fälle von sekundärer Gicht gesehen (je einen bei Polycythaemia vera und bei myeloischer Metaplasie bei Osteomyelosklerose — einer davon mit Steinen), bei denen erhöhte Plasmaharnsäurewerte bei einer nur sehr gering erhöhten Tagesausscheidung bestanden, einer Tagesausscheidung, bei der im akuten Versuch keine Erhöhung der Plasmaharnsäure zustandegekommen wäre. Ähnliche Beobachtungen finden sich an mehreren Stellen der Literatur.

3. Pathogenese der Gichtniere

Harnsäure diffundiert durch alle extracellulären Flüssigkeitsräume und findet sich im Interstitium in der gleichen Konzentration wie im Plasma (THANNHAUSER u. CZONICZER, 1921; ZÖLLNER, 1960a). Steigt bei der üblichen Natriumkonzentration die der Harnsäure über einen Grenzwert von ungefähr 6,5 mg-%, so kommt es bei pH 7,4 zur Ausfällung von Natriumurat. In einigen Geweben (z.B. der Synovia oder dem Schleimbeutel) folgt darauf eine entzündliche Reaktion, der Gichtanfall. Aus anderen Geweben, z.B. den Gefäßwänden oder der Muskulatur, werden die Mikrokristalle offensichtlich rasch eliminiert, da sie dort nur ausnahmsweise histologisch nachzuweisen sind. Letzten Endes gibt es Gewebe, wie Knorpel, Knochen und Teile der Subcutis, wo Harnsäure, ohne eine klinisch faßbare akute Reaktion hervorzurufen, liegen bleibt. Zu letzteren scheint auch die Niere zu gehören.

Das klassische Beispiel einer renalen interstitiellen Harnsäureausfällung ist der (weiße) „Harnsäureinfarkt" des Neugeborenen. SOKOLOFF (1957) hat gezeigt, daß eine der häufigsten Formen der Gichtniere des Erwachsenen ähnlich aussieht. Es handelt sich um weiße kristalline Harnsäureablagerungen im Nierenmark, besonders in den Pyramiden, die in mehr als 80% der sezierten Gichtfälle gefunden wurden.

Im Gegensatz zu den übrigen Geweben dürfte die interstitielle Harnsäurekonzentration in der Niere — ebenso wie die interstitielle Konzentration anderer Ionen — nicht nur von der Uratkonzentration im Plasmawasser abhängen, sondern auch von der intratubulären Konzentration; die Tendenz zur Harnsäureablagerung in den Pyramiden wäre damit zu erklären. Zum genaueren Verständnis der Erscheinungsformen der Gichtniere ist an dieser Stelle ein kurzer Abriß von Physiologie und Pathologie der renalen Harnsäureausscheidung am Platz.

a) Physiologie und Pathologie der renalen Harnsäureausscheidung

Für den Mechanismus der renalen Harnsäureausscheidung gilt heute die Theorie, daß Filtration, Rückresorption und tubuläre Sekretion beteiligt sind (GUTMAN u. YÜ, 1961), als gesichert, nachdem bereits 1959 von GUTMAN et al. gezeigt worden war, daß der Mensch unter bestimmten Bedingungen Harnsäure tubulär sezernieren kann, und NUGENT u. TYLER (1959) ebenso wie ZÖLLNER (1958, 1960) darauf hingewiesen hatten, daß die Besonderheiten der renalen Harnsäureausscheidung bzw. die Hyperuricämie bei Gichtkranken durch eine Störung der tubulären Harnsäuresekretion erklärt werden können. Während YÜ u. GUTMAN (1953) jedoch eine vollständige Ultrafiltrierbarkeit von Harnsäure annahmen, machen dies neuere, allerdings größtenteils in vitro durchgeführte Untersuchungen über eine gewisse Eiweißbindung von Harnsäure (<5% der Plasmaharnsäure) weniger wahrscheinlich (ALVSAKER, 1966; KLINENBERG u. KIPPEN, 1970; CAMPION et al., 1973; KIPPEN et al., 1974). Der wegen Eiweißbindung nicht filtrierbare Anteil ist dementsprechend gering. Neben der Niere erfolgt in geringem Ausmaß eine Ausscheidung von Harnsäure auch über den Magen-Darm-Trakt. Hierbei unterliegen täglich ca. 50—100 mg der bakteriellen Uricolyse.

Von der filtrierten Harnsäure wird der größte Teil zurückresorbiert; wenn man keine Sekretion annimmt, errechnet sich eine Rückresorption von 95%. Die Harnsäureclearance von Personen mit normaler Plasmaharnsäurekonzentration liegt um 9 ml/min. Über die Harnsäureclearance von Gichtkranken bestand keine Einigkeit. Ältere amerikanische Autoren gaben sie als normal an, europäische Arbeiten von MUGLER et al. (1956) sowie VILLA et al. (1958) widersprachen diesen Befunden. LAUDAT et al. (1962) fanden Normalwerte für die Harnsäureclearance von 9,5 ml/min, bei Gichtpatienten 5,8 ml/min. Da von den meisten Gichtpatienten normale Tagesmengen Harnsäure ausgeschieden werden, die Plasmaharnsäurespiegel bei der Gicht aber erhöht sind, war eine Verringerung der Harnsäureclearance bei Gicht von vornherein wahrscheinlich. SEEGMILLER et al. (1962) haben die Clearance von Normalen und Gichtkranken unter Berücksichtigung der Harnsäurebildung noch einmal nachgeprüft und die theoretisch zu erwartenden Befunde erhoben.

Für genauere Vergleiche der Harnsäureausscheidung Gesunder und Gichtkranker entscheidend wurde die Entdeckung von NUGENT u. TYLER (1959), daß bei gleichem Plasmaharnsäurespiegel (beim Gesunden durch orale Nucleinsäuregabe angehoben) die Harnsäureclearance des Gichtkranken wesentlich niedriger ist als die des Normalen. Dieser Befund, der eine ältere Feststellung von BRØCHNER-MORTENSEN (1940) über die Zunahme der Harnsäureclearance nach oraler Purinzufuhr beim Gesunden, aber nicht beim Gichtiker, in eine präzisere Form bringt, ist anschließend mehrfach bestätigt worden (vgl. WYNGAARDEN, 1960; OGRYZLO, 1960; SEEGMILLER et al., 1962; LATHEM u. RODNAN, 1962; REUBI u. VORBURGER, 1962) und gilt heute als allgemein anerkannt. Lediglich YÜ et al. (1962) kamen zu der Schlußfolgerung, daß Gichtiker eine Harnsäurebelastung ebensogut ausscheiden können wie Gesunde, doch finden sich Hyperuricämiker in ihrer Gruppe gesunder Versuchspersonen. Ihr weiterer Einwand, daß die Harnsäureausscheidung im akuten Versuch (Anhebung der Plasmaharnsäurekonzentration der normalen Kontrollpersonen durch mehrtägige Nucleinsäurezufuhr) nicht mit der Harnsäureausscheidung bei der chronischen Hyperuricämie der Gichtpatienten vergleichbar sei, wird durch Versuche von NUGENT et al. (1964) widerlegt, die einigen Kontrollpersonen monatelang sehr purinreiche Kost verabreichten und danach immer noch die gleichen charakteristischen Unterschiede zu der Harnsäureausscheidung Gichtkranker fanden.

Versuche, die Mechanismen der Harnsäureausscheidung im Rahmen der Filtrations-Rückresorptions-Theorie zahlenmäßig zu beschreiben, führten zur Angabe einer maximalen tubulären Rückresorption (T_m) von 15 mg/min/1,73 m² durch BERLINER et al. (1950), doch zeigten die Kurven, mit deren Hilfe T_m abgeschätzt wurde, sehr viel "Splay". 1957 berichteten dann GUTMAN und YÜ über ihre Bestimmungen der Filtration und Rückresorption von Harnsäure bei Gichtpatienten. Im untersuchten Bereich war die Beziehung zwischen filtrierter und rückresorbierter Harnsäuremenge konstant, die Rückresorption betrug unabhängig von der filtrierten Menge 88—95%. Ein Vergleich der Ergebnisse dieser Untersuchungen mit den Resultaten von BERLINER et al. führte zu dem Ergebnis, daß mit zunehmender Filtration zwar beim Normalen die Rückresorption (in mg/min)

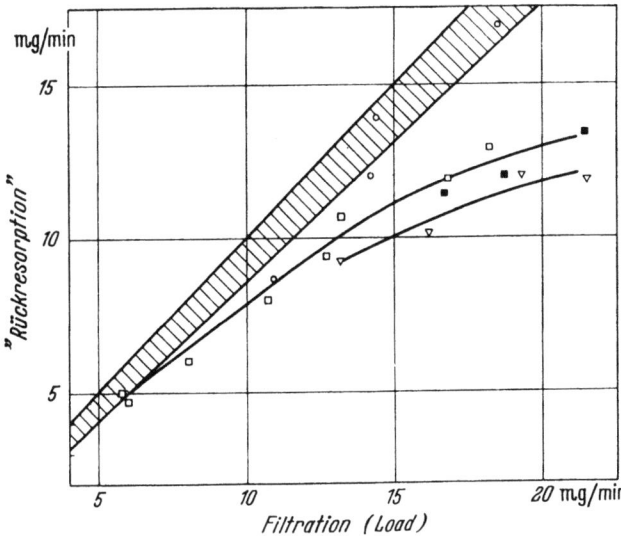

Abb. 2. Die Beziehung zwischen filtrierter und rückresorbierter Harnsäure beim Gichtkranken und beim Normalen. Filtration berechnet aus Inulinclearance und Plasmaharnsäure, „Rückresorption" als Differenz zwischen Filtration und Ausscheidung. Der Bereich aller Werte bei über 200 Gichtkranken (schraffiertes Gebiet unterhalb der Diagonalen für vollständige Rückresorption) ist einer Arbeit von GUTMAN u. YÜ (1957) entnommen; bei gesunden Kontrollpersonen unter Ruhebedingungen fanden diese Autoren Filtrationen unter 8 mg/min. Die Werte für Normalpersonen, denen Lithiumurat infundiert oder injiziert wurde, entstammen einer Untersuchung von BERLINER et al. (1950). Die im Gichtkerbereich liegenden Punkte der Versuchsperson o wurden bei rasch ansteigender Plasmaharnsäure gewonnen

ihrem Maximum (T_m) zustrebt, beim Gichtkranken dagegen kein T_m-Wert erkennbar wird (Abb. 2). Für die Deutung dieser Ergebnisse gibt es zwei Möglichkeiten, nämlich die Annahme einer Fähigkeit des Normalen, die (tatsächliche) Rückresorption bei Zunahme der filtrierten Menge (oder der Plasmaharnsäurekonzentration) zu vermindern, oder die Annahme, daß die errechnete Rückresorption keinem physiologischen Vorgang entspricht, daß vielmehr eine tubuläre Sekretion existiert, die mit steigendem Plasmaharnsäurespiegel zunimmt. Dem Gichtkranken würde dementsprechend entweder die Fähigkeit, die Rückresorption von Urat zu vermindern oder die Fähigkeit, die Sekretion ausreichend zu erhöhen, fehlen.

Eine tubuläre Sekretion von Harnsäure ist bei einer Reihe von Säugetieren nachgewiesen worden, zuerst beim Dalmatiner Hund durch FRIEDMAN u. BYERS (1948). Während bei dieser Rasse der Nachweis einfach war, mußten bei anderen Arten besondere experimentelle Bedingungen eingehalten werden. Dies gelang zuerst POULSEN u. PRAETORIUS (1954), die bei Kaninchen während intravenöser Harnsäureinfusionen für die Harnsäureclearance höhere Werte als für die Kreatininclearance erreichen konnten. Beim Menschen wiesen GUTMAN et al. (1959) eine tubuläre Sekretion bei Personen mit eingeschränkter glomerulärer Filtrationsrate nach, denen zur Hemmung der Harnsäurerückresorption Sulfinpyrazon, zur Steigerung der Diurese Mannit und zur Lieferung ausreichender Harnsäuremengen Urat infundiert wurde. Bei osmotischer Diurese und Uratinfusion gelang kurz darauf der Nachweis einer Sekretion auch beim Hund (LATHEM et al., 1960). Versuche, den Ort der tubulären Harnsäuresekretion festzulegen, hat-

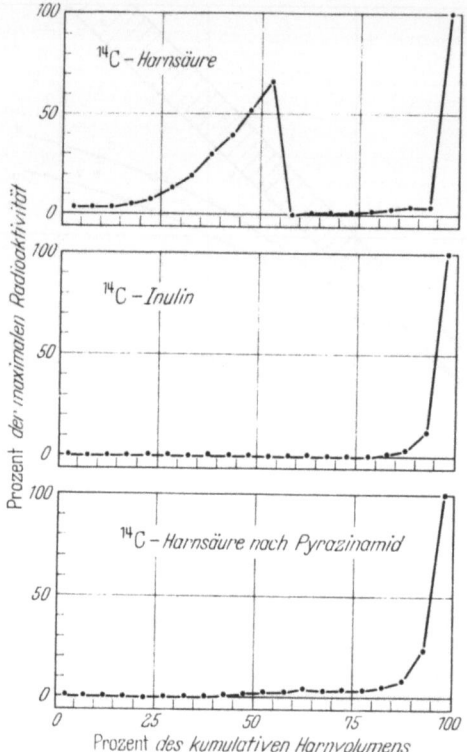

Abb. 3. Demonstration einer tubulären Harnsäureausscheidung mit Hilfe der Stop-flow-Methode. 10—15 sec vor Freigabe des Harnflusses wurde radioaktive Harnsäure bzw. radioaktives Inulin in die Nierenarterie injiziert. Das Volumen der Einzelproben betrug ungefähr 0,5 ml, die gesamte Harnsammlung dauerte 3 min bzw. bis zu einem Gesamtvolumen von 20 ml. Der frühe Gipfel der Harnsäureausscheidung bzw. sein Ausbleiben nach Pyrazinamid weist auf eine distale tubuläre Sekretion hin.
(Darstellung nach Zahlen von DAVIS et al., 1965)

ten zu nicht ganz einheitlichen Ergebnissen geführt. YÜ et al. (1960) fanden zwar mit der stop-flow-Analyse eine Harnsäuresekretion im distalen Tubulus, die durch das Hyperuricämie erzeugende Pyrazinamid verhindert werden kann (DAVIS et al., 1965), doch konnten KESSLER et al. (1959) außer beim Dalmatiner mit der gleichen Technik keine tubuläre Sekretion nachweisen. Bei Berücksichtigung der angewandten Methodik wird man den Ergebnissen von DAVIS et al. (Abb. 3) die meiste Beweiskraft zuerkennen.

In der Rattenniere fanden GREGER et al. (1971) sowie LANG et al. (1972) im proximalen Tubulus eine Sekretion von Harnsäure oberhalb der Rückresorptionsstelle. Beim Menschen vermuten STEELE u. BONER (1973) sowie DIAMOND u. PAOLINO (1973) ebenfalls eine Sekretion von Harnsäure proximal des Rückresorptionsortes. Ihre Untersuchungen schließen jedoch nicht aus, daß Rückresorption und Sekretion an derselben Stelle lokalisiert sind. FANELLI u. WEINER (1973) kommen zu der Schlußfolgerung, daß wenigstens beim Schimpansen die Harnsäuresekretion nicht distal der Resorption stattfindet.

Faßt man die Ergebnisse zusammen, so muß man die Harnsäureausscheidung der Säugetiere (ausschließlich der Dalmatiner Hunde) als die Folge des Zusammenwirkens von glomerulärer Filtration, fast vollständiger Rückresorption im

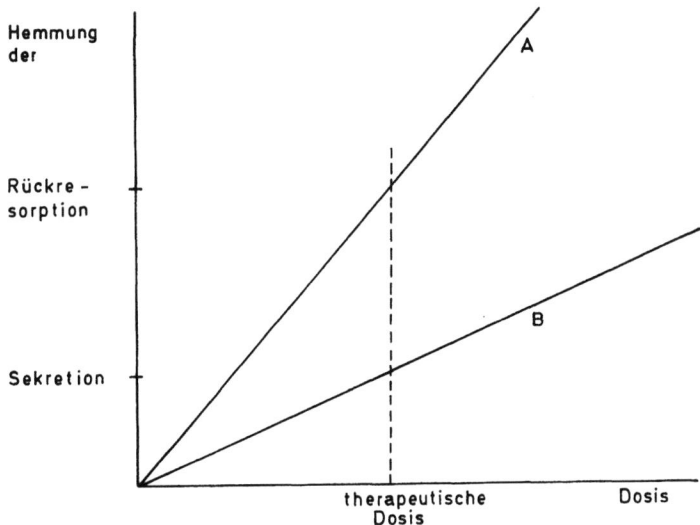

Abb. 4. Schematische Beziehung zwischen der therapeutischen Dosis eines Arzneimittels und seiner Wirkung auf den tubulären Harnsäuretransport. Bei der Substanz A (Beispiel Uricosurica) wird in therapeutischen Dosen nicht nur die Sekretion, sondern auch die Rückresorption gehemmt, während die Verbindung B (Beispiel Pyrazinamid) in therapeutischer Dosis nur die Sekretion hemmt

proximalen Tubulus und einer von der Höhe des Harnsäurespiegels im Plasma abhängigen Sekretion im proximalen, wahrscheinlich auch distalen Tubulus ansehen. Es wird weiter unten gezeigt werden, daß diese Hypothese für eine Zahl klinischer Betrachtungen, speziell auch der Gichtniere, einen brauchbaren Standpunkt gibt. Hier sei erwähnt, daß Arzneimittel, welche in therapeutischen Dosen den Harnsäurespiegel im Plasma senken (Uricosurica) als Hemmstoffe der proximalen tubulären Rückresorption angesehen werden können. In niedriger Dosierung führen sie (z. B. Probenecid) dagegen zu einer Erhöhung des Serumharnsäurespiegels, so daß anzunehmen ist, daß niedrige Dosen die Harnsäuresekretion, höhere Dosen zusätzlich die Rückresorption hemmen. Es hängt somit von der therapeutischen Dosis einer den tubulären Harnsäuretransport beeinflussenden Verbindung ab, ob nur die Harnsäuresekretion oder zusätzlich die Harnsäurerückresorption beeinflußt wird (Abb. 4).

Betrachtet man die Ergebnisse der stop-flow-Analysen, zusammen mit den erwähnten nierenphysiologischen Befunden, so wird man zu dem Ergebnis kommen, daß die Befunde bei der Gicht durch eine Verringerung der Fähigkeit zur tubulären Harnsäuresekretion, oder durch die Unfähigkeit zu einer ausreichenden Steigerung der Harnsäuresekretion im Tubulus bei Zunahme der Harnsäurekonzentration im Glomerulusfiltrat bzw. im Plasma zu erklären sind.

Die Fortschritte der Genetik haben wiederholt gezeigt, daß angeborene Stoffwechseldefekte, gleichgültig ob es sich um Enzymopathien oder Transportstörungen handelt, auch dann generalisiert vorkommen können, wenn ihre Nachweisbarkeit auf einige Organe beschränkt bleibt. In diesem Sinne war auch die Leistung anderer Harnsäure sezernierender Epithelien zu prüfen, nachdem im Anschluß an ältere Autoren vor allem SORENSEN (1960) auf die quantitative Bedeutung der enteralen Harnsäureausscheidung hingewiesen hatte. Es gelang nachzuweisen, daß die (im Rahmen der enteralen Harnsäureausscheidung am leichtesten zu prüfende) Sekretion im Speichel mit steigender Harnsäurekonzentration im

Plasma zunimmt (ZÖLLNER, 1963a) und damit den Beweis zu führen, daß durch Variation der Sekretion die Harnsäureausscheidung sich auch in anderen Organen als der Niere dem Plasmaspiegel anpassen kann. Bei Gichtpatienten sowie einer Versuchsperson mit gichtischer Familienanamnese war bei gleicher Harnsäurekonzentration im Plasma die Ausscheidung im Speichel deutlich geringer als bei nicht gichtischen Versuchspersonen (ZÖLLNER, 1965a).

Über die metabolischen Vorgänge beim tubulären Harnsäuretransport ist noch sehr wenig bekannt. Eine Reihe von Arzneimitteln hemmt Sekretion oder (und) Rückresorption, doch kann dieser Befund biochemisch noch nicht gedeutet werden, da keine ausreichenden Kenntnisse über die Wirkung der Verbindungen vorliegen. Eine Ausnahme bilden die Vitamin K-Antagonisten vom Dicumarol- und Phenylindandiontyp, die durch Blockierung der Harnsäurerückresorption uricosurisch wirken, und von denen man annehmen darf, daß sie Reaktionen hemmen, an denen Vitamin K-haltige Coenzyme beteiligt sind. Die uricosurische und die hypoprothrombinämische Wirkung der Vitamin K-Antagonisten gehen dabei nicht immer parallel. Das Phenprocumarol z. B. hat eine bemerkenswert geringe uricosurische Wirkung, während das von PASERO u. MARINI (1958) eingeführte 2-Phenyl-5-brom-1,3-indandion bei guter uricosurischer Aktivität die Prothrombinspiegel kaum verringert (PASERO, 1960).

Unter den Stoffen, welche die Harnsäureausscheidung beeinflussen, sind auch solche, die im Körper in großem Maße entstehen können, wie Milchsäure, Brenztraubensäure, β-Hydroxybuttersäure und Acetessigsäure (GIBSON u. DOISY, 1923; MICHAEL, 1944; YÜ et al., 1957). Besonders Milchsäure verringert die Harnsäureausscheidung sehr stark (Abfall der Clearance auf etwa 1 ml/min!), ähnlich β-Hydroxybuttersäure. Die Ketonsäuren scheinen die Ausscheidung zu erhöhen, und es ist deshalb zu vermuten, daß die Transportleistung der Tubuluszellen für Harnsäure von ihrem Redoxpotential, wahrscheinlich vom extramitochondrialen $\frac{NADH}{NAD^+}$-Quotienten abhängt.

Für die Praxis bedeuten diese Ergebnisse eine Erklärung des Harnsäureanstieges bei körperlicher Belastung (Milchsäureanstieg, NICHOLS et al., 1951), nach Alkoholgenuß (Milchsäureanstieg, LIEBER et al., 1962) und bei der Ketose des Hungernden und des Diabetikers.

b) Löslichkeit der Harnsäure

Am Beginn der Gichtniere steht immer die Ausfällung von Harnsäure oder Urat. Gelöste Harnsäure und das Uration sind nicht toxisch und kommen als materia peccans nicht in Frage.

Harnsäure ist eine zweiwertige Säure. Innerhalb physiologischer Wasserstoffionenkonzentrationen bilden sich jedoch nur einwertige Salze. Je nach pH-Wert kommen in den Körperflüssigkeiten freie Harnsäure oder (und) Urate vor. Dementsprechend bestehen Ausfällungen aus freier Harnsäure oder Uraten, vorwiegend Mononatriumurat.

Die Dissoziationskonstante pK' der Harnsäure beträgt 5,8 (BERNOULLI u. LOEBENSTEIN, 1940). Bei pH 7,4 liegen also nach

$$pH = pK' + \log \frac{Urat}{Harnsäure}$$

97,5% als Uration vor, bei pH 4,8 immer noch beinahe 10%. Daraus folgt, daß freie Harnsäure im Körper nur im Gemisch mit Uraten vorkommen kann

Tabelle 1. Löslichkeit von Gesamtharnsäure in Abhängigkeit vom pH, berechnet aus der Annahme, daß die Löslichkeit der freien Harnsäure pH-unabhängig 0,39 mMol/l beträgt und daß kein Überschuß von Natriumionen vorliegt, der die Löslichkeit verringert

pH	Gesamtharnsäure	
	mMol/l	mg/l
5,0	0,48	80
6,0	1,3	220
6,88	7,1	1190
7,0	9,4	1580
8,0	90,4	15200

und daß Überlegungen über die Harnsäureausfällung von Beobachtungen über das Verhalten von Uratlösungen bezüglich Dissoziation und Löslichkeit der verschiedenen ionisierten Formen bei verschiedenen pH-Werten ausgehen müssen.

Die Löslichkeit der Harnsäure in Wasser beträgt nach GUDZENT (1928) bei 37° 65 mg in 1 Liter Wasser. Die Löslichkeit des Natriumurates in reinem Wasser liegt nach Angaben des gleichen Autors bei Körpertemperatur bei 1,3 g pro Liter Wasser. Wegen des sehr kleinen Löslichkeitsproduktes für Natriumurat, das von HARPUDER u. ERBSEN (1924) mit $4,9 \times 10^{-5}$ angegeben wurde, ist die Löslichkeit von Uraten in Salzlösungen wesentlich geringer und beträgt nach GUDZENT in einprozentiger Kochsalzlösung bei 37° nur 130 mg/l. Für das Plasma berechneten PETERS u. VAN SLYKE (1946) eine Löslichkeit von 64 mg/l, in guter Übereinstimmung mit der klinischen Beobachtung, daß bei unbehandelter Gicht Anfälle erst bei Harnsäurekonzentrationen im Plasma über 6,5 mg-% beobachtet werden.

Die Verhältnisse im Harn liegen komplizierter, weil hier die Schwankungen sowohl im pH als auch in der Salzkonzentration wesentlich größer sind. Nimmt man den theoretischen Fall an, daß ein (Modell)-Harn nur soviel Kationen wie Urationen enthält, so können in ihm bei zunehmendem pH nach der Henderson-Hasselbach-Gleichung steigende Mengen Gesamtharnsäure in Lösung gehen, nämlich die (bei jedem pH-Wert gleiche) lösliche Menge freier Harnsäure und die zunehmende Menge Urat, die in Abwesenheit von Salzen gut löslich ist. PETERS u. VAN SLYKE (1946) berechnen, im wesentlichen aus Daten von GUDZENT (1928), die in Tab. 1 aufgeführten Werte.

Die Tabelle zeigt die zwischen pH 6 und 7 rasch zunehmende Löslichkeit; der bei pH 8 errechnete Wert ist dagegen nicht reell, da eine Uratlösung nur durch Alkaliüberschuß auf pH 8 gebracht werden kann, so daß die Löslichkeit verringert wird. Tatsächlich ist für den normalen Harn die eingesetzte Löslichkeit ohnehin zu hoch veranschlagt, da der Harn reichlich Alkaliionen enthält.

Während die Voraussetzungen für die Ausfällung von Harnsäure im Harn noch etwas komplizierter sind als aus der bisherigen Darstellung hervorgeht, da die Neigung der Urate, übersättigte Lösungen zu bilden, noch berücksichtigt werden muß (s. unten), eignen sich die beschriebenen Beziehungen, die für eine Wiederauflösung von ausgefällter Harnsäure möglichen Verfahren, nämlich Verringerung der Ausscheidung, Alkalisierung und Verdünnung, gegeneinander abzuwägen; mit einer Wiederauflösung ist nur zu rechnen, wenn die Konzentration der im Harn (oder Körperwasser) vorhandenen freien Harnsäure und Urate geringer als die echte Löslichkeit ist.

Eine Verringerung der Harnsäureausscheidung und damit ihrer Konzentration im Harn läßt sich durch diätetische oder medikamentöse Maßnahmen erreichen. An dieser Stelle bringt ihre Besprechung keine wichtigen Gesichtspunkte.

Alkalisierung durch Zufuhr z.B. von Natrium- und Kaliumcitrat führt eine Verbesserung der Gesamtlöslichkeit herbei. Dabei ist eine Alkalisierung über pH 7 (6,5—7,5) unnötig, da jenseits dieses Bereiches der notwendigerweise zunehmende Alkaliionenüberschuß die Löslichkeit von Urat zunehmend verringert.

Theoretisch interessanter ist die Verringerung der Harnsäurekonzentration durch Wasserzufuhr. Da die Löslichkeit der Urationen, wie erwähnt, durch das Löslichkeitsprodukt K_s, begrenzt ist:

$$(Na^\oplus) \times (Urat^\ominus) = K_s,$$

kann durch Senkung der Konzentration der Natriumionen (im Beispiel auf die Hälfte, zunächst ohne Änderung des Volumens) die Uratkonzentration erhöht (im Beispiel verdoppelt) werden:

$$\frac{(Na^\oplus)}{2} \times 2\,(Urat^\ominus) = K_s.$$

Wurde die Senkung der Natriumkonzentration durch Zugabe von Wasser (durch Diurese) erreicht (wurde also im Beispiel das Volumen verdoppelt), so kann im größeren (doppelten) Volumen noch mehr (noch einmal doppelt so viel) Urat gelöst werden; insgesamt ist also bei Verdoppelung der Harnmenge durch Diurese viermal so viel Urat lösbar wie in der Ausgangsmenge. Wie man sich leicht überzeugen kann, ist das berechnete Beispiel ein Sonderfall der Regel, daß im Rahmen der Gesamtharnsäurelöslichkeit die Uratlöslichkeit bei Harnverdünnung mit dem Quadrat des Volumens zunimmt.

Urate haben die Eigentümlichkeit, übersättigte Lösungen zu bilden, die recht stabil sind, und in denen — selbst bei Anwesenheit von Alkaliionen — die Löslichkeit des Natriumurates im Wasser überschritten werden kann. Alkalische Reaktionen begünstigen das Auftreten dieser übersättigten Lösungen, doch werden sie auch bei den üblichen pH-Werten des Harns gebildet. Kommt es bei Stehen solcher übersättigter Lösungen zur Aufhebung des metastabilen Zustandes, so verschiebt sich das Gleichgewicht in der folgenden Beziehung nach rechts und je nach pH-Wert und Alkaliionenkonzentration kommt es zur Ausfällung von Uraten oder freier Harnsäure.

Urate in über-   ⟶ Urate in echter Lösung   ⇌ abhängig   freie Harnsäure
sättigter Lösung   ↓   vom pH   in echter Lösung
                         Ausfällung bei höherer   ↓
                         Alkaliionenkonzentra-   Ausfällung bei
                         tion und höheren pH-   niederen pH-
                         Werten   Werten

In einem Harn mit einem pH = pK'_{Urat} = 5,8 sind die Konzentrationen von Uraten und freier Harnsäure gleich. Ist die Natriumkonzentration so groß wie die im Plasma, so ist auch die Löslichkeit von Uraten und freier Harnsäure ungefähr gleich. Unterhalb von pH 5,8 überwiegt unter diesen Bedingungen die freie Harnsäure, so daß bei zu hoher Gesamtharnsäurekonzentration vorwiegend die freie Form ausfällt, oberhalb liegen mehr Urate vor, die dann den Niederschlag bilden. Ist die Alkaliionenkonzentration geringer, so verschiebt sich unter Zunahme der Gesamtlöslichkeit der Harnsäure die pH-Grenze, die bestimmt, ob Harnsäure oder Urate ausfallen, nach oben.

c) Spezielle Fragen der Entstehung der Gichtniere

Die Gichtniere ist gekennzeichnet durch interstitielle und intratubuläre Harnsäureausfällungen, glomeruläre und tubuläre Veränderungen verschiedener Art, Pyelonephritis, Hyalinose und Sklerose der Nierengefäße sowie Nephrolithiasis.

Die zur Gichtniere führenden Harnsäureausfällungen kommen sowohl im Tubuluslumen als auch im Interstitium zustande (MAYNE, 1956; SOKOLOFF, 1957; TALBOTT u. TERPLAN, 1960; MUNCK, 1966). Es hat zwar nicht an Stimmen gefehlt, die auf Grund gewisser Experimente die Ansicht verfochten, daß die Harnsäureausfällungen in der Niere primär immer intratubulär erfolgen, aber das Schwergewicht der Argumente spricht doch für zwei verschiedene Orte und Arten. Schon ASCHOFF hat klar beschrieben, daß die interstitielle Harnsäureausfällung weiß, die in den harnbereitenden Tubuli gelblich ist. SOKOLOFF (1957) gibt an, daß die gelben, vornehmlich bei Leukämie auftretenden Ablagerungen amorph, die bei Gicht dagegen kristallin seien. Aus den oben diskutierten Gründen (pH, interstitielle Natriumkonzentrationen) ist es wahrscheinlich, daß die interstitiellen Ablagerungen aus Natriumurat bestehen, die intratubulären Niederschläge vorwiegend aus freier Harnsäure (PRIEN u. FRONDEL, 1947).

Kommt es bei akuter Ausfällung von Harnsäure zur Tubulus-Blockade durch zylinderartige Ausgüsse der Sammelröhren, so führt dies zur Hemmung der glomerulären Filtration und selbst zur Anurie. In akuten, experimentell erzeugten Läsionen bei Hunden und Ratten fanden DUNCAN et al. (1963) Dilatation der distalen Tubuli und selbst der Glomerula, nachdem früher bereits DUNN u. POLSON (1926) sowie SMITH u. LEE (1957) an Kaninchen entsprechende Befunde erhoben hatten. Die injizierten Mengen waren jedoch immer erheblich (100—1000 mg/kg); entsprechend viel Harnsäure wird beim Menschen höchstens gelegentlich während der energischen Behandlung einer Hämoblastose freigesetzt. Dennoch glauben DUNCAN et al. (1963), daß ihre Versuche auch ein Modell für die Gichtniere seien und geben an, daß die primär intraluminären Niederschläge durch Degeneration des Tubulusepithels mit nachfolgender Fibrose zu interstitiellen Uratablagerungen werden können. Ähnliche Ansichten äußern WALLACE u. BERNSTEIN (1963).

Die Uratausfällung im Interstitium der Niere ist sicher ein komplizierterer Vorgang als in den extracellulären Räumen anderer Gewebe, in denen sowohl die Uratkonzentration als auch die Konzentrationen von Natrium und Kalium denen im Plasmawasser entsprechen und verhältnismäßig konstant sind. Ob die Uratkonzentration an allen Stellen des Interstitiums der Niere vorwiegend von der Harnsäurekonzentration im Plasma oder im Tubuluslumen abhängt, ist noch unbestimmt. Darüber hinaus kann die Ausfällung durch zwei weitere Variable beeinflußt werden, nämlich die Konzentrationen von Natrium und Wasserstoffionen.

Die Pyelonephritis wird gewöhnlich als Folge einer Nephrolithiasis, eventuell einer intratubulären Harnsäureausfällung angesehen, so z. B. von BROWN u. MALLORY (1950), welche annehmen, daß die in den Sammelröhrchen bzw. Tubuli vorhandenen Uratkristalle zur Pyelonephritis prädisponieren. Tatsächlich gelingt es auch, durch Tierversuche diese Annahme wahrscheinlich zu machen; SMITH u. LEE (1957) fanden bei der experimentellen „Harnsäurenephritis" die ersten Veränderungen an den Sammelröhren. RICHET et al. (1961) gaben an, die am besten definierten Veränderungen der Gichtniere, nämlich eine „aufsteigende interstitielle Nephritis" zusammen mit Tubulusatrophie und interstitieller Fibrose vornehmlich bei Nephrolithiasis festgestellt zu haben. Trotz dieser guten Argumente müssen die Schlußfolgerungen, denen sich viele Pathologen angeschlossen haben, bezweifelt werden, da einerseits, wie bereits erwähnt, die experimentellen Läsionen unter Bedingungen zustandekommen, die den bei der Gicht herrschenden nicht entsprechen, andererseits autoptische Befunde erfahrungsgemäß leicht zur Überwertung der finalen Ereignisse führen. Tatsächlich wurde im autoptischen Material von TALBOTT u. TERPLAN (1960) die Pyelonephritis auch bei Fällen mit minimalen Nierenveränderungen, wo sie schwer als Folge chronischer Harnstauung zu erklären ist, fast immer gefunden.

LOUYOT et al. (1959) beobachteten in Nierenpunktionen interstitielle Entzündungen mit cellulären Infiltraten in 12 von 22 Fällen, von denen bei dreien die Tubulusepithelien normal waren; bei den übrigen bestand dagegen eine gute Übereinstimmung zwischen dem Vorkommen entzündlicher Veränderungen im Interstitium und abgeplatteten Epithelien bzw. Dilatation der Tubuli. Bei der Punktion sehr früher Fälle fanden GREENBAUM et al. (1961) dagegen ausschließlich eine interstitielle Fibrose. Faßt man diese Befunde zusammen, so wird man die Häufigkeit der Pyelonephritis eher einer primären Schädigung der Niere durch die interstitielle Harnsäureablagerung als einer Nephrolithiasis bzw. anderen, die Tubuli obstruierenden Harnsäureausfällungen zuschreiben, man nehme denn an, daß die Obstruktion der intrarenalen Harnwege bei der Gicht ein nahezu obligatorisches Ereignis sei.

Glomeruläre Veränderungen fanden GREENBAUM et al. (1961) in neun von zwölf Fällen, LOUYOT et al. (1963) in 21 von 22 Fällen. Im allgemeinen stimmen die Prüfungen der Nierenfunktion gut mit den Punktionsergebnissen überein, leichte glomeruläre Veränderungen gehen mit normaler Nierenfunktion einher, während bei schweren Veränderungen bereits Einschränkungen der Nierenfunktion festgestellt werden können.

Die Pathogenese der Harnsäureausfällung bei der Gicht wird in den meisten Fällen nicht, wie man zunächst annehmen mag, durch eine vermehrte Harnsäureausscheidung und eine dadurch erhöhte Harnsäurekonzentration im Endharn erklärt: Bei der Mehrzahl der Gichtiker ist die Tagesausscheidung von Harnsäure normal oder wenig erhöht, GUTMAN u. YÜ (1957) fanden nur bei 6% der Gichtiker eine Tagesausscheidung über 800 mg. (Damit steht die Harnsäuresteinbildung in einem Gegensatz zu der Harnsäureurolithiasis bei Leukämien und anderen, mit vermehrtem Zellumsatz einhergehenden Hämoblastosen.) Die erwähnte Häufigkeit des anatomischen Befundes einer intratubulären Harnsäureausfällung spricht dafür, daß die entscheidenden Präcipitationsvorgänge weiter harnstromaufwärts erfolgen. (Da der Endharn ohnehin eine übersättigte Harnsäurelösung darstellt, ist mit einer Wiederauflösung einmal ausgefallener Harnsäure bei üblichen pH-Werten und Harnmengen nicht zu rechnen.)

Der für die Harnsäureausfällung verantwortliche Unterschied zwischen Normalpersonen und Patienten mit familiärer Hyperuricämie besteht wahrscheinlich in der höheren Harnsäurekonzentration im Primärharn der letzteren. Folgt man der Theorie, daß bei der familiären Hyperuricämie ein Defekt der tubulären Harnsäuresekretion vorliegt und normalerweise Harnsäure sowohl im proximalen als auch distalen Tubulus sezerniert wird, so müssen zwischen Normalpersonen und familiären Hyperuricämikern nicht nur in den proximalen Tubulusabschnitten, sondern auch in den Schleifen deutliche Unterschiede der Harnsäurekonzentration angenommen werden (Abb. 5).

Als weiterer pathogenetischer Mechanismus für die Harnsäureausfällung kommt eine im Vergleich zum Gesunden stärkere Säuerung des Harns in Frage. COTTET (1961) hat bei Gicht den pH-Wert des Harns von Patienten mit Harnsäurelithiasis im Mittel um 0,2 niedriger als bei Patienten ohne Steine gefunden, doch sind die Unterschiede nicht überzeugend und andere Ursachen nicht ausgeschlos-

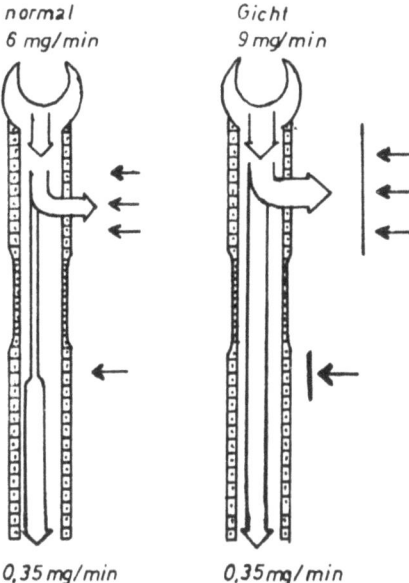

Abb. 5. Schema der renalen Harnsäureausscheidung bei der Gicht (familiäre Hyperuricämie) im Vergleich zu den normalen Verhältnissen

sen. Es mag dennoch sein, daß eine alimentär bedingte Harnacidose bei der Gicht am Zustandekommen der Harnsäureausfällung mitwirkt; als alleiniger Faktor kommt sie aber wohl nicht in Frage.

Anders mögen die Verhältnisse bei der von HENNEMAN et al. (1962) beschriebenen nicht gichtischen, vererblichen Harnsäurelithiasis liegen, bei der im Harn sehr niedrige pH-Werte regelmäßig gefunden werden. Weitere Untersuchungen zu diesem interessanten Krankheitsbild stammen von ATSMON et al. (1960) sowie DE VRIES et al. (1962). Trotz intensiver Bemühungen konnte der metabolische Defekt, der zu dem niedrigen pH-Wert führt, aber noch nicht aufgeklärt werden. HENNEMAN et al. machen eine erniedrigte Ammoniumausscheidung dafür verantwortlich, während DE VRIES et al. Vermehrungen der Phosphatausscheidung bei ihren Patienten fanden.

Als Zusatzursache für die Bildung von Harnsäuresteinen bei der Gicht und anderen Leiden werden immer wieder Besonderheiten einer Matrix beschrieben. Inwiefern es bei einem klar definierten metabolischen Grundleiden bzw. im Zusammenhang mit anderen, zur Hyperuricämie führenden Krankheiten, gleichzeitig zur typischen Bildung einer Matrix kommen soll, ist nicht recht verständlich.

4. Mutmaßlicher Verlauf der Gichtniere

Die Nierenbiopsien zeigen, daß morphologisch faßbare Veränderungen der Niere bei der Gicht schon frühzeitig auftreten können, bei einer Reihe von Fällen wahrscheinlich bereits vor dem ersten Gelenkanfall. Dabei ist die Nierenfunktion zunächst meist normal, um später, mit dem Fortschreiten der histologisch faßbaren Veränderungen, sich zu verschlechtern.

Hyalinisierung oder selbst Sklerose der Glomerula sowie tubuläre Veränderungen dürften die erste Läsion sein, die sich in der Niere des Gichtikers entwickelt, denn diese Veränderungen werden am häufigsten gefunden, kommen bereits bei verhältnismäßig jungen Patienten vor und treten in Nieren auf, in denen weder Gefäßveränderungen noch interstitielle entzündliche Reaktionen nachweisbar sind. Für solche Fälle hat TUROLLA (1960) den Begriff der gichtischen Glomerulonephrose eingeführt.

Die Gefäßveränderungen treten im allgemeinen später auf, wenngleich auch Fälle vorkommen, in denen sie das Bild beherrschen und vermutlich von vornherein beherrscht haben. Die Mehrzahl der Patienten, bei denen das vorkommt, sind jedoch verhältnismäßig alte Personen (über 55 Jahre mit langer Gichtanamnese). Ihre frühere Ansicht (1959), daß Gefäßveränderungen frühzeitig auftreten, haben LOUYOT et al. zurückgenommen.

Der Befall des Interstitiums hängt offensichtlich von der Dauer der Gicht ab, selbst wenn manchmal bei kurzer Gichtanamnese Veränderungen gefunden werden. Gelegentlich beherrscht die interstitielle Reaktion sogar das Bild und der Ausdruck interstitielle Gichtnephritis wird berechtigt. Von LOUYOT et al. (1963) wird bezweifelt, ob die Entwicklung der interstitiellen Nephritis mit Gefäßveränderungen, mit Harnsäureausfällungen im Interstitium bzw. mit einer Mikrolithiasis oder Uratablagerung im Mark und darauffolgender Harnstauung in Zusammenhang gebracht werden kann. Die Autoren halten es für wahrscheinlicher, daß die Reaktion des Bindegewebes dem Auftreten von Harnsäuredepots in Form größerer Ablagerungen vorausgeht und sehen in ihr eine direkte Folge der hohen interstitiellen Harnsäurekonzentration. Gemeinsam mit FAHR (1925) sowie TALBOTT u. TERPLAN (1960) halten wir es für wahrscheinlich, daß Mikrokristalle auftreten, welche für die Irritation und anschließende Reaktion des interstitiellen Gewebes und der Tubuluszellen verantwortlich sind.

II. Symptomatologie und Diagnose

1. Symptomatologie

Von den meisten Autoren wird eine strenge Unterteilung zwischen den Befunden bei Kranken ohne und mit Nierensteinen gemacht, speziell von LOUYOT et al. (1963). Im Kollektiv scheinbar steinfreier Gichtkranker ist jedoch ein mehr oder weniger großer Prozentsatz von Patienten mit Nierensteinen enthalten, ohne daß man beim Auftreten der ersten Kolik sagen könnte, wie lang vorher bereits eine Nephrolithiasis bestanden hat. Aus diesem Grund hat die genannte Aufteilung nur begrenzten Wert.

a) Häufigkeit der Nephrolithiasis bei Gicht

Die Angaben über die Häufigkeit der Nephrolithiasis bei der Gicht liegen zwischen 5 und 40%. Die Mehrzahl der Autoren gibt etwa 20% an.

Der Vergleich der Angaben ist schwierig. Wird der röntgenologische Steinnachweis der Beurteilung zugrundegelegt, so entgehen viele Fälle der Diagnose, da kleine Harnsäurekonkremente weder einen positiven noch, bei der Pyelographie, einen negativen Kontrast geben. Auch die Angaben über die Häufigkeit von Steinkoliken sind, speziell bei späterer Auswertung von Krankenblättern, unzuverlässig und führen zu niederen Ergebnissen, es sei denn, daß nach der Steinsymptomatik gezielt gefragt wird. Aber selbst bei gezielter Anamneseerhebung sind Angaben über die Häufigkeit der Nephrolithiasis zum Zeitpunkt der ersten Untersuchung des Patienten seltener als in einem über längere Zeit beobachteten Krankengut, da erfahrungsgemäß viele Patienten ohne typische Kolikanamnese früher oder später doch noch an Nierensteinen mit Koliken erkranken. Angaben über eine Steinhäufigkeit von 5% sind sicher zu nieder, haben doch HAUGE u.

Tabelle 2. Häufigkeit wichtiger, auf die Niere verweisender Befunde bei Gicht in Prozenten der in Klammern angegebenen Zahl der Fälle

	Protein-urie	Hämat-urie	Leuko-cyturie	Cylin-drurie	Hyper-azotämie	Hyper-tonie
Williamson (1920)	45 (116)					
Schnitker u. Richter (1936)	31 (55)				38 (45)	
Brøchner-Mortensen (1941)	25 (100)				11 (100)	
Talbott u. Terplan (1960) (nach Krankengeschichten autoptischer Fälle)						
klinisch leichte Gicht	77 (69)	43 (69)			54 (65)	57 (68)
schwere tophöse Gicht	81 (32)	50 (32)			78 (32)	61 (33)
Ravault u. Viala (1960)	29 (103)					
Louyot et al. (1963)	42 (150)	63 (27)	74 (27)	17 (150)	19 (136)	40 (140)
Eigene Werte bis 1965	35 (122)	45 (122)	33 (122)	4 (122)		28 (122)
Zöllner u. Schattenkirchner (1966)	36 (22)	41 (22)	55 (22)	0 (22)		55 (22)
Tcherdakoff (1973)	11,4 (42)	6 (28)	9,4 (32)			23 (30)

Harvald (1955) in der Verwandtschaft (!) von Gichtkranken bereits eine Häufigkeit von 9% festgestellt; bei den hyperuricämischen, eventuell gichtischen Familienmitgliedern muß die Häufigkeit wesentlich höher liegen. In unserem Krankengut ist die klinisch aus der Kolikanamnese diagnostizierte Nephrolithiasis mit 41% von 122 Fällen häufiger als in den meisten anderen Statistiken. Spezielle Erwähnung verdient dennoch die Häufigkeit der Steinanamnese bereits beim ersten Gichtanfall; hier ist es allerdings besonders nötig, nach Einleitung der ersten Therapie, die natürlich vorgeht, eine genaue Anamnese zu erheben. Eine Nachuntersuchung dieser Frage von Zöllner u. Schattenkirchner ergab in einer 1965 begonnenen Serie von 22 Patienten eine Häufigkeit von 41% (vgl. Tab. 2).

Inwieweit unsere eigenen Zahlen für alle Patientenkollektive beweisen, daß die Nephrolithiasis bei Gicht häufiger ist als dies meist angegeben wird, ist noch eingehender zu prüfen. Die Gicht im Nachkriegsdeutschland stellt einen Sonderfall dar, insofern als bei der bis zur Währungsreform ausgehungerten Bevölkerung eine reichliche Purinzufuhr nach diesem Zeitpunkt eine größere Rolle als üblich gespielt haben dürfte und man deshalb eine besonders hohe Purinzufuhr als zusätzliche Ursache der Steinkrankheit diskutieren muß.

b) Proteinurie

Eine geringe Proteinurie ist häufig, sie wird in etwa einem Drittel der Fälle gefunden. Nicht in allen Fällen ist sie konstant festzustellen, sie kann kommen und gehen.

Proteinurie vor dem ersten Gichtanfall ist in der Literatur mehrfach beschrieben, und auch wir verfügen über eine einschlägige Beobachtung. Es ist deshalb

Tabelle 3. Häufigkeit von wichtigsten Harnbefunden und Blutdruckerhöhungen bei Gichtkranken mit und ohne Urolithiasis (Fälle von ZÖLLNER u. SCHATTENKIRCHNER, 1966)

	Gichtkranke mit Urolithiasis	Gichtkranke ohne Urolithiasis	Gesamtes Krankengut mit Gicht
Zahl der Patienten	9	13	22
Eiweiß			
Spur	1 (11,1%)	2 (15,4%)	3 (13,6%)
reichlich	4 (44,4%)	1 (7,7%)	5 (22,5%)
zusammen	5 (55,5%)	3 (23,1%)	8 (36,1%)
Zylinder	0 (0 %)	0 (0 %)	0 (0 %)
Erythrocyten			
vereinzelt	3 (33,3%)	2 (15,4%)	5 (22,5%)
reichlich	4 (44,4%)	0 (0 %)	4 (18,2%)
zusammen	7 (77,7%)	2 (15,4%)	9 (40,7%)
Leukocyten	5 (55,5%)	7 (53,9%)	12 (54,6%)
Blutdruckerhöhung systolisch über 150 oder diastolisch über 95 mm Hg	5 (55,5%)	7 (53,9%)	12 (54,6%)

vermutlich zweckmäßig, bei der Suche nach der Ursache für eine anderweitig nicht erklärte Proteinurie den Harnsäurespiegel im Plasma bestimmen zu lassen und eine genaue Familienanamnese bezüglich Gichtanfällen und Steinkoliken in der Verwandtschaft zu erheben.

Von einigen Autoren wird auch die beim Gichtanfall auftretende Proteinurie auf die Gichtniere bezogen. So richtig es ist, daß die Proteinurie Schwankungen unterliegt, so wenig darf man eine ausschließlich während des Anfalles auftretende Eiweißausscheidung als Teil der Gichtnierensymptomatik ansehen; hier kommt ebenso eine febrile Albuminurie bzw. die Reaktion der Niere auf die akute Arthritis, die ja auch anderweitig schwere Allgemeinsymptome hervorrufen kann, in Frage.

c) Hämaturie

Die Häufigkeit der Hämaturie bei der nicht durch Steine komplizierten Gichtniere wird sehr unterschiedlich eingeschätzt. LOUYOT et al. (1963) fanden bei 17 von 27 Personen vermehrt Erythrocyten im Harn, bei drei davon war die Erythrocytenausscheidung reichlich. REUBI u. VORBURGER (1962) geben an, daß eine Mikrohämaturie auch im Harn von Patienten ohne Lithiasis „eventuell" auftreten könne. Wir (ZÖLLNER u. SCHATTENKIRCHNER, 1966) fanden bei Patienten ohne Hinweis auf das Vorliegen von Steinen in 15% der Fälle vereinzelte Erythrocyten (Tab. 3).

Ob die bei der Gichtniere beobachtete Hämaturie Vorbote der Lithiasis oder Ausdruck einer Glomerulumschädigung ist, läßt sich im Einzelfall nur durch längere Krankenbeobachtung klären. Von vielen französischen Autoren wird die Hämaturie bereits als Beweis für das Vorliegen einer Mikrolithiasis angesehen. Andere französische Autoren leugnen diesen Zusammenhang und beziehen Fälle von Hämaturie auf die „Gichtnephritis".

d) Leukocyturie

Auch über den Zeitpunkt des Auftretens der Leukocyten im Harn besteht keine Einigkeit. REUBI u. VORBURGER (1962) halten die Leukocyturie für das

Symptom einer Pyelonephritis, für deren Auftreten nach ihrer Ansicht eine Nephrolithiasis notwendig ist, während LOUYOT et al. bei 20 von 27 Personen vermehrt Leukocyten, wenn auch in 16 davon keine ausgeprägte Leukocyturie als Ausdruck der „Gichtnephritis" finden. Unserer eigenen Erfahrung nach findet man Leukocyturie bei Patienten mit und ohne Steinen gleich häufig (Tab. 3). Grundsätzlich ist, wenn man die pathologischen Befunde erwägt, gar nicht zu erwarten, daß bei allen Fällen von gichtischer Pyelonephritis ein Steinbefall vorliegt.

e) Cylindrurie

Auch dieses Symptom kann verhältnismäßig früh auftreten. Die Häufigkeitsangaben in der Literatur liegen unter 20%, wir fanden Cylinder nur selten, möglicherweise weil wir unsere Patienten zu reichlicher Flüssigkeitsaufnahme anhalten.

Die Cylinder sind im allgemeinen hyalin oder granuliert, gelegentlich kommen Erythrocytencylinder vor, welche selbstverständlich eine andere Bedeutung haben.

Nach REUBI u. VORBURGER (1962) werden die Cylinder bei Albuminurie gefunden, während LOUYOT et al. (1963) in einem Drittel ihrer Fälle mit Cylindern keine Albuminurie feststellen konnten. Ein Zusammentreffen von Cylindrurie und Leukocyturie bzw. Hämaturie scheint nicht häufiger zu sein, als es dem Zufall entspricht.

Trotz der nicht vollständigen Koinzidenz mit der Albuminurie wird man dem Befund von Cylindern wohl die gleiche Bedeutung zumessen. Dementsprechend ist es empfehlenswert, in Fällen ungeklärter Cylindrurie an eine Gichtniere zu denken.

f) Nierenfunktionsproben

Von den meisten Autoren wird betont, daß Einschränkungen der Nierenfunktion verhältnismäßig spät auftreten. Nur rund ein Viertel der Patienten starben früher an der Niereninsuffizienz (TALBOTT u. TERPLAN, 1960). Ödeme kommen bei der unkomplizierten Gichtniere nicht vor, sondern treten nur im Zusammenhang mit einer Herzinsuffizienz auf.

Die Angaben der verschiedenen Untersucher über die Häufigkeit einer Harnstofferhöhung im Blut liegen zwischen 7 und 38%, sieht man von den Angaben von TALBOTT u. TERPLAN (1960) ab. Diese Prozentwerte hängen offensichtlich von den besonderen Interessen der jeweiligen Untersucher ab; verständlicherweise sind sie bei Patienten aus Arthritiskliniken niedriger als bei den Fällen von Nephrologen.

Über die Clearance verschiedener Substanzen bei der Gicht liegt ein reiches Material vor auf Grund der vielen Untersuchungen zur Frage der renalen Pathogenese der Krankheit. GUTMAN u. YÜ (1957) haben bei 150 Gichtkranken ohne erkennbarer Nierenbeteiligung die Inulinclearance bestimmt; in einem Drittel der Fälle lag sie unter 90 ml/min, in einem Sechstel unter 80 ml/min. Auch die PAH-Clearance wurde häufig verringert gefunden. GUTMAN u. YÜ (1957) glauben allerdings, daß die Einschränkung der Inulinclearance das altersübliche Maß bei ihren verhältnismäßig alten Patienten nicht überschreitet, während sie für die Verringerung der PAH-Clearance die gichtischen Nierenveränderungen verantwortlich machen.

Im Gegensatz zu den Clearance-Untersuchungen ist die Phenolrotprobe bei der Gichtniere bisher kaum systematisch untersucht worden. LOUYOT et al. (1963) geben eine verringerte Phenolrotausscheidung in 41% der Fälle an.

g) Symptome der akuten Pyelonephritis

Symptome der akuten Pyelonephritis wie Leukocyturie, Empfindlichkeit der Nierenlager, rasche Blutkörperchensenkung sind selten. Häufigkeit und Symptome der chronischen Pyelonephritis wurden bereits abgehandelt. Zu ergänzen bleibt der Hinweis, daß eine chronisch leicht beschleunigte Blutkörperchensenkung das Augenmerk in diese Richtung lenken sollte, während Pyelogramme wegen der Häufigkeit der Lithiasis nicht immer eindeutig zu beurteilen sind.

h) Hypertonie

Die Angaben über die Häufigkeit der Hypertonie hängen wieder weitgehend von der Frage ab, ob das ausgezählte Krankengut im Querschnitt beurteilt wurde oder ob der Beurteilung Verlaufsbeobachtungen zugrunde liegen. Hierauf weist GUDZENT (1928) hin, der 17 Kranke beschreibt, die er über viele Jahre beobachtet hat. Von diesen Kranken hatten bei der ersten Untersuchung fünf eine Hypertonie. Von den zwölf Kranken mit normalem Blutdruck entwickelten sieben eine unter seiner Beobachtung allmählich ansteigende Blutdruckerhöhung; der Anteil der Hypertoniker bei diesen Patienten stieg also von 30% auf 70%. Für sein Gesamtkrankengut von 78 Fällen (ausschließlich Männer) gibt GUDZENT eine Hypertoniehäufigkeit von 40% bei der Erstuntersuchung an. Keiner der Hypertoniker war jünger als 40 Jahre, aber bereits im 6. Lebensjahrzehnt überwogen die Hypertoniker die Normotoniker im Verhältnis 19:15, im 7. Lebensjahrzehnt 13:5. Neuere Statistiken s. Hypertoniekapitel.

Die Häufigkeit der Hypertonie bei der Gicht wird weiterhin durch die Tatsache unterstrichen, daß ein großer Prozentsatz der Gichtiker an Gefäßkomplikationen stirbt (TALBOTT u. LILIENFELD, 1959; REUBI u. VORBURGER, 1962; SCHNITKER u. RICHTER, 1936). Wahrscheinlich spielen beim Zustandekommen der gichtischen Arteriosklerose auch Störungen des Lipoidstoffwechsels eine Rolle. Fettstoffwechselstörungen werden bei Gichtpatienten gehäuft angetroffen (s. Kapitel Klinische Wertigkeit der Hyperuricämie, Beziehung zu anderen Krankheiten).

2. Diagnose

Bis vor etwa 25 Jahren war es vornehmlich von akademischem Interesse, die Diagnose einer Gichtniere rechtzeitig zu stellen, da eine kausale Behandlung nicht möglich und für eine symptomatische Behandlung die Diagnose nicht nötig war. Dies hat sich bereits durch die Einführung der Uricosurica geändert (PHILLIPS, 1955; TALBOTT u. TERPLAN, 1960; ZÖLLNER, 1963a), so daß heute die rechtzeitige Erkennung der Ätiologie einer „renalen Arteriosklerose", einer Pyelonephritis, einer Urolithiasis für die Gesundheit des Patienten von Bedeutung ist.

Bei jedem der genannten Nierenleiden sollte man die Gichtniere in die differentialdiagnostischen Erwägungen aufnehmen. Ganz besonders gilt dies, wenn eine anderweitig nicht erklärte Hämaturie besteht, wenn der Patient ein verhältnismäßig junger Mann ist oder wenn gar die Anamnese eines Gichtanfalles erhoben werden kann. Leider vergessen viele Patienten ihre Gicht im Intervall oder halten deren Angabe dem Nephrologen gegenüber für unwichtig. Nicht selten stehen klassische Gichtanfälle unter anderer Bezeichnung oder unter Fehldiagnosen in Behandlung, so daß es nötig ist, ganz allgemein nach akuten Gelenk- oder Fußbeschwerden zu fragen. Manchmal ist die Anamnese selbst dann leer; die Gichtniere geht der gichtischen Arthritis voraus. Hier kann eine Familienanamnese, in der gehäuft Gicht oder Urolithiasis vorkommen, noch wichtige diagnostische Fingerzeige ergeben. Zum mutmaßlichen Ausschluß der Diagnose Gichtniere kann dienen, daß bei Frauen vor der Menopause die Hyperuricämie sehr selten ist (RAKIC et al., 1964).

Die wichtigste diagnostische Maßnahme ist die Bestimmung der Serumharnsäure. Genaue Werte sind ausschließlich von einer enzymatischen Methode zu erwarten (ZÖLLNER, 1963b). Erhöhte Harnsäurewerte bei normalen oder nahezu normalen Nierenfunktionen sind, wenn man von einigen seltenen Stoffwechselkrankheiten absieht (vgl. ZÖLLNER, 1960), Ausdruck der familiären Hyperuricämie oder Folge vermehrten Zellumsatzes bei Hämoblastosen, proliferierenden Krankheiten des RHS, Bestrahlung oder Chemotherapie von Leukämien und Tumoren, massiver Chemotherapie anderer Krankheiten, sowie ausgedehnten entzündlichen Prozessen. Bei all diesen Krankheiten kann, vorausgesetzt, daß die Hyperuricämie längere Zeit anhält, die eine oder andere Form der Nierenschädigung durch Harnsäure entstehen.

Letzte Klarheit kann nur die Nierenbiopsie bringen. Hierzu hat man sich bislang nur selten entschlossen, da aus der Sicherstellung der Diagnose keine wesentlichen therapeutischen Konsequenzen erwuchsen. Seitdem die Gichtniere einer kausalen Therapie zugänglich ist, mag man sich etwas häufiger zur Nierenpunktion entschließen. Richtlinien hierzu sind erst nach weiteren Erfahrungen möglich.

Steht die klassische Gicht mit Gelenkbefall im Vordergrund der Beschwerden, so ist eine Nierendiagnostik dennoch indiziert. Wiederholte Analysen des Harns und bei Verdacht auf Nierensteine auch eine Pyelographie sind grundsätzliche Anforderungen, die gegebenenfalls durch Nierenfunktionsprüfungen zu ergänzen sind. Aus der Art der Befunde wird man gewisse Rückschlüsse auf die Art der vorherrschenden Läsion ziehen dürfen; wie zuverlässig diese Rückschlüsse sind, werden erst weitere klinisch-pathologische Studien mit Nierenbiopsien ergeben.

Bei fortgeschrittener Gichtniere mit einer Einschränkung der glomerulären Filtrationsrate auf weniger als 50% finden sich im i.v.-Pyelogramm nach KRÖPELIN u. MERTZ (1972) charakteristische röntgenologische Zeichen. Typisch sind nach diesen Autoren im Hilusbereich um die Kelche verlaufende, bis zur Rindenregion reichende unregelmäßig begrenzte rinnenförmige Aufhellungsbezirke. Ihnen entspricht pathologisch-anatomisch eine — besonders im inneren Markraum vorhandene — diffuse zellarme Sklerose. Weiterhin weisen die Autoren auf spezielle röntgenologische Papillenveränderungen bei der Gichtniere hin, die die Abgrenzung von einer infektiös-toxischen Papillennekrose erlauben sollen.

III. Verlauf und Prognose

Der Verlauf der Gichtniere kann als verhältnismäßig gutartig bezeichnet werden, da die Lebensdauer vom Auftreten der ersten Symptome bis zu den zum Tode führenden finalen Komplikationen meist lang ist; die Hälfte aller Patienten mit Gichtniere stirbt nicht an dieser Krankheit oder kardiovasculären Ereignissen, sondern an anderen Krankheiten (TALBOTT u. TERPLAN, 1960). Welcher Prozentsatz der kardiovasculären Ereignisse auf die Gichtniere zurückzuführen ist, ist schwer zu entscheiden. Da kein Hinweis auf andere zur Hypertonie führende Mechanismen bei der Gicht gefunden werden kann, wird man die mit der Hypertonie in Verbindung stehenden Kreislaufkrankheiten der Gichtiker als renal bedingt ansehen dürfen. Andererseits ist bei der Gicht auch die Hyperlipoidämie häufig. Weiterhin hängt bei den meisten Patienten die Manifestation der Gicht von einem gewissen Wohlleben ab, welches auch auf andere Weise die Gefäßprognose ungünstig beeinflussen kann.

Die Lebenserwartung von Patienten mit Gichtniere wird von GUDZENT (1928) anhand von 43 Fällen (unter Ausschluß von Patienten, die an interkurrenten Krankheiten starben, bei denen von 39 Fällen die Todesursache mit der Niere in Zusammenhang gestanden hatte) als deutlich verkürzt angegeben. Sechs seiner Patienten starben vor dem 44. Lebensjahr, 19 vor dem 55. und nur 11 überschritten das 65. Von den 19 Gichtkranken, die nur das 55. Lebensjahr erreichten, starben 11 an „Schrumpfniere" und 3 an Gefäßsklerose mit starker Nierenbeteiligung. Patienten ohne erkennbare Nierenbeteiligung (im zitierten Material eine kleine Minderzahl) wurden wesentlich älter. Im Gegensatz zu GUDZENT geben COOMBS et al. (1940) an, daß das Fortschreiten zur kritischen Niereninsuffizienz extrem langsam sei und die Lebensdauer wenig beeinträchtige. Zu einer ähnlichen Stellungnahme kommen aus dem gleichen Arbeitskreis TALBOTT und LILIENFELD (1959). Auch CURSCHMANN (1944) beurteilt die Prognose der Gicht als sehr günstig, wenngleich seine Angaben mehr auf der Beobachtung von Einzelfällen zu beruhen scheinen. Bis zur Mitteilung zuverlässiger Ergebnisse wird man es bei diesen Angaben bewenden lassen müssen. Die Angaben der amerikanischen Autoren berechtigen aber wohl doch zu dem Schluß, daß bei jeweils ähnlicher Symptomatologie die Gichtniere eine günstigere Prognose als andere chronische Nierenaffektionen hat. Neuere Ergebnisse s. Prognosekapitel.

IV. Therapie

Sieht man von den Maßnahmen ab, welche sich gegen die Folgen der Gichtniere, Infektion, chirurgische Komplikationen der Lithiasis und Hypertonie richten, so bleiben als spezielle Behandlung der Gichtniere Verordnungen, die darauf hinzielen, die Harnsäurekonzentrationen im Plasma und Interstitium, im Tubuluslumen und im Harn zu senken mit dem Ziel, Ausfällungen im Gewebe und im Tubuluslumen sowie Steine in den Kelchen und im Becken wieder aufzulösen; die bloße Verhinderung weiterer Ablagerungen ist nur ein Zwischenziel.

Durch Erfahrungen mit der den Plasmaharnsäurespiegel senkenden uricosurischen Therapie ist sichergestellt, daß im Gewebe ausgefallene Harnsäure wieder aufgelöst und abtransportiert werden kann, selbst wenn die Tophi großen Umfang erreicht haben. Auch Harnsäuresteine im Nierenbecken können durch geeignete Maßnahmen vollständig aufgelöst werden.

1. Erniedrigung der Harnsäurekonzentrationen im Plasma und Interstitium

Für die Verringerung der Harnsäurekonzentration im Plasma und im Interstitium stehen grundsätzlich drei Möglichkeiten zur Verfügung, nämlich eine Einschränkung der Zufuhr von Harnsäurevorläufern mit der Nahrung, eine Beschleunigung der Harnsäureausscheidung durch die Niere und eine Hemmung der Harnsäurebildung aus ihren Vorläufern Hypoxanthin und Xanthin.

a) Einfluß der Diät auf den Harnsäurespiegel

Über die Bedeutung der Kostzusammensetzung für die Manifestation der Gicht kann kein Zweifel bestehen, nachdem die Erfahrungen vieler Kriege und Notzeiten in den meisten Gegenden der Erde die heilende Wirkung strenger Diät klar beweisen. Untersuchungen von GRIEBSCH u. ZÖLLNER (1970) zeigten, daß der Einfluß der Nahrungspurine auf Serumharnsäure und renale Harnsäureausscheidung von ihrem Gehalt an Ribonucleinsäure und Desoxyribonucleinsäure abhängt. Die mathematische Berechnung ihrer Ergebnisse ergab, daß bei gesunden Personen die orale Gabe von 1 g Ribonucleinsäure zu einer Erhöhung der Serumharnsäure um 0,9 mg-% führt, während unter der gleichen Dosis Desoxyribonucleinsäure der Anstieg nur 0,4 mg-% beträgt. Die Harnsäureausscheidung im Urin stieg dabei unter 1 g Ribonucleinsäure um 113 mg tgl., unter 1 g Desoxyribonucleinsäure dagegen nur um 68 mg tgl. an. Berücksichtigt man noch dazu, daß der Puringehalt meist für 100 g des Nahrungsmittels und nicht für 100 kcal (420 kJ) angegeben wird, so zeigt sich, daß die Lebensmitteltabellen im Hinblick auf die Purine nur begrenzten Wert haben.

ZÖLLNER u. KURZ (1966) beobachteten unter einer extrem eiweiß- und fettarmen Diät bei gesunden Personen einen Abfall der Serumharnsäure von 4,8 auf 3,1 mg-%. Nachuntersuchungen von GRÖBNER u. ZÖLLNER (1971) ergaben unter einer streng purinarmen isocalorischen Diät mit einem Purin-N von weniger als 10 mg/1000 kcal (10 mg/4200 kJ) und einer Eiweißzufuhr von 10 Energieprozent innerhalb von 10 Tagen einen Abfall des Serumharnsäurespiegels von 5,0 auf 3,8 mg-% sowie der renalen Harnsäureausscheidung von 500 auf 328 mg tgl. Die Diät reicht jedoch nur in seltenen Fällen aus, den Harnsäurespiegel von Gichtikern zu normalisieren, ganz abgesehen davon, daß wenige Patienten mit leichter Gicht (und für diese käme eine ausschließliche Diätbehandlung in erster Linie in Frage) eine Diät regelmäßig einhalten. So ist es zu erklären, daß zahlreiche Autoren (BAUER u. KLEMPERER, 1944; TALBOTT, 1957) auf die Diät zur Senkung der Harnsäurekonzentration im Plasma verzichten, wenn keine besonderen Umstände ihre Vorschrift nötig machen. Soll die Harnsäureausscheidung verringert werden, so kommt der Diät allerdings größere Bedeutung zu.

Überreichliche Fettzufuhr sowie langdauerndes Fasten führen im Zusammenhang mit der sich entwickelnden Ketose zur Verringerung der Harnsäureausscheidung und damit zu einer Hyperuricämie. Analoges gilt für die Zufuhr von Alkohol, durch die der Milchsäurespiegel erhöht und eine Hyperuricämie erzeugt wird.

b) Uricosurische Maßnahmen zur Senkung der Plasmaspiegel

Einfachste Maßnahme zur Vermehrung der renalen Harnsäureausscheidung ist die Erzeugung einer Wasserdiurese, da die Harnsäure bis zu einem "augmentation limit" von ca. 1 ml Harn pro Minute mit zunehmendem Harnvolumen zunehmend ausgeschieden wird. Die Flüssigkeitszufuhr muß also eine dermaßen hohe Harnproduktion während aller Tagesstunden erreichen. Abhängig von Beruf, Wohnung, Jahreszeit und Kost sind hierfür 1,5—2,5 Liter Trinkmenge täglich nötig.

Eine größere Zahl von Medikamenten erhöht durch Hemmung der tubulären Rückresorption die renale Harnsäureausscheidung. Unter diesen uricosurisch wirksamen Verbindungen haben Probenecid (Benemid®) und Sulfinpyrazon (Anturano®) schon lange festen Fuß in der Therapie gefaßt (ZÖLLNER, 1963c). Eine ausreichende und langanhaltende Wirkung wird auch durch Benzbromaronum (Uricovac®) erreicht (ZÖLLNER et al., 1968, 1970a, b, c; MERTZ, 1969). Diese Mittel senken den Plasmaharnsäurespiegel, wobei es, je nach Größe der Harnsäuredepots, zu einer kürzer oder länger dauernden Vermehrung der renalen Harnsäureausscheidung kommt (Abb. 6). Bei Normalpersonen mit einem Harnsäurepool von etwa 1000 mg dauert die Mehrausscheidung von Harnsäure bei fortgesetzter Gabe von Uricosurica nur einen, höchstens wenige Tage; anschließend halten sich der erreichte niedrigere Plasmaspiegel und die durch ihn bedingte Verminderung der Harnsäuremenge im Primärfiltrat einerseits und die Verringerung der Rückresorption andererseits in einem Gleichgewicht. Werden bei der Gicht durch

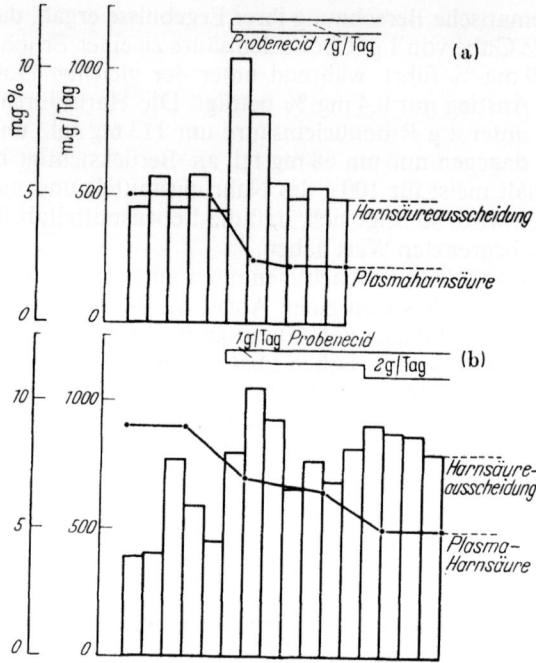

Abb. 6. Senkung der Plasmaharnsäure und Vermehrung der Harnsäureausscheidung unter der Verabreichung von Probenecid bei einer gesunden freiwilligen Versuchsperson (a) und bei einem Patienten mit Gicht (b) (eigene Versuche)

den Abfall der Plasmaharnsäure unter die Löslichkeitsgrenze laufend Depots mobilisiert, so bleibt für die Dauer dieser Mobilisierung eine Hyperuricurie bestehen und kann gelegentlich sehr hohe Werte erreichen. Mehrausscheidungen von 75 g innerhalb von 5 Monaten sind beobachtet worden, das sind etwa 500 mg pro Tag. Unserer Erfahrung nach ist diese speziell bei schwerer Gicht geringer. Eine Mehrausscheidung von 200 bis 300 mg pro Tag ist als guter Erfolg zu werten und führt im Verlauf längerer Zeit ebenfalls zu erwünschten therapeutischen Ergebnissen.

Die Dosierung der Mittel ist individuell verschieden. Im allgemeinen liegen die wirksamen täglichen Dosen bei 2—3 g Probenecid, 200—400 mg Sulfinpyrazon bzw. 100 mg Benzbromaronum. Die Verabreichung muß *einschleichend* erfolgen, um renale Harnsäureausfällungen bei zu starker Vermehrung der Ausscheidung zu vermeiden. Die Literatur enthält einige eindrucksvolle Schilderungen von Anurie bei zu rascher Steigerung der Probeneciddosierung (z. B. FRITZE u. MÜLLER, 1962), doch kann man solche Mißgeschicke sicher verhindern, wenn man die Dosis erst dann steigert, wenn unter der ersten Dosierung kein weiterer Abfall des Plasmaharnsäurespiegels erfolgt und außerdem der Harnsäureausfällung durch Verdünnung und Neutralisierung des Harns entgegengewirkt wird. Probenecid hemmt den tubulären Transport auch anderer Substanzen, z. B. des Penicillins oder der PAS, und erhöht dadurch deren Plasmaspiegel. Toxische Nebenerscheinungen bei Probenecidtherapie sind selten, doch kommen Magenbeschwerden vor und zwingen zu vorübergehendem Absetzen. Das gleiche gilt für Sulfinpyrazon. Unter Benzbromaronum werden gelegentlich gastrointestinale Beschwerden beobachtet. Sorgfältige Berichte über Langzeiterfahrungen mit Benz-

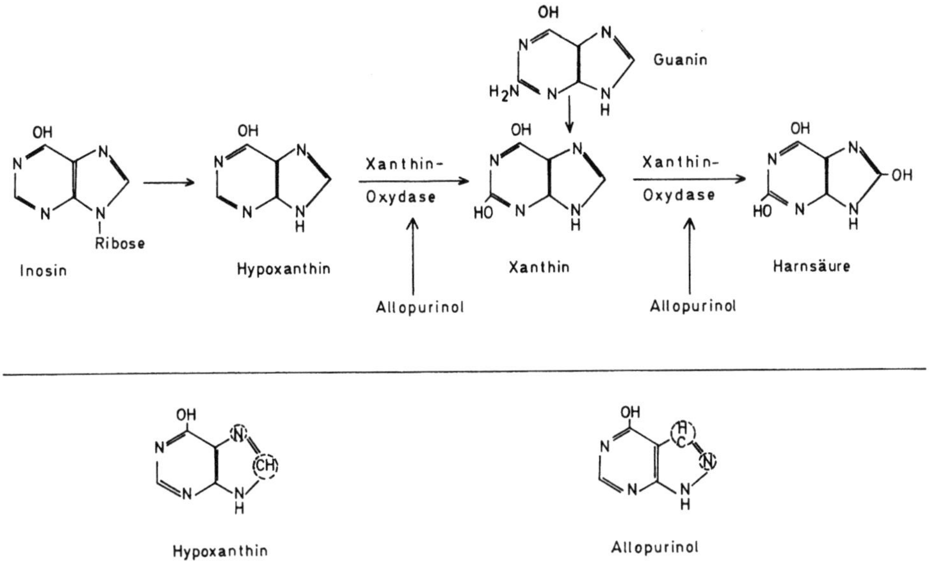

Abb. 7. Allopurinol und die durch Allopurinol hervorgerufene Hemmung der Xanthinoxydase

bromaronum stehen noch aus. Gelegentlich treten nach Einleitung einer uricosurischen Therapie zunächst vermehrt Gelenkanfälle auf, weswegen TALBOTT (1957) empfiehlt, die Behandlung anfangs mit prophylaktischen Colchicindosen (wir geben meist 0,5—1 mg tgl.) zu kombinieren.

Salicylate hemmen die Wirkung der Uricosurica Probenecid und Sulfinpyrazon und sind deshalb bei der Behandlung mit diesen Uricosurica zu vermeiden. Die Wirkung des Benzbromaronums soll allerdings durch Salicylate nicht beeinflußt werden.

c) Medikamente zur Hemmung der Harnsäurebildung

Einige cytostatisch wirksame Medikamente hemmen die Harnsäuresynthese. Für die Gichtbehandlung kommen cytostatisch wirksame Verbindungen natürlich nicht in Frage, doch wurde bei der Durchtestung einschlägiger Präparate eine Substanz gefunden, das Allopurinol, welches die Harnsäurebildung hemmt, ohne das normale Zellwachstum zu beeinflussen.

Die Wirkung des Allopurinols, das in seiner Struktur vom Hypoxanthin nur durch die Vertauschung eines Kohlenstoffatoms mit einem Stickstoffatom im Fünferring verschieden ist, beruht auf der kompetitiven Hemmung der Xanthinoxydase, des Enzyms, welches die Oxydation von Hypoxanthin und Xanthin zu Harnsäure katalysiert (Abb. 7).

Daneben besitzt Allopurinol auch einen unmittelbaren Einfluß auf die Purinsynthese de novo (Zusammenfassung: GRÖBNER u. ZÖLLNER, 1975) sowie auf den Pyrimidinstoffwechsel. Als Folge der Hemmung der Pyrimidinsynthese kommt es zum Auftreten einer Orotacidurie (Zusammenfassung: GRÖBNER u. ZÖLLNER, 1975).

Die klinische Erprobung des Präparates in den Händen von RUNDLES et al. (1963), YÜ u. GUTMAN (1964), HALL et al. (1964) ergab eine Senkung der Harnsäurespiegel unter gleichzeitiger Verringerung der Harnsäureausscheidung, während

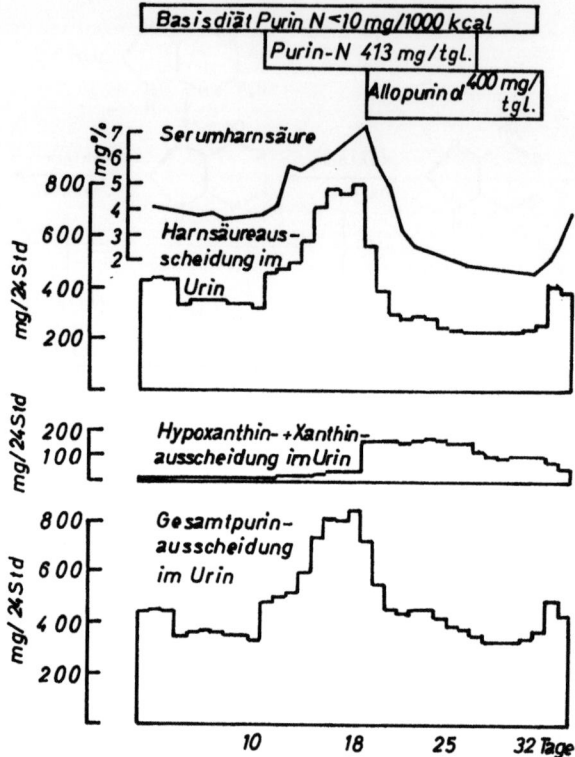

Abb. 8. Serumharnsäure, renale Tagesausscheidung von Harnsäure, Hypoxanthin und Xanthin sowie der Gesamtpurine unter purinarmer Basisdiät und nach Zulage von RNS, RNS und Allopurinol sowie Allopurinol allein. (Modifiziert nach ZÖLLNER u. GRÖBNER, 1970)

die Ausscheidung von Hypoxanthin und Xanthin zunimmt (Abb. 8). Bei den meisten Patienten wird dabei die Verringerung der renalen Harnsäureausscheidung nicht durch die vermehrte Oxypurinelimination ersetzt (Abb. 8) (RUNDLES et al., 1963; DELBARRE et al., 1966; RUNDLES et al., 1966; HITCHINGS, 1966; ZÖLLNER u. GRÖBNER, 1970). Dies wird auf die zusätzliche Hemmung der Purinsynthese de novo zurückgeführt. Eine unterschiedliche Beeinflussung der endogenen und exogenen Uratquote durch Allopurinol bietet eine alternative Erklärung des „Purindefizits" (ZÖLLNER u. GRÖBNER, 1970).

In der Anwendung gibt Allopurinol (Zyloric®, Urosin®, Foligan®, Allopurinol®) in Dosen von 200—800 mg tgl. eine wesentlich zuverlässigere Senkung des Harnsäurespiegels als die Uricosurica (ZÖLLNER, 1966; ZÖLLNER u. SCHATTENKIRCHNER, 1967). Es gelingt in nahezu allen Fällen, die Harnsäurespiegel durch 300—400 mg Allopurinol täglich zu normalisieren; und bei Gabe von 800 mg erreichen alle Patienten einen tiefen normalen Harnsäurespiegel (Abb. 9).

Nebenwirkungen unter Allopurinoltherapie sind selten. Gastrointestinale Beschwerden, allergische Hautreaktionen, gelegentlich Fieber, Blutbildveränderungen, Leberfunktionsstörungen und Vasculitis sind beobachtet worden (YÜ u. GUTMAN, 1964; KLINENBERG et al., 1965; JARZOBSKI et al., 1970). Xanthinsteine unter Allopurinolbehandlung traten lediglich bei zwei Kindern mit Lesch-Nyhan-Syndrom sowie einem Patienten mit Lymphosarkom auf (GREENE et al., 1969; SORENSEN u. SEEGMILLER, 1968; BAND et al., 1970).

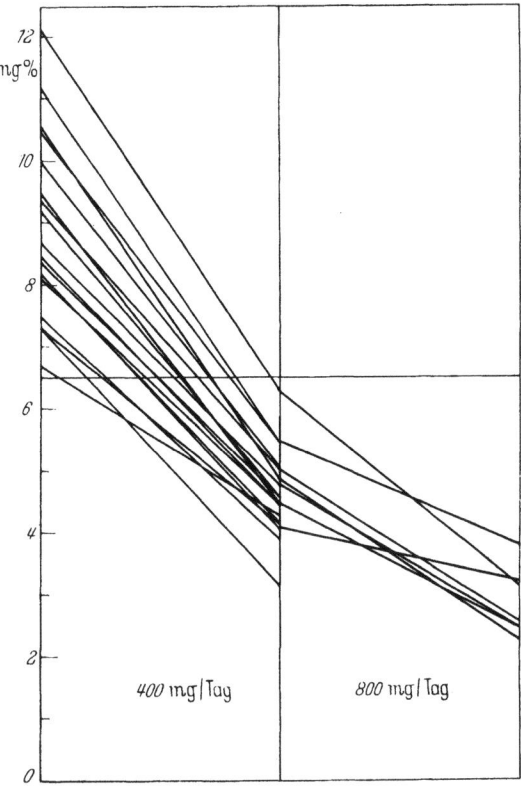

Abb. 9. Senkung der Plasmaharnsäure unter der Verabreichung von Allopurinol (jeweils 5 Tage Verabreichung). (Eigene Versuche)

2. Erniedrigung der tubulären Harnsäurekonzentration

Alle Maßnahmen, welche eine Erniedrigung der Harnsäurekonzentration im Plasma zu erzielen vermögen, sind auch geeignet, die Harnsäurekonzentration im Glomerulumfiltrat, d.h. im Anfangsteil des proximalen Tubulus zu verringern. Andererseits wird bei allen Behandlungsmethoden, welche die Harnsäurebildung nicht beeinflussen — bei gleichem Harnzeitvolumen — die Harnsäurekonzentration im Sammelröhrchen gegenüber der Periode vor der Behandlung unverändert sein, bzw. erhöht, wenn es unter der Behandlung zur Mobilisation und Ausscheidung von Harnsäuredepots kommt. In den übrigen Abschnitten des Nephrons kommen verminderte, aber auch erhöhte Harnsäurekonzentrationen vor, die von den Mechanismen der physiologischen bzw. pathologischen Harnsäureausscheidung einerseits und ihrer Beeinflussung durch die getroffenen Maßnahmen andererseits abhängen.

a) Einfluß von Diät oder Medikamenten, welche die Harnsäurebildung hemmen, auf die intratubuläre Harnsäurekonzentration

Eine Verringerung der Harnsäureausscheidung durch diätetische oder medikamentöse Maßnahmen führt, proportional der Verringerung der Plasmakonzentration, nicht nur zu einer Verringerung der Konzentration im Anfangsteil des proximalen Tubulus, sondern auch zu einer proportionalen Verringerung in den Sammelröhrchen. Auch in den dazwischen liegenden Abschnitten des Nephrons dürften die Harnsäurekonzentrationen im Vergleich zu der Periode vor der Behandlung proportional vermindert sein. Gelingt diese Senkung der Harnsäurekonzentration in ausreichender Weise, so werden weitere Ausfällungen im Tubuluslumen oder im Interstitium nicht mehr stattfinden können, und gleichzeitig werden die Voraussetzungen für eine Wiederauflösung von Präcipitaten bzw. interstitiellen Harnsäureablagerungen geschaffen.

b) Einfluß uricosurischer Medikamente auf die intratubuläre Harnsäurekonzentration

Während der Behandlung mit Uricosurica wird die unter der Wirkung des Medikamentes erniedrigte Harnsäurekonzentration in den Anfangsabschnitten des proximalen Tubulus im Verlauf der Harnbereitung auf die normale bzw. während der uricosurischen Wirkung erhöhte Konzentration im Sammelröhrchen angehoben. Da die Uricosurica durch die Blockierung der Harnsäurerückresorption wirken, findet diese Konzentrationserhöhung bereits am Ort der Rückresorption, als welcher der proximale Tubulus angesehen wird, statt. Dies gilt sowohl für Patienten mit dem renalen Defekt der familiären Hyperuricämie (also eingeschränkter Fähigkeit zur Harnsäuresekretion) als auch Personen mit normalem Harnsäureausscheidungsmechanismus, weil die Uricosurica auch die Harnsäuresekretion hemmen (YÜ u. GUTMAN, 1955). Unter der Wirkung der Uricosurica ist also vom Ort der Harnsäurerückresorption bis zum Sammelröhrchen die intratubuläre Harnsäurekonzentration nicht verringert, möglicherweise erhöht (im Vergleich zu unbehandelten Personen mit gleichem Harnsäurespiegel im Plasma). Kommt es unter der Wirkung des Medikamentes zur Mobilisation von Depots, so muß diese Erhöhung der Harnsäurekonzentration — im Vergleich zur Vorperiode — jedenfalls zustande kommen. Somit ist es nicht verwunderlich, daß unter der Uricosuricabehandlung intratubuläre Harnsäureausfällungen, die zu Anurie führen können, vorkommen. Uricosurica sind deshalb einschleichend zu dosieren; gleichzeitig sollten reichliche Flüssigkeitszufuhr und Neutralisierung, d.h. Maßnahmen zur Verhütung der Harnsäureausfällung, verordnet werden. COTTET (1961) hat als maximal anzustrebende Harnsäuretagesausscheidung 1,2 g angegeben, wir sind, wenn keine Nephrolithiasis vorliegt, nicht zurückhaltend, bei Vorliegen von Konkrementen dagegen noch vorsichtiger. Eine Anurie haben wir dabei nie gesehen. Das Auftreten einer Hämaturie, ebenfalls selten, kann durch Eintauchstreifen heute vom Patienten selbst kontrolliert werden (ZÖLLNER, 1965c).

Aufgrund des Gesagten kommen Uricosurica zur Behandlung der Gicht und Verhütung der gichtischen Nephrolithiasis heute nur noch in zweiter Linie in Frage. Bei langfristiger Behandlung mit Uricosurica darf aber vielleicht doch erwartet werden, daß nach Ausscheidung der Depots und der damit erfolgten Normalisierung der Harnsäureausscheidung auch die Gichtniere günstig beeinflußt wird, speziell wenn man durch reichliche Flüssigkeitsgaben für eine Verringerung der Harnsäurekonzentration im Endharn sorgt (PHILLIPS, 1955; TALBOTT u. TERPLAN, 1960; ZÖLLNER, 1963a).

Bei fortgeschrittener Nierenschädigung sind die Uricosurica oft wenig wirksam. Hier sollte dem Allopurinol der Vorzug gegeben werden. Das gleiche gilt für die Behandlung der Harnsäurenephrolithiasis.

c) Weitere Maßnahmen zur Verhütung der Harnsäureausfällung

Die Bedeutung der Wasserzufuhr bzw. der Neutralisierung wurde bereits erwähnt; sie wird im nächsten Abschnitt ausführlicher behandelt. Intratubuläre Harnsäureausfällungen, wie sie bei zu energischer Uricosuricatherapie, aber auch bei raschem Anstieg der Harnsäureausscheidung bei Chemo- bzw. Radiotherapie von Hämoblastosen vorkommen, können durch Alkali meist wieder aufgelöst werden, die entsprechende Anurie ist bei rechtzeitiger Therapie gelegentlich reversibel. Zu dieser Therapie bedient man sich am besten einer Infusion von Mannit (20%) und Natriumlactat oder Natriumbicarbonat. Es werden auch Tris-Puffer verwendet, jedoch ohne erkennbaren Vorteil.

3. Erniedrigung der Harnsäurekonzentration im Harn und Maßnahmen zur Verhütung der Harnsäureausfällung

Es wurde schon besprochen, daß die Steinbildung in der Gichtniere in den meisten Fällen nicht die Folge einer vermehrten Harnsäureausscheidung sein kann, weil die Harnsäureausscheidung in mehr als der Hälfte aller Fälle normal ist und nur äußerst selten 1 g pro Tag überschreitet. Die Ausfällungsvorgänge werden vielmehr durch die intratubuläre Erhöhung der Harnsäurekonzentration eingeleitet, so daß es zuerst zur Bildung kleinerer und größerer Konkremente innerhalb des Tubuluslumens kommt. Maßnahmen, die auf eine Verringerung der Harnsäurekonzentration im Harn zielen, haben deshalb bei der familiären Hyperuricämie nur dann prophylaktischen Wert, wenn sie bereits im Tubuluslumen wirksam werden, während sie bei den anderen Formen von Harnsäurenephrolithiasis in jedem Fall von prophylaktischer Bedeutung sind. Sollen Harnsäuresteine im Nierenbecken aufgelöst werden, so sind die zu besprechenden Maßnahmen bei beiden Patientengruppen von gleichem therapeutischem Wert.

a) Verringerung der Harnsäurekonzentration durch Verringerung der Harnsäurebildung

Hier kommen die erörterten Maßnahmen ebenso wie die Hemmung der Harnsäurebildung durch Allopurinol in Frage. Die Wirkung einer streng purinarmen und mäßig eiweißarmen Kost auf die renale Harnsäureausscheidung läßt sich dabei deutlich demonstrieren: Die bei unbeschränkter Kost bis zu 900 mg Harnsäure pro Tag betragende Ausscheidung (eigene Messungen in Münchener Kliniken) geht in die Nähe der endogenen Harnsäurequote, also in den Bereich von 300—400 mg pro Tag zurück. Über die Bedeutung nicht purinhaltiger Eiweiße haben BIEN et al. (1953) Untersuchungen angestellt. Ihre Ergebnisse zeigen, daß eine Mehrzufuhr von Eiweißstickstoff zu einer Mehrausscheidung von Harnsäurestickstoff führt, doch ist diese Mehrausscheidung gering, etwa ein Prozent des Eiweißstickstoffes. Die Zulage von 10 g Eiweiß (etwa ein Viertelliter Milch) bringt dennoch eine Mehrausscheidung von 16 mg Harnsäure-N, entsprechend 50 mg Harnsäure, eine nicht zu vernachlässigende Menge.

Bei der Zusammenstellung einer purinarmen Kost darf man nicht nur vom Puringehalt der Nahrungsmittel ausgehen, sondern muß auch die Mengen, in denen sie verzehrt werden, berücksichtigen. Leider bleibt in den meisten einschlägigen Diätvorschriften einerseits der relativ niedrige Harnsäuregehalt mancher reichlich verwendeter Nahrungsmittel, z.B. vieler Gemüse, unberücksichtigt, während andererseits Nahrungsmittel mit hohem Harnsäuregehalt, die aber nur in geringem Maße verwendet werden, z.B. Fleischextrakt, verboten sind (ZÖLLNER, 1965b). Die Folge ist eine langweilige Kostzusammenstellung, die nur wenig Aussichten auf Einhaltung hat.

Allopurinol sollte in der Therapie dann eingesetzt werden, wenn Diätvorschriften allein nicht ausreichen. Bei der Allopurinolbehandlung tritt an die Stelle der sich verringernden Harnsäureausscheidung eine Ausscheidung von Hypoxanthin und Xanthin. Abgesehen davon, daß sich damit die Ausscheidung der Hydroxypurine auf drei Verbindungen verteilt, also bereits ein deutlicher Gewinn erzielt ist, ist das Xanthin in Wasser mehr als dreimal, das Hypoxanthin nahezu 30mal löslicher als die Harnsäure (BENDICH, 1955).

b) Verringerung der Harnsäurekonzentration durch Diurese

Die minimale Harnmenge, die für eine nennenswerte Harnsäureverdünnung im Harn erzielt werden sollte, beträgt 1,5 Liter pro Tag, weil bis zu dieser Größe der Harnsäureausscheidung auch noch ein gewisser uricosurischer Effekt der Wasserzufuhr zur Wirkung kommt. Die meisten Autoren (z.B. COTTET, 1961) fordern jedoch größere Harnmengen, 2 Liter bzw. 2,5 Liter in 24 Std. Die hierzu nötige Trinkmenge hängt von vielen äußeren Umständen ab, speziell dem Klima und der Art der körperlichen Betätigung. Dem Patienten muß deshalb die Messung der Harnmenge, nicht der Trinkmenge, vorgeschrieben werden. Entscheidend wichtig ist auch, daß die Diurese nicht auf den Tag beschränkt bleibt, sondern auch nachts fortbesteht. Hierzu verordnen wir reichlich Flüssigkeitszufuhr vor dem Schlafengehen sowie einen halben Liter Wasser in der Mitte der Schlafperiode. Die Patienten gewöhnen sich rasch an die Notwendigkeit, einen Wecker zu stellen sowie an die auftretende Nykturie.

c) Beeinflussung der Harnsäurelöslichkeit durch Alkalizufuhr

Es wurde schon gezeigt, daß im alkalischen Milieu mehr Harnsäure gelöst werden kann als im saueren, und daß darüber hinaus Urate übersättigte Lösungen bilden können. Durch Alkalisierung wird also eine Neuausfällung von Harnsäure hintangehalten. Andererseits wurde dargetan, daß ein Überschuß an Alkaliionen die Uratlöslichkeit wieder zurückdrängt.

Für die Alkalisierung, besser Neutralisierung, eignet sich in Anlehnung an ATSMON et al. (1959) seit einigen Jahren Eisenbergsche Lösung (bestehend aus 40 g Citronensäure, 60 g Natriumcitrat, 66 g Kaliumcitrat, 6 g Pomeranzenextrakt, die in gewöhnlichem Sirup gelöst werden, Endvolumen 600 ml). Die notwendige Dosis, um den pH-Wert des Harnes regelmäßig in den Bereich zwischen 6,5 und 7,0 anzuheben, beträgt im allgemeinen 4 Eßlöffel täglich, am besten in Säften. Es empfiehlt sich, den Patienten ein Merck-Testpapier für den pH-Bereich von 6—8 zu verschreiben und sie anzuhalten, die Dosierung selbst so einzurichten, daß die Werte aus dem gewünschten Bereich weder nach oben noch nach unten abweichen. Die üblicherweise notwendige Dosierung der Eisenbergschen Lösung führt zur Zufuhr von etwa 40 g Rohrzucker, eine Menge, die zwar calorisch wenig zu Buch schlägt, dagegen bei Patienten mit schwerem Diabetes berücksichtigt werden muß, oft aber auch aus geschmacklichen Gründen abgelehnt wird. In dem Handelspräparat Uralyt-U® sind die wesentlichen Bestandteile, ohne Zucker, in Form eines Granulats zusammengefaßt, was für viele Patienten einen Vorteil bedeutet. Selbstverständlich sind alle anderen Formen einer adäquaten Neutralisierung ebenfalls zweckmäßig, entscheidend ist die laufende pH-Kontrolle durch den Patienten selbst (ZÖLLNER, 1963a).

Die Spätrisiken chronischer Alkalisierung dürften sich auch bei der Behandlung der Harnsäurelithiasis ergeben. Wir betrachten deswegen die Alkalisierung als Maßnahme zur Steinauflösung (bzw. zur Verhinderung der Ausfällung der Harnsäure bei Einleitung einer uricosurischen Therapie), während wir als Dauerprophylaxe der Steinbildung diätetische Maßnahmen, Allopurinol sowie eine reichliche Flüssigkeitszufuhr ansehen.

4. Vermeidung von Harnsäurespiegelerhöhungen in der Prophylaxe der Gichtniere

Die Rolle der Kost für die Harnsäurekonzentration im Interstitium, im Tubuluslumen und im Endharn wurde bereits besprochen. Darüber hinaus bleibt zu erwägen, ob gewissen Medikamenten, speziell den Saluretica sowie den metabolischen Effekten der Alkoholzufuhr und der Ketoacidose, welche die Plasmaharnsäurespiegel erhöhen und Gichtanfälle auslösen können, auch in der Genese der Gichtniere Bedeutung zukommt. Statistiken hierüber liegen nicht vor; auch weiß man nicht, ob es unter den genannten Bedingungen zu vermehrtem Auftreten der Nephrolithiasis kommt. Ob dies darauf beruht, daß die erwähnten Medikamente bzw. Stoffwechselsituationen nur vorübergehend auf den Patienten einwirken oder ob doch grundsätzliche funktionelle Unterschiede bestehen, bleibt deshalb zunächst offen. Es dürfte dennoch richtig sein, bei schlecht eingestelltem Diabetes bzw. chronischer Behandlung mit Saluretica nicht nur auf die Hyperuricämie zu achten, sondern auch die Möglichkeit einer Gichtniere bzw. von Nierenveränderungen, welche ihr ähneln, zu erwägen.

Bestehen bei einer Gicht keinerlei Symptome einer Nierenbeteiligung, so kann die Niere nahezu unberücksichtigt bleiben. Die Einleitung einer uricosurischen Therapie muß dennoch unter langsamer Steigerung der Dosierung des gewählten Medikamentes, am besten unter gleichzeitiger reichlicher Flüssigkeitsgabe und eventuell Alkaligabe, gegebenenfalls Colchicinprophylaxe, erfolgen. Ist die Plasmaharnsäure normalisiert, so wird die uricosurische Therapie fortgesetzt; eine weitere Neutralisierung ist aber nicht notwendig und sollte angesichts der möglichen ungünstigen Folgen sehr lang dauernder Alkalizufuhr unterbleiben; selbstverständlich bleibt reichliche Flüssigkeitszufuhr zweckmäßig.

Bestehen bei der Gicht Symptome einer Nierenbeteiligung, so sollte die Harnsäureausscheidung verringert werden. Bei Harnsäurenephrolithiasis ist die Einschränkung der Harnsäureausscheidung eine grundlegende therapeutische Maßnahme. Neben die energische Diättherapie tritt die Behandlung mit Allopurinol, und zwar in einer Dosis, die ausreicht, die Plasmaharnsäure unter 4,5 mg-% bzw. die Harnsäureausscheidung auf etwa 50% des Ausgangswertes zu senken (ZÖLLNER u. SCHATTENKIRCHNER, 1966). Besonders reichliche Flüssigkeitszufuhr und eine ausreichende Neutralisierung des Harns sind bei dieser Patientengruppe unerläßlich. Die Neutralisierung wird bis zur Beseitigung der Konkremente durchgeführt; eine sehr reichliche Flüssigkeitszufuhr sollte bei Patienten, die an einer Harnsäurelithiasis gelitten haben, lebenslänglich geübt werden.

Maßnahmen gegen die Folgen der Gichtniere müssen, solange sie indiziert sind, wie in bisher üblicher Weise auch weiterhin angewendet werden. Dies gilt speziell für die Behandlung der Hypertonie (wobei Saluretica allerdings zu vermeiden sind) und der Pyelonephritis. In der Behandlung der Nephrolithiasis dagegen ist heute eine konservative Haltung erlaubt; besteht keine dringende Indikation zur Operation, so ist zunächst der Versuch einer Steinauflösung durch Zufuhr von reichlich Flüssigkeit und Alkali in Kombination mit Allopurinol die Behandlung der Wahl.

Literatur

ATSMON, A., FRANK, M., LAZEBNIK, J., KOCHWA, S., DE VRIES, A.: Uric acid stones, a study of 58 patients. J. Urol. (Baltimore) **84**, 167 (1960).

ATSMON, A., DE VRIES, A., LAZEBNIK, J., SALINGER, H.: Dissolution of renal uric acid stones by oral alkalinization and large fluid intake in a patient suffering from gout. Amer. J. Med. **27**, 167 (1959).

ALVSAKER, J. O.: Uric acid in human plasma. Isolation and Identification of plasma proteins interacting with urate. Scand. J. clin. Lab. Invest. **18**, 227 (1966).

BAND, P. R., SILVERBERG, D. S., HENDERSON, J. F., ULAN, R. A., WENSEL, R. H., BANERGIE, T. K., LITTLE, A. S.: Xanthine nephropathy in a patient with lymphosarcoma treated with allopurinol. New Engl. J. Med. **283**, 354 (1970).
BAUER, W., KLEMPERER, F.: The treatment of gout. New Engl. J. Med. **231**, 681 (1944).
BECKER, M. A., MEYER, H. J., SEEGMILLER, J. E.: Purineoverproduction and gout due to increased phosphoribosylpyrophosphate synthetase activity. Israel J. med. Sci. **9**, 4 (1973).
BENDICH, A.: Chemistry of purines and pyrimidines. In: The nucleic acids, Vol. I, p. 81. New York: Academic Press 1955.
BERLINER, R. W., HILTON, J. G., YÜ, T. F., KENNEDY, T. J., JR.: The renal mechanism for urate excretion in man. J. clin. Invest. **29**, 396 (1950).
BERNOULLI, A. L., LOEBENSTEIN, A.: Dissoziationskonstanten der Harnsäure. Helv. chim. Acta **23**, 245 (1940).
BIEN, E. J., YÜ, T. F., BENEDICT, J. D., GUTMAN, A. B., STETTEN, D., JR.: The relation of dietary nitrogen consumption to the rate of uric acid synthesis in normal and gouty man. J. clin. Invest. **32**, 778 (1953).
BRØCHNER-MORTENSEN, K.: Uric acid content in blood and urine in health and disease. Medicine (Baltimore) **19**, 161 (1940).
BRØCHNER-MORTENSEN, K.: 100 gouty patients. Acta med. scand. **106**, 81 (1941).
BROWN, J., MALLORY, G. K.: Renal changes in gout. New Engl. J. Med. **243**, 325 (1950).
CAMPION, D. S., BLUESTONE, R., KLINENBERG, J. R.: Uric acid characterization of its interaction with human serum albumin. J. clin. Invest. **52**, 2383 (1973).
COOMBS, F. S., PECORA, L. D., THOROGOOD, E., CONSOLAZIO, W. V., TALBOTT, J. H.: Renal function in patients with gout. J. clin. Invest. **19**, 525 (1940).
COTTET, J.: Confrontations Thérapeutique. Comment traiter la goutte lorsqu'elle est compliquée de lithiase? Presse méd. **69**, 1557 (1961).
CURSCHMANN, H.: Lehrbuch der speziellen Prognostik innerer Krankheiten. Stuttgart: Enke 1944.
DAVIS, B. B., FIELD, J. B., RODNAN, G. P., KEDES, L. H.: Localization and pyrazinamide inhibition of distal transtubular movement of uric acid-2-C^{14} with a modified stop-flow technique. J. clin. Invest. **44**, 716 (1965).
DELBARRE, F., AMOR, B., AUSCHER, C., DEGERY, A.: Treatment of gout with allopurinol, a study of 106 cases. Ann. rheum. Dis. **25**, 627 (1966).
DIAMOND, H. S., PAOLINO, J. S.: Evidence for a postsecretory reabsorption site for uric acid in man. J. clin. Invest. **52**, 1491 (1973).
DICKINSON, W. H.: Disease of the kidney. Med.-Chir. Transact., London **26**, 169 (1861).
DUNCAN, H., WAKIM, K. G., WARD, L. E.: Renal lesions resulting from induced hyperuricemia in animals. Proc. Mayo Clin. **38**, 411 (1963).
DUNN, J. S., POLSON, C. L.: Experimental uric acid nephritis. J. Path. Bact. **29**, 337 (1926).
EBSTEIN, W.: Natur und Behandlung der Gicht, 2. Aufl. Wiesbaden: Bergmann 1906.
FAHR, T.: Pathologische Anatomie des Morbus Brightii. In: HENKE, F., LUBARSCH, O.: Handbuch der speziellen pathologischen Anatomie und Histologie, Bd. VI/1, S. 156. Berlin: Springer 1925.
FANELLI, G. M., WEINER, J. M.: Pyrazinoate excretion in the chimpanzee. Relation to urate disposition and the actions of uricosuric drugs. J. clin. Invest. **52**, 1946 (1973).
FRIEDMAN, M., BYERS, S. O.: Observations concerning the causes of the excess excretion of uric acid in the dalmatian dog. J. biol. Chem. **175**, 272 (1948).
FRITZE, E., MÜLLER, H. O.: Zur Probenecid-Behandlung der chronischen Gicht. Dtsch. med. Wschr. **87**, 82 (1962).
GARROD, A. B.: A treatise on gout and rheumatic gout. London: Longmans Greene 1876.
GIBSON, H. V., DOISY, E. A.: A note on the effect of some organic acids upon the uric acid excretion of man. J. biol. Chem. **55**, 605 (1923).
GREENBAUM, D., ROSS, J. H., STEINBERG, V. L.: Renal biopsy in gout. Brit. med. J. **1961 I**, 1502.
GREENE, M. L., FUJIMOTO, W. Y., SEEGMILLER, J. E.: Urinary Xanthine stones—a rare complication of allopurinol therapy. New Engl. J. Med. **280**, 426 (1969).
GREGER, R., LANG, F., DEETJEN, P.: Handling of uric acid in the rat kidney. I. Microanalysis of uric acid in proximal tubular fluid. Pflügers Arch. ges. Physiol. **324**, 279 (1971).
GRIEBSCH, A., ZÖLLNER, N.: Über die dosisabhängige Wirkung oral verabreichter DNS und RNS auf Harnsäurespiegel und Harnsäureausscheidung des Gesunden und des Hyperurikämikers. Hoppe Seylers Z. physiol. Chem. **351**, 1297 (1970).
GRÖBNER, W., ZÖLLNER, N.: Epidemiologie und Pathophysiologie der Gicht. In: BOECKER: Fettsucht-Gicht. Stuttgart: Thieme 1971.

GRÖBNER, W., ZÖLLNER, N.: Zur Beeinflussung der Purin- und Pyrimidinsynthese durch Allopurinol. Klin. Wschr. **53**, 255 (1975).
GRÖBNER, W., ZÖLLNER, N.: Störungen des menschlichen Pyrimidinstoffwechsels. Münch. med. Wschr. **117**, 1453 (1975).
GUDZENT, F.: Gicht und Rheumatismus. Berlin: Springer 1928.
GUTMAN, A. B.: Primary and secondary gout. Ann. intern. Med. **39**, 1062 (1953).
GUTMAN, A. B., YÜ, T. F.: Current principles in the management of gout. Amer. J. Med. **13**, 744 (1952).
GUTMAN, A. B., YÜ, T. F.: Renal function in gout. Amer. J. Med. **23**, 600 (1957).
GUTMAN, A. B., YÜ, T. F.: A three component system for regulation of renal excretion of uric acid in man. Trans. Ass. Amer. Phycns **74**, 353 (1961).
GUTMAN, A. B., YÜ, T. F., BERGER, L.: Tubular secretion of urate in man. J. clin. Invest. **38**, 1778 (1959).
HALL, A. P., HOLLOWAY, V. P., SCOTT, J. T.: 4-Hydroxypyrazolo-(3,4-d)-pyrimidine (HPP) in the treatment of gout. Preliminary observations. Ann. rheum. Dis. **23**, 439 (1964).
HARPUDER, K., ERBSEN, H.: Untersuchungen zur „Löslichkeit der Harnsäure". Biochem. Z. **148**, 344 (1924).
HARRIS, H.: The "inborn errors" today. In GARROD: Inborn errors of metabolism, p. 120. New York and Toronto: London and Oxford University Press 1963.
HAUGE, M., HARVALD, B.: Heredity in gout and hyperuricemia. Acta med. scand. **152**, 247 (1955).
HENNEMAN, PH. H., WALLACH, ST., DEMPSEY, E. F.: The metabolic defect responsible for uric acid stone formation. J. clin. Invest. **41**, 537 (1962).
HITCHINGS, G. H.: Effects of allopurinol in relation to purine biosynthesis. Ann. rheum. Dis. **25**, 601 (1966).
JARZOBSKY, JR., FERRY, J., WOMBOLT, D., FITCH, D. M., EGAN, J. D.: Vasculitis with allopurinol therapy. Amer. Heart J. **79**, 116 (1970).
KELLEY, W. N., ROSENBLOOM, F. M., MILLER, J., SEEGMILLER, J. E.: An enzymatic basis for variation in response to allopurinol. HGPRT deficiency. New Engl. J. Med. **278**, 287 (1968).
KESSLER, R. H., HIERHOLZER, K., GURD, R. S.: Localization of urate transport in the nephron and dalmatian dog kidney. Amer. J. Physiol. **197**, 601 (1959).
KIPPEN, J., KLINENBERG, J. R., WEINBERGER, A., WILCOX, W. R.: Factors affecting urate solubility in vitro. Ann. rheum. Dis. **33**, 313 (1974).
KLINENBERG, J. R., GOLDFINGER, S. E., SEEGMILLER, J. E.: The effectiveness of the xanthine oxidase inhibitor allopurinol in the treatment of gout. Ann. intern. Med. **62**, 639 (1965).
KLINENBERG, J. R., KIPPEN, J.: The binding of urate to plasma proteins determined by means of equilibrium dialysis. J. Lab. clin. Med. **75**, 503 (1970).
KÖNIG, E., ZÖLLNER, N.: Sekundäre Gicht bei Osteomyelosklerose und bei Polycythaemia vera. Med. Klin. **57**, 1741 (1962).
KRÖPELIN, T., MERTZ, D. P.: Zur Röntgendiagnostik der Gichtniere. Dtsch. med. Wschr. **97**, 71 (1972).
LANG, F., GREGER, R., DEETJEN, P.: Handling of uric acid by the rat Kidney. II. Microperfusion studies on bidirectional transport of uric acid in the proximal tubule. Pflügers Arch ges. Physiol. **335**, 257 (1972).
LATHEM, W., DAVIS, B. B., RODNAN, G. P.: Renal tubular secretion of uric acid in the mongrel dog. Amer. J. Physiol. **199**, 9 (1960).
LATHEM, W., RODNAN, G. P.: Impairment of uric acid excretion in gout. J. clin. Invest. **41**, 1955 (1962).
LAUDAT, M.-H., RYCKEWAERT, A., LAGRUE, G., MILLIEZ, P., SÈZE, S.: Le rôle de l'suffisance rénale urico-eliminatoire dans la goutte primitive. Rev. franç. Etud. clin. biol. **7**, 155 (1962).
LIEBER, CH. S., JONES, D. P., LOSOWSKY, M. S., DAVIDSON, C. S.: Interrelation of uric acid and ethanol metabolism in man. J. clin. Invest. **41**, 1863 (1962).
LOUYOT, P., RAUBER, G., GAUCHER, A., HURIET, C., PETERSCHMITT, J.: Le rein du goutteux. In: La goutte. Rapports Présentés au XXXIVe Cong. Franç. de Médicine. Paris: Masson 1963.
LOUYOT, P., RAUBER, G., HURIET, C., GAUCHER, A.: Rein goutteux et ponction-biopsie. J. Urol. méd. chir. **65**, 628 (1959).
MAYNE, J. G.: Pathological study of the renal lesions found in 27 patients with gout. Ann. rheum. Dis. **15**, 61 (1956).
MERTZ, D. P.: Veränderungen der Serumkonzentration von Harnsäure unter der Wirkung von Benzbromaronum. Münch. med. Wschr. **111**, 491 (1969).
MUGLER, A., PERNET, J. L., PERNET, A., FRIEDRICH, S.: Le pouvoir d'épuration du rein pour l'acide urique chez l'hyperuricémique d'après l'étude de 400 clearances. Contemp. Rheum. **1956**, 574.
MUNCK, A.: Die Niere bei Gicht. Beitr. path. Anat. **133**, 409 (1966).

NICHOLS, J., MILLER, A. T., JR., HIATT, E. P.: Influence of muscular exercise on uric acid excretion in man. J. appl. Physiol. **3**, 501 (1951).

NUGENT, C. A., MACDIARMID, W. D., TYLER, F. H.: Renal excretion of urate in patients with gout. Arch. intern. Med. **133**, 115 (1964).

NUGENT, C. A., TYLER, F. H.: The renal excretion of uric acid in patients with gout and in nongouty subjects. J. clin. Invest. **38**, 1890 (1959).

OGRYZLO, M. A.: The renal factor in the etiology of primary gout. Canad. med. Ass. J. **83**, 1326 (1960).

PASERO, G.: Über die urikosurische Wirkung antiprothrombinämischer Substanzen und einiger neuer Indandionderivate und über die Beziehung zwischen Vitamin K und tubulärer Harnsäurerückresorption. Dtsch. med. Wschr. **85**, 854 (1960).

PASERO, G., MARINI, N.: Sull'azione uricuria del 2-fenil-5-bromo-1,3-indandione. Gazz. med. ital. **117**, 561 (1958).

PETERS, J. P., VAN SLYKE, D. D.: Quantitative clinical chemistry interpretations, Vol. I. Baltimore: Williams & Wilkins 1946.

PHILLIPS, R. W.: Reversal of renal insufficiency in gout, report of a case treated with probenecid (Benemid). Arch. intern. Med. **66**, 823 (1955).

POULSEN, H., PRAETORIUS, E.: Tubular excretion of uric acid in rabbits. Acta pharmacol. (Kbh.) **10**, 371 (1954).

PRIEN, E. L., FRONDEL, C.: Studies in urolithiasis; composition of urinary calculi. J. Urol. (Baltimore) **57**, 949 (1947).

RAKIC, M. T., VALKENBERG, H. A., DAVIDSON, R. T., ENGELS, J. P., MIKKELSEN, W. M., NEEL, J. V., DUFF, I. F.: Observations on the natural history of hyperuricemia and gout. Amer. J. Med. **37**, 826 (1964).

RAVAULT, P. P., VIALA, J. J.: Considérations cliniques et étiopathologiques sur les manifestations renales de la goutte. Rev. lyon. Méd. **9**, 1069 (1960).

REUBI, F., VORBURGER, C.: Die Gichtniere. Münch. med. Wschr. **104**, 2152 (1962).

REUTTER, F., SCHAUB, F.: Harnsäurestoffwechsel und Salidiuretika. Dtsch. med. Wschr. **89**, 1101 (1964).

RICHET, G., ARDAILLON, R., DE MONTÉRA, H., SLAMA, R., BONGAULT, T.: Le rein goutteux. Étude de 31 cas de néphropathie associée à la goutte. Presse méd. **69**, 644 (1961).

RUNDLES, R. W.: Metabolic effects of allopurinol and allo-xanthine. Ann. rheum. Dis. **25**, 615 (1966).

RUNDLES, R. W., WYNGAARDEN, J. B., HITCHINGS, G. H., ELION, G. B., SILBERMAN, H. R.: Effects of a xanthine oxidase inhibitor on thiopurine metabolism, hyperuricemia and gout. Trans. Ass. Amer. Phycns **76**, 126 (1963).

SCHNITKER, M. A., RICHTER, A. B.: Nephritis in gout. Amer. J. med. Sci. **192**, 241 (1936).

SEEGMILLER, J. E., GRAYZEL, A. I., HOWELL, R. R., PLATO, C.: The renal excretion of uric acid in gout. J. clin. Invest. **41**, 1094 (1962).

SMITH, J. F., LEE, Y. CH.: Experimental uric acid nephritis in the rabbit. J. exp. Med. **105**, 615 (1957).

SOKOLOFF, L.: The pathology of gout. Metabolism **6**, 230 (1957).

SØRENSEN, L. B.: The elimination of uric acid in man. Studies by means of C^{14}-labeled uric acid. Uricolysis. Scand. J. clin. Lab. Invest. **12**, Suppl. 54, 3 (1960).

SØRENSEN, L., SEEGMILLER, J. R.: Seminars on the Lesch-Nyhan-Syndrome: Management and treatment discussion. Ped. Proc. **27**, 1097 (1968).

SPERLING, O., BOER, P., PESSKY-BROSH, S., KANAREK, E., DE VRIES, A.: Altered kinetic property of erythrocyte phosphoribosylpyrophosphate synthetase in excessive purine production. Rev. Europ. Étud. clin. biol. **17**, 703 (1972).

STEELE, T. H., BONER, G.: Origins of the uricosuric response. J. clin. Invest. **52**, 1368 (1973).

TALBOTT, J. H.: Gout. New York and London: Grune & Stratton 1957.

TALBOTT, J. H., LILIENFELD, A.: Longevity in gout. Geriatrics **14**, 409 (1959).

TALBOTT, J. H., TERPLAN, K. L.: The kidney in gout. Medicine (Baltimore) **39**, 405 (1960).

THANNHAUSER, S. J.: Lehrbuch des Stoffwechsels und der Stoffwechselkrankheiten. München: Bergmann 1929.

THANNHAUSER, S. J.: Über die Pathogenese der Gicht. Dtsch. med. Wschr. **81**, 492 (1956).

THANNHAUSER, S. J., CZONICZER, G.: Kennen wir Erkrankungen des Menschen, die durch eine Störung des intermediären Purinstoffwechsels verursacht werden? Dtsch. Arch. klin. Med. **135**, 224 (1921).

TCHERDAKOFF, P.: Rene e'iperuricemia. Minerva med. **64**, 4039 (1973).

Turolla, E.: Contributio critico e casistico sul coridetto „rene gottso". Arch. De Vecchi Anat. pat. 34, 391 (1960).
Villa, L., Robecchi, A., Ballabio, C. B.: Physiopathology, clinical manifestation and treatment of gout. Part 1, physiopathology and pathogenesis. Ann. rheum. Dis. 17, 9 (1958).
De Vries, A., Frank, M., Atsmon, A.: Inherited uric acid lithiasis. Amer. J. Med. 33, 880 (1962).
Wallace, St. L., Bernstein, D.: The relationship between gout and the kidney. Metabolism 12, 440 (1963).
Wyngaarden, J. B.: On the dual etiology of primary gout. Arthr. and Rheum. 3, 414 (1960).
Wyngaarden, J. B.: Gout. Advanc. Metab. Dis. 2, 2 (1965).
Yü, T. F., Berger, L., Gutman, A. B.: Renal function in gout. II. Effect of uric acid loading on renal excretion of uric acid. Amer. J. Med. 33, 829 (1962).
Yü, T. F., Berger, L., Kupfer, S., Gutman, A. B.: Tubular secretion of urate in the dog. Amer. J. Physiol. 199, 1199 (1960).
Yü, T. F., Gutman, A. B.: Ultrafiltrability of plasma urate in man. Proc. Soc. exp. Biol. (N.Y.) 84, 21 (1953).
Yü, T. F., Gutman, A. B.: Paradoxical retention of uric acid by uricosuric drugs in low dosage. Proc. Soc. exp. Biol. (N.Y.) 90, 542 (1955).
Yü, T. F., Gutman, A. B.: Effect of allopurinol (4-Hydroxy-pyrazolo-(3,4-d)pyrimidine) on serum and urinary uric acid in primary and secondary gout. Amer. J. Med. 37, 885 (1964).
Yü, T. F., Sirota, J. H., Berger, L., Halpern, M., Gutman, A. B.: Effect of sodium lactate infusion on urate clearance in man. Proc. Soc. exp. Biol. (N.Y.) 96, 809 (1957).
Zöllner, N.: Angeborene Stoffwechselstörungen. Dtsch. med. Wschr. 83, 609 (1958).
Zöllner, N.: Moderne Gichtprobleme, Ätiologie, Pathogenese, Klinik. Ergebn. inn. Med. Kinderheilk. 14, 321 (1960a).
Zöllner, N.: Gicht. Internist (Berl.) 1, 333 (1960b).
Zöllner, N.: Der Purinstoffwechsel und seine Störungen. Verh. dtsch. Ges. Urol. 20, 15 (1963a).
Zöllner, N.: Eine einfache Modifikation der enzymatischen Harnsäurebestimmung. Z. klin. Chem. 1, 178 (1963b).
Zöllner, N.: Pathogenese, Klinik und Therapie der Gicht. Therapiewoche 13, 129 (1963c).
Zöllner, N.: Physiologie und Pathologie der Harnsäure. Praxis 53, 1122 (1965a).
Zöllner, N.: Diät bei Gicht und Harnsäureleiden. In: Thienemanns Diätkochbücher, H. 5. Stuttgart: Thienemann 1965b.
Zöllner, N.: Untersuchungen über die Brauchbarkeit kombinierter Schnelldiagnostika zur Harnanalyse. Med. Klin. 60, 248 (1965c).
Zöllner, N.: Die Behandlung der Gicht und der Uratnephrolithiasis mit Allopurinol. Verh. dtsch. Ges. inn. Med. 72, 781 (1966).
Zöllner, N., Dofel, W., Gröbner, W.: Die Wirkung von Benzbromaronum auf die renale Harnsäureausscheidung Gesunder. Klin. Wschr. 48, 426 (1970).
Zöllner, N., Griebsch, A.: Diet and Gout. Purine Metabolism in Man, Vol. 41 B, p. 435. New York: Plenum Publishing Corporation 1974.
Zöllner, N., Griebsch, A., Fink, J. K.: Über die Wirkung von Benzbromaronum auf den Serumharnsäurespiegel und die Harnsäureausscheidung des Gichtkranken. Dtsch. med. Wschr. 95, 2405 (1970).
Zöllner, N., Griebsch, A., Gröbner, W., Hector, G., Schattenkirchner, M.: Klinische Erfahrungen mit dem neuen Uricosuricum Benzbromaronum. Verh. dtsch. Ges. inn. Med. 76, 853 (1970).
Zöllner, N., Gröbner, W.: Der unterschiedliche Einfluß von Allopurinol auf die endogene und exogene Uratquote. Europ. J. clin. Pharmacol. 3, 56 (1970).
Zöllner, N., Kurz, G.: Unveröffentlicht.
Zöllner, N., Schattenkirchner, M.: Unveröffentlicht (1966).
Zöllner, N., Schattenkirchner, M.: Allopurinol in der Behandlung der Gicht und der Harnsäure-Nephrolithiasis. Dtsch. med. Wschr. 92, 654 (1967).
Zöllner, N., Stern, G., Gröbner, W., Dofel, W.: Über die Senkung des Harnsäurespiegels im Plasma durch Benzbromaronum. Klin. Wschr. 46, 1318 (1968).

bb) Harnsäurelithiasis

Von

P. May

Mit 10 Abbildungen

Vorkommen und Häufigkeit

Die Harnsteinbildung ist zwar über die ganze Welt verbreitet, häuft sich jedoch in Gebieten, die geomedizinisch als „Steingürtel" bezeichnet werden.

Die ätiologischen Faktoren der Harnsteinentstehung sind vielschichtig. Zum Teil sind die Ursachen aufgeklärt. Dazu zählen vor allem Stoffwechselstörungen sowie die Folgen von Harnstauung und Infektion. Als weitere ursächliche Faktoren werden geographische und rassische Eigentümlichkeiten, Vererbung, konstitutionelle Faktoren sowie die Ernährung und Streßwirkung diskutiert.

Nach ALKEN (1971 b) besteht kein Zweifel an einer steigenden Frequenz der Urolithiasis in Deutschland. Derartige „Steinwellen" wurden nach dem ersten und zweiten Weltkrieg beobachtet und auf die Ernährungsumstellung in den Nachkriegsjahren zurückgeführt.

Im Zusammenhang mit der zunehmenden Häufigkeit der Nephrolithiasis ist besonders das prozentuale Ansteigen von Harnsäuresteinen bemerkenswert.

Die zunehmende Häufigkeit von Harnsäuresteinträgern innerhalb des letzten Jahrzehnts wird aus der Tab. 1 deutlich.

Die veränderten Lebens- und Ernährungsgewohnheiten mögen zwar kausalpathologisch eine Rolle spielen, die Weiterentwicklung der klinisch-chemischen und röntgenologischen Diagnostik trägt jedoch sicherlich auch zu einer besseren Erfassung von Harnsäuresteinbildnern bei.

Während sich die Angaben der meisten Autoren auf qualitative Untersuchungsmethoden stützen, zeigen die quantitativen Analysen beispielsweise von SCHNEIDER et al. (1969) mit 38,8% einen besonders hohen Anteil reiner Harnsäuresteine.

Die Zunahme von Harnsäuresteinträgern kann auch mit dem vermehrten Auftreten der primären Gichterkrankung in Zusammenhang gebracht werden. So erwartet MERTZ (1971), daß die Morbidität an Gicht unter der männlichen erwachsenen Bevölkerung bis auf 1—2% ansteigt, während ZÖLLNER (1970) sogar damit rechnet, daß in Zukunft 3% aller Männer, die das 65. Lebensjahr erreichen, an dieser Erkrankung leiden werden. Der gleiche Verfasser fand bei 40% seiner gichtkranken Patienten Harnsäuresteine.

Unter Zugrundelegung der zum Teil schwankenden Literaturangaben kann heute angenommen werden, daß rund 25% aller Harnsteine aus reiner Harnsäure oder zu einem so hohen Prozentsatz aus einem Harnsäureanteil bestehen, daß eine konservativ-medikamentöse Therapie mit dem Ziel der Litholyse in Frage kommt.

Die Pathogenese der Harnsäuresteinbildung

Die Entstehung von Harnsteinen ist ein komplexes Geschehen.

Die Formalpathogenese ist teilweise noch ungeklärt. Die zahlreich in Frage kommenden intra- und extrarenalen Faktoren der Steinentstehung sind bei einer klinisch manifesten Steinkrankheit häufig nicht faßbar, da es sich meist um bio-

Tabelle 1. Häufigkeit von Harnsäuresteinen

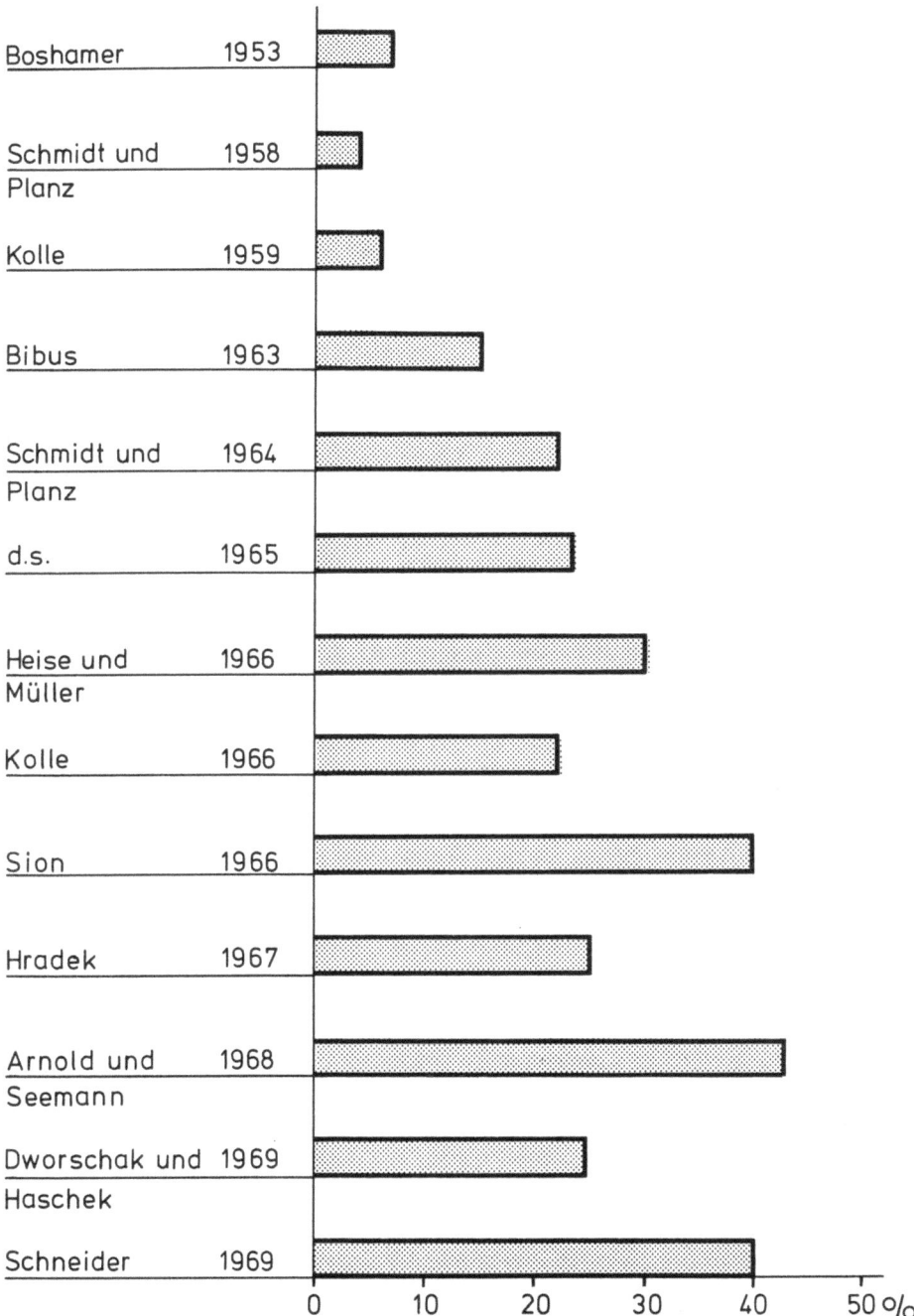

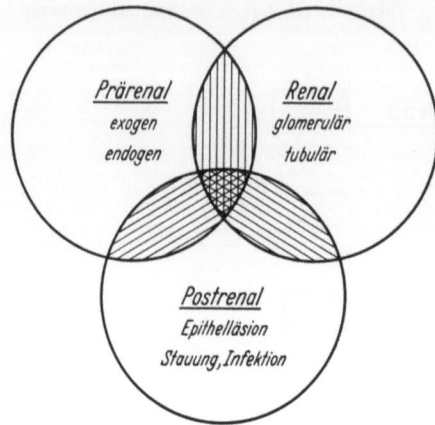

Abb. 1. Faktoren der Harnsteinpathogenese.
(Nach: ALKEN, Leitfaden der Urologie. Stuttgart: Thieme 1971)

chemische und im Mikrobereich sich abspielende Abläufe handelt, die zur Zeit der klinischen Diagnose bereits längere Zeit zurückliegen.

Für die Harnsteinbildung werden gegenwärtig zwei übergeordnete Theorien diskutiert: Die Kristallisations- und die Kolloidtheorie.

Die Kristallisationstheorie wurde bereits 1860 von HELLER vertreten. Sie sieht in der Steinbildung ein reines Kristallisationsproblem. Den im Harn vorliegenden organischen Kolloiden wird kein aktiver Anteil bei der Steinbildung zuerkannt.

Als wichtigste Voraussetzung wird eine pathologische Übersättigung des Harns mit Steinkomponenten und eine Instabilität des Urins angesehen (SCHULTHEIS, 1950). Im gleichen Sinne postuliert HAMMARSTEN (1946): „Ohne Übersättigung keine Steine!"

Die zweite Voraussetzung ist das Vorhandensein eines Kristallisationszentrums, von dem aus die Kristalle radiärwärts wachsen können.

Als Kristallisationszentrum kommt eine organische Matrix in Frage, die aus Uromucoiden, Mikrokristallen, Bakterien, Epithelschäden oder Fremdkörpern bestehen kann.

Auf Grund der Kristallisationstheorie beginnt die Steinbildung mit der Ausfällung von Harnsalzen, die durch Eiweißkolloide des Harns zu einem Konkrement geformt werden (VERMEULEN et al., 1965).

STAEMMLER (1958) fand Harnsäurekristalldrusen in den Markkanälchen, im Papillenbereich sowie im Nierenbecken mantelförmig von Mucoproteiden umgeben.

Er hält daher entsprechend der Kristallisationstheorie die Ausfällung der Kristalle für den primären, die Eiweißumhüllung für den sekundären Vorgang.

Auf die Bedeutung der kristallinen Uratpräcipitation wird von DE VRIES et al. (1965) und COTTET et al. (1955) eingegangen.

Bei histologischen Untersuchungen kindlicher Nieren fand bereits ASCHOFF (1900) Harnsäurekristalle in den Sammelröhrchen, die als sogenannte Harnsäureinfarkte beschrieben wurden. Der gleiche Verfasser wies entsprechend der Kristallisationstheorie auf Harnsäureinfarkte als Steinbildungszentren hin.

Das Auftreten von Harnsäureinfarkten bei Neugeborenen und Kindern wird von ALLEN (1951) mit einem Mangel des Enzyms Urease erklärt. Kristallinisch und auch aufbaumäßig besteht nach STAEMMLER (1958) kein wesentlicher Unterschied gegenüber echten Konkrementen, die wie die Harnsäureinfarkte von Mucoproteinen umgeben sind.

MITCHELL (1951) fand bei 500 Konkrementen von Kindern in 58% der Fälle einen Aufbau aus Harnsäure bzw. Uraten.

Auf Grund dieser Ergebnisse können Harnsäureinfarkte auch für die Genese kindlicher Konkremente bedeutungsvoll sein.

Nach BOSHAMER (1961) ist im Zusammenhang mit der Kristallisationstheorie die Auffassung vom Harn als übersättigter Lösung entscheidend.

Im Gegensatz zur Kristallisationstheorie gehen die Kolloidtheorien vom Vorhandensein einer sogenannten Gerüstsubstanz aus.

Der Ausfall der Steinmatrix, bestehend aus organischen Substanzen, wird als primärer, die Steinbildung bestimmender Vorgang bezeichnet, während das Auskristallisieren der Harnsalze, die Entwicklung zum Konkrement, als sekundärer Vorgang aufgefaßt wird.

Die schon von EBSTEIN (1884) vertretene Auffassung, daß Steine nur entstehen, wenn organisches Bindemittel von Versteinerungsmasse durchdrungen wird, baute LICHTWITZ (1944) zur entscheidenden Kolloidtheorie aus, die nach BOSHAMER (1961) die Betrachtungsweise des Steinproblems bis in die neueste Zeit beeinflußt hat.

Die Kristalloide werden angeblich durch die Harnkolloide in Lösung gehalten. Diese „Schutzkolloide" sollen die schwerlöslichen Ionen vor dem Ausfallen schützen.

Neuere Ergebnisse über die Beschaffung der Harnkolloide basieren auf Untersuchungen von ALKEN et al. (1957a, b), ALKEN u. HERMANN (1957), DULCE (1958) sowie von KEUTEL et al. (1959).

Zu den organisierten Harnkolloiden zählen die Uroproteine, die Uromucoide und bestimmte saure Mucopolysaccharide.

BOYCE et al. (1958) fanden eine wesentlich stärkere Ausscheidung von Uroproteinen im Harn von Steinkranken.

DULCE (1956) macht eine sogenannte „aktive" Matrix für die Entstehung aller anorganischen kristallinen Steinformen verantwortlich, während für die Bildung organischer Konkremente, insbesondere für die Entstehung von Harnsäuresteinen, eine „inaktive" Matrix erforderlich sei. Sie soll den Kristallisationskern abgeben und als semipermeable Membran den Ausfall der Kristalle bewirken.

Eine Übersättigung des Harns mit dem Steinbildner, d.h. im speziellen Fall mit Harnsäure, ist Voraussetzung.

BOSHAMER (1961) vermutet auch auf Grund der Matrixuntersuchungen von DULCE (1958) für Harnsäuresteine eher eine Entwicklung entsprechend der Kristallisationstheorie als nach den Theorien von BOYCE bzw. nach den älteren Kolloidtheorien. Die zahlreichen experimentellen und klinischen Ergebnisse über Harnsäuresteinbildung lassen nämlich darauf schließen, daß einer relativen Übersättigung des Urins mit Harnsäure bei gleichzeitiger Änderung des Lösungsvermittlers eine zentrale Bedeutung zukommt.

Folgende Ursachen der Harnsäuresteinbildung sind kausal-pathogenetisch bekannt:
1. Eine vermehrte Ausscheidung von Harnsäure im Endharn.
2. Veränderte Mechanismen der tubulären Rückresorption und Sekretion von Harnsäure, wie sie von ZÖLLNER (1967b) beim Krankheitsbild der familiären Hyperurikämie bzw. Gicht beschrieben werden.
3. Eine Verringerung des Lösungsvermögens von Harnsäurekristallen durch vermehrte Harnkonzentrierung bzw. Harnsäuerung im Sinne einer sog. „Säurestarre des Urins", die bei der idiopathischen Harnsäuresteindiathese beobachtet wird.

Eine nicht gichtige, sogenannte sekundäre Hyperurikämie mit vermehrter Ausscheidung von Harnsäure im Endharn kann durch verschiedene Grundleiden ausgelöst werden:

Eine sekundäre Hyperurikämie tritt bei Patienten mit myeloproliferativen Prozessen wie Polycythaemia vera, Polyglobulie, Paraproteinämien, infektiöser Mononucleose, Thalassaemia maior, Pneumonie, Psoriasis und Sarkoidose auf. Weiterhin kann eine sekundäre Hyperurikämie durch radiologi-

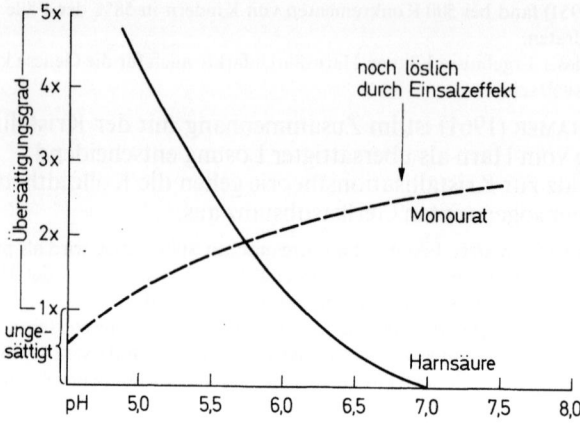

Abb. 2. pH und Übersättigungsgrad von Harnsäure und Monourat im Harn. (Nach BRESSEL, modifiziert nach DULCE)

sche und cytostatische Behandlung, durch einen hämorrhagischen Schockzustand und durch Gabe von 2-Äthylamino-1,3,4-thiadiazol oder durch Verabreichung von Sulfonamidsaluretica hervorgerufen werden. Ebenso können Ketosen (z. B. bei dekompensiertem Diabetes mellitus), arterielle Hypertension, respiratorische Acidose und bestimmte endokrine Erkrankungen wie Akromegalie, Hypo- und Hyperparathyreoidismus eine sekundäre Hyperuricämie und eine eventuelle Harnsäuresteinbildung auslösen (MERTZ, 1971).

Bei sekundärer Hyperuricämie kommt es durch einen erhöhten Umsatz von Nucleinsäuren zu einer vermehrten Produktion von Harnsäure und anderen Purinen.

So beschrieben bereits BEDRNA u. POLCACK (1929) sowie KRITZLER (1958) bei Leucämien infolge des gesteigerten Zellumsatzes eine Hyperuricämie, die zur Verlegung der Harnleiter mit Uratkristallen führte.

Die bei sekundärer Hyperuricämie gültige Erklärung einer Harnsäuresteinbildung infolge einer gesteigerten Harnsäurekonzentration im Endharn bzw. im ausgeschiedenen Urin, trifft für das Krankheitsbild der Gicht nicht zu. Untersuchungen von ZÖLLNER (1967b) ergaben, daß die überwiegende Mehrzahl der Gichtpatienten nicht mehr Harnsäure ausscheidet als die Normalbevölkerung; andererseits wird der enge Zusammenhang zwischen Gicht und Harnsäuresteinbildung durch zahlreiche Statistiken untermauert:

So fanden ARMSTRONG und GREENE (1953) bei 13%, HENCH et al. (1928) bei 12%, PAILLARD u. FAUVERT (1956) bei 18%, ZÖLLNER u. LÜHRS (1967) sogar bei 40% der Gichtpatienten Harnsäuresteine.

Auf die Pathogenese der gichtigen Hyperuricämie soll hier nur insoweit eingegangen werden, als es für das Verständnis der Steinbildung erforderlich ist.

Die normale Regulation der renalen Harnsäureausscheidung beim Menschen schließt glomeruläre Filtration, tubuläre Reabsorption und tubuläre Sekretion ein (GUTMAN et al., 1959).

YÜ et al. (1962) diskutieren eine vollständige Rückresorption des glomerulär filtrierten Harnsäureanteils. Weitere zahlreiche Untersuchungen dienten dem Ziel, den Ort der tubulären Harnsäuresekretion festzulegen.

YÜ et al. (1960) sowie DAVIS et al. (1965) fanden mit Hilfe der Stopflowmethode normalerweise eine Harnsäuresekretion nur im Bereich des distalen Tubulusanteils, die durch Pyracinamid gehemmt werden konnte.

Über die der familiären Hyperuricämie zugrundeliegenden Stoffwechselstörungen werden zwei Theorien diskutiert: Die Überproduktionstheorie und die Ausscheidungstheorie.

Die sogenannte Überproduktionstheorie basiert auf Untersuchungen von BENEDICT et al. (1952), die bei Gichtkranken eine rasche Ausscheidung vermehrter Mengen markierter Harnsäure nach Gabe des markierten Vorläufers 15-N-Glycin gefunden hatten. Danach soll die Hyperuricämie die Folge einer gesteigerten Harnsäuresynthese sein. Nach ZÖLLNER (1960) und WYNGAARDEN (1965) zeigen diese Ergebnisse keine gesteigerte Harnsäurebildung, sondern nur eine Besonderheit des Purinstoffwechsels auf, die zudem angeblich nur bei einem Teil der Gichtpatienten zu beobachten sei.

Die Ausscheidungstheorie macht im Gegensatz zur Überproduktionstheorie eine Funktionsstörung der Niere für das Zustandekommen der Hyperuricämie verantwortlich.

NUGENT u. TYLER (1959) fanden, daß bei gleichem Plasmaharnsäurespiegel die Harnsäureclearance bei Gichtpatienten niedriger ist als bei Gesunden. Dieses Ergebnis wurde in der Folge von zahlreichen Autoren bestätigt (WYNGAARDEN, 1960; OGRYZLO, 1960; SEEGMÜLLER et al., 1962; LATHEM u. RODNAN, 1962; REUBI u. VORBURGER, 1962).

Untersuchungen von ZÖLLNER (1967b) über den Mechanismus der Harnsäureausscheidung bei Gichtikern zeigen, daß die Uratkonzentration im Plasma bzw. im Glomerulusfiltrat zunimmt, während gleichzeitig ein Defekt der tubulären Harnsekretion vorzuliegen scheint. Durch die erhöhte Harnsäurekonzentration im Primärharn und damit auch in den proximalen Tubulusabschnitten soll es zur tubulären Harnsäureausfällung kommen.

Als weiterer zusätzlicher Faktor der Steinbildung wird neben der Harnsäureübersättigung des Urins eine stärkere Säuerung diskutiert.

Nach COTTET (1961) liegt der pH-Wert des Harns bei Gichtpatienten mit Steinen um durchschnittlich 0,2 unter dem gemessenen pH-Wert von Patienten ohne Harnsäuresteine.

Zahlreiche Untersuchungen zeigten, daß in fast allen Gichtnieren Harnsäureablagerungen zu finden sind.

ZOLLINGER u. MUNK (1966) stellten in Gichtnieren nicht nur intratubuläre, sondern auch interstitielle Harnsäureausfällungen fest. PRIEN u. FRONDEL (1947) beschrieben, daß die interstitiellen Ablagerungen aus Natriumurat, die intratubulären aber aus freier Harnsäure bestehen sollen.

Die Harnsäureausfällungen im Bereich der Nieren können kristallin oder amorph sein. Sie finden sich in Papillennähe sowie in den Henleschen Schleifen und in den Sammelröhrchen. Die genaue Ursache von Uratausfällen im Interstitium der Niere scheint jedoch noch nicht hinreichend geklärt.

Das Krankheitsbild der sogenannten idiopathischen Harnsäuresteinbildung ist durch einen normalen Serumharnsäurespiegel, in der Regel auch durch eine normale Harnsäureausscheidung im 24 Std-Urin gekennzeichnet. Es wird lediglich ein stark acidifizierter Harn mit einem Urin-pH unter 5,5 beobachtet.

Auf Grund der Untersuchungsergebnisse von ATSMON et al. (1959), GUTMAN u. YÜ (1965) sowie von SPERLING et al. (1966) soll die Harnsäuerung auf einer gestörten Ammoniumgenese beruhen. MATOUSCHEK u. BÖWERING (1968) diskutieren als Ursache der Harnacidität bei Uratsteindiathese eine verminderte Ammoniakausscheidung.

Die sogenannte „Säurestarre" des Urins ist ein weiterer wichtiger pathogenetischer Faktor der Uratsteinbildung, der sowohl die Löslichkeit der Harnsäure herabsetzt als auch die Kristallisation fördert.

Symptomatik

Koliken und Dauerschmerz finden sich als charakteristische Symptome bei Harnsteinen.

Der Kolikanfall setzt ein mit stechenden krampfartigen Beschwerden in der Nierenloge, die entlang dem Ureter in die Blasen-, Leisten- und Genitalgegend ausstrahlen. Die Dauer variiert zwischen wenigen Minuten und vielen Stunden. Mit kurzen Unterbrechungen können sich die Kolikanfälle von wechselnder Stärke aber auch über Tage hinziehen. Typisch für die Steinkolik sind die Unruhe des Patienten sowie reflektorische Auswirkungen auf Herz, Kreislauf und Magen. Der Höhepunkt des Kolikanfalls ist häufig durch Erbrechen gekennzeichnet; ein reflektorisch bedingter Meteorismus wirkt sich bei Röntgenuntersuchungen besonders störend aus.

Über die pathophysiologischen Veränderungen, die einen Kolikanfall auslösen können, existieren verschiedene Theorien. Durch den Dehnungsreiz des Konkrements soll es zu einem Spasmus der glatten Harnleitermuskulatur kommen, der eine Ektasie des vorgeschalteten Hohlsystems herbeiführt. Harnrückstauung in die Niere mit gleichzeitiger Dehnung der Nierenkapsel sind die Folge (MAY et al., 1969).

Diese Vorstellung über den kolikauslösenden Mechanismus erklärt, warum selbst kleinste Oxalatsteine mit ihrer die Harnleiterwand reizenden zackigen Oberfläche wesentlich öfter Koliken verursachen, als glattwandige Harnsäuresteine. Ebenso ist verständlich, daß häufiger bewegliche Konkremente zur Kolik führen, wenn es auch viele Ausnahmen von dieser Regel gibt.

Die Mehrzahl der langsam wachsenden Harnsäuresteine im Nierenbeckenkelchsystem oder der mit den Kelchpapillen verwachsenen Konkremente wird oft nur durch eine Urographie als Zufallsbefund entdeckt, wenn ein chronischer Harnwegsinfekt oder eine Hämaturie den Patienten zum Arzt führt.

Leichtere subjektive Beschwerden in Form von Druckgefühl in der Lenden- oder Oberbauchgegend sowie diffuse Kreuzschmerzen werden oft wenig beachtet oder fehlgedeutet.

Verursacht ein Harnleiterkonkrement eine chronische Harnrückstauung, so tritt das „gastrointestinale Syndrom" nicht selten in den Vordergrund. Es handelt sich dabei um Abdominalerscheinungen verschiedener Art, wobei eine dyspeptische, eine hepatische und eine pseudoappendicitische Form unterschieden wird. Es empfiehlt sich daher auch eine urologische Untersuchung im Zusammenhang mit den genannten Symptomen.

Das Einsetzen von Koliken erleichtert die Diagnose.

Differentialdiagnostisch ist auf der rechten Seite eine Appendicitis auszuschließen; der retrorenale Reflex kann in seltenen Fällen eine Schmerzempfindung auf der Gegenseite auslösen, wodurch die Kolik in der kontralateralen Niere verspürt wird. Ebenfalls relativ selten sind ausstrahlende Schmerzen in die Schulterblattgegend, wodurch eine Gallenkolik vorgetäuscht werden kann. Das Auftreten einer Reflexanurie bei schweren Kolikanfällen infolge eines einseitigen Ureterverschlußsteines haben wir vereinzelt beobachtet.

Bei der großen Variationsbreite kolikauslösender Faktoren läßt sich die Differentialdiagnose häufig erst durch laborchemische und röntgenologische Untersuchungen abklären.

In der urologischen Praxis wird nicht selten eine Anurie als Folge der Verlegung beider Ureteren oder der Harnröhre mit Harnsäurekonkrementen oft in Form von Steingrieß beobachtet, ohne daß Schmerzen oder andere Symptome vorausgingen. Insbesondere glattwandige Harnsäuresteine gelangen oft völlig symptomlos von der Niere bis in die Blase, um die Harnleiterostien oder den Blasenausgang zu verschließen. Dumpfes, unbestimmtes Druckgefühl in der Flanke oder im Bereich der Costovertebralgegend weist mitunter auf eine chronische Harnstauung hin.

Objektive Symptome

Die Steinanalyse nach Spontanabgang eines Konkrements beweist die Ursache der Beschwerden. Harnsäuresteine bleiben jedoch nicht selten in der Blase und wachsen weiter, insbesondere wenn ein Prostata-Adenom oder eine Harnröhrenstriktur den Spontanabgang erschwert. Die Geburt des Steins in die Blase führt meist zu einem sofortigen Sistieren aller Beschwerden. Ödeme und entzündliche Schwellung des traumatisierten Harnleiterostiums können jedoch später zu erneuten Koliken führen; daher ist auch bei nachweislich abgegangenem Konkrement eine Röntgenkontrolle erforderlich.

Makrohämaturien sind häufiger Folge einer Arrosion der Harnleiterschleimhaut durch den wandernden Stein, seltener Folge einer Fornixruptur infolge pathologischer Harndrucksteigerung im gestauten Hohlsystem.

Makrohämaturien werden daher öfter bei zackigen Calciumoxalat-Steinen als bei Harnsäuresteinen mit glattwandiger Oberfläche beobachtet. Eine Mikrohämaturie ist bei Konkrementen im ableitenden Hohlsystem fast immer nachweisbar. Harnsäurekristalle im Blasenurin sind kein Beweis für Steinbildung, haben jedoch für die Verdachtsdiagnose Bedeutung.

Die Harninfektion, die häufig als sekundäre Begleiterscheinung der Steinbildung durch Harnstauung und Traumatisierung des Hohlsystems verursacht wird, schafft veränderte Voraussetzungen für die Harnsäureausfällung. Die Häufigkeit einer Harnwegsinfektion bei Harnsäuresteinen wird unterschiedlich angegeben (VAHLENSIECK, 1970; KOHLICEK, 1967; ARNOLD u. SEEMANN, 1968). Auf Grund eigener Erfahrungen gehört die Harnsäurelithiasis zur Gruppe der primär aseptischen Harnsteine.

Diagnostik

Für die Verdachtsdiagnose eines Harnsäuresteins sind anamnestische Angaben über frühere Konkrementabgänge sowie über familiäre Grundkrankheiten wie Gicht oder familiäre Hyperuricämie entscheidend. Koliken und andere typische Symptome akuter Harnsteinbeschwerden fehlen häufig. Die Verdachtsdiagnose wird durch röntgenologische und klinisch-chemische Untersuchungen gesichert.

Röntgenuntersuchungen

Jede Röntgenuntersuchung der Harnwege beginnt mit der Leeraufnahme. Sie muß den gesamten oberen Harntrakt, einschließlich Nieren- und Blasengegend erfassen. Reine Harnsäuresteine geben im Gegensatz zu kalkhaltigen Konkrementen keinen röntgendichten Schatten.

Der nicht schattengebende Harnsäurestein wird bei der intravenösen Urographie als Aussparung oder Umfließungsfigur sichtbar.

Der urographische Nachweis eines Harnsäuresteins verlangt eine gute Vorbereitung des Patienten. Der Darm muß entleert sein, Darmgasüberlagerungen können eine Kontrastmittelaussparung im Bereich der Harnwege vortäuschen. Um eine ausreichende Kontrastschärfe zu erreichen, hat der Patient vor der Untersuchung eine 12stündige Flüssigkeitskarenz einzuhalten. Eine intravenöse Kontrastmittelinfusion verbessert die Bildqualität und läßt auch bei eingeschränkter Nierenfunktion noch eine urographische Aussage zu. Bei ektatischem oder hydronephrotisch erweitertem Nierenbeckenkelchsystem läßt sich oft durch Spätaufnahmen nach Kontrastmittelinfusion noch eine befriedigende Darstellung erreichen. Auf das Anlegen einer Bauchdeckenkompression wird zur Abklärung von Harnsäuresteinen verzichtet, da eine Prallfüllung des Nierenbeckenkelchsystems mit Kontrastmittel zur Kontrastmittelüberlagerung des Konkrements führen kann. Häufig läßt sich die Konfiguration nicht schattengebender Aussparungsbezirke sowie ihre Beziehungen zur Wand des Hohlsystems durch eine retrograde Pyelographie mit Kontrastmittel oder Luft, mitunter auch durch gleichzeitige Schichtaufnahmen näher abgrenzen.

Aseptische Bedingungen sind insbesondere bei der retrograden Pyelographie beispielsweise durch Verwendung von Nebacetin als Spüllösung von entscheidender Bedeutung, da durch eine Sekundärinfektion des oberen Hohlsystems ein durch Chemolitholyse auflösbarer Harnsäurestein zum nicht mehr auflösbaren Infektstein mit Phosphatmantel werden kann.

Oft ist auf Grund röntgenologischer Untersuchungen allein die entscheidende differentialdiagnostische Frage nicht befriedigend zu beantworten, ob ein Aussparungseffekt durch einen Harnsäurestein oder durch einen Tumor im Bereich des Nierenbeckenkelchsystems oder des Harnleiters hervorgerufen wird. Im allgemeinen handelt es sich um ein vom Uroepithel ausgehendes Papillom. Typische klinisch-chemische Befunde oder anamnestische Angaben über frühere Harnsäuresteinabgänge erleichtern in diesem Fall die Diagnose. VAHLENSIECK (1970) weist darauf hin, daß bei röntgenologischem Verdacht auf ein Harnsäurekonkrement und bei gleichzeitig nachgewiesenen Harnsäurekristallen im Urin und saurem Urin-pH eventuell eine „diagnostische alkalisierende Behandlung" in Frage kommt. Sorgfältige Verlaufskontrollen sind in solchen Fällen besonders wichtig, um einen Nierenbeckentumor auszuschließen. KIERFELD (1968), SCHÖLL (1968), HARTUNG (1966) und BRESSEL et al. (1969) warnen dringend vor einer kritiklosen alkalisierenden Dauertherapie nicht sicher abgeklärter vermeintlicher Harnsäuresteine, da nicht nur maligne Tumoren, sondern auch tuberkulöse Prozesse auf diese Weise der unbedingt erforderlichen Frühbehandlung entzogen werden. Falls laborchemische und röntgenologische Untersuchungsmethoden keine befriedigende Klärung bringen, sollte im Zweifelsfall durch eine operative Freilegung die Diagnose gesichert werden.

Der klinisch-chemische Befund und seine Beurteilung

Für die klinisch-chemische Diagnostik einer Harnsäuresteindiathese sind der Urin-pH-Wert, die Höhe des Serumharnsäurespiegels und die Menge der Harnsäureexkretion im 24 Std-Urin von entscheidender Bedeutung.

Der Urin-pH-Wert liegt normalerweise zwischen 5,8 und 6,6. Ein pH-Wert unter 5,5 läßt auf eine idiopathische Harnsäuresteinbildung, ein gleichzeitig erhöhter Harnsäurewert im Serum auf eine familiäre Hyperuricämie oder Gicht schließen; allerdings kann ein sekundärer Infekt den Urin alkalisieren. Bei proliferierenden Erkrankungen liegt der Urin-pH-Wert im Normbereich, die Serumharnsäure, normal bis 6,5 mg-%, ist aber ebenso wie bei familiärer Hyperuricämie erhöht.

Proliferierende Erkrankungen sowie die Verabreichung von Uricosurica steigern die Harnsäureexkretion im 24 Std-Urin. Nach COTTET (1961) handelt es sich um eine idiopathische Harnsäuresteindiathese, wenn die Serumharnsäurekonzentration und die Harnsäureexkretion im Normbereich liegen. Einziges klinisch-chemisch nachweisbares Symptom bei idiopathischer Harnsäurelithiasis ist die „Säurestarre des Urins".

Therapie

Die Harnsäuresteinbildung ist das „Symptom" einer Stoffwechselstörung, deren Ursache vielseitig sein kann. Welche Faktoren zur Steinbildung führen, ist letztlich noch nicht geklärt. Bekanntlich sind nicht alle Patienten, die vermehrt

Harnsäure ausscheiden, Steinbildner. Bei operativer Entfernung des Konkrements wird zwar das Symptom beseitigt, nicht aber die Steinerkrankung. Das Rezidiv ist schon da, bevor die Operationswunde verheilt ist (ALKEN, 1966). Nach DWORSCHAK u. HASCHEK (1969) liegt die Rezidivgefahr bei Patienten mit Hyperuricämie bei fast 80%.

Die Methode der Wahl bei Harnsäuresteinen ist heute eine orale medikamentöse Behandlung mit dem Ziel der Auflösung und Rezidivprophylaxe. Zur konservativen Therapie und Prophylaxe von Harnsäuresteinpatienten bieten sich heute folgende Möglichkeiten an:

1. Die Korrektur der Harnacidität durch Alkalisierung, um eine verbesserte Löslichkeit der Harnsäure im Urin zu erzielen.
2. Senkung der Harnsäurekonzentration im Urin durch Diuresesteigerung.
3. Senkung der Konzentration von Harnsäure im Urin und im Serum durch Diätmaßnahmen und medikamentöse Therapie.

Die sogenannte idiopathische Harnsäuresteindiathese ist durch eine Säuerung des Urins mit einem pH unter 5,5 gekennzeichnet. Die Harnsäureausscheidung sowie die Harnsäurekonzentration im Blutserum liegen meist im Normbereich.

Bereits im Jahre 1861 hat HOWSHIP auf die Bedeutung der Alkalisierung des Urins zur Behandlung der Harnsäuresteine hingewiesen.

1955 gaben EISENBERG et al. eine Citronensäure-, Natrium- und Kaliumcitratlösung, die sogenannte Eisenbergsche Lösung zur Harnsäuresteinauflösung an. Seit dem Erfahrungsbericht von BIBUS (1955) über eine erfolgreiche diätetische Behandlung von Harnsäuresteinpatienten mit Zitronensaft machte die Entwicklung der Alkalisierungstherapie ständige Fortschritte. Als bestgeeignetes Präparat zur Alkalisierung des Urins steht heute Uralyt-U[1] (in 100 g Granulat: 46,3 g Kalium citr. sicc., 39 g Natrium citr. sicc., 14,5 g Acid. citr. sicc.) zur Verfügung. Das zur Steinauflösung und Rezidivprophylaxe günstige Urin-pH soll zwischen 6,4 und 6,7 liegen. Werte über 7,0 sind zu vermeiden, da ein Ausfall von Phosphaten zu befürchten ist. Dem Präparat liegt ein Spezialindikatorpapier und eine Tabelle bei; so kann der Patient selbst den pH-Wert seines Harns bestimmen und registrieren. Er ist dadurch in der Lage, unter geeigneter Überwachung seine individuelle Dosierung richtig einzupendeln. Im allgemeinen dauert eine konstante pH-Einstellung des Urins mit Hilfe von Uralyt-U etwa 1 Woche. Wenn Farbuntüchtigkeit zu einer falschen Beurteilung des Spezialindikatorpapiers führt, müssen die Angehörigen entsprechend unterrichtet werden. Ambulante Kontrollen erfolgen in 3 wöchentlichem Abstand und müssen die Protokollierung der pH-Werte, den Urinstatus sowie die Infekttherapie berücksichtigen. Eine Bestimmung der Serumelektrolytwerte und der Serumharnsäure ist in 2 monatigem Abstand erforderlich.

Kriterien für den Therapieerfolg sind das Nachlassen subjektiver Beschwerden, wie Druckgefühl im Nierenbereich oder Koliken, Normalisierung des Sediments sowie in erster Linie röntgenologisch eine Verkleinerung oder ein Verschwinden der Konkremente.

Seit Einführung der Alkalisierungsbehandlung und insbesondere seit dem Einsatz des Präparats Uralyt-U nehmen die positiven Erfahrungsberichte über eine medikamentöse Harnsäuresteinauflösung ständig zu (ATSMON et al., 1963; KOLLWITZ, 1964; ORZECHOWSKI, 1965; HARTUNG, 1966; KAPLAN, 1966; LOEBENSTEIN, 1966; PLANZ, 1966; SCOTT, 1966; BREITWIESER et al., 1967; KOLLE, 1967; WLESS, 1967; HRADEC et al., 1969; MAKRIGIANNIS u. GACA, 1970).

Bis 1971 konnten nach statistischen Erhebungen der Firma Dr. Madaus in Köln insgesamt 711 publizierte Fälle mit Uralyt-U aufgelöst werden. Nur bei

---

[1] Firma Madaus.

weniger als 5% der behandelten Patienten war keine erfolgreiche Therapie möglich. Dieser geringe Prozentsatz entspricht in etwa dem Anteil von Fehldiagnosen und calciumhaltigen Mischsteinen. Ein Verkleinerungseffekt wurde zwar auch bei Mischsteinen mit überwiegendem Harnsäureanteil beobachtet. Insbesondere bei extrem alkalischem Harnmilieu ist jedoch die Gefahr eines apositionellen Wachstums der Konkremente durch Ausfällung von Phosphat gegeben. In solchen Fällen ist daher eine besonders sorgfältige Überwachung angezeigt.

Der Einsatz von Uralyt-U bei Harnsäurelithiasis gehört heute zur Standardtherapie des Urologen. Die Zahl der erfolgreich aufgelösten Harnsäuresteine liegt daher sicherlich wesentlich höher als die im Schrifttum erfaßten Fälle.

Routinemäßig ist vor Einleitung der Alkalisierungstherapie bei Harnsäuresteindiathese eine wiederholte Bestimmung des Urin-pH-Wertes nötig. Bei alkalischem Harn ist ein Infekt die Ursache.

Untersuchungen von KOLLWITZ (1965) zeigten einen Anstieg der ausgefällten Harnsäuremenge in Abhängigkeit von der Füllungszeit sowie eine Induktionswirkung durch Fibrinflocken. FRANK et al. (1965) beobachteten bei Harnsäuresteinpatienten mit Begleitinfekt zum Teil eine vermehrte Wirkung der peroralen Chemolitholyse. Derartige Untersuchungsergebnisse unterstreichen die Notwendigkeit einer gezielten antibiotischen Langzeitbehandlung neben der Alkalisierungstherapie.

Analyse der eigenen Behandlungsergebnisse bei Harnsäuresteinbildnern mit und ohne Hyperuricämie

Durch die erfolgreiche konservativ medikamentöse Therapie ist es heute möglich geworden, die meisten Harnsäuresteinbildner vorwiegend ambulant zu behandeln. Voraussetzung ist allerdings eine konsequente urologische Kontrolle, insbesondere während der Auflösungsphase.

Bei den konsequent behandelten unkomplizierten Fällen konnten wir auch beim eigenen Krankengut in rund 90% eine erfolgreiche Chemolitholyse durch Alkalisierung und Allopurinol erzielen.

Ein wesentlich problematischeres, streng selektiertes Krankengut stellen unsere stationär behandelten Harnsäuresteinbildner dar. Eine stationäre Behandlung führen wir durch bei Anurie und Harnstauung bzw. bei röntgenologisch stummer oder stark funktionsgeschädigter Niere, bei teilcalcifizierten oder großen Konkrementen mit therapieresistentem Harnwegsinfekt und bei eingeklemmten Harnleitersteinen.

Von insgesamt 203 Harnsäuresteinpatienten, bei denen wegen eines der genannten Befunde eine stationäre Behandlung zwischen 1965 und 1971 erforderlich war, konnten 153 regelmäßig kontrolliert werden.

Erwartungsgemäß fand sich bei 116 Patienten eine Säurestarre des Urins, bei über einem Drittel der Fälle war wegen eines bakteriell nachgewiesenen Harnwegsinfektes eine antibiotische Behandlung notwendig. Dieser relativ hohe Prozentsatz infizierter Harnsäuresteine mag mit dem ebenfalls hohen Prozentsatz von Abflußstörungen zusammenhängen.

Bei 81 der insgesamt 153 Patienten hatte das Konkrement zu einer Stauung des vorgeschalteten Hohlsystems geführt, davon 16 mal einseitig. In fast 10% der Fälle fanden wir bei der Aufnahme eine Anurie mit Serumkreatininwerten über 10 mg-%, die sich in 6 Fällen bis zur Entlassung normalisiert hatten. 44 mal kam es allein unter konservativ medikamentöser Therapie zu einer raschen Rückbildung der Stauungszeichen mit Verkleinerung oder Abgang der Konkremente. In 32 Fällen mit totalem beidseitigem oder einseitigem Ureterverschluß konnten wir ebenfalls auf ein operatives Eingreifen verzichten. Ein Ureterenkatheter wurde an

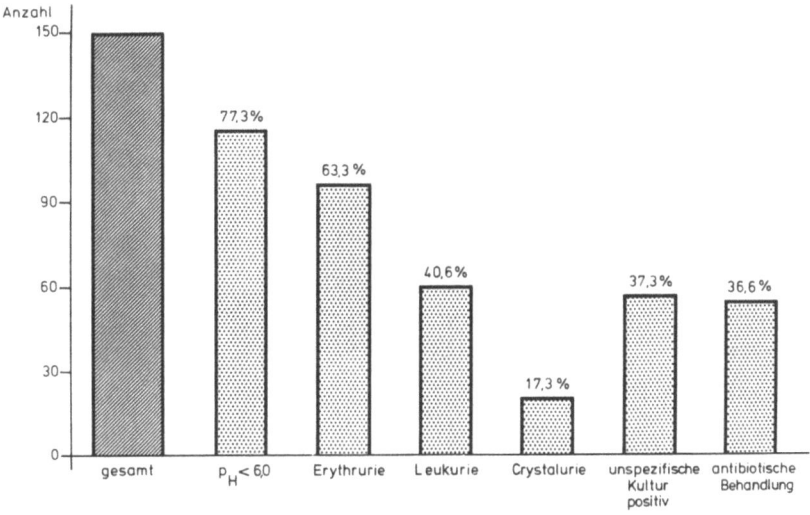

Abb. 3. Urinanalysen bei Harnsäurelithiasis

Harnsäureverschlußsteinen vorbeigeführt und durchschnittlich 14 Tage lang bei liegendem Katheter und Antibioticaschutz sowie gleichzeitiger antiphlogistischer Therapie eine konservative Behandlung durchgeführt.

Nur bei 21 Fällen, die instrumentell nicht entlastet werden konnten, war ein akutes operatives Eingreifen notwendig, in erster Linie um die akute Stauung zu beseitigen und damit die Entwicklung einer Hydronephrose zu vermeiden.

Vor Beginn der Behandlung untersuchten wir in der Regel mindestens 3mal bei jedem Patienten den Harnsäurespiegel im Blutserum und fanden in 84,5% der Fälle eine Hyperuricämie, in 40% eine Hyperuricurie. Diese Zahlen liegen über den Vergleichsergebnissen der einschlägigen Literatur. Erwähnenswert ist auch der relativ hohe Prozentsatz von Patienten mit Hypercalcämie und Hypercalcurie bei gleichzeitiger Hyperuricurie. Umgekehrt finden sich in der Literatur in letzter Zeit zahlreiche Beobachtungen, die ein gehäuftes Vorkommen von Hyperuricurie und Calciumoxalat-Steinbildung mitteilen.

Bei Harnsäuresteinbildung mit Hyperuricämie kombinieren wir, wie schon betont, grundsätzlich eine Alkalisierungsbehandlung mit einer Allopurinoltherapie.

Insgesamt war bei 83 von 117 Patienten eine rein medikamentöse Therapie innerhalb durchschnittlich 48 Tagen erfolgreich, in 34 Fällen mußte zusätzlich instrumentell eine akute Abflußstörung beseitigt werden, entweder zu Anfang der Behandlung oder wenn ein medikamentös verkleinerter Nierenbeckenstein den Harnleiter verlegt hatte.

Drei typische Fälle aus unserem Krankengut sollen abschließend den Erfolg einer Chemolitholyse durch Alkalisierung und Allopurinoltherapie bei Harnsäurelithiasis demonstrieren.

Der Einsatz einer Alkalisierungsbehandlung bei Hyperuricämie, kombiniert mit Allopurinol, ist heute die Therapie der Wahl bei Harnsäuresteinen. Operative oder instrumentelle Maßnahmen sind in der Regel nur bei großen Blasenkonkrementen, doppelseitigem Vorkommen und Verschluß des ableitenden Systems, also bei vitaler Indikation erforderlich.

Analyse der eigenen Behandlungsergebnisse bei Harnsäuresteinbildnern

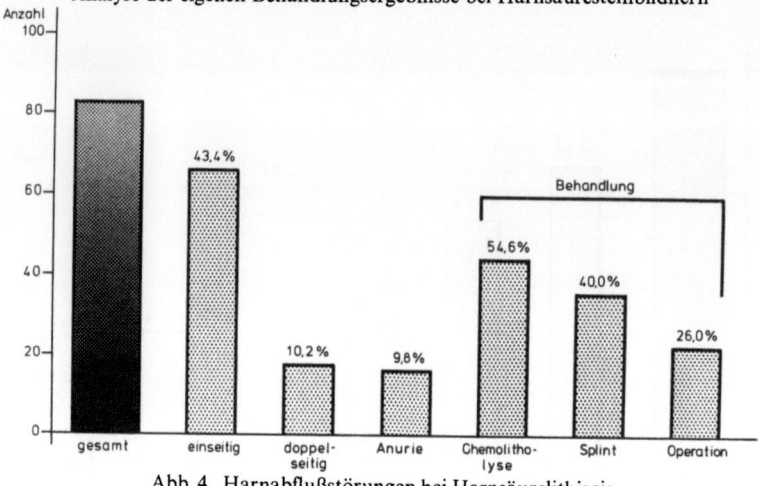

Abb. 4. Harnabflußstörungen bei Harnsäurelithiasis

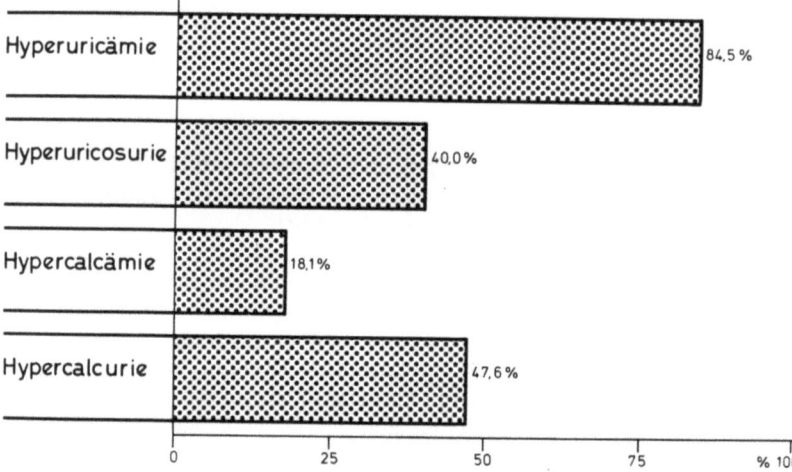

Abb. 5. Laborchemische Ergebnisse bei Harnsäurelithiasis

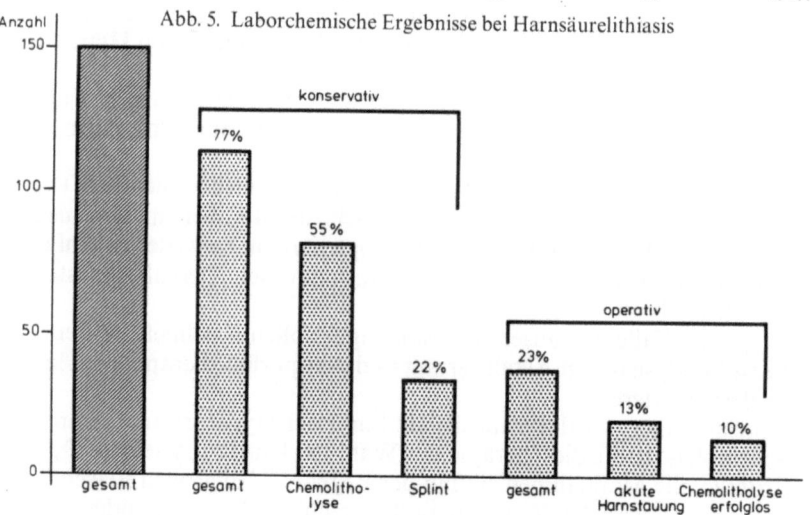

Abb. 6. Eigene Behandlungsergebnisse

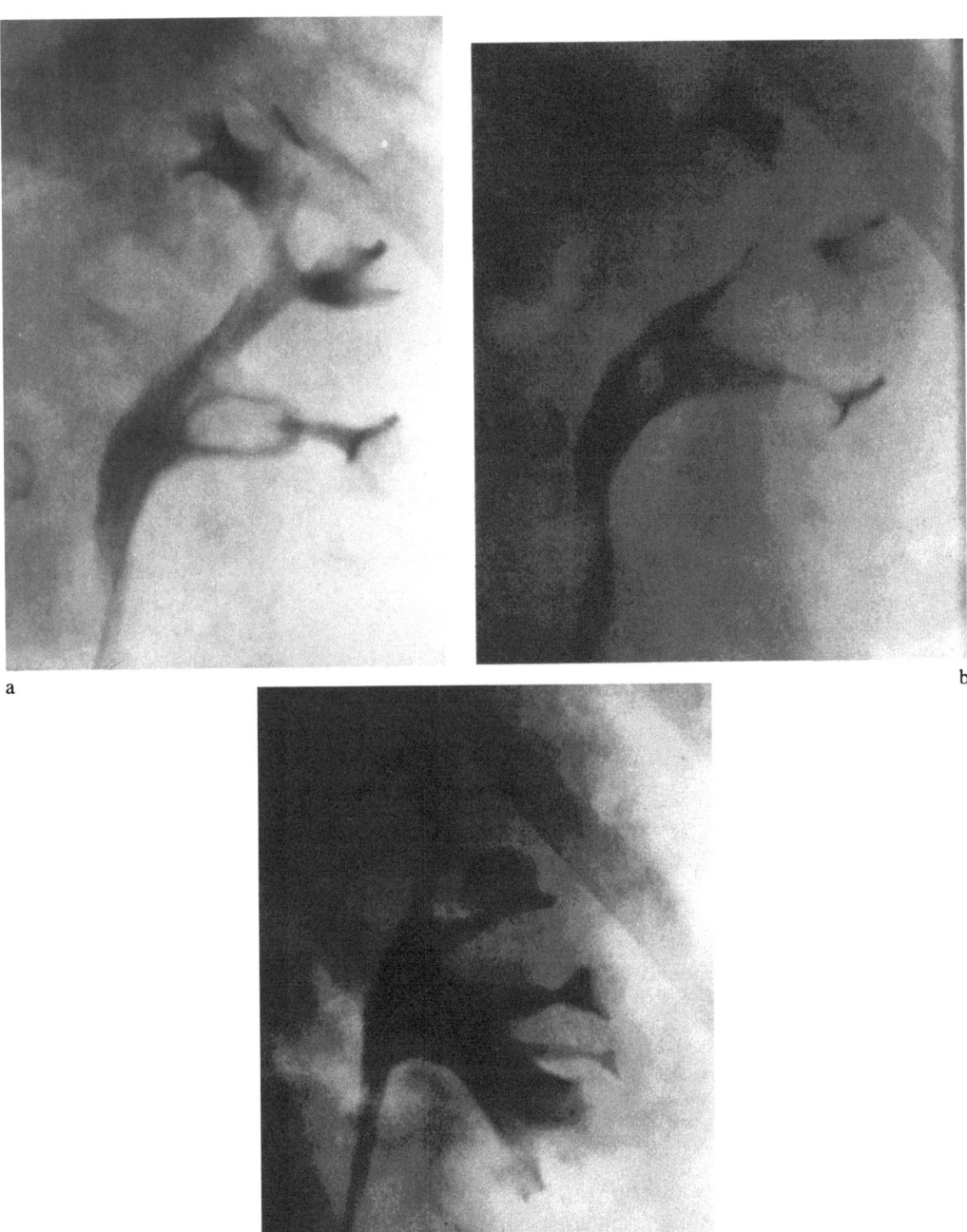

Abb. 7a—c. A.W. 61 Jahre. Seit August 1964 rezidivierende spontane Steinabgänge links. Steinanalyse: Harnsäure. Mai 1971 eintägige Nierenkolik links mit Makrohämaturie. (a) Retrogrades Pyelogramm (21. 5. 1971): Haselnußgroßer, nicht schattengebender Nierenbeckenstein links. Harnsäurewert im Serum normal.. Harn-pH: 5,4. Sediment: massenhaft Erythrocyten, vereinzelt Leukocyten, Harnsäurekristalle. Bakterien negativ. (b) Retrogrades Pyelogramm (1. 6. 1971): Der Stein hat sich um ca. die Hälfte verkleinert. Harn-pH: 6,7. (c) Retrogrades Pyelogramm (12. 6. 1971): Völlige Auflösung des Steines. Harn-pH: 6,6. Harnsediment o. B. Der Patient ist beschwerdefrei

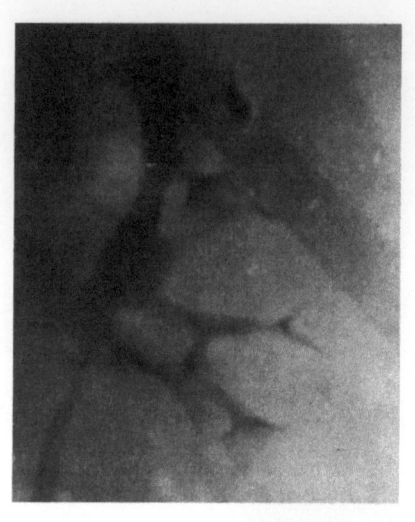
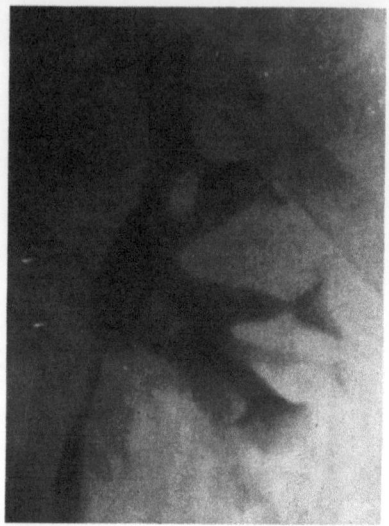
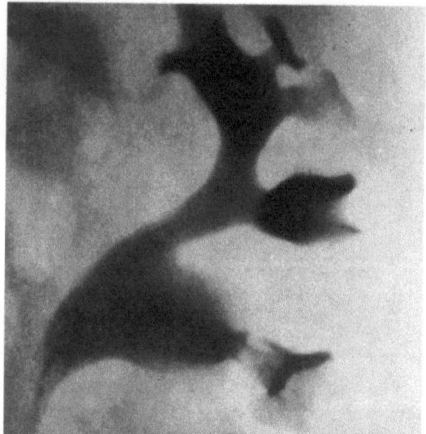

Abb. 8a—c. H.A. 42 Jahre. Am 24. 12. 1961 Pyelolithotomie rechts. Steinanalyse: Harnsäure. Seither rezidivierende Steinabgänge. Stationäre Aufnahme am 12. 8. 1970 wegen linksseitiger Kolik und Makrohämaturie. (a) Retrogrades Pyelogramm (13. 8. 1970): Bohnengroßer, nicht schattengebender Nierenbeckenstein links. Harnsäure im Serum normal. Harn-pH: 5,5. Sediment: Massenhaft Ery, vereinzelt Leuko, keine Bakterien. (b) Retrogrades Pyelogramm (25. 8. 1970): Deutliche Verkleinerung des Konkrements. Harn-pH: 6,7. (c) Retrogrades Pyelogramm (1. 9. 1970): Totalauflösung des Konkrements, der Patient ist beschwerde- und infektfrei

Erfahrungsgemäß können durch ständige orale Alkalisierung auch Rezidive zuverlässig verhindert werden. Eine chronische Alkalizufuhr kann allerdings in besonders gelagerten Fällen mit unerwünschten Nebenwirkungen verbunden sein. Beispielsweise ist bei manifester Herzinsuffizienz oder Hypertonie die erhöhte Natriumzufuhr kontraindiziert; auch die verabreichte Kaliummenge muß bei Patienten mit Niereninsuffizienz oder bei gleichzeitiger Digitalisierung beachtet werden.

Bei der Rezidivprophylaxe ist es erforderlich, daß sie über Jahrzehnte durchgeführt wird.

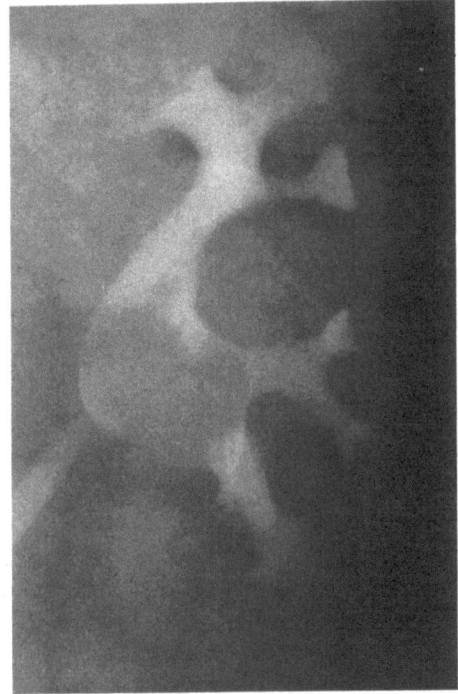
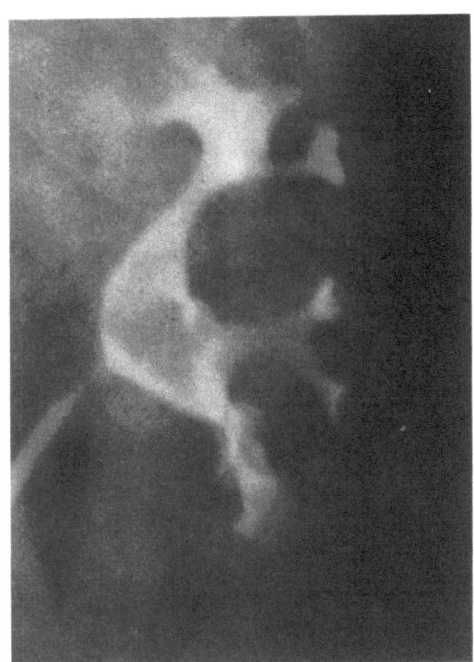
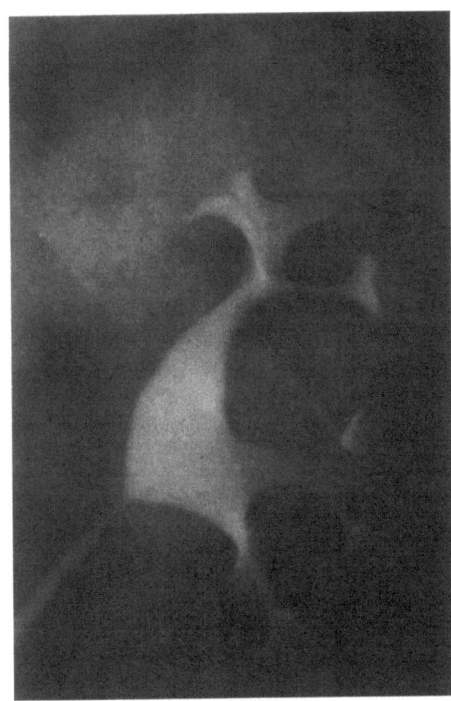

Abb. 9a—c. J. N. 63 Jahre. Seit 3 Wochen rezidivierende linksseitige Flankenkoliken mit Makrohämaturie. Stationäre Aufnahme am 12.2.1970. (a) Urogramm (14.12.1970): Walnußgroßer, unregelmäßig begrenzter, nicht schattengebender Nierenbeckenstein links. (Röntgenologisch Differentialdiagnose: Nierenbeckentumor!) Harnsäure im Serum 6,9 mg-%. Harn-pH: 5,3. Sediment: massenhaft Erythrocyten, vereinzelt Leuko, vereinzelt Plattenepithelien, Harnsäurekristalle. Bakterien negativ. (b) Urogramm (4.1.1971): Deutliche Verkleinerung des Konkrements. (c) Urogramm (30.3.1971): Totalauflösung des Konkrements, der Patient ist beschwerde- und infektfrei

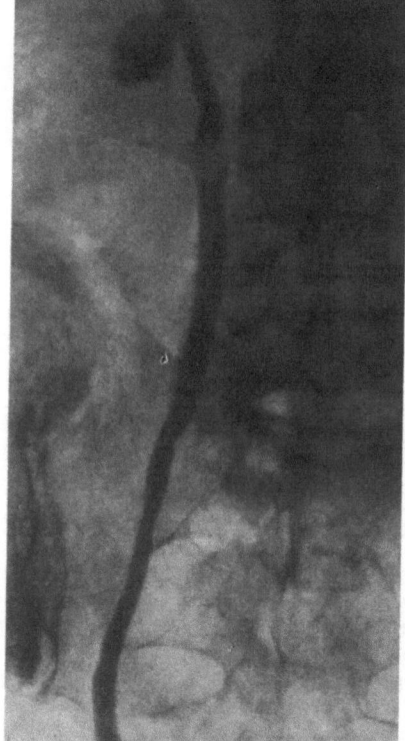
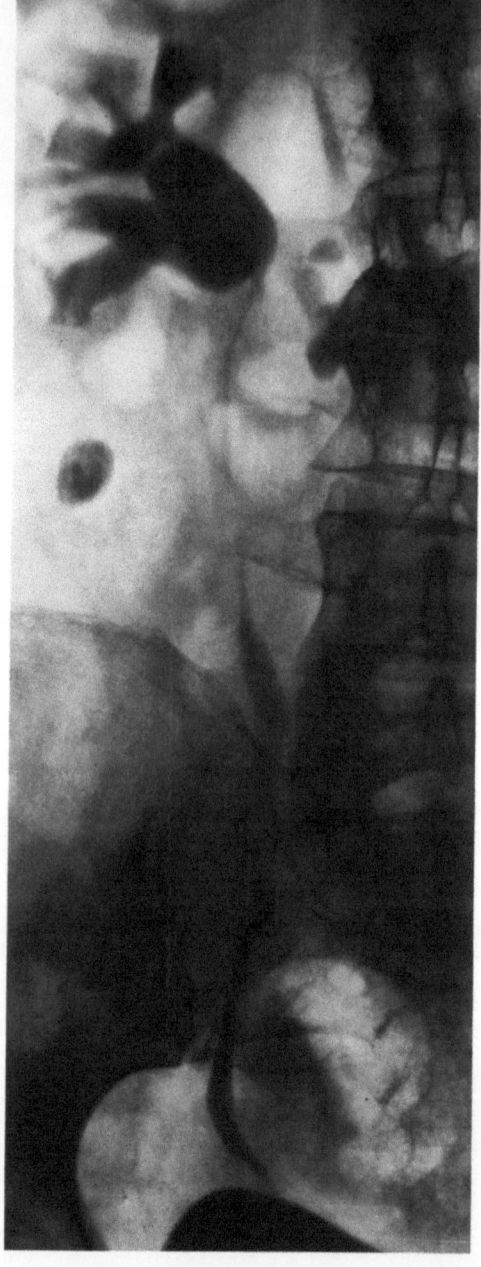

Abb. 10a u. b. H.W. 64 Jahre. Seit 5 Wochen rezidivierende rechtsseitige Flankenkoliken. Stationäre Aufnahme am 16. 7. 1971. (a) Retrogrades Pyelogramm (1. 7. 1971): Bohnengroßer, glattbegrenzter Verschlußstein im Bereich des rechten oberen Harnleiterdrittels bei extremer Nierenbeckenkelchektasie. (b) Urogramm (16. 7. 1971): Zustand nach Spontanabgang des verkleinerten Konkrements 15 Tage nach oraler Medikation von Uralyt-U während gleichzeitiger Entlastung der Niere durch einen Ureterenverweilkatheter

Nach einjähriger rezidivfreier Zeit kann vorübergehend die Alkalisierungsbehandlung abgesetzt werden. In dieser therapiefreien Zeit kommt im Rahmen der Prophylaxe diätetischen Maßnahmen sowie der Zitronensaftbehandlung und einer Diuresesteigerung große Bedeutung zu. In jedem Fall sollte der Harnsäuresteinbildner den Urin-pH-Wert weiterhin kontrollieren.

Zur Erhöhung der Harndilution halten wir die Verordnung alkalisierender Heilwässer wie Vichy-Wasser oder Wildunger Helenenquelle für nützlich. Pilsner-Bier, das bekanntlich eine stark säuernde Wirkung hat, sollte vermieden werden.

Unter dem Eindruck der guten Ergebnisse einer rein konservativen Therapie bei Harnsäurelithiasis sollte die hohe Rezidivneigung, die sich sehr oft symptomlos ankündigt, nicht unterschätzt und vernachlässigt werden. In diesem Zusammenhang sei auch erwähnt, daß die purinarme Ernährung zwar heute an Bedeutung zurücktritt, doch sollten Harnsäuresteinbildner purinreiche Nahrungsmittel meiden. Ausreichende Flüssigkeitsaufnahme, die eine tägliche Harnausscheidung von 1500 ml in 24 Std garantiert, ist auch heute noch entscheidend für den Therapieerfolg.

Literatur

ABESHOUSE, B. S., WEINBERG, T.: Experimental study of solvent action of "versene" on urinary calculi. J. Urol. (Baltimore) **65**, 316—332 (1951).

ALBRIGHT, F., SULKOWITCH, H. W., CHUTE, R.: Non-surgical aspects of the kidnes stone problem. J. Amer. med. Ass. **113**, 2049 (1939).

ALKEN, C. E.: Gedanken zur Klinik der Nephrolithiasis. Urologe **5**, 161—163 (1966).

ALKEN, C. E.: Gedanken zur Nephrolithiasis. Urologe **8**, 179—180 (1969).

ALKEN, C. E.: Jeder dritte Nierenstein auflösbar? Dtsch. Ärztebl. **68**, 13—15 (1971b).

ALKEN, C. E.: Leitfaden für Urologie. Stuttgart: Thieme 1971.

ALKEN, C. E., HERMANN, G.: Untersuchungen über die Urolithiasis unter besonderer Berücksichtigung der Bevölkerungsstatistik. Urol. int. (Basel) **4**, 335—344 (1957).

ALKEN, C. E., HERMANN, G., WEBER, B.: Eine Methode zur lichtelektrischen Bestimmung der Gesamtstabilität des Harns. Z. Urol. **50**, 335—341 (1957).

ALKEN, C. E., HERMANN, G., WEBER, B.: Zur Frage der Beziehung von Schutzkolloiden und Oberflächenspannung im menschlichen Urin. Z. Urol. **50**, 423—433 (1957a).

ALLEN, A. C.: The kidney. New York: Grune und Stratton 1951.

AMSTRONG, W. A., GREENE, L. F.: Uric acid calculi: With particular reference to determination of uric acid content of blood. J. Urol. (Baltimore) **70**, 545—546 (1953).

ARNOLD, W., SEEMANN, N.: Therapie des Harnsäuresteinleidens. Dtsch. med. Wschr. **93**, 1791—1794 (1968).

ASCHOFF, L.: Histologische Untersuchungen über die Harnsäureablagerungen. Verh. dtsch. Ges. Path., Meran 1900.

ATSMON, A., DE VRIES, A., FRANK, M.: Uric acid lithiasis. J. Urol. (Baltimore) **84**, 167—175 (1960).

ATSMON, A., DE VRIES, A., LAZEBNIK, J., SALINGER, H.: Dissolution of renal uric acid stones by oral alkalinization and large fluid intake in a patient suffering from gout. Amer. J. Med. **27**, 167—172 (1959).

BAUER, K. M.: Harnsteingenese und -prophylaxe. Medizinische **52**, 1939—1941 (1957).

BEDRNA, J., POLCACK, J.: Harnsäuresteinbildung bei Leucämie. Med. Klin. **25**, 1700—1705 (1929).

BENEDICT, J. D., ROCHE, M., YU, T. F., BIEN, E. J., GUTMAN, A. B., DE SETTEN, W., JR.: Incorporation of clycine nitrogen into uric acid in normal and gouty man. Metabolism **1**, 3—14 (1952).

BIBUS, B.: Die konservative Therapie der Harnsäuresteine. Verh. dtsch. Ges. Urol. 20. Tagg. September 1963 (Wien).

BLESS, K. D.: Unsere bisherigen Erfahrungen in der Behandlung der Uratsteinbildung und der Uratsteindiathese mit Uralyt-U. Therapiewoche **17**, 7—10 (1967).

BOEMINGHAUS, H.: Harnsteine. Z. Urol. **29**, 14—26 (1935).

BOEMINGHAUS, H.: Steingenese, Steinauflösung, konservative Behandlung Steinkranker und Prophylaxe nach operativer Steinentfernung. Konkrementbildung und Nebenschilddrüse. Medizinische **1953**, 369—375.

BOSHAMER, K.: Morphologie und Genese der Harnsteine. In: Handb. d. Urologie, Bd. X. Berlin-Heidelberg-New York: Springer 1961.

BOSHAMER, K.: Lehrbuch der Urologie, 7. Aufl. Stuttgart: Fischer 1968.

BOYCE, W. H., GARVEY, K.: The amount and nature of the organic matrix in Urinary calculi. A Review. J. Urol. (Baltimore) **76**, 213—229 (1956a).

BOYCE, W. H., GARVEY, F. K., NORFLETT, C. M.: Ion binding properties of electrophoretically homogenous mucoproteins of urine in normal subjects and in patients with renal calculus disease. J. Urol. (Baltimore) **72**, 1019—1031 (1954a).

BOYCE, W. H., GARVEY, F. K., NORFLETT, C. M.: Proteins and other biocolloids of urine in health and in calculus disease. I. Electrophoretic studies at ph 4,5 and 8,6 of those components suluble in molar sodium chloride. J. clin. Invest. **33**, 1287—1299 (1954).

BOYCE, W. H., KING, J. S.: Cystal-Matrix-Interrelations in calculi. J. Urol. (Baltimore) **81**, 351—367 (1959).

BOYCE, W. H., POOL, C. S., MESCHEN, J., KING, J. S.: Organic matrix of urinary calculi. Acta radiol. (Stockh.) **50**, 543—551 (1958).

BOYCE, W. H., SULKIN, N. M.: Biocolloids of urin in health and in calculous disease. J. clin. Invest. **35**, 1067—1091 (1956).

BREITWASSER, P., RUILE, K., PLATT, O.: Konservative Behandlung der Harnsäurediathese. Med. Welt (Stuttg.) **18**, 2130—2135 (1967).

BRESSEL, M., HOPPE-SEYLER, G. F., HORN, H. D.: Diagnostik und konservative Therapie der Urolithiasis. Internist (Berl.) **9**, 184—195 (1968).

BRINKMANN, W.: Zur Prophylaxe des postoperativen Harnsteinrezidivs unter Berücksichtigung medikamentöser Möglichkeiten. Medizinische **36**, 1300—1304 (1957).

CHAUVIN, E., COLAS, R.: Calcul coralliforme du veni extrait per pyélotomie e'larpie. J. Urol. Néphrol. **60**, 72—73 (1954).

COTTET, J.: Confrontations Thérapeutiques, Comment traiter la goutte lorsqu'elle est compliquée de lithiase? Presse méd. **96**, 1557—1569 (1961).

COTTET, J., MIKOL, G.: Le syndrome biochimique de la lithiase urique. In: La lithiase urinaire, Tome I. Paris: Vigot 1955.

DAVIS, B. B., FIELD, J. B., RODMAN, G. P., KEDES, L. H.: Localization and pyrazinamide inhibition of distal transtubular movement of uric acid-2-Cl 4 with a modified stop-flow technique. J. clin. Invest. **44**, 716—720 (1965).

DIX, V. W.: Harnleitersteine. Ann. roy. Coll. Surg. Engl. **11**, 137—156 (1962).

DULCE, H. J.: Untersuchungen über die Bedeutung der Schutzkolloide und Kristalloide für die Löslichkeit von Calciumoxalat im Harn. Ärztl. Wschr. **11**, 445—450 (1956).

DULCE, H. J.: Über die Harnkolloide, Urol. int. (Basel) **7**, 65—72 (1958).

DULCE, H. J.: Harnsteine und Ernährung. Urologe **1**, 233—238 (1962).

DWORSCHAK, W., HASCHEK, H.: Konservative Behandlung von Nierensteinen. Med. Klin. **64**, 273—278 (1969).

EBSTEIN, W. V.: Die Natur und Bedeutung der Harnsteine. Wiesbaden: Bergmann 1884.

EISENBERG, H., CONNOR, T. B., HOWARD, J. E. A.: Useful agent for alkali therapy. J. clin. Endocrin. **15**, 503—507 (1955).

FROHMÜLLER, H.: Die Entstehung von Harnsteinen. Med. Klinik **64**, 269—273 (1969).

GASSER, G., BRAUNER, K., PREISINGER, A.: Das Harnsteinproblem. Z. Urol. **49**, 148—159 (1956).

GEHRES, R. F., RAYMOND, S.: A new chemical approach to the dilution of urinary calculi. J. Urol. (Baltimore) **65**, 474—483 (1951).

GEINITZ, W.: Tierversuche zur Verhinderung der Harnsteinbildung. Münch. med. Wschr. **98**, 895—897 (1956).

GUNST, W.: Ein Beitrag zur intrarenalen Steinauflösung. Medizinische **1956**, 226, 227—228.

GUTMAN, A. B., YU, T. F.: Renal function in gout. Amer. J. Med. **23**, 600—610 (1957).

GUTMAN, A. B., YU, T. F.: Uric acid metabolism in normal man and in primary gout. New Engl. J. Med. **273**, 252—270 (1965).

GUTMAN, A. B., YU, T. F.: A three component system for regulation of renal excretion of uric acid in man. Trans. Ass. Amer. Phycns **74**, 353—359 (1961).

GUTMAN, A. B., YU, T. F., BERGER, C.: Tubular secretion of urate in man. J. clin. Invest. **38**, 1778—1781 (1959).

HAMMARSTEN, G.: Formation of aseptic stones in urinary tract. Nord. Med. **30**, 911—925 (1946).

HARTUNG, F.: Fortschritte und Erfolge in der Behandlung der Urat-Urolithiasis. Med. Welt **17**, 2759—2762 (1966).
HEISE, G. W., MÜLLER, G. W.: Beiträge zur Entstehung und Auflösung von Harnsteinen. Urologe **5**, 171—177 (1966).
HELLER, F.: Die Harnkonkretionen. Wien 1860.
HENCH, T. S., VANZANT, F. R., NOMLAND, R.: Basis for early differential diagnosis of gout; clinical comparison of 100 cases each of gout, rheumatic fever and infections arthritis. Trans. Ass. Amer. Physiol. **43**, 217—229 (1928).
HERMAN, J. R.: Recent advances in the study and treatment of Urolithiasis. N. Y. St. J. Med. **57**, 17—29 (1957).
HEUSSER, H.: Die Prophylaxe der Urolithiasis vom pharmakologischen Standpunkt aus. Praxis **1955**, 1062—1069, 1087—1091.
HIGGINS, C. C.: Dietary control in calculous disease. Mod. Hosp. **51**, 84 (1938).
HIRSCH, H. H., VOIT, E.: Experimentelle Untersuchungen über die Verhinderung der Harnsteinbildung durch Schutzkolloidvermehrung im Harn. Klin. Wschr. **32**, 651—654 (1954).
HRADEK, E., PETRIK, R., SRAMEK, F., SIMON, V.: Uratsteinleiden in Böhmen. Urologe **8**, 193—198 (1969).
KAPLAN, F.: Urinary stones. Medical grand Rounds. Berichte Parkland Memorial Hospital 21.4, 1966.
KEUTEL, H. J., HERMANN, G., LICHT, W.: Immunoelektrophotometrische Untersuchungen über den serumidentischen Anteil der Harn-Kolloide und ihre Bedeutung bei der Harnsteinbildung. Clin. chim. Acta **4**, 665—672 (1959).
KIERFELD, G.: Indikationsstellung zur konservativen Uratsteintherapie und -prophylaxe. Dtsch. med. Wschr. **93**, 1547—1549 (1968).
KOCH, F. E.: Experimentelle Therapie der Nierensteinkrise. Therapiewoche **1951**, Folge 9, 507.
KOHLICEK, J.: Konservative Behandlung der Harnsäuresteine. Med. Klin. **62**, 1919—1920 (1967).
KOLLE, P.: Der Harnsäurestein. Neue Wege der Therapie. Münch. med. Wschr. **109**, 243—248 (1967).
KOLLWITZ, A. A.: Die Behandlung und Prophylaxe von Harnsäuresteinen der Niere durch orale Alkalisierung. Dtsch. med. Wschr. **91**, 1257—1259 (1966).
KRITZLER, R. A.: Uric acid lithiasis. Amer. J. Med. **25**, 532 (1958).
LATHEM, W., RODMAN, G. P.: Impairment of uric acid excretion in gout. J. clin. Invest. **41**, 1955—1967 (1962).
LICHTWITZ, L.: Formation of concretions. In: J. Alexander's Colloid Chemistry, Vol. 5, p. 1063. New York: Reinhold 1944.
LOEBENSTEIN, H.: Der Wandel in der Indikationsstellung durch die perorale Litholyse von Harnsteinen. Urologe **5**, 178—181 (1966).
MACRIGIANNIS, D., GACA, A.: Orale Auflösung und Rezidivprophylaxe von Harnsäuresteinen der Niere. Dtsch. med. Wschr. **26**, 1383—1387 (1970).
MATOUSCHEK, E., BÖWERING, R.: Citronensäure- und Harnsäureausscheidung im Urin Gesunder und Harnsäuresteinträgern vor und nach Einnahme eines citronensäurecitrathaltigen Granulats. Klin. Wschr. **46**, 1011—1012 (1968).
MATOUSCHEK, E., BÖWERING, R.: Über die Harnsäuerung bei Harnsäuresteinträgern. Klin. Wschr. **46**, 1012—1014 (1968).
MERTZ, D. P.: Gicht, Grundlagen, Klinik und Therapie. Stuttgart: Thieme 1971.
MIDDLETON, R. E., GRUA, O. E.: Überblick über die Erfahrungen während eines Jahres mit dem Johnson-Extraktor in der Behandlung von Harnleitersteinen. J. Urol. (Baltimore) **68**, 125—136 (1952).
MITCHELL, N.: Zit. nach: CAMPBELL, M.: Clinical pediatr. urology, p. 639. Philadelphia: Saunders 1951.
MOORE, T. D., SWEETSER, T. H., JR.: Die Entstehung von Steinen aus dem Nierenbecken mit Hilfe von Fibrinkoagula. J. Urol. (Baltimore) **67**, 579—584 (1952).
NUGENT, C. A., TYLER, F. H.: The renal excretion of uric acid in patients with gout and in nongouty subject. J. clin. Invest. **38**, 1890—1905 (1959).
OGRYZLO, M. A.: The renal factor in the etiology of primary gout. Canad. med. Ass. J. **83**, 1326—1329 (1960).
PAILLARD, H., FAUVERT, R.: La Goutte, Vol. I. Paris: Bailliere 1956.
PLANZ, K.: Die Therapie der Uratsteindiathese. Ther. d. Gegenw. **12**, 1518—1523 (1966).
PRIEM, E. C., FRONDEL, C.: Studies in urolithiasis. I. Composition of urinary calculi. J. Urol. (Baltimore) **57**, 949—954 (1947).
PRIEM, E. C., FRONDEL, C.: II. Relationship between pathogenesis, structure and compositions of calculi. J. Urol. (Baltimore) **61**, 820—824 (1949).

PRIEN, E. L., WALKER, B. S.: Studies in urolithiasis. J. Urol. (Baltimore) **74**, 440—446 (1955).
REUBI, F., VORBURGER, C.: Die Gichtniere. Münch. med. Wschr. **104**, 2154—2161 (1962).
SCHMIDT, A. W., PLANZ, K.: Prophylaxe und konservative Therapie der Uratsteindiathese. Urologe **4**, 156—162 (1965).
SCHNEIDER, H. J., KLOTZ, L., HORN, H.: Die Herstellung eines Titratgranulats und seine Verwendung in der Therapie der Harnsäurelithiasis. Z. Urol. Nephrol. **62**, 351—355 (1969).
SCHÖLL, H.: Behandlung der Harnsäuresteine. Wien. med. Wschr. **118**, 883—891 (1968).
SCHULTHEIS, T.: Über die Entstehung von Harnsteinen als Folge der Änderung der Stabilität des Harnes. Sonderh. Z. Urol. (1949).
SCOTT, J. T.: Dissolution of renal uric acid stones by oral alkalinization. Brit. med. J. **1966 II**, 317—325.
SEEGMÜLLER, J. F., GRAYZEL, A. J., HOWEL, R. R., PLATO, C.: The renal excretion of uric acid in gout. J. clin. Invest. **41**, 1094—1099 (1962).
SORRENTINO, F.: Experimentelle Untersuchungen über Möglichkeiten einer biologischen Behandlung der Harnsäuresteine. Z. Urol. **52**, 281—292 (1959).
SPERLING, M., FRANK, M., DE VRIES, A.: L'excretion urinaire d'amminoniae an cours de la goutte. Revue franç. Étud. clin. biol. **11**, 401—404 (1966).
STAEHLER, W.: Zur Auflösung der Nierensteine durch Zitronensäure mittels Harnleiterkatheter (Instrumentelle Litholyse). Med. Welt **37**, 1—7 (1951).
STAEMMLER, M.: Beitrag zur Entstehung von Nierensteinen. Z. Urol. **52**, 3—18 (1959).
STAEMMLER, M.: Die Entstehung von Nierensteinen in morphologischer Sicht. Tagg. Nordrh.-Westf. Urol. Ges. Aachen 22. Nov. 1958.
SUBY, H. I., ALBRIGHT, F., WAYNE, J., DEMPSY, E.: Dissolution of urinary calculi: Experiments with ethylene and diamine tetra-acetic-acid with and without "wetting agent". J. Urol. (Baltimore) **66**, 527—532 (1951).
SUBY, H., SUBY, R. M., ALBRIGHT, F.: Dissolution of urinary calculs. J. Urol. (Baltimore) **68**, 96—104 (1952).
UEBELHÖR, R.: Tinkturen bei Nierensteinleiden. Wien. med. Wschr. **107** (35), 699—703 (1957).
VAHLENSIECK, W.: Methodik der peroralen Chemolitholyse und Dauer der Prophylaxe bei Harnsäuresteinen. Med. Welt **36**, 1559—1566 (1970).
VERMEULEN, C. W., LYON, E. S., FRIED, F. A.: On the nature of the stone forming process. J. Urol. (Baltimore) **94**, 176—194 (1965).
VRIES DE, A., SPERLING, O., FRANK, M., ORA, K.: Apercu sur les facteurs metaboliques de la lithiase ueique. Vie méd. **46**, 923—933 (1965).
WYNGAARDEN, J. B.: On the dual etiology of primary gout. Arthr. and Rheum. **3**, 414—421 (1960).
YU, T. F., BERGER, L., KUPFER, S., GUTMAN, A. B.: Tubular excretion or urate in the dog. Amer. J. Physiol. **199**, 1199—1205 (1960).
YU, T. F., BERGER, F., KUPFER, S., GUTMAN, A. B.: Renal function in gout. II. Effect of uric acid loading in renal excretion of uric acid. Amer. J. Med. **33**, 829—833 (1962).
ZÖLLNER, N.: Die Gichtniere. In: Handbuch der Inneren Medizin, S. 77. Berlin-Heidelberg-New York: Springer 1967.
ZÖLLNER, N.: Die Behandlung der Gicht und die internistische Behandlung der Harnsäurenephrolithiasis. Dtsch. med. Wschr. **93**, 310—312 (1968).
ZÖLLNER, N.: Die interne Behandlung des Harnsäuresteinleidens. Urologe **7**, 46—50 (1968a).
ZÖLLNER, N.: Fortschritte auf dem Gebiet der Gicht. Orthop. Prax. **5**, 167—176 (1969).
ZÖLLNER, N.: Erfolgsbeurteilung bei der Gichtbehandlung. Therapiewoche **34**, 1655—1658 (1970).
ZÖLLNER, N., LÜHRS, M.: Der Mechanismus der Harnsäuresteinbildung aus der Sicht des Internisten. Urol. int. (Basel) **22**, 492—505 (1967a).
ZÖLLNER, N., SCHATTENKIRCHNER, M.: Die Behandlung der Gicht und der Harnsäurenephrolithiasis mit Allopurinol. Dtsch. med. Wschr. **92**, 654—659 (1967b).
ZOLLINGER, H.: Niere und ableitende Harnwege. In: Doerr-Uehlinger, Spezielle pathologische Anatomie, Bd. 3. Berlin-Heidelberg-New York: Springer 1966.

cc) Hyperuricämie und Hypertonie

Von

H. Lydtin

Koincidenz von Gicht und Hochdruck

Das Thema dieses Beitrages stellt einleitend die Frage, ob arterieller Hochdruck und Gicht bzw. Hyperurikämie nach allgemeiner ärztlicher Erfahrung überdurchschnittlich häufig gemeinsam auftreten.

In zahlreichen *Hochdruckkollektiven* fand sich wesentlich häufiger als in Kontrollgruppen gleicher Alterszusammensetzung eine Hyperurikämie (Dollery et al., 1960; Kinsey et al., 1961; Breckenridge, 1966; Cannon et al., 1966). Iskovitz und Sellers (1963) stellten bei 1% von 3396 Hochdruckpatienten Gicht fest. Im übrigen Krankengut lag die Gichthäufigkeit bei 0,2%. Die Untersuchungsreihe von Kinsey et al. an 400 Hochdruckpatienten ergab bei 3,4% eine typische Gichtanamnese. Der Anteil von Patienten mit Hyperurikämie erreichte in einem Hochdruckkollektiv von 217 Patienten 47% (Cannon et al.); bei Patienten ohne medikamentöse Vorbehandlung wurden in 38% und bei behandelten Patienten in 58% erhöhte Harnsäurewerte festgestellt. Bei Patienten, die Thiazid-Saluretica erhielten, erreichte der Prozentsatz der Hyperurikämiker 67%.

Untersuchungen, die von Patienten mit *manifester Gicht* oder mit *Hyperurikämie* ausgehen, liefern weitere Indizien für Zusammenhänge zwischen Hochdruck und Hyperurikämie. Die Angaben über die Häufigkeit erhöhter Blutdruckwerte bei Patienten mit Gicht gehen im Schrifttum weit auseinander (s. Tab. 1). Ein Vergleich der einzelnen Studien macht deutlich, daß sich die Ergebnisse von Querschnitt- und von Längsschnittuntersuchungen wesentlich voneinander unterscheiden. Für ein ausschließlich männliches Krankengut von 78 Patienten gibt Gudzent (1928) eine Hypertoniehäufigkeit von 40% bei der ersten Untersuchung an. 17 der Patienten wurden von ihm z.T. über viele Jahre beobachtet. Von diesen wiesen in der initialen Beobachtungszeit 5 einen erhöhten Blutdruck auf, 7 von den übrigen 12 Patienten entwickelten mit der Zeit eine zunehmende Blutdruckerhöhung. Der Anteil von Hochdruckkranken stieg somit in diesem Kollektiv von etwa 30% (bei Betrachtung im Querschnitt) auf 70% im Längsschnittprofil. Trotz dieser verhältnismäßig kleinen Fallzahl steckt diese Studie in repräsentativer Weise den Bereich ab, in dem die Mehrheit der Häufigkeitsangaben für Hochdruck bei Gicht liegt. Nur wenige Autoren fanden Hochdruck bei Gicht in weniger als 30% des Krankengutes (Ravault u. Viala 20%; Kuzell et al. 25,7% (bei Männern), 35,8% (bei Frauen); Desèze und Ryckewaert: 28%). Bei zusammenfassender Beurteilung der nach Alter, Beobachtungszeit, Hochdruckkriterien und Fallzahl sehr unterschiedlichen Studien ist die Annahme gerechtfertigt, daß bei mindestens der Hälfte aller Patienten mit manifester Gicht eine Erhöhung des arteriellen Blutdruckes vorliegt. Die Häufigkeit des Hochdruckes steigt mit zunehmender Schwere der Nierenfunktionseinschränkung (Schnitker u. Richter, 1936). Mit Zunahme des Lebensalters bei der Erstmanifestation der Gicht steigt die Häufigkeit einer mäßiggradigen Hypertension, schwere Hypertonien und Niereninsuffizienz werden jedoch bei jüngeren Gichtpatienten verhältnismäßig häufig angetroffen (Mertz, 1973).

Bei *Hyperurikämie ohne typische Gichtanamnese* werden allgemein niedrigere Angaben für die Hochdruckhäufigkeit gemacht: Van Peenen: 19% (9% in der Vergleichsgruppe); Thorpe u. Daley: 26,3% (Hochdruck: mehr als 160/

Tabelle 1. Hypertonie bei Gicht (systolische und/oder diastolische Druckerhöhung)

	Hochdruck	Gicht	%
BROGSITTER	16	18	89
CANNON et al.	102	217	47
COOMBS et al.	8 (12)	22	36 (54)
GONICK et al.	43	70	62
GRAHAME u. SCOTT	184	354	52
GREENBAUM et al.	3	12	25
HENNINGES u. MERTZ	33	50	66
KOLLER u. ZOLLINGER	3	5	60
KUZELL et al.	♂ 96	373	25,7
	♀ 47	131	35,8
LOUYOT et al.	56	140	40
MERTZ u. BABUCKE	♂ 51	71	71,8
	♀ 45	62	72,6
MOELLER	17	27	62,9
RÜCKERT u. CHOWANETZ	29	44	65,9
SCHNITKER u. RICHTER	30	55	53,5
TALBOTT u. TERPLAN	104	191	54,4
	40	70 (leicht)	
	34	61 (mittel)	
	30	60 (schwer)	50,0
THORPE u. DALEY	10	30	33,3
WEISS u. SEGALOFF	126	280	45
ZÖLLNER u. SCHATTENKIRCHENER	12	22	55
ZÖLLNER	34	122	28

95 mm Hg). In der Vergleichsgruppe von THORPE u. DALEY mit normalen Harnsäurespiegeln fanden sich nur bei 8,1% erhöhte Blutdruckwerte. In einem hyperurikämischen Kollektiv von 50 jüngeren Patienten (Durchschnittsalter 29,8 Jahre) ergab sich zum Zeitpunkt der Untersuchung 23mal eine typische Gichtanamnese. Von den übrigen 27 Patienten hatten 10 eine vorher nicht bekannte Nephropathie; innerhalb des Gesamtkollektives lagen die Blutdruckwerte bei 33 Patienten über 140/100 mm Hg (HENNINGES u. MERTZ, 1971).

Mögliche pathogenetische Zusammenhänge zwischen Hochdruck und Gicht bzw. Hyperuricämie

Eine unvoreingenommene Analyse der Gründe für ein gehäuftes Zusammentreffen von Hochdruck und Gicht bzw. Hyperuricämie muß zunächst die Möglichkeit erörtern, daß die erhöhten Harnsäurewerte *Folge des Hochdruckes und/oder seiner Behandlung* sind.

Eine Einschränkung der Nierenfunktion infolge hypertoner Gefäßveränderungen kann mit dem Anstieg harnpflichtiger Substanzen auch zu erhöhten Harnsäurespiegeln führen. Die arteriosklerotische Schrumpfniere ist jedoch nur für wenige finale Hyperuricämien bei Hochdruckpatienten verantwortlich zu machen. Bei essentieller Hypertonie wurden überhöhte Serumlactatspiegel beobachtet und zur Erklärung einer verminderten tubulären Urataussscheidung herangezogen (CANNON et al., 1966). Die Saluretica der Thiazidgruppe dürften in der Hochdruckbehandlung am häufigsten als Ursache erhöhter Harnsäurespiegel in

Betracht kommen. Daneben können auch andere Saluretica wie Azetazolamid, Furosemid und Etacrynsäure die Harnsäurespiegel im Serum erhöhen. Kaliumsparende Diuretica wie Spironolacton, Triamteren und Amilorid induzieren keine klinisch relevanten Harnsäureanstiege (MERTZ, 1973).

Die klinische Bedeutung der durch Thiazidgaben induzierten Harnsäureanstiege wird unterschiedlich beurteilt. Nach allgemeiner klinischer Erfahrung gehört das erstmalige Auftreten eines Gichtanfalles, das Manifestwerden der Gicht unter saluretischer Therapie einer Hypertonie zu den seltenen Beobachtungen. Die bei längerer Thiazidgabe zu beobachtenden Anstiege der Serumharnsäure sind bei normalen Ausgangswerten verhältnismäßig klein (KUSUS et al., 1969). Die Serumharnsäurewerte steigen unter saluretischer Therapie in den ersten 3 Monaten, um sich dann auf einem erhöhten Niveau einzustellen oder unter Umständen wieder abzusinken (HEIMSOTH u. HARTMANN, 1965). Saluretica erhöhen die Serumharnsäure bei längerer Verabreichung an Hochdruckpatienten wahrscheinlich sowohl durch intrarenale als auch durch extrarenale Mechanismen. Die Verminderung des extracellulären Flüssigkeitsvolumens und eine evtl. Erhöhung des Serumlactatspiegels wirken dabei gleichsinnig. Für die Beteiligung extrarenaler Mechanismen spricht u.a. das Auftreten einer Hyperuricämie nach Kochsalzrestriktion (SUKI et al., 1967). Zusammenfassend läßt sich feststellen, daß sowohl der Hochdruck allein als auch seine Therapie durch Saluretica und durch Kochsalzrestriktion erhöhte Harnsäurespiegel im Serum hervorrufen können; die saluretische Therapie löst jedoch im allgemeinen nur bei vorher manifester Gicht einen Anfall aus (HUTCHINSON, 1963; KUSUS et al., 1969; PRIDDLE et al., 1970; SFIKAKIS, 1970; WALCOTT et al., 1970).

Die überzufällig hohe Koincidenz von Hyperuricämie und Hochdruck an nicht vorbehandelten Patienten, wie sie z.B. durch die Studie von CANNON et al. (1966) belegt wird, weist auf die Möglichkeit weiterer ätiopathogenetischer Zusammenhänge zwischen Hochdruck und Hyperuricämie hin. Dabei sind sowohl ein gemeinsamer Mechanismus, der dem Hochdruck und der Gicht zugrundeliegt, als auch die Verursachung des Hochdruckes durch die Hyperuricämie zu diskutieren.

Da arteriosklerotische extra- und/oder intrarenale Gefäßstenosen über eine renale Ischämie zur Hypertonie führen können, ist Ausgangspunkt der Suche nach einem *gemeinsamen pathogenetischen Mechanismus* die Koincidenz der Gicht mit anderen die vorzeitige Entwicklung einer Arteriosklerose begünstigenden „Risikofaktoren": Hyperlipidämie, Diabetes mellitus und Übergewicht.

Bereits 1920 beschrieb CHAUFFARD (zit. nach GUDZENT, 1928) das Vorkommen einer Hypercholesterinämie bei Gichtpatienten und wies damit auf die Störungen im Fettstoffwechsel bei Gicht hin. Erhöhte Triglyceridspiegel wurden in 38—100% verschiedener Kollektive von Patienten mit Gicht beobachtet (FELDMANN u. WALLACE, 1964; BENEDEK, 1967; MERTZ et al., 1970; RONDIER et al., 1970; THIELE et al., 1970). Zwischen der Höhe der Triglyceridspiegel und dem Serumcholesterin scheint dabei keine sichere Beziehung zu bestehen (MERTZ, 1973). Auch andere Untersucher fanden keine Beziehung zwischen der Höhe des Harnsäurespiegels und dem Serumcholesterin (MYERS et al., 1968).

Vermehrt wurden Hyperlipoproteinämien des Typs IV nach FREDRICKSON et al. (1967) bei hyperlipidämischen Gichtkranken beobachtet (MERTZ u. BABUCKE, 1971); allerdings müssen diese Befunde noch erweitert und an größeren Kollektiven bestätigt werden. Da in den bisher vorliegenden Studien mit meist kleinen Fallzahlen u.a. Ernährungsgewohnheiten, Alkoholkonsum und Körpergewicht nicht berücksichtigt wurden, lassen sich vorerst über die Feststellung einer Koincidenz zwischen Hypertriglyceridämie und Hyperuricämie hinaus keine sicheren

Aussagen über direkte Verbindungen zwischen Harnsäure- und -Fettstoffwechsel machen.

Ähnlich ungeklärt sind die Beziehungen zwischen Hyperuricämie und Kohlenhydratstoffwechsel. Je nach Größe der untersuchten Kollektive und nach ihrer Zusammensetzung variieren die Häufigkeitsangaben über einen weiten Bereich. GUDZENT (1928) fand nur bei 2,5% seiner Gichtpatienten einen klinisch manifesten Diabetes mellitus. HALL et al. (1967) beobachteten bei 240 Hyperuricämikern 1,7% manifeste Diabetiker und unter 76 Gichtpatienten keinen Zuckerkranken. MYERS et al. (1968) fanden keine Beziehung zwischen Serumharnsäurespiegel und Diabeteshäufigkeit. An kleineren Gicht- bzw. Hyperuricämiekollektiven werden meist höhere Prozentsätze für manifesten oder latenten Diabetes angegeben (HERMANN, 1958; BERNHEIM, 1968; THIELE et al., 1970; MERTZ, 1973).

Es ist durchaus möglich, daß eine Überernährung mit entsprechendem Übergewicht und Hypertriglyceridämie die Voraussetzung für die Manifestation von zwei voneinander unabhängigen Stoffwechselkrankheiten darstellt (THORPE u. DALEY, 1971; VAN PEENEN, 1971). Jedenfalls ist damit zu rechnen, daß die Kombination einer Hyperuricämie mit Diabetes mellitus und Hyperlipidämie die vorzeitige Ausbildung einer Arteriosklerose und damit auch die Entstehung von extra- und intrarenalen Gefäßstenosen begünstigt.

Vor allem die pathologisch-anatomischen Befunde an der Niere sprechen für eine *führende Rolle der Hyperuricämie* in der Pathogenese der Hypertonie. In sehr hohen Prozentsätzen werden bei Gichtkranken histologische Veränderungen an der Niere gefunden (TALBOTT u. TERPLAN, 1960/1963; Richet et al., 1961; GONICK et al., 1965; PRUNIER, 1967; TALBOTT, 1967; ZOLLINGER, 1967; ZÖLLNER, 1968).

Das Spektrum histologisch faßbarer Nierenveränderungen bei Gicht umfaßt die infektiöse und die nichtinfektiöse interstitielle Nephritis, die Nephrolithiasis mit und ohne Pyelonephritis, die renalen Gefäßveränderungen und die extracapillären Glomerulosklerosen. Die Häufigkeitsangaben für die einzelnen Veränderungen variieren in weiten Bereichen je nach Patientenkollektiv und Methodik der Untersuchung (Sektion oder Nierenbiopsie).

Dementsprechend wird das Hauptgewicht entweder mehr auf die primäre Verlegung des Tubuluslumens mit entzündlicher Begleitreaktion des Interstitiums (GREENBAUM et al., 1961), auf entzündliche Veränderungen im Interstitium (mit und ohne bakterielle Komponente; MERTZ, 1973) oder auf die Glomerulosklerose (KOLLER u. ZOLLINGER, 1945) gelegt. Mit Ausnahme der Glomerulosklerose handelt es sich dabei um Veränderungen, die in direkten Zusammenhang mit den erhöhten Harnsäurespiegeln gebracht werden können. Die 1945 von KOLLER u. ZOLLINGER bei Gichtpatienten beschriebene Glomerulosklerose zeigt eine weitgehende Ähnlichkeit mit den Veränderungen am Glomerulum bei Diabetes mellitus.

KOLLER u. ZOLLINGER vertraten die Meinung, daß es sich bei der gichtischen Glomerulosklerose um eine der Stoffwechselstörung subordinierte Störung handelt, d.h. daß die Hyperuricämie die Ausbildung der Veränderungen nicht nur begünstigt, sondern überhaupt erst ermöglicht. Dabei wird von den Autoren eine direkte Beziehung zwischen Glomerulosklerose und Hypertonie hergestellt.

Diese Vorstellungen werden in der Übersichtsarbeit von LÖFFLER u. KOLLER (1955) wieder aufgenommen. Danach soll die Glomerulosklerose in Zusammenhang mit der Sklerose der Arterien und Arteriolen stehen. TALBOTT u. TERPLAN (1960, 1963) schließen sich aufgrund ihrer eigenen histologischen Ergebnisse dieser Vorstellung an und betonen die Häufigkeit des histologischen Nachweises einer die Arteriolen einbeziehenden Nephrosklerose bei Gicht. Über den Mechanismus einer direkten Wirkung der Harnsäure auf die Gefäße gibt es bisher lediglich Spekulationen.

EBSTEIN (1906) hat Nierenveränderungen, die pathologisch-anatomisch einer Gichtniere gleichen, bei Patienten, die nie an einer Gelenkgicht erkrankt waren, beschrieben und als „primäre Nierengicht" bezeichnet. Durch neuere Untersuchungen wurde bestätigt, daß pathologisch-anatomische Veränderungen an der Niere dem eigentlichen Gelenkbefall bei Hyperuricämie vorausgehen können (GONICK et al., 1965). Damit läßt sich eine Blutdruckerhöhung auch bei Hyperuricämie ohne Gicht auf renale Mechanismen zurückführen (CANNON et al., 1966).

Arteriosklerotische Gefäßveränderungen, interstitielle Nephritis infolge Uratablagerung und aufsteigende Entzündung können gemeinsam zu einer verminderten Durchblutung des Nierenparenchyms führen. Die Mehrheit der Indizien spricht somit für eine renal-ischämische Verursachung des Hochdruckes bei der Hyperuricämie. Allerdings ist der Indizienbeweis noch lückenhaft. Bei jedem einzelnen Patienten ist das gesamte Spektrum möglicher Zusammenhänge zwischen Hyperuricämie und Hypertonie zu berücksichtigen (REUBI u. VORBURGER, 1962). Sorgfältige Untersuchungen der Hämodynamik, des Renin-Angiotensin-Aldosteron-Systems, der Nierenfunktion unter Einbeziehung der histologischen Befunde stehen bisher ebenso aus wie gut geplante prospektive Langzeitstudien an genügend großen hyperuricämischen Kollektiven.

Bei der bereits im Kindesalter manifesten Gicht infolge eines Mangels von Hypoxanthin-Guanin-Phosphoribosyltransferase, dem sogenannten Lesch-Nyhan-Syndrom, ist bisher das Auftreten von Hochdruck nicht beschrieben worden (KELLEY u. WYNGAARDEN, 1972). Allerdings erreichen diese Patienten nur im Ausnahmefall das Erwachsenenalter.

Behandlung des Hochdrucks bei Gicht und Hyperuricämie

Aus der besonderen Gefährdung des Gichtkranken durch Herzinfarkt und Apoplex (SCHETTLER, 1962) und aus dem multifaktoriellen Risikoprofil dieser Patienten ergibt sich die Notwendigkeit einer energischen antihypertensiven Behandlung bei gemeinsamem Auftreten von Gicht bzw. Hyperuricämie und Hochdruck. Die Behandlung des Hochdrucks bei der Hyperuricämie folgt grundsätzlich den gleichen Prinzipien wie die sonstige Hochdrucktherapie. Sie beginnt mit einer allgemeinen Regelung der Lebensführung, Einschaltung längerer Ruhezeiten in den Tagesablauf, Einhaltung ausreichender Nachtruhe, sinnvolle Freizeitgestaltung, diätetische Kochsalzbeschränkung und führt zu den spezifischen Formen der medikamentösen Hochdrucktherapie. Grundsätzlich ist die Einhaltung einer natriumarmen Kost (entsprechend etwa 3 g NaCl) gegenüber der Verabreichung von Saluretica zu bevorzugen. Beim therapeutischen Einsatz der Saluretica ist zu berücksichtigen, daß der Hyperuricämiker ebenso wie der Gesunde mit einem signifikanten Anstieg der Serumharnsäurewerte reagiert. Gichtpatienten, die mit Allopurinol behandelt werden, reagieren ebenfalls auf Saluretikagabe mit einem Anstieg der Serumharnsäurewerte. Unter Umständen muß die Allopurinoldosis nach Beginn einer Hochdruckbehandlung mit Thiazidsaluretica erhöht werden (MERTZ, 1973). Allerdings kann der Anstieg der Serumharnsäure unter Saluretikabehandlung nicht nur durch Allopurinol, sondern auch durch Uricosurica aufgehoben werden (KUSUS et al., 1969). Da der Hochdruck bei Hyperuricämikern als Indiz für eine Beteiligung der Niere am Krankheitsgeschehen gewertet werden muß, läßt sich eine Bevorzugung von Allopurinol gegenüber Uricosurica vertreten, da durch letztere einer vorgeschädigten Niere eine erhöhte Harnsäureausscheidung aufgezwungen wird. Da es sich bei der Hochdruckbehandlung meist um eine lebenslängliche Therapie handelt und die Erfahrungen mit Allopurinol erst über wenige Jahre gehen, kann die Allopurinolbehandlung von hyperuricämischen Hochdruckpatienten nicht vorbehaltlos vertreten werden (SFIKAKIS, 1970). Grundsätzlich kann auch auf eine salureticafreie Hochdrucktherapie übergegangen werden; letztere führt im allgemeinen nicht zu einem klinisch relevanten Anstieg der Serumharnsäure (WALCOTT et al., 1970). Der therapeutische Einsatz anderer Antihypertonica wie Reserpin, Hydralazin, α-Methyl-Dopa, Clonidin, Guanethidin, Diazoxid und β-Receptorenblocker erfolgt nach den für die allgemeine Hochdrucktherapie geltenden Prinzipien. Durch Kombination der einzelnen Substanzen wird versucht, die Wirkung zu potenzieren und dosisabhängige Nebenwirkungen auf ein Minimum zu beschränken. Bei allen Patienten mit eingeschränkter Nierenfunktion ist zu berücksichtigen, daß eine stärkere Blutdrucksenkung über eine weitere Verminderung der Nierenfunktion zu einem Anstieg der harnpflichtigen Substanzen und auch der Serumharnsäure führen kann.

Werden Hochdruckpatienten mit Hyperuricämie durch Saluretica behandelt, kann durch Verabreichung kleiner Colchicindosen eine Anfallsprophylaxe der Gicht durchgeführt werden (PRIDDLE et al., 1970).

Literatur

BENEDEK, TH. G.: Correlations of serum uric acid and lipid concentrations in normal, gouty and atherosclerotic men. Ann. intern. Med. **66**, 851—861 (1967).
BERNHEIM, C.: Goutte et diabète. Schweiz. med. Wschr. **98**, 327—334 (1968).
BRECKENRIDGE, A.: Hypertension and hyperuricaemia. Lancet **1966 I**, 15.
BRØCHNER-MORTENSEN, K.: Hundred gouty patients. Acta med. scand. **106**, 81 (1941).
BROGSITTER, A. M.: Histopathologie der Gelenkgicht. Leipzig: Vogel 1927
CANNON, P. J., STASON, W. B., DEMARTINI, F. E., SOMMERS, S. C., LARAGH, J. H.: Hyperuricemia in primary and renal hypertension. New. Engl. J. Med. **275**, 457 (1966).
CHIANG, B. N., PERLMAN, L. V., EPSTEIN, F. H.: Overweight and Hypertension. Circulation **39**, 403—421 (1969).
COOMBS, F. S., PECORA, L. J., THOROGOOD, E., CONSOLAZIO, W. V., TALBOTT, J. H.: Renal function in patients with gout. J. clin. Invest. **19**, 525—534 (1940).
DESÈZE, S., RYCKEWAERT, A.: La goutte. Paris: L'expansion scientifique française 1960.
DOLLERY, C. T., DUNCAN, H., SCHUMER, B.: Hyperuricaemia related to treatment of hypertension. Brit. med. J. **1960 II**, 832.
EBSTEIN, W.: Natur und Behandlung der Gicht, 2. Aufl., Wiesbaden: J. F. Bergmann 1906.
FELDMAN, E. B., WALLACE, ST. L.: Hypertriglyceridemia in gout. Circulation **29**, 508—514 (1964).
FISHBERG, A. M.: Hypertension and Nephritis. London: Baillière-Tindall 1939.
FREDRICKSON, D. S., LEVY, R. J., LEES, R. S.: Fat transport in lipoproteins — an integrated approach to mechanisms and disorders. New Engl. J. Med. **276**, 33—34, 94—103, 148—156, 215—225, 273—281 (1967).
GONICK, H. C., RUBINI, M. E., GLEASON, I. O., SOMMERS, SH. C.: The renal lesion in gout. Ann. intern. Med. **62**, 667—674 (1965).
GRAHAME, R., SCOTT, J. T.: Clinical survey of 354 patients with gout. Ann rheum. Dis. **29**, 461—468 (1970).
GREENBAUM, D., ROSS, J. H., STEINBERG, V. L.: Renal biopsy in gout. Brit. med. J. **1961 I**, 1502—1504.
GUDZENT, F.: Gicht und Rheumatismus. Berlin: Springer 1928.
HALL, A. P., BARRY, P. E., DAWBER, T. R., MCNAMARA, P. M.: Epidemiology of gout and hyperuricemia. A long-term population study. Amer. J. Med. **42**, 27—37 (1967).
HALL, A. P.: Correlations among hyperuricemia, hypercholesterolemia, coronary disease and hypertension. Arthr. and Rheum. **8**, 846 (1965).
HEIMSOTH, V., HARTMANN, F.: Untersuchungen zur Störung des Harnsäure-Stoffwechsels nach Salureticaverabreichung. Dtsch. med. Wschr. **90**, 1905—1908 (1965).

HENNINGES, D., MERTZ, D. P.: Zum klinischen Bild der juvenilen Gicht. Verh. dtsch. Ges. inn. Med. **77**, 180—183 (1971).
HERMAN, J. B.: Gout and diabetes. Metabolism **7**, 703 (1958).
HUTCHINSON, J. C.: Metabolic and hypotensive effects of a new rauwolfia-thiazide combination. Geriatrics **24**, 68—74 (1969).
ISKOVITZ, H. D., SELLERS, A. M.: Gout and hyperuricemia after adrenalectomy for hypertension. New. Engl. J. Med. **268**, 1105 (1963).
KELLEY, W. N., WYNGAARDEN, J. B.: The Lesch-Nyhan syndrome. In: The metabolic basis of inherited disease (Eds. STANBURY, J. B., WYNGAARDEN, J. B., FREDRICKSON, D. S.), 3. Ed. New York: McGraw Hill 1972.
KINSEY, D., WALTHER, R., SISE, H. S., WITHLAW, G., SMITHWICK, R.: Incidence of hyperuricemia in 400 hypertensive patients. Circulation **24**, 972—973 (1961).
KOLLER, F., ZOLLINGER, H. U.: Gichtische Glomerulosklerose. Schweiz. med. Wschr. **75**, 97—105 (1945).
KUSUS, T., LYDTIN, H., ZÖLLNER, N.: Saluretische Behandlung der Hypertonie und der Harnsäurespiegel im Serum. Arzneimittel-Forsch. **19**, 1887—1889 (1969).
KUZELL, W. C., SCHAFFARZICK, R. W., NAUGLER, W. E., KOETS, P., MANKLE, E. A., BROWN, B., CHAMPLIN, B.: Some observations on 520 gouty patients. J. chron. Dis. **2**, 645—669 (1955).
LÖFFLER, W., KOLLER, F.: Die Gicht. In: Handbuch der inneren Medizin, 4. Aufl., Band VII, 2. Teil: Stoffwechsel-Krankheiten. Berlin-Göttingen-Heidelberg: Springer 1955.
LOUYOT, P., RAUBER, G., GAUCHER, A., HURIET, C., PETERSCHMITT, J.: Le rein du Goutteux. La Goutte, Rapport du 34 ème Congrès Français de Medecine. Paris: Masson 1963.
MERTZ, D. P.: Gichtniere und Nierengicht. Dtsch. med. J. **19**, 413—421 (1968).
MERTZ, D. P.: Wirkung von Spironolacton und Thiabutazid auf die Serumkonzentrationen von Harnsäure und Lipiden bei Gichtkranken und Stoffwechselgesunden. Dtsch. med. Wschr. **98**, 11—15 (1973).
MERTZ, D. P.: Gicht — Grundlagen, Klinik und Therapie, 2. Aufl., Stuttgart: Thieme 1973.
MERTZ, D. P., BABUCKE, G.: Epidemiologie und klinisches Bild der primären Gicht — Beobachtungen zwischen 1948 und 1968. Münch. med. Wschr. **113**, 617—624 (1971).
MERTZ, D. P., SARRE, H.: Gicht und Hypertonie. In: Hypertonie (Hrsg. SARRE, H.). Stuttgart: Schattauer 1969.
MERTZ, D. P., SULZBERGER, I., KLÖPFER, M.: Diabetes mellitus, Hyperlipidämie, Fettleber, Hypertension bei primärer Gicht und deren Beeinflussung durch Benzbromaronum. Münch. med. Wschr. **112** 241—247 (1970).
MIKKELSEN, W. M., DODGE, H. J., VALKENBURG, H.: The distribution of serum uric acid values in a population unselected as to gout and hyperuricemia. Amer. J. Med. **39**, 242 (1965).
MOELLER, J.: Nierenbioptische Untersuchungen zur Bedeutung der Gichtniere. Med. Welt (Stuttg.) **19**, 1052—1059 (1968).
MYERS, A. R., EPSTEIN, F. H., DODGE, H. J. MIKKELSEN, W. M.: The relationship of serum uric acid to risk factors in coronary heart disease. Amer. J. Med. **45**, 520—528 (1968).
PRIDDLE, W. W., LIU, S. F., BREITHAUPT, D. J.: Management of hypertension — further sodium and potassium studies. J. Amer. Geriat. Soc. **18**, 861—892 (1970).
PRUNIER, PH.: Complications renales de la goutte. Presse méd. **75**, 139—141 (1967).
RAVAULT, P. P., VIALA, J. J.: Considérations cliniques et étiopathologiques sur les manifestations rénales de la goutte. Rev. lyon. Méd. **9**, 1069—1085 (1960).
REUBI, F., VORBURGER, C.: Die Gichtniere. Münch. med. Wschr. **104**, 2152—2155 (1962).
RICHET, G., ARDAILLOU, R., DE MONTÈRA, H., SLAMA, R., BOUGAULT, T.: Le rein goutteux. Presse méd. **69**, 644—647 (1961).
RONDIER, J., TRUFFERT, J., LE GO, A., BROULLHET, H., SAPORTA, L., DE GENNES, J. L., DELBARRE, F.: Goutte et Hyperlipidémies. Rev. Europ. Etudes clin. biol. **15**, 959—968 (1970).
ROSENBLOOM, J.: The blood pressure in gout. J. Amer. med. Ass. **70**, 2000 (1918).
RÜCKERT, K.-H., CHOWANETZ, W.: Die übersehene Gicht. Münch. med. Wschr. **114**, 663—665 (1972).
SCHETTLER, G.: Krankheiten des Wohlstandes. Dtsch. med. Wschr. **87**, 1221—1227 (1962).
SCHNITKER, M. A., RICHTER, A. B.: Nephritis in gout. Amer. J. med. Sci. **192**, 241 (1936).
SFIKAKIS, P.: Diuretics and hyperuricemia. New. Engl. J. Med. **282**, 1047—1048 (1970).
SUKI, W. N., HULL, A. R., RECTOR, F. C., JR., SELDIN, D. W.: Mechanism of the effect of thiazide diuretics on calcium and uric acid (Abstract). J. clin. Invest. **46**, 1121 (1967).
TALBOTT, J. H.: Gout, 3. Ed. New York: Grune and Stratton 1967.

TALBOTT, J. H., TERPLAN, K. L.: The kidney in gout. Medicine (Baltimore) **39**, 405—466 (1960).
TALBOTT, J. H., TERPLAN, K. L.: The kidney in gout. In: Diseases of the kidney (Hrsg. STRAUSS, M. B., WELT, L. G.). Boston: Little Brown 1963.
THIELE, P., HEIDELMANN, G., GÄRTNER, A., SCHNEIDER, V., TELLKAMP, F.: Aktuelle Gichtprobleme. Z. ges. inn. Med. **25**, 458—463 (1970).
THORPE, J. J., DALEY, J. M.: Hyperuricemia and gout in an employee population. J. occup. Med. **13**, 524—534 (1971).
VACHTENHEIM, J., SRAMEK, F.: Clinical symptoms and progress of the gout complicated by urolithiasis. Fysiat. Věstn. **49**, 171—178 (1971).
VAN PEENEN, H. J.: The Causes of Nonazotemic Hyperuricemia. Amer. J. clin. Path. **55**, 698—700 (1971).
WALCOTT, G., OWEN, G. C., END, J. A., ROSENBAUM, F. F., KLINK, D. D.: Management of the mild hypertensive. Wis. med. J. **69**, 231—236 (1970).
WEISS, T. E., SEGALOFF, A.: Gouty Arthritis and Gout. Springfield/Ill.: Ch. C. Thomas 1959.
ZOLLINGER, H. U.: Die entzündlichen interstitiellen Nierenerkrankungen. In: Spezielle pathologische Anatomie, Bd. III (Hrsg. DOERR, W., UEHLINGER, E.). Berlin-Heidelberg-New York: Springer 1966.
ZÖLLNER, N., SCHATTENKIRCHNER, M.: Allopurinol in der Behandlung der Gicht und der Harnsäure-Nephrolithiasis. Dtsch. med. Wschr. **92**, 654—660 (1967).
ZÖLLNER, N.: Die Gichtniere. In: Handbuch der inneren Medizin, 5. Aufl., Bd. 8 (Hrsg. SCHWIEGK, H.). Berlin-Heidelberg-New York: Springer 1968.

VII. Therapie und Prophylaxe der Gicht

1. Die Therapie des Gichtanfalles

Von

M. SCHATTENKIRCHNER

Das Ziel der Behandlung des Gichtanfalles ist eine möglichst schnelle und anhaltende Beseitigung einer akuten, sehr schmerzhaften gichtischen Entzündung. WALLACE et al. (1967) fordern als Kriterien des Erfolges einer Anfallbehandlung eine Beseitigung der Beschwerden bzw. eine entscheidende Besserung innerhalb von 48 Std nach Behandlungsbeginn und ein Anhalten des Erfolges von über sieben Tagen. Will man nach dieser Forderung die Wirksamkeit der in Frage kommenden Anfallmittel prüfen, dann ist die bekannte Tatsache zu berücksichtigen, daß ein beginnender Anfall, den ein erfahrener Gichtpatient häufig schon an Prodromalzeichen erkennt, oder ein frischer Anfall, der etwa am Morgen nach nächtlichem Beginn diagnostiziert wird, viel sicherer, rascher und mit geringeren Dosen eines brauchbaren Mittels erfolgreich behandelt werden kann als ein über Tage bestehender Anfall. WALLACE (1961) hält einen Verzug der Behandlung von nur wenigen Stunden schon für wesentlich entscheidend bezüglich der Dauer bis zum Wirkungseintritt. Andererseits aber klingen die meisten Gichtanfälle nach ein bis zwei Wochen auch spontan ab. So ist es verständlich, daß die Wirksamkeit eines Anfallsmittels, angegeben in Prozentzahlen des Ansprechens bzw. Versagens für die einzelnen Mittel, in der Literatur unter nicht gleichen Voraussetzungen unterschiedlich angegeben wird. Entscheidend für den Erfolg ist nicht nur die Wahl eines brauchbaren Mittels und eine ausreichende Dosierung, sondern vor allem sein entschlossener sofortiger Einsatz.

Folgende Stoffe stehen uns zur Behandlung des Gichtanfalles zur Verfügung: Colchicin, Phenylbutazon und Oxyphenbutazon, Indomethacin. Adrenocorticotrope Hormone (ACTH) und Corticosteroide kommen primär nicht zum Einsatz.

Colchicin

Colchicin wird schon seit 1500 Jahren zur Behandlung des Gichtanfalles verwendet (HARTUNG, 1954). GARROD (1863) wies vor über 100 Jahren bereits auf die große therapeutische Sicherheit des Colchicins und seine Spezifität hin. Im Jahre 1939 machte LOCKIE erneut auf den Wert des Colchicins als diagnostische Hilfe bei der Gicht aufmerksam.

An der *Sicherheit* seiner Wirkung wurde nie gezweifelt. Mit großer Übereinstimmung wird eine Quote des Ansprechens des Gichtanfalles auf eine Colchicintherapie mit Werten zwischen 75% und über 95% in der Literatur angegeben:

GUTMAN u. YÜ	(1952)	75%
SMYTH	(1953)	über 95%
KUZELL et al.	(1955)	80%
DE SÉZE et al.	(1958)	75%
ZÖLLNER	(1960)	über 90%
GUTMAN	(1965)	80%
WALLACE et al.	(1967)	75%

Seine *strenge Spezifität* ist jedoch in den letzten Jahren öfter in Zweifel gezogen oder verneint worden. KAPLAN berichtete im Jahre 1960 über 4 Fälle von akuter Sarkoidose mit Gelenkbeteiligung. Die begleitenden Arthritiden sprachen ausgezeichnet auf eine Colchicintherapie an. Auch BUNIM et al. (1962) und ZVAIFLER u. PEKIN (1963) berichteten über solche Beobachtungen.

ZUCKNER (1962) prüfte die Wirkung von Colchicin bei der chronischen Polyarthritis. 30 Patienten, 24 bezüglich des Rheumafaktors serologisch positiv und 6 serologisch negative, mit akuten Arthritiden erhielten eine maximale Dosis von 7,2 mg Colchicin per os. 10 der 30 Patienten gaben eine gute bis ausgezeichnete Besserung der Beschwerden an. Bei 4 dieser Patienten war auch innerhalb von 24 Std ein Erfolg objektiv festzustellen, der sich auch zu einem späteren Zeitpunkt reproduzieren ließ. Allerdings war die Besserung jeweils nur kurzfristig. Es ließen sich aber auch 3 von 8 Patienten mit chronischer Polyarthritis durch orale Placebogaben bessern. Eine intravenöse Gabe von 2—3 mg Colchicin brachte 7 von 14 Patienten eine Besserung, eine intravenöse Placebogabe 2 von 4 Patienten. Diese beiden konnten wenige Tage vorher durch Colchicingaben ebenfalls gebessert werden. ZUCKNER stellt nach diesen Beobachtungen die diagnostische Bedeutung der positiven Antwort auf einen Behandlungsversuch mit Colchicin in Frage. Auch WALLACE et al. (1967) sind der Frage der diagnostischen Zuverlässigkeit des sog. Colchicin-Tests nachgegangen. Sie fordern von einem idealen diagnostischen Test einen therapeutischen Effekt bei allen Gichtpatienten und ein Fehlen des Ansprechens bei anderen Erkrankungen. Außerdem postulieren sie, wie bereits erwähnt, eine Besserung innerhalb von 48 Std nach Behandlungsbeginn und ein Anhalten des Erfolges anschließend auf mindestens eine Woche. Sie fanden ein Ansprechen bei 44 von 58 Patienten mit Gichtanfällen (etwa 75%). In keinem einzigen Fall von 28 Patienten mit chronischer Polyarthritis mit akuten Schüben an einzelnen Gelenken war nach diesen Kriterien ein Ansprechen zu erkennen, ebensowenig zeigte sich ein Einfluß bei 6 Patienten mit akuter Sarkoidose mit Arthritiden, bei 6 Fällen mit rheumatischem Fieber, bei 2 Fällen von M. Reiter, bei 4 Fällen von akuten Arthritiden im Rahmen eines Lupus erythematodes disseminatus. Ein deutliches Ansprechen fanden sie bei einem Fall von Erythema nodosum ohne Anhalt für Sarkoidose und bei 2 von 11 Fällen mit unklaren akuten Arthritiden.

Bei einer Untersuchung an 58 Gichtpatienten und 64 Patienten mit anderen Arthritiden waren also drei „falsch positive" Ergebnisse zu verzeichnen. Die „falsch negativen" Ergebnisse führen die Autoren vorwiegend auf eine Verzögerung des Behandlungsbeginnes zurück. Es handelte sich nicht in jedem Falle um frische Gichtattacken. WALLACE et al. glauben, daß der sog. Colchicin-Test nützlich, aber nicht untrüglich sei.

KANTOR u. BROWN (1966) dagegen sind aufgrund ihrer Untersuchungen der Meinung, daß Colchicin streng spezifisch wirke. Sie gaben Colchicin intravenös bei 20 Gichtanfällen und 31 anderen akuten Arthritiden. Die Gichtanfälle sprachen alle schnell und eindrucksvoll, die anderen Arthritiden entweder gar nicht oder nur langsam und fraglich an.

Colchicin wirkt bei der Pseudogicht bzw. bei akuten Arthritiden im Rahmen einer Chondrocalcinose, wie MCCARTY (1965) feststellte, nicht, was erstaunlich ist, nachdem in diesem Falle ebenso wie bei der Gicht eine Kristallphagocytose durch polymorphkernige Leukocyten im Gelenkspunktat bei der akuten Entzündung nachzuweisen ist und die Wirkungsweise des Colchicin nach mehreren Hypothesen in einer Hemmung der Phagocytose der Leukocyten beruht. Hingegen konnten MCCARTY u. GATTER (1966) ebenso wie THOMPSON et al. (1968) eine deutliche und prompte Wirkung des Colchicin bei sog. calcifizierenden Tendinitiden und lokalen Weichteilcalcifikationen mit akuten entzündlichen Reaktionen feststellen. Solche Veränderungen kommen bei Patienten im chronischen Dialyseprogramm vor.

Nach allen Berichten der Literatur und unseren eigenen Erfahrungen ist Colchicin ein hochwirksames und ziemlich spezifisches, wenn auch nicht absolut spezifisches Mittel zur Behandlung des Gichtanfalles. Abgesehen davon, daß die bezüglich des Ansprechens auf Colchicin noch in Frage kommenden Erkrankungen mit akuten Arthritiden gegenüber der Gicht keine bedeutenden differentialdiagnostischen Schwierigkeiten bieten, ist das prompte Ansprechen auf Colchicin meist kein noch fehlendes beweisendes Kriterium für die Diagnose, sondern stellt nur eine erfreuliche Bestätigung der ohnehin schon gesicherten Diagnose dar.

Entscheidend für die Wahl des Colchicin zur Behandlung des Gichtanfalles ist also weniger seine Spezifität, sondern vielmehr die hohe Rate des Ansprechens und eine im wesentlichen geringe Gefahr durch Nebenwirkungen.

Nebenwirkungen treten zwar häufig auf und sind z.T. auch lästig, bei richtigem Vorgehen jedoch nie gefährlich. Bekannt sind vor allem die gastrointestinalen Nebenwirkungen wie Durchfälle, Übelkeit, Inappetenz, Bauchschmerzen. Der behandelnde Arzt oder der Patient selbst wird die Behandlung abbrechen, wenn diese Nebenwirkungen zu unangenehm werden, braucht aber dann keine ernsteren Schädigungen wie Knochenmarkstörungen, Blutungen, Neuritiden, Haarausfall mehr zu befürchten. Die Gefahr von Knochenmarkschädigungen ist jedoch bei Phenylbutazon, wenn auch selten, ohne andere für den Arzt oder Patienten erkennbare Erscheinungen vorhanden, was besonders bei der im allgemeinen üblichen ambulanten Behandlung des Gichtanfalles ins Gewicht fällt.

Eine echte Überempfindlichkeit auf Colchicin, d.h. eine Situation, bei der auf geringe Colchicindosen die schwersten toxischen Erscheinungen auftreten, ist extrem selten. MC LEOD u. PHILLIPS (1947) berichten von einem Fall, bei dem insgesamt 7 mg oral über einen Zeitraum von 4 Tagen verabreichtes Colchicin zum Tode führte. Bei langfristiger Colchicingabe in einer Dosis von 1—2 mg täglich sind keine sicheren Nebenwirkungen bekannt geworden.

YÜ u. GUTMAN (1961) fanden bei über 200 Patienten, die unter Colchicin-Dauerprophylaxe standen, über einen Beobachtungszeitraum von durchschnittlich 5,4 Jahren hinweg keine pathologischen Befunde, die auf Colchicin zurückzuführen gewesen wären. Bei höheren Dosen auf längere Zeit verabreicht, wie sie zur Behandlung maligner Prozesse versuchsweise gegeben wurden, um die cytostatische Wirkung des Colchicin zu verwenden, kam es zu Leukopenie, Anämie und Haarausfall (SEED et al. 1940).

Für das Auftreten genetischer Schäden bei länger dauernder niedrig dosierter Colchicintherapie (sog. Colchicinprophylaxe) oder häufigeren Anfallsbehandlungen liegen keine sicheren Hinweise vor. LOCKIE (1965) berichtete von einer 37jährigen Frau, die 9 Jahre lang fälschlicherweise täglich 1,5 mg Colchicin eingenommen hatte und in dieser Zeit drei gesunde Kinder zur Welt gebracht hatte. CESTARI et al. (1969) vermuteten einen kausalen Zusammenhang zwischen der Geburt eines mongoloiden Kindes und der Colchicinprophylaxe seines Vaters. HOEFNAGEL (1969) gibt zu bedenken, daß Trisomie bei Eltern mit Gicht nicht häufiger sei als bei gesunden Eltern. Er fordert zur Klärung dieser Frage eine vergleichende Untersuchung über die Häufigkeit von Trisomie bei Kindern gichtischer Väter, die unter Colchicinbehandlung stehen, und Kindern, deren Väter an Gicht leiden, jedoch keine Colchicinbehandlung zur Zeit der Zeugung hatten.

TIMSON (1969) glaubt wohl mit Recht, daß es sich bei dem beschriebenen Fall um ein zufälliges Zusammentreffen handelt. WALKER (1969) fand unter den Eltern von 200 mongoloiden Kindern keinen zur Zeit der Zeugung oder zuvor unter einer Colchicintherapie stehenden Elternteil.

HAWKINS et al. (1965) beschrieben bei einem Patienten mit excessiver tophöser Gicht, die neben harnsäuresenkenden Medikamenten auch mit Colchicin dauernd behandelt werden mußte, eine megaloblastäre Anämie. WEBB et al. (1968) zeigten eine deutliche Abnahme der Vitamin B_{12}-Resorption beim Menschen nach oraler Colchicingabe über mehrere Tage hinweg. RACE et al. (1966) fanden bei täglichen Gaben von 2,6—3,9 mg Colchicin nach 4—6 Tagen einen Anstieg des fäkalen Fettes, Stickstoffes, Natrium und Kalium und einen Abfall der d-Xylose-Ausscheidung beim Menschen. Eine Biopsie aus dem Dünndarm ergab eine Verminderung der intestinalen Lactase-, Saccharase- und Maltase-Aktivität, d. h. es wurde eine Malabsorption induziert.

Klinische Berichte über häufigeres Vorkommen von megaloblastären Anämien bei Gichtpatienten, die unter Colchicin-Dauerbehandlung stehen, fehlen jedoch in der Literatur. Auch in unserem umfangreichen Krankengut an Gichtpatienten konnten wir keine häufigeren megaloblastären Anämien beobachten. Allerdings verwenden wir bei einer prophylaktischen Behandlung immer Dosen unter 2,6 mg Colchicin täglich. Auch erstreckt sich eine prophylaktische Behandlung selten über 3 Monate hinaus.

Das Vorgehen bei der Anfallsbehandlung mit Colchicin variiert bei den einzelnen Autoren. Wir verwenden immer Colchicin als Reinsubstanz (Colchicinum purissimum) und rezeptieren es als Pillen zu $1/2$ mg. Die Analyse von Dragee-Fertigpräparaten hat einen sehr unterschiedlichen Wirkstoffgehalt ergeben, vermutlich erklärbar durch eine relativ kurze Haltbarkeit des Colchicin in der Drageeverarbeitung (ZÖLLNER, 1960).

GUTMAN (1951), WALLACE (1961) empfehlen beim Gichtanfall stündlich 0,5 mg oder alle 2 Std 1 mg Colchicin. SMYTH (1953) empfiehlt sogar nur 0,5 mg Colchicin alle 2 Std. Wir geben in den ersten 4 Std der Behandlung 4 mg insgesamt, also jede Stunde 1 mg, anschließend stündlich 0,5 mg. Es wird dann im allgemeinen fortgefahren bis zur eindeutigen Besserung oder bis zum Eintritt nicht mehr tolerierbarer Nebenwirkungen von seiten des Gastrointestinaltraktes oder bis zum Erreichen einer Gesamtdosis von 8 mg in den ersten 24 Std. Im Falle einer Besserung wird dann in den darauffolgenden Tagen schrittweise reduziert und unter Umständen eine mehrere Wochen dauernde Prophylaxe mit einer täglichen Dosis von 1,5 mg angeschlossen. Zur Verhütung bzw. Behandlung von Durchfällen verschreiben wir routinemäßig Tinctura opii simplex und empfehlen eine Dosierung von 3—4 × 10 Tropfen täglich.

Die benötigte Colchicindosis bis zum Ansprechen sollte beim einzelnen Patienten registriert werden. Bei einem späteren Anfall kann dann die Hälfte bis zwei Drittel dieser Dosis zu Beginn auf einmal gegeben werden und der Rest verteilt auf die folgenden Stunden. Damit wird eine schnellere Schmerzfreiheit erreicht (WALLACE, 1961).

Ein häufig empfohlenes Vorgehen ist die Gabe einer intravenösen Dosis von 2—3 mg zu Beginn, der Rest wird dann in stündlichen Dosen oral verabreicht. Zur intravenösen Injektion eignen sich sowohl Colchicin als auch seine Derivate (z. B. Desoxymethylacetylcolchicin) (KORFMACHER u. ZÖLLNER, 1960).

Durch intravenöse Verabreichung von Colchicin zu Beginn der Behandlung wird die Zeit bis zum Ansprechen verkürzt und das Risiko gastrointestinaler Nebenwirkungen vermindert, das bedeutet auch, daß die Ansprechquote erhöht wird. DAVIS u. BARTFELD (1954) berichten ein Ansprechen auf i.v.-Gaben bei einigen Patienten innerhalb von 5—15 min nach der Injektion. DE SÈZE et al. (1958), die initial 3 mg Colchicin intravenös gaben, stellten ebenso wie GRAHAM u. ROBERTS (1953) ein durchschnittliches Ansprechen nach 3—4 Std fest. Sie erlebten jedoch einige Male Phlebitiden und bei fehlerhaften Injektionen Gewebsnekrosen, was auch RODNAN (1964) zu bedenken gibt.

Es ist häufiger, daß wegen gastrointestinaler Nebenwirkungen die Therapie abgebrochen werden muß und deshalb kein Erfolg eintritt, als daß ohne besondere Nebenwirkungen die Maximaldosis gegeben werden kann, ohne daß es zum Therapieerfolg kommt.

Im letzteren Falle kann nach 3 Tagen erneut ein Therapieversuch mit Colchicin nach dem gleichen Vorgehen durchgeführt werden. Wir sehen jedoch in solchen Fällen eine Indikation für den Einsatz von ACTH, je 75—100 IE an zwei aufeinanderfolgenden Tagen, bzw. 30—50 mg Prednisolon oder der Äquivalenzdosis eines anderen Corticosteroids ebenfalls an zwei aufeinanderfolgenden Tagen in Kombination mit der laufenden, in langsamen Schritten wieder zu reduzierenden Colchicinbehandlung. Die Reduktion des Colchicin muß in diesem Falle jedoch langsamer erfolgen, da die Gefahr von Rezidivattacken bei hormonbehandelten Gichtanfällen größer ist. Im allgemeinen geben wir dann Colchicin mindestens 10 Tage nach Abklingen des Gichtanfalles weiter.

Für die reine ACTH-Behandlung des Gichtanfalles wird von KUZELL et al. (1955) aufgrund einer Beobachtung an 520 Gichtpatienten, wovon ein Teil im Anfall mit ACTH behandelt worden war, eine Ansprechquote von 93% angegeben.

Phenylbutazon

Phenylbutazon ist ebenfalls ausgezeichnet wirksam beim Gichtanfall. KUZELL et al. (1955) finden eine Ansprechbarkeit von 91% und geben Phenylbutazon gegenüber dem Colchicin den Vorzug. DE SÈZE et al. (1958) kamen an einem großen Patientengut zu einer nahezu gleichen Zahl (92%). Das Ansprechen war meist schon in den ersten 2 Std nach Behandlungsbeginn zu beobachten. GUTMAN (1951) zeigt für Phenylbutazon aufgrund einer Studie an 233 Gichtanfällen nur eine Quote des Ansprechens von 79%. Für Colchicin nennt er bei 429 behandelten Anfällen unter den gleichen Beurteilungskriterien eine Ansprechquote von 80%.

Als Dosierung wird entweder am ersten Tage eine intramuskuläre Injektion von 1000 mg Phenylbutazon und an den folgenden Tagen abfallende orale Dosen, oder zu Beginn oral 200 mg und dann alle 3 Std 100 mg bis zu einer Tagesgesamtdosis von 800 mg empfohlen, an den darauffolgenden Tagen dann ebenfalls abfallende orale Dosen (400 mg, 200 mg). BOYLE u. BUCHANAN (1971) geben ein Schema von 200 mg oral alle 6 Std an. Spätestens nach 48 Std sei dabei der Anfall coupiert.

Oxyphenbutazon hat nach GUTMAN (1951) gegenüber Phenylbutazon keine Vorzüge bezüglich Quote der Ansprechbarkeit und Risiko von Nebenwirkungen.

DE SÈZE et al. (1958) beobachteten in 3 von 89 Fällen von Gichtattacken, die mit Phenylbutazon behandelt worden waren, Ödeme. Ähnlich wie nach einer Corticosteroid- oder ACTH-Behandlung kommt es auch bei Phenylbutazon häufig zu Rezidivattacken (PLOTZ, 1965). Außerdem beeinflußt Phenylbutazon wegen seiner uricosurischen Wirkung den Plasmauratspiegel. Ein zwar seltener, aber gefürchteter Nachteil des Phenylbutazon ist seine Schädigung des hämatopoëtischen Gewebes. Sie kann bereits bei kleinen Dosen und nach einmaliger Gabe ohne Vorzeichen in Gang kommen.

Indometacin

SMYTH et al. (1963) behandelten Gichtanfälle bei zehn Patienten mit hohen Dosen von 600—800 mg Indometacin am ersten Tage und objektivierten in allen Fällen innerhalb von 2—4 Std eine deutliche Besserung, in 24—48 Std eine völlige Remission. Ernste Nebenwirkungen waren nicht zu berichten. BOARDMAN u. HART (1965) erzielten ein ausgezeichnetes Ansprechen schon mit geringeren Dosen von 75—100 mg täglich.

EMMERSON (1967) schildert ein Ansprechen in praktisch 100% der Fälle. Er beobachtete 22 Gichtpatienten über 2 Jahre. Die Wirkung trat meist in den ersten vier Std des Anfalles ein und war nach 24 Std voll erreicht. Vier der behandelten Patienten klagten über Kopfschmerzen und Konzentrationsschwäche. EMMERSON gibt folgendes Dosierungsschema an: 100 mg alle 4 Std bis zur Schmerzerleichterung, dann 100 mg alle acht Std für 24 Std, dann 75 mg alle acht Std für weitere 24 Std, dann 50 mg alle acht Std für nochmals 24 Std.

STEELE u. PHELPS (1971) stellten in einer Doppelblindstudie unter strengen Beurteilungskriterien bei zehn indometacin-behandelten Gicht- und Pseudogichtanfällen ein ausgezeichnetes oder sehr gutes Ansprechen fest (weitgehendes Verschwinden der Entzündungssymptomatik in 0—36 bzw. 37—72 Std). Bei den placebobehandelten Patienten trat in keinem Falle eine Besserung ein. Die gegebene Indometacin-Dosis war 100 mg zu Beginn, dann fortlaufend alle sechs Std 50 mg. Ernstere Nebenwirkungen traten nicht auf.

SCHILLING (1965) hat ebenfalls bei 22 Patienten mit 31 Gichtanfällen keinen Therapieversager. Das Ansprechen war meist in den ersten 6 Std nach Behandlungsbeginn zu registrieren. Als Dosis wird von ihm 300 mg für den ersten Tag angegeben. Die Gesamtdosis kann sowohl oral als auch rectal oder auch aufgeteilt in Kapseln und Suppositorien gegeben werden. Auch wir haben in den letzten Jahren ein sicheres und promptes Ansprechen auf Indometacin beim Gichtanfall gesehen. Die optimale Dosierung stellt u. E. das von EMMERSON angegebene Schema dar. Eine Dosis von 300 mg pro Tag wird dabei nicht überschritten.

Die hauptsächlichsten Nebenwirkungen sind Unverträglichkeit von seiten des Magen-Darm-Traktes, Kopfschmerzen, Benommenheit, Konzentrationsschwäche, Schwindel, Exantheme, Ödeme. Bei etwa einem Sechstel bis zu einem Drittel der Patienten kommt es zumindest bei mehrere Tage dauernder Therapie zu irgendeiner oder mehreren dieser Nebenwirkungen. Die Quote der Nebenwirkungen ist bei einer Dosierung über 200 mg täglich entschieden höher als etwa bei einer Tagesdosis von 75 mg (BOARDMAN u. HART, 1967). Für eine nur wenige Tage dauernde Therapie, bei der nur am ersten Tage eine Dosis von über 200 mg Indometacin gegeben werden muß, ist auf jeden Fall die Gefahr einer Ulcusentstehung im unteren Oesophagus, Magen oder Dünndarm, die bei Dauertherapie mit Indometacin gegeben ist, unbedeutend. Leber-, Nieren- oder Knochenmarkschädigungen sind bei Indometacinbehandlung so selten, daß sie nach HEALEY (1967) vielleicht nur eine Koinzidenz darstellen.

Indometacin stellt unseres Erachtens neben Colchicin das brauchbarste Mittel zur Bekämpfung des Gichtanfalles dar: Es wirkt sehr sicher, es beeinflußt den Plasmauratspiegel nicht, ernste Nebenwirkungen sind bei einer kurzfristigen Behandlung nicht zu erwarten.

Weitere Arzneimittel

Es ist noch zu erwähnen, daß natürlich die verschiedensten sogenannten Antirheumatica auf ihre Wirkung beim Gichtanfall untersucht wurden. Ihre Ansprechquote kommt jedoch nicht an die Quote der besprochenen Mittel heran. Ihre möglichen Nebenwirkungen sind in jedem Falle nicht unerheblich.

Von SLONIM et al. (1962) wurde das fungistatische Mittel Griseofulvin in einer Dosierung von 4—16 g innerhalb 24 Std untersucht. Es brachte bei 16 von 23 Gichtanfällen eine Remission, bei einer Kontrollgruppe mit Placebo kam es in keinem Falle zu einer Besserung. Als Anfallstherapeuticum hat Griseofulvin jedoch nie zur Diskussion gestanden.

Bezüglich der Verwendung von ACTH und Corticosteroiden soll nochmals betont werden, daß sich nur in seltenen Fällen eine Indikation für eine alleinige Behandlung mit einem Hormonpräparat ergibt. In der Regel werden ACTH oder Corticosteroide bei Patienten, deren Anfälle nicht auf Colchicin ansprechen, in Kombination mit Colchicin verwendet. Der therapeutische Effekt beruht auf der starken antiphlogistischen Wirkung der Nebennierenrindenhormone. In der Literatur finden sich weder Argumente noch Beobachtungen, nach denen ACTH und Corticosteroide unterschiedliche Wirksamkeit haben könnten. Vorauszusetzen ist natürlich eine normale Funktion der Nebennierenrinde bei der Gabe von ACTH. Eine sogenannte ausschleichende Behandlung ist nach einer zweitägigen Corticoidbehandlung des Gichtanfalles nicht erforderlich, da eine Atrophie der Nebennierenrinde nach einer zweitägigen Behandlung nicht eintritt. Corticosteroide kommen in seltenen Fällen intraarticulär beim Gichtanfall zur Anwendung.

Neben der medikamentösen Therapie sind keine definierten weiteren Maßnahmen bei der Behandlung des Gichtanfalles erforderlich. Das betroffene Gelenk wird vom Patienten wegen der starken Schmerzen unbeweglich gehalten. Ein berufstätiger Patient wird für einige Tage sich schonen müssen.

Diätetische Maßnahmen, außer Alkoholverbot und vielleicht der Anweisung, leichte Kost und ausreichend Flüssigkeit zu sich zu nehmen, sind nicht erforderlich.

Eine physikalische Therapie, außer vorsichtigen Kälteanwendungen, falls sie vertragen werden, verbietet sich bei einer hochakuten Arthritis.

Insgesamt kann gesagt werden, daß die Behandlung des Gichtanfalles im allgemeinen ein elegant zu lösendes Problem ist. Für den Patienten ist das gezielte und entschlossene Handeln des Arztes, das ihn innerhalb von wenigen Stunden von unerträglichen Schmerzen befreit, ein sehr eindrucksvolles Erlebnis. Unter dem Eindruck dieses Erlebnisses gelingt es auch dem behandelnden Arzt, den schnell vergessenden und außerhalb seiner Anfälle sich völlig gesund fühlenden Gichtpatienten von der Bedeutung einer konsequent durchzuführenden medikamentösen Dauerbehandlung zu überzeugen.

Literatur

BOARDMAN, P. L., HART, F. D.: Indomethacin in the treatment of acute gout. Practitioner **194**, 560—565 (1965).

BOARDMAN, P. L., HART, F. D.: Side-effects of indomethacin. Ann. rheum. Dis. **26**, 127—132 (1967).

BOYLE, J. A., BUCHANAN, W. W.: Clinical Rheumatology, pp. 219—261. Oxford and Edinburgh: Blackwell Scientific Publications 1971.

BUNIM, J. J., KIMBERG, D. V., THOMAS, L. B., VAN SCOTT, E. J., KLATSKIN, G.: The syndrome of sarcoidosis, psoriasis and gout. Ann. intern. Med. **57**, 1018—1040 (1962).

CESTARI, A. N., BOTELHO, J. P., FILHO, VIEIRA, YONENAGO, Y., MAGNELLI, N., IMADA, J.: A case of human reproductive abnormalities possibly induced by colchicine treatment. Rev. brasil. Biol. **25**, 253 (1965). Zit. n. WALLACE, S. L., ERTEL, N. H.: Colchicine, Current problems. Bull. rheum. Dis. **20**, 582—587 (1969).

Davis, J. S., Bartfeld, H.: The effect of intravenous colchicine on acute gout. Amer. J. Med. 16, 218—219 (1954).
De Sèze, S., Ryckewaert, A., Levernieux, J., Marteau, R.: Physiopathology, clinical treatment of gout. II Clinical and therapeutical studies. Ann. rheum. Dis. 17, 15—22 (1958).
Emmerson, B. T.: Regimen of indomethacin therapy in acute gouty arthritis. Brit. med. J. **1967 II**, 272—274.
Garrod, A. B.: The Nature and Treatment of Gout and Rheumatic Gout, 2. Ed. London: Walton and Marbery 1863. Zit. n. Wallace, S. L., Ertel, N. H.: Colchicine, current problems. Bull. rheum. Dis. 20, 582—587 (1969).
Graham, W., Roberts, J. B.: Intravenous colchicine in treatment of gouty arthritis. Ann. rheum. Dis. 12, 16—19 (1953).
Gutman, A. B.: Management of gouty arthritis. Bull. rheum. Dis. 1, 11—15 (1951).
Gutman, A. B.: Treatment of primary gout: the present status. Arthr. and Rheum. 8, 911—920 (1965).
Gutman, A. B., Yu, T. F.: Current principles of management in gout. Amer. J. Med. 13, 744—759 (1952).
Hartung, E. F.: History of the use of colchicine and related medicaments in gout. Ann. rheum. Dis. 13, 190—200 (1954).
Hawkins, C. F., Ellis, H. A., Rawson, A.: Malignant gout with tophaceous small intestine and megaloblastic anaemia. Ann. rheum. Dis. 24, 224—233 (1965).
Healey, L. A.: An appraisal of indomethacin. Bull. on the Rheum. Dis. 18, 483—486 (1967).
Hoefnagel, D.: Trisomy after colchicine therapy. Lancet **1969 I**, 1160.
Kantor, T. G., Brown, R.: Test of non-specific anti-inflammatory activity of colchicine. Arthr. Rheum. 9, 862 (1969); Vortrag Interim Meeting der Amer. Rheum. Ass., Dez. 1966, Cincinnati/Ohio.
Kaplan, H.: Sarcoid Arthritis with Response to Colchicine. N. Engl. J. Med. 263, 778—781 (1960).
Korfmacher, I., Zöllner, N.: Vor- und Nachteile der Behandlung des Gichtanfalles mit dem Colchicinabkömmling Demecolcin. Münch. med. Wschr. 102, 550—551 (1960).
Kuzell, W. C., Schaffarzick, R. W., Naugler, E. W., Koets, P., Mankle, E. A., Brown, B., Camplin, B.: Some observations on 520 gouty patients. J. chron. Dis. 2, 645—669 (1955).
Lockie, L. M.: A discussion of a therapeutic test and a provocative test in gouty arthritis. Ann. intern. Med. 13, 755—760 (1939).
Lockie, L. M.: Diskussion zur Arbeit: Robinson, W. D.: The present status of colchicine and uricosuric agents in management of primary gout. Arthr. and Rheum. 8, 865—882 (1965).
McCarty, D. J.: Crystal deposition diseases. J. Amer. med. Ass. 193, 129—132 (1965).
McCarty, D. J., Gatter, R. A.: Recurrent acute inflammation associated with focal apatite crystal deposition. Arthr. and Rheum. 9, 804—819 (1966).
McLeod, J. G., Phillips, L.: Hypersensitivity to colchicine. Ann. rheum. Dis. 6, 224 (1947), zit. n. Wallace, S. L.
Plotz, C. M.: Diskussion zur Arbeit: Robinson, W. D.: The present status of colchicine and uricosuric agents in management of primary gout. Arthr. and Rheum. 8, 865—882 (1965).
Race, T. F., Paes, J. C., Faloon, W. W.: Intestinal malabsorption induced by oral colchicine. Clin. Res. 14, 480 (1966).
Rodnan, G. P.: Treatment of gout. Mod. Treatm. 1, 1203—1220 (1964).
Schilling, F.: Erfahrungen mit Indomethacin, insbesondere bei der Spondylitis ankylopoetica und im Gichtanfall. Münch. med. Wschr. 107, 2176—2180 (1965).
Seed, L., Slaughter, D. P., Limarzi, L. R.: Effect of colchicine on human carcinoma. Surgery 7, 696 (1940), zit. n. Wallace, S. L.
Slonim, R. R., Howell, D. S., Brown, H. E., jr.: Influence of griseofulvin upon acute gouty arthritis. Arthr. and Rheum. 5, 397—404 (1962).
Smyth, C. J.: Current therapy of gout. J. Amer. med. Ass. 152, 1106—1112 (1953).
Smyth, C. J., Velayos, E. E., Amoroso, L.: A method for measuring swelling of hands and feet. Part II: Influence of a new antiinflammatory drug, indomethacin, in acute gout. Acta rheum. scand. 9, 306—322 (1963).
Steele, A. D., Phelps, P.: Double-blind evaluation of indomethacin and BLR-743 versus placebo in gout and pseudogout. Arthr. and Rheum. 14, 415 (1971); Interim Scientific Session Amer. Rheum. Ass. Juni 1971.
Thompson, G. R., Ting, Y. M., Riggs, G. A., Fenn, M. E., Denning, R. M.: Calcific tendinitis and soft tissue calcification resembling gout. J. Amer. med. Ass. 203, 464—470 (1968).

TIMSON, J.: Trisomy after colchicine therapy. Lancet **1969 I**, 370.
WALKER, F. A.: Trisomy after colchicine therapy. Lancet **1969 I**, 257—258.
WALLACE, S. L.: Colchicine: clinical pharmalogy. Amer. J. Med. **30**, 439—448 (1961).
WALLACE, S. L., BERNSTEIN, D., DIAMOND, H.: Diagnostic value of colchicine therapeutic trial. J. Amer. med. Ass. **199**, 525—528 (1967).
WEBB, D. J., CHODOS, R. B., MAHAS, C. Q., FALOON, W. W.: Mechanism of Vitamin B-12-malabsorption in patients receiving colchicine. N. Engl. J. Med. **279**, 845—850 (1968).
YU, T. F., GUTMAN, A. B.: Efficacy of colchicine in prophylaxis in gout. Ann. intern. Med. **55**, 179—192 (1961).
ZÖLLNER, N.: Moderne Gichtprobleme. In: Erg. d. Inn. Med. und Kinderheilkunde, Bd. 14. S. 321—389. Berlin-Göttingen-Heidelberg: Springer 1960.
ZUCKNER, J.: Response to colchicine therapeutical trial in rheumatoid arthritis. N. Engl. J. Med. **267**, 682—686 (1962).
ZVAIFLER, N. J., MED. **111**, 99—102 (1963). Significance of urate crystals in synovial fluids. Arch. intern. Med. **111**, 99—102 (1963).

2. Die Pharmakologie der Anfallsmittel

Von

U. Trabert

Mit 10 Abbildungen

Colchicin

Einleitung

Colchicin ist das Hauptalkaloid der Herbstzeitlose (Colchicum autumnale) aus der Familie der Liliengewächse (Liliaceae). Semen Colchici enthält etwa 0,4% Colchicin. Die Pflanze verdankt ihren Namen dem griechischen Arzt Dioscorides (1.Jahrhundert nach Christi) nach der kleinasiatischen Landschaft Kolchis am Schwarzen Meer, wo sie, wie auch in Mitteleuropa, verbreitet vorkommt. Schon seit fast 2000 Jahren dienen Zubereitungen als Heilmittel bei Gicht und rheumatischen Erkrankungen.

HARTUNG (1953) gibt einen umfassenden Überblick über die Historie dieser uralten Heilpflanze, deren wesentlichster Inhaltsstoff in der Mitte dieses Jahrhunderts ungeahnte Aktualität für die experimentelle Zellforschung und nach wie vor für die Behandlung der Gichtarthritis erhalten hat.

Chemie

1883 gelang ZEISEL die Isolierung der Reinsubstanz und die Bestimmung der Summenformel. Die 1924 von WINDAUS vorgeschlagene Strukturformel entspricht der des Allo-Colchicins. Die heute gültige Formel wurde 1945 von DEWAR gefunden. Sie wurde durch die Totalsynthese bestätigt, die 1959 ESCHENMOSER gelang (WERNER u. DÖNGES, 1973). Colchicin entspricht in einem wesentlichen Punkt nicht der Definition eines Alkaloids — das Molekül besitzt keine basischen Eigenschaften. Das Stickstoffatom liegt in einer Amidbindung vor. Außerdem ist Colchicin wasserlöslich, eine Eigenschaft, die DEWAR veranlaßte, für den Ring C eine Tropolonstruktur zu postulieren (Abb. 1). WINDAUS hatte noch ein Phenanthrengerüst mit einem Methylester in der Seitenkette angenommen.

Colchicin hat die Summenformel $C_{22}H_{25}NO_6$, das Molekulargewicht 399,4. Das DAB 7 verlangt eine Reinheit von 97% und beschreibt ein gelblich-weißes, amorphes Pulver, das sich in etwa 25 Teilen Wasser löst und in Äthanol und Chloroform leicht löslich ist. Die Substanz schmilzt zwischen 160° und 164° C, die spezifische Drehung $[\alpha]_D^{20°}$ der alkoholischen Lösung liegt zwischen $-235°$ und $-245°$.

Das Tropolon selbst ist eine Säure, deren Stärke zwischen der des Phenols und der der Essigsäure liegt. Die Methoxygruppe an Ring C hat deshalb den Charakter einer Esterbindung und ist damit wesentlich reaktiver als die Methoxygruppen des Ringes A. Phenoläther sind gegen Alkalien beständig. Dagegen lassen sich bereits durch Erhitzen von Colchicin mit Ammoniak oder Alkylaminen die entsprechenden Säureamide bzw. substituierten Aminoderivate des Tropolonrings darstellen (WERNER u. DÖNGES, 1973).

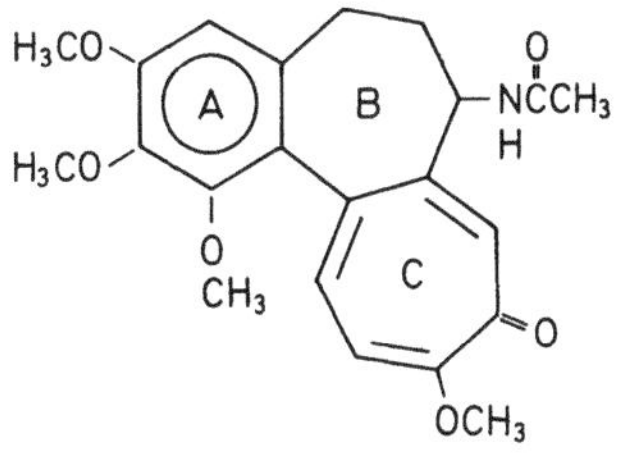

Abb. 1. Colchicin, Tropolon: Die gewählte Abbildungsweise verdeutlicht, daß die benachbarten CO-Gruppen des α-Tropolons gleichberechtigt das H$^+$ Ion binden, weil hierdurch ein energetisch begünstigtes aromatisches System entsteht. Auch bei Carbonsäuren läßt sich die Bindung des Wasserstoffions nicht einem der beiden Sauerstoffatome zuordnen

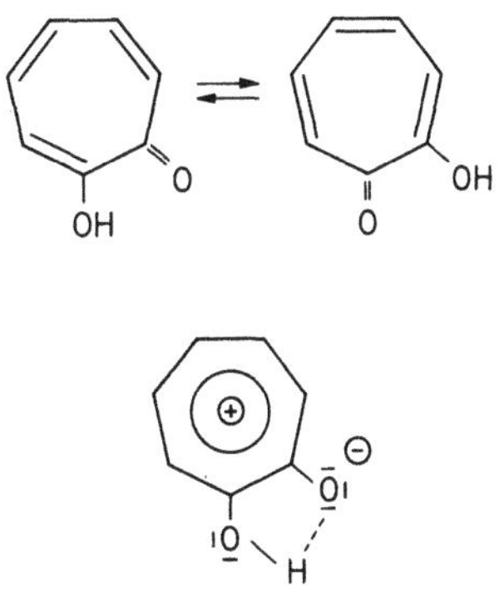

Fragen der optischen Isomerie und Konformation sollen hier nur angedeutet werden. Colchicin besitzt ein asymmetrisches Kohlenstoffatom im Ring B, das die Acetylaminogruppe trägt. Wirksam ist das linksdrehende (-) optische Isomer. Die Anordnung von Ring A und Ring C zueinander, also die Konformation des Moleküls, ist jedoch ebenfalls von ganz entscheidender Bedeutung für die Wirksamkeit der Substanz. Bei Wegfall des Asymmetriezentrums im Desacetylaminocolchicin resultiert eine Verbindung mit noch stärkerer Wirkung als die linksdrehende Substanz. Im allgemeinen entspricht die Wirkung einer Substanz nach Verlust des Asymmetriezentrums der des schwächer wirksamen optischen Antipoden. Wird eine freie Drehbarkeit der Ringe A und C zueinander dadurch ermöglicht, daß Ring B gesprengt wird (eine solche Verbindung wurde von dem japanischen Chemiker NOZOE synthetisiert), entsteht eine wirkungslose Verbindung (WERNER u. DÖNGES, 1973). Die vorgenannten Autoren haben die antimitotische Wirksamkeit einer ganzen Reihe verschiedener Colchicin-Derivate untersucht und werten die eben beschriebenen Verhältnisse als Hinweis darauf, daß die Konformation des Moleküls die Reaktion mit dem Receptor selbst ermöglicht, während optische Isomere bzw. die Art der Substitution die Wirkung des Moleküls auf dem Wege einer unterschiedlichen Penetrationsfähigkeit in die Zelle beeinflussen. ZWEIG u. CHIGNELL (1973) zeigten jedoch durch Untersuchungen im zellfreien Medium, daß die Affinität zum Receptor (Tubuline, s. S. 440) auch von der jeweiligen Substitution abhängt.

Vor 100 Jahren hat erstmals STRUVE (1873) im Zusammenhang mit einer forensischen Fragestellung darauf hingewiesen, daß gelöstes Colchicin durch Sonnenlicht verändert wird. GREWE u. WULF (1951) gelang die Isolierung und Charakterisierung dreier Substanzen, die als α-, β- und γ-Lumicolchicine bezeichnet wurden. FORBES (1955) und GARDNER et al. (1957) konnten β- und γ-Lumicolchicin als Stereoisomere einer tetracyclischen Verbindung charakterisieren, die durch Verlagerung einer Doppelbindung im Tropolonring zustandekommt (Abb. 2). α-Lumicolchicin ist ein dimeres, oktacyclisches Molekül. Die Lumicolchicine besitzen weder antimitotische (ARONSON u. INOUÉ, 1970; SAGORIN et al., 1972), noch antientzündliche Wirksamkeit (MALAWISTA et al., 1972).

Abbildung 3 zeigt einige Colchicin-Derivate, von denen Desacetylmethylcolchicin (Demecolcin, Colcemid) eine gewisse Bedeutung auch in der Anfallsbehandlung besaß. Trimethylcolchicinsäure (TMCA) wurde besonders von WALLACE (1961a) als Anfallsmittel propagiert, das nebenwirkungsärmer sei. Auch

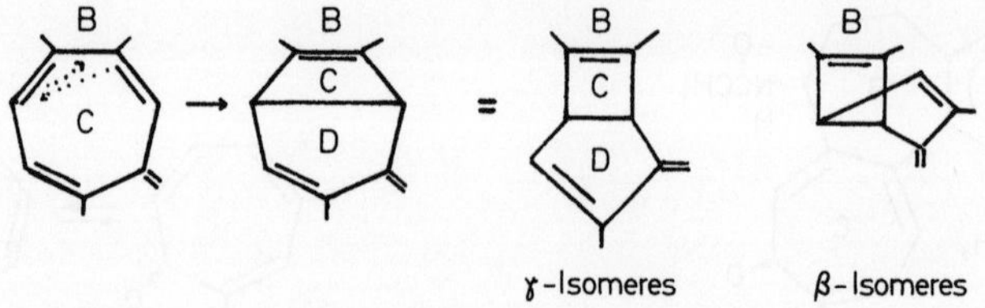

γ-Isomeres   β-Isomeres

Abb. 2. Lumicolchicine: Diese Substanzen sind Photoisomerisationsprodukte des Colchicins. Die Umlagerung zweier Doppelbindungen im Ring C führt zur Bildung zweier tetracyclischer stereoisomerer Verbindungen — β- und γ-Lumicolchicin. Das nicht dargestellte α-Lumicolchicin entsteht durch Dimerisation von β- und γ-Lumicolchicin

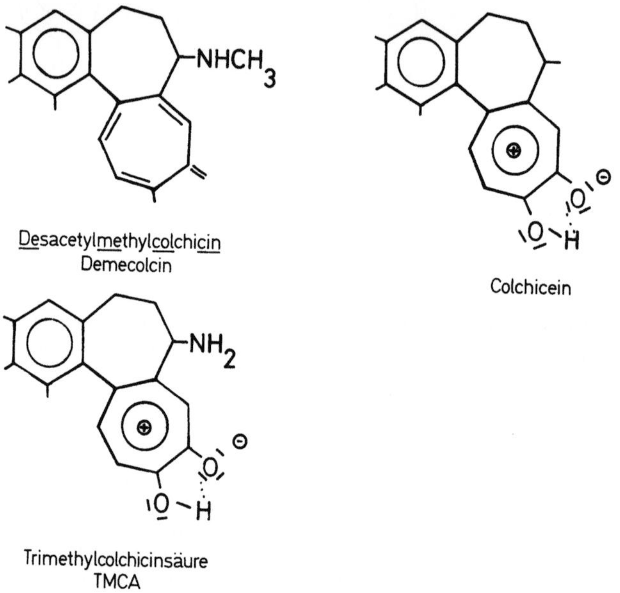

Desacetylmethylcolchicin
Demecolcin

Colchicein

Trimethylcolchicinsäure
TMCA

Abb. 3. Derivate des Colchicins: Das erste, Demecolcin, entsteht nicht im Organismus, erlangte aber eine gewisse Bedeutung in der Anfallsbehandlung. Die beiden anderen Derivate entstehen wahrscheinlich im Organismus durch Hydrolyse der jeweiligen Amid- oder (und) Esterbindung (Desacetylierung an Ring B und Demethylierung an Ring C). Es wurde lediglich das gemeinsame Grundgerüst dargestellt, seine Substitution jedoch nur, wenn sie von derjenigen beim Colchicin abweicht

Thio-Verbindungen, die anstelle der Methoxy-Gruppe an Ring C eine Methylmercapto-Gruppe enthalten, wurden klinisch getestet. Gegenüber der Muttersubstanz konnten sie sich bisher alle nicht durchsetzen. Colchicein ist unwirksam.

Pharmakokinetik

Nach oraler Applikation wird Colchicin sicher gut resorbiert, zumal experimentelle Daten von WALASZEK et al. (1960) Anhaltspunkte geben, daß ein Teil des in den Darm ausgeschiedenen Colchicins reabsorbiert wird.

LETTRE u. LUTZE (1944) haben die Verteilung von Colchicin in den einzelnen Organen des Meerschweinchens nach intraperitonealer Applikation untersucht. Sie entwickelten hierzu eine recht empfindliche biologische Methode — sie bestimmten den Mitosehemmeffekt der wäßrigen Organextrakte an Fibroblastenkulturen. Damit ließen sich noch Colchicinkonzentrationen von 10—40 ng/ml zuverlässig erfassen. BACK et al. (1951) konnten mit radioaktiv markiertem Colchicin diese Ergebnisse im wesentlichen bestätigen und besser quantifizieren. Vier Std nach Applikation des Pharmakons an der Maus fanden sie Hirn, Muskulatur, Herz und Blut frei von Radioaktivität, dagegen 39% in der Milz, 30% in der Niere, 21% im Intestinum und 10% in der Leber.

Tumorgewebe hat ebenfalls eine hohe Affinität zu Colchicin — die gleichen Autoren fanden bei tumortragenden Mäusen 17% im Sarkomgewebe, die Milz blieb dagegen bei sämtlichen Versuchstieren frei von Colchicin.

BORISY u. TAYLOR (1967) haben in vitro die Affinität von ^{3}H-markiertem Colchicin in verschiedenen Geweben untersucht und hierbei die bei weitem stärkste Bindung von Colchicin an Kaninchen-, Schweine- und Rattenhirn, noch dreifach höhere an Tintenfischaxoplasma gefunden. Nachdem CAVANAGH u. LEWIS (1969) beobachteten, daß intraperitoneal appliziertes Colchicin bei der Ratte weder nach 2 Std, noch nach 4 Std die Mitoserate der Subependymalplatte beeinflußte, postulierten sie die Existenz einer Blut-Hirn-Schranke. WALLACE u. ERTEL (1969) sprechen von einer „frühen" Blut-Hirnschranke, die aus bisher unbekannten Gründen, abhängig von der Dosis, nach einer gewissen Zeit durchbrochen werden kann (s. auch Toxikologie, S. 444). Auch für andere Organe besteht keine klare Beziehung der Colchicin-Affinität des entsprechenden Gewebes in vitro — das von seinem Gehalt an Mikrotubuli abhängt — und dem Organgehalt in vivo (WALLACE u. ERTEL, 1969).

Die genaue qualitative und quantitative Erfassung von Colchicin und seinen Metaboliten erfordert die Verwendung von radioaktiv markierten Substanzen, die zu erfassenden Konzentrationen in vivo liegen in Größenordnungen von einigen µg-% und weit darunter. Über Struktur und zeitliches Auftreten der Abbauprodukte des Colchicins und ihre Wirksamkeit ist wenig bekannt.

WALLACE et al. (1970) fanden in den ersten Std nach i.v. Applikation von 2 mg Colchicin keine Abbauprodukte im Plasma. WALASZEK et al. (1960) konnten nachweisen, daß gerade initial zum Zeitpunkt hoher Plasmakonzentrationen des Pharmakons wahrscheinlich in der Leber beträchtliche Mengen desacetyliert werden. Während der ersten 67 min nach i.v. Applikation von 3 mg ^{14}C-Colchicin, dessen Carboxyl-C der Acetylgruppe an Ring B markiert war (WZ in Tab. 1), wurden 4% als $^{14}CO_2$ abgeatmet. Dieser Wert erlaubt natürlich nur eine grobe Schätzung, wieviel Colchicin in diesem Zeitraum desacetyliert wurde, die tatsächliche Menge kann wesentlich höher liegen.

Die Bestimmung der biologischen HWZ des Colchicins bereitet über die eben angedeuteten Probleme hinaus deshalb große Schwierigkeiten, weil Colchicin rasch und nachhaltig an intracelluläre Strukturen gebunden wird. Die biologische HWZ läßt sich deshalb nicht am Verlauf der Plasmakonzentrationen ablesen. Darüber hinaus könnte der Konzentrationsverlauf in den einzelnen Organen ebenso differieren, wie die jeweiligen Maximalkonzentrationen, die hier gefunden werden können. Nach WALLACE (1972) erreicht die Colchicinkonzentration in den Leukocyten rasch ein Maximum und bleibt hier nach der einmaligen intravenösen Applikation von 3 mg hoch und stabil über 24 Std lang.

Die Messung der Ausscheidung im Urin gibt gewisse Anhaltspunkte für das Verhalten des Gesamtkörperpools. Es werden unterschiedliche Mengen in den Faeces ausgeschieden, abhängig von der Species des Versuchstiers. Die Ausscheidung über die Faeces kommt hauptsächlich über die Galle, teilweise auch direkt über die Darmwand zustande. Beim Menschen fehlen bisher vollständige Bilanzierungen.

Tabelle 1 faßt den Hauptteil der Ergebnisse von Isotopenuntersuchungen am Menschen durch WALASZEK et al. (1960) und WALLACE et al. (1970) zusammen.

Tabelle 1. Zusammenstellung von Ergebnissen, die WALASZEK et al. (1960) (WZ) und WALLACE et al. (1970) (W) gewonnen haben. Für die Art der radioaktiven ^{14}C-Markierung wurden folgende Symbole gewählt: 1. bio — es handelt sich um biosynthetisch gewonnenes Colchicin, dessen markiertes C-Atom an beliebiger Stelle des Moleküls sitzt. 2. B — das Carboxyl-C der Acetylgruppe an Ring B ist markiert. 3. C — die Markierung erfolgte an der Methoxygruppe an Ring C

Erkrankung der Patienten	Anzahl der Patienten	Autor	applizierte Dosis mg i.v.	radioaktive Markierung	Plasma Anfangskonzentration μg%	mittleres Verteilungs-Volumen l/kg	HWZ min	Urin 6 Std	12 Std	24 Std	48 Std	HCCl$_3$-lösliche Metaboliten	Atemluft ^{14}CO$_2$ in 67 min in % der applizierten Dosis
								in % der applizierten Dosis					
I. Asthma ohne E.	2 2	WZ	2–3 2–3	bio	—	—	—	7,7	10,4	19,7	27,5	7,6	—
II. Verschiedene Erkrankungen	5	W	2	C	1,8±0,7	2,2±0,8	19 ± 7,5			9,2			
III. Gicht	1 1 4	WZ WZ W	3 3 2	bio B C	1,5±0,6	2,1±0,8	29 ±11	0,8 0,4	2,9 0,8	3,3 2,4	3,8 3,2	17,0 8,1	4
IV. Chronische Leber-Erkrankungen	3	W	2	C	2,8±0,3	1,2±0,3	9,3± 0,5			10,4 10,4			
V. Chronische Nieren-Erkrankungen	4	W	2	C	1,9±1,3	1,8±1,1	40 ±26			1,1			
VI. Carcinom	5 1	WZ	3 3	bio B				2,9 0,07	3,3 0,1	3,9 0,19	4,3 0,2	1,5 0,1	

Der Aussagewert ist durch die geringen Patientenzahlen der einzelnen Gruppen und die teilweise beträchtlichen Abweichungen der Resultate innerhalb der Patientenkollektive beschränkt. Außerdem differieren die Ergebnisse z.T. zwischen den Untersuchern, wozu die unterschiedliche Art der radioaktiven Markierung beiträgt (s. Legende zur Tab. 1). Einige Aussagen lassen sich trotzdem treffen:

1. Bereits 10 min nach Injektion verteilt sich das Pharmakon auf etwa 2 l/kg Körpergewicht, berechnet aus der Plasmakonzentration, d.h. bereits zu diesem Zeitpunkt übertrifft die intracelluläre Konzentration diejenige des Extracellulärraums. Dies übrigens trotz einer relativ weitgehenden, wenn auch sehr lockeren Bindung an Plasmaalbumin (WALLACE et al., 1970).

2. Die Plasmahalbwertszeiten übersteigen im Mittel nie 40 min, als Extremwert wurde bei einem Patienten mit schwerer Nierenfunktionseinschränkung 75 min bestimmt. Im „Normalkollektiv" betrug das Mittel 20 min und überstieg nur bei einem Patienten 30 min, so daß hiernach Colchicin bereits weitgehend eliminiert sein müßte, wenn es nach Überdosierung erst beginnt, toxisch zu wirken.

3. Dagegen werden bis zu 18% des über die Nieren in 48 Std ausgeschiedenen Colchicins erst während der zweiten 24 Std im Urin gefunden.

4. Der Vergleich der einzelnen Patientengruppen ergibt:

a) Einen höheren Plasmainitialspiegel, kleineres Verteilungsvolumen, kürzere Plasma-HWZ und raschere Ausscheidung über die Nieren bei den Patienten mit schwerem Leberzellschaden. Offenbar fallen bei diesen Patienten Leber und bei Vorliegen portaler Hypertension auch teilweise die Milz mit ihrer an sich hohen Affinität für Colchicin für die initiale Aufnahme der Substanz aus (Initialspiegel, Verteilungsraum). Damit ist der Ausscheidungsweg über die Galle ebenfalls blockiert, die Ausscheidung über die Nieren erfolgt rascher (HWZ) und in größerem Umfange.

b) Carcinomträger scheiden wesentlich weniger über die Niere aus; WALASZEK et al. (1960) fanden bei tumortragenden Mäusen, im Vergleich zu Normaltieren, relativ höhere Mengen in den Faeces.

c) Die verlängerte Plasma-HWZ und verminderte renale Ausscheidung bei Patienten mit schwerer Niereninsuffizienz bedürfen keines Kommentars.

d) Bemerkenswerte Abweichungen gegenüber den Patienten mit unterschiedlichen Erkrankungen finden sich bei Gicht-Patienten. Diese Abweichungen betreffen bei WALASZEK et al. (1960) die Ausscheidung im Urin, bei WALLACE et al. (1970) die Plasma-HWZ, während die Ausscheidung im Urin bei diesem Autorenkollektiv mit dem „Normalkollektiv" praktisch übereinstimmt. Erklärungsversuche hierfür müßten vorerst rein spekulativ bleiben.

Auf die Beziehung dieser Befunde zu den im Kapitel Toxicität geschilderten Vergiftungsfällen sei bereits an dieser Stelle hingewiesen.

Wirkungsweise

Die Wirkung von Colchicin als Anfallsmittel ist auch heute noch nicht in allen Einzelheiten aufgeklärt. Die milden unspezifisch antiphlogistischen Eigenschaften der Substanz stehen in keiner Relation zu ihrer Potenz bei der Behandlung der Gichtarthritis. Neben dieser seit etwa 2 Jahrtausenden bekannten Wirkung beschäftigt Colchicin etwa seit Mitte der Dreißiger Jahre dieses Jahrhunderts die experimentellen Zellforscher als Mitosegift (Metaphasengift). Unter anderem wird von HARTUNG (1953) die Frage aufgeworfen, ob beide Eigenschaften etwas miteinander zu tun haben könnten. 15 Jahre später vertritt dies MALAWISTA (1968) als Arbeitshypothese.

Den polymorphkernigen Leukocyten (PMN im angloamerikanischen Schrifttum) oder Granulocyten kommt eine Schlüsselrolle in der Pathogenese des Gichtanfalls zu — aleukämische Individuen zeigen keine arthritische Reaktion auf intraarticuläre Uratablagerungen (PHELPS u. MCCARTY, 1966).

Um die zentrale Funktion der Phagocytose gruppiert sich eine Reihe von Teilfunktionen, die Voraussetzung, Begleit- oder Folgereaktionen darstellen. WALLACE u. ERTEL (1969) haben diese Einzelfunktionen und ihre Beeinflußbarkeit durch Colchicin zusammengestellt. Hiervon sollen zunächst solche geschildert werden, die der eigentlichen Phagocytose vorausgehen: hierzu gehören ungerichtete Spontanbewegungen der Leukocyten ("random motility"), deren Ausmaß die Wahrscheinlichkeit bestimmt, daß ein Leukocyt zufällig auf ein Uratkristall trifft.

PHELPS (1969a) fand eine Zunahme dieser Art von Leukocytenbewegungen unter dem Einfluß von Uratkristallen und gelöstem Urat und konnte gleichzeitig nachweisen, daß dieser Effekt durch Colchicin (10^{-8} M) teilweise aufgehoben wird.

Leukocyten, die Uratkristalle phagocytiert haben, bilden eine nicht dialysierbare Substanz, die auf andere Leukocyten chemotaktisch wirkt. Die Bildung dieser Substanz kann durch Colchicin in einer Konzentration von 10^{-7} bis 10^{-6} M sicher unterdrückt werden (PHELPS, 1969b, 1970). CANER (1965) konnte zeigen, daß etwa entsprechende Konzentrationen des Pharmakons die Reaktion von Leukocyten auf einen chemotaktisch wirksamen Reiz, also die Chemotaxis selbst, zu unterdrücken vermögen. In der Versuchsanordnung von CANER, in der Staphylococcus albus als chemotaktisch wirksames Agens fungierte, sind die Bakterien selbst ebenfalls der Colchicinwirkung ausgesetzt.

Zur Frage der Relevanz experimenteller Ergebnisse sei folgendes angemerkt: Die biologische HWZ des Colchicins ist nicht genau bestimmbar, und die Substanz besitzt eine hohe Affinität zu intracellulären Strukturen, auch zu denen der Leukocyten. Insofern läßt sich nicht fordern, daß die von WALLACE et al. (1970) bestimmten kurzzeitigen maximalen Plasmakonzentrationen von bis zu 10^{-8} M als verbindlich für den Aussagewert des *in vitro* Experiments zu gelten haben. Eine kritische Wertung der jeweils benötigten Konzentration ist jedoch gerade beim Colchicin zu fordern. Sie differieren bei den einzelnen Untersuchern um Größenordnungen von mehreren Zehner-Potenzen.

Einer der wenigen *in vivo*-Versuche sei hier erwähnt:

FRUHMAN (1960) konnte mit 0,2 mg Colchicin subcutan pro Ratte die Mobilisierung von Leukocyten nach intraperitonealer Injektion von Endotoxin hemmen.

Eine Blockierung der Phagocytose durch Colchicin als entscheidendes Wirkprinzip in der Anfallsbehandlung wird von der überwiegenden Anzahl neuerer Untersucher verneint (MALAWISTA u. BODEL, 1967; MALAWISTA, 1971a; ZURIER et al., 1973). Gegenteilige Ergebnisse benötigten relativ hohe Colchicinkonzentrationen, die jeweils über 10^{-5} M lagen (GOLDFINGER et al., 1965; FRITZE et al., 1967). Diese Aussage kann jedoch nur getroffen werden, wenn man den Begriff der Phagocytose entsprechend eng faßt und von den bereits eingangs erwähnten Begleitreaktionen abtrennt:

Der *eigentliche Vorgang besteht lediglich in der Umscheidung eines Stücks Extracellulärraums*, der die zu phagocytierende Substanz enthält, *durch die Plasmamembran, die sich an dieser Stelle* schließlich von der Zelloberfläche als phagocytotische Vacuole oder Phagosom *abschnürt* und sich Richtung Zellinneres bewegt. Diese Phagosomen werden dann mit lysosomalen Enzymen beladen, die in sogenannten primären Lysosomen abgepackt bzw. in den Granula der polymorphkernigen Leukocyten enthalten sind. Damit ist eine Verdauungsvacuole (ein Phagolysosom, ein secundäres Lysosom) entstanden. Dieses Phagolysosom kann als sogenannter Restkörper (residual body) in der Zelle verbleiben, es kann seinen Inhalt wieder, verdaut oder unverdaut, mit den Enzymen in den Extracellulärraum abgeben, die Membran des Phagolysosomen kann aber auch rupturieren. Die sauren Hydrolasen gelangen in diesem Fall in das umgebende Cytoplasma, das führt zum Zelltod, die Plasmamembran wird ebenfalls zerstört, der gesamte Zellinhalt wird frei. Dies trifft für die Uratphagocytose zu (s. u. a. SCHUMACHER u. PHELPS, 1971; SOBERMAN et al., 1973). Dem oben gezeichneten Bild der Phagocytose mit einem Teil ihrer intracellulären Folgereaktionen liegen im wesentlichen die Vorstellungen von DEDUVE u. WATTIAUX (1965) zugrunde. Es gibt hiervon Abweichungen, insbesondere muß es nicht in jedem Fall zur vollständigen Abschnürung von Phagosomen von der Zelloberfläche kommen, damit lysosomale Enzyme freigesetzt werden (ZURIER et al., 1973).

Subcelluläre Partikel, wie die oben beschriebenen Phagosomen, primären oder sekundären Lysosomen oder Mitochondrien bewegen sich nicht zufällig im Sinne der BROWNschen Bewegung frei im Cytoplasma, sondern folgen hierbei filamentären Leitstrukturen. Diese Form der Bewegung von intracellulärem Material oder subcellulären Strukturen wurde von FREED u. LEBOWITZ (1970) als "long saltatory movements" (LSM) beschrieben. BHISEY u. FREED (1971) haben den Einfluß von Colchicin auf diese LSM in Peritonealmakrophagen beschrieben, MALAWISTA (1971) am Melanocytenmodell der Froschhaut.

Unter diesen filamentären Leitstrukturen lassen sich Mikrotubuli und Mikrofilamente unterscheiden. Die Mikrofilamente sind u. a. für den oben geschilderten Vorgang der eigentlichen Phagocytose verantwortlich und werden durch Cytochalasin B zerstört. Cytochalasin B ist Stoffwechselprodukt eines Pilzes. Für die Colchicinwirkung von möglicherweise entscheidender Bedeutung sind die Mikrotubuli, weil sie diese Substanz spezifisch zu binden vermögen. MALAWISTA (1968) entwickelte angesichts dieses Colchicinbindungsvermögens, der Beteiligung der Mikrotubuli am Aufbau der Metaphasenspindel und der bereits damals bekannten Funktionen der Mikrotubuli in der Interphasezelle die Arbeitshypothese, der entzündungshemmenden und antimitotischen Wirkung des Colchicins lägen ein gemeinsamer Mechanismus zugrunde.

Mikrotubuli wurden mit der Einführung der Glutaraldehydfixationstechnik (SABATANI et al., 1963) der elektronenmikroskopischen Beobachtung zugänglich. Als Vorlage für die folgende Beschreibung dieser zur Zeit intensiv beforschten subcellulären Strukturen dienten Übersichtsarbeiten von PORTER (1966), OLMSTED u. BORISY (1973) und vor allem BARDELE (1973). Auf eine kurze Übersicht von BUCHER (1972) sei ebenfalls hingewiesen.

Mikrotubuli sind Hohlzylinder mit einem Außendurchmesser von 240 ± 20 Å, einem Innendurchmesser von 150 Å und einer Länge bis zu mehreren µ. Die Wand besteht aus 50 Å dicken Protofilamenten. Diese Protofilamente bauen sich aus globulären Proteinen auf, die als Vorstufen reichlich im Cytoplasma vorkommen. Etwa 1—2% der Gesamtzellproteine und 6—12% der Kernspindelproteine sind Proteine der Mikrotubuli. Die Mikrotubuli und ihre Vorstufen stehen in einem dauernden Prozeß des Auf- und Abbaus ("assambly — disassambly"), der gegebenenfalls in Sekundenfrist ablaufen kann. Ein Beispiel hierfür demonstriert BARDELE (1973) am Umbau der Axopodien von Helioflagellaten.

Die Mikrotubuli aufbauenden Proteine werden nach einem Vorschlag von MOHRI (1968) *Tubuline* genannt. Sie gehören zu den Strukturproteinen, unterscheiden sich aber von solchen anderer Provenienz durch ihre Aminosäurezusammensetzung, z. B. dem Actin und Myosin der Muskulatur, dem Flagellin der Bakteriengeißeln oder dem Filarin der Neurofilamente. Die Zusammensetzung der Tubuline verschiedener Species stimmt nicht überein. Es handelt sich um elektronenoptisch nicht darzustellende 6 S-Proteine vom Molekulargewicht 110000, die sich aus zwei nur unwesentlich verschiedenen Proteinuntereinheiten aufbauen. Diese Heterodimeren können sich zu längsorientierten Protofilamenten zusammenfügen, von denen meist 13 einen Mikrotubulus bilden. Die helicale Anordnung eines oder weniger Protofilamente ist ebenfalls möglich. Die Abbildung von BARDELE (1973) gibt eine mögliche Vorstellung wieder (Abb. 4).

Die Mikrotubuli bzw. ihre Untereinheiten binden bestimmte Substanzen sehr spezifisch, Colchicin und eine große Anzahl seiner Derivate (ZWEIG u. CHIGNELL, 1973) sowie Vincaalkaloide, Griseofulvin, Podophyllotoxin, Guanosintriphosphat. Bindungsstelle, Stöchiometrie, Intensität und Effekt dieser Bindung differieren (s. auch Abb. 5). Colchicin wird im Verhältnis 1:1 (Molekül/Heterodimeres) gebunden. Diese Bindung ist so spezifisch, daß sich der Gehalt einer Zelle

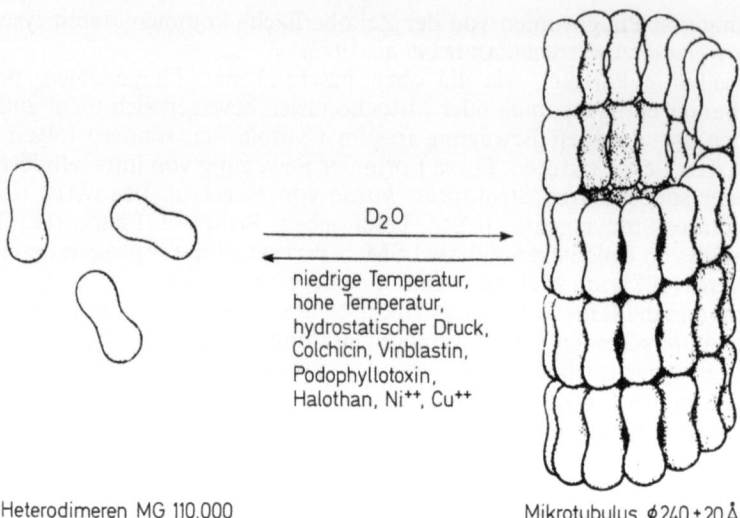

Abb. 4. Die hier wiedergegebene Abbildung von BARDELE (1973) trägt der filamentären und der helicalen Organisation der Mikrotubuli Rechnung

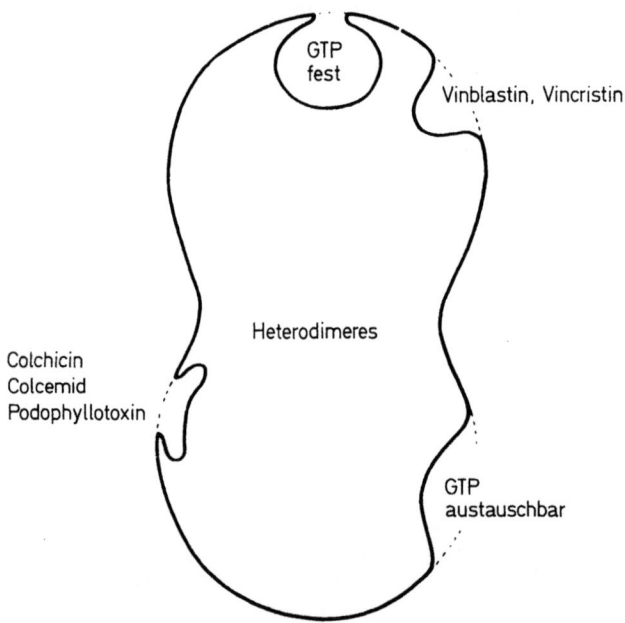

Abb. 5. Bindungsort für Nucleotide und Mitosegifte am Tubulin-Heterodimeren (BARDELE, 1973)

an mikrotubulären Proteinen mit markiertem Colchicin bestimmen läßt (WERNER u. DÖNGES, 1973). Die Bildung dieses Komplexes diente der Isolierung und Charakterisierung dieser Proteine. Colchicin blockiert durch seine Bindung an die Tubuline nicht nur deren Polymerisation (assambly), sondern führt auch zu einer mehr oder weniger raschen und vollständigen Depolymerisation (disassambly) der Mikrotubuli.

Dieser Komplex mit Colchicin ist stabiler als z.B. derjenige mit Vinblastin, die Bindung löst sich erst nach 12stündigem Spülen mit einer alkaloidfreien Salzlösung (BHISEY u. FREED, 1971). Es hängt von der Konformation des Tubulins ab, ob diese Bindung zustandekommt. Eine A-, B- und C-Konformation der Tubuline unterscheiden sich durch den Anteil von α-Helix und Faltblattstruktur bzw. zufälliger Wicklung ("random coil"). Sie gehen durch Änderung von Temperatur und pH ineinander über. Die B-Konformation, stabil bei 37° C, besitzt ein optimales Colchicinbindungsvermögen bei pH 6,8 bis 7,0. Die B-Konformation wird durch ihre Bindung an Colchicin, Vinblastin und bestimmte Nucleotide bis zu einem gewissen Grad stabilisiert. Die Bindung an Colchicin löst sich durch Bestrahlung mit langwelligem UV-Licht, die entstehenden Lumicolchicine (s. S. 434) besitzen keine Affinität zu den Tubulinen. Die Beteiligung der Tubuline an anderen Zellstrukturen als den Mikrotubuli wird diskutiert. WUNDERLICH et al. (1973) konnten durch eine Colchicinkonzentration von 10^{-3} M Funktionen der Zellmembran beeinflussen.

Der Bindungsort für Podophyllotoxin könnte dem für Colchicin entsprechen — beide hemmen sich kompetitiv. Die Vinca-Alkaloide werden an anderer Stelle gebunden, sie hemmen die Bindung von Colchicin nicht kompetitiv (ZWEIG u. CHIGNELL, 1973). Die Bindung der Vinca-Alkaloide führt zu einer Aggregation zu hexagonalen Kristallen (BENSCH u. MALAWISTA, 1969), die bis zu einem gewissen Grade ihr Colchicinbindungsvermögen behalten. Der Bindung von GTP könnte eine wesentliche Rolle für den Assamblyprozeß zufallen.

Die Funktion der Mikrotubuli (nach OLMSTED u. BORISY, 1973) betrifft:
1. die Bewegung der Chromosomen bei der Zellteilung,
2. den intracellulären Transport von Material,
3. die Entwicklung und Erhaltung der Zellform als eine Art Skeletfunktion,
4. die Zellbewegung,
5. die sensorische Transduktion.

Ein Teil dieser Funktionen setzt in besonderer Weise die Fähigkeit zu raschem "assambly" und "disassambly" ("transient functions") voraus, wie z.B. die Bildung der Mitosespindel oder jewels mit lokalen Sol-Gel-Transformationen des Cytoplasmas verbundene kurzfristige Änderungen der Zellform.

Die Bedeutung der Mikrotubuli für intracelluläre Transportvorgänge sei besonders hervorgehoben. Für sämtliche derartige Transportvorgänge ist bislang völlig unklar, ob die Mikrotubuli hierfür lediglich als passive Leitstrukturen fungieren oder ein aktives Transportsystem darstellen, das gleichzeitig hierfür die Energie liefert. Die Bewegung von Substanzen an den Mikrotubuli betreffen u.a. die Sekretion von Stoffwechselprodukten, wie des Insulins durch die β-Zellen des Pankreas (LACY et al., 1968) oder der Lipoproteine durch die Leber (ORCI et al., 1973), die Freisetzung lysosomaler Enzyme (u.a. ZURIER et al., 1973) und den Axontransport im Neuriten der Nervenzelle (BARDELE, 1973).

Wie bereits erwähnt, ist die Ordnung und die gerichtete Bewegung von Zellorganellen, aber auch von phagocytiertem Material (FREED u. LEBOWITZ, 1970; BHISEY u. FREED, 1971) ebenfalls von einem intakten System der Mikrotubuli abhängig. Intracelluläre Partikel werden dabei "long saltatory movements" (LSM) unterworfen. Die gleichen Autoren vermuten, daß auf diesem Wege die Fusion primärer Lysosomen mit phagocytotischen (oder pinocytotischen) Vacuolen zustande kommt.

BHISEY u. FREED (1971) zeigen, daß Peritonealmakrophagen unter Colchicineinfluß von einer auf der Unterlage gleitenden Bewegung in eine amöboide Form der Motilität übergehen. Dabei verlieren die Zellen ihre innere Ordnung völlig und Mitochondrien und Lysosomen verfallen statt LSM der Brownschen Bewegung. MALAWISTA (1971) wies am Melanocytenmodell der Froschhaut die hohe Selektivität solcher Transportprozesse nach — hier für die Melaningranula bei der Hell- und Dunkelstellung. Damit einher ging die bereits erwähnte Sol-Gel-Transformation des Cytoplasmas.

SCHUMACHER u. PHELPS (1971) haben in einer ausführlichen elektronenmikroskopischen Untersuchung die Vorgänge in Leukocyten bei der Uratphagocytose untersucht, SOBERMAN et al. (1973) den gleichen Prozeß lichtoptisch mit Cinemikroskopie an Leukocyten des Hundehais (Mustelus canis). Besonders die letzteren Untersucher demonstrierten eindrucksvoll, daß die Membran der Phagosomen, in denen die Uratkristalle ja zunächst enthalten sind, erst dann rupturiert, wenn sie mit lysosomalen Enzymen der Leukocytengranula beladen wurden.

MALAWISTA u. BODEL (1967) sowie MALAWISTA (1971a) beobachteten unter Colchicineinfluß ($2,5 \times 10^{-6}$ M) bzw. nach Präinkubation mit Vinblastin ($2,5 \times 10^{-5}$ M) nicht nur eine „Dissoziierung von Phagocytose und erhöhtem Sauerstoffverbrauch", sondern auch ein vermindertes Auftreten cytoplasmatischer Vacuolen ("digestive vacuoles" = Phagolysosom) mit entsprechend verminderter Degranulierung des Cytoplasmas. Die eigentliche Phagocytose der verwendeten Staphylo- bzw. Streptokokken blieb selbst bei Konzentrationen von $2,5 \times 10^{-4}$ M unbeeinflußt.

Die während der letzten fünf Jahre erschienenen Veröffentlichungen sprechen in der Mehrzahl für die Richtigkeit der Arbeitshypothese von MALAWISTA (1968), daß der antientzündlichen und antimitotischen Wirkung des Colchicins ein gleicher Wirkungsmechanismus zugrunde liegt: die Beeinflussung des mikrotubulären Apparates.

Entsprechendes gilt für eine große Anzahl von Colchicin-Derivaten und für die Vincaalcaloide, Podophyllotoxin und Griseofulvin (ZWEIG u. CHIGNELL, 1973). Diese Autoren haben antiphlogistische und antimitotische Wirkung der genannten Verbindungen in Beziehung gesetzt zu deren Fähigkeit, die Bindung von ^{3}H-Colchicin an die Neurotubuli im zellfreien System zu hemmen und fanden jeweils eine eindrucksvolle Relation von entzündungshemmender und antimitotischer Potenz und Affinität zu den Neurotubuli.

Die Untersuchungen der eben genannten Autoren könnten dazu beitragen, einem Einwand gegen die Hypothese von MALAWISTA zu begegnen: Die (scheinbare?) Dissoziierung der antiphlogistischen und antimitotischen Wirkung bei der Trimethylcolchicinsäure, auf die u.a. WALLACE (1961a, 1961b) und MALAWISTA (1968) ausdrücklich hinweisen. Trimethylcolchicinsäure (TMCA) ist ein durchaus potentes Gichtmittel, wie bereits oben erwähnt, besitzt aber praktisch keine antimitotische Wirkung. ZWEIG u. CHIGNELL (1973) konnten dies bestätigen, vermißten aber gleichzeitig eine lokale antientzündliche Wirkung an der Rattenhaut, in die vorher Uratkristalle injiziert worden waren. Gleichzeitig fehlte eine Affinität zu den Neurotubuli. Gänzlich andersartig verhielt sich eine Substanz, deren freie Hydroxylgruppe am Tropolonring methyliert war. Diese Substanz zeigte kompetitive Hemmung der Colchicinbindung, antimitotische und entzündungshemmende Wirkung. Das legt den Schluß nah, daß TMCA im Organismus zumindest teilweise methyliert wird und deshalb die Gichtarthritis zum Abklingen bringt. Die antimitotische Wirkung wurde dagegen jeweils in vitro getestet. Schon WECHSLER et al. (1965) wiesen nach, daß TMCA im Gegensatz zu Colchicin in vitro nicht die mit der Phagocytose durch Leukocyten verbundene Mehrproduktion von Lactat hemmt.

Es ist bis heute nicht möglich, eine sichere Zuordnung sämtlicher Einzeleffekte des Colchicins zum mikrotubulären Apparat zu treffen, zumal eine ganze Reihe von Funktionen des mikrotubulären Apparates diesem lediglich auf Grund ihrer Unterdrückbarkeit durch Colchicin zugeschrieben wurde. Es ist aber durchaus vorstellbar, daß verschiedene Konzentrationen des Pharmakons jeweils in der Lage sind, nur bestimmte Teilfunktionen des mikrotubulären Apparates zu unterdrücken, ohne daß jeweils auch ein morphologisches Verschwinden der Mikrotubuli gefordert werden müßte. MALAWISTA u. BENSCH (1967) benötigten hierfür bei Leukocyten Colchicinkonzentrationen von $2,5 \times 10^{-5}$ bis $2,5 \times 10^{-4}$ M.

Toxikologie

Die Colchicinsensitivität verschiedener Versuchstiere schwankt stark. Die DL_{50} bei Ratten nach i.v. Applikation beträgt 1,7 mg/kg, diejenige bei Katzen 0,25 mg/kg (FERGUSON, 1952). Bemerkenswert ist das Intervall zwischen Applikation der tödlichen Dosis und dem Auftreten toxischer Erscheinungen. Mit höchsten Dosen (4 mg/kg Körpergewicht) betrug dieses Intervall mindestens 6 Std, nach niedrigeren Dosen konnten 24 Std vergehen. Die Ratten wurden lethargisch und schwächlich, verweigerten das Futter, bekamen Durchfälle und zeigten eine vorübergehende Überempfindlichkeit gegen Geräusche, ein ungepflegtes Aussehen und verloren zwischen 10% und 30% an Gewicht. Einige entwickelten eine Paralyse der Hinterpfoten 48 Std nach Colchicinapplikation. Ein Ascites bildete sich am Ende der ersten Woche nach intraperitonealer und intravenöser Applikation und blieb bei den überlebenden Tieren zwei Wochen lang bestehen.

Der Tod trat ohne spezifische Symptome ein — die Ratten wurden immer schwächer und zunehmend dehydratisiert, erlitten Verlust von Reflexen und Gehfähigkeit, wurden völlig kraftlos und starben schließlich nach Atemstillstand. Krämpfe wurden nicht beobachtet. Der Tod trat nie plötzlich ein, frühestens nach 12 Std, unter Umständen erst in der zweiten Woche. Die Mehrzahl der toxischen Symptome verschwand innerhalb von 2—7 Tagen bei den überlebenden Tieren. Eine gewisse Toleranz gegenüber dem Pharmakon durch allmählich ansteigende Dosen war nicht nachzuweisen.

Bei den wesentlich empfindlicheren Katzen standen die gastrointestinalen Erscheinungen im Vordergrund, wobei die Erbrechen auslösende mit der individuell tödlichen Dosis korrelierte. Der Autor deutet das Erbrechen als zentralen Colchicineffekt, da es unter Barbituratnarkose ausblieb, dagegen bei gastrektomierten Tieren in der gleichen Frequenz beobachtet wurde.

Colchicin hat seine Potenz in der Therapie des Gichtanfalls und relative Nebenwirkungsarmut tausendfach bewiesen. Trotzdem soll nicht unerwähnt bleiben, daß die DL_{50} bei der Katze (Ratten sind wesentlich weniger empfindlich) größenordnungsmäßig in einem Bereich liegt, der einem Anfallspatienten in den ersten 48 Std gegebenenfalls appliziert wird. WALLACE (1961 b) referiert eine Anzahl von Todesfällen mit therapeutischen Dosen bei Carcinom-Patienten. MCLEOD u. PHILLIPS (1947) berichten über einen Todesfall nach 7 mg innerhalb 3 Tagen, der als ein Beispiel von Hypersensitivität gegenüber dem Medikament gewertet wurde. BORUCHOW (1966) berichtet vom Tod eines Patienten mit Pankreas-Carcinom, der in 11 Tagen insgesamt 14 mg Colchicin erhalten hatte. Dieser Patient (11,6 mg-% Gesamtbilirubin) konnte das Pharmakon nicht mit der Galle ausscheiden.

Den bisher wohl einzigen bekannt gewordenen Fall einer massiven Colchicinvergiftung, die überlebt wurde, berichtete CARR (1965) von einem nierenkranken Gichtpatienten, der mit einem Serumcreatinin von 3,7 mg-% stationär aufgenommen wurde und dessen Creatininspiegel während der nächsten Tage auf 6 mg-% anstieg. Nach einer intermittierenden peroralen Behandlung mit Colchicin während 18 Tagen (am 18. Tag 4 mg i.v., die Gesamtdosis während dieser 18 Tage lag bei etwa 45 mg) wurde kein Colchicin mehr gegeben, da jetzt massive Nebenwirkungen in Form von Schwäche, Schwindel, Erbrechen, Durchfall, Fieber und Verwirrungszuständen auftraten. Dem Patienten fielen die Haare aus, und es entwickelte sich eine nach weiteren 18 Tagen voll reversible Pancytopenie, die mehrfache Bluttransfusionen erforderte. Leber und Nervensystem waren in die toxischen Colchicinwirkungen einbezogen. Ein Anstieg der alkalischen Phosphatase und der SGOT normalisierte sich nach 15 Tagen, während einiger Tage bestand eine Hepatomegalie. Die zentralnervösen Symptome gipfelten in generalisierten tonisch-klonischen Krämpfen um den 10. Tag. Verwirrungszustände und Krämpfe schwanden dann innerhalb weniger Tage, während die Sehnenreflexe erst am 40. Tag nach Auftreten der ersten Intoxikationserscheinungen wieder auszulösen waren. Unter ähnlichen Erscheinungen starb ein Patient, der 15 mg Colchicin in suicidaler Absicht eingenommen hatte (zitiert nach WALLACE, 1961 b).

Auch die Bedeutung des mikrotubulären Systems für Morphogenese und Spermiohistogenese kann klinisch relevant werden. MERLIN (1971) berichtet einen Fall von Azoospermie unter Colchicinlangzeitbehandlung. Der Patient hatte mehrere Jahre lang 1/100 grain (0,65 mg) Colchicin täglich zur Anfallsprophylaxe eingenommen, das Spermatogramm normalisierte sich allmählich innerhalb von etwa 6 Monaten nach Absetzen des Präparates, zeigte aber noch nach 3 Monaten eine Oligospermie II. Grades. Nachdem der Patient Vater eines gesunden Kindes geworden war, ließ sich die Azoospermie einige Jahre später reproduzieren. Hierzu waren eine tägliche Einnahme von 0,65 mg über 4 Monate und von 1,3 mg über weitere 7 Monate erforderlich.

Zusammenfassung

Colchicin wird gut resorbiert, verläßt rasch die Blutbahn, um sich in entsprechenden Organen, zu denen auch die peripheren Leukocyten gehören, anzureichern. Es wird über Galle, Intestinum und Nieren ausgeschieden. Die biologische HWZ des Colchicins ist bisher ebensowenig exakt bestimmbar, wie Anzahl, chemische Konstitution und pharmakologische Wirksamkeit seiner Metaboliten im menschlichen Organismus. Als entscheidendes Wirkprinzip darf die Beeinflussung des mikrotubulären Apparates gelten. Die Mikrotubuli besitzen u. a. vielfältige Funktionen bei der Bewegung von Zellen und ihrer subcellulären Strukturen. Wahrscheinlich hängt die Mehrzahl der mit der Phagocytose verknüpften Vorgänge von einem intakten mikrotubulären System ab — ausgenommen die eigentliche Phagocytose. Die Substanz besitzt eine relativ zu anderen Antiphlogistica geringe therapeutische Breite. Es besteht offenbar eine Blut-Hirnschranke, die unter therapeutischen Bedingungen in der Regel vor den fatalen Folgen der hohen Affinität zum Nervengewebe bewahrt.

Antirheumatica

(Phenylbutazon, Oxyphenbutazon, Indometacin)

Einleitung

Die in der Überschrift genannten Substanzen haben sich in der Therapie des Gichtanfalles bewährt. Aus pharmakologischer Sicht vertreten sie eine ganze Substanzgruppe, die chemisch gewisse saure Eigenschaften verbindet, pharmakologisch die Trias antiphlogistischer, analgetischer und antipyretischer Wirkung. Die relative Ausprägung dieser Eigenschaften zueinander unterscheidet sich bei den einzelnen Substanzen teilweise stark.

Das Oxyphenbutazon soll als Metabolit des Phenylbutazons mit nur unwesentlich verschiedener Wirksamkeit mit diesem gemeinsam besprochen werden. Ebenfalls gemeinsam dargestellt wird die entzündungshemmende Wirkung der nicht steroidalen Antiphlogistica mit ihren hier genannten Vertretern.

Phenylbutazon

Chemie

Phenylbutazon wurde 1946 von H. STENZL synthetisiert. Es ist 1,2-Diphenyl-3,5-dioxo-4n-butyl-pyrazolidin, läßt sich aber auch als Derivat des 3-Hydroxypyrazolons auffassen, wenn man die Enolform zugrundelegt.

Phenylbutazon reagiert sauer — das Enolat-Anion ist resonanzstabilisiert (Abb. 6). Der pK_a-Wert beträgt 4,5. Mit starken Basen entstehen stabile Salze. Das Natriumsalz diente zunächst als Lösungsvermittler für Aminophenazon (Irgapyrin®). Die Summenformel lautet $C_{19}H_{20}O_2N_2$, das Molekulargewicht beträgt

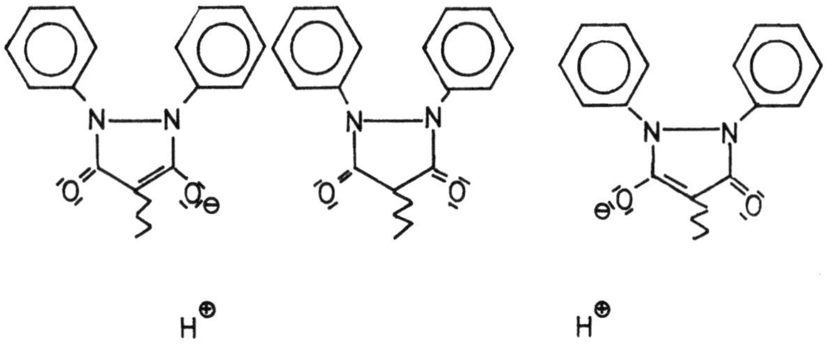

Enolat-Form   Dicarbonyl-Form   Enolat-Form

Abb. 6. Phenylbutazon: die für ein heterocyclisches Ringsystem unübliche Schreibweise will die symmetrische Struktur des Moleküls mit zwei gleichberechtigten Carbonylfunktionen verdeutlichen

308,4. Es handelt sich um ein weißes Pulver von schwach bitterem Geschmack. In reinem Wasser löst sich die Substanz nur bis zu einer Konzentration von 1,5 mg-%, die Löslichkeit — bedingt durch Übergang der Dicarbonyl- in die Enolatform — steigt mit Ionenstärke und pH stark an. Ein m/15 Phosphatpuffer von pH 7 löst bereits 188 mg-% (PULVER et al., 1956). Aus vergleichenden Messungen der Gefrierpunktserniedrigung schließen die gleichen Autoren, daß Phenylbutazon beim Blut-pH als einwertiges Anion, also in der Enolatform vorliegt. Die Dicarbonylform ist dagegen gut in organischen Solventien löslich. Wäßrige saure Lösungen sind auf diese Weise gut extrahierbar.

Pharmakokinetik

Phenylbutazon liegt als Natriumsalz zur Injektion und in der Dicarbonylform zur enteralen *Applikation* in Tabletten und Suppositorien vor.

Nach GLADTKE (1968) wird es nach oraler Applikation zu 85%, nach rectaler Applikation zu etwa 50% *resorbiert*. Die enterale Resorption wird durch Antacida erschwert (AZARNOFF u. HURWITZ, 1970; PRESCOTT, 1973). Das trifft für alle sauer reagierenden Pharmaka zu, die bei hohen pH-Werten dissoziieren, aber nur in der lipophilen (hier Dicarbonyl-)Form resorbiert werden.

Im Plasma wird Phenylbutazon zu 98% an *Plasmaalbumin* gebunden (BURNS et al., 1953; WUNDERLY, 1956). Dieser Prozentsatz fällt jedoch mit der Höhe der Gesamtkonzentration, da diese Proteinbindung offenbar gesättigt wird, wenn Konzentrationen von ca. 15 mg-% überschritten werden. Nach BURNS et al. (1953) beträgt die Plasmaeiweißbindung bei einer Gesamtkonzentration von 25 mg-% nur noch 88%.

Das Verteilungsvolumen ist kleiner als der Extracellulärraum — etwa ein Drittel einer Einzeldosis von Phenylbutazon wird im Plasma gefunden (BRODIE et al., 1954). Auch nach längerdauernder Gabe des Pharmakons übertrifft die Plasmakonzentration diejenige in den Körperorganen beträchtlich. Nach GLADTKE (1968) besteht eine numerische Beziehung des Verteilungsvolumens zum EZV bei Kindern in verschiedenen Lebensaltern. WILHELMI u. PULVER (1955) fanden in entzündetem Gewebe eine höhere Konzentration als im Normalgewebe.

Phenylbutazon kann aus biologischem Material durch eine colorimetrische Methode von PULVER (1950) bestimmt werden, bei der Oxyphenbutazon nicht mit erfaßt wird, die aber relativ aufwendig ist. BURNS et al. (1953) verwendeten ein spektrophotometrisches Verfahren, ohne die Metaboliten abzutrennen. Sie ermit-

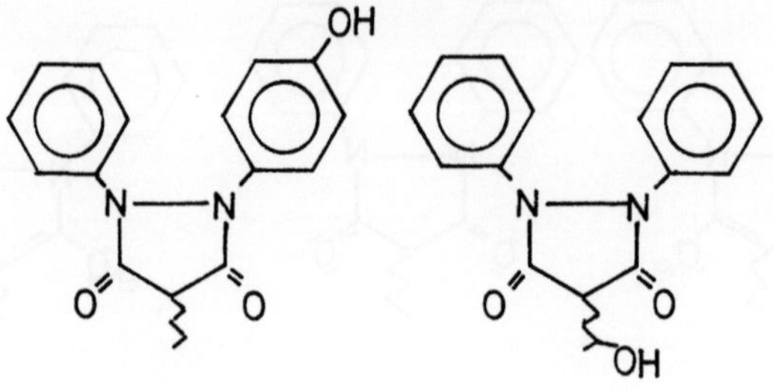

Metabolit I   Metabolit II

Abb. 7. Die Metaboliten des Phenylbutazons: Metabolit I, 1-Phenyl-2-(p-hydroxyphenyl)-3,5-dioxo-4n-butyl-pyrazolidin; Metabolit II, 1,2-Diphenyl-3,5-dioxo-4n-(3′-hydroxybutyl)-pyrazolidin

telten mit dieser Methode *Plasmahalbwertszeiten* von 72 Std beim Menschen, 6 Std für Hund und Ratte, 5 Std beim Meerschweinchen und 3 Std beim Kaninchen. HERRMANN (1959) modifizierte diese Methode. Er bestimmte Plasmahalbwertszeiten für Phenylbutazon zwischen 24 und 48 Std beim Menschen, für Oxyphenbutazon um 72 Std. Es darf angenommen werden, daß spätere Untersucher die Methode von BURNS et al. (1953) verwendeten, da Stammsubstanz und Metabolit I sich weitgehend in ihrer Wirkung entsprechen, es also durchaus sinnvoll erscheint, die Pharmakokinetik beider Substanzen gemeinsam zu erfassen. VESELL u. PAGE (1968) sowie VESELL et al. (1971) bestimmten die Plasmahalbwertszeit bei Zwillingen. Bei homozygoten stimmten sie überein, bei heterozygoten nicht. Die gefundenen Werte streuten zwischen 1,2 Tagen und 7,3 Tagen. WHITTAKER u. EVANS (1970) postulierten eine polygenetische Kontrolle mit einer gewissen Beziehung zur Körpergröße. Sie fanden bei einem Durchschnittswert von gleichfalls etwa 3 Tagen in Einzelfällen solche von über 2 Wochen.

Die Frage, ob Phenylbutazon kumuliert, ist nicht einfach zu beantworten. Die lange HWZ des Medikaments bzw. von Metabolit I legt diese Vermutung natürlich nahe. Andererseits haben BURNS et al. (1953) nachweisen können, daß ein individuell verschieden hoher Plasmaspiegel über längere Zeit durch eine weitere Dosiserhöhung nicht mehr wesentlich angehoben werden kann — offenbar wird der nichtproteingebundene Anteil wesentlich rascher abgebaut, als der gemessenen HWZ entspricht. Die gleichen Autoren weisen praktisch identische Eliminationskurven des Präparates nach 10 tägiger Behandlung mit 800 bzw. 1600 mg/tgl. für den jeweiligen Patienten vor. Diese Eliminationskurven sind nicht mit einer Erhöhung des Gesamtkörperpools durch die zweifach höhere Phenylbutazondosis zu vereinbaren. Der individuell verschieden hohe maximal erreichbare Dauerplasmaspiegel ist mit einer Dosierung von etwa 800 mg/tgl. erreicht, auch die Verdoppelung einer täglichen Dosis von 400 mg/tgl. bewirkt keine äquivalente Erhöhung des Serumplasmaspiegels (bis zu etwa 50%).

BURNS et al. (1955) haben die Metaboliten des Phenylbutazons isoliert. Es handelt sich um zwei Hydroxylierungsprodukte, das Hydroxyphenylderivat (Metabolit I) und das γ-Hydroxybutylderivat (Metabolit II) (Abb. 7). Metabolit I repräsentiert 30—50% des Gesamtblutspiegels (HERRMANN, 1959). Metabolit II findet sich im Plasma dagegen nur in unbedeutenden Konzentrationen. Dagegen erscheinen 15% einer applizierten Phenylbutazondosis als Metabolit II im Urin, 3% als Metabolit I und nur Spuren als unverändertes Phenylbutazon. Der Abbauweg über Metabolit II ist also offenbar nicht unbedeutend, die niedrige Plasmakonzentration des Metaboliten folgt aus der relativ kurzen Plasmahalbwertszeit von 10 Std (YÜ et al., 1958). Wahrscheinlich wird der größte Anteil zu gut wasserlöslichen, bisher nicht bekannten Metaboliten abgebaut.

Phenylbutazon und Oxyphenbutazon werden im endoplasmatischen Reticulum der Leber durch Cytochrom P 450, eine mischfunktionelle Oxydase, oxydiert

(DAVIES u. THORGEIRSSON, 1971); hierbei ist die Aktivität der Cytochrom P 450-Reductase geschwindigkeitsbestimmend. Dieses Enzym wird offenbar biphasisch durch Phenylbutazon induziert, d. h. der Enzyminduktion geht eine Phase dosisabhängiger, nicht-kompetitiver Hemmung des Enzyms voraus.

Phenylbutazon induziert auch die Metabolisierung anderer lipophiler Substanzen, wie Phenobarbital, Diphenylhydantoin, Tolbutamid, Digitoxin (SOLOMON u. ABRAMS, 1972; PRESCOTT, 1973). PRESCOTT (1973) weist auf die Möglichkeit hin, daß die Wirkung der genannten Pharmaka durch Phenylbutazon abgeschwächt wird bzw. toxische Effekte möglich sind, wenn eine längerdauernde Therapie mit Phenylbutazon abgebrochen wird, die unter Gaben dieser Substanz erforderlichen Dosierungen der genannten Pharmaka jedoch beibehalten werden. Auf die möglichen Konsequenzen der Proteinbindung von Phenylbutazon sei an dieser Stelle ebenfalls bereits hingewiesen — bekanntestes Beispiel sind die Verstärkung der Dicumarol- und der oralen Antidiabeticawirkung (SOLOMON et al., 1968). Auch freie Fettsäuren verdrängen Phenylbutazon und Warfarin aus ihrer Plasmaproteinbindung.

Allgemeine Pharmakologie

Antipyretische und analgetische Wirkung des Phenylbutazons werden bei der Besprechung der antientzündlichen Wirkung erwähnt. Eine allgemeine Vorbemerkung soll das Verhältnis der pharmakologischen Wirkung von Phenylbutazon und Metabolit I, Oxyphenbutazon, betreffen. Die pharmakologischen Eigenschaften beider Substanzen stimmen tatsächlich weitgehend überein, die entzündungshemmende Wirkung des Phenylbutazons hängt nicht etwa von der Bildung seines Metaboliten ab. Es liegt eine ganze Reihe von *in vitro* Untersuchungen vor, in denen die Muttersubstanz wenigstens ebenso wirksam wie ihr Metabolit ist. Die längere biologische HWZ des Oxyphenbutazons erlaubt andererseits eine etwas niedrigere Dosierung.

Es gibt einige definierte pharmakologische Eigenschaften des Phenylbutazons, deren Mechanismus nicht vollständig bekannt ist, mit denen der Kliniker aber als Nebenwirkung zu rechnen hat.

Der Einfluß auf das hämatopoetische System, den inzwischen jeder Therapeut fürchtet, der aber vergleichsweise selten beobachtet wird, wird hierbei nicht berücksichtigt. Nicht zuletzt deswegen, weil hierbei im Einzelfall der pathogenetische Mechanismus jeweils unterschiedlich sein mag und keine eindeutige Relation zur Dosierung erkennen läßt.

Von besonderer klinischer Relevanz sind: die ulcerogene Wirkung, die Beeinflussung des Salz-Wasserhaushaltes, die uricosurische Wirkung, der strumigene Effekt.

Die *ulcerogene* Wirkung ist allen potenten Antiphlogistica gemeinsam. Eine vermehrte Salzsäureproduktion als wesentlicher pathogenetischer Faktor ließ sich nicht verifizieren. PAULUS u. WHITEHOUSE (1973) referieren sogar tierexperimentelle Ergebnisse über eine verminderte Salzsäureproduktion nach Acetylsalicylsäuregaben (beim Menschen nicht bestätigt). HEMMATI (1969) konnte beim Menschen nach Phenylbutazon keine wesentliche Steigerung der Säureproduktion nachweisen. Dagegen bleibt die cytostatische Wirkung als Ursache der Ulcusentstehung in der Diskussion. BUCCIARELLI et al. (1968) fanden eine Minderung der Mitoserate der Antrumzellen des Rattenmagens. KARZEL (u.a. 1967) hat den cytostatischen Effekt mit therapeutischen Konzentrationen *in vitro* mehrfach belegt. Dagegen hat NICOLOFF (1968) für Indometacin bei Hunden keine Änderung der Mitoserate der Antrumzellen gefunden, auch die Sekretion von Salzsäure war trotz Ulcusentstehung bei den betreffenden Tieren nicht vermehrt. Die *in vitro*-Ergebnisse von KARZEL (1967) waren jedoch auch mit Indometacin zu reproduzieren.

Die Magenschleimproduktion ist von JOHANSSON u. LINDQUIST (1971) vermindert gefunden worden, besonders ihr Gehalt an Mucopolysacchariden. Auch diese Befunde stimmen mit *in vitro* gewonnenen Ergebnissen überein (s. S. 454). JOHANSSON und LINDQUIST halten den Befund für wesentlich und diskutieren gleichzeitig die Frage, inwieweit die Applikationsart die Ulcerogenität beeinflußt. Sie begründen, daß lokale *und* Einwirkung über die Blutbahn an der Ulcusentstehung beteiligt seien. PAULUS u. WHITEHOUSE (1973) referieren für die Acetylsalicylsäure Untersuchungen, die für diese Substanz eine ausschließlich lokale Wirkung für die Entwicklung von Ulcera wahrscheinlich machen.

LEWIS et al. (1971) diskutieren eine vermehrte Freisetzung lysosomaler Enzyme durch hohe lokale Konzentrationen der Antiphlogistica als Mitursache zur Ulcusentstehung.

Zur Frage der Beeinflussung des *Salz- und Wasserhaushaltes* findet sich bereits bei von RECHENBERG (1961) eine umfangreiche Literaturzusammenstellung. Grundlegende Arbeiten stammen u.a. von YÜ et al. (1953), BRODIE et al. (1954) und YÜ et al. (1958). Phenylbutazon und Oxyphenbutazon bewirken eine Retention von Kochsalz und Wasser bereits bei Plasmaspiegeln, die für einen Therapieeffekt gefordert werden (etwa ab 5 mg-%). Die Verminderung der Kochsalz- und Wasserausscheidung hält etwa 3—5 Tage an, um sich dann auch unter Fortdauer der Therapie zu normalisieren. Die entstandene normotone Hyperhydratation normalisiert sich jedoch erst nach Abbruch der Therapie durch die dann vorübergehend überschießende Diurese. Die Retention bewirkt Hämodilution mit Abnahme des Hämatokrits und des onkotischen Drucks (Anämie und Ödemneigung). Eine Gewichtszunahme ist über die erwähnte Hämodilution hinaus durch die Vergrößerung des EZV bedingt. Während MEIERS u. WETZELS (1964) in Übereinstimmung mit einer ganzen Reihe von Voruntersuchern annehmen, daß die Nierenfunktion im Bereich des proximalen Tubulus beeinflußt wird, postulieren BARTELHEIMER u. SENFT (1968) eine Wirkung am aufsteigenden Schenkel der Henleschen Schleife. Die Ausscheidung von Kalium wird nicht beeinflußt.

Auch die *uricosurische* Wirkung wird in erster Linie als Beeinflussung der tubulären Funktion gedeutet (s. Kapitel Uricosurica). WHITEHOUSE et al. (1971) vertreten die Auffassung, die Freisetzung von Natriumurat aus seiner Plasmaeiweißbindung sei an der uricosurischen Wirkung beteiligt. Nach CAMPION et al. (1973) sind bei Körpertemperatur etwa 20% Natriumurat an Plasmaalbumine gebunden.

Über die *strumigene* Wirkung sind bei von RECHENBERG (1961) eine Reihe experimenteller Daten verschiedener Autoren zusammengestellt — übereinstimmend wird von einer Hemmung der ^{131}J-Aufnahme durch die Schilddrüse berichtet, die sich allerdings bei Fortdauer der Therapie normalisiert. Offenbar besteht noch keine Klarheit über die genaue Pathogenese der Phenylbutazon-Struma (WOODBURY, 1970). Es ist beeindruckend, wie gut sich die entstandene euthyreote Struma nach Absetzen des Pharmakons auch ohne zusätzliche Medikation zurückbildet (WESSEL, 1967).

Indometacin

Chemie

Indometacin ist 1-(p-Chlorbenzoyl)-5-methoxy-2-methylindol-3-essigsäure (Abb. 8). Die Substanz wurde in der Vorstellung, einen Serotoninantagonisten therapeutisch nutzen zu können, unter 350 synthetisierten Indolderivaten als wirksam gefunden (sie entbehrt übrigens einer serotoninantagonistischen Wirkung). Die Synthese wurde von SHEN et al. (1963) bekanntgegeben.

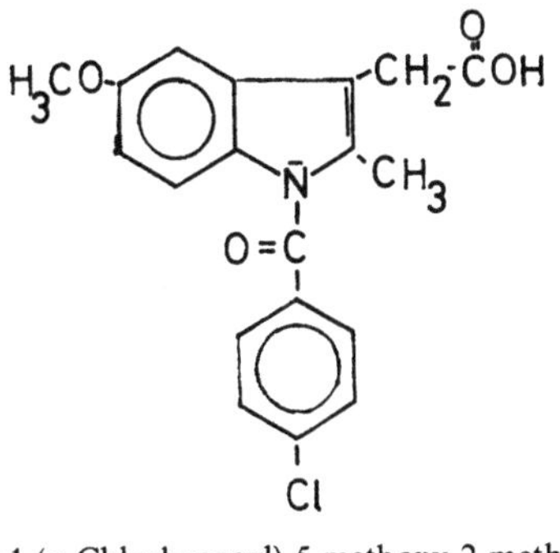

Abb. 8. Indometacin: 1-(p-Chlorbenzoyl)-5-methoxy-2-methyl-indol-3-essigsäure

Die Summenformel lautet $C_{19}H_{16}NO_4Cl$, das Molekulargewicht beträgt 357,78. Indometacin ist ein gelbliches Pulver, das zwischen 156 und 160° C schmilzt. Die Substanz löst sich gut in Laugen und polaren organischen Lösungsmitteln. Die Amidbindung zwischen Indol-N und p-Chlorbenzoesäure wird in alkalischer Lösung allmählich hydrolysiert, so daß haltbare wäßrige Lösungen bisher nicht im Handel sind.

Pharmakokinetik

Indometacin wird nach oraler Gabe schnell resorbiert und erreicht maximale Plasmaspiegel nach einer Std (HUCKER et al., 1966). Nach rectaler Applikation erfolgt die Resorption noch etwas rascher und beträgt etwa 75% derjenigen nach oraler Gabe (HOLT u. HAWKINS, 1965). 90% der Substanz werden an Plasmaproteine gebunden. Das Verteilungsvolumen ist größer als das EZV, die Plasma-HWZ liegt bei nur zwei Std. Bereits Plasmakonzentrationen unter 0,1 mg-% sind deutlich analgetisch und antiphlogistisch wirksam (HOLT u. HAWKINS, 1965).

Die Metabolisierung von Indometacin erfolgt als Demethylierung der Methoxygruppe und als Hydrolyse am Indol-N. Stammsubstanz und Metabolite werden in freier Form und als Glucuronide in Urin und Faeces ausgeschieden. Ausscheidungsform und -wege differieren bei den verschiedenen Tierspecies beträchtlich. Beim Menschen wird ausschließlich das Glucuronid des unveränderten Indometacins im Urin gefunden (HARMAN et al., 1964). HUCKER et al. (1966) fanden bei zwei von drei Versuchspersonen auch eine Ausscheidung über die Faeces. Im Gegensatz zu Versuchstieren verschiedener Species scheint beim Menschen die Ausscheidung über die Gallenwege nur eine geringe Rolle zu spielen (HUCKER et al., 1966).

Allgemeine Pharmakologie

Die antiphlogistischen, antipyretischen und analgetischen Eigenschaften des Indometacins werden zusammen mit Phenylbutazon und Oxyphenbutazon auf S. 451 besprochen. Der *ulcerogene* Effekt ist ebenfalls sämtlichen Antiphlogistica gemeinsam, es darf hierzu auf die allgemeine Pharmakologie des Phenylbutazons (S. 448) verwiesen werden. NICOLOFF (1968) hat die Ulcusentstehung in Experimenten bei Hunden untersucht, als Ursache jedoch weder eine vermehrte Säureproduktion noch eine Mitosehemmung im Antrumbereich finden können.

Die übrigen Nebenwirkungen des Indometacins (s. klinischer Teil) betreffen hauptsächlich das ZNS. ROTHERMICH (1966) konnte nachweisen, daß eine enge Relation zur maximalen Höhe des Plasmaspiegels unter den jeweiligen Therapiebedingungen besteht. Die Ursache dieser nie bedrohlichen, aber u. U. höchst lästigen Nebenwirkungen, ist nicht bekannt.

Die Cooperating Clinics of the ARA (1967) stellten fest, daß Indometacin bei Patienten, die gleichzeitig mit Salicylaten behandelt werden, lediglich einen Placeboeffekt zeigt. CHAMPION et al. (1971) fanden keine wechselseitige Beeinflussung der Plasmaspiegel bei gleichzeitiger Gabe beider Substanzen. Die Beobachtung der American Rheumatism Association bedarf weiterhin der Abklärung.

Die gerinnungshemmende Wirkung von Cumarinderivaten wird nach FROST u. HESS (1966) und MÜLLER u. ZOLLINGER (1966) nicht verstärkt.

Zur antiphlogistischen Wirksamkeit

Der eigentliche Wirkungsmechanismus der Antiphlogistica ist nach wie vor unbekannt. Man kennt nur eine große Anzahl verschiedener Effekte, die durch die fraglichen Substanzen zu erzielen sind und die eine mehr oder weniger enge Beziehung zum Entzündungsvorgang aufweisen. Die Aufklärung der mit der Entzündung verbundenen biochemischen, immunologischen und zellbiologischen Vorgänge wird auch die eigentliche Wirkungsweise der Antirheumatica erkennen helfen. PAULUS u. WHITEHOUSE (1973) mußten in einer kritischen Würdigung der gegenwärtigen Vorstellungen und Ergebnisse feststellen, daß ein entscheidender Durchbruch bislang trotz intensiver Bemühungen nicht gelungen sei.

Hier sollen zunächst einige Möglichkeiten vorgestellt werden, eine antientzündliche Wirkung nachzuweisen. Hierzu dienen seit etwa 25 Jahren Entzündungsmodelle am Versuchstier, die gleichzeitig eine begrenzte Differenzierung hinsichtlich Auslösungsmodus und Entzündungsstadium erlauben. Eine gewisse Übersicht vermitteln hierzu WINTER (1966a, 1966b), WILHELMI (1966), KROHS et al. (1972). Inzwischen wurden in dem Bestreben, den Wirkungsmechanismus auf molekularer Ebene aufzuklären, eine Reihe brauchbarer *in vitro*-Teste entwickelt, die im zweiten Teil dieses Abschnittes dargestellt werden sollen. Zuletzt wird anhand einer Übersicht von DOMENJOZ (1971) ein grober Abriß über neuere Vorstellungen zum eigentlichen Wirkungsmechanismus gegeben.

Nur einige *Entzündungsmodelle am Ganztier* sollen hier vorgestellt werden, die sich als besonders geeignet für die Prüfung entzündungshemmender Substanzen erwiesen haben — d.h. in erster Linie, daß die mit der betreffenden Methode gewonnenen Ergebnisse gut mit den klinischen Erfahrungen korrelieren.

Die Ausbildung eines Ödems der Rattenpfote wird schon sehr lange zur Testung herangezogen. Dabei wird eine entzündungserregende Substanz unter die Plantaraponeurose injiziert und die Volumenzunahme, z.B. wie in Abb. 9 gezeigt, bestimmt. Als ödemauslösende Substanzen kommen u.a. Kaolin, Aerosil, Eiklar, Dextran, Bradykinin und Carrageen in Frage. Die betreffende antientzündlich wirkende Substanz wird im allgemeinen etwa 30—60 min vor Applikation des Phlogisticums gegeben. Das durch Carrageen (Irländisch Moos) ausgelöste Ödem läßt sich besonders gut durch Antiphlogistica beeinflussen. Abbildung 10 zeigt entsprechende Dosis-Wirkungsbeziehungen (WINTER, 1966b).

WINTER (1966b) beschreibt außerdem die Wirkung von Antiphlogistica auf das "cotton pellet" Granulom und die Adjuvans-Arthritis. Der erste Test untersucht die Hemmung der Granulombildung nach Implantation eines Wattebausches unter die Haut, der dort eine Woche lang belassen wird. Die Tiere werden dann getötet, die Granulome herauspräpariert und ihre Größe mit derjenigen unbehandelter Tiere verglichen.

Die Adjuvansarthritis stellt ein Polyarthritismodell dar. Hierbei werden abgetötete Tuberkelbazillen in Paraffin-Suspension intradermal oder subcutan (WINTER u. NUSS, 1966) in den Rattenschwanz injiziert.

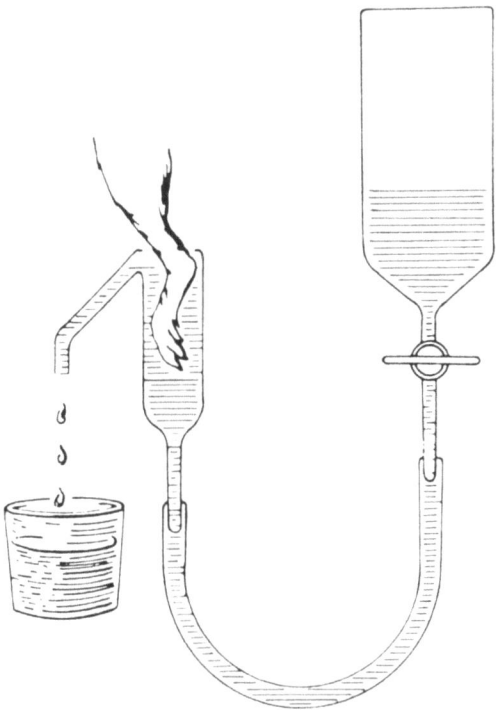

Abb. 9. Prinzip der Bestimmung des Rattenpfotenödems (Nach KROHS et al., 1972)

Nach etwa 10—12 Tagen entwickelt sich eine Polyarthritis zusammen mit entzündlichen Läsionen und granulomatösen Veränderungen an verschiedenen Körperstellen. Die Tiere verlieren an Gewicht. Die Beeinflussung des Körpergewichts, der Gelenkschwellung und der Konzentration eines anormalen Serumproteins — nach ihrem Erstbeschreiber als Glenn-Einheiten bezeichnet — kann bestimmt werden.

Bei den hier angeführten pharmakologischen Tests zeigt Indometacin eine etwa 10-100fach stärkere Wirkung als Phenylbutazon. Ein derartiger Wirkungsunterschied widerspricht der klinischen Erfahrung. Er wird aber erklärlich, wenn man die unterschiedlichen Halbwertszeiten der Substanzen bei Versuchstier und Mensch berücksichtigt. Die HWZ des Indometacins ist bei der Ratte doppelt so lang wie beim Menschen, nämlich 4 Std; dagegen beträgt diejenige des Phenylbutazons bei der Ratte nur 6 Std, während sie beim Menschen (s. S. 447) im Durchschnitt etwa 3 Tage beträgt.

STEELE u. MCCARTY, JR. (1966) haben im Doppelblindversuch die artifizielle Uratarthritis beim Menschen durch Methylprednisolon, Phenylbutazon, Aspirin und Colchicin eindrucksvoll beeinflußt.

In vitro-screening-Tests ermöglichen unter anderem die protektive Wirkung der Antiphlogistica auf die Hitzekoagulation bestimmter Serumproteine (MIZUSHIMA, 1965; MIZUSHIMA u. SUZUKI, 1965) und die hypotone Hämolyse (INGLOT u. WOLNA, 1968). Möglicherweise werden diese protektiven Effekte durch die Bindung der Antiphlogistica an die ε-Aminogruppe des Lysins vermittelt, da sie durch Reagenzien aufhebbar sind (2,4,6-Trinitrobenzolsulfonsäure), die diese Bin-

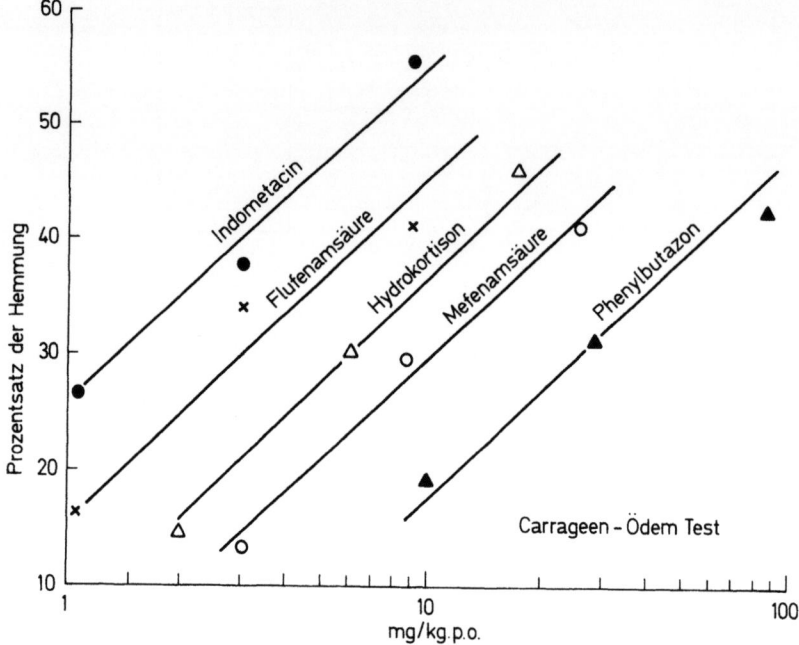

Abb. 10. Dosis-Wirkungsbeziehung am Carrageen-Ödem der Rattenpfote (Nach WINTER, 1966)

dungsstelle blockieren (MIZUSHIMA u. SAKAI, 1969). Andererseits vermögen Antiphlogistica die Bindung von Trinitrobenzaldehyd an die ε-Aminogruppe des Lysins zu verhindern. Die Hemmung der Bildung dieses Komplexes, der farbig ist und zwei definierte Absorptionsmaxima aufweist, dient ebenfalls als *in vitro*-screening-Test (SKIDMORE u. WHITEHOUSE, 1965).

Der *eigentliche Wirkungsmechanismus* der Antiphlogistica ist nach wie vor Gegenstand intensiver Forschungsarbeiten. Die zitierten Übersichtsarbeiten geben hiervon eine Vorstellung (WINTER, 1966, 1971; DOMENJOZ, 1971; PAULUS u. WHITEHOUSE, 1973). Die Ausführungen von DOMENJOZ (1971) sollen hier in sehr gedrängter Form wiedergegeben werden. Einige der vom Autor zitierten Arbeiten werden kurz referiert. Die Auswahl dieser Publikationen konnte nicht nach ihrer Wertigkeit erfolgen — sie soll lediglich dazu dienen, wenigstens einige Aspekte des Problems zu veranschaulichen.

DOMENJOZ berichtet zunächst über Untersuchungen, die den Einfluß der Antiphlogistica auf Schmerzperception und Temperaturregulation betreffen. Für die analgetische Wirkung scheint eine Interferenz mit schmerzproduzierenden Substanzen am Receptor eine wesentliche Rolle zu spielen. Jedenfalls läßt sich der Mechanismus der analgetischen Wirkung antirheumatischer Substanzen von derjenigen des Morphintyps eindeutig differenzieren. Auch bei der Unterdrückung einer Fieberreaktion scheinen periphere Wirkungen wesentlich beteiligt zu sein.

DOMENJOZ setzt sich anschließend mit dem Einfluß der Antiphlogistica auf das adreno-hypophyseale System und das Nebennierenmark bzw. die Catecholamine auseinander. Danach sprechen zahlreiche Untersuchungen gegen eine Mittlerrolle der Corticosteroide für die Wirkung der nichtsteroidalen Antiphlogistica. Dagegen bestehen Anhaltspunkte, daß eine Beeinflussung des Adenylcyclase-Systems ähnlich der antientzündlichen Catecholaminwirkung beteiligt sein könnte, die durch β-Receptorenblocker antagonisiert wird.

Die am Ort der Entzündung selbst ablaufenden Prozesse, die durch Antiphlogistica beeinflußt werden, unterteilt DOMENJOZ in katabole, reaktive und anabole. Katabole Prozesse lassen sich durch stabilisierende Effekte auf Proteine und Membranstrukturen sowie die Hemmung kataboler Enzyme beeinflussen.

Stabilisierende Effekte wurden bereits bei der Besprechung von screening-Tests zur Wirkung der Antiphlogistica erwähnt (s. S. 452). Die Steigerung kataboler Prozesse während des Entzündungsablaufs kann nicht überraschen, da den Lysosomen eine wesentliche Rolle im Entzündungsgeschehen zufällt. MÖRSDORF (1966) hat nachgewiesen, daß Proteine und organische Ester in entzündetem Gewebe vermehrt hydrolysiert werden. Diese Steigerung der Hydrolysrate vermögen Antiphlogistica zu unterdrücken, abhängig vom verwendeten Substrat (MÖRSDORF, 1969). Als Substrate dienten N-α-benzoyl-D,L-arginin-p-nitroanilid (DL-BAPA), L-Lysin-p-nitroanilid (LPA) und Rinderserumalbumin. Die Hydrolyse der beiden erstgenannten Substanzen blieb unbeeinflußt, während die von Serumalbumin gehemmt wurde und zwar kompetitiv. Das spricht wieder für eine stabilisierende Wirkung auf Proteine — hier gegen enzymatischen Abbau. Dagegen konnte DOMENJOZ (1966) eine Hemmung der ATEE (Acetyl-L-tyrosin-äthylester)-Esterase in therapeutischen Konzentrationen nachweisen.

In der „reaktiven Phase" der Entzündung werden eine ganze Anzahl verschiedenster Verbindungen gebildet bzw. freigesetzt, die als „Entzündungsmediatoren" gelten. DOMENJOZ führt hier folgende Substanzen an: Histamin, Serotonin, verschiedene biologisch definierte Permeabilitätsfaktoren, aktivierte Gerinnungsfaktoren (z. B. den Hageman-Faktor) mit proteolytischen Eigenschaften, das Enzym Kallikrein, die Plasmakinine Bradykinin und Kallidin, basische Polypeptide aus Zellkernen und Leukocytenlysosomen, die Prostaglandine E_2 und $F_{2\alpha}$, die "slow reacting substances" SRS C und SRS A und möglicherweise die "rabbit aorta contracting substance" RCS und ihr Releasing-Faktor.

Der Einfluß der Antiphlogistica auf Bildung und Wirkung dieser Entzündungsmediatoren ist nach wie vor Gegenstand umfangreicher Untersuchungen.

Im letzten Abschnitt seiner Ausführungen befaßt sich DOMENJOZ mit der Einwirkung der Antiphlogistica auf anabole Prozesse. Der Effekt auf ATP-Gehalt der Zelle, Mucopolysaccharidbiosynthese und Zellproliferation wird diskutiert.

Umfangreiche Untersuchungen galten dem erstgenannten Problem vor allem deshalb, da Mitte der sechziger Jahre die *in vitro* nachweisbare Entkopplung der oxydativen Phosphorylierung als ein wesentliches Wirkprinzip der Antiphlogistica angesehen wurde (WHITEHOUSE, 1964, 1965). Unter anderen konnten KALBHEN u. DOMENJOZ (1969) jedoch ausschließen, daß eine Erniedrigung des in der entzündeten Zelle erhöhten ATP-Gehaltes mit der konventionell meßbaren Entzündungshemmung (Rattenpfotenödem) korreliert ist.

Die Mucopolysaccharidbiosynthese ist auf verschiedenen Stufen hemmbar. SCHÖNHÖFER u. PERREY (1967) fanden eine Aktivitätsminderung des Glucose-6-Phosphat synthetisierenden Enzyms in der Rattenmagenmucosa, jedoch nicht in der Rattenleber (vergleiche ulcerogene Phenylbutazonwirkung S. 449). Die hierfür erforderliche orale Dosis von 200 mg/kg Phenylbutazon war allerdings hoch. KALBHEN et al. (1967) konnten den Einbau von ^{14}C-Glucosamin in die durch Fibroblasten *in vitro* gebildeten Mucopolysaccharide in Konzentrationen hemmen, die unterhalb therapeutischer Serumspiegel lagen (1 mg-% Phenylbutazon, 0,2 mg-% Indometacin). Diese Konzentrationen lagen auch noch unterhalb der cytostatisch wirksamen Konzentrationen, die KARZEL (1967) an Mastocytomzellen und Fibroblastenkulturen getestet hat. BREULL u. KARZEL (1970) halten es auf Grund eines Vergleichs von Zellvolumen, Protein- und DNS-Gehalt von Ehrlich-Ascites-Tumor-Zellen für möglich, daß eine Hemmung der DNS-Synthese für den cytostatischen Effekt anzuschuldigen sei.

Auch die Funktion der *Leukocyten* ist durch Antiphlogistica zu beeinflussen: CHANG (1968) hemmte die Phagocytose mit therapeutischen Konzentrationen, DIROSA et al. (1972) verminderten die Emigration von Monocyten in das Dextran-induzierte Pleuraexsudat der Ratte, YARON et al. (1971) blockierten die vermehrte Produktion von Hyaluronsäure in Fibroblastenkulturen, die durch Frieren und Auftauen aufgeschlossenen Leukocyten ausgesetzt waren. PHELPS (1969a) beobachtete eine Verminderung der „random motility" der Leukocyten durch kleine Indometacindosen, wie er dies gleichzeitig für Colchicin nachgewiesen hatte. Die Wechselwirkung von nicht-steroidalen Antiphlogistica und *Lysosomen* wird ausführlich an Hand einer umfassenden Literaturübersicht bei PAULUS u. WHITEHOUSE (1973) diskutiert. Trotz der „Plethora" von Publikationen zu diesem Thema fordern die genannten Autoren nach einer kritischen Würdigung von etwa 40 Literaturstellen zusätzliche Daten, die besonders an Lysosomen menschlicher Herkunft zu gewinnen wären, um eine definitive Beziehung experimenteller Einzelergebnisse zum therapeutischen Effekt herstellen zu können.

In jüngster Zeit beschäftigen sich FAMAEY (1973a) und FAMAEY u. WHITEHOUSE (1973b) mit der Einwirkung von Antiphlogistica auf biologische Membranen — zunächst die der Mitochondrien, deren Permeabilität für Ionen und kleine Moleküle verändert wird. Nicht unerwähnt soll zum Schluß noch eine interessante Arbeitshypothese von MCARTHUR et al. (1971, 1972) bleiben, die L-Tryptophan und bestimmte Dipeptide durch Antirheumatica aus ihrer Plasmaalbuminbindung verdrängen konnten. Sie postulierten daraufhin die Existenz antientzündlich wirkender Polypeptide im Serum, deren Nachweis ihnen tatsächlich gelang. Allerdings steht der Beweis noch aus, daß es diese Polypeptide sind, die durch Antiphlogistica aus ihrer Plasmaalbuminbindung freigesetzt werden, und die genannten Autoren sind bestrebt, bei Patienten mit chronischer Polyarthritis einen erniedrigten Serumspiegel dieser Polypeptide nachzuweisen.

Literatur

ARONSON, J., INOUÉ, S.: Reversal by light of the action of N-methyl, N-desacetyl colchicine on mitosis. J. Cell Biol. **45**, 470—477 (1970).

AZARNOFF, D. L., HURWITZ, A.: Drug interactions. Pharmacol. Physicians **4**, 1—7 (1970).

BACK, A., WALASZEK, E. J., UMEKI, E.: Distribution of radioactive colchicine in some organs of normal and tumor-bearing mice. Proc. Soc. exp. Biol. (N.Y.) **77**, 667—669 (1951).

BARDELE, D. F.: Struktur, Biochemie und Funktion der Mikrotubuli. Cytobiology **7**, 442—488 (1973).

BARTELHEIMER, H. K., SENFT, G.: Zur Lokalisation der tubulären Wirkung einiger antirheumatisch wirkender Substanzen. Arzneimittel-Forsch. **18**, 567—570 (1968).

BENSCH, K. G., MALAWISTA, S. E.: Microtubular crystals in mammalian cells. J. Cell Biol. **40**, 95—107 (1969).

BHISEY, A. N., FREED, J. J.: Ameboid movement induced in cultured macrophages by colchicine or vinblastine. Exp. Cell Res. **64**, 419—429 (1971).

BORISY, G. G., TAYLOR, E. W.: The mechanism of action of colchicine-H_3 to cellular protein. J. Cell Biol. **34**, 525—533 (1967).

BORUCHOW, I. B.: Bone marrow depression associated with acute colchicine toxicity in the presence of hepatic dysfunction. Cancer Res. **19**, 541—543 (1966).

BREULL, W., KARZEL, K.: Action of phenylbutazone in cytostatic concentrations on cell volume, protein and DNA content of Ehrlich ascites tumor cells cultured *in vitro*. Arch. int. Pharmacodyn. **184**, 317—327 (1970).

BRODIE, B. B., LOWMAN, E. W., BURNS, J. J., LEE, P. R., CHENKIN, TH., GOLDMAN, A., WEINER, M., STEELE, J. M.: Observations on the antirheumatic and physiological effects of phenylbutazone (Butazolidin) and some comparisons with cortisone. Amer. J. Med. **16**, 181—190 (1954).

BUCCIARELLI, G., BILLIOTTI, G., ANDREOLI, F., MASI, C., MICHELI, E.: The action of phenylbutazone on the mitotic activity of gastric antrum cells. Sperimentale **118**, 469—474 (1968).

BUCHER, N. L. R.: Microtubules. N. Engl. J. Med. **287**, 195—197 (1972).

BURNS, J. J., ROSE, K. R., CHENKIN, TH., GOLDMAN, A., SCHULERT, A., BRODIE, B. B.: The physiological disposition of phenylbutazone (Butazolidin) in man and a method for its estimation in biological material. J. Pharmacol. exp. Ther. **109**, 346—357 (1953).

BURNS, J. J., ROSE, R. K., GOODWIN, S., REICHENTHAL, J., HORNING, E. C., BRODIE, B. B.: The metabolic fate of phenylbutazone (Butazolidin) in man. J. Pharmacol. exp. Ther. **113**, 481—489 (1955).

CAMPION, S. D., BLUESTONE, R., KLINENBERG, J. R.: Binding of Na-urate to human serum albumin under physiological conditions. Arthr. and Rheum. **15**, (Abstr.) 537 (1973).

CANER, J. E. Z.: Colchicine inhibition of chemotaxis. Arthr. and Rheum. **8**, 757—764 (1965).

CARR, A. A.: Colchicine toxicity. Arch. intern. Med. **115**, 29—33 (1965).

CAVANAGH, J. B., LEWIS, P. D.: Perfusion-fixation, colchicine and mitotic activity. J. Anat. (Lond.) **104**, 341—350 (1969).

CHAMPION, D., MONGAN, E., PAULUS, H., SARKISSIAN, E., OKUM, R., PEARSON, C.: Effect of concurrent aspirin (ASA) administration on serum concentrations of indomethacin. Arthr. and Rheum. **14**, 375 (1971).
CHANG, Y. H.: The effect of anti-inflammatory drugs on phagocytosis in vitro. Arthr. and Rheum. **11**, 473 (1968).
Cooperating Clinics of the American Rheumatism Association: Three-month trial of indomethacin in rheumatoid arthritis with special reference to analysis and inference. Clin. Pharmacol. Ther. **8**, 11—37 (1967).
DAVIES, D. S., THORGEIRSSON, S. S.: Mechanism of hepatic drug oxidation and its relationship to individual differences in rates of oxidation in man. Ann. N. Y. Acad. Sci. **179**, 411—420 (1971).
DE DUVE, CH., WATTIAUX, R.: Functions of lysosomes. Physiol. Rev. **28**, 435—492 (1965).
DI ROSA, M., SORRENTINO, L., PARENTE, L.: Non-steroidal anti-inflammatory drugs and leucocyte emigration. J. Pharm. Pharmacol. **24**, 575—577 (1972).
DOMENJOZ, R.: Comparison of therapeutically important antirheumatics on the basis of experimental results. Med. Pharmacol. exp. **14**, 321—331 (1966).
DOMENJOZ, R.: The pharmacology of antirheumatic agents. In: Rheumatoid Arthritis. New York-London: Academic Press 1971.
FAMAEY, J. P.: Interactions between non-steroidal anti-inflammatory drugs and biological membranes. — I. High amplitude pseudo-energized mitochondrial swelling and membrane permeability changes induced by various non-steroidal anti-inflammatory drugs. Biochem. Pharmacol. **22**, 2693—2705 (1973a).
FAMAEY, J. P., WHITEHOUSE, M. W.: Interactions between non-steroidal anti-inflammatory drugs and biological membranes. — II. Swelling and membrane permeability changes induced in some immunocompetent cells by various non-steroidal anti-inflammatory drugs. Biochem. Pharmacol. **22**, 2707—2717 (1973b).
FERGUSON, F. C. J.: Colchicine I. General pharmacology. J. Pharmacol. exp. Ther. **106**, 261—270 (1952).
FORBES, E. J.: Colchicine and related compounds. Part. XIV. Structure of β- and α-lumicolchicine. J. chem. Soc., 3864—3870 (1955).
FREED, J. J., LEBOWITZ, M. M.: The association of a class of saltatory movements with microtubules in cultured cells. J. Cell Biol. **45**, 334—354 (1970).
FRITZE, E., KALLWEIT, C., MÜLLER, H. O.: Die Uratphagozytose der Granulozyten und ihre Beeinflussung durch Colchicin. Z. Rheumaforsch. **26**, 44—56 (1967).
FROST, H., HESS, H.: Gleichzeitige Verabreichung von Indometacin und Anticoagulantien. In: Die Entzündung; Grundlagen und pharmakologische Beeinflussung. München: Urban und Schwarzenberg 1966.
FRUHMAN, G. J.: Inhibition of neutrophil mobilization by colchicine. Proc. Soc. exp. Biol. (N. Y.) **104**, 284—286 (1960).
GARDNER, BRANDON, P. D. R. L., HAYNES, C. R.: The structures of β and γ lumicolchicine. Ring D elaboration products. J. Amer. chem. Soc. **79**, 6334—6337 (1957).
GLADTKE, E.: Pharmacokinetic studies on phenylbutazone in children. Farmaco **10**, 897—906 (1968).
GOLDFINGER, S. E., HOWELL, R. R., SEEGMILLER, J. E.: Suppression of the metabolic accompaniments of phagocytosis by colchicine. Arthr. and Rheum. **8**, 1112—1122 (1965).
GREWE, R., WULF, W.: Die Umwandlung des Colchicins durch Sonnenlicht. Chem. Ber. **84**, 621—623 (1951).
HARMANN, R. E., MEISINGER, M. A. P., DAVIS, G. E., KNEHL, F. A., JR.: The metabolites of indomethacin, a new anti-inflammatory drug. J. Pharmacol. exp. Ther. **143**, 215—220 (1964).
HARTUNG, E. F.: History of the use of colchicine and related medicaments in gout with suggestions for further research. Ann. rheum. Dis. **13**, 190—200 (1953).
HEMMATI, A.: Der Einfluß von Phenylbutazon und Oxyphenbutazon auf die Magensäureproduktion. Arzneimittel-Forsch. **19**, 1130—1132 (1969).
HERRMANN, B.: Über den Stoffwechsel des Butazolidin®. Med. exp. (Basel) **1**, 170—178 (1959).
HOLT, L. P. J., HAWKINS, C. F.: Indomethacin: Studies of absorption and of the use of indomethacin suppositories. Brit. Med. J. **1965 I**, 1354—1356.
HUCKER, H. B., ZACCHEI, A. G., COX, S. V., BRODIE, D. A., CANTWELL, N. H. R.: Studies on the absorption, distribution and excretion of indomethacin in various species. J. Pharmacol. exp. Ther. **153**, 237—249 (1966).
INGLOT, A. D., WOLNA, E.: Reactions of non-steroidal anti-inflammatory drugs with the erythrocyte membrane. Biochem. Pharmacol. **17**, 269—279 (1968).

JOHANSSON, H., LINDQUIST, B.: Anti-inflammatory drugs and gastric mucus. Scand. J. Gastroent. **6**, 49—54 (1971).
KALBHEN, D. A., DOMENJOZ, R.: in vivo and in vitro studies on the influence of antirheumatic drugs on the energy level. In: Inflammation Biochemistry and Drug Interaction. Amsterdam: Excerpta Medica Foundation 1969.
KALBHEN, D. A., KARZEL, K., DOMENJOZ, R.: The inhibitory effects of some antiphlogistic drugs on the glucosamine incorporation into mucopolysaccharides synthesized by fibroblast cultures. Med. Pharmacol. exp. **16**, 185—189 (1967).
KARZEL, K.: Der Einfluß von Antiphlogistika auf Lebens- und Vermehrungsfähigkeit normaler und neoplastischer Zellen in vitro. Arch. int. Pharmacodyn. **169**, 70—82 (1967).
KLINENBERG, J. R., BLUESTONE, R., SCHLOSSTEIN, L., WAISMAN, J., WHITEHOUSE, M. W.: Urate deposition disease; how is it regulated and how can it be modified? Ann. intern. Med. **78**, 99—111 (1973).
KROHS, W., FICKERT, R., GRANZER, E., ALPERMANN, H.-G.: Schwache Analgetica (Antipyretica, Antiphlogistica). In: Arzneimittel; Entwicklung, Wirkung, Darstellung; Band I: Therapeutica mit Wirkung auf das zentrale Nervensystem. Weinheim/Bergstr.: Verlag Chemie 1972.
LACY, P. E.: The pancreatic beta cell. N. Engl. J. Med. **276**, 187—195 (1967).
LACY, P. E., HOWELL, S. L., YOUNG, D. A., FINK, C. J.: New hypothesis of insulin secretion. Nature **219**, 1177—1179 (1968).
LETTRÉ, H., LUTZE, M.: Beitrag zur Verteilung und Wirkung der Colchicine im Tierkörper. Z. physiol. Chem. **281**, 58—64 (1944).
LEWIS, D. A., CAPSTICK, R. B., ANCILL, R. J.: The action of azapropazone, oxyphenbutazone and phenylbutazone on lysosomes. J. Pharm. Pharmacol. **23**, 931—935 (1971).
MALAWISTA, S. E.: The action of colchicine in acute gout. Arthr. and Rheum. **8**, 752—756 (1966).
MALAWISTA, S. E.: Colchicine: A common mechanism for its antiinflammatory and anti-mitotic effects. Arthr. and Rheum. **11**, 191—197 (1968).
MALAWISTA, S. E.: Vinblastine: colchicine-like effects on human blood leucocytes during phagocytosis. Blood **37**, 519—529 (1971 a).
MALAWISTA, S. E.: The melanocyte model. Colchicine-like effects of other antimitotic agents. J. Cell Biol. **49**, 848—855 (1971 b).
MALAWISTA, S. E., BENSCH, K. G.: Human polymorphonuclear leucocytes: demonstration of microtubules and effect of colchicine. Science **156**, 521—522 (1967).
MALAWISTA, S. E., BODEL, P. T.: The dissociation by colchicine of phagocytosis from increased oxygen consumption in human leucocytes. J. clin. Invest. **46**, 786—796 (1967).
MALAWISTA, S. E., CHANG, Y. H., WILSON, L.: Lumicolchicine: Lack of anti-inflammatory effect. Arthr. and Rheum. **15**, 641—642 (1972).
MCARTHUR, J. N., DAWKINS, P. D., SMITH, M. J. H.: The displacement of L-tryptophan and dipeptides from bovine albumin in vitro and from human plasma in vivo by antirheumatic drugs. J. Pharm. Pharmacol. **23**, 393—398 (1971).
MCARTHUR, J. N., SMITH, M. J. H., FREEMAN, P. C.: Antiinflammatory substance in human serum. J. Pharm. Pharmacol. **24**, 669—671 (1972).
MCLEOD, J. G., PHILLIPS, L.: Hypersensitivity to colchicine. Ann. rheum. Dis. **6**, 224—229 (1947).
MEIERS, H. G., WETZELS, E.: Phenylbutazon und Nierenfunktionen. Arzneimittel-Forsch. **14**, 252—258 (1964).
MERLIN, H. E.: Azoospermia caused by colchicine — a case report. Fertil. and Steril. **23**, 180—181 (1971).
MIZUSHIMA, Y.: Simple screening test for antirheumatic drugs. Lancet **1965 I**, 169—170.
MIZUSHIMA, Y., SAKAI, S.: Stabilization of erythrocyte membrane by non-steroid anti-inflammatory drugs. J. Pharm. Pharmacol. **21**, 327—328 (1969).
MIZUSHIMA, Y., SUZUKI, H.: Interaction between plasma proteins and antirheumatic or new antiphlogistic drugs. Arch. int. Pharmacodyn. **157**, 115—124 (1965).
MOHRI, H.: Amino-acid composition of "tubulin" constituting microtubules of sperm flagella. Nature **217**, 1053—1054 (1968).
MÖRSDORF, K.: Proteolytische und esterolytische Prozesse im entzündeten Gewebe. In: Die Entzündung; Grundlagen und pharmakologische Beeinflussung. München: Urban und Schwarzenberg 1966.
MÖRSDORF, K.: The inhibition of protein catabolism by anti-inflammatory drugs. In: Inflammation Biochemistry and Drug Interaction. Amsterdam: Excerpta Medica Foundation 1969.
MÜLLER, G., ZOLLINGER, W.: Der Einfluß von Indometacin auf die Blutgerinnung unter besonderer Berücksichtigung der Interferenz mit Antikoagulantien. In: Die Entzündung; Grundlagen und pharmakologische Beeinflussung. München: Urban und Schwarzenberg 1966.

Nicoloff, D. M.: Indomethacin. Effect on gastric secretion, parietal cell population and ulcer provocation in the dog. Arch. Surg. **97**, 809—815 (1968).

Olmsted, J. B., Borisy, G. G.: Microtubules. Ann. Rev. Biochem. **42**, 507—540 (1973).

Orci, L., Le Marchand, Y., Singh, A., Assimacopoulos-Jeannet, F., Roiller, Ch., Jeaurenaud, B.: Microtubules — role in lipoprotein secretion by the liver. Nature **244**, 30—32 (1973).

Paulus, H. E., Whitehouse, M. W.: Nonsteroid anti-inflammatory agents. Ann. Rev. Pharmacol. **13**, 107—125 (1973).

Phelps, P.: Polymorphonuclear leucocyte motility *in vitro*. II. Stimulatory effect of monosodium urate crystals and urate in solution; partial inhibition by colchicine and indomethacin. Arthr. and Rheum. **12**, 189—196 (1969a).

Phelps, P.: Polymorphonuclear leucocyte motility in vitro. III. Possible release of a chemotactic substance after phagocytosis of urate crystals by polymorphonuclear leucocytes. Arthr. and Rheum. **12**, 197—204 (1969b).

Phelps, P.: Polymorphonuclear leucocyte motility in vitro. IV. Colchicine inhibition of chemotactic activity formation after phagocytosis of urate crystals. Arthr. and Rheum. **13**, 1—9 (1970).

Phelps, P., McCarty, D. J.: Crystal-induced inflammation in canine joints. II. Importance of polymorphonuclear leucocytes. J. exp. Med. **124**, 115—125 (1966).

Porter, K. R.: Cytoplasmic microtubules and their functions. In: Ciba Found. Symp. on principels of biomolecular organization. London: Churchill 1966.

Prescott, L. F.: Clinically important drug interactions. Drugs **5**, 161—186 (1973).

Pulver, R.: Über Irgapyrin, ein neues Antirheumaticum und Analgeticum. Schweiz. med. Wschr. **80**, 308—310 (1950).

Pulver, R., Exer, B., Herrmann, B.: Über die Beeinflussung enzymatischer Reaktionen durch Phenylbutazon und die Übertragbarkeit fermentchemischer Befunde auf die Stoffwechselprozesse der Zelle. Schweiz. med. Wschr. **86**, 1080—1085 (1956).

v. Rechenberg, H. K.: Butazolidin. Stuttgart: Thieme 1961.

Rothermich, N. O.: An extended study of indomethacin. I. Clinical Pharmacology. J. Amer. med. Ass. **195**, 531—536 (1966).

Sabatani, D. D., Bensch, K., Barrnett, R. J.: Cytochemistry and electron microscopy. The preservation of cellular ultrastructure and enzymatic activity by aldehyde fixation. J. Cell. Biol. **17**, 19—58 (1963).

Sagorin, C., Ertel, N. H., Wallace, S. L.: Photoisomeration of colchicine: Loss of significant antimitotic activity in human lymphocytes. Arthr. and Rheum. **15**, 213—217 (1972).

Schönhöfer, P., Perrey, K. H.: The effect of a single large dose of salicylate and phenylbutazone on the glucosamine-6-phosphate synthesis *in vivo* by the liver and by the gastric mucosa of rats. Med. Pharmacol. exp. **17**, 175—182 (1967).

Schumacher, R. H., Phelps, P.: Sequential changes in human polymorphonuclear leucocytes after urate crystal phagocytosis. An electron microscopic study. Arthr. and Rheum. **14**, 513—526 (1971).

Shen, T. Y., Windholz, T. B., Rosegay, A., Witzel, B. E., Wilson, A. N., Willett, J. D., Holtz, W. J., Ellis, R. L., Matzuk, A. R., Lucas, S., Stammer, C. H., Holly, F. W., Sarett, L. H., Risley, E. A., Nuss, G. W., Winter, C. A.: Non-steroid anti-inflammatory agents. J. Amer. chem. Soc. **85**, 488 (1963).

Skidmore, I. F., Whitehouse, M. W.: Effect of non-steroid anti-inflammatory drugs on aldehyde binding to plasma albumen: a novel *in vitro* assay for potential anti-inflammatory activity. J. Pharm. Pharmacol. **17**, 671—673 (1965).

Soberman, R. J., Hoffstein, S., Weissmann, G.: Direct evidence for "suicide sac" hypothesis of lysosomal enzyme release by monosodium urate. Arthr. and Rheum. **16**, 132—133 (1973).

Solomon, H. M., Abrams, W. B.: Interaction between digitoxin and other drugs in man. Amer. Heart J. **83**, 277—280 (1972).

Solomon, H. M., Schrogie, J. J., Williams, D.: The displacement of phenylbutazone-^{14}C and warfarin-^{14}C from human albumin by various drugs and fatty acids. Biochem. Pharmacol. **17**, 143—151 (1968).

Steele, D., McCarty, D. J., jr.: An experimental model of acute inflammation in man. Arthr. and Rheum. **9**, 430—442 (1966).

Struve, R.: Erfahrungen auf dem Gebiet der gerichtlichen Chemie. Z. analyt. Chemie **12**, 164—176 (1873).

Vesell, E. S., Page, J. G.: Genetic control of drug levels in man: Phenylbutazone. Science **159**, 1479—1480 (1968).

Vesell, E. S., Passananti, G. T., Greene, F. E., Page, J. G.: Genetic control of drug levels and of the induction of drug metabolizing enzymes in man: individual variability in the extent of allopurinol and nortriptyline inhibition of drug metabolism. Ann. N.Y. Acad. Sci. **179**, 752—773 (1971).

Walaszek, E. J., Kocsis, J. J., Leroy, G. V., Geiling, E. M. K.: Studies on excretion of radioactive colchicine. Arch. int. Pharmacodyn. **125**, 371—382 (1960).

Wallace, S. L.: Trimethylcolchicinic acid in the treatment of acute gout. Ann. intern. Med. **54**, 274—279 (1961a).

Wallace, S. L.: Colchicine. Clinical pharmacology in acute gouty arthritis. Amer. J. Med. **30**, 439—448 (1961b).

Wallace, S. L.: The treatment of gout. Arthr. and Rheum. **15**, 317—323 (1972).

Wallace, S. L., Ertel, N. H.: Colchicine: current problems. Bull. Rheum. Dis. **20**, 582—587 (1969).

Wallace, S. L., Omokoku, B., Ertel, N. H.: Colchicine plasma levels. Implications as to pharmacology and mechanism of action. Amer. J. Med. **48**, 443—448 (1970).

Wechsler, R., Wallace, S. L., Gerber, D., Scherer, J.: Colchicine and trimethylcolchicinic acid: a comparison of their effects on human white blood cells in vitro. Arthr. and Rheum. **8**, 1104—1111 (1965).

Werner, D., Dönges, K. H.: Chemie und Wirkungsmechanismus des Colchicins und seiner Derivate. Arzneimittel-Forsch. **22**, 306—315 (1973).

Wessel, G.: Zur strumigenen Wirkung des Phenylbutazons. Dtsch. Gesundh.-Wes. **22**, 1640—1642 (1967).

Whitehouse, M. W.: Uncoupling of oxidative phosphorylation by some arylacetic acids (anti-inflammatory of hypocholesterolemic drugs). Nature **4919**, 629—630 (1964).

Whitehouse, M. W.: Some biochemical and pharmacological properties of anti-inflammatory drugs. Prog. Drug. Res. **8**, 301—429 (1965).

Whitehouse, M. W., Kippen, I., Klinenberg, J. R.: Biochemical properties of anti-inflammatory drugs — XII. Inhibition of urate binding to human albumin by salicylate and phenylbutazone analogues and some novel anti-inflammatory drugs. Biochem. Pharmacol. **20**, 3309—3320 (1971).

Whittaker, J. A., Price Evans, D. A.: Genetic control of phenylbutazone metabolism in man. Brit. med. J. **1970 IV**, 323—328.

Wilhelmi, G.: Zur Methodik der Antiphlogistika — Prüfung im Tierexperiment. In: Die Entzündung; Grundlagen und pharmakologische Beeinflussung. München: Urban und Schwarzenberg 1966.

Wilhelmi, G., Pulver, R.: Untersuchungen zur Frage eines peripheren Angriffspunktes der Pyrazole bei der antiphlogistischen Wirkung. Arzneimittel-Forsch. **5**, 221—224 (1955).

Winter, C. A.: Nonsteroid anti-inflammatory agents. Ann. Rev. Pharmacol. **6**, 157—174 (1966).

Winter, C. A.: Die Beurteilung der entzündungshemmenden Wirkung bei Tieren: In: Die Entzündung; Grundlagen und pharmakologische Beeinflussung. München: Urban und Schwarzenberg 1966a.

Winter, Ch. A.: Der Wirkungsmechanismus nichtsteroider entzündungshemmender Präparate. Arzneimittel-Forsch. **21**, 1805—1811 (1971).

Winter, C. A., Nuss, G. W.: Treatment of adjuvant arthritis in rats with anti-inflammatory drugs. Arthr. and Rheum. **9**, 394—403 (1966b).

Woodbury, D. M.: Analgesics, antipyretics, anti-inflammatory agents and inhibitors of uric acid synthesis. In: The pharmacological basis of therapeutics. London: Collier-Macmillan 1970.

Wunderlich, F., Müller, R., Speth, V.: Direct evidence for colchicine-induced impairment in the mobility of membrane components. Science **182**, 1136—1138 (1973).

Wunderly, Ch.: Die Proteinbindung von 3,5-Dioxo-1,2-diphenyl-4-n-butyl-pyrazolidin und weiteren Pharmaka. Arzneimittel-Forsch. **6**, 731—734 (1956).

Yaron, M., Yaron, I., Allalouf, D.: Effect of some anti-inflammatory drugs on fibroblast-leucocyte interaction *in vitro*. Ann rheum. Dis. **30**, 613—618 (1971).

Yu, T. F., Burns, J. J., Paton, B. C., Gutman, A. B., Brodie, B. B.: Phenylbutazone metabolites: antirheumatic, sodium retaining and uricosuric effects in man. J. Pharmacol. exp. Ther. **123**, 63—69 (1958).

Yu, T. F., Sirota, J. H., Gutman, A. B.: Effect of phenylbutazone (3,5 Dioxo-1,2-diphenyl-4n-butylpyrazolidine) on renal clearance of urate and other discrete renal functions in goutry subjects. J. clin. Invest. **32**, 1121—1132 (1953).

Zurier, R. B., Hoffstein, S., Weissmann, G.: Mechanism of lysosomal enzyme release from human leucocytes. I. Effect of cyclic nucleotides and colchicine. J. Cell Biol. **58**, 27—41 (1973).

Zweig, M. H., Chignell, C. F.: Interaction of colchicine analogs vinblastine and podophyllotoxin with rat brain microtubule protein. Biochem. Pharmacol. **22**, 2141—2150 (1973).

3. Dauertherapie

a) Einleitung

Von

N. ZÖLLNER

Ziel der Dauerbehandlung ist die Beseitigung der Gicht und ihrer Folgen, einschließlich der Hypertonie und der cardialen Folgeerkrankungen. Um dieses ideale Ziel zu erreichen, wird als Nahziel zunächst die Normalisierung des Harnsäurespiegels angesehen.

Mit den heutigen therapeutischen Möglichkeiten können die der Gicht zugrundeliegenden renalen bzw. metabolischen Mechanismen nicht beeinflußt werden, zumindest nicht bei der „primären" Gicht. Die Besonderheiten in der renalen Harnsäureausscheidung und auch die jeweiligen zur Überproduktion führenden metabolischen Mechanismen bleiben fortbestehen. Bei der Dauertherapie ist auch die beste Behandlung nicht kausal im üblichen Sinne des Wortes; die Unterbrechung der Therapie führt zum Wiederauftreten der Gicht.

Bei den „sekundären" Gichtformen ist die Grundlage der Dauertherapie die Behandlung der Ursache, wenn immer dies möglich ist, z.B. bei der arzneimittelbedingten Hyperurikämie oder bei der diabetischen Ketoacidose. Interessanterweise kann bei manchen Krankheiten des blutbildenden Apparates die Gicht bestehen bleiben, wenn die Blutkrankheit beherrscht ist, z.B. bei der Polycythämie. Hier, wie in den Fällen, wo das Grundleiden nicht angegangen werden kann, sind die Prinzipien der Dauerbehandlung der „primären" Gichtformen angezeigt.

Als leicht zu bestimmendes Ziel der Dauerbehandlung wird die Normalisierung des Harnsäurespiegels im Plasma im allgemeinen in den Vordergrund geschoben. Dabei wird übersehen, daß einige Folgeerscheinungen der Gicht, speziell Nierensteine und Hypertonie, mit den Besonderheiten der Harnsäureausscheidung wahrscheinlich enger zusammenhängen, und daß der Erfolg ihrer Behandlung dementsprechend von einer Verringerung der Harnsäureausscheidung abhängt. Die zuverlässige Bestimmung der Harnsäureausscheidung ist äußerst schwierig und wird deshalb nur selten angestrebt; eine gewisse Hilfe bei der Beurteilung der Therapie dürfte die Bestimmung der Relation zwischen den Ausscheidungen von Harnsäure und Kreatinin im Nachtharn bedeuten.

Bei der Wahl der Dauertherapie für einen Patienten spielen im allgemeinen vier Gesichtspunkte eine Rolle, nämlich

die Fähigkeit des Patienten mitzuarbeiten,
die Wirkung der gewählten Therapie auf Harnsäurespiegel und Harnsäureausscheidung,
die Nebenwirkungen,
die Wirtschaftlichkeit.

Keine der im folgenden geschilderten Therapieformen erfüllt alle vier Forderungen in idealer Weise, so daß, in Kenntnis des Patienten, individuelle Entscheidungen notwendig sind. Wo immer durchführbar, empfiehlt sich die Diätbehandlung, die aber in der Regel durch eine medikamentöse Behandlung mit Allopurinol oder Uricosurica ergänzt werden muß.

Einige früher in der Dauerbehandlung der Gicht eingesetzte Arzneimittel, wie z.B. die Orotsäure, sind wieder aufgegeben worden. Neue Arzneimittel stehen in der Erprobung. Ihre Einführung wird davon abhängen, ob die heute bereits große Sicherheit der Dauertherapie und ihre Wirtschaftlichkeit (gemessen an den Kosten der unbehandelten Gicht) dadurch verbessert werden können.

b) Pharmakologische Hemmung der Purin- und Harnsäuresynthese

Von

W. KAISER

Mit 4 Abbildungen

Zur Behandlung der Hyperurikämie kommen im allgemeinen folgende Therapiemaßnahmen in Betracht, die entweder die Bildung von Harnsäure vermindern oder ihre Elimination erhöhen:

1. Senkung der Serumharnsäure mit Hilfe diätetischer Maßnahmen (z.B. purinarme Ernährung, Vermeiden von Alkohol).
2. Erhöhung der renalen Harnsäureexkretion unter Verwendung verschiedener urikosurischer Medikamente. Die Nettoexkretion der Harnsäure wird dabei durch Änderung der tubulären Harnsäurereabsorption erhöht.
3. Hemmung der Purin- und Harnsäuresynthese durch Substanzen, die
   a) direkt die *de novo*-Purinsynthese hemmen,
   b) die Umwandlung der Oxypurinvorstufen in Harnsäure durch Hemmung der Xanthin-Oxydase verhindern und
   c) beide Mechanismen aufweisen.

Für die Anwendung dieser verschiedenen Therapiemaßnahmen ergeben sich auch unterschiedliche Indikationen.

Die Behandlung eines Gichtpatienten ist im allgemeinen indiziert entweder bei wiederholten Gichtanfällen, dem Nachweis einer Gichtniere, dem Auftreten von Tophi oder bei Serumharnsäurewerten über 9,0 mg/100 ml.

Die Differenzierung in der Anwendung von Urikosurica bzw. Hemmstoffen der Purin- und Harnsäuresynthese ist bei dem breiten Wirkungsspektrum beider Gruppen schwierig. Urikosurica bergen vor allem die Gefahr der Bildung von Harnsäuresteinen in sich, bei Gichtniere oder Niereninsuffizienz sind sie deshalb meist kontraindiziert. Für den klinischen Gebrauch kommt von den Substanzen, die die Purin- und Harnsäuresynthese hemmen, in erster Linie Allopurinol in Betracht.

In der Purin- und Harnsäuresynthese spielen zwei Stoffwechselwege eine Hauptrolle (s. Abb. 2). Die Nucleotide und deren Abbauprodukt, die Harnsäure, werden in den meisten Zellen entweder aus einfachen Vorstufen über einen *de novo*-Stoffwechselweg oder durch Wiederverwendung bzw. Einschleusung präformierter Purinbasen oder Nucleoside in einem Reutilisationsstoffwechsel gebildet.

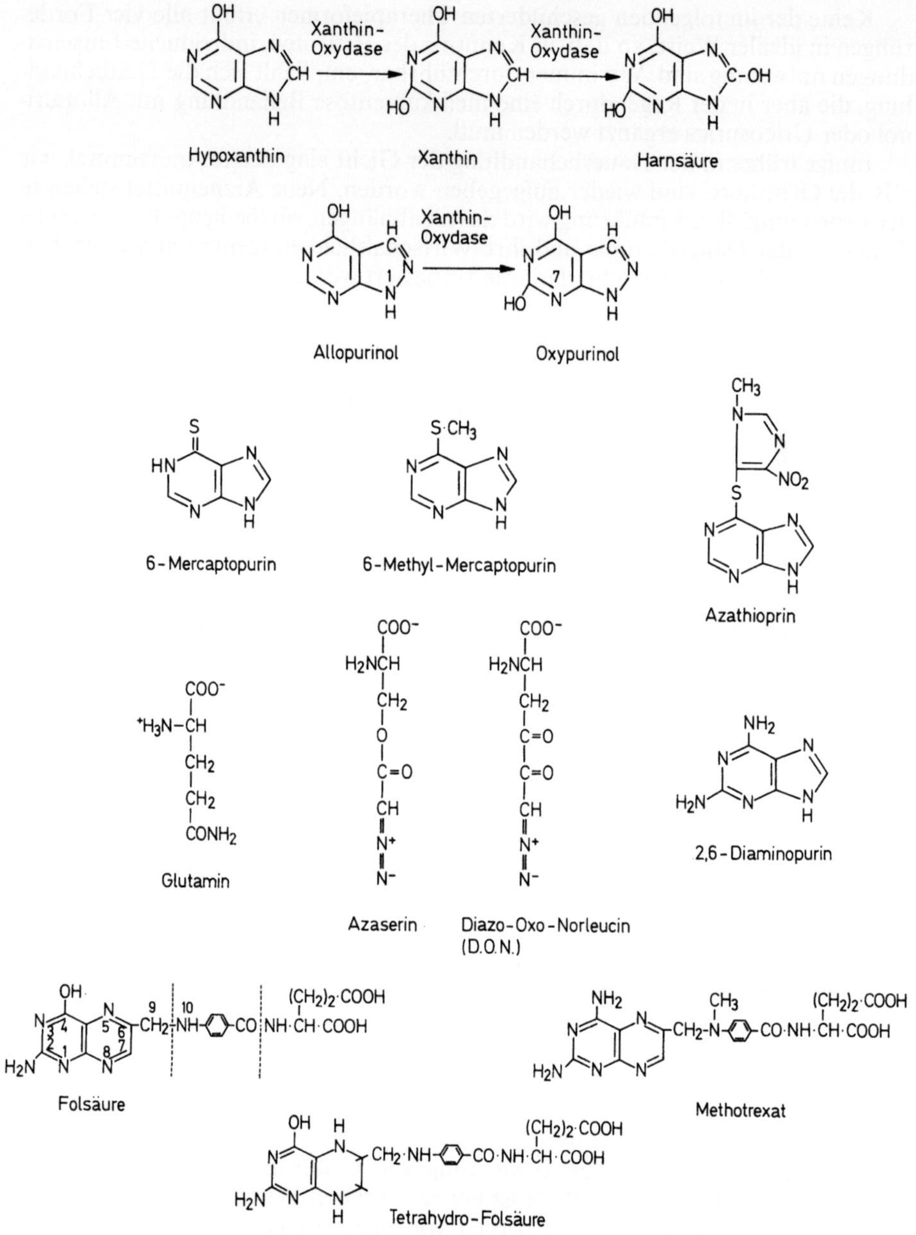

Abb. 1. Hemmer der Purin- und Harnsäuresynthese

Die Harnsäure entsteht aus Purinribonucleotiden durch Dephosphorylierung, Desaminierung, Spaltung der Glykosidbindungen und Oxydation im sog. Purinkatabolismus. Alle Zellen sind abhängig von einer ausgewogenen Bereitstellung an Nucleotiden, dementsprechend erfordert die Sicherstellung optimaler intracellulärer Nucleotidkonzentrationen normalerweise eine feine Regulation verschiedener Prozesse im Purinstoffwechsel. Die Hauptkontrolle des *de novo*-Stoffwechselweges geschieht über eine Endproduktregulation oder Feedback-Hemmung der Aktivität von Enzymen. Ein Endprodukt des Stoffwechselweges übt somit eine negative Kontrolle auf sich selbst aus. Nach der Synthese des ersten komplett in dem *de novo*-Stoffwechselweg gebildeten Nucleotids IMP folgt eine weitere metabolische Regulation (Interkonversionsstoffwechsel der Nucleotide), die die Kontrolle über die für die Zellen geeignete Gleichgewichtseinstellung der verschiedenen Nucleotidklassen übernimmt (Adeninnucleotide und Guaninnucleotide).

Die Geschwindigkeit der *de novo*-Purinsynthese wird limitiert durch die zur Verfügung stehenden Substratkonzentrationen in den verschiedenen Reaktionen (Glutamin, Glycin, Aspartat, 5,10-Methenyl-H_4-Folsäure, 10-Formyl-H_4-Folsäure, PRPP und ATP). Der erste Schritt der *de novo*-Purinsynthese, die Reaktion mit der PRPP-Amidotransferase, wird heute allgemein als eine Schlüsselreaktion für die Regulation des gesamten Purinstoffwechselweges angesehen, weil hier die Hemmwirkung der Endprodukte dieser Synthesekette angreift. Bei Zugabe von Purinen zu isolierten Zellen oder nach Injektion bei Tieren wird die Purinbiosynthese durch Hemmung an einem frühen Schritt der Synthese vermindert. In verschiedenen Untersuchungen konnte gezeigt werden, daß die Geschwindigkeit der Phosphoribosylamin-Synthese durch die Konzentration der Purinnucleotide kontrolliert wird.

Um ihre Hemmwirkung entfalten zu können, müssen die Purine intracellulär zuerst in Nucleotide umgewandelt werden. Nach heutiger Kenntnis kommen für das Entstehen einer Hemmwirkung durch Purinbasen und ihre folgende Umwandlung in Nucleotide am ersten Schritt der *de novo*-Purinsynthese drei Möglichkeiten in Frage: Eine Hemmung der PRPP-Amidotransferase durch Purinnucleotide, eine Hemmung der PRPP-Synthese durch Purinnucleotide und ein „Abziehen" von PRPP aus der *de novo*-Synthese, indem es vorwiegend bei der Bildung von Nucleotiden aus präformierten Purinbasen verbraucht wird.

Die Mehrzahl der Medikamente, die die *de novo*-Purinbiosynthese hemmen, sind Antimetabolite, d.h. Verbindungen, die strukturell mit einem Stoffwechselprodukt der Synthesekette nahe verwandt sind (strukturanaloge Antimetabolite) und die durch Kompetition mit diesem die weitere Verwendung des natürlichen Metaboliten in dem biosynthetischen Stoffwechselweg verhindern. Das physiologische Substrat oder Co-Faktoren werden von ihrem Bindungsplatz am Enzymprotein verdrängt. Der Antimetabolit muß dabei vom Metaboliten chemisch so differieren, daß das in einer Enzymreaktion gebildete Analogon zu keiner weiteren enzymatischen Reaktion in der Folge führen kann.

Eine Vielzahl von Antimetaboliten der Purinsynthese haben ihre Nützlichkeit vor allem bei der Behandlung von Tumoren und Leukämien sowie bei der Therapie bakterieller Infektionen erwiesen.

Für die Behandlung von Patienten, die eine übermäßige Purin- und Harnsäuresynthese aufweisen, scheint als logische Folgerung die Therapie mit Medikamenten am günstigsten, die diese erhöhte Produktion durch Hemmung der *de novo*-Purinbiosynthese zu hemmen vermögen. Aus diesem Grunde wurde seit langer Zeit nach solchen exogenen, nichttoxischen Hemmern der Purin- und Harnsäuresynthese gesucht.

Im wesentlichen kann eine pharmakologische Kontrolle der Purin- und Harnsäuresynthese in drei verschiedene Arten von Hemmwirkungen eingeteilt werden bzw. drei Gruppen von Chemotherapeutica haben als künstliche, exogene Regulatoren der *de novo*-Purinbiosynthese Bedeutung:

I. Analoge des Glutamins: Azaserin (O-Diazoacetyl-L-Serin) und DON (Diazo-Oxo-Norleucin) können als klassische kompetitive Hemmstoffe angesehen werden. Ihre Hemmwirkung kommt auf Grund ihrer strukturellen Ähnlichkeit zu Glutamin zustande.

II. *Analoge der Folsäure:* Methotrexat (Amethopterin) und Aminopterin hemmen die Reduktion der Folsäure zur aktiven Coenzym-Form.

III. Verschiedene Nucleotide von Basenanalogen können die Wirkung der natürlichen Purinribonucleotide auf die Phosphoribosylamin-Synthese imitieren. Dadurch kommt es zu einer Feedback-Hemmung auf die *de novo*-Purinbiosynthese.

In diese Gruppe gehören z. B. das Allopurinol, das 6-Mercaptopurin, 6-Methylmercaptopurin-Ribonucleosid, 6-Thioguanin, 2,6-Diaminopurin (Basenanaloge).

Die Reihenfolge, in der die einzelnen Antimetabolite hier behandelt werden, ist nicht nach ihrer klinischen Wertigkeit aufgestellt, sondern nach deren Eingriff in der Synthesekette der Purin- und Harnsäuresynthese.

In Abb. 2 sind die Wirkorte der verschiedenen Inhibitoren auf die Purin- und Harnsäuresynthese zusammengestellt.

I. Analoge des Glutamins

Azaserin (O-Diazoacetyl-L-Serin) und DON (Diazo-Oxo-Norleucin) (s. Abb. 1) sind die beiden wichtigsten Antibiotica mit antimetabolischer Wirkung auf Glutamin. Sie wurden aus Streptomyces und verwandten Organismen als wachstumshemmende Stoffe isoliert. In einer Reihe von Untersuchungen an tierischen Geweben konnte die Hemmung der Purinbiosynthese durch diese beiden Antibiotica nachgewiesen werden (BENETT *et al.*, 1956; HENDERSON *et al.*, 1957; FRANKLIN Z. COOK, 1969; BROCKMAN u. CHUMLEY, 1965). Diese beiden Glutaminanaloge können jeden einzelnen der drei Schritte der Purinbiosynthese hemmen, in dem L-Glutamin als Substrat verwendet wird. Die Hauptwirkung dieser beiden Glutaminanaloge auf Mikroorganismen und tierische Zellen wird an die Phosphoribosyl-Formylglycinamidin-Synthetase-Reaktion lokalisiert, wodurch es zur Akkumulation von FGAR kommt. Beim Menschen fanden GRAYZEL *et al.* (1960) durch DON eine Hemmung des ^{14}C-Glycineinbaus in die renale Harnsäure, die Serumharnsäurekonzentrationen und die renale Harnsäureausscheidung waren dabei vermindert. ZUCKERMAN *et al.* (1959) fanden unter Azaserin ähnliche Ergebnisse. Trotz der hochgradigen Spezifität und Wirksamkeit von Azaserin in *in vitro*-Tests zeigten klinische Untersuchungen mit Azaserin bei neoplastischen Erkrankungen wenig therapeutischen Effekt (ELLISON, 1954). Dies hängt vermutlich mit einer raschen *in vivo*-Inaktivierung zusammen. Deshalb, und wegen sonstiger toxischer Nebenwirkungen, kommt diesen beiden Substanzen als Therapeuticum zur Hemmung der Purinsynthese beim Menschen keine Bedeutung zu. Zur Anwendung kommen sie vornehmlich bei der *in vitro*-Bestimmung der Purinbiosynthese. So wird z. B. in Fibroblastenkulturen der Einbau von ^{14}C-Glycin oder ^{14}C-Formiat in das Akkumulationsprodukt FGAR, nach Blockierung des Folgeschritts mittels Azaserin oder DON, als Maß für die Geschwindigkeit der frühen Reaktionen des Purinbiosyntheseweges betrachtet.

II. Analoge der Folsäure

Die Umwandlung der Folsäure in ihre verschiedenen aktiven Coenzym-Formen geschieht durch eine initiale Reduktion zur Tetrahydro-Folsäure mittels zweier Enzyme, der Folsäure- und der Dihydrofolsäure-Reduktase. Die Analoge der Folsäure verhindern nun diese Reduktion zur Tetrahydro-Folsäure, indem sie mit der Folsäure um die beiden Enzyme konkurrieren. Da manche Antagonisten oft eine um ein Vielfaches stärkere Affinität zu den Reduktaseenzymen besitzen, ist die Hemmung meist irreversibel.

Die Analoge der Folsäure *Amethopterin* (Methotrexat) und *Aminopterin* verhindern also den Einbau von Folsäure und üben dadurch ihren hemmenden Einfluß auf die Purinbiosynthese aus. So hemmt Amethopterin den Einbau von ^{14}C-Formiat in die Purine der Leukocyten bei undifferenzierter, akuter Leukämie und bei chronischer Granulocytenleukämie des Menschen. Keinen Effekt zeigt es aber *in vitro* bei normalen Leukocyten oder bei Leukocyten von Patienten mit chronischer lymphatischer Leukämie (WELL u. WINZLER, 1959).

Methotrexat hat klinisch eine große Bedeutung als Antitumor-Medikament. Bei einigen Patienten mit akuter Leukämie kommt es während der Therapie mit Methotrexat (allein oder in Kombination mit anderen Cytostatica) zu — allerdings meist nur vorübergehenden — Remissionen. Gute Erfolge haben sich bei der Therapie des Burkitt-Lymphoms und beim Choriocarcinom gezeigt.

Die Folsäure-Antimetabolite haben also ihre Hauptindikationen bei der Behandlung der akuten Leukämien, für die Behandlung einer primären oder sekundären Hyperurikämie kommen sie nicht in Frage.

III. Analoge und Derivate von Purinbasen oder Nucleosiden

Die Hemmung der Purinbiosynthese durch einige Purinanaloge und -derivate (s. Abb. 1 u. 2) kommt direkt durch Nachahmung der normalen Endprodukthemmung natürlicher Purine zustande, d.h. sie wirken auf die gleiche Weise wie die natürlich vorkommenden Nucleotide durch Feedback-Hemmung oder indem sie PRPP für ihre eigene Umwandlung in Nucleotide verbrauchen und damit für die Purinbiosynthese einen Substratmangel schaffen. Diese Stoffe finden ihre Verwendung bei der Chemotherapie des Krebses, der Chemotherapie einiger parasitärer und viraler Infektionen, zur Suppression der Immunantworten und bei der Behandlung der Hyperurikämie.

Extracelluläre Purinbasen und ihre entsprechenden Ribonucleoside werden von den Zellen aufgenommen und dort in die verschiedenen Ribonucleotide umgewandelt. Purinanaloge können nun gleichfalls als freie Basen verabreicht und über den gleichen Stoffwechselweg über das Ribonucleosid zum Ribonucleotid umgewandelt werden bzw. direkt zum Ribonucleotid über ein Phosphoribosyl-Transferase-Enzym. Bei Verabreichung eines Ribonucleosids wird dieses entweder direkt von der Zelle aufgenommen und zum Ribonucleotid umgewandelt oder zuerst zur freien Base gespalten und dann zum Ribonucleotid metabolisiert. Die biologische Wirkung nach Verabreichung eines Purinanalogs kommt also erst nach Umwandlung in die Ribonucleotidform zustande und nicht durch die freie Base. Diese „Aktivierung" der Medikamente, d.h. die Umwandlung in die pharmakologisch aktive Form geschieht letzten Endes mit Hilfe der Purinphosphoribosyl-Transferasen. Hiermit ist auch zu erklären, warum Zellen, denen das entsprechende Enzym zur Aktivierung des Pharmakons fehlt (z. B. mangelhafte Hemmung der *de novo*-Synthese beim Lesch-Nyhan-Syndrom mit HG-PRT-Mangel durch Allopurinol) therapieresistent sind.

Auch bei der Krebstherapie mit Analogen von Nucleosiden ist für deren pharmakologische Aktivität die Umwandlung in die entsprechenden Ribonucleotide erforderlich. Dies geschieht mit Hilfe von Purinribonucleosid-Kinasen, meist der Adenosin-Kinase.

Es wurden nun eine Reihe von Purinanalogen synthetisiert, vor allem solche der Purinbasen Adenin und Guanin (s. Abb. 1 u. 2), und auf ihre antimetabolische

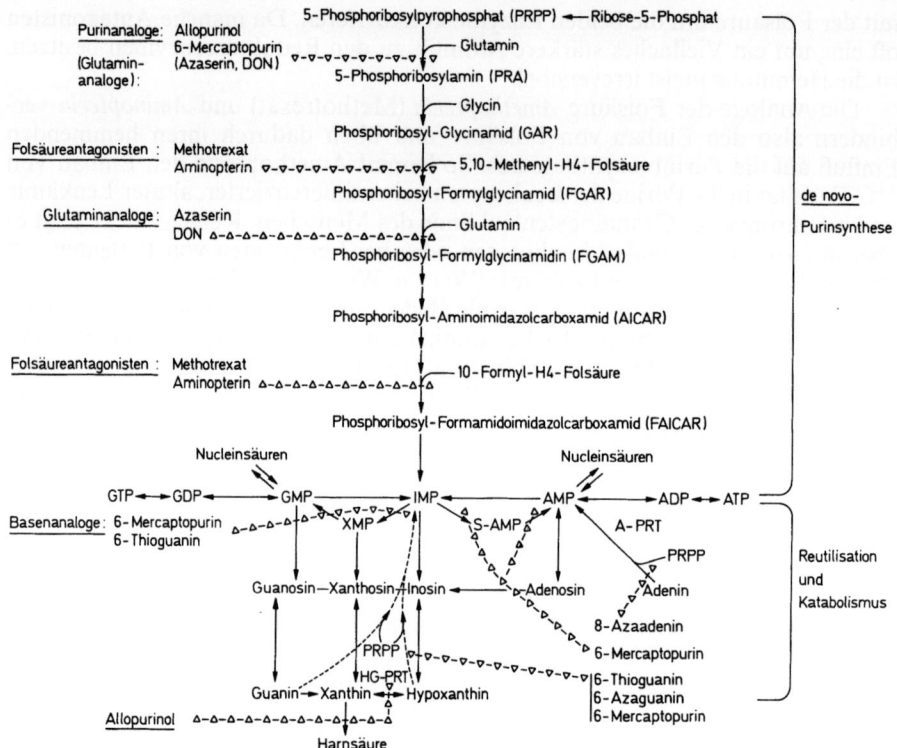

Abb. 2. Angriffspunkte verschiedener Hemmer in der Purin- und Harnsäuresynthese

Wirksamkeit getestet. Bei einigen wurden nur Gruppen außerhalb des Ringes ersetzt, wie z. B. bei 6-Mercaptopurin und 6-Thioguanin, bei anderen wurde der Imidazolring isosterisch geändert, wie z. B. beim 8-Azaguanin. Bei einigen wurde der Zuckeranteil des Purinribonucleosids modifiziert, wie z. B. beim Arabinosid des Adenins. Alle diese Änderungen führen zu einer gewissen antimetabolischen Wirksamkeit.

Als mögliche Wirkorte bzw. Mechanismen für die Inhibition der Purin- und Harnsäuresynthese durch Purinanaloge kommen verschiedene Stellen in Betracht (s. Abb. 2):

a) Hemmung der PRPP-Synthese.

Keine große Rolle spielen klinisch Antimetabolite, die zur Hemmung der *de novo*-Purinbiosynthese infolge Verminderung der PRPP-Synthese führen. Die antitumoröse Wirkung der Triphosphate einiger Adenosinanaloge (z. B. Xylosyladenin, 3-Desoxyadenosin, Tubercidin, Formycin) wird auf die Hemmung der PRPP-Synthetase zurückgeführt.

b) Hemmung der PRPP-Amidotransferase.

Die meisten Purinanaloge, die die Purinbiosynthese hemmen, sind zumindest teilweise Inhibitoren der PRPP-Amidotransferase. Hierzu gehören unter anderem Allopurinol, 6-Mercaptopurin und die verwandten Verbindungen Azathioprin, 6-Methylmercaptopurin-Ribonucleosid und Thioguanin.

Basenanaloge, die in Phosphoribosyltransferase-Reaktionen zum erhöhten PRPP-Verbrauch führen, können indirekt durch den dadurch herbeigeführten PRPP-Mangel für die PRPP-Amidotransferase-Reaktion zur Verminderung der

Purinbiosynthese führen. Hierher gehören neben Allopurinol und 2,6-Diaminopurin auch Orotsäure und Adenin.

Von allen diesen Substanzen ist bekannt, daß sie die intracellulären PRPP-Spiegel senken, experimentell nachgewiesen ist dies *in vivo* in Erythrocyten und *in vitro* in Fibroblastenkulturen.

c) Hemmung im Bereich des Interkonversionsstoffwechsels.

Als Inhibitoren im Bereich des Interkonversionsstoffwechsels der Purinribonucleotide greifen vor allem die 6-Thio- und 6-Chloropurine sowie einige Analoge von Aminosäuren an. In Bakterien und in Säugetierzellen hemmen die Ribonucleotide von 6-Mercaptopurin und 6-Thioguanin die IMP-Dehydrogenase (HENDERSON u. PATERSON, 1973); die Adenylosuccinat-Synthetase und die Adenylosuccinat-Lyase werden gleichfalls durch 6-Mercaptoribonucleotid gehemmt (NICHOL et al., 1967; HAMPTON, 1963).

d) Hemmung im Bereich des Reutilisationsstoffwechselwegs oder im Bereich des Purinkatabolismus.

Der "salvage"- oder Reutilisationsstoffwechselweg der Nucleotidbiosynthese hat bei der antimetabolischen Wirkung auf die Purin- und Purinnucleotidbiosynthese eine besondere Bedeutung. Einmal vermögen nur die Enzyme dieses Stoffwechselweges die Umwandlung der Antimetabolite in ihre entsprechenden Nucleotidderivate durchzuführen, und dies sind in den meisten Fällen allein die aktiven Formen der Substanzen. Zweitens ist dieser Stoffwechselweg durch die Abhängigkeit einiger Zellsysteme von präformierten Purinen hemmenden Einflüssen besonders zugänglich (s. Abb. 2).

Als Inhibitoren der Harnsäuresynthese — also im Bereich des Purinkatabolismus — spielen besonders Substanzen eine Rolle, die die Xanthin-Oxydase hemmen. Dieses Enzym katalysiert die Oxydation von Hypoxanthin zu Xanthin und von Xanthin zu Harnsäure. Als Hemmer der Xanthinoxydase sind eine Reihe von Purinanaloge (sowie 6-Pteridylaldehyd) bekannt. Hierher gehören Adenin und 2,6-Diaminopurin (WYNGAARDEN, 1957), 6-Thiopurin (BERGMANN u. UNGAR, 1960; SILBERMAN u. WYNGAARDEN, 1961), 6-Chloropurin (DUGGAN u. TITUS, 1959), 4-Diazoimidazol-5-Carboxamid (IWATA et al., 1969) und symmetrische Triazine (FRIDOVICH, 1965).

Die größte klinische Verwendung zur Behandlung der familiären Hyperuricämie und zur Kontrolle der renalen Harnsäureausfällung bei leukämischen Patienten, die mit Cytostatica behandelt werden, hat hier Allopurinol, ein Analoges von Hypoxanthin, gefunden.

1. Allopurinol (4-Hydroxy-Pyrazolo-[3,4-d]Pyrimidin)

Allopurinol wurde ursprünglich als ein Medikament zur Chemotherapie von Tumoren synthetisiert, zeigte aber als solches keinen Effekt auf die Hemmung des Tumorwachstums (WHITE, 1959; SHAW et al., 1960). Klinisch wurde es von RUNDLES et al. (1963) erst als eine Zusatztherapie bei Patienten verwendet, die zur Behandlung einer Leukämie 6-Mercaptopurin erhielten. Bei Verabreichung von 6-Mercaptopurin werden etwa 25—30% des Pharmakons durch die Xanthin-Oxydase zu dem inerten Metaboliten Thioharnsäure umgewandelt, d.h. inaktiviert. Deshalb suchte man nach einem wirksamen Inhibitor für die Xanthin-Oxydase, der den starken Verlust in der Wirksamkeit dieses Medikamentes verhindern und so als nützliches therapeutisches Adjuvans zur Leukämietherapie Verwendung finden könnte. Sollte es möglich sein, die Xanthin-Oxydase *in vivo* durch eine Substanz zu hemmen, würde man eine metabolische Inaktivierung von 6-Mercaptopurin verringern können. Von den verschiedenen in diesem Zusammenhang geprüften Pyrazolopyrimidinen schien Allopurinol, ein Strukturanaloges von Hypoxanthin, am besten geeignet. ELION et al. (1963) konnten nämlich zeigen, daß Allopurinol *in vitro* ein starker Hemmer der Xanthin-Oxydase ist. Bei Mäusen und bei Menschen wurde die Umwandlung von 6-Mercaptopurin in 6-Thioharnsäure reduziert und damit dessen antitumoröse und immunsuppressive Wirkungen um ein Mehrfaches verstärkt, bzw. die 6-Mercaptopurin-Dosis konnte bei gleichzeitiger Gabe von Allopurinol gesenkt werden. Bei den daraufhin mit Allopurinol behandelten Patienten wurde aber nun auch eine starke Erniedrigung der Serumharnsäurewerte und der renalen Harnsäureexkretion festgestellt, d.h. eine Verminderung der Harnsäurebildung. Danach wurde diese Substanz bei Gichtpatienten geprüft und als therapeutisches Mittel mit neuem Wirkungsprinzip zur Behandlung der primären und sekundären Hyperurikämie empfohlen (RUNDLES et al., 1963; WYNGAARDEN et al. 1963).

Besondere Indikationsgebiete für Allopurinol sind vor allem die Hyperurikämie und Gicht, die durch eine bereits bestehende Nierenerkrankung kompliziert sind, sekundäre Hyperurikämien (besonders bei Hämoblastosen) und Unverträglichkeiten von Urikosurica.

a) Klinik

Langjährige Erfahrung und ausgedehnte Studien lassen an der Nützlichkeit und Wirksamkeit von Allopurinol bei der Behandlung der primären und sekundären Gicht keinen Zweifel (YÜ u. GUTMAN, 1964; RUNDLES et al., 1964; RUNDLES et al., 1966; KLINENBERG et al., 1965; WYNGAARDEN et al., 1965; DELBARRE et al., 1966; ALEXANDER u. BRENDLER, 1967; SCOTT, 1966; RUNDLES et al., 1969).

Während der Verabreichung von Allopurinol an Normalpersonen und den meisten Gichtpatienten führt die partielle Hemmung der Xanthin-Oxydase zu einer Senkung der Serumharnsäure und der renalen Harnsäureausscheidung. Diese Wirkung tritt bereits innerhalb von 24—48 Std auf, mit einem Maximum zwischen 4 Tagen und 2 Wochen. Gleichzeitig mit diesen Änderungen ist ein Anstieg der Oxypurinvorstufen Xanthin und Hypoxanthin in Serum und Urin, und zwar bereits innerhalb von ca. 4—6 Std, zu beobachten. Die Serumharnsäurekonzentration kann durch entsprechende Allopurinoldosierung auf jeden gewünschten Wert (bis zu 2—3 mg/100 ml) eingestellt werden. Bei den meisten Patienten können mit einer Dosis von 200—300 mg/die normale Serumharnsäurespiegel erreicht werden, bei schwerer Gicht mit ausgeprägten Tophi werden 400—600 mg und selten 700—1000 mg/die benötigt. Die Standarddosierung liegt im allgemeinen zu Beginn bei 300 mg/die, bei Langzeitbehandlung um 200 mg täglich, die tägliche Maximaldosis liegt bei 800 mg/die, bei Kindern um 8 mg/kg/Tag. Die stärkste Senkung der Serumharnsäurespiegel ist also bereits einige Tage nach Therapiebeginn erreicht, sie bleibt relativ konstant über lange Zeit. Nach Beendigung der Allopurinoltherapie steigen die Serumharnsäurewerte innerhalb einer Woche, unabhängig von der Dauer der Therapie, wieder zu den Werten vor Beginn der Therapie an (FYFE et al., 1974; ELION u. NELSON, 1974).

Aus zwei Gründen kommt es bei der partiellen Blockierung der Xanthin-Oxydase während der Allopurinoltherapie nicht zu einer übermäßigen Akkumulation von Hypoxanthin und Xanthin. Erstens ist deren renale Clearance sehr hoch (entspricht etwa der glomerulären Filtrationsrate), zweitens werden diese beiden Oxypurine im Reutilisationsstoffwechsel wieder zu IMP aufgebaut. Es kommt also zu einer nur geringen Erhöhung der Oxypurine im Serum (0,5—1 mg/100 ml, selten bis 2 mg/100 ml [KLINENBERG et al., 1965; RUNDLES et al., 1963; YÜ u. GUTMAN, 1964]).

Bei einer Hemmung der Harnsäurebildung durch die Hemmung der Xanthin-Oxydase würde man eine entsprechende Erhöhung der Vorstufen der gehemmten Reaktion, Xanthin und Hypoxanthin erwarten. Tatsächlich können diese beiden Substanzen auch in erhöhtem Ausmaß unter Allopurinoltherapie im Urin nachgewiesen werden, die Erhöhung der Oxypurine im Serum ist jedoch gering [etwa $^1/_{10}$ der reduzierten Serumharnsäurefraktion wird durch Oxypurine ersetzt (HITCHINGS, 1969b)]. Als ein Faktor für die begrenzte Erhöhung der Serumoxypurine ist dementsprechend die hohe renale Clearance dieser Substanzen anzusehen. Der Hauptfaktor, der eine Erhöhung der Serum- und Gewebeoxypurine limitiert, kommt jedoch zustande über eine Verminderung des Gesamt-Purin-Endprodukts auf etwa 35—65% (HITCHINGS, 1966). In der Bilanz ist also die Oxypurinausscheidung geringer als die entsprechende Verminderung der Harnsäureausscheidung, d.h. die Erhöhung der Oxypurinausscheidung ist nicht äquimolar, es ist ein Defizit festzustellen. Neben der sehr hohen Clearance der Oxypurine wird dies mit einer Hemmung der *de novo*-Purinsynthese durch Allopurinol erklärt (RUNDLES et al., 1963; RUNDLES et al., 1966; YÜ u. GUTMAN, 1964; GOLDFINGER et al., 1965; ELION et al., 1968). Der Anteil von Xanthin ist etwa 4mal höher, vermutlich durch die bevorzugte Reutilisation von Hypoxanthin zu IMP durch die HG-PRT (HITCHINGS, 1969, WYNGAARDEN u. KELLEY, 1972).

Werden durch die Allopurinoltherapie über längere Zeit normale Serumharnsäurewerte erreicht, kommt es zur Auflösung der Gichttophi, zur Besserung der destruktiven Gichtarthritis, die Bildung von Harnsäuresteinen sowie das Fortschreiten der Gichtnephropathie werden verhindert. Eine gleichzeitige Verabreichung von Urikosurica führt zu einer Vermehrung der Harnsäureexkretion und einer weiteren Senkung der Serumharnspiegel (RUNDLES et al., 1966). Allopurinol beeinflußt die Wirksamkeit urikosurischer Medikamente nicht, desgleichen wird die Clearance von Allopurinol durch gleichzeitige Verabreichung von Urikosurica nicht verändert, so daß man eigentlich eine additive Wirksamkeit annehmen müßte. Da die Clearance des aus Allopurinol entstehenden Oxypurinol jedoch durch urikosurisch wirksame Medikamente erhöht wird, wird der Hemmeffekt auf die Harnsäurebildung zu einem gewissen Grad vermindert. Damit wird auch die Ausscheidung der Oxypurine durch Urikosurica vermindert (ELION et al., 1968; GOLDFINGER et al., 1965).

Neben der guten therapeutischen Wirksamkeit bei der primären Hyperurikämie zeigt Allopurinol seine große Effektivität bei der Beseitigung bzw. Verhinderung der bei der cytostatischen Therapie von Leukämien oder Lymphomen oft auftretenden exzessiven sekundären Hyperurikämie mit ihren Folgeerscheinungen (RIESELBACH et al., 1964; KRAKOFF, 1965; WATTS et al., 1966).

Für die Kontrolle des Harnsäurespiegels unter Allopurinoltherapie ist im allgemeinen zu Beginn ein etwa 2wöchiger, in der Dauertherapie ein etwa 1—3monatiger Abstand erforderlich. Bei der Therapie einer Gichtniere, bzw. von Harnsäuresteinen, ist unbedingt für eine ausreichende Harnmenge von mindestens zwei Litern zu sorgen. Um eine Präcipitation von Harnsäure zu vermeiden, wird oft eine zusätzliche Neutralisierung des Harns vorgeschlagen (pH 6,4-6,8). Bei Vorliegen einer schweren Niereninsuffizienz sollte die Allopurinoldosis reduziert werden.

Da ein großer Teil der therapeutischen Wirksamkeit des Allopurinols durch die länger anhaltende Aktivität des Oxypurinols zustande kommt (s. S. 473, Pharmakokinetik), prüften RODNAN et al. (1974), ob sich eine einmal täglich verabreichte Allopurinoldosis (300 mg) therapeutisch gleich effektiv auf die Serumharnsäuresenkung auswirken könnte wie mehrere kleinere Dosen (3 × 100 mg). Auf Grund ihrer Kurzzeitstudie (über 2 Wochen täglich 1 × 300 mg) ist nicht auszu-

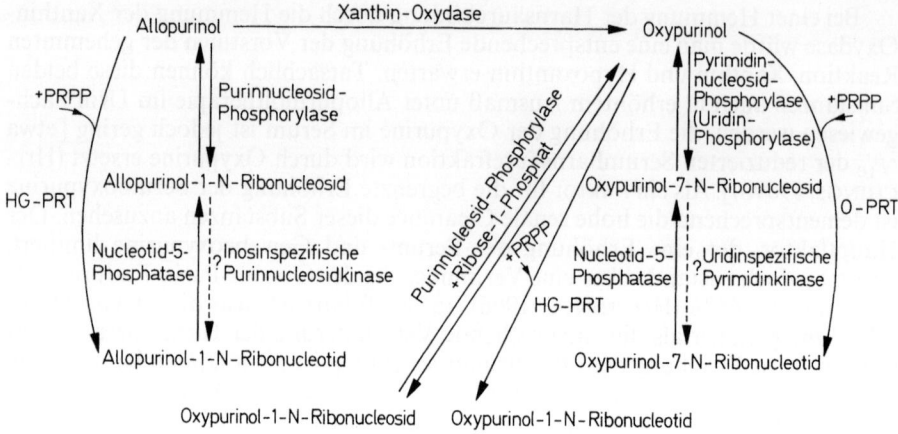

Abb. 3. Metabolismus von Allopurinol und Oxypurinol

schließen, daß diese Dosierung therapeutisch ähnlich gut wirksam ist wie die Gabe von 3 × 100 mg pro Tag. Eine endgültige Beurteilung sollte jedoch von einer breiteren Untersuchungsserie abhängig gemacht werden.

Für Allopurinol gibt es im Handel nur die orale Verabreichungsform. Von KANN et al. (1968) wurde zur Behandlung ihrer Patienten mit sekundärer Hyperurikämie bei neoplastischen Prozessen — wegen der bei diesen Patienten vorhandenen Schwierigkeiten die orale Medikation einzunehmen — eine Präparation zur parenteralen Zufuhr von Allopurinol entwickelt. Dazu wurde das löslichere Natriumsalz von Allopurinol verwendet. Die Präparation war ohne Schwierigkeiten zu verabreichen, gut wirksam und nicht toxisch, ist jedoch relativ instabil. Intravenöse Gaben von bis zu 420 mg pro qm Körperoberfläche pro 24 Std wurden hiervon an einzelne Patienten verabreicht und wurden gut toleriert. Keine wesentlichen Unterschiede ergaben sich bei Vergleich der Wirksamkeit von oral und intravenös verabreichtem Allopurinol.

b) Metabolismus und Pharmakokinetik von Allopurinol

Metabolismus (s. Abb. 3)

Allopurinol, ein Analoges von Hypoxanthin, ist in erster Linie ein synthetischer Hemmer der Xanthin-Oxydase. Bei der Clearance von Allopurinol aus dem Blutkreislauf spielen zwei Prozesse eine Rolle, 1. die renale Elimination und 2. die Metabolisierung. Allopurinol wird durch die Xanthin-Oxydase *in vivo* zum entsprechenden Xanthinanalog Oxypurinol (Oxoallopurinol, Alloxanthin) umgewandelt (ELION, 1966), und zwar beträgt diese Umwandlung *in vivo* etwa 45—65% des verabreichten Allopurinols (verabreichte Dosis in diesen Untersuchungen: 2 × 400 mg/die (KRENITSKY et al., 1967). Ein geringer Teil des Allopurinols wird durch die Purinnucleosid-Phosphorylase mit Ribose-1-Phosphat direkt zu Allopurinol-1-N-Ribonucleosid (KRENITSKY et al., 1967) und vermutlich wiederum direkt durch die HG-PRT zu Allopurinol-1-N-Ribonucleotid umgewandelt. KRENITSKY et al. (1967) gelang der Nachweis für die Bildung von Allopurinol- oder Oxypurinolribonucleotid *in vivo* nicht, obgleich sie nach Allopurinolgabe im Urin eines Patienten Allopurinol-1-N-Ribonucleosid und Oxypurinol-7-N-Ribonucleosid nachweisen konnten. Vor allem die Ergebnisse von Fox et al.

(1971) und KELLEY et al. (1971 a) wiesen aber darauf hin, daß in vivo Ribonucleotide von Allopurinol und Oxypurinol gebildet werden müssen. Mit der von KRENITSKY et al. (1967) angewendeten Methode war die untere Grenze der Nachweisbarkeit für die Ribonucleotide nur 10^{-6} M. Mit empfindlicheren Nachweismethoden wurden kürzlich auch in Rattengeweben die Ribonucleotide aller drei bekannten Ribonucleoside von Allopurinol und Oxypurinol nachgewiesen (FYFE et al., 1974; ELION u. NELSON, 1974).

Der weitaus größte Teil des aus Allopurinol durch die Xanthin-Oxydase entstehenden Oxypurinols wird als solches renal ausgeschieden. Ein geringer Teil des Oxypurinols wird durch die Pyrimidinnucleosid-Phosphorylase zu Oxypurinol-7-N-Ribonucleosid und durch die Purinnucleosid-Phosphorylase auch zu Oxypurinol-1-N-Ribonucleosid umgewandelt (ELION et al., 1968). Oxypurinol-7-N-Ribonucleotid wird direkt durch die O-PRT gebildet, Oxypurinol-1-N-Ribonucleotid vermutlich durch die HG-PRT (BEARDMORE u. KELLEY, 1971a).

Nach Bildung von Oxypurinol-7-N-Ribonucleotid durch die O-PRT scheint es durch die Nucleotid-5-Phosphatase zur Bildung von Oxypurinol-7-N-Ribonucleosid zu kommen. Dieses wird dann beim Menschen im Urin ausgeschieden (KRENITSKY et al., 1967; GREENE et al., 1969).

In Isotopenstudien mit $6-^{14}$C-Allopurinol wird bis zu 20% der verabreichten Radioaktivität nicht in Allopurinol oder seinen Metaboliten im Urin wiedergefunden (SIMMONDS, 1969). Nach den Untersuchungen von FOX et al. (1970b) soll ein Teil des Allopurinols in Nucleinsäuren des Gewebes eingebaut werden. ELION et al. (1966) konnten jedoch in ihren ersten Untersuchungen mit ^{14}C-Allopurinol bei Mäusen in vivo keinen Einbau der Radioaktivität in den untersuchten Geweben feststellen. Das würde bedeuten, daß jener Teil des ^{14}C, der nach Verabreichung von ^{14}C-Allopurinol nicht im Urin wiedergefunden werden kann (bis zu 20%), entweder aus dem Darm nicht resorbiert wird oder in das Dünndarmlumen sezerniert und mit den Faeces ausgeschieden wird. Nach oraler Gabe von 169 mg $6-^{14}$C-Allopurinol konnten ELION et al. (1966) innerhalb von 48 Std nach der Verabreichung 19,9% des ^{14}C in den Faeces wiederfinden.

Pharmakokinetik

Allopurinol wird schnell aus dem Darm resorbiert. Allopurinol selbst hat eine Halbwertszeit von etwa 2—3 Std (ELION et al., 1966b). Im Urin werden etwa 3—10% des verabreichten Allopurinols in 24 Std unverändert ausgeschieden (verabreichte Dosis 2×400 mg/die [ELION et al., 1966b]), etwa 70% als Oxypurinol (KRENITSKY et al., 1967) und ein geringerer Teil als Allopurinol-1-N-Ribonucleosid (KRENITSKY et al., 1967) sowie vermutlich als Allopurinol-1-N-Ribonucleotid (Fox et al., 1970).

Bei intravenöser Gabe einer Einzeldosis von 140 mg ^{14}C-Allopurinol als Natriumsalz fanden ELION et al. (1968) im Plasma eine Halbwertszeit für das verabreichte ^{14}C von 8 Std während der initialen 8 Std-Periode, danach erhöhte sich die Halbwertszeit auf 16 Std. Bei der Fraktionierung der Radioaktivität ergab sich, daß bereits nach 1 Std 65% der Radioaktivität im Plasma in der Oxypurinolfraktion nachzuweisen war, nach 2 Std waren es 85% und nach 6 Std 100%. Demnach wäre die Clearance von Allopurinol aus dem Plasma nach einer einmaligen intravenösen Gabe durch Oxydation und Exkretion bereits nach 6 Std abgeschlossen. Die Gesamtausscheidung von ^{14}C im Urin betrug nach 1 Std 8,2%, nach 2 Std 14%, nach 6 Std 38% und nach 24 Std 47,5% der verabreichten Dosis. Bei Fraktionierung der Urinausscheidung waren nach 1 Std 43%, nach 2 Std 15% der Radioaktivität im Allopurinol, nach 12 Std die gesamte Radioaktivität nur noch in der Oxypurinolfraktion nachzuweisen. Die Clearance für Oxypurinol wurde für die Periode von 6—12 Std nach intravenöser Verabreichung von Allopurinol auf etwa 28 ml/min berechnet.

Bei *oraler* Verabreichung von 160 mg ^{14}C-Allopurinol konnte nach 30 min noch keine Radioaktivität nachgewiesen werden. Nach 1 Std entsprach die Radioaktivität im Plasma einer Allopurinolkonzentration von 2,2 µg/ml. Nach 2— 6 Std wurde ein Plateau erreicht, danach fiel sie langsam — innerhalb von 48 Std — auf etwa 1 µg/ml (Oxypurinol) ab. Das Maximum der Urinexkretion war nach 2—3 Std erreicht, nach 6 Std konnte die gesamte Radioaktivität im ausgeschiedenen Oxypurinol nachgewiesen werden. Die kumulative ^{14}C-Ausscheidung im Urin betrug 9,5% in 6 Std, 25% in 24 Std und 38,5% in 48 Std. Die Halbwertszeit für Oxypurinol aus dem Plasma wurde auf 28 Std berechnet, als renale Clearance konnten 15 ml/min errechnet werden.

Nach einer Einzeldosis von 300 mg Allopurinol ist der Plasmaspiegel beim Menschen 1—3 Std nach der Verabreichung unter 10 µM, nach 6 Std ist im Plasma kein Allopurinol mehr nachweisbar (ELION u. NELSON, 1974). Die Plasma-Oxypurinolspiegel sind bei Verabreichung von 300 mg täglich konstant bei etwa 65 µM. Diese relative Konstanz kommt zustande durch die Reabsorption von Oxypurinol in den Nierentubuli und der damit zusammenhängenden geringeren Clearance. Allopurinol wird also von der menschlichen Niere in einer der Glomerulumfiltration ähnlichen Geschwindigkeit eliminiert und damit ähnlich wie die natürlichen Oxypurine Hypoxanthin und Xanthin. Die Clearance von Oxypurinol dagegen ist wesentlich geringer, was für eine Reabsorption in den renalen Tubuli spricht. Oxypurinol verhält sich demnach in der Clearance eher wie ein Analoges der Harnsäure und nicht von Xanthin, was auch zum Ausdruck kommt in der in gleicher Weise erfolgenden Beeinflussung der Oxypurinolexkretion durch Substanzen, die die Harnsäureausscheidung erhöhen (Urikosurica, wie z.B. Probenecid). Beim Menschen entspricht die Oxypurinolclearance in etwa dem Dreifachen der Harnsäureclearance und die Plasmaspiegel können nach ELION *et al.* (1968) bei Kenntnis der Harnsäureclearance und der Allopurinoldosierung vorausberechnet werden.

Da sowohl Allopurinol als auch Oxypurinol die Oxydation von Allopurinol verhindern, erhöht sich die Halbwertszeit für Allopurinol bei steigender Xanthin-Oxydase-Hemmung. Dies kann nun entweder herbeigeführt werden durch Dosiserhöhung oder durch Akkumulation von Oxypurinol während der Dauertherapie. Diese Akkumulation von Oxypurinol während der Langzeittherapie scheint nach ELION *et al.* (1966b) wesentlich zur therapeutischen Wirksamkeit des Medikaments beizutragen. Oxypurinol scheint ähnlich wie Harnsäure reabsorbiert zu werden und zeigt bei hohen Konzentrationen in der renalen Exkretion eine kompetitive (d.h. urikosurische) Wirkung auf die Harnsäureausscheidung (ELION *et al.*, 1968).

Bei Allopurinolgabe bleibt so der Oxypurinolspiegel längere Zeit bestehen und zwar in einer direkten Relation zur Allopurinoldosis und einer umgekehrten Relation zu seiner renalen Clearance. Die Plasmaspiegel von Oxypurinol steigen deshalb auch bei chronischer Niereninsuffizienz an.

Allopurinol und Oxypurinol sind im gesamten Körperwasser gleichmäßig verteilt (außer im Gehirn, wo die Spiegel etwa halb so hoch wie die Serumspiegel sind [ELION *et al.*, 1966b]). RUNDLES *et al.* (1969) konnten eine wesentliche Serumproteinbindung von Allopurinol und Oxypurinol nicht nachweisen. Die maximale Löslichkeit für Oxypurinol im Urin bei pH 7,0 beträgt 70 mg/100 ml (LEVIN u. ABRAHAMS, 1966). Diese Konzentration wird praktisch nie erreicht.

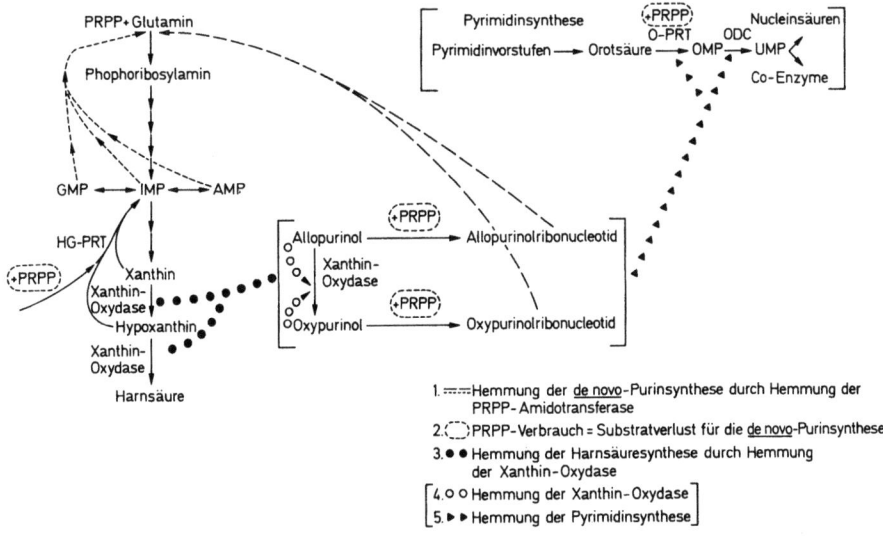

Abb. 4. Wirkungen von Allopurinol auf die Purin- und Harnsäuresynthese

c) Wirkungsmechanismus von Allopurinol auf die Purin- und Harnsäuresynthese

Für die Wirkung von Allopurinol auf den Purin- und Harnsäurestoffwechsel kommen zwei verschiedene Mechanismen in Betracht.
1. Die Hauptwirkung auf die Hemmung der Xanthin-Oxydase.
2. Die Hemmwirkung auf die *de novo*-Purinsynthese.

Hemmung der Xanthin-Oxydase (s. Abb. 4)

Xanthin-Oxydase katalysiert die Oxydation verschiedener natürlicher Purinsubstrate und Purin-Antimetabolite. Allopurinol und Oxypurinol hemmen die Oxydation von Hypoxanthin zu Xanthin und von Xanthin zu Harnsäure *in vitro* (FEIGELSON et al., 1957) und *in vivo* (RUNDLES et al., 1963), indem sie die Xanthin-Oxydase pseudo-irreversibel inaktivieren; d.h. die Inaktivierung kommt zustande, wenn das Enzym und Allopurinol in Abwesenheit von Substrat inkubiert werden, kann jedoch durch längere Dialyse wieder aufgehoben werden. Beim Menschen scheint es nicht zu einer irreversiblen Aktivierung der Xanthin-Oxydase zu kommen, deshalb ist auch keine Enzyminduktion nachweisbar. Die Michaeliskonstante von Allopurinol ist etwa 30mal niedriger als die des natürlichen Substrats der Xanthin-Oxydase, des Xanthins. Die Michaeliskonstante für Oxypurinol ist etwas höher als die von Allopurinol und ähnlich derjenigen von Xanthin (ELION, 1966b). Es ist auch diskutiert worden, ob die *in vivo*-Hemmung der Xanthin-Oxydase primär durch Oxypurinol und nicht durch Allopurinol zustande kommt. Bei direktem Vergleich der beiden Substanzen ist Allopurinol jedoch wirksamer als Inhibitor der Xanthin-Oxydase *in vitro* (ELION et al., 1964), *in vivo* bei Mäusen (ELION et al., 1963) und wenn beim Menschen Einzeldosen von Allopurinol verabreicht werden (ELION et al., 1968). Allopurinol ist sowohl Inhibitor als auch Substrat für die Xanthin-Oxydase und das Produkt seiner durch das Enzym katalysierten Oxydation, das Oxypurinol ist wiederum selbst ein Hemmer der Xanthin-Oxydase. Allopurinol ist also auch ein Substrat für die Xanthin-Oxydase, es wird langsam zu Oxypurinol oxydiert. Oxypurinol ist ein strukturelles Isomer von Xanthin und ein nichtkompetitiver Hemmer der Xanthin-Oxydase

(ELION et al., 1964). Dies erklärt die komplexe Enzymkinetik, die *in vitro* bei der Hemmung der Xanthin-Oxydase durch Allopurinol vorliegt. Oxypurinol scheint (CHALMERS et al., 1968) auch *in vivo* eine geringere Hemmwirkung auf die Xanthin-Oxydase auszuüben als Allopurinol, möglicherweise bedingt durch schlechte Resorption. Die Synthese von Xanthin-Oxydase soll nach ELION et al. (1966) durch Oxypurinol weder induziert noch deprimiert werden. Die Wirkungen von Allopurinol auf den Serumharnsäurespiegel bleiben über lange Zeit konstant. Daraus kann man schließen, daß eine begrenzte Induzierbarkeit der Xanthin-Oxydase vorhanden sein muß, oder wenn eine Induzierbarkeit überhaupt besteht, muß sie ihr Maximum bereits zu einem frühen Zeitpunkt während der Therapie erreicht haben.

Eine totale Hemmung der Xanthin-Oxydase durch Allopurinol wurde beim Menschen nicht durchgeführt. Da sich eine lineare logarithmische Dosis-Wirkungskurve ergibt, kann man durch Extrapolation errechnen, daß beim Menschen zur kompletten Hemmung der Xanthin-Oxydase eine Allopurinoldosis von 5 g/Tag erforderlich wäre (HITCHINGS, 1966). Bei dieser hohen Dosierung würden jedoch vermutlich die Absorption und auch die Löslichkeit von Oxypurinol ein limitierender Faktor sein (SIMMONDS et al., 1973). Von SWEETMAN (1968) wurde Allopurinol in steigender Dosierung an Kinder mit einem Gewicht von 15 kg verabreicht. Dabei ergab sich eine Sättigung der Xanthin-Oxydase bei einer Dosis von 1000 mg/Tag.

Diese Eigenschaft — Hemmung der Xanthin-Oxydase — führte dazu, Allopurinol als therapeutisches Mittel zur Reduzierung der Harnsäureproduktion einzuführen (RUNDLES et al., 1963; HALL et al., 1964; YÜ u. GUTMAN, 1964; KLINENBERG et al., 1965; WATTS et al., 1966; SCOTT et al., 1966; ANDERSON et al., 1967).

Hemmwirkung von Allopurinol auf die de novo-Purinsynthese

Außer dem Hemmeffekt auf die letzten Schritte des Purinkatabolismus hat Allopurinol bei den meisten Personen noch einen zusätzlichen Hemmeffekt auf die *de novo*-Purinsynthese (s. Abb. 4). RUNDLES et al. (1963) wiesen als erste auf die Diskrepanz der Gesamtpurinexkretion (Harnsäure plus Oxypurine) vor und während der Allopurinolbehandlung hin. Sie vermuteten deshalb, daß es durch Allopurinol, neben der hemmenden Wirkung auf die Xanthin-Oxydase, gleichzeitig zu einer Hemmung der *de novo*-Purinsynthese kommen müßte. Tatsächlich wurde in mehreren Untersuchungen (RUNDLES et al., 1963; DELBARRE et al., 1966; RUNDLES et al., 1966; HITCHINGS, 1966) nachgewiesen, daß es bei der Behandlung zu einer Verminderung in der renalen Harnsäureexkretion, aber nicht zu einer äquivalenten Ausscheidung von Oxypurinen kommt. Das Defizit in dieser Bilanz reicht von 10—60%. Einen weiteren Hinweis auf die Hemmung der *de novo*-Purinsynthese durch Allopurinol ergaben Untersuchungen von EMMERSON (1966). Die bei Allopurinolgabe verminderte Harnausscheidung der Gesamtpurine geht einher mit einer Reduktion des ^{14}C-Einbaus von Glycin, der jedoch nur nachzuweisen ist bei Patienten mit intakter HG-PRT. Für die Wirksamkeit von Allopurinol auf die *de novo*-Purinsynthese scheint das Enzym HG-PRT notwendig zu sein. Dies ergibt sich aus Untersuchungsergebnissen vor allem an Patienten mit Lesch-Nyhan-Syndrom. Obwohl auch bei diesen Patienten die Allopurinolwirkung auf die Xanthin-Oxydase vorhanden ist, kommt es nicht zur Hemmung der *de novo*-Purinsynthese. Die Verminderung der renalen Harnsäureausscheidung wird also ersetzt durch eine sich stöchiometrisch nicht entsprechende Erhöhung der Hypoxanthin- und Xanthinausscheidung (KELLEY et al., 1968; KELLEY et al., 1969; SORENSEN et al., 1970).

Für die Entstehung der Hemmwirkung auf die *de novo*-Purinsynthese durch Allopurinol kommen verschiedene Mechanismen in Frage, für die die Anwesenheit der HG-PRT Voraussetzung ist.

α) Die Feedback-Hemmung auf die PRPP-Amidotransferase durch natürliche Ribonucleotide (Abb. 2)

Durch eine vermehrte Umwandlung des bei Hemmung der Xanthin-Oxydase akkumulierten Hypoxanthins zu IMP im Reutilisationsstoffwechsel und der darauffolgenden Metabolisierung im Interkonversionsstoffwechsel von IMP zu AMP und GMP, kommt es zur allosterischen Hemmwirkung auf die *de novo*-Purinsynthese im Bereich des ersten geschwindigkeitsbestimmenden Schritts, der PRPP-Amidotransferase-Reaktion.

β) Pseudo-Feedback-Hemmung durch Allopurinol- und Oxypurinolribonucleotide

Nach der Umwandlung von Allopurinol zu Allopurinol-1-N-Ribonucleotid bzw. Oxypurinol-7-N-Ribonucleotid, kommt es direkt durch diese Ribonucleotide zur Hemmwirkung auf die PRPP-Amidotransferase im Sinne einer Feedback-Hemmung durch allosterische Mechanismen (Pseudo-Feedback-Hemmung).

γ) Substratverarmung von PRPP für die de novo-Purinsynthese

Durch den vermehrten Verbrauch von PRPP bei der Bildung von Allopurinol- bzw. Oxypurinolribonucleotiden und/oder der erhöhten Reutilisation des akkumulierten Hypoxanthins und Xanthins zu IMP, kommt es zu einem intracellulären PRPP-Defizit. Da die PRPP-Konzentration entscheidend für die Geschwindigkeit am ersten Schritt der *de novo*-Purinsynthese ist, kann die Purinsynthese durch Substratmangel von PRPP vermindert werden.

ad α) Die Feedback-Hemmung auf die PRPP-Amidotransferase durch natürliche Ribonucleotide

Beim Menschen konnte ein solcher Ablauf des Mechanismus zur Hemmwirkung nicht direkt nachgewiesen werden. In Untersuchungen an Mäusen fanden jedoch POMALES et al. (1963 u. 1965) nach Allopurinolverabreichung einen signifikant höheren Einbau von radioaktiv markiertem Hypoxanthin in die löslichen Nucleotide und in Adenin und Guanin von Nucleinsäuren, was als Hinweis für einen derartigen Mechanismus gelten könnte. Darüber hinaus konnten RUNDLES et al. (1966) beim Menschen nachweisen, daß Allopurinol die Reutilisation von Hypoxanthin aus exogen zugeführtem Inosin erhöht. ELION u. NELSON (1974) versuchten Änderungen in der Poolgröße natürlicher Purinnucleotide nach Allopurinolverabreichung nachzuweisen. Nach einmaliger intravenöser Gabe von Allopurinol (20 mg/kg) ergab sich nach 1 Std in Rattenlebern ein vorübergehender Abfall in den Spiegeln von AMP, GMP, GDP und ATP, nach 3 und 24 Std waren diese Spiegel wieder normal oder geringfügig höher als die Ausgangswerte. Die Nucleotidpools änderten sich nach einer einmaligen Gabe einer hohen Allopurinoldosis also nur kurzzeitig. Auch bei Langzeitverabreichung von Allopurinol zeigten die Purinnucleotidspiegel von Rattenlebern keine wesentliche Beeinflussung. Die IMP-Spiegel zeigten dabei eine geringe, jedoch statistisch nicht eindeutig signifikante Erhöhung. Diese Tatsache der Konstanthaltung der Purinnucleotidspiegel kann jedoch allein damit erklärt werden, daß es durch Allopurinol zu einer vermehrten Reutilisation von Hypoxanthin und Xanthin zur Nucleotidsynthese kommt. Eine Feedback-Hemmung der *de novo*-Purinsynthese durch Allopurinol, infolge einer Erhöhung der natürlichen Purinnucleotide, erscheint deshalb wohl möglich, eine definitive Aussage aber, ob diesem Mechanismus eine wesentliche Rolle zufällt, läßt sich bei kritischer Wertung der experimentellen Daten bis heute nicht treffen.

ad β) Pseudo-Feedback-Hemmung durch Allopurinol- und Oxypurinolribonucleotide

WYNGAARDEN vermutete als erster (1965), daß Allopurinol in sein Ribonucleotid umgewandelt werden könnte und dieses durch Pseudo-Feedback-Hemmung die PRPP-Amidotransferase hemmen würde. Er konnte diese Theorie untermauern, indem er enzymatisch geringe Mengen Allopurinolribonucleotid synthetisierte und damit eine Hemmwirkung auf die Purinbiosynthese erzielen konnte.

Die Bildung von Allopurinolribonucleotid konnte in anderen *in vitro*-Untersuchungen nachgewiesen werden (ELION et al., 1966; Fox et al., 1970), hier hemmt es auch deutlich die *de novo*-Purinsynthese durch Hemmung des Enzyms PRPP-Amidotransferase (MCCOLLISTER et al., 1964). Daraus konnte geschlossen werden, daß Allopurinol die Purinsynthese über einen Mechanismus hemmt, der unabhängig von seinem Effekt auf die Xanthin-Oxydase ist. *In vivo* konnte die Bildung von Allopurinolribonucleotid zuerst nie direkt nachgewiesen werden, indirekt gab es jedoch Hinweise auf eine *in vivo*-Bildung beim Menschen. Nach Allopurinolgabe wird nämlich im Urin normalerweise Allopurinolribonucleosid ausgeschieden, bei Patienten mit Lesch-Nyhan-Syndrom, bei denen die Bildung von Allopurinolribonucleotid durch das Fehlen der HG-PRT unmöglich ist, beobachtet man keine Ausscheidung von Allopurinolribonucleosid, gleichzeitig kommt es auch zu keiner Reduktion in der Gesamtpurinausscheidung (SWEETMAN, 1968).

Allopurinol-1-N-Ribonucleotid ist für die PRPP-Amidotransferase aus Taubenleber ein wirksamer Hemmer, während Allopurinol selbst keinen Einfluß zeigt (MCCOLLISTER et al., 1964). Nach den Untersuchungen von ELION u. NELSON (1964) an Ratten scheint es unwahrscheinlich, daß Allopurinol-1-N-Ribonucleotid für die Feedback-Hemmung auf die *de novo*-Purinsynthese verantwortlich zu machen ist. Die Untersuchungsergebnisse von KAISER u. STOCKER (1974) an Kulturen von menschlichen Fibroblasten sprechen andererseits dafür, daß Allopurinol-1-N-Ribonucleotid und Oxypurinol-7-N-Ribonucleotid Hemmeffekte auf die Purin- und Pyrimidin-Synthese ausüben. Auch KELLEY u. WYNGAARDEN (1970) nehmen auf Grund ihrer Untersuchungen an menschlichen Fibroblasten am ehesten an, daß die Hemmwirkung auf die *de novo*-Synthese als Konsequenz der Umwandlung von Allopurinol in seine Ribonucleotid-Form anzusehen ist. Nach ihren Untersuchungen ist für Oxypurinol (allerdings in relativ hohen Konzentrationen in Fibroblastenkulturen) ein ähnlicher Wirkungsmechanismus auf die *de-novo*-Synthese anzunehmen.

ad γ) Substratverarmung von PRPP für die *de novo*-Purinsynthese

Nach Verabreichung von Allopurinol (2—4 mg/kg per os) kann innerhalb von 3—5 Std ein deutlicher PRPP-Abfall in den Erythrocyten der Versuchspersonen nachgewiesen werden (Fox et al., 1970b). Da die Erythrocyten keine Xanthin-Oxydase besitzen, kommt es hier bei Allopurinolgabe auch nicht direkt zur Akkumulation von Hypoxanthin und Xanthin. Ein vermehrter PRPP-Verbrauch durch erhöhte IMP-Bildung in der Reutilisation ist in den Erythrocyten damit kaum wahrscheinlich. Der PRPP-Abfall wird nach *in vivo*- und *in vitro*-Untersuchungen mit größter Wahrscheinlichkeit durch den Verbrauch an PRPP während der Umwandlung von Allopurinol zu Allopurinolribonucleotid erklärt (Fox et al., 1970b), denn bei Inkubation von Allopurinol mit Erythrocyten von Patienten mit HG-PRT-Mangel kommt es nicht zur Senkung des intracellulären PRPP (Fox et al., 1970b). Der durch die Umwandlung von Allopurinol zu Allopurinol-1-N-Ribonucleotid entstehende intracelluläre PRPP-Mangel könnte nun durch Substratmangel am ersten Schritt der *de novo*-Purinsynthese zu der bei Allopurinolgabe beobachteten verminderten Purinbiosynthese beitragen. Nach Oxypurinolverabreichung konnte dagegen kein PRPP-Abfall in Erythrocyten beobachtet werden (Fox et al., 1970b), obwohl auch hier zur Bildung von Oxypurinol-7-N-Ribonucleotid PRPP (in der Reaktion mit O-PRT) verbraucht wird. Es könnte sein, daß Untersuchungen am Erythrocyten für die Betrachtung der Gesamtsituation nicht relevant sind, da die Erythrocyten keinen *de novo*-Stoffwechselweg für die gesamte Purinsynthese aufweisen. In Fibroblasten, die eine vollständige *de-novo*-Purinsynthese haben, kommt es nämlich nicht zu einem signifikanten Abfall in der PRPP-Konzentration bei Allopurinolkonzentrationen von 0,1 mM (KELLEY et al., 1971a), und diese Konzentrationen sind 10—100mal höher als die Plasmaspiegel beim Menschen (ELION u. NELSON, 1974). Trotzdem wäre es z.B. in der Rattenleber möglich, daß bei hohen Allopurinoldosierungen genügend Allopurinol- und Oxypurinolribonucleotid gebildet würde, um zu einem kurzzeitigen Abfall der PRPP-Spiegel zu führen (ELION u. NELSON, 1974). Eine direkte Einwirkung auf die PRPP-Synthese durch Allopurinol scheidet nach *in vitro*-Untersuchungen von Fox et al. (1970b) mit größter Wahrscheinlichkeit als Ursache des PRPP-Abfalls aus. Aus Untersuchungen über den Einfluß von Allopurinol auf den Purinstoffwechsel bei einem Patienten mit kongenitalem Xanthin-Oxydase-Mangel (ENGELMAN et al., 1964) konnte geschlossen werden, daß der Effekt von Allopurinol nur indirekt über Änderungen der Hypoxanthin-Konzentration zustande kommen kann. Bei fehlender Xanthin-Oxydase muß die Hauptwirkung von Allopurinol (Bildung von Hypoxanthin und Xanthin statt Harnsäure) ausbleiben, mögliche Einflüsse bei Allopurinolgabe könnten dann nur durch eine direkte Wirkung auf die Purinbiosynthese entstehen. Nachdem sich bei diesem Patienten jedoch nach Gabe von Allopurinol kein Einfluß auf die Purinsynthese nachweisen ließ, wäre ein direkter Einfluß von Allopurinol oder Allopurinolribonucleotid auf die *de novo*-Purinsynthese eigentlich ausgeschlossen. In Fibroblasten von Patienten mit HG-PRT-Mangel hemmen hohe Konzentrationen von sowohl Allopurinol als auch Oxypurinol einen frühen Schritt der *de novo*-Purinsynthese (KELLEY u. WYNGAARDEN, 1970). Dies dürfte auf die Wirkung von Oxypurinol-7-N-Ribonucleotid zurückzuführen sein, welches unmittelbar aus Oxypurinol (durch die O-PRT) entsteht.

Auch wenn nicht alle experimentellen Daten eindeutig belegen können, daß die Ursache für die *in vivo*-Hemmwirkung von Allopurinol auf die *de novo*-Purinbiosynthese über einen primären PRPP-Abfall mit nachfolgender Substratverarmung zu erklären ist, spricht doch die Mehrzahl zumindest für eine teilweise Beteiligung dieses Mechanismus.

d) *Einfluß von Allopurinol auf die intestinale Absorption exogener Purine*

Allopurinolgabe scheint die Absorption von mit der Diät zugeführten Purinen zu vermindern bzw. die Re-Exkretion von Purinen in das Dünndarmlumen zu fördern. Für den Pyrimidintransport (zumindest Uracil) konnte *in vitro* am Rattendünndarm eine starke Hemmung nachgewiesen werden (SCHANKER et al., 1963). Allopurinolgabe führt beim Menschen zu einer signifikanten Verminderung der durch exogene RNA-Zufuhr (aus Hefe) erhöhten Purinausscheidung (KRAKOFF u. MEYER, 1965; BOWERING et al., 1969; DELBARRE et al., 1966; ZÖLLNER et al., 1972). Diese Wirkung kann nicht allein mit einer Feedback-Hemmung der Purinsynthese durch Allopurinol erklärt werden. Eine Erklärung hierfür wäre aber eine durch Allopurinol herbeigeführte verminderte Absorption bzw. erhöhte Exkretion von exogenen Purinen in das intestinale Lumen. Die quantitative Elimination der exogenen Uratquote bei Allopurinol-Verabreichung wäre evtl. zu erklären mit einer Anreicherung von Allopurinol im Dünndarmepithel während seiner Resorption (GRÖBNER u. ZÖLLNER, 1970). Ein Teil der durch Allopurinol herbeigeführten Verminderung der Purinexkretion könnte demnach bei Patienten, die sich nicht purinarm ernähren, durch intestinale Elimination der mit der Diät zugeführten Purine zustande kommen.

e) Einfluß von Allopurinol auf die Pyrimidinsynthese

Bei Patienten, die mit Allopurinol behandelt werden, kommt es zu einer erhöhten renalen Exkretion von Orotsäure und Orotidin (Fox et al., 1970). Die renale Orotsäure- und Orotidinausscheidung beträgt dabei zwischen 14,1 und 65,2 mg/24 Std (KELLEY u. BEARDMORE, 1970; BEARDMORE et al., 1972), d.h. es kommt zu einer 7—10fachen Erhöhung der renalen Ausscheidung dieser beiden Metaboliten des Pyrimidinstoffwechsels. Nach den Untersuchungen von BEARDMORE und KELLEY (1971b) und KELLEY et al. (1971) hemmt Oxypurinol und in geringerem Ausmaß Allopurinol die Umwandlung von Orotsäure zu UMP *in vivo* und in Zellkulturen. Oxypurinol-7-N-Ribonucleotid dürfte vermutlich der einzige Metabolit sein, der bei Lesch-Nyhan-Syndrom die auch bei diesen Patienten zu beobachtende Hemmung der *de novo*-Pyrimidinsynthese bewirkt (BEARDMORE u. KELLEY, 1971b).

Für die Hemmung der Pyrimidinsynthese durch Allopurinol kommen 2 Wirkungsmechanismen in Betracht: entweder direkt eine Feedback-Hemmung an den *ersten* Schritten der Pyrimidinsynthese oder eine verminderte PRPP-Synthese durch vermehrten Verbrauch von PRPP bei den Reaktionen mit Allopurinol. Damit würde ähnlich wie bei der Purinsynthese ein PRPP-Substratmangel für die späteren Schritte der *de novo*-Pyrimidinsynthese auftreten. Die Hemmwirkung auf die Pyrimidinsynthese scheint in erster Linie auf eine Hemmung der OMP-Decarboxylase durch Allopurinol-7-N-Ribonucleotid zurückzuführen zu sein (KELLEY u. BEARDMORE, 1974). In Erythrocyten von Patienten, die mit Allopurinol behandelt werden, ist die Aktivität sowohl der O-PRT als auch der OMP-Decarboxylase auf etwa das 5—8fache erhöht (BEARDMORE u. KELLEY, 1971a). Diese beiden Enzyme bilden einen Proteinkomplex, der unter bestimmten Bedingungen zur Assoziation bzw. Dissoziation fähig sein soll (BROWN et al., 1972). Die gleichzeitige, koordinierte Erhöhung der beiden Enzymaktivitäten unter Allopurinolgabe scheint teilweise durch eine Stabilisierung des Komplexes, infolge Bildung einer stärker aggregierten Form (z.B. ein Trimer des ursprünglichen Enzymkomplexes), zustande zu kommen, eine Induktion der *de novo*-Enzymprotein-Synthese konnte bis jetzt aber nicht sicher ausgeschlossen werden (BROWN et al., 1972).

Nach den Untersuchungen von KELLEY und BEARDMORE (1970) hemmen sowohl Allopurinol-1-N-Ribonucleotid und Xanthinribonucleotid als auch Oxypurinol-7-N-Ribonucleotid die OMP-Decarboxylase-Reaktion. Das erklärt auch, warum Allopurinol bei HG-PRT-Mangel (hier ist keine Bildung von Allopurinol-1-N-Ribonucleotid möglich) zu einer Orotsäureausscheidung führen kann (BEARDMORE et al., 1970). Allopurinol und Oxypurinol hemmen also nach den Untersuchungen von BEARDMORE u. KELLEY (1974) die *de novo*-Pyrimidinsynthese durch Hemmung der OMP-Decarboxylase. Diese Hemmung scheint über die Ribonucleotidderivate von Oxypurinol und Allopurinol (Allopurinol-1-N-Ribonucleotid, Oxypurinol-1-N-Ribonucleotid und Oxypurinol-7-N-Ribonucleotid) und Xanthosin-5-Monophosphat zustande zu kommen. Die Wirkung von Allopurinol auf den Pyrimidinstoffwechsel simuliert teilweise eine Form der Orotacidurie, bei der im Urin als Hauptmetabolit Orotidin ausgeschieden wird, die Orotsäureausscheidung ist dabei nur gering erhöht. Der entscheidende metabolische Block soll bei diesem Enzymdefekt an dem Enzym OMP-Decarboxylase lokalisiert sein (BROWN et al., 1972). Die Hemmung der Pyrimidinsynthese durch Allopurinolgabe könnte diesen Enzymdefekt nachahmen. Nachdem Defekte bei der Pyrimidinsynthese durch mangelhafte Synthese von UMP zu Störungen in der Synthese von Nucleinsäuren und Coenzymen führen könnten, wären theoretisch durch langzeitige Allopurinolgaben auch Störungen in diesem System nicht ganz auszuschließen. Bis jetzt konnten jedoch bei Therapie mit Allopurinol keine wesentlichen, klinisch signifikanten Abnormitäten im Pyrimidinstoffwechsel festgestellt werden.

f) Einflüsse von Allopurinol auf andere Enzymsysteme

Vermutlich infolge Hemmung der Xanthin-Oxydase und einem evtl. dadurch bedingten H_2O_2-Defizit kommt es durch Allopurinolgabe zu einer Hemmung der Tryptophanpyrrolase (CHYTIL, 1968; GHOSH u. FORREST, 1967). Bei Hühnern, denen längere Zeit Allopurinol verabreicht wurde, fanden WEIR u. FISHER (1970) eine starke Verminderung der Xanthin-Oxydase-Aktivität in der Leber und im Pankreas; wenn das Allopurinol jedoch aus den Leberextrakten entfernt wurde, betrug die Enzymaktivität das Doppelte der Kontrolltiere. Die Geschwindigkeit der Xanthin-Oxydase-Synthese war proportional erhöht, was diese Autoren mit einer verminderten Feedback-Repression der Xanthin-Oxydase-Synthese durch Harnsäure oder mit einer Induzierung der Enzymsynthese durch z. B. Allopurinol oder Xanthin und Hypoxanthin erklärten. Nach HITCHINGS et al. (1950) ist jedoch keine signifikante Induktion der Xanthin-Oxydase während Allopurinoltherapie nachzuweisen. Die Purinnucleosid-Phosphorylase (KRENITSKY et al., 1967; KRENITSKY et al., 1968) sowie die Pyrimidin-Desoxyribosyltransferase (GALLE et al., 1968) werden in vitro von Allopurinol gehemmt. Die Urat-Oxydase wird bei niedrigen Allopurinolkonzentrationen gehemmt, bei hohen aktiviert (TRUSEVE u. WILLIAMS, 1968).

g) Nebenwirkungen von Allopurinol

Ernsthafte Komplikationen während einer Allopurinoltherapie sind selten. KUZELL et al. (1966) fanden bei etwa 20% ihrer Patienten geringe Nebenwirkungen, bei etwa 5% ihrer Patienten setzten sie das Medikament wegen stärkerer Nebenwirkungen ab. Diese Zahlen sind nach unserer Erfahrung sicher zu hoch.

Zu Beginn der Allopurinoltherapie werden vermehrt Gichtanfälle beobachtet (YÜ u. GUTMAN, 1964). Das dürfte damit zusammenhängen, daß bei jeder raschen Änderung der Serumharnsäure, sowohl zu hohen als auch zu niedrigen Werten ("uric acid on move") häufiger Gichtanfälle auftreten. Aus diesem Grunde wird gerne empfohlen, während der ersten Monate der Allopurinoltherapie zusätzlich täglich Colchicin zu verabreichen. Eine direkte Erhöhung der Entzündungsbereitschaft durch Allopurinol ist nicht anzunehmen; auf Grund tierexperimenteller Untersuchungen ist sogar vermutet worden, daß Allopurinol selbst eine direkte, wenn auch geringe antiphlogistische Wirkung entfaltet. In verschiedenen Tiermodellen wurde eine iatrogen verstärkte vasculäre Permeabilität durch Allopurinol gehemmt (RIESTERER u. JAQUES, 1969; JAQUES u. HELFER, 1971). Da es während einer Therapie mit Allopurinol zu einer geringen Erhöhung in der Oxypurinkonzentration kommt und vor allem Xanthin in neutralem und saurem Urin schlecht löslich ist (KLINENBERG et al., 1965) wäre daran zu denken, daß es während der Allopurinolbehandlung zur Ausfällung von Xanthinkristallen oder Xanthinsteinen im harnableitenden System kommen könnte (Löslichkeit im Urin 8,0 mg/100 ml bei pH 5,0 13 mg/100 ml bei pH 7,0). Unter normalen Umständen wurden solche Ausfällungen nicht beobachtet, da die kritische Löslichkeit von Xanthin bei 10 mg/100 ml Serum und diejenige von Hypoxanthin bei 115 mg/100 ml Serum liegt; darüber hinaus ist die Clearance von Oxypurinen etwa 10mal höher als die der Harnsäure. Bei exzessiver Harnsäureexkretion jedoch, z. B. beim Lesch-Nyhan-Syndrom (SORENSEN u. SEEGMILLER, 1968; GREENE et al., 1969), mit einer Harnsäureexkretion um 1500 mg/24 Std oder bei cytostatischer Therapie (BAND et al., 1970), kann es jedoch auch unter Allopurinoltherapie zur Entwicklung von Xanthinsteinen kommen.

Von WATTS et al. (1971) wurden bei Patienten, die unter Allopurinoltherapie standen, in den Muskeln Xanthin-, Hypoxanthin- und Oxypurinolkristalle gefunden, ohne daß klinische Manifestationen einer Muskelerkrankung nachgewiesen werden konnten. Selten werden während einer Allopurinoltherapie vermehrt Kopfschmerzen und verschiedene gastrointestinale Symptome (Übelkeit, Brechreiz und Diarrhoen) beobachtet (YÜ u. GUTMAN, 1964). Diese können teilweise vermieden werden durch Einnahme der Tabletten mit genügend Flüssigkeitsmenge oder nach dem Essen. Weitere seltene toxische Nebenwirkungen sind Überempfindlichkeitsreaktionen an der Haut wie Juckreiz und Exantheme, manchmal mit Temperaturerhöhungen (KLINENBERG et al., 1966). Nach Untersuchungen an der Universität Boston (JICK et al., 1972) scheint bei Allopurinolgabe besonders häufig eine Überempfindlichkeitsreaktion der Haut auf Ampicillin aufzutreten (in 22,4% gegenüber 7,5% bei Personen ohne gleichzeitige Allopurinolgabe, d.h., das relative Risiko war bei Kombination von Allopurinol und Ampicillin 3mal höher). Leukopenien, Thrombocytopenien, Hepatitis und Vasculitis wurden gelegentlich unter Allopurinoltherapie beobachtet (JARZOBSKY et al., 1970). Kontraindiziert ist vorerst die Therapie mit Allopurinol während der Schwangerschaft und Stillzeit, obwohl im Tierversuch keine Zunahme an Mißbildungen der Totgeburten beobachtet wurde. Bei dringender Indikation scheint die Gabe von Allopurinol vom 4. Schwangerschaftsmonat an erlaubt. Auf Grund früherer Untersuchungen wurden Einflüsse von Allopurinol auf die Absorption, Speicherung oder Utilisation von Eisen angenommen. Dies scheint jedoch nicht signifikant zu sein (HITCHINGS, 1964; RUNDLES et al., 1966). Bei Ratten wurde unter Allopurinolgabe eine Vermehrung des Eisengehaltes in der Leber festgestellt. Da mögliche Einflüsse auf den Eisenstoffwechsel durch Allopurinol nicht ganz ausgeschlossen werden können, wird empfohlen, Allopurinol- und Eisentherapie nicht zu kombinieren; an Patienten mit idiopathischer Hämochromatose oder deren nahen Blutsverwandten sollte Allopurinol nur bei dringendster Indikation verabreicht werden.

Die enzymatische Oxydation von 6-Mercaptopurin zum Endprodukt 6-Thioharnsäure wird durch Allopurinol gehemmt. Bei gleichzeitiger Gabe von Allopurinol und 6-Mercaptopurin bzw. Azathioprin muß also zur Vermeidung von Überdosierungserscheinungen die Dosis der letzteren um etwa 75% vermindert werden (KELLEY, 1968). Da Allopurinol die Pharmakokinetik von Cumarinderivaten beeinflußt, sollte bei gleichzeitiger Gabe beider Medikamente die Blutgerinnung besonders sorgfältig kontrolliert werden. Nach VESELL et al.(1971) betrug z.B. die mittlere Halbwertszeit für Dicumarol im Plasma von Normalpersonen 51,0±9 Std, nach zweiwöchiger Allopurinolgabe (2,5 mg/kg per os pro Tag) hatte sich dieser Wert auf das Dreifache (152,5±72,6 Std) erhöht. In gleicher Weise verlängert Allopurinol die Halbwertszeit von Antipyrin (VESELL et al. 1971). Als Mechanismus für diese Wirkungen von Allopurinol wird von den Autoren (auf Grund ihrer Untersuchungen an Rattenlebern) eine verminderte hepatische Metabolisierung dieser beiden Substanzen angenommen.

2. Hemmung der de novo-Purinsynthese durch verschiedene andere Purinanaloge

Die antimetabolische Wirkung dieser Pharmaka wird vor allem bei der cytostatischen Therapie von Tumoren eingesetzt. Ihre primäre Anwendung liegt in der Wachstumshemmung leukämischer Zellen. Da sie keine qualitativen biochemischen Unterschiede zwischen normalen und malignen Zellen machen, ist ihre direkte Anwendung bei der Behandlung der primären Hyperurikämie oder Gicht wegen ihrer toxischen Nebenwirkungen nicht angezeigt.

Mit 6-Mercaptopurin, Azathioprin, 6-Thioguanin, 8-Azaguanin, 6-Mercaptopurin-Ribonucleotid und 6-Methylmercaptopurin-Ribonucleosid konnte an verschiedenen Geweben eine Hemmung der *de novo*-Purinsynthese nachgewiesen werden (s. Abb. 2). Bei Blockierung mit Azaserin kommt es jeweils zur verminderten Akkumulation von FGAR (BROCKMAN u. ANDERSON, 1963). Zur Hemmung der *de novo*-Purinsynthese in Form einer Pseudo-Feedback-Hemmung auf die PRPP-Amidotransferase ist die vorherige Umwandlung dieser Substanzen in die jeweilige Ribonucleotidform durch das Enzym HG-PRT erforderlich (BROCKMAN u. ANDERSON, 1963; BROCKMAN, 1969; MCCOLLISTER et al., 1964).

6-Mercaptopurin

Diese Substanz wurde 1952 synthetisiert (ELION et al.) und 1953 klinisch eingesetzt (BURCHENAL et al., 1953; MINER u. RHOADS, 1954). 6-Mercaptopurin, ein Strukturanaloges von Hypoxanthin, verhindert die celluläre Hypoxanthinaufnahme und vermindert damit die Synthese von Inosin. Normalerweise ist dies von geringerer Bedeutung, da Inosin in der *de novo*-Synthese aus IMP entstehen kann. Im Gesamtkörper scheint jedoch auch eine Hemmung dieses Stoffwechselweges eine gewisse Bedeutung zu haben. Die Hauptwirkung von 6-Mercaptopurin tritt nach seiner Umwandlung zum Ribonucleotid Thio-IMP auf. Durch diese Substanz werden verschiedene Stoffwechselwege der Purinsynthese beeinflußt. Als Hauptwirkung wird die Hemmung der Umwandlung von IMP zu S-AMP und XMP und die weitere Umwandlung von S-AMP zu AMP und von XMP zu GMP angesehen (s. Abb. 2). So hemmt also 6-Mercaptopurin nicht nur den Einbau bzw. die Reutilisation von IMP, sondern auch durch sein Nucleotid die Stoffwechselwege die von Hypoxanthin zu AMP und GMP führen. Die dadurch entstehende Akkumulation von IMP führt zur Feedback-Hemmung an der PRPP-Amidotransferase. Eine weitere Hemmung an diesem Schritt kommt darüber hinaus direkt durch negative Feedback-Hemmung mit dem gebildeten Thio-IMP zustande. Eine gewisse Resistenz gegenüber 6-Mercaptopurin tritt bei HG-PRT-Mangel auf, da dieses Enzym zur Umwandlung von 6-Mercaptopurin zu Thio-IMP benötigt wird. Die höchste Wirksamkeit weist 6-Mercaptopurin in jenen Zellen auf, die besonders abhängig von Hypoxanthin als Purinnucleotidquelle sind. Etwa 25—30% des 6-Mercaptopurin wird normalerweise durch Xanthin-Oxydase zu dem inerten Metaboliten 6-Thioharnsäure, der dann im Urin ausgeschieden wird, umgewandelt (HAMILTON u. ELION, 1954; ELION et al., 1962).

In vitro sind sowohl 6-Mercaptopurin als auch 6-Thioharnsäure noch kompetitive Hemmer der Xanthin-Oxydation durch das Enzym Xanthin-Oxydase (SILBERMAN u. WYNGAARDEN, 1961). Da Allopurinol die Oxydation von 6-Mercaptopurin zu 6-Thioharnsäure durch die Xanthin-Oxydase hemmt, muß, bei gleichzeitiger Gabe von Allopurinol, die Dosierung von 6-Mercaptopurin bzw. Azathioprin zur Vermeidung toxischer Nebenwirkungen dieser Substanzen um etwa 75% gesenkt werden. Allopurinol potenziert also den cytotoxischen Effekt von 6-Mercaptopurin auf die Zellproliferation.

Azathioprin (6-[1-methyl-4-nitro-5-imidazolyl]-thiopurin)

Azathioprin ist ein Derivat von 6-Mercaptopurin. Azathioprin und 6-Mercaptopurin wirken in hoher Dosierung antileukämisch, in niedriger Dosierung immunsuppressiv. Klinisch hat es besondere Bedeutung als Immunsuppressivum, als solches wird es vor allem zur Kontrolle der Abstoßungsreaktion von Transplantaten und bei Autoimmunerkrankungen verwendet. Azathioprin scheint weniger toxisch als 6-Mercaptopurin zu sein, vermutlich durch die langsame Freisetzung von 6-Mercaptopurin (ELION, 1967). Die aktive Form entsteht durch eine nichtenzymatische Spaltung in die freie Mercapto-Verbindung und eine daraufhin erfolgende Umwandlung in 6-Mercaptoribonucleotid. Aus der Tatsache, daß bei Patienten mit HG-PRT-Mangel nach Gabe von Azathioprin keine Hemmung der *de novo*-Synthese auftritt, darf man schließen, daß diese Form die aktive Hemmsubstanz bei der Pseudo-Feedback-Hemmung sein muß (SORENSEN, 1963); KELLEY et al., 1967a; SORENSEN u. BENKE, 1967). Die Senkung der Plasmaharnsäurekonzentration, der renalen Harnsäureausscheidung (um etwa 40%) bei Gichtpatienten während Azathiopringabe, wurde erstmals 1966 von SORENSEN beobachtet. Als Wirkungsmechanismus wurde eine Hemmung der *de novo*-Purinsynthese angesehen. Ähnliche Ergebnisse wurden von anderen Untersuchern gefunden (KELLEY et al., 1967a).

Da weder im Serum noch im Urin während der Therapie mit Azathioprin die Oxypurine ansteigen, darf man annehmen, daß die verminderte Harnsäurebildung nicht auf einer Hemmung der Xanthin-Oxydase beruht. Azathioprin hemmt demnach die *de novo*-Purinsynthese. Die Hemmung ist bei jenen Gichtpatienten am größten, die eine erhöhte *de novo*-Harnsäure- bzw. Purinsynthese aufweisen. Als Hemm-Mechanismus nimmt man eine Pseudo-Feedback-Hemmung auf die PRPP-Amidotransferase an (SORENSEN, 1966; KELLEY et al., 1967a). Die erforderliche Dosierung zur Senkung der Serumharnsäure beim Menschen ist relativ hoch.

6-Methylmercaptopurin-Ribonucleosid (6-Methyl-thioinosin)

1965 fand HENDERSON, daß diese Substanz ein sehr starker *in vitro*-Hemmer der Phosphoribosyl-Formylglycinamid-Synthese in Ehrlich-Ascites-Tumorzellen war. Seine Hemmung betrug ungefähr das 500fache des stärksten natürlichen Hemmers Adenin. Diese Hemmung der *de novo*-Purinsynthese wurde auch an menschlichen Fibroblastenkulturen (ROSENBLOOM et al., 1968) und *in vivo* an verschiedenen Geweben der Maus beobachtet (HENDERSON u. MERCER, 1966). 6-Methylmercaptopurin-Ribonucleosid scheint der stärkste Hemmer der PRPP-Amidotransferase in Zellextrakten (MCCOLLISTER et al., 1964) und intakten Zellen (HENDERSON, 1963) zu sein. Der Wirkungsmechanismus auf die Purinbiosynthese ist jenem von 6-Mercaptopurin ähnlich, es wird *in vivo* durch eine Kinase in die Nucleotidform umgewandelt.

6-Thioguanin

6-Thioguanin ist in seinem klinischen Anwendungsbereich und in seinen antimetabolischen Eigenschaften dem 6-Mercaptopurin ähnlich. Es unterscheidet sich vom 6-Mercaptopurin chemisch durch die Aminogruppe am C-Atom 2. 6-Thioguanin hemmt nach seiner Umwandlung zum Ribonucleotid (durch die HG-PRT) eine Reihe von Stoffwechselwegen, die zur Bildung von Purinnucleotiden führen. Nachgewiesen ist die Hemmung der *de novo*-Purinsynthese von Mäusetumoren. Ähnlich wie für 6-Mercaptopurin ist eine Feedback-Hemmung auf die PRPP-Amidotransferase zu beobachten.

8-Azaguanin

Die Wirkungsweise dieses Antimetaboliten ähnelt derjenigen von 6-Mercaptopurin und 6-Thioguanin. Einige seiner antimetabolischen Effekte kommen darüber hinaus sicher durch seinen Einbau als Guaninanaloges in RNA zustande, wodurch es zur Hemmung der Proteinsynthese kommen kann.

5-Aminoimidazol-4-Carboxamid(AICAR)

AICAR hemmt in hoher Dosierung gleichfalls die *de novo*-Purinsynthese beim Menschen (SEEGMILLER et al., 1955). Seine Wirkungsweise kommt wahrscheinlich durch die Umwandlung dieses Stoffwechsel-Zwischenprodukts in normale Nucleotide und die danach erfolgende Aktivierung endogener Feedback-Mechanismen zustande. Eine Folge dieser Umwandlung ist jedoch der Abbau dieser auf solche Weise gebildeten Nucleotide zu Harnsäure; damit wird die Hemmung der Purinsynthese in der Gesamtbilanz der Harnsäuresynthese teilweise wieder aufgehoben (SEEGMILLER et al., 1955; SORENSEN, 1966).

Antibiotica

Eine Reihe von Antibiotica beeinflussen die Purinsynthese (z.B. Psicofuranin, Cordycepin und Tubercidin). Alle sind chemisch verwandt mit Adenosin, weshalb sie auch vor allem jene Enzyme hemmen, die Adenin und seine Derivate metabolisieren.

Hadacidin (N-Formyl-Hydroxylamino-Essigsäure)

Hadacidin, ein Analoges von L-Aspartat, hemmt die Umwandlung von IMP zu N-Succinyl-Adenylsäure und XMP. Die toxischen Nebenerscheinungen dieser Substanz schließen eine klinische Anwendung aus.

Adenin

Adenin hemmt vermutlich durch Aktivierung des Feedback-Kontrollmechanismus an der PRPP-Amidotransferase (FOX et al., 1970b) oder durch Verminderung der intrazellulären PRPP-Konzentration die Purinbiosynthese. Zumindest könnte man dies aus einer signifikanten Hemmung des ^{15}N-Glycineinbaus in die renale Harnsäure nach Adeninverabreichung sowohl bei Normalpersonen als auch bei Gichtpatienten schließen (SEEGMILLER et al., 1968).

Orotsäure

Durch Verabreichung von Orotsäure (2—6 g/die) kann beim Menschen eine Senkung des Harnsäurespiegels im Serum erreicht werden (STANDERFER u. HANDLER, 1959; KELLEY et al., 1970a). Diese Wirkung kommt sowohl durch vermehrte Harnsäureausscheidung als auch durch eine Hemmung der Purinbiosynthese zustande (KELLEY et al., 1970b). Dies letztere vermutlich wiederum durch Verminderung des für die PRPP-Amidotransferase essentiellen Substrats PRPP (Verbrauch von PRPP bei der Umwandlung von Orotsäure zu OMP durch das Enzym O-PRT).

So kommt es auch nach der Verabreichung von Orotsäure zu einem intraerythrocytären PRPP-Abfall (2 g Orotsäure führen bereits 4 Std nach Verabreichung zu einem Abfall des intrazellulären PRPP auf 45%). Die Verminderung des ^{14}C-Glycineinbaus in die renale Harnsäure beträgt nach KELLEY et al. (1970a) 21—38%. Bei Patienten mit HG-PRT-Mangel ist hingegen kein Effekt nachweisbar. Gegen eine risikolose klinische Verwendung von Orotsäure zur Senkung des Serumharnsäurespiegels spricht in erster Linie die bei der Ratte beobachtete rasche Entwicklung einer Fettleber (STANDERFER u. HANDLER, 1969; CREASEY et al., 1961).

IV. Abbau der Harnsäure innerhalb des Körpers durch Injektion von Urikase

Durch Infusion bzw. Injektion von hoch gereinigter Urikase kann eine vorübergehende Senkung des Serumharnsäurespiegels erreicht werden (ALTMAN et al., 1949; LANDON u. HUDSON, 1957; KISSEL et al., 1968). Zur Therapie der Hyperurikämie ist Uricase jedoch nicht geeignet, da sich bei intravenöser Verabreichung sehr schnell Antikörper gegen das Enzymprotein entwickeln, wodurch die Wirksamkeit in kurzer Zeit aufgehoben wird (VILLIAUMEY, et al., 1972).

V. Stimulation der Purinbiosynthese durch Medikamente

1956 beobachteten KRAKOFF u. MAGILL beim Menschen nach Anwendung von 2-Ethylamino-1,2,3-Thiadiazol (EAT) eine Erhöhung des Serumharnsäurespiegels von z. B. 6 auf 15 mg/100 ml und eine Erhöhung der renalen Harnsäureausscheidung um das 4—5fache. Da der Einbau von radioaktiv markiertem Glycin und Formiat in die renale Harnsäure durch EAT erhöht und die Erhöhung der renalen Harnsäureausscheidung bei Gabe von EAT durch Azaserin und DON verhindert werden konnte, lag der Verdacht nahe, daß dieses Medikament die *de novo*-Purinsynthese erhöht. Sogar bei Patienten mit Lesch-Nyhan-Syndrom, bei denen die Geschwindigkeit des Glycineinbaus in die renale Harnsäure bereits 20mal höher als bei Normalpersonen war, konnten NYHAN et al. (1968) eine Erhöhung des Glycineinbaus auf das 30fache des Normalen beobachten; die Serumharnsäurekonzentration stieg von 11 auf 25,4 mg/100 ml, die renale Harnsäureexkretion von 900 auf 4000 mg/die. Das bedeutet, daß die Wirkung von EAT auf die Purinbiosynthese unabhängig von der Aktivität der HG-PRT ist. Interessanterweise kann die Erhöhung der *de novo*-Purinsynthese mit EAT durch gleichzeitige Gabe hoher Dosen Nikotinamid (oder Nikotinsäure) verhindert werden (SEEGMILLER et al., 1959).

Literatur

ALEXANDER, S., BRENDLER, H.: Treatment of uric acid urolithiasis with allopurinol, a xanthine oxidase inhibitor. J. Urol. **97**, 340—343 (1967).

ALTMAN, K. I., SMULL, K., GUZMAN-BARRON, E. S.: A new method for the preparation of uricase and the effect of uricase on the blood uric acid levels of the chicken. Arch. Biochem. **21**, 158—165 (1949).

ANDERSON, E. E., RUNDLES, R. W., SOLBERMAN, H. R., METZ, E. N.: Allopurinol control of hyperuricosuria: a new concept in the prevention of uric acid stones. J. Urol. **97**, 344—347 (1967).

AUSCHER, C., MERCIER, N., PASQUIER, C., DELBARRE, F.: Allopurinol and thiopurinol: effect *in vivo* on uricary oxypurine excretion and rate of synthesis of their ribonucleotides in different enzymatic deficiencies. In: SPERLING, O., DE VRIES, A., WYNGAARDEN, J. B. (Eds.): Advances in Experimental Medicine and Biology. Vol. 41 B. Purine metabolism in man, pp. 657—662. New York-London: Plenum Press 1974.

BAND, P. R., SILVERBERG, D. S., HENDERSON, J. F., ULAN, R. A., WENSEL, R. H., BANERJEE, T. K., LITTLE, A. S.: Xanthine nephropathy in a patient with lymphosarcoma treated with allopurinol. New. Engl. J. Med. **283**, 354—357 (1970).

BEARDMORE, T. D., CASHMAN, J., KELLEY, W. N.: Mechanism of allopurinol mediated increase in enzyme activity in man. J. clin. Invest. **51**, 1823—1832 (1972).

BEARDMORE, T. D., FOX, I. H., KELLEY, W. N.: Effect of allopurinol on pyrimidine metabolism in the Lesch-Nyhan syndrome. Lancet **1970 II**, 830—831.

BEARDMORE, T. D., KELLEY, W. N.: Studies on the mechanism of allopurinol-induced inhibition of pyrimidine metabolism. Clin. Res. **19**, 27 (1971a).

BEARDMORE, T. D., KELLEY, W. N.: Mechanism of allopurinol mediated inhibition of pyrimidine biosynthesis. J. Lab. clin. Med. **78**, 696—704 (1971b).

BEARDMORE, T. D., KELLEY, W. N.: Effects of allopurinol and oxipurinol on pyrimidine biosynthesis in man. In: SPERLING, O., DE VRIES, A., WYNGAARDEN, J. B. (Eds.): Advances in Experimental Medicine and Biology. Vol. 41 B. Purine metabolism in man, pp. 609—619. New York-London: Plenum Press 1974.

BENNETT, L. L., JR., SCHABEL, F. M., JR., SHIPPER, H. E.: Studies on the mode of action of azaserine. Arch. Biochem. Biophys. **64**, 423—436 (1956).

BERGMANN, F., UNGAR, H.: The enzymatic oxidation of 6-mercaptopurine to 6-thiouric acid. J. Amer. chem. Soc. **82**, 3957—3960 (1960).

BOWERING, J., MARGEN, S., CALLOWAY, D. H., RHYNE, A.: Suppression of uric acid formation from dietary nucleic acid with allopurinol. Amer. J. clin. Nutr. **22**, 1426—1428 (1969).

BROCKMAN, R. W.: Metabolism and mechanisms of action of purine analogues. In: Exploitable Molecular Mechanism and Neoplasia, pp. 435—464. Baltimore: Williams & Wilkins 1969.

BROCKMAN, R. W., ANDERSON, E. P.: Biochemistry of cancer (metabolic aspects). Ann. Rev. Biochem. **32**, 463—512 (1963).

BROCKMAN, R. W., CHUMLEY, S.: Inhibition of formylglycinamide ribonucleotide synthesis in neoplastic cells by purines and analogues. Biochim. biophys. Acta (Amst.) **95**, 365—379 (1965).

Brown, G. K., Fox, R. M., O'Sullivan, W. J.: Alteration of quaternary structural behaviour of an hepatic orotate phosphoribosyltransferase-orotidine-5′-phosphate-decarboxylase complex in rats following allopurinol therapy. Biochem. Pharmacol. **21**, 2469—2477 (1972).

Burchenal, J. H., Murphy, M. L., Ellison, R. R., Sykes, M. P., Tan, T. C., Leone, L. A., Karnofsky, D. A., Crarer, L. F., Dargeon, H. W., Rhoads, C. P.: Clinical evaluation of a new antimetabolite, 6-mercaptopurine, in the treatment of leukemia and allied diseases. Blood **8**, 965—999 (1953).

Chalwers, R. A., Krömer, H., Scott, J. T., Watts, R. W. E.: A comparative study of the xanthine oxidase inhibitors, allopurinol and oxipurinol in man. Clin. Sci. **35**, 353—362 (1968).

Chytil, F.: Activation of liver tryptophan oxygenase by adenosine 3′, 5′-phosphate and by other purine derivatives. J. Biol. Chem. **243**, 893—899 (1968).

Creasey, W. A., Hankin, L., Handschumacher, R. E.: Fatty livers induced by orotic acid. I. Accumulation and metabolism of lipids. J. biol. Chem. **236**, 2064—2070 (1961).

Delbarre, F., Amer, B., Auscher, C., De Gery, A.: Treatment of gout with allopurinol, a study of 106 cases. Ann. rheum. Dis. **25**, 627—633 (1966).

Delbarre, F., Auscher, C., De Gery, A., Brouilhet, H., Olivier, J.-L.: Le traitement de la dyspurine goutteuse par la mercaptopyrazolo-pyrimidine (MPP: thiopurinol). Presse méd. **76**, 2329—2332 (1968).

Duggan, D. E., Titus, E.: 6-chloropurine and 6-chlorouric acid as substrates and inhibitors of purine-oxidizing enzymes. J. biol. Chem. **234**, 2100—2104 (1959).

Elion, G. B.: Enzymatic and metabolic studies with allopurinol. Ann. rheum. Dis. **25**, 608—614 (1966).

Elion, G. B.: Biochemistry and pharmacology of purine analogues. Fed. Proc. **26**, 898—903 (1967).

Elion, G. B., Burgi, E., Hitchings, G. H.: Studies on condensed pyrimidine systems. IX. The synthesis of some 6-substituted purines. J. Amer. chem. Soc. **74**, 411—414 (1952).

Elion, G. B., Callahan, S. W., Hitchings, G. H., Rundles, R. W., Laszlo, J.: Experimental, clinical and metabolic studies of thiopurines. In: Cancer Chemother. Rep. No. 16, p. 197 (1962).

Elion, G. B., Callahan, S., Nathan, H., Bieber, S., Rundles, R. W., Hitchings, G. H.: Potentiation by inhibition of drug degradation: 6-substituted purines and xanthine oxidase. Biochem. Pharmacol. **12**, 85—93 (1963).

Elion, G. B., Kovensky, A., Hitchings, G. H., Metz, E., Rundles, R. W.: Metabolic studies of allopurinol, an inhibitor of xanthine oxidase. Biochem. Pharmacol. **15**, 863—880 (1966).

Elion, G. B., Nelson, D. J.: Ribonucleotides of allopurinol and oxipurinol in rat tissues and their significance in purine metabolism. In: Sperling, O., De Vries, A., Wyngaarden, J. B. (Eds.): Advances in Experimental. New York-London: Plenum Press 1974.

Elion, G. B., Taylor, T. J., Hitchings, G. H.: Binding of substrates and inhibitors to xanthine oxidase from different species. Abstracts of Communications to the 6th International Congress of Biochemistry, New York, p. 305 (1964).

Elion, G. B., Yu, T. F., Gutman, A. B., Hitchings, G. H.: Renal clearance of oxipurinol, the chief metabolite of allopurinol. Amer. J. Med. **45**, 69—77 (1968).

Ellison, R. R., Karnofsky, D. A., Sternberg, S. S., Murphy, M. L., Burchenal, J. H.: Clinical trials of o-diazoacetyl-1-serine (azaserine) in neoplastic disease. Cancer **7**, 801—814 (1954).

Emmerson, B. T.: Discussion — Symposium on allopurinol. Ann. rheum. Dis. **25**, 621—622 (1966).

Engelman, K., Watts, R. W. E., Klinenberg, J. R., Sjoerdsma, A., Seegmiller, J. E.: Clinical, physiological and biochemical studies of a patient with xanthinuria and pheochromocytoma. Amer. J. Med. **37**, 839—861 (1964).

Feigelson, P., Davidson, J. D., Robius, R. K.: Pyrazolopyrimidines as inhibitors and substrates of xanthine oxidase. J. biol. Chem. **226**, 993—1000 (1957).

Fox, R. M., Royse-Smith, D., O'Sullivan, W. J.: Orotidinuria induced by allopurinol. Science **168**, 861—862 (1970a).

Fox, R. M., Wood, M. H., O'Sullivan, W. J.: Studies on the coordinate activity and lability of orotidylate phosphoribosyltransferase and decarboxylase in human erythrocytes and the effects of allopurinol administration. J. clin. Invest. **50**, 1050—1060 (1971).

Fox, I. H., Wyngaarden, J. B., Kelley, W. N.: Depletion of erythrocyte phosphoribosylpyrophosphate in man, a newly observed effect of allopurinol. New. Engl. J. Med. **283**, 1177—1182 (1970).

Franklin, T. J., Cook, J. M.: The inhibition of nucleic acid synthesis by mycophenolic acid. Biochem. J. **113**, 515—524 (1969).

FRIDOVICH, I.: A new class of xanthine oxidase inhibitors isolated from guanidinium salts. Biochemistry (Wash.) **4**, 1098 (1965).

FYFE, J. A., NELSON, D. J., HITCHINGS, G. H.: The molecular basis for the effects of allopurinol on pyrimidine metabolism. In: SPERLING, O., DE VRIES, A., WYNGAARDEN, J. B. (Eds.): Advances in Experimental Medicine and Biology. Vol. 41 B. Purine metabolism in man, pp. 621—628. New York-London: Plenum Press 1974.

GALLO, R. D., PERRY, S., BREITMAN, T. R.: Inhibition of human leukocyte pyrimidine deoxynucleoside synthesis by allopurinol and 6-mercaptopurine. Biochem. Pharmacol. **17**, 2185—2191 (1968).

GHOSH, D., FORREST, H. S.: Inhibition of tryptophan pyrrolase by some naturally occurring pteridines. Arch. Biochem. **120**, 578—582 (1967).

GOLDFINGER, S., KLINENBERG, J. R., SEEGMILLER, J. E.: The renal excretion of oxypurines. J. clin. Invest. **44**, 623—628 (1965).

GRAHAME, R., SIMMONDS, H. A., CADENHEAD, A., DEAN, B. M.: Metabolic studies of thiopurinol in man and the pig. In: SPERLING, O., DE VRIES, A., WYNGAARDEN, J. B. (Eds.): Advances in Experimental Medicine and Biology. Vol. 41 B. Purine metabolism in man, pp. 597—605. New York-London: Plenum Press 1974.

GRAYZEL, A. I., SEEGMILLER, J. E., LOVE, E.: Suppression of uric acid synthesis in the gouty human by the use of 6-diazo-5-oxo-l-norleucine. J. clin. Invest. **39**, 447—454 (1960).

GREENE, M. L., FRYIMOTO, W. Y., SEEGMILLER, J. E.: Urinary xanthine stones—a rare complication of allopurinol therapy. New Engl. J. Med. **280**, 426—427 (1969).

GRÖBNER, W., ZÖLLNER, N.: Das unterschiedliche Verhalten der endogenen und exogenen Uratquote nach Verabreichung von Allopurinol. Hoppe-Seylers Z. physiol. Chem. **351**, 1305—1306 (1970).

HALL, A. P., HOLLOWAY, V. P., SCOTT, J. T.: 4-hydroxypyrazolo (3,4 −d)pyrimidine (HPP) in the treatment of gout. Preliminary observations. Amer. rheum. Dis. **23**, 439—446 (1964).

HAMILTON, L., ELION, G. B.: The fate of 6-mercaptopurine in man. Ann. N.Y. Acad. Sci. **60**, 304—314 (1955).

HAMPTON, A.: Reactions of ribonucleotide derivatives of purine analogues at the catalytic site of inosine-5′-phosphate dehydrogenase. J. biol. Chem. **238**, 3068—3074 (1963).

HENDERSON, J. F.: Feedback inhibition of purine biosynthesis in ascites tumor cells by purine analogues. Biochem. Pharmacol. **12**, 551—556 (1963).

HENDERSON, J. F., LE PAGE, G. A., McIVER, F. A.: Observations on the action of azaserine in mammilian tissues. Cancer Res. **17** (6), 609—612 (1957).

HENDERSON, J. F., MERCER, N. J. H.: Feedback inhibition of purine biosynthesis *de novo* in mouse tissues *in vivo*. Nature (London) **212**, 507—508 (1966).

HENDERSON, J. F., PATERSON, A. R. P.: Nucleotide Metabolism, pp. 148—149. New York-London: Academic-Press 1973.

HITCHINGS, G. H.: In: PLATTNER, P. A. (Ed.): Chemotherapy of Cancer, p. 77. Amsterdam: Elsevier 1964.

HITCHINGS, G. H.: Effects of allopurinol in relation to purine biosynthesis. Ann. rheum. Dis. **25**, 601—607 (1966).

HITCHINGS, G. H.: Chemotherapy and comparative biochemistry: G. H. A. CLOWES memorial lecture. Cancer Res. **29**, 1895—1903 (1969a).

HITCHINGS, G. H.: Allopurinol, an inhibitor of xanthine oxidase; physiological and biochemical studies. FEBS Symposium **16**, 11—22 (1969b).

HITCHINGS, G. H., ELION, G. B., FALLO, E. A., RUSSELL, P. B., VAN DER WERFF, H.: Studies on analogues of purines and pyrimidines. Ann. N.Y. Acad. Sci. **52**, 1318—1335 (1950).

IWATA, H., YAMAMOTO, I., MURAKI, K.: Potent xanthine oxidase inhibitors—4(or 5)-diazo-imidazole-5(or 4)—carboxamide and two related compounds. Biochem. Pharmacol. **18**, 955—957 (1969).

JAQUES, R., HELFER, H.: The antinociceptive and anti-exudative action of a xanthine oxidase inhibitor (allopurinol) and of xanthine. Pharmacology **5**, 49—54 (1971).

JARZOBSKY, J., FERRY, J., WOMBOLT, D., FITCH, D. M., EGAN, J. D.: Vasculitis with allopurinol therapy. Amer. Heart J. **79**, 116—121 (1970).

JICK, H., SLONE, D. et al. (Boston Collaborative Drug Surveillance Program.): Excess of ampicillin rashes associated with allopurinol or hyperuricemia. New Engl. J. Med. **286**, 505—507 (1972).

KAISER, W., STOCKER, K.: Purine and pyrimidine biosynthesis in neurospora crassa and human skin fibroblasts. Alteration by ribosides and ribotides of allopurinol and oxipurinol. In: SPERLING, O., DE VRIES, A., WYNGAARDEN, J. B. (Eds.): Advances in Experimental Medicine and Biology. Vol. 41 B. Purine metabolism in men, pp. 629—635. New York-London: Plenum Press 1974.

KANN, H. E., JR., WELLS, J. H., GALLELLI, J. F., SCHEIN, P. S., COONEY, D. A., SMITH, E. R., SEEGMILLER, J. E., CARBONE, P. P.: The development and use of an intravenous preparation of allopurinol. Amer. J. med. Sci. **256**, 53—63 (1968).

KELLEY, W. N.: Hypoxanthine-guanine phosphoribosyl transferase deficiency in the Lesch-Nyhan syndrome and gout. Fed. Proc. **27**, 1047—1052 (1968).

KELLEY, W. N., BEARDMORE, T. D.: Allopurinol: alteration in pyrimidine metabolism in man. Science **169**, 388—390 (1970).

KELLEY, W. N., BEARDMORE, T. D., FOX, I. H., MEADE, J. C.: Effect of allopurinol and oxipurinol on pyrimidine synthesis in cultured human fibroblasts. Biochem. Pharmacol. **20**, 1471—1478 (1971 a).

KELLEY, W. N., FOX, I. H., WYNGAARDEN, J. B.: Regulation of purine biosynthesis in cultured human cells. I. Effects of orotic acid. Biochim. biophys. Acta (Amst.) **215**, 512—516 (1970 b).

KELLEY, W. N., GREENE, M. L., FOX, I. H., ROSENBLOOM, F. M., LEVY, R. I., SEEGMILLER, J. E.: Effects of orotic acid on purine and lipoprotein metabolism in man. Metabolism **19** (12), 1025—1035 (1970).

KELLEY, W. N., GREENE, M. L., ROSENBLOOM, F. M., HENDERSON, J. F., SEEGMILLER, J. E.: Hypoxanthine-guanine phosphoribosyltransferase deficiency in gout. Ann. intern. Med. **70**, 155—206 (1969).

KELLEY, W. N., ROSENBLOOM, F. M., HENDERSON, J. F., SEEGMILLER, J. E.: A specific enzyme defect in gout associated with overproduction of uric acid. Proc. nat. Acad. Sci. (Wash.) **57**, 1735—1739 (1967).

KELLEY, W. N., ROSENBLOOM, F. M., MILLER, J., SEEGMILLER, J. E.: An enzymatic basis for variations in response to allopurinol: hypoxanthine-guanine phosphoribosyltransferase deficiency. New Engl. J. Med. **278**, 287—293 (1968).

KELLEY, W. N., ROSENBLOOM, F. M., SEEGMILLER, J. E.: The effects of azathioprine (Imuran) on purine synthesis in clinical disorders of purine metabolism. J. clin. Invest. **46**, 1518—1529 (1967).

KELLEY, W. N., WYNGAARDEN, J. B.: Effects of allopurinol and oxipurinol on purine synthesis in cultured human cells. J. clin. Invest. **49**, 602—609 (1970).

KLINENBERG, J. R., GOLDFINGER, S. E., SEEGMILLER, J. E.: The effectiveness of the xanthine oxidase inhibitor allopurinol in the treatment of gout. Ann. intern. Med. **62**, 639—647 (1965).

KISSEL, P., LAMARCHE, M., ROYER, R.: Modification of uricemia and the excretion of uric acid nitrogen by an enzyme of fungal origin. Nature (London) **217**, 72—74 (1968).

KRAKOFF, I. H.: Xanthine oxidase inhibition in the management of hyperuricemia in leukemias and lymphomas. Arthr. and Rheum. **8**, 896—898 (1965).

KRAKOFF, I. H., MAGILL, G. B.: Effects of 2-ethylamino-1,3,4-thiadiazole HCl on uric acid production in man. Proc. Soc. exp. Biol. (N.Y.) **91**, 470—472 (1956).

KRAKOFF, I. H., MEYER, R. L.: Prevention of hyperuricemia in leukemia and lymphoma: use of allopurinol, a xanthine oxidase inhibitor. J. Amer. med. Ass. **193**, 1 (1965).

KRENITSKY, T. A., ELION, G. B., HENDERSON, A. M., HITCHINGS, G. H.: Inhibition of human purine nucleoside phosphorylase: Studies with intact erythrocytes and the purified enzyme. J. biol. Chem. **243**, 2876—2881 (1968).

KRENITSKY, T. A., ELION, G. B., STRELITZ, R. A., HITCHINGS, G. H.: Ribonucleosides of allopurinol and oxoallopurinol. J. biol. Chem. **242**, 2675—2682 (1967).

KUZELL, W. C., SEEBACK, L. M., GLOVER, R. P., JACKMAN, A. E.: Treatment of gout with allopurinol and Sulphinpyrazone in combination and with allopurinol alone. Ann. rheum. Dis. **25**, 634—642 (1966).

LANDON, M., HUDSON, P. B.: Uricolytic activity of purified uricase in two human beings. Science **125**, 937—938 (1957).

LEVIN, N. W., ABRAHAMS, O. L.: Allopurinol in patients with impaired renal function. Ann. rheum. Dis. **25**, 681—687 (1966).

MCCOLLISTER, R. J., GILBERT, W. R., ASHTON, D. H., WYNGAARDEN, J. B.: Pseudofeedback inhibition of purine synthesis by 6-mercaptopurine ribonucleotide and other purine analogues. J. biol. Chem. **239**, 1560—1563 (1964).

MEYSKENS, F. L., WILLIAMS, H. E.: Concentration and synthesis of phosphoribosylpyrophosphate in erythrocytes from normal, hyperuricemic and gouty subjects. Metabolism **20**, 731—742 (1971).

MINER, R. W., RHOADS, C. P. (Eds.): 6-Mercaptopurine. Ann. N.Y. Acad. Sci. **60**, 183—507 (1954).

NICHOL, A. W., NOMURA, A., HAMPTON, A.: Studies on phosphate binding sites of inosinic acid dehydrogenase and adenylosuccinate synthetase. Biochemistry **6**, 1008—1015 (1967).

NYHAN, W. L., SWEETMAN, L., LESCH, M.: Effects of the uricogenic agent, 2-ethylamino-1,3,4-thiadiazole in hypoxanthine-guanine phosphoribosyltransferase deficiency. Metabolism **17**, 846—853 (1968).

Pomales, R., Bieber, S., Friedman, R., Hitchings, G. H.: Augmentation of incorporation of hypoxanthine into nucleic acids by the administration of an inhibitor of xanthine oxidase. Biochim. biophys. Acta (Amst.) **72**, 119—120 (1963).

Pomales, R., Elion, G. B., Hitchings, G. H.: Xanthine as precursor of nucleic acid purines in mouse. Biochim. biophys. Acta (Amst.) **95**, 505—506 (1965).

Rieselbach, R. E., Bentzel, C. J., Cotlove, E., Frei, E., Freireich, E. J.: Uric acid excretion and renal function in the acute hyperuricemia of leukemia: Pathogenesis and therapy of uric acid nephropathy. Amer. J. Med. **37**, 872—883 (1964).

Riesterer, L., Jaques, R.: The anti-inflammatory action of a xanthine oxidase inhibitor (allopurinol). Pharmacology **2**, 288—294 (1969).

Rodman, G. P., Robin, J. A., Tolchin, S. F.: Efficacy of single day dose allopurinol in gouty hyperuricemia. In: Sperling, O., de Vries, A., Wyngaarden, J. B. (Eds.): Advances in Experimental Medicine and Biology. Vol. 41 B. Purine metabolism in man, pp. 571—575. New York-London: Plenum Press 1974.

Rosenbloom, F. M., Henderson, J. F., Kelley, W. N., Seegmiller, J. E.: Accelerated purine biosynthesis *de novo* in skin fibroblasts deficient in hypoxanthine-guanine phosphoribosyltransferase activity. Biochim. biophys. Acta (Amst.) **166**, 258—260 (1968).

Rundles, R. W., Metz, E. N., Silberman, H. R.: Allopurinol in the treatment of gout. Ann. intern. Med. **64**, 229—258 (1966).

Rundles, R. W., Silberman, H. R., Hitchings, G. H., Elion, G. B.: Effects of xanthine oxidase inhibitor on clinical manifestations and purine metabolism in gout. Ann. intern. Med. **60**, 717—718 (1964).

Rundles, R. W., Wyngaarden, J. B., Hitchings, G. H., Elion, G. B., Silberman, H. R.: Effects of a xanthine oxidase inhibitor on thiopurine metabolism, hyperuricemia and gout. Trans. Ass. Amer. Phycns. **76**, 126—140 (1963).

Rundles, R. W., Wyngaarden, J. B., Hitchings, G. H., Elion, G. B.: Drugs and uric acid. Ann. Rev. Pharmacol. **9**, 345—362 (1969).

Schanker, L. S., Jeffrey, J. J., Tocco, D. J.: Interaction of purines with the pyrimidine transport process of the small intestine. Biochem. Pharmacol. **12**, 1047—1053 (1963).

Scott, J. T.: Comparison of allopurinol and probenecid. Ann. rheum. Dis. **25**, 623—626 (1966).

Scott, J. T., Hall, A. P., Grehame, R.: Allopurinol in the treatment of gout. Brit. med. J. **1966 II**, 321—327.

Scott, J. T., Loebl, W. Y.: Withdrawal of allopurinol in patients with gout. In: Sperling, O., de-Vries, A., Wyngaarden, J. B. (Eds.): Advances in Experimental Medicine and Biology. Vol. 41 B. Purine metabolism in man, pp. 577—579. New York-London: Plenum Press 1974.

Seegmiller, J. E., Grayzel, A. I., Liddle, L.: Excessive uric acid production in the human induced by 2-ethylamino-1,3,4-thiadiazole. Nature (London) **183**, 1463—1464 (1959).

Seegmiller, J. E., Klinenberg, J. R., Miller, J., Watts, R. W. E.: Suppression of glycine-N^{15}-incorporation into urinary uric acid by adenine-8-C^{13} in normal and gouty subjects. J. clin. Invest. **47**, 1193—1203 (1968).

Seegmiller, J. E., Lester, L., Stetten, De W., Jr.: Incorporation of 4-amino-5-imidazolecarboxamide-4 ^{13}C into uric acid in the normal human. J. biol. Chem. **216**, 653—662 (1955).

Shaw, R. K., Shulman, R. N., Davidson, J. D., Rall, D. P., Frei, E.: Studies with the experimental antitumor agent 4-aminopyrazolo-(3,4-d)pyrimidine. Cancer **13**, 482—489 (1960).

Silberman, H. R., Wyngaarden, J. B.: 6-mercaptopurine as substrate and inhibitor of xanthine oxidase. Biochim. biophys. Acta (Amst.) **47**, 178—180 (1961).

Simmonds, H. A.: Urinary excretion of purines, pyrimidines and pyrazolopyrimidines in patients treated with allopurinol or oxipurinol. Clin. chim. Acta **23**, 353 (1969).

Simmonds, H. A., Hatfield, P. J., Cameron, J. S., Jones, A. S., Cadenhead, A.: Metabolic studies of purine metabolism in the pig during the oral administration of guanine and allopurinol. Biochem. Pharmacol. **22**, 2537—2551 (1973).

Skipper, H. E.: On the mechanism of action of 6-mercaptopurine. Ann. N.Y. Acad. Sci. **60**, 315 (1954).

Skipper, H. E., Robins, R. K., Thomson, J. R., Cheng, C. C., Brockman, R. W., Schabel, F. M., Jr.: Structure-activity relationships observed on screening a series of pyrazolopyrimidines against experimental neoplasms. Cancer Res. **17**, 579—596 (1957).

Sorensen, L. B.: Suppression of the shunt pathway in primary gout by azathioprine. Proc. nat. Acad. Sci. (Wash.) **55**, 571—575 (1966).

Sorensen, L. B., Benke, P. J.: Biochemical evidence for a distinct type of primary gout. Nature (London) **213**, 1122—1123 (1967).

Sorensen, L. B., Kawahara, F., Chow, D., Benke, P. J., Coben, L.: Excessive purine synthesis and neurologic dysfunction in children. Arthr. and Rheum. **13**, 835 (1970).

Sorensen, L., Seegmiller, J. E.: Seminars on the Lesch-Nyhan syndrome: Management and treatment, discussion. Fed. Proc. **27**, 1097—1104 (1968).

Standorfer, S. B., Handler, P.: Fatty liver induced by orotic acid feeding. Proc. Soc. exp. Biol. Med. (N.Y.) **90**, 270 (1955).

Sweetman, L.: Urinary and cerebrospinal fluid oxypurine levels and allopurinol metabolism in the Lesch-Nyhan syndrome. Fed. Proc. **27**, 1055—1059 (1968).

Truscoe, R., Williams, V.: The effect of allopurinol on urate oxidase activity. Biochem. Pharmacol. **17**, 165—167 (1968).

Vessell, E. S., Passananti, S. T., Greene, F. E., Page, J. G.: Genetic control of drug levels and of the induction of drug-metabolizing enzymes in man: individual variability in the extent of allopurinol and nortryptiline inhibition of drug metabolism. Ann. N.Y. Acad. Sci. **179**, 752—773 (1971).

Villiaumey, J., Larget-Piet, B., Rotterdam, H.: Quelques donnés sur les variations de l'uricémie et de l'uraturie sous l'effet d'une urate-oxydase. Rev. Rheumatisme **39**, 138—140 (1972).

Watts, R. W. E., Scott, J. T., Chalmero, R. A., Bitensky, L., Chayen, J.: Microscopic studies on skeletal muscle in gout patients treated with allopurinol. Quart. J. Med. **157**, 1—14 (1971).

Watts, R. W. E., Snedden, W., Parker, R. A.: A quantitative study of skeletal-muscle purines and pyrazolo (3,4-d) pyrimidines in gout patients treated with allopurinol. Clin. Sci. **41**, 153—158 (1971).

Watts, R. W. E., Watkins, P. J., Mathias, J. Q., Gibbs, D. A.: Allopurinol and acute uric acid nephropathy. Brit. med. J. **1966 I**, 205—208.

Weir, E., Fisher, J. R.: The effect of allopurinol on the excretion of oxypurines by the chick. Biochim. biophys. Acta (Amst.) **222**, 556—557 (1970).

Wells, W., Winzler, R. J.: Metabolism of human leukocytes in vitro. III. Incorporation of formate-C^{14} into cellular components of leukemic human leukocytes. Cancer Res. **19**, 1086—1090 (1959).

White, F. R.: 4-Aminopyrazolo(3,4-d) pyrimidine and three derivatives. Cancer Chemother. Rep. **3**, 26 (1959).

Wyngaarden, J. B.: 2,6-Diaminopurine as substrate and inhibitor of xanthine oxidase. J. biol. Chem. **224**, 453—462 (1957).

Wyngaarden, J. B.: Xanthine oxidase inhibitors in the management of gout. Arthr. and Rheum. **8**, 883—890 (1965).

Wyngaarden, J. B., Kelley, W. N.: In: The Metabolic Basis of Inherited Disease. 3rd Ed., p. 889. New York: McGraw-Hill 1972.

Wyngaarden, J. B., Rundles, R. W., Metz, E. N.: Allopurinol in the treatment of gout. Ann. intern. Med. **62**, 842—847 (1965).

Wyngaarden, J. B., Rundles, R. W., Silberman, H. R., Hunter, S.: Control of hyperuricemia with hydroxy pyrazolopyrimidine, a purine analogue which inhibits uric acid synthesis. Arthr. and Rheum. **6**, 306 (1963).

Yü, T. F., Gutman, A. B.: Effects of allopurinol (4-hydroxy pyrazolo [3,4-d] pyrimidine) on serum and urinary uric acid in primary and secondary gout. Amer. J. Med. **37**, 885—898 (1964).

Zöllner, N., Griebsch, A., Gröbner, W.: Einfluß verschiedener Purine auf den Harnsäurestoffwechsel. Ernähr.-Umschau **3**, 79—82 (1972).

Zuckerman, R., Drell, W., Levin, Y. H.: Urinary purines in gout: effect of azaserine. Arthr. and Rheum. **2**, 46—47 (1959).

c) Uricosurica

Von

W. GRÖBNER und N. ZÖLLNER

Mit 24 Abbildungen

Die Behandlung der chronischen Hyperuricämie muß eine dauerhafte Senkung des Serumharnsäurespiegels anstreben. Neben diätetischen Maßnahmen stehen hierzu Arzneimittel zur Verfügung, die entweder die Harnsäuresynthese hemmen oder durch Erhöhung der renalen Harnsäureausscheidung den Serumharnsäurespiegel senken (Uricosurica).

Physiologie und Pathologie der Harnsäure

Normaler Harnsäurespiegel und Hyperuricämie

Harnsäure ist eine schwache Säure und liegt im physiologischen pH-Bereich des Plasmas zu 97,5% als Uration vor, während sie bei den niedrigeren pH-Werten, die innerhalb des Ausscheidungssystems der Niere vorherrschen, zum großen Teil in freier Form eliminiert wird. Da das Hauptkation der extracellulären Flüssigkeit Natrium ist, werden die Löslichkeitseigenschaften im Körper vorwiegend jene des Mononatriumurats sein. Für das Plasma berechneten PETERS u. VAN SLYKE (1946) eine Löslichkeit von 6,4 mg-%. Im Harn liegen die Verhältnisse etwas komplizierter, da hier Schwankungen im pH und der Salzkonzentration sowie die Neigung der Urate zur Bildung übersättigter Lösungen berücksichtigt werden müssen (Zusammenfassung bei ZÖLLNER, 1968).

Die Höhe des Serumharnsäurespiegels wird vom Alter, Geschlecht, Ernährung und zahlreichen weiteren Faktoren beeinflußt. In der Tecumseh-Studie, in der an einem großen auslesefreien Material enzymatische Serumharnsäurebestimmungen durchgeführt wurden, fanden MIKKELSEN et al. (1965) einen mittleren Serumharnsäurespiegel von 4,9 mg-% ± 1,4 (S) bei Männern bzw. 4,2 mg-% ± 1,16 (S) bei Frauen. Ähnliche Ergebnisse wurden auch von HALL et al. in Framingham (1967) sowie ZÖLLNER (1963) (Untersuchungen an 384 Blutspendern) mitgeteilt. Nach neueren Untersuchungen von GRIEBSCH u. ZÖLLNER (1973) betragen die mittleren Serumharnsäurespiegel in Süddeutschland bei Männern 6,00 ± 1,22 mg/ 100 ml, bei Frauen 4,35 ± 1,06 mg/100 ml. Geänderte Ernährungsgewohnheiten dürften hierbei die wahrscheinlichste Ursache für den Anstieg der Plasmaharnsäure im letzten Jahrzehnt bei den Männern sein (GRIEBSCH u. ZÖLLNER).

Überprüft man die in den epidemiologischen Studien gewonnenen Verteilungskurven der Harnsäurewerte im Serum, so läßt sich statistisch keine eindeutige Grenze zwischen normalen und erhöhten Werten festlegen. Schwankungen der Serumharnsäure jeder Einzelperson und andere Faktoren sind ursächlich anzuschuldigen. Nach klinischer Erfahrung gelten im allgemeinen als obere Grenze der Norm für enzymatische Methoden Werte von 7,0 mg-% für Männer bzw. 6,0 mg-% für Frauen. Diese Werte sind insofern auch interessant, als im gleichen Bereich die Löslichkeit des Natriumurats im Plasmawasser liegt. Eine Erhöhung der Serumharnsäurekonzentration auf Werte oberhalb dieser Grenze bedeutet das Vorliegen einer übersättigten Lösung mit der Neigung zur Harnsäureausfällung bei Auftreten von entsprechenden physikalischen Voraussetzungen.

Harnsäurebildung und -ausscheidung sowie deren Störung bei der familiären Hyperuricämie

Ausgangssubstanz der Purinsynthese ist 5-Phosphoribosyl-1-Pyrophosphat, das mit Glutamin-Phosphoribosylpyrophosphat-Amidotransferase zum 5-Phosphoribosyl-1-Amin reagiert. Über eine Reihe weiterer Zwischenstufen entsteht schließlich Inosinsäure (IMP), aus der die anderen Nucleotide, nämlich Adenyl- und Guanylsäure (AMP, GMP) gebildet werden. Sie wiederum hemmen im Sinne eines Rückkoppelungsprozesses den ersten Schritt der Purinsynthese, nämlich die Aminierung von 5-Phosphoribosyl-1-Pyrophosphat zu 5-Phosphoribosyl-1-Amin ebenso wie die Bildung der eigentlichen Nucleotide aus Inosinsäure. Störungen dieser Feedback-Regulation der Purinsynthese, eine Veränderung der Enzymaktivität der Glutamin-Phosphoribosylpyrophosphat-Amidotransferase sowie ein Anstieg der Substratkonzentration von Glutamin oder 5-Phosphoribosyl-1-Pyrophosphat werden als mögliche Ursachen einer gesteigerten Purinsynthese diskutiert. Eine bedeutende Rolle in der Regulation der Purinsynthese spielt auch die Hypoxanthin-Guanin-Phosphoribosyltransferase. Dieses Enzym katalysiert die Umwandlung von Hypoxanthin und Guanin zu ihren entsprechenden Nucleotiden. Guanylsäure und Inosinsäure sind wiederum Feed-back-Inhibitoren der de novo-Purinsynthese (KELLEY et al., 1968). Ein Fehlen der Hypoxanthin-Guanin-Phosphoribosyltransferase führt somit zu einer Störung der Feed-back-Regulation und Steigerung der Purinsynthese [1].

Der Abbau der Inosinsäure erfolgt über Inosin, Hypoxanthin und Xanthin zu Harnsäure.

Harnsäure ist das Endprodukt des Purinstoffwechsels, dessen sich der Körper nur durch Ausscheidung entledigen kann. Von der Harnsäure im Körper unterliegen nach Sekretion in den Magen-Darm-Kanal täglich etwa 100 mg der bakteriellen Uricolyse. Der Rest, bei purinarmer Kost etwa 400—500 mg täglich, wird durch die Niere eliminiert (ZÖLLNER, 1960). Der Mechanismus der renalen Harnsäureausscheidung ist durch Filtration, fast vollständige Rückresorption im proximalen und Sekretion im proximalen und distalen Tubulus gekennzeichnet. Durch das Zusammenwirken von Filtration, Rückresorption und Sekretion ergibt sich eine normale Harnsäureclearance von $8,7 \pm 2,5$ ml/min. LAUNDAT et al. (1962) fanden bei Gesunden einen Wert von 9,5 ml/min, bei Gichtpatienten dagegen 5,8 ml/min. Da die Mehrzahl der Gichtiker bei erhöhtem Serumharnsäurespiegel normale Mengen Harnsäure ausscheidet, bedeutet dies, daß bei der Gicht Eigentümlichkeiten der Harnsäureausscheidung bestehen. Zahlreiche Untersuchungen führten zu dem Ergebnis, daß die familiäre Hyperuricämie durch eine Verminderung der Fähigkeit, die Harnsäuresekretion ausreichend zu erhöhen, zustande kommt (Zusammenfassung ZÖLLNER, 1960). Unterstützt wird diese Schlußfolgerung auch durch die Beobachtung ZÖLLNERs (1964), daß bei gleichem Harnsäurespiegel bei Gichtkranken auch die saliväre Harnsäuresekretion niedriger als bei Normalpersonen ist, der Sekretionsdefekt also nicht auf die Niere allein beschränkt zu sein scheint.

Uricosurische Maßnahmen zur Senkung des Serumharnsäurespiegels

Wasserdiurese

Einfachste Maßnahme zur Vermehrung der Harnsäureausscheidung im Urin ist die Erzeugung einer Wasserdiurese, da Harnsäure bis zu einem "Augmentation limit" von 1 ml Harn pro min mit zunehmendem Harnvolumen vermehrt ausge-

---

[1] In den letzten Jahren gesellten sich noch weitere Enzymanomalien als Ursache einer gesteigerten Purinsynthese hinzu.

schieden wird (BRØCHNER-MORTENSEN, 1937; SALA et al., 1956). Es ist deshalb notwendig, durch ausreichende Flüssigkeitszufuhr während aller Tagesstunden eine hohe Harnproduktion (2—3 Liter) zu erreichen.

Uricosurica

Die Wirkung der Uricosurica beruht auf einer Hemmung der tubulären Harnsäurerückresorption, in deren Gefolge es bis zur Einstellung eines neuen Plasmaspiegels und vollständiger Ausschwemmung eventueller Harnsäuredepots zu einer vermehrten renalen Harnsäureausscheidung kommt. Dieser Effekt wird von strukturell verschiedenartigen Substanzen hervorgerufen, die sich zu folgenden Stoffgruppen zusammenfassen lassen:

a) Salicylate: Salicylsäure, Acetylsalicylsäure, Natriumsalicylat.

b) Benzoesäurederivate: Alkylsulfonamidobenzoesäure: Carinamid. N-Alkylsulfamylbenzoesäuren: Probenecid, Longacid.

c) Pyrazolidinderivate: Phenylbutazon und seine Metaboliten, Ketophenylbutazon, G-25671 (1,2-Diphenyl-4-(phenyl-thioäthyl)-3,5-dioxo-pyrazolidin, Sulfinpyrazon.

d) Benzofuranderivate: Benzaronum, Benziodaronum, Benzbromaronum.

e) Cumarin- und Indandionderivate.

f) Zoxazolamin.

g) Uricosurisch wirksame Verbindungen unterschiedlicher Struktur: Phenylchinolincarbonsäure, Niridazol, Clofibrat, MK-185, Röntgenkontrastmittel usw.

Von den zahlreichen uricosurisch wirksamen Pharmaka haben in der Langzeitbehandlung der Hyperuricämie nur Probenecid und Sulfinpyrazon festen Fuß gefaßt. Eine zuverlässige und langanhaltende Senkung des Serumharnsäurespiegels wird auch mit Benzbromaronum erreicht (DELBARRE et al., 1967; STERNON et al., 1967; ZÖLLNER et al., 1968, 1970a, b; KOTZAUREK u. HUEBER, 1968; MERTZ, 1969; MERTZ et al., 1970; MASBERNARD u. FRANCOZ, 1969; MASBERNARD u. VACCON, 1970; GROSS u. GIRARD, 1972). Die Möglichkeiten zur Dauertherapie mit den anderen uricosurischen Verbindungen sind begrenzt, da viele von ihnen entweder potentiell toxisch sind oder in wirksamer Dosierung unerwünschte Nebenerscheinungen aufweisen.

Allgemeine Eigenschaften der Uricosurica

Mit Ausnahme von Zoxazolamin, einer schwachen Base, besitzen die meisten Uricosurica schwach saure Eigenschaften. Die Erhöhung der renalen Harnsäureausscheidung ist Folge einer Hemmung der tubulären Harnsäurerückresorption. In niedriger Dosierung können mehrere uricosurisch wirksame Verbindungen die tubuläre Harnsäuresekretion blockieren, so daß eine verminderte renale Harnsäureausscheidung resultiert. Diese sog. paradoxe Harnsäureretention beruht auf einem kompetitiven Hemmechanismus, da Harnsäure gemeinsam mit anderen organischen Säuren über denselben sekretorischen Transportmechanismus ("Organic acid system") ausgeschieden wird (WEINER u. MUDGE, 1964). Wird durch die Steigerung der verabreichten Dosis zusätzlich die tubuläre Harnsäurerückresorption blockiert, so resultiert als „Netto-Effekt" eine Erhöhung der renalen Harnsäureausscheidung. Eine paradoxe Harnsäureretention wurde von YÜ u. GUTMAN (1955) für Phenylbutazon, Probenecid und Natriumsalicylat nachgewiesen. So führen orale Salicylatdosen von 1—2 g/tgl. zu einem Anstieg der Serumharnsäurekonzentration, während die Verabreichung von 4—5 g/tgl. eine Harnsäuremehrausscheidung im Urin und Abfall des Serumharnsäurespiegels verursacht. Mittlere Salicylatdosen lassen die Serumharnsäure und renale Harnsäure-

Tabelle 1. Additive und antagonistische Wirkungen einiger Uricosurica. (Nach SEEGMILLER u. GRAYZEL, 1960)

Versuchs-personen	Arzneimittel	Dosis g/tgl.	Harnsäureausscheidung im Urin mg/24 Std	
			Nach Gabe des einzelnen Uricosuricums	Nach kombinierter Gabe
1	Probenecid	3,0	576	897
	Zoxazolamin	0,75	729	
2	Probenecid	3,0	673	114
	Na-Salicylat	6,0	909	
3	Na-Salicylat	6,0	281	30
	Sulfinpyrazon	0,6	527	
4	Zoxazolamin	1,5	1195	740
	Na-Salicylat	4,8	632	

ausscheidung unbeeinflußt (YÜ u. GUTMAN, 1959). Sulfinpyrazon, Zoxazolamin und Benzbromaronum führen dagegen in niederer Dosierung zu keiner Harnsäureretention.

Die molekularen Vorgänge beim tubulären Harnsäuretransport bzw. die Art seiner Beeinflussung durch Uricosurica sind noch weitgehend unbekannt. Lediglich von den Vitamin K-Antagonisten vom Dicumarol- und Phenylindandiontyp, die durch Blockierung der Harnsäurerückresorption uricosurisch wirken, darf man annehmen, daß sie Reaktionen hemmen, an denen Vitamin K-haltige Coenzyme beteiligt sind (ZÖLLNER, 1968; ZÖLLNER u. GRÖBNER, 1969). Dies würde für eine Rolle des Vitamins K in diesen Transportvorgängen sprechen; diese Hypothese wird durch die Feststellung einer Erhöhung der Harnsäureclearance beim Vitamin K-Mangel des Verschlußikterus gestützt (PASERO u. MASINI, 1958).

Werden Uricosurica kombiniert verabreicht, so können additive oder antagonistische Effekte auftreten (Tab. 1). So führt die gleichzeitige Gabe von Zoxazolamin und Probenecid zu einer Erhöhung der renalen Harnsäureausscheidung, während Salicylate die Wirkung des Probenecids, Sulfinpyrazons und Zoxazolamins antagonistisch beeinflussen (SEEGMILLER u. GRAYZEL, 1960). Die Ursache dieser Effekte ist noch weitgehend unbekannt.

Bei Normalpersonen können uricosurische Pharmaka zu einer Harnsäuremehrausscheidung führen, die durch die Verringerung des Harnsäurepools nicht zu erklären ist. So fanden BISHOP et al. (1951) während einer Abnahme des Harnsäurepools von 964 auf 466 mg unter Probenecid eine Mehrausscheidung von 2705 mg. WYNGAARDEN (1955) beobachtete bei einer Versuchsperson während 9 tägiger uricosurischer Phenylbutazontherapie eine Mehrausscheidung von 1630 mg bei einer gleichzeitigen Verringerung des Pools von 1272 auf 716 mg, weist jedoch in diesem Fall auf die Ausnahme hin. ZÖLLNER et al. (1970) errechneten nach Verabreichung von Benzbromaronum, einem Benzofuranderivat, eine Differenz zwischen Harnsäuremehrausscheidung und errechneter Poolabnahme von im Mittel 186 mg, bei einer Versuchsperson z.B. 493 mg. Die wahrscheinlichste Erklärung ist die, daß bei abnehmendem Harnsäurespiegel die enterale Ausscheidung zugunsten der renalen Harnsäureausscheidung abnimmt (ZÖLLNER, 1960). Bei Hyperuricämikern und Patienten mit Gicht kann unter uricosurischer

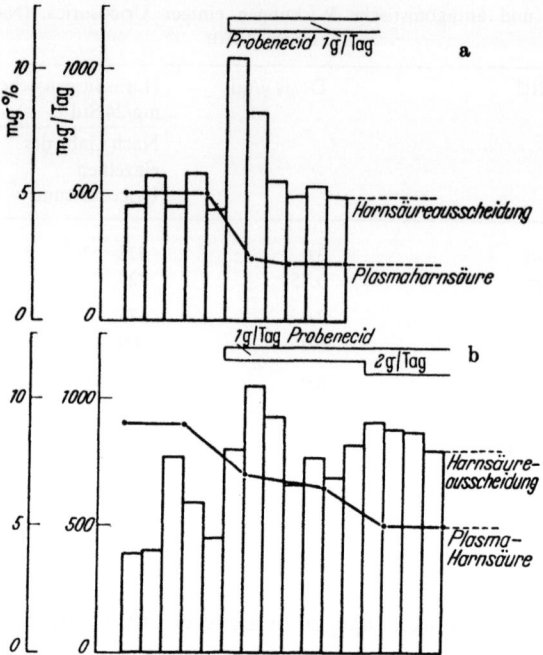

Abb. 1a u. b. Senkung der Plasmaharnsäure und Vermehrung der Harnsäureausscheidung unter der Verabreichung von Probenecid bei einer gesunden freiwilligen Versuchsperson (a) und bei einem Patienten mit Gicht (b). (Nach ZÖLLNER, 1968)

Therapie eine Harnsäuremehrausscheidung, die größer als die errechnete Poolabnahme ist, auch auf eine Mobilisation von Harnsäure aus den Ablagerungen (z. B. Gelenke, Tophi) zurückgeführt werden (TALBOTT, 1967).

Die Harnsäuremehrausscheidung nach Verabreichung eines Uricosuricums hält in Abhängigkeit von der Größe des Harnsäurepools mehr oder weniger lange an (Abb. 1). Während bei Normalpersonen die Harnsäuremehrausscheidung nach Einleitung der Therapie nur einen oder höchstens wenige Tage anhält, beobachtet man bei Hyperuricämikern Harnsäuremehrausscheidungen, die über Monate andauern. Sie beruhen auf einer ständigen Mobilisation von Harnsäure aus den Depots, hervorgerufen durch den Abfall der Plasmaharnsäure unter die Löslichkeitsgrenze. So wurden Harnsäuremehrausscheidungen von 75 g innerhalb von 5 Monaten beobachtet. Dadurch entsteht, vor allem zu Beginn einer uricosurischen Therapie, die Gefahr einer tubulären Harnsäureausfällung und möglicherweise Anurie, wenn nicht besondere Vorsichtsmaßnahmen ergriffen werden.

Die uricosurische Therapie ist eine Dauertherapie, die durch Beobachtung des Serumharnsäurespiegels verfolgt wird. Unter Verwendung der Uricasemethode wird dabei ein Wert von 5 mg-% angestrebt. Die einmal festgestellte medikamentöse Tagesdosis ist eine Dauerdosis. Nebenwirkungen wie Kopfschmerzen, gastrointestinale Beschwerden und Arzneimittelexantheme treten bei etwa 5—10% aller Patienten, die mit Probenecid oder Sulfinpyrazon behandelt werden, auf (YÜ u. GUTMAN, 1967; GUTMAN, 1968). Ernstere toxische Erscheinungen wie nephrotisches Syndrom (SCOTT u. O'BRIEN, 1968) sowie die Beeinflussung des hämatopoetischen Systems wurden nur vereinzelt beschrieben (YÜ et al., 1958; PERSELLIN u. SCHMID, 1961). REYNOLDS et al. (1957) beobachteten unter Probene-

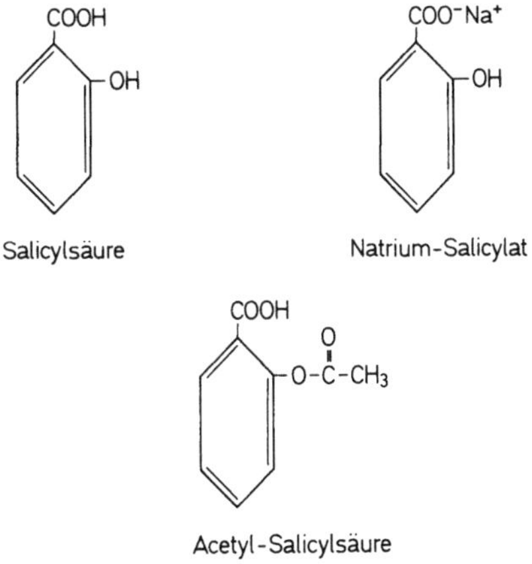

Abb. 2. Salicylsäure und ihre Derivate

cid das Auftreten einer akuten Leberdystrophie. Allerdings wurde dieses Arzneimittel trotz Zeichen einer allergischen Reaktion nicht rechtzeitig abgesetzt. Gichtanfälle zu Beginn einer uricosurischen Therapie sowie das mögliche Auftreten einer Nephrolithiasis sind Nebenwirkungen jedes Uricosuricums, wenn nicht besondere Vorsichtsmaßnahmen wie Colchicinprophylaxe bzw. ausreichende Flüssigkeitszufuhr und Harnneutralisierung getroffen werden.

Die einzelnen Uricosurica

Salicylate

Salicylsäure, Natrium-Salicylat und Acetylsalicylsäure sind die wichtigsten uricosurisch wirksamen Salicylate (Abb. 2). Nach oraler Einnahme werden sie im Magen und oberen Dünndarm rasch resorbiert. Meßbare Plasmakonzentrationen finden sich bereits innerhalb von 30 min. Etwa 50—80% der resorbierten Salicylatdosis ist im Serum an Eiweiß, hauptsächlich Albumin, gebunden. Hypalbuminämie geht mit einem Anstieg von freier, nicht gebundener Salicylsäure im Serum einher (GOODMAN u. GILMAN, 1970). Die Ausscheidung erfolgt hauptsächlich renal, wobei etwa 10% als freie Salicylsäure, 69% als Salicylursäure, 20% als Salicyl-phenol- und Salicyl-acyl-glucuronid und 1% als Gentisinsäure eliminiert werden (GOODMAN u. GILMAN, 1970). In alkalischem Urin steigt die Ausscheidung von freiem Salicylat an, während sie mit absinkendem Urin-pH infolge einer passiven Rückdiffusion der undissoziierten Form abnimmt. Salicylate können die renale Harnsäureausscheidung sowohl vermindern als auch erhöhen (BAUER u. KLEMPERER, 1944; YÜ u. GUTMAN, 1955, 1959). So sahen YÜ u. GUTMAN (1959) bei 23 Gichtikern nach täglicher oraler Verabreichung von 1, 2, 3 und 5,2 g Acetylsalicylsäure Veränderungen der Harnsäuretagesausscheidung von −21%, −14%, +16% und +37%. Renale Clearanceuntersuchungen derselben Autoren zeigten, daß diese reversiblen Effekte eng mit der Salicylatkonzentration im Plasma bzw. Urin korreliert sind. Unter langsamer Dauerinfusion von Natriumsalicylat beobachteten sie bei acht Gichtkranken, daß niedrige Plasmasalicylatkonzentrationen (1,5—10 mg-%) und niedrige Ausscheidungsraten von freiem Salicylat (0,05—0,5 mg/min) gewöhnlich mit einem Abfall der Harnsäureclearance einhergehen. Höhere Konzentrationen (Plasmasalicylat > 10 oder 12 mg-%; renale Ausscheidungsrate von freiem Salicylat 0,5—1,0 mg und mehr/min) sind mit einem Anstieg der Harnsäureclearance verbunden. Untersuchungen nach Alkalisierung und Ansäuerung des Urins ergaben, daß diese Salicylatwirkung auf die Harnsäureausscheidung im Urin eng mit der tubulären Konzentration von freiem Salicylat und damit dem Urin-pH verknüpft ist. Alkalisierung des Urins vergrößert die uricosurische Salicylatwirkung (YÜ u. GUTMAN, 1959).

Die paradoxe Harnsäureretention nach Zufuhr niedriger Salicylatdosen wird auf eine Blockierung der tubulären Harnsäuresekretion zurückgeführt (YÜ u. GUTMAN, 1955, 1959). Höhere Dosen führen durch zusätzliche Hemmung der Harnsäurerückresorption zu einer vermehrten Harnsäureausscheidung im Urin. Mittlere Dosen in der Größenordnung von 2—3 g/tgl. verändern die renale Harnsäureausscheidung nicht, da sich möglicherweise unter dieser Dosierung die Effekte der Harnsäurerückresorptionshemmung und der Harnsäuresekretionsblokkierung gegenseitig aufheben, so daß daraus keine oder nur geringe Nettoänderungen der Harnsäureausscheidung resultieren (YÜ u. GUTMAN, 1959). Von BLUESTONE et al. (1969) wird auf Grund von in vitro-Untersuchungen eine uricosurische Salicylatwirkung zum Teil auf eine Verdrängung von Urat aus einer Plasma-Eiweißbindung mit folgender Erhöhung der glomerulären Harnsäurefiltrationsrate zurückgeführt. Dieser Befund steht jedoch im Widerspruch zu den Untersuchungen von YÜ u. GUTMAN (1953) sowie anderen Autoren, die keine Proteinbindung der Serum-Harnsäure nachweisen konnten.

Salicylate heben die uricosurische Wirkung von Probenecid (GUTMAN u. YÜ, 1951; PASCALE et al., 1952; SEEGMILLER u. GRAYZEL, 1960; BRØCHNER-MORTENSEN, 1958; YÜ u. GUTMAN, 1959), Zoxazolamin (BURNS et al., 1958) und Phenylbutazonderivaten (OGRYZLO u. HARRISON, 1957; KERSLEY et al., 1958) auf. Lediglich MARSON (1954) konnte keine eindeutige Hemmwirkung finden. Die Verschiedenheit der Beobachtungen mag jedoch auf experimentelle Unterschiede zurückzuführen sein.

Der Einfluß der Salicylate auf die renale Harnsäureausscheidung war schon Ende des vorigen Jahrhunderts bekannt, auch die ersten Empfehlungen, Salicylsäure zur Behandlung der chronischen Gicht zu verwenden, sind jahrzehntealt (SÉE, 1877; CAMPBELL, 1878). Das Auftreten von Nebenwirkungen unter der erforderlichen hohen Dosierung begrenzte jedoch die Anwendung der Salicylate in der Gichttherapie. JENNINGS (1937) empfahl deshalb eine intermittierende Arzneimitteleinnahme. Nach Verabreichung der uricosurisch wirksamen Dosen an drei bis vier aufeinanderfolgenden Tagen pro Woche beobachtete er eine Normalisierung des Serumharnsäurespiegels. BAUER u. KLEMPERER (1944) konnten diese Befunde jedoch nicht bestätigen. Im Gegensatz zu anderen Autoren stellten sie außerdem fest, daß die Wirkung von Acetylsalicylsäure bei fortgesetzter Gabe innerhalb weniger Monate abklingt.

Die ersten eindrucksvollen Erfolge unter Salicylatdauertherapie wurden von YÜ u. GUTMAN (1951) sowie MARSON (1952, 1953, 1954) mitgeteilt. Der fast regelmäßig auftretende Salicylismus soll in den meisten Fällen innerhalb weniger Wochen toleriert werden (MARSON, 1953), so daß die notwendigen Salicylatmengen täglich eingenommen werden können. Nach MARSON (1954) üben 6 g Natriumsalicylat, in drei Dosen über den Tag verteilt, oder eine Einzeldosis von 6,5 g einen stärkeren uricosurischen Effekt als 2 g Probenecid, in der gleichen Weise verabreicht, aus. Bei Dauerbehandlung mit Salicylat (6 g/tgl.) gelang es demselben Autor, den Serumharnsäurespiegel bei 17 Patienten durchschnittlich auf 50% des Ausgangswertes zu senken. Die tägliche Verabreichung von 2 g Probenecid bei sechs Gichtikern führte im Mittel zu einer Senkung des Serumharnsäurespiegels auf 68% des Ausgangswertes. Der Autor schloß daraus, daß die Salicylatwirkung der Probenecidwirkung überlegen ist. Im übrigen entsprach der Verlauf der Behandlung den Erfahrungen mit Probenecid, d.h. die Anfälle verschwanden erst nach Monaten, die Tophi nahmen nur langsam ab (MARSON, 1953).

Nebenwirkungen unter langdauernder Salicylattherapie treten nicht selten auf. Am häufigsten werden Salicylismus, gastrointestinale Blutungen, allergische Reaktionen und eine Hemmung der Prothrombinbildung beobachtet. Hypoprothrombinämische Blutungen wurden von MARSON (1953) nicht gesehen. Orale Vitamin K-Zufuhr führte jeweils zu einem Anstieg niedriger Quickwerte.

Mit der Einführung neuer Uricosurica wurde die Salicylatbehandlung der chronischen Gicht allgemein verlassen. Die Harnsäureretention bei niedriger Dosierung, welche eine strenge Befolgung der Behandlungsvorschrift durch die oft eigenwilligen Gichtkranken notwendig macht, und die unangenehmen, wenn auch angeblich vorübergehenden Erscheinungen des Salicylismus erweisen sich als wesentliche Nachteile in der Dauertherapie der Gicht.

Derivate der Benzoesäure

Carinamid und Probenecid wurden zunächst in die Therapie eingeführt, um durch Hemmung der tubulären Sekretion von Penicillin eine höhere Konzentration dieses Arzneimittels im Blut zu gewährleisten. Auf die uricosurische Wirkung des Carinamids wiesen erstmals WOLFSON et al. (1948) hin. GUTMAN (1950) konnte diese Beobachtung bei Gichtkranken bestätigen. Das häufige Auftreten von Nebenwirkungen unter der erforderlichen hohen Dosierung erwies sich jedoch als wesentlicher Nachteil für die Gichtbehandlung. Mit der Einführung des wirksameren Probenecids wurde die Carinamidtherapie wieder verlassen.

Carinamid

Nach oraler Gabe wird Carinamid (Abb. 3) trotz seiner geringen Wasserlöslichkeit schnell und fast vollständig aus dem Gastrointestinaltrakt resorbiert. Der größte Teil ist im Plasma an Eiweiß gebunden. Die Ausscheidung erfolgt durch die Nieren, wobei 60% der verabreichten Dosis unverändert, der Rest in Form von noch nicht identifizierten Metaboliten im Urin aufgefunden wird (Zusammenfassung bei GUTMAN, 1966).

Im Jahre 1948 beobachteten WOLFSON et al. nach einmaliger oraler Gabe von 4,6 g Carinamid bei Normalpersonen einen Anstieg der renalen Harnsäureausscheidung um 50—120% des Ausgangswertes. Ihm entsprach ein Abfall des Serumharnsäurespiegels. GUTMAN (1950), der die Wirkung dieses Arzneimittels bei 13 Gichtkranken untersuchte, stellte unter einer täglichen Dosis von 12—13,5 g eine mittlere Harnsäuremehrausscheidung von 61% fest. Die in kurzen Zeitintervallen notwendige Einnahme von hohen Dosen, die zur Aufrechterhaltung wirksamer Blutspiegel erforderlich sind, sowie das häufige Auftreten von Nebenwirkungen (Arzneimittelexantheme, gastrointestinale Störungen) machen Carinamid für die Langzeitbehandlung der Gicht ungeeignet.

Probenecid [2]

Probenecid (Abb. 4) wird schnell und fast vollständig aus dem Gastrointestinaltrakt resorbiert (BOGER et al., 1950; DAYTON et al., 1963). Nach Zufuhr von 1,0 g per os werden meßbare Plasmakonzentrationen schon innerhalb von 30 min beobachtet (BOGER et al., 1950).

Die höchsten Serumspiegel finden sich 1—5 Std nach oraler Verabreichung. Eine Einzeldosis von 2 g Probenecid per os führt innerhalb von 4 Std zu Plasma-

---

[2] Benemid®.

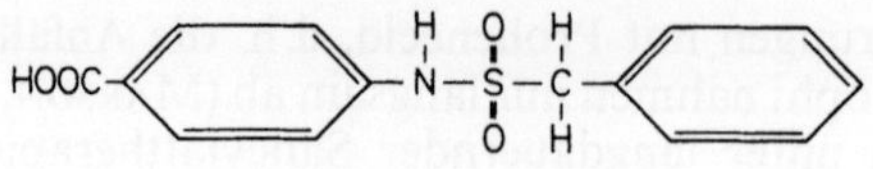

Abb. 3. Carinamid

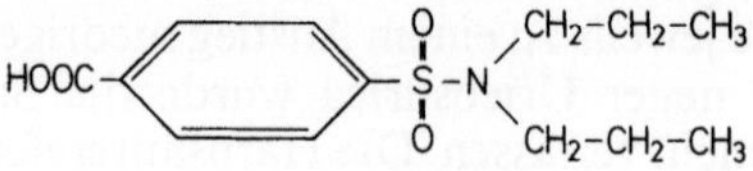

Probenecid

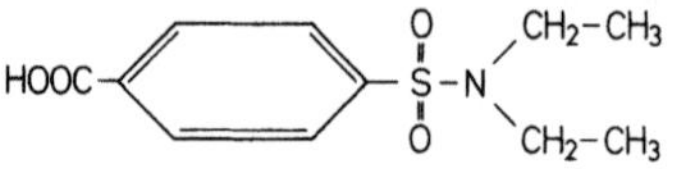

Longacid

Abb. 4. Probenecid und Longacid

spiegeln von 15—20 mg-% (BOGER et al., 1950; DAYTON et al., 1963). Die Plasmahalbwertszeit ist dosisabhängig und beträgt durchschnittlich 6—12 Std (DAYTON et al., 1963). Von DAYTON et al. (1963) wurden jedoch in zwei Fällen auch Halbwertszeiten von 4 bzw. 17 Std beobachtet.

Bei Plasmakonzentrationen von 2—10 mg-% sind etwa 90% des Probenecids an Eiweiß, hauptsächlich Albumin, gebunden (DAYTON et al., 1963). Der Verteilungsraum beschränkt sich somit im wesentlichen auf den Extracellulärraum. Die Ausscheidung erfolgt renal, wobei innerhalb von 48 Std nur etwa 4% der verabreichten Dosis unverändert im Urin aufgefunden werden (PEREL et al., 1970). Hauptmetabolit ist das Probenecid-Mono-Acyl-Glucuronid. Die restlichen im Urin aufgefundenen Metaboliten entstehen durch Oxydationsvorgänge an der n-Propylseitenkette (Abb. 5). Etwa 4,6—8,0% der verabreichten Probeneciddosis wird als N-Depropyl-Metabolit eliminiert (PEREL et al., 1970).

Infolge eines pKa von 3,4 (SHORE et al., 1957) ist das Ausmaß der renalen Elimination von Probenecid vom Urin-pH abhängig. In saurem Urin ist die Ausscheidung infolge einer passiven Rückdiffusion niedrig, mit steigendem Urin-pH nimmt sie zu. Dabei kann bei hohem Urinvolumen das Verhältnis von ausgeschiedenem/filtriertem Probenecid einen Wert von 1,0 überschreiten, so daß eine tubuläre Sekretion für Probenecid angenommen werden muß. DAYTON et al. (1963) beobachteten bei einem Gichtpatienten nach intravenöser Zufuhr von 1,0 g Natriumbicarbonat ein Verhältnis von ausgeschiedenem/filtriertem Probenecid von 3,41.

Zwei Eigenschaften des Probenecids sind von wesentlicher Bedeutung:
1. Die Beeinflussung der renalen Ausscheidung einer Reihe organischer Verbindungen.
2. Seine uricosurische Wirkung.

Die Hemmung der tubulären Sekretion von Penicillin und Paraaminosalicylsäure erlangte durch die Gewährleistung höherer Blutspiegel dieser wichtigen Therapeutica Bedeutung. So führt die Verabreichung von 1,0—2,0 g Probenecid/tgl., auf mehrere Einzeldosen verteilt, zu einem Anstieg des Serumpenicillinspiegels um das 2—3fache (BOGER et al., 1950). Unter denselben Bedingungen stieg nach Gabe von 2,0 g Probenecid der Plasmaspiegel von Paraaminosalicylsäure

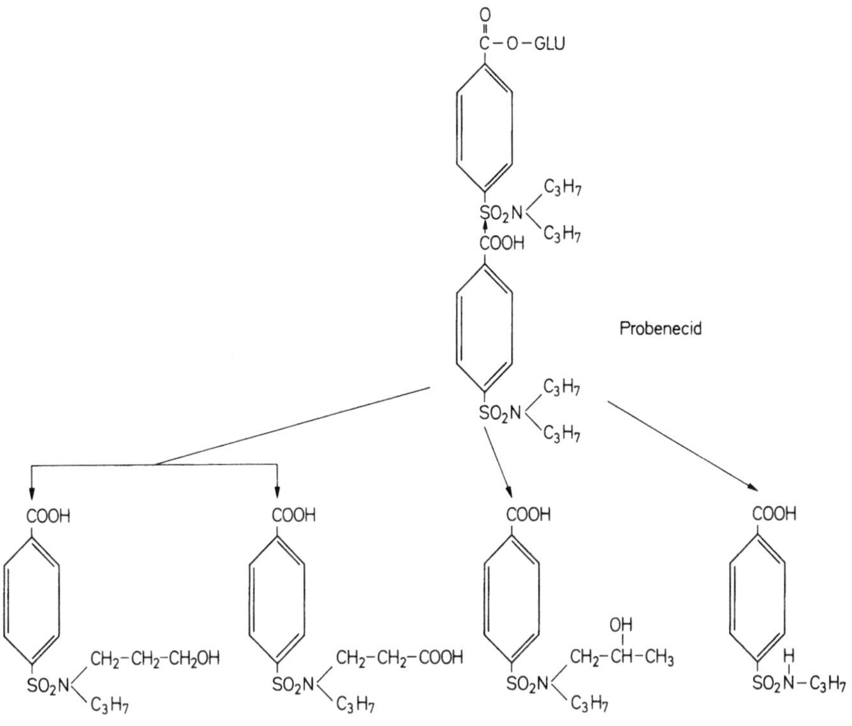

Abb. 5. Metabolismus von Probenecid. (Nach PEREL et al., 1970)

um das 2,3—4,1fache an (BOGER et al., 1950). Zahlreiche weitere Verbindungen wie p-Aminohippursäure, Phenolsulphthalein, Salicylsäure und seine Acyl- und Phenolglucuronide, Pantothensäure, Androsteron, Corticotropin, Dijodthyrosin, Phloricin und seine konjugierten Glucuronide sowie Acetazolamid werden in ihrer Ausscheidung durch Probenecid beeinflußt (Zusammenfassung bei GUTMAN, 1966). Von Bedeutung ist auch die Blockierung der tubulären Sekretion von Indometacin, so daß es bei gleichzeitiger Gabe von Probenecid und hohen Indometacindosen zu Intoxikationserscheinungen durch Indometacin kommen kann (GOODMAN u. GILMAN, 1970). Die Erhöhung der Insulinclearance (SETAISHI et al., 1970) sowie der Alloxanthinclearance sind zusätzliche Eigenschaften des Probenecids. Weiterhin ist bekannt, daß mehrere enzymatische Prozesse, vor allem die Konjugation von Benzoesäurederivaten mit Glycin durch Probenecid gehemmt werden (BEYER et al., 1950).

Probenecid verändert nicht die renale Elektrolytausscheidung (BEYER et al., 1951; SIROTA et al., 1952). Lediglich bei einigen Personen beobachteten SIROTA et al. (1952) einen Anstieg der Natrium- und Chloridclearance. Einen vorübergehenden Abfall des Serumphosphorspiegels bei 4 Patienten mit idiopathischer Hypercalciurie nach Gabe von Probenecid stellten GARCIA u. YENDT (1970) fest. PASCALE et al. (1954) sowie KOLB u. RUKES (1954) beschrieben unter Probenecid eine Senkung des Phosphatspiegels bei Hypoparathyreoidismus. FORD u. SPURR (1953) beobachteten einen Anstieg der fäkalen Phosphatausscheidung.

Nach der Mitteilung von WOLFSON et al. (1948) über die uricosurischen Eigenschaften des Carinamids lag es nahe, auch das strukturähnliche Probenecid auf seine uricosurische Wirkung zu prüfen. Die ersten Erfahrungen wurden von GUT-

Tabelle 2. Der Einfluß einer langsamen Probenecidinfusion auf die renale Harnsäureclearance. (Mod. nach YÜ u. GUTMAN, 1955)

Periode (min)	Probenecid-infusion (mg/min)	Plasma-harnsäure (mg/100 ml)	Harnsäure-clearance (ml/min)
Kontroll-	0	7,3	8,73
periode	0	7,2	9,14
	0	7,0	8,07
(Probenecidinfusion 0,1 g/500 ml 5% Glucose)			
15	0,2	7,4	8,07
15	0,2	7,6	5,46
19	0,2	7,2	6,15
16	0,4	7,0	7,17
16	0,4	6,9	7,63
13	0,4	7,0	8,03
19	0,6	7,1	7,42
20	0,6	7,0	8,45
23	1,2	7,0	10,6
17	1,2	7,0	12,0

MAN (1950) sowie GUTMAN u. YÜ (1951) mitgeteilt. Sie und andere Autoren stellten außerdem fest, daß die Wirkung von 2 g Probenecid der Wirkung von 12 g Carinamid äquivalent ist.

Der uricosurische Wirkungsmechanismus des Probenecids beruht auf einer Hemmung der tubulären Harnsäurerückresorption. Die glomeruläre Filtration wird nicht beeinflußt (SIROTA et al., 1952). Niedrige Dosen führen durch Hemmung der tubulären Harnsäuresekretion zu einer paradoxen Harnsäureretention. So beobachteten YÜ u. GUTMAN (1955) bei einem Gichtkranken unter langsamer Infusion von 0,2 mg Probenecid/min einen Abfall der Harnsäureclearance. Nach Steigerung der Infusionsrate auf 0,4 mg/min ließ sich eine Clearanceeinschränkung nicht mehr nachweisen, während noch höhere Dosen zu einer Uricurie führten (Tab. 2).

Entsprechend der kurzen Resorptionszeit tritt der harnsäuresenkende Effekt des Probenecids rasch ein. Ein Clearanceanstieg ist in den meisten Fällen innerhalb von 40 min nachweisbar (SIROTA et al. 1952). Nach Verabreichung von 2 g Probenecid per os beobachteten SIROTA et al. (1952) bei Gichtkranken einen mittleren Anstieg der Harnsäureclearance von 8,55 auf 32,9 ml/min. Diese Befunde stehen mit den Ergebnissen von ZÖLLNER et al. (1970) in Einklang, die bei einer gesunden Versuchsperson bereits 1 Std nach oraler Gabe von 1,5 g Probenecid bei Abnahme des Plasmaspiegels eine stark erhöhte renale Harnsäureausscheidung fanden. Die Harnsäureclearance stieg innerhalb von 4 Std bis auf 35,70 ml/min an und war 8,75 Std nach Arzneimittelgabe noch deutlich erhöht (Abb. 6). Lediglich BISHOP et al. (1954) konnten bei 2 Patienten mit rheumatischer Arthritis nach oraler Gabe von 1,5 g Probenecid trotz Abnahme der Serumharnsäure und des Harnsäurepools keine signifikante Harnsäuremehrausscheidung im Urin feststellen. Nach TALBOTT (1967) sind zur Senkung der Plasmaharnsäure Probenecidkonzentrationen im Serum von 1—5 mg/100 ml erforderlich (Abb. 7). Höhere Spiegel bewirken in der Regel keinen stärkeren Effekt.

Niedrige Salicylatdosen heben die uricosurische Wirkung des Probenecids auf (GUTMAN u. YÜ, 1951; BRØCHNER-MORTENSEN, 1958; YÜ u. GUTMAN, 1959). Die

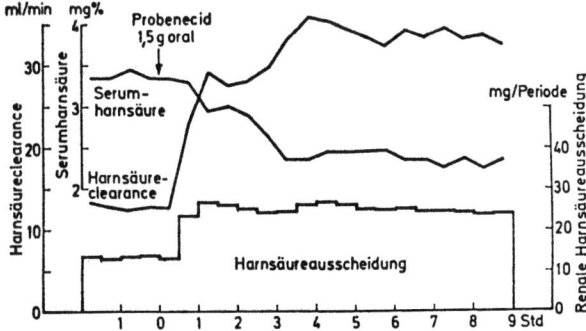

Abb. 6. Serumharnsäurespiegel, Harnsäureausscheidung und Harnsäureclearance nach einmaliger oraler Gabe von 1,5 g Probenecid bei einer gesunden Versuchsperson. (Nach ZÖLLNER et al., 1970)

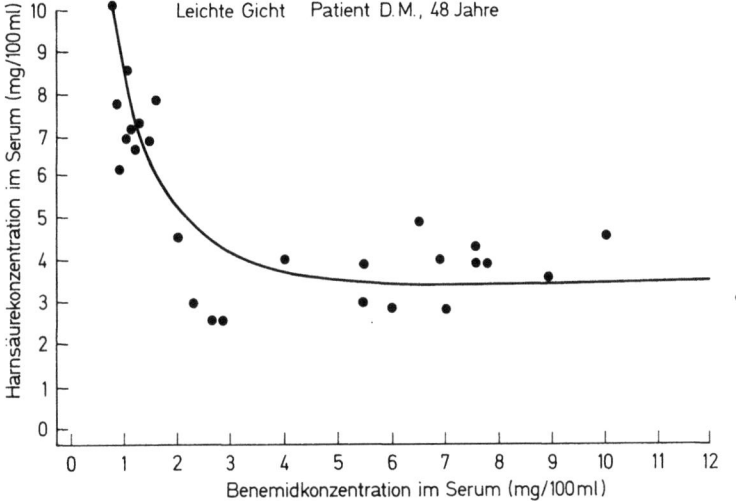

Abb. 7. Die Serumharnsäurekonzentration als eine Funktion des Benemidgehaltes im Serum. (Aus: TALBOTT, J. H.: Die Gicht, S. 99, Abb. 11. Stuttgart: Hippokrates-Verlag 1967)

Ursache ist noch weitgehend unbekannt. Von YÜ u. GUTMAN (1959) wurde angenommen, daß sich möglicherweise die Effekte der Harnsäurerückresorptionshemmung durch Probenecid und der Sekretionsblockierung durch Salicylate gegenseitig aufheben. Andererseits zeigen auch große Salicylatdosen, die selbst uricosurisch wirken, einen Antagonismus gegen Probenecid (PASCALE et al., 1952; YÜ u. GUTMAN, 1959). Lediglich MARSON (1954) konnte keine eindeutige Beeinflussung der uricosurischen Probenecidwirkung durch Salicylate feststellen. Im Vergleich zu den Salicylaten ist der antagonistische Effekt des Probenecids gegen die durch Salicylate hervorgerufene Harnsäuremehrausscheidung weitaus geringer (YÜ u. GUTMAN, 1959). Er geht mit einem Abfall der freien Salicylatkonzentration im Tubulusharn einher. Eine Hemmung der tubulären Salicylatsekretion durch Probenecid ist ursächlich anzuschuldigen. Additive Effekte werden dagegen beobachtet, wenn Probenecid in Kombination mit Zoxazolamin, Benzbromaronum oder Sulfinpyrazon verabreicht wird (YÜ u. GUTMAN, 1959a; SEEGMILLER u. GRAYZEL, 1960; DOFEL, 1971). PEREL et al. (1969) stellten außerdem fest, daß Probenecid in saurem wie auch alkalischem Urin die tubuläre Sekretion von Sulfinpyrazon und

Parahydroxysulfinpyrazon blockiert. Umgekehrt wird die Probenecidausscheidung durch Sulfinpyrazon nicht beeinflußt.

Probenecid besitzt keine antiphlogistische Wirkung und wird hauptsächlich zur Normalisierung der Serumharnsäure eingesetzt. Die Dosierung richtet sich nach der Wirkung auf die Plasmaharnsäure, die in den Normbereich oder zumindest in dessen Nähe gesenkt werden soll. Da zu Beginn der Behandlung Harnsäuremengen ausgeschieden werden, die zu Kristallurie und Hämaturie führen können, ist es erforderlich, anfangs niedrige Dosen (2 × 0,25 g/tgl.) zu wählen und gleichzeitig Alkali in Form von Eisenbergscher Lösung oder Uralyt-U® sowie reichliche Flüssigkeitszufuhr zu verordnen. Die durchschnittliche Tagesdosis beträgt 0,5—3,0 g. In dem Krankengut von GUTMAN u. YÜ (1957) betrug die optimale Dosis bei 10% der Patienten 0,5 g/tgl., bei 50% 1,0 g/tgl., bei 25% 1,5—2,0 g/tgl. und bei 15% 2,5—3,0 g/tgl.

Erfahrungen mit Probenecid in der Gichtbehandlung wurden von GUTMAN (1950, 1965), GUTMAN u. YÜ (1951, 1952), YÜ u. GUTMAN (1967), TALBOTT et al. (1951), TALBOTT (1959), PASCALE et al. (1952), KUZELL et al. (1955), BARTELS (1955), BARTELS u. MATOSSIAN (1959), OGRYZLO u. HARRISON (1957), BRØCHNER-MORTENSEN (1958), EMMERSON (1963), FROST (1965) sowie zahlreichen anderen Autoren mitgeteilt. GUTMAN u. YÜ (1951) beobachteten bei 18 Patienten nach Gabe von 2,0 g Probenecid per os im Verlauf der ersten Woche einen mittleren Abfall des Serumharnsäurespiegels um 42% bzw. um 47% nach weiteren 7 Tagen. 1,0 g/tgl. (24 Patienten) führten innerhalb des gleichen Zeitraums zu einem mittleren Abfall um 33% bzw. 34%. Unter einer Dosis von 0,5 g/tgl. (20 Personen) betrug der mittlere Abfall 27% des Ausgangswertes in der ersten bzw. 28% in der zweiten Woche. In den meisten Fällen konnte die Senkung des Serumharnsäurespiegels unter fortgesetzter Therapie aufrechterhalten werden. Dem Abfall der Serumharnsäure entsprach ein Anstieg der renalen Harnsäureausscheidung. Nach Zufuhr von 2,0 g Probenecid/tgl. betrug die durchschnittliche Harnsäuremehrausscheidung in 12 Fällen in der ersten Woche 67%, in der zweiten Woche 35,7% des Ausgangswertes. Die entsprechenden Werte unter 1,0 g (16 Fälle) betrugen +52,2% bzw. +22,2%, unter 0,5 g/tgl. (11 Fälle) +46,6% bzw. +23,5%. Die höchsten Harnsäurewerte im Urin wurden unmittelbar nach Einleitung der Therapie gemessen. Dabei kann die Harnsäuremehrausscheidung unter fortgesetzter Behandlung in Abhängigkeit von der Größe des Harnsäurepools über Monate anhalten. So wurden von GUTMAN u. YÜ (1952) Harnsäuremehrausscheidungen von insgesamt 100 g beschrieben. PASCALE et al. (1952) untersuchten die Wirkung des Probenecids bei 20 Gichtkranken, wobei die Therapie bei 10 Patienten bis zu 7½ Monate verfolgt wurde. Unter einer Tagesdosis von 2,0 g Probenecid fiel innerhalb von 72 Std die Serumharnsäure auf durchschnittlich 55% des Ausgangswertes ab, während die entsprechende mittlere Harnsäureausscheidung bis auf 200% der Kontrollperiode anstieg. Die Zahl der Gichtanfälle verringerte sich unter fortgesetzter Therapie. Lediglich in drei Fällen mit eingeschränkter Nierenfunktion konnte kein Abfall des Serumharnsäurespiegels erzielt werden. Diese Erfahrungen von GUTMAN u. YÜ (1951), PASCALE et al. (1952) sowie zahlreichen weiteren Autoren konnten auch von BARTELS (1955) bestätigt werden, der 42 Gichtiker über 12—30 Monate mit Probenecid behandelte. In 38 Fällen konnte eine Normalisierung des Serumharnsäurespiegels erreicht werden. 15 Patienten waren nach Behandlungsbeginn anfallsfrei, bei 24 Patienten verliefen die Gichtanfälle während der ersten 6—9 Behandlungsmonate milder. In drei Fällen war der Therapieerfolg unbefriedigend.

Im allgemeinen werden unter konsequenter Probenecidtherapie nach einer kürzeren oder längeren Zeit, die von der Größe der Harnsäuredepots abhängt, keine Gichtanfälle mehr beobachtet. Tophi werden kleiner oder können ganz verschwinden. Hinsichtlich der Beeinflussung der Gichtniere können z.Z. jedoch keine Aussagen gemacht werden, wie denn Probenecid bei Gichtkranken mit Niereninsuffizienz gelegentlich versagt. Lediglich PHILLIPS (1955) konnte bei einem 31jährigen Patienten mit Niereninsuffizienz während einer 34monatigen Probenecidbehandlung eine wesentliche Besserung der Nierenfunktion beobachten. Heute wird man bei Patienten mit eingeschränkter Nierenfunktion allerdings Allopurinol den Vorzug geben.

Die Toxicität von Probenecid ist gering. Im Tierversuch führten hohe Dosen zu zentralnervösen Erscheinungen in Form von Muskelzucken sowie tonischklonischen Krämpfen. Der Tod trat wahrscheinlich infolge Atemversagens ein (MCKINNEY et al., 1951). Beim Menschen wurden von RIZZUTO et al. (1965) nach Einnahme von 47 g Probenecid (Suicidversuch) Krämpfe und Koma beobachtet. Unter der gewöhnlichen therapeutischen Dosierung von 0,5—2,0 g wird Probenecid gut toleriert. Nebenwirkungen in Form von Magen-Darmstörungen mit gelegentlicher Reaktivierung eines Ulcus oder allergischen Reaktionen treten bei etwa 10% aller behandelten Patienten auf (GUTMAN, 1965, 1968). Nach BOGER u. STRICKLAND (1955) werden Magen-Darmstörungen bei 3,1% und allergische Reaktionen, vor allem Exantheme, bei 2% aller Patienten beobachtet. Allerdings wurde in den meisten Fällen Probenecid in Kombination mit Penicillin verabreicht, so daß die Exantheme zum größten Teil einer Penicillinallergie zugeschrieben werden müssen.

Unter 169 Gichtikern stellten GUTMAN u. YÜ (1957) in 13 Fällen (8%) Magen-Darm-Störungen schweren Grades, in 8 Fällen (5%) allergische Reaktionen fest. Berichte über das Auftreten einer Lebernekrose (REYNOLDS et al., 1957) sowie nephrotisches Syndrom (SCOTT u. O'BRIEN, 1968, HERTZ et al., 1972) betreffen Einzelbeobachtungen. Eine erfolgreiche Desensibilisierung bei Probenecidallergie wurde von AUSTRIAN u. BOGER (1956) mitgeteilt. Das Auftreten von Gichtanfällen zu Beginn einer uricosurischen Therapie sowie Harnsäureausfällungen in der Niere mit Nierenkoliken und Hämaturie (Häufigkeit etwa 1% nach BOGER u. STRICKLAND, 1955) sind Nebenwirkungen jedes Uricosuricums, wenn nicht besondere Vorsichtsmaßnahmen wie Colchicinprophylaxe bzw. ausreichende Flüssigkeitszufuhr und Neutralisierung des Harns getroffen werden.

Longacid

Uricosurische Eigenschaften besitzen auch das p-Carboxybenzolsulfodibutylamid sowie das p-Carboxybenzolsulfodiäthylamid (Abb.4), die sich vom Probenecid nur durch die Länge der Seitenketten unterscheiden und früher als Longacid im Handel waren. Mit der Dibutylamid-Verbindung fanden BUCHBORN u. WENK (1954) bei 12 Versuchspersonen eine durchschnittliche Herabsetzung der tubulären Harnsäurerückresorption um 25%. Bei einem Gichtkranken ergab sich allerdings unter der Behandlung mit 2 g Longacid nur ein vorübergehender Abfall der Serumharnsäure. GAMP (1957) hat an Gichtkranken die Wirkung der Diäthylamid-Verbindung mit der des Probenecids verglichen. Aus seinen Untersuchungen ergibt sich eine annähernd gleiche Wirksamkeit der beiden Substanzen, möglicherweise ist die erforderliche Longacid-Dosis etwas höher. Langfristige Beobachtungen von Longacid-behandelten Gichtikern liegen nicht vor.

Pyrazolidinderivate

Phenylbutazon und seine Metaboliten

Phenylbutazon (Abb.8) wird rasch und vollständig aus dem Gastrointestinaltrakt resorbiert. Nach oraler Zufuhr werden die höchsten Plasmakonzentrationen

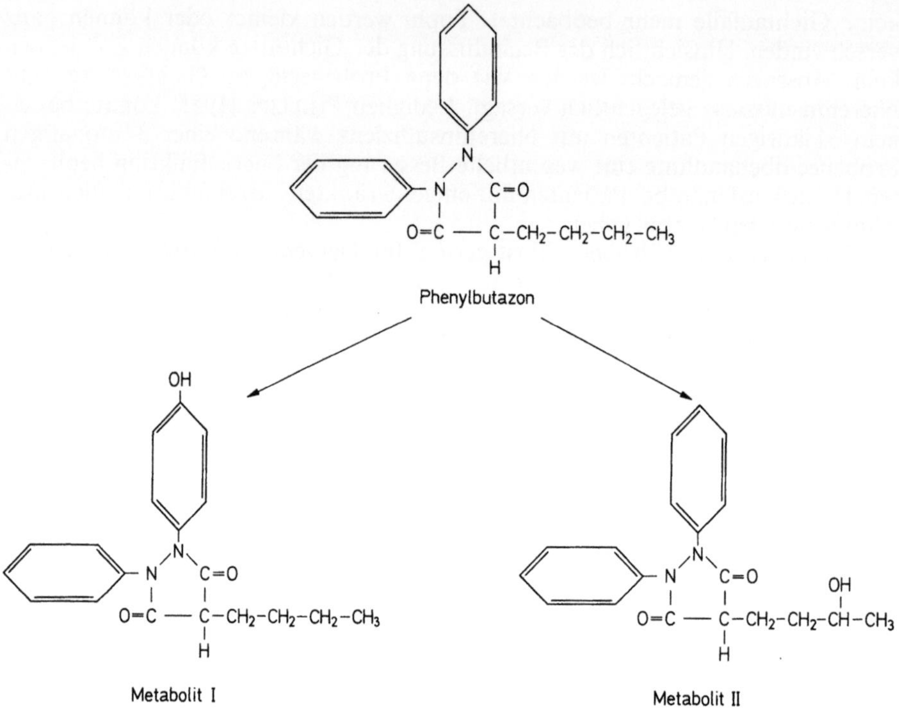

Abb. 8. Phenylbutazon und seine Metaboliten

innerhalb von 2 Std, nach intramuskulärer Gabe jedoch erst nach 6—10 Std erreicht. Eine verzögerte Freisetzung des Arzneimittels aus der Injektionsstelle ist ursächlich anzuschuldigen (BURNS et al., 1953). Im Plasma ist Phenylbutazon bei einer Konzentration von 5—15 mg-% zu 98% an Eiweiß gebunden. Höhere Spiegel setzen das Ausmaß der Proteinbindung herab. So beobachteten BURNS et al. (1953) bei einer Phenylbutazonkonzentration von 25 mg-% nur eine Proteinbindung von 88%. Die Halbwertszeit beim Menschen beträgt durchschnittlich 72 Std. Sie unterliegt jedoch beträchtlichen individuellen Variationen, was auf einer unterschiedlichen Metabolisierungsgeschwindigkeit beruht, da nur ein minimaler Anteil des Arzneimittels unverändert im Urin aufgefunden wird. Metaboliten sind das Oxyphenbutazon (Metabolit I) sowie das 3'-Hydroxyphenylbutazon (Metabolit II) (Abb. 8).

Der renale Ausscheidungsmechanismus von Phenylbutazon ist beim Menschen noch nicht vollständig geklärt, da nur geringe Mengen im Urin aufgefunden werden (GUTMAN, 1966). Beim Hund konnten GUTMAN et al. (1960) eine tubuläre Nettorückresorption in saurem sowie eine aktive tubuläre Sekretion in alkalischem Urin nachweisen.

Für die Gichtbehandlung sind zwei Eigenschaften des Phenylbutazons von Bedeutung:

1. Eine ausgeprägte antiphlogistische Wirkung, die sich die Therapie des akuten Gichtanfalles zunutze macht.
2. Eine mäßige uricosurische Wirkung.

In der Anfallsbehandlung ist Phenylbutazon nach Ansicht zahlreicher Autoren hochwirksam (BAUER u. SINGH, 1957; KUZELL et al., 1954; DE SEZE et al., 1958). Die notwendige Dosis beträgt durchschnittlich 1 g/tgl. über 3—5 Tage.

Tabelle 3. Der Einfluß von Phenylbutazon auf die renale Harnsäureclearance. (Mod. nach YÜ u. GUTMAN, 1955)

Plasmaphenylbutazon- konzentration mg/100 ml	Plasmaharnsäure mg/100 ml	Harnsäureclearance ml/min
0	9,2	8,02
2,3	9,5	6,15
3,0	9,4	6,04
10,0	9,5	10,4
12,0	9,5	12,7
15,5	9,3	13,9
16,7	9,0	24,4

Mitteilungen über eine Senkung des Serumharnsäurespiegels durch Phenylbutazon liegen von KUZELL u. SCHAFFARZICK (1952), GUTMAN u. YÜ (1952), KIDD et al. (1953), JOHNSON et al. (1954), WYNGAARDEN (1955) und anderen Autoren vor. Der Mechanismus der Harnsäuresenkung im Serum war jedoch lange Zeit ungeklärt. So beschrieben einige Autoren einen uricosurischen Effekt (GUTMAN u. YÜ, 1952; YÜ et al., 1953; WYNGAARDEN, 1955); andere Autoren (KUZELL u. SCHAFFARZICK 1952, KIDD et al., 1953, JOHNSON et al., 1954) beobachteten nur unbedeutende bzw. keine Änderungen der renalen Harnsäureausscheidung nach Phenylbutazongabe. Diese sich widersprechenden Befunde sind darauf zurückzuführen, daß erstens der uricosurische Effekt des Phenylbutazons erst bei einer Plasmakonzentration von 10 mg-% und darüber einsetzt, zweitens eine gewisse Senkung der Serumharnsäure auch auf die durch Phenylbutazon hervorgerufene Vergrößerung des Extracellulärraumes zurückzuführen ist. So beobachteten YÜ et al. (1953) bei drei Gichtpatienten nach intravenöser Phenylbutazonverabreichung eine ausgeprägte Hemmung der renalen NaCl-Ausscheidung, die nach Absetzen der Medikation noch drei Tage lang anhielt.

Die uricosurische Wirkung des Phenylbutazons beruht auf einer Hemmung der tubulären Harnsäurerückresorption. Eine Harnsäuremehrausscheidung ist jedoch erst bei Plasmaphenylbutazonkonzentrationen von 10 mg-% und darüber nachweisbar. Niedrige Konzentrationen gehen mit einer Einschränkung der Harnsäureclearance einher (Tab. 3).

Phenylbutazon besitzt keinen Einfluß auf die glomeruläre Filtrationsrate. Die PAH-, Na^+- und Cl-Clearance sowie die tubuläre Sekretion von Phenolsulphthalein werden dagegen deutlich vermindert (YÜ et al., 1953; BRODIE et al., 1954). Ein Antagonismus gegen Sulfinpyrazon oder Probenecid wird nicht beobachtet. Bei Gichtkranken, die unter Probenecidtherapie (1,0 g/tgl.) standen, konnten YÜ et al. (1953) nach zusätzlicher Verabreichung von 600 mg Phenylbutazon per os lediglich in den beiden ersten Tagen eine geringe Verminderung der renalen Harnsäureausscheidung feststellen.

Nach intravenöser Zufuhr von 12—27 mg Phenylbutazon/kg Körpergewicht steigt nach Untersuchungen von YÜ et al. (1953) bei Gichtkranken die Harnsäureclearance von durchschnittlich 6,3 auf 19,3 ml/min an. Die höchsten Werte werden dabei innerhalb der ersten 4 Std erreicht. Untersuchungen derselben Autoren zeigten, daß der uricosurische Wirkungseintritt dabei eng mit der Plasmaphenylbutazonkonzentration verknüpft ist. Erst bei Spiegeln von 10 mg-% und darüber ist mit einem uricosurischen Effekt zu rechnen.

WYNGAARDEN berichtete 1955 über das Verhalten von Serumharnsäure, Harnsäurepool und Harnsäureausscheidung im Urin bei 2 Versuchspersonen, die

Tabelle 4. Prozentuale Veränderung von $C_{HS}C_{Inulin}$ unter niedrigen Oxyphenbutazonkonzentrationen. (Mod. nach YÜ u. GUTMAN, 1955)

Versuchspersonen	Oxyphenbutazonkonzentration im Plasma mg/100 ml	Prozentuale Veränderung des Quotienten C_{HS}/C_{Inulin}
1	0,5	−32,8
2	3,6	−31,8
3	7,0	−24,8
4	5,9	−22,0
5	4,3	−20,7
6	1,3	−20,7
7	5,0	−18,0

mehrere Tage lang 0,8 g Phenylbutazon einnahmen. Während bei der einen Person dieses Arzneimittel zu einer Harnsäuremehrausscheidung führte, die größer als die Abnahme des Harnsäurepools war, setzte unter denselben Bedingungen bei der zweiten Versuchsperson trotz ausgeprägtem Abfall der Serumharnsäure nur eine mäßige renale Harnsäuremehrausscheidung ein. Auf eine derartige Diskrepanz zwischen Serumharnsäureabfall und renaler Harnsäureausscheidung wurde auch von BISHOP et al. (1954) hingewiesen. Bei 2 Patienten mit rheumatoider Arthritis konnten sie nach oraler Verabreichung von 400 mg Phenylbutazon trotz Abnahme des Harnsäurepools, gesteigerter Turn over-Rate und Senkung der Serumharnsäurekonzentration keinen signifikanten Anstieg der renalen Harnsäureausscheidung feststellen. Die Autoren schlossen aus ihren Befunden, daß dieses Arzneimittel nur bei Patienten mit erhöhtem Harnsäurepool zu einer Harnsäuremehrausscheidung führt.

Die wirksame Phenylbutazondosis zur Anfallskupierung beträgt 1 g/tgl. über drei bis fünf Tage, eine uricosurische Wirkung setzt erst bei täglichen oralen Dosen von durchschnittlich 600—800 mg ein. Der uricosurische Effekt ist jedoch dem des Probenecids, Sulfinpyrazons und Benzbromaronums deutlich unterlegen. Außerdem rechtfertigen die zahlreichen Nebenwirkungen keine Langzeitbehandlung mit diesem Arzneimittel.

Oxyphenbutazon (Metabolit I)

Oxyphenbutazon unterscheidet sich vom Phenylbutazon durch eine Hydroxylgruppe in der para-Position des Benzolrings (Abb. 8). Nach oraler Zufuhr wird die Verbindung rasch und fast vollständig aus dem Gastrointestinaltrakt resorbiert; bei Plasmaspiegeln von 5—15 mg-% entspricht der Grad der Proteinbindung dem der Muttersubstanz. Die Halbwertszeit beim Menschen beträgt durchschnittlich drei Tage. Die renale Ausscheidung an unveränderter Substanz ist gering, so daß eine Metabolisierung zu zum Teil bis jetzt noch unbekannten Stoffwechselprodukten angenommen werden muß (Zusammenfassung bei GUTMAN, 1966).

Wie Phenylbutazon besitzt Oxyphenbutazon antiphlogistische und uricosurische Eigenschaften. Bei geringen Plasmaoxyphenbutazonkonzentrationen wird die Harnsäureclearance erniedrigt (Tab. 4), Plasmaspiegel über 10 mg-% führen durch Hemmung der tubulären Harnsäurerückresorption zu einer Harnsäuremehrausscheidung.

Abgesehen von einer besseren Magenverträglichkeit entsprechen die toxischen Eigenschaften des Oxyphenbutazons denen des Phenylbutazons (GOODMAN u. GILMAN, 1970).

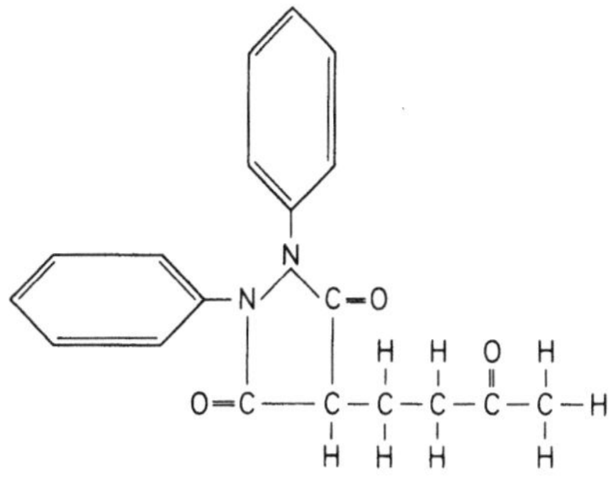

Abb. 9. Ketophenylbutazon

Der *Metabolit II*, 3'-Hydroxyphenylbutazon, entsteht durch Einführung einer Hydroxylgruppe in die Position 3 der Butylseitenkette (Abb. 8). Im Gegensatz zu Phenylbutazon und Oxyphenbutazon ist nach oraler Zufuhr die Resorption aus dem Gastrointestinaltrakt gering. Bei Plasmaspiegeln von 5—15 mg-% beträgt die Proteinbindung beim Menschen etwa 93%, die durchschnittliche Halbwertszeit der Verbindung zehn Stunden. Die uricosurischen Eigenschaften des 3'-Hydroxyphenylbutazons sind denen des Phenylbutazons und Oxyphenbutazons überlegen. So sahen YÜ et al. (1958) bei 3'-Hydroxyphenylbutazonspiegeln im Serum von 5—9 mg-% einen drei- bis fünffachen Anstieg des Quotienten C_{Hs}/C_{GFR} gegenüber der Kontrollperiode (zitiert bei GUTMAN, 1966).

Ketophenylbutazon

Über seine Erfahrungen mit diesem Phenylbutazonderivat in der Gichtbehandlung berichtete MUGLER (1971). Ketophenylbutazon (Abb. 9) besitzt antiphlogistische und uricosurische Eigenschaften. MUGLER (1971) behandelte 43 Gichtkranke mit einer Ketophenylbutazondosis von 250—750 mg/tgl.

Die Behandlungsdauer erstreckte sich in 80% der Fälle über 10—18 Tage. Bei allen Patienten stieg die renale Harnsäureausscheidung bei Abfall des Serumharnsäurespiegels signifikant an. In 37% der Fälle betrug dabei der Anstieg mehr als 100%.

Die Magenverträglichkeit war im Vergleich zu Phenylbutazon bemerkenswert gut. Eine Wasserretention wurde in einem Fall beobachtet, Störungen des Blutbildes traten nicht auf. Gichtanfälle wurden allerdings in neun Fällen beobachtet, so daß die antiphlogistische Wirkung unter dieser Dosis zu gering ist.

1,2-Diphenyl-4-(2-phenylthioäthyl)-3,5-dioxopyrazolidin = G-25671

Die uricosurischen Eigenschaften von Phenylbutazon und die seiner Metaboliten gaben Anlaß zur Suche nach weiteren uricosurisch wirksamen Verbindungen ähnlicher Struktur, aber mit geringeren Nebenwirkungen. Auf diese Weise wurde G-25671 entdeckt, eine Verbindung, in der die Butylseitenkette des Phenylbutazons durch eine Phenylthioäthylgruppe ersetzt ist (Abb. 10).

Wie Phenylbutazon wird G-25671 fast vollständig aus dem Gastrointestinaltrakt resorbiert. Die Halbwertszeit beträgt jedoch nur etwa 3 Std, weshalb dieses Arzneimittel zur Aufrechterhaltung eines konstanten Blutspiegels in verteilten Tagesdosen verabreicht werden muß. Ursache dieser kurzen Halbwertszeit ist eine rasche Metabolisierung; die Ausscheidung der unveränderten Substanz im Urin ist minimal.

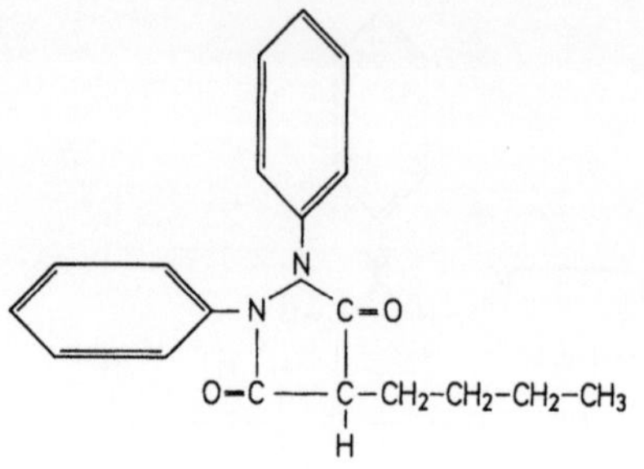

Abb. 10. Phenylbutazon und G-25671

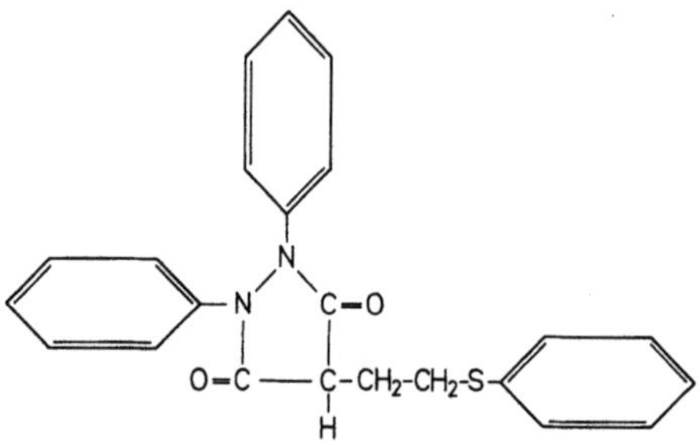

Bis auf einige Ausnahmen verändert G-25671 nicht die Inulinclearance. Die PAH-Clearance sowie die Phenolsulphthaleinausscheidung wird jedoch verringert. Das Ausmaß der NaCl- und Wasserretention ist im Vergleich zu Phenylbutazon wesentlich geringer (YÜ et al., 1956). Eine Beeinflussung der renalen Kalium- und Phosphatausscheidung wird nicht beobachtet.

G-25671 besitzt antiphlogistische und uricosurische Eigenschaften. Die entzündungshemmende Wirkung ist jedoch der des Phenylbutazons und Oxyphenbutazons deutlich unterlegen. Während YÜ et al. (1956) nach Verabreichung von 800 mg Phenylbutazon/tgl. unter 103 Gichtanfällen bei einer „Versagerquote" von 12% in 74% der Fälle innerhalb von 1—2 Tagen und in 14% innerhalb der ersten Behandlungswoche eine vollständige Remission beobachteten, war unter zehn Anfällen nach Zufuhr von täglich 1 g G-25671 innerhalb von 24—48 Std nur in 30% eine komplette Remission zu erzielen.

Die uricosurische Wirkung von G-25671 beruht auf einer Hemmung der tubulären Harnsäurerückresorption und setzt nach intravenöser Arzneimittelgabe innerhalb von 40 min ein. Dabei führen bereits Plasmakonzentrationen von 1 mg-% zu einem Anstieg der Harnsäureclearance (Tab. 5). Nach rascher intravenöser Infusion von 16 mg G-25671/kg/KG beobachteten YÜ et al. (1956) bei sieben Versuchspersonen einen Anstieg des Quotienten aus Harnsäure- und Inulinclearance von durchschnittlich 6,15 auf 30,6%. Diesem Anstieg der renalen Harnsäureausscheidung entsprach ein Abfall der Serumharnsäure um 2,3±0,5 mg-%. Die mehrtägige orale Verabreichung von 1,0 g G-25671, auf fünf Tagesdosen verteilt, führte bei fünf Gichtkranken nach 48 Std zu einer Harnsäuremehrausscheidung von 97%. Ihr entsprach ein Abfall des Serumharnsäurespie-

Tabelle 5. Der Einfluß der Serumkonzentration von G-25671 auf die Harnsäureclearance.
(Mod. nach YÜ et al., 1956)

Serumkonzentration von G-25671 (mg/100 ml)	Inulinclearance (ml/min)	Serumharnsäure (mg/100 ml)	Harnsäureclearance (ml/min)
0	89,1	7,5	9,54
0,2	82,3	7,8	9,28
1,0	92,8	7,6	11,4
1,2	90,0	7,3	12,6
2,7	92,8	7,4	16,3

gels (Untersuchungen an 13 Gichtkranken) von 9,6 mg-% auf 4,2 mg-%. Diese Ergebnisse stimmen mit den Erfahrungen von OGRYZLO u. HARRISON (1957) überein. Nach täglicher oraler Zufuhr von 1,0 g G-25671 fiel bei einem Gichtiker die Serumharnsäure innerhalb von sechs Tagen von 10,0 mg-% auf 4,2 mg-%, bei einem weiteren Gichtkranken von 10,0 auf 5,7 mg-% ab. Vergleichsuntersuchungen an derselben Versuchsperson ergaben, daß die Dosen von 1 g G-25671/tgl., 1 g Phenylbutazon/tgl., 0,5 g Sulfinpyrazon/tgl., 3 g Probenecid/tgl. und 6 g Acetylsalicylsäure/tgl. bezüglich ihrer uricosurischen Wirkung äquivalent sind. Niedrige Salicylatdosen beeinflussen die harnsäuresenkende Wirkung von G-25671 und Sulfinpyrazon antagonistisch, weshalb die kombinierte Verabreichung von Salicylaten mit diesen Pharmaka vermieden werden sollte.

Die Toxicität von G-25671 wurde von YÜ et al. (1956) an 28 Gichtkranken untersucht, wobei sich die Beobachtungsdauer allerdings nur bei sieben Personen über 3—10 Monate erstreckte. Bei drei Patienten entwickelten sich ein bis zwei Tage nach Therapiebeginn allergische Reaktionen, bei drei weiteren Patienten traten infolge des uricosurischen Wirkungsmechanismus renale Komplikationen auf. Gastrointestinale Störungen wurden nur in zwei Fällen beobachtet. Die sorgfältige, regelmäßige Überwachung der sieben Patienten, die über längere Zeit G-25671 erhielten, ließ keine Knochenmarksdepression, Neuro- oder Hepatotoxicität erkennen. Keine gastrointestinalen Beschwerden wurden von OGRYZLO u. HARRISON (1957) beobachtet, die 25 Patienten G-25671 über durchschnittlich sechs Monate verabreichten. In drei Fällen trat ein maculopapulöses Exanthem auf. Bei einigen Patienten nahm die Leucocytenzahl geringgradig ab. Trotz dieser günstigen Mitteilungen ist bei der Strukturverwandtschaft von G-25671 mit Phenylbutazon eine uricosurische Langzeittherapie nicht zu rechtfertigen. Außerdem wurde mit Sulfinpyrazon, einem Metaboliten von G-25671, ein wesentlich wirksameres und praktisch nebenwirkungsfreies Uricosuricum gefunden.

Sulfinpyrazon [3]

Sulfinpyrazon, 1,2-Diphenyl-3,5-dioxo-4-(2-phenyl-sulfinyläthyl)-pyrazolidin, ist der Sulfoxydmetabolit von G-25671 (Abb. 11). Er wurde von BURNS et al. im Jahre 1957 aus dem Urin isoliert. Es handelt sich um eine starke Säure (pKa 2,8), die ausgeprägte uricosurische, jedoch keine antiphlogistische Eigenschaften besitzt und in Form von 2 optisch aktiven Isomeren vorkommt. Die aus dem Urin gewonnene Verbindung stellt ein Gemisch aus beiden Isomeren, vorwiegend der D-Form dar (DAYTON et al., 1961).

---

[3] Anturano®.

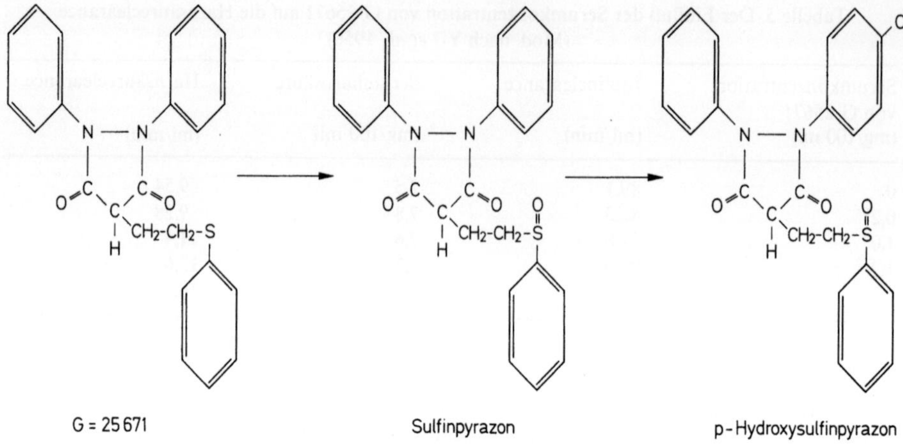

G = 25 671   Sulfinpyrazon   p-Hydroxysulfinpyrazon

Abb. 11. G-25671, Sulfinpyrazon und p-Hydroxysulfinpyrazon

Sulfinpyrazon wird schnell und fast vollständig aus dem Gastrointestinaltrakt resorbiert. Die intravenöse oder orale Zufuhr einer Dosis von 600 mg führt innerhalb von zwei Stunden zu fast gleichen Plasmakonzentrationen (BURNS et al., 1957). Bei einem Plasmaspiegel von 10 mg-% sind annähernd 98% an Eiweiß gebunden (DAYTON et al., 1961). Die Halbwertszeit beträgt im Vergleich zu Phenylbutazon nur etwa 3 Std, weshalb die tägliche Gesamtmenge in Form von mehreren Einzeldosen eingenommen werden muß (BURNS et al., 1957). Die Ausscheidung erfolgt durch die Nieren, wobei innerhalb von 24 Std etwa 25% der verabreichten Dosis im Urin aufgefunden werden (BURNS et al., 1957). Die Gesamtausscheidung an unveränderter Substanz beträgt 90% (GOODMAN u. GILMAN, 1970). Hauptmetabolit ist das ebenfalls uricosurisch wirksame p-Hydroxysulfinpyrazon (DAYTON et al., 1961).

Der Mechanismus der renalen Elimination von Sulfinpyrazon ist vorwiegend durch eine tubuläre Sekretion gekennzeichnet, da auf Grund einer starken Plasma-Eiweißbindung nur wenig glomerulär filtriert wird. Das Ausmaß einer tubulären Rückresorption in saurem Urin, durch passive Rückdiffusion, ist gering, weil der größte Teil dieser Verbindung in dissoziierter Form vorliegt (GOODMAN u. GILMAN, 1970). Alkalisierung des Urins führt zu keiner bedeutenden Zunahme der Sulfinpyrazonausscheidung (GUTMAN et al., 1960).

Sulfinpyrazon beeinflußt nicht die glomeruläre Filtrationsrate sowie die renale Elektrolytausscheidung (BURNS et al., 1957). Dagegen wird die PAH-Clearance sowie die Phenolsulphthaleinausscheidung eingeschränkt. Die uricosurische Wirkung beruht auf einer Hemmung der tubulären Harnsäurerückresorption. Sie übertrifft die der übrigen Phenylbutazonderivate. So steigt der Quotient C_{HS}/C_{Inulin} nach intravenöser Zufuhr von 5 mg Sulfinpyrazon/kg/KG um das Siebenfache an (BURNS et al., 1957), während vergleichsweise nach intravenöser Verabreichung von 16 mg G-25671/kg/KG bzw. 12—27 mg Phenylbutazon/kg/KG nur ein Anstieg um das Fünf- bzw. Dreifache des Ausgangswertes zu beobachten ist (YÜ et al., 1953, 1956). Nach OGRYZLO u. HARRISON (1957) werden vergleichbare Effekte bezüglich der Serumharnsäuresenkung und renalen Harnsäureausscheidung mit 1 g Phenylbutazon/tgl., 1 g G-25671/tgl. und 0,5 g Sulfinpyrazon/tgl. erzielt. Bei gleicher Dosierung übertrifft Sulfinpyrazon die uricosurische Wirkung des Probenecids um das Sechsfache (OGRYZLO u. HARRISON, 1957).

Tabelle 6. Der Einfluß von Acetylsalicylsäure auf die durch Sulfinpyrazon hervorgerufene Harnsäuremehrausscheidung. (Mod. nach KERSLEY et al., 1958)

	Serumharnsäure (mg/100 ml)	Harnsäureausscheidung im Urin (mg/24 Std)
Kontrollperiode	7,7	576
Sulfinpyrazon 400 mg/tgl. per os	4,8	947
Sulfinpyrazon 400 mg/tgl. per os + 3,5 g Acetylsalicylsäure per os	8,8	401

Die minimale intravenöse Dosis, die zur Erzielung eines uricosurischen Effektes erforderlich ist, beträgt 35 mg (BURNS et al., 1957). Ein ausgeprägter Clearanceanstieg ist dabei innerhalb von 2 Std zu verzeichnen. Die wirksamen oralen Tagesdosen liegen bei 200—400 mg, wobei infolge der kurzen Halbwertszeit die Gesamtdosis auf 3—4 Einzelportionen verteilt werden sollte. Um renale Harnsäureausfällungen zu vermeiden, muß dabei zu Beginn der Therapie auf eine einschleichende Dosierung, Neutralisierung des Harns sowie ausreichendes Urinvolumen geachtet werden.

Sulfinpyrazon sollte nicht in Kombination mit Salicylaten verabreicht werden, da sich die uricosurischen Wirkungen gegenseitig aufheben (OGRYZLO u. HARRISON, 1957; KERSLEY et al., 1958; SEEGMILLER u. GRAYZEL, 1960; YÜ et al., 1963). KERSLEY et al. (1958) beobachteten bei Gichtpatienten, die mit Sulfinpyrazon eingestellt waren, nach Zulage von Acetylsalicylsäure in den meisten Fällen eine Verminderung der renalen Harnsäureausscheidung unter die Werte der Kontrollperiode (Tab. 6). Diese Ergebnisse konnten von YÜ et al. (1963) mittels Clearanceuntersuchungen an Gichtpatienten, denen zuerst Sulfinpyrazon (anfangs 300 mg, dann 10 mg/min), anschließend zusätzlich Natriumsalicylat (anfangs 3 g, dann 10—20 mg/min) infundiert wurde, bestätigt werden. Mit der Aufhebung des uricosurischen Sulfinpyrazoneffektes ging eine Abnahme der Plasmasulfinpyrazonkonzentration einher, obwohl die renale Ausscheidung dieses Uricosuricums nicht zunahm. Die Autoren führten diese Erscheinung auf eine partielle Verdrängung des Sulfinpyrazons aus seiner Plasmaeiweißbindung durch Natriumsalicylat bei gleichzeitiger Vergrößerung des Sulfinpyrazonverteilungsraumes zurück. Das in umgekehrter Reihenfolge durchgeführte Experiment ging ebenfalls mit einer Abnahme der renalen Harnsäureausscheidung einher. Gleichzeitig nahm jedoch die tubuläre Salicylatsekretion ab. Die Autoren schlossen aus diesen Befunden, daß Plasmaeiweißbindung und renaler Tubulus als Orte der gegenseitigen Beeinflussung dieser Verbindungen anzusehen sind.

Die Wirksamkeit von Sulfinpyrazon als Uricosuricum wurde von zahlreichen Autoren unterstrichen (BURNS et al., 1957; OGRYZLO u. HARRISON, 1957; YÜ et al., 1958; KERSLEY et al., 1958; PERSELLIN u. SCHMID 1961; MELLINGHOFF u. GROSS, 1962; THOMPSON et al., 1962; EMMERSON, 1963; etc.). KERSLEY et al. (1958) stellten bei 7 Gichtpatienten unter 400 mg Sulfinpyrazon/tgl. im Verlauf einer Woche einen mittleren Anstieg der renalen Harnsäureausscheidung von 581 auf 914 mg/tgl. fest. Die Dosiserhöhung auf 800 mg/tgl. führte bei 5 Patienten nach weiteren 7 Tagen zu einer durchschnittlichen Tagesharnsäureausscheidung von 1042 mg. Die bei 11 Patienten bestimmte Serumharnsäure fiel im Mittel von 7,8 auf 4,0 mg-% ab. PERSELLIN u. SCHMID (1961) verfolgten bei 17 Gichtikern unter einer Tagesdosis von 400 mg Sulfinpyrazon die Serumharnsäure über insgesamt 14 Monate. Sie fanden dabei einen mittleren Abfall um 3,3 mg-%. Diese Befunde

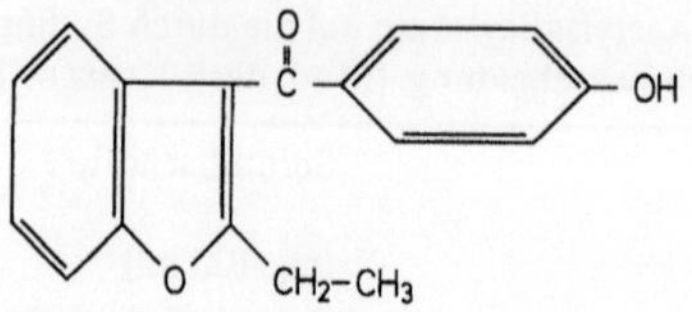

Benzaronum

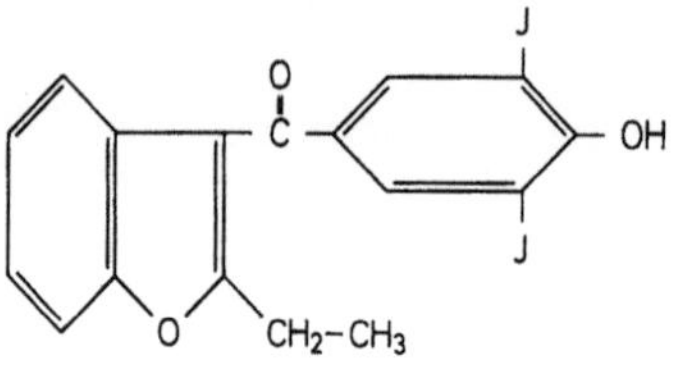

Benziodaronum

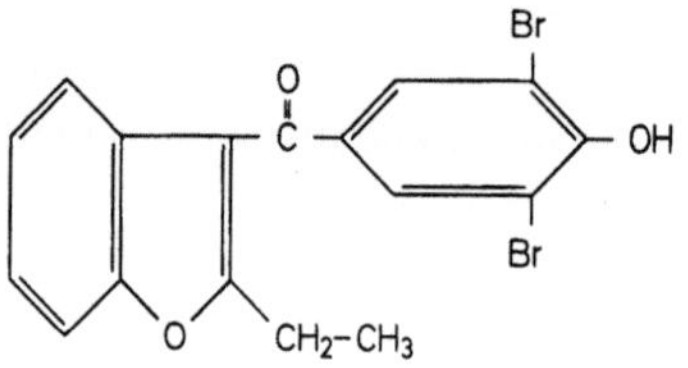

Benzbromaronum

Abb. 12. Benzaronum, Benzbromaronum und Benziodaronum

stehen auch mit den Ergebnissen von THOMPSON et al. (1962) in Einklang, die 15 Gichtpatienten über längere Zeit mit 300 mg Sulfinpyrazon/tgl. behandelten. In 3 Fällen fiel die Serumharnsäure um etwa 15%, in 4 Fällen um 16—29%, in 6 Fällen um 30—45% und in 2 Fällen um 46 und mehr Prozent ab. Die Serumharnsäuresenkung ging jeweils mit einem Anstieg der renalen Harnsäureausscheidung einher.

Die Toxicität des Sulfinpyrazons entspricht in ihrer Häufigkeit der des Probenecids. Nebenwirkungen treten bei etwa 10—15% aller behandelten Patienten auf (YÜ et al., 1958; EMMERSON, 1963; GOODMAN u. GILMAN, 1970). Am häufigsten wird über Magen-Darmstörungen geklagt, vereinzelt kommt es zur Reaktivierung eines alten Ulcus. Allergische Reaktionen treten in etwa 3% der Fälle auf (FRIEND, 1968). Gelegentlich wird eine Leukopenie beobachtet (YÜ et al., 1958; PERSELLIN u. SCHMID, 1961), weshalb regelmäßige Blutbildkontrollen durchgeführt werden sollten.

Uricosurisch wirksam ist auch p-Hydroxysulfinpyrazon (Abb. 11), ein Metabolit des Sulfinpyrazons (GUTMAN et al., 1960). Dies ist nicht überraschend, da diese Verbindung ebenfalls eine starke Säure ist und unter den Phenylbutazonanalogen eine Relation zwischen pKa und uricosurischer Wirkung besteht. Die stark sauren Verbindungen sind wirksame Uricosurica (BURNS et al., 1958a; BURNS et al., 1960).

Benzofuranderivate

Unter den Benzofuranabkömmlingen steigern nur Benzaronum, Benziodaronum und Benzbromaronum (Abb. 12) die renale Harnsäureausscheidung. Untersuchungen von DELBARRE et al. (1965) ergaben, daß die orale Verabreichung von 400 mg Benzaronum bereits nach ein bis zwei Stunden zu einem deutlichen Anstieg der Harnsäureclearance führt (Tab. 7). Gegenüber den halogenierten Derivaten besitzt diese Verbindung jedoch nur einen verhältnismäßig geringen uricosurischen Effekt. So fanden DELBARRE et al. (1967) bei drei Personen 2 Std nach oraler Gabe von 400 mg Benzaronum einen Anstieg der Harnsäureclearance von durchschnittlich 8,55 ml/min auf 22,18 ml/min, während dieselbe Dosis Benzioda-

Tabelle 7. Harnsäureclearance ml/min bei 5 Versuchspersonen nach oraler Verabreichung von 400 mg Benzaronum. (Mod. nach DELBARRE et. al., 1965)

Vp	Harnsäureclearance ml/min		
	Kontrollperiode	1 Std	2 Std
		nach Gabe von 400 mg Benzaronum per os	
1	11,1	24,4	23,8
2	9,0	9,0	23,0
3	8,0	20,9	18,1
4	7,9	18,0	24,0
5	6,3	12,7	22,0

ronum bzw. Benzbromaronum zum selben Zeitpunkt die Harnsäureclearance von im Mittel 9,50 ml/min auf 40,57 ml/min bzw. von 8,09 ml/min auf 32,83 ml/min erhöhte.

Benziodaronum

Nach Untersuchungen von BROEKHUYSEN et al. (1961) mittels radioaktiv markiertem Benziodaronum werden nach oraler Zufuhr 30—40% der verabreichten Dosis resorbiert. Mit steigender Dosierung nimmt dabei die Plasmakonzentration von Benziodaronum sowie die seiner Metaboliten zu. Der Abfall des Benziodaronumspiegels im Serum erfolgt rasch, wobei schon nach kurzer Zeit außer der Reinsubstanz drei zusätzliche, noch nicht identifizierte iodierte organische Metaboliten im Plasma nachgewiesen werden können. Die Ausscheidung des Benziodaronums erfolgt vorwiegend enteral. Auf Grund ihrer Untersuchungen vermuten BROEKHUYSEN et al. (1961), daß dieses Arzneimittel vor seiner endgültigen Eliminierung einen enterohepatischen Kreislauf durchläuft.

Benziodaronum wird im Organismus nur geringgradig dehalogeniert. In vitro-Experimente ergaben, daß diese Verbindung in einer molaren Konzentration von 10^{-5} bis 10^{-6} in Gegenwart von Leber-, Nieren- oder Schilddrüsengewebshomogenaten nicht dehalogeniert wird (BROEKHUYSEN et al., 1961).

Auf die harnsäuresenkende Wirkung von Benziodaronum, das als Coronardilatator in die Therapie eingeführt wurde, wiesen erstmals NIVET et al. (1965) hin. Nach täglicher, überwiegend intravenöser Verabreichung von 300 mg Benziodaronum beobachteten sie bei 13 Patienten innerhalb von 9 Tagen einen mittleren Abfall des Serumharnsäurespiegels von 6,89 auf 3,13 mg-%. Die bei 12 Patienten gemessene renale Harnsäureausscheidung stieg allerdings nur um durchschnittlich 56 mg/tgl. an, so daß die Autoren neben einem uricosurischen einen zweiten, die Harnsäuresynthese beeinflussenden Wirkungsmechanismus in Erwägung zogen. Dies würde auch mit Untersuchungen von MÜLLER u. BRESNIK (1972) in Einklang stehen, die unter Benziodaronumtherapie einen Anstieg der Aktivitäten von Adenin- und Hypoxanthin-guanin-phosphoribosyltransferase beobachteten. Über eine gesteigerte Bildung von Purinnucleotiden aus den entsprechenden freien Basen und damit verstärkte Rückkopplungshemmung der Glutamin-Phosphoribosyl-1-Pyrophosphat- Amidotransferase sowie andere Mechanismen käme es auf diesem Wege zu einer Beeinflussung der de novo Purinsynthese.

Zahlreiche weitere Autoren bestätigten den harnsäuresenkenden Effekt des Benziodaronums (DELBARRE et al., 1965, 1965a, 1967; RICHET et al., 1966, 1966a; MEDVEDOWSKY u. MARCOVICI, 1966; NIVET et al., 1967; PODEVIN et al., 1967). Im Gegensatz zu NIVET et al. (1965, 1967) konnten jedoch DELBARRE et al. (1965,

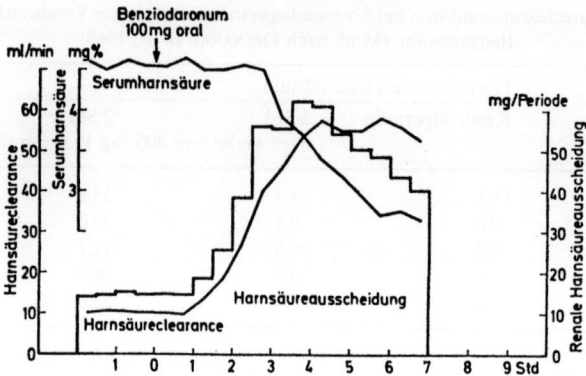

Abb. 13. Serumharnsäurespiegel, Harnsäureausscheidung und Harnsäureclearance nach einmaliger oraler Gabe von 100 mg Benziodaronum bei einer gesunden Versuchsperson. (Nach ZÖLLNER et al., 1970)

1965a), GROSS et al. (1967) sowie PODEVIN et al. (1967) den Serumharnsäureabfall jeweils mit einem entsprechenden Anstieg der renalen Harnsäureausscheidung erklären.

Untersuchungen zur Frage des uricosurischen Wirkungseintritts ergaben, daß während intravenöser Infusion von 5 mg Benziodaronum/min bereits nach 10 min ein Anstieg der Harnsäureclearance festzustellen ist (PODEVIN et al., 1967). Die orale Verabreichung einer Dosis von 200 bzw. 300 mg führte dagegen erst nach 3 Std zu einer Senkung der Serumharnsäure. Diese Ergebnisse stimmen mit den Beobachtungen von ZÖLLNER et al. (1970) überein. Nach einmaliger Gabe von 100 mg Benziodaronum per os begann die Serumharnsäure bei einer gesunden Versuchsperson 3,25 Std nach Arzneimittelgabe abzufallen. Dem Abfall entsprach ein Anstieg der renalen Harnsäureausscheidung bis auf maximal 61,80 mg/ 30 min. 6,75 Std nach Arzneimittelverabreichung war die Harnsäureclearance noch deutlich erhöht (Abb. 13).

Benziodaronum beeinflußt nicht die glomeruläre Filtrationsrate sowie die renale NaCl-Ausscheidung. Möglicherweise steigt die Kaliumelimination geringgradig an (PODEVIN et al., 1967). Der Oxalsäuregehalt des Urins wird dagegen deutlich vermehrt (MUGLER, 1967). Serumcalcium, -phosphor und Blutzucker zeigen unter Benziodaronum keine Veränderungen (GROSS et al., 1967). Der uricosurische Wirkungsmechanismus des Benziodaronums dürfte auf einer Hemmung der tubulären Harnsäurerückresorption beruhen. Eine paradoxe Harnsäureretention nach Zufuhr niedriger Dosen wird nicht beobachtet (PODEVIN et al., 1967). Ebenso läßt sich eine Hemmung der Xanthinoxydase nur in vitro nachweisen. Außerdem zeichnet sich diese Verbindung durch den fehlenden Antagonismus gegen Salicylate aus (COTTET u. VITTU, 1967).

Die uricosurisch wirksamen Dosen von Benziodaronum liegen bei 100— 300 mg täglich. Nur gelegentlich muß die Dosis erhöht werden. Erfahrungen in der Behandlung von Gichtkranken unter dieser Dosierung wurden von zahlreichen Autoren mitgeteilt (RICHET et al., 1966a; MEDVEDOWSKY u. MARCOVICCI, 1966; DELBARRE et al., 1967; OLMER u. LAFON, 1967; COTTET u. VITTU, 1967; MUGLER, 1967; GERBAUX, 1968; MASBERNARD et al., 1968, 1969; RYCKEWAERT et al., 1969). Übereinstimmend wurde dabei die ausgeprägte harnsäuresenkende Wirkung des Benziodaronums hervorgehoben. MASBERNARD et al. (1968), die 73 Hyperuricämiker mit diesem Arzneimittel behandelten, konnten in allen Fällen einen raschen, monatelang anhaltenden Abfall der Serumharnsäure sowie einen

Anstieg der renalen Harnsäureausscheidung erzielen. Über ähnliche Erfolge berichteten auch RYCKEWAERT et al. (1969), die 40 Gichtiker 12—15 Monate lang mit Benziodaronum therapierten. Bei 36 Patienten konnte der Serumharnsäurespiegel auf einen Wert unter 6,0 mg-% gesenkt werden. In 8 Fällen kam es zur völligen Rückbildung vorhandener Tophi. Gichtanfälle traten allerdings trotz Colchicinprophylaxe in den ersten 3 Behandlungsmonaten relativ häufig auf. Auf die günstige uricosurische Wirkung von Benziodaronum bei Patienten mit eingeschränkter Nierenfunktion wurde von RICHET et al. (1966, 1966a) sowie OLMER u. LAFON (1967) hingewiesen. Allerdings sollte in diesen Fällen besser Allopurinol zur Behandlung eingesetzt werden. Nebenwirkungen werden während der Behandlung mit Benziodaronum selten beobachtet. Gelegentlich treten gastrointestinale Beschwerden (Nausea, Diarrhoe) oder Jodallergien auf. MASBERNARD et al. (1968) mußten aus diesen Gründen bei 5% ihrer Patienten die Therapie vorzeitig abbrechen. Die Beeinflussung bestimmter Schilddrüsenfunktionsteste durch Benziodaronum stellt einen gewissen Nachteil dar.

Benzbromaronum[4]

Bei der Untersuchung weiterer Benzofuranabkömmlinge wurde im strukturanalogen Benzbromaronum (Abb. 12) ein Uricosuricum von gleicher Wirkung gefunden, das sich bei niederer Dosierung durch zuverlässige und langfristige Senkung des Serumharnsäurespiegels auszeichnet (DELBARRE et al., 1967; STERNON, 1967; ZÖLLNER et al., 1968, 1970a,b; KOTZAUREK u. HUEBER, 1968; MERTZ, 1969; MERTZ et al., 1970; MASBERNARD u. FRANCOZ, 1969; MASBERNARD u. VACCON, 1970; GROSS u. GIRAD, 1972). Infolge des fehlenden Jodgehaltes besitzt diese Verbindung darüber hinaus den Vorteil, Schilddrüsenfunktionsteste nicht zu beeinflussen.

Nach Untersuchungen von BROEKHUYSEN et al. (1972), die zehn Versuchspersonen eine orale Dosis von 100 mg Tritium-markiertem Benzbromaronum verabreichten, werden etwa 50% der gegebenen Dosis aus dem Gastrointestinaltrakt resorbiert. Eine maximale Radioaktivität läßt sich nach sechs Stunden nachweisen. Diesem Maximum folgt ein geringer Abfall der Radioaktivität, anschließend stellt sich ein Plateau ein, das bis zu 48 Std nach oraler Gabe des Arzneimittels nachweisbar ist. Während der Plateauphase ist die Radioaktivität vorwiegend auf Benzaronum zurückzuführen, da Benzbromaronum in der Leber größtenteils dehalogeniert wird.

Die Ausscheidung erfolgt vorwiegend via Galle enteral; nur etwa 8% der resorbierten Dosis werden renal eliminiert.

Der harnsäuresenkende Wirkungsmechanismus von Benzbromaronum entspricht dem eines Uricosuricums. Damit vereinbar ist auch die Angabe von MERTZ (1969), daß bei einer glomerulären Filtrationsrate unter 20 ml/min mit einer Wirkung von Benzbromaronum nicht mehr gerechnet werden kann. Eine paradoxe Harnsäureretention nach Zufuhr niedriger Dosen, eine antagonistische Beeinflussung durch Salicylate sowie Veränderungen der Kreatininclearance oder Diurese durch Benzbromaronum werden nicht beobachtet (DANCHOT, 1968; ZÖLLNER et al., 1970, 1970a; GROSS u. GIRARD, 1972). Eine Hemmung der Xanthinoxydase ließ sich bisher nur in vitro nachweisen (DELTOUR et al., 1967). GREILING (1969) beobachtete in einem Fall unter Benzbromaronum eine verminderte Hypoxanthin- und Xanthinausscheidung im Urin. Er vermutet, daß dieser Befund auf eine Aktivierung der Hypoxanthin-Guanin-Phosphoribosyltransferase zurückzuführen ist.

---

[4] Uricovac®.

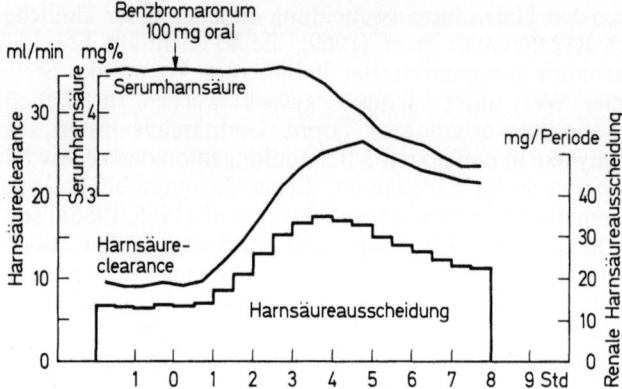

Abb. 14. Das Verhalten der Mittelwerte von Serumharnsäure, Harnsäureausscheidung und Harnsäureclearance bei sieben gesunden männlichen Versuchspersonen vor und nach einmaliger oraler Gabe von 100 mg Benzbromaronum. (Nach ZÖLLNER et al., 1970)

Pharmakodynamische Untersuchungen von ZÖLLNER et al. (1970) über die Wirkung von Benzbromaronum auf Serumharnsäure, renale Harnsäureausscheidung und Harnsäureclearance ergaben, daß bei gesunden Personen durchschnittlich 1 Std nach oraler Verabreichung einer Dosis von 100 mg die Harnsäureausscheidung im Urin ansteigt (Abb. 14, Tab. 8). Dabei wird der höchste Wert pro Sammelperiode von 30 min zwischen 3,50 und 4 Std nach Arzneimittelgabe erzielt. Der Serumharnsäureabfall setzt dagegen erst nach 3,25 Std ein und verringert den Harnsäurespiegel im Verlauf von 7,75 Std um durchschnittlich 26,8%. Die mittlere Harnsäureclearance steigt bis auf 26,54 ml/min an, wobei in Einzelfällen Werte von 40 ml/min erreicht werden (Abb. 15). Diese Befunde stimmen grundsätzlich mit den Ergebnissen von MASBERNARD u. VACCON (1970) überein, die bei Normo- und Hyperuricämikern nach Verabreichung derselben Dosis innerhalb von zwei Std eine Verdoppelung der renalen Harnsäureausscheidung feststellten. Der Maximaleffekt wurde bei Normouricämikern nach 3—6, bei Hyperuricämikern nach 3—9 Std beobachtet. Dem Anstieg der renalen Harnsäureausscheidung entsprach ein Abfall des Serumharnsäurespiegels, der 2—4 Std nach Arzneimittelgabe einsetzte und nach 12—15 Std sein Minimum erreichte. ZÖLLNER et al. (1970) beobachteten den tiefsten Serumharnsäurewert nach 16, einen Wiederanstieg nach 20 Std.

Normo- und Hyperuricämiker (mit oder ohne Gicht) verhalten sich unter Benzbromaronum nach MASBERNARD u. VACCON (1970) grundsätzlich gleich. ZÖLLNER et al. (1970a) stellten dagegen bei Gichtkranken unter einer Dosis von 100 mg einen verzögerten Wirkungseintritt fest. Der maximale Effekt, gemessen an der Harnsäureclearance, wurde erst in der 7. und 8. Stunde erreicht. DELBARRE et al. (1967) wiederum konnten bei Gichtkranken unter einer Dosierung von 400 mg bereits innerhalb von 60 min einen deutlichen Clearanceanstieg nachweisen. Möglicherweise hängt somit der Zeitpunkt des uricosurischen Wirkungseintritts auch von der Höhe der gewählten Dosis ab.

Im Vergleich zu Benzbromaronum entfaltet Benziodaronum eine stärkere Wirkung (Abb. 16). Dies stimmt auch mit den Ergebnissen von DELBARRE et al. (1967) überein. MASBERNARD u. VACCON (1970) dagegen sahen nach Verabreichung beider Präparate keine Wirkungsunterschiede.

Tabelle 8. Einzel- und Mittelwerte der Harnsäureausscheidung (mg pro Sammelperiode von 30 min) Benzbromaronum. (Aus

	−4	−3	−2	−1	1	2	3	4	5	6
K. T., 34 J.	11,28	12,18	11,90	13,68	13,30	12,92	12,52	17,00	28,20	33,00
G. O., 19 J.	12,40	12,20	12,60	12,65	12,45	12,80	18,70	21,60	27,00	31,20
W. S., 25 J.	15,85	16,50	16,80	16,80	16,80	17,05	19,80	26,10	34,00	40,40
M. S., 27 J.	12,45	12,90	12,35	12,60	12,75	14,30	17,40	21,45	26,80	30,00
J. H., 54 J.	14,00	13,60	13,30	13,60	13,80	14,70	17,30	17,10	18,80	21,30
A. U., 56 J.	13,10	12,95	12,25	12,95	13,20	13,70	17,20	21,80	24,00	27,70
M. C., 37 J.	—	10,16	10,75	12,27	10,48	10,68	15,70	20,70	23,40	31,22
$\bar{x}$		12,93	12,85	13,51	13,25	13,74	16,95	20,82	26,03	30,69

Einzel- und Mittelwerte der Serumharnsäure (mg-%) während der Sammelperioden von je 30 min bei Benzbromaronum

	−4	−3	−2	−1	1	2	3	4	5	6
K. T., 34 J.	5,40	5,40	5,40	5,50	5,35	5,25	5,25	5,40	5,45	5,45
G. O., 19 J.	3,50	3,55	3,50	3,65	3,60	3,50	3,65	3,60	3,65	3,70
W. S., 25 J.	4,25	4,25	4,15	4,25	4,25	4,30	4,20	4,30	4,25	4,25
M. S., 27 J.	5,90	6,00	5,90	5,85	5,95	5,90	5,85	5,90	5,90	5,95
J. H., 54 J.	3,30	3,25	3,25	3,30	3,40	3,35	3,30	3,30	3,20	3,30
A. U., 56 J.	5,20	5,30	5,25	5,20	5,20	5,30	5,25	5,25	5,30	5,25
M. C., 37 J.	4,35	4,30	4,30	4,25	4,25	4,25	4,30	4,25	4,25	4,30
$\bar{x}$	4,56	4,57	4,54	4,57	4,57	4,55	4,54	4,57	4,57	4,60

Einzel- und Mittelwerte der Harnsäureclearance (ml/min) während der Sammelperioden von je 30 min 100 mg

	−4	−3	−2	−1	1	2	3	4	5	6
K. T., 34 J.	6,88	7,40	7,22	8,16	8,16	8,08	7,83	10,30	17,00	20,00
G. O., 19 J.	11,10	10,75	10,95	10,80	10,75	11,35	16,00	18,70	23,00	27,70
W. S., 25 J.	10,20	10,70	11,10	10,85	10,85	10,90	13,00	16,65	21,50	26,10
M. S., 27 J.	6,35	6,45	6,30	6,50	6,45	7,30	8,90	10,90	13,60	15,10
J. H., 54 J.	13,70	13,50	12,80	13,20	13,10	14,20	16,80	16,70	18,95	20,80
A. U., 56 J.	8,20	7,95	7,55	8,05	8,20	8,40	10,60	13,40	15,20	17,05
M. C., 37 J.	—	7,30	7,70	8,90	7,74	7,75	10,90	15,05	16,90	21,80
$\bar{x}$	—	9,15	9,09	9,49	9,32	9,71	12,00	14,53	18,02	21,22

Vergleichbare Effekte werden erzielt, wenn 100 mg Benzbromaronum bzw. 1,5 g Probenecid als Einzeldosis verabreicht werden (Abb. 17). Im Gegensatz zu Benzbromaronum setzt die uricosurische Wirkung des Probenecids jedoch früher ein. So ist bereits 1 Std nach oraler Gabe von 1,5 g Probenecid die Harnsäureclearance bei Abnahme des Plasmaspiegels stark vermehrt. Die Erhöhung der Harnsäureausscheidung ist von der dritten Sammelperiode an maximal und nimmt nicht mehr weiter zu. Ganz anders der Ablauf unter Benzbromaronum. Drei Std nach oraler Verabreichung, einem Zeitpunkt, zu dem nach Probenecid die medikamentös bedingte Senkung des Serumharnsäurespiegels ihr maximales Ausmaß beinahe erreicht hat, läßt sich an der Serumharnsäure noch kein Benzbromaro-

bei sieben gesunden männlichen Versuchspersonen vor und nach einmaliger oraler Gabe von 100 mg ZÖLLNER et al., 1970)

7	8	9	10	11	12	13	14	15	16	17	18
30,40	33,30	30,70	28,60	27,70	26,00	25,80	23,50	21,40	22,80	20,90	22,00
36,60	32,80	31,20	27,40	23,10	23,90	20,40	20,60	21,50	19,50	18,90	18,15
40,40	42,70	38,40	41,00	38,60	35,40	35,70	31,20	27,30	29,90	28,90	28,30
33,70	38,00	43,00	40,30	39,20	35,60	35,00	31,70	29,75	25,00	—	—
24,80	23,70	25,30	27,00	23,40	22,40	20,20	21,80	19,65	17,90	18,90	17,05
34,60	37,80	35,70	34,00	29,50	28,20	26,20	23,80	22,10	23,20	22,55	20,00
34,90	35,70	33,90	33,40	27,10	23,60	21,80	19,80	19,20	20,70	16,86	18,00
33,63	34,86	34,03	33,10	29,80	27,87	26,44	24,63	22,99	22,71	—	—

sieben gesunden männlichen Versuchspersonen vor und nach einmaliger oraler Gabe von 100 mg

7	8	9	10	11	12	13	14	15	16	17	18
5,45	5,50	5,50	5,25	5,05	5,00	4,75	4,70	4,65	4,55	4,00	4,00
3,60	3,50	3,35	2,85	2,70	2,75	2,60	2,50	2,60	2,65	2,60	2,55
4,00	4,00	3,25	3,35	3,25	3,25	3,30	3,25	3,15	3,25	3,30	3,25
5,90	5,50	5,15	4,95	4,85	4,75	4,85	4,80	4,30	4,15	—	—
3,35	2,90	2,85	2,95	2,75	2,65	2,65	2,45	2,35	2,25	2,35	2,30
5,25	5,20	4,70	4,60	4,25	4,15	3,90	3,80	3,70	3,60	3,60	3,65
4,25	4,30	4,30	3,90	3,40	3,15	3,00	2,80	2,80	2,90	2,80	2,70
4,54	4,41	4,16	3,98	3,75	3,67	3,58	3,47	3,36	3,34	—	—

bei sieben gesunden männlichen Versuchspersonen vor und nach einmaliger oraler Gabe von Benzbromaronum

7	8	9	10	11	12	13	14	15	16	17	18
18,30	19,85	18,30	18,00	18,00	17,00	17,80	16,40	15,15	15,90	17,10	18,20
31,80	29,20	27,70	30,00	26,70	27,10	24,40	25,80	25,70	23,00	22,80	22,25
27,70	29,40	32,50	33,60	32,70	29,90	29,60	26,40	23,70	25,20	24,10	23,90
17,10	20,70	25,00	24,40	24,20	22,55	21,60	19,85	20,70	18,05	—	—
23,90	26,40	28,60	29,40	27,40	27,20	24,60	26,50	26,80	25,60	25,90	23,90
21,40	23,50	24,70	24,00	21,50	21,90	21,70	20,30	19,35	20,90	20,20	17,70
25,35	25,70	24,30	26,40	24,70	23,15	22,30	21,80	21,20	22,00	18,60	20,55
23,65	24,97	25,87	26,54	25,03	24,11	23,14	22,44	21,80	21,52	—	—

numeffekt erkennen. Ähnlich deutlich ist der sehr viel langsamere Wirkungseintritt auch bei Betrachtung von Harnsäureausscheidung und -clearance. Langsame Resorption, lange Bindung der wirksamen Substanzen an die Plasmaproteine oder die Bildung von Metaboliten als wirksamer Komponente kommen als Erklärung dieses Benzbromaronumeffektes in Frage (ZÖLLNER et al., 1970).

Die einmalige Gabe von 100 mg Benzbromaronum per os führt im Laufe des 1. Tages zu einem Abfall des Serumharnsäurespiegels um durchschnittlich 28% (MERTZ, 1969). ZÖLLNER et al. (1970) beobachteten bei 18 Versuchspersonen nach Verabreichung derselben Dosis innerhalb des gleichen Zeitraumes eine Senkung der Serumharnsäure auf durchschnittlich 66,5% des Ausgangswertes. Erst am

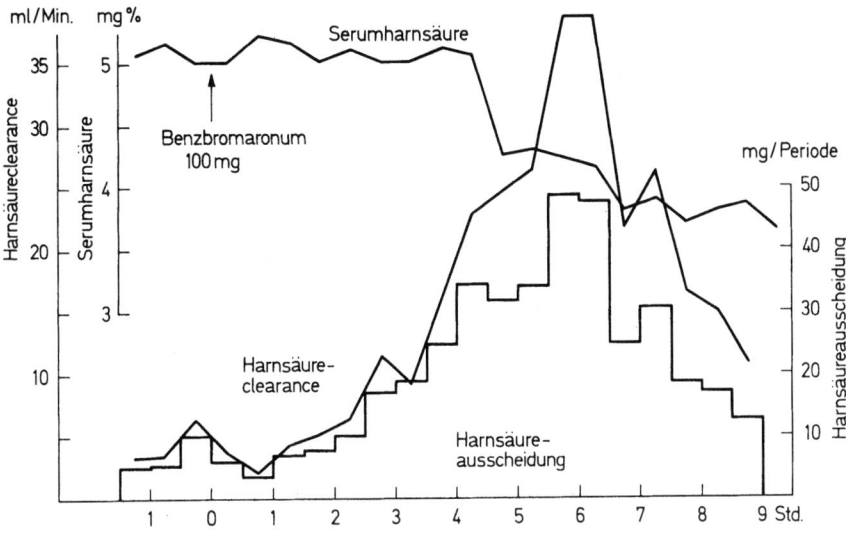

Abb. 15. Serumharnsäurespiegel, Harnsäureausscheidung und Harnsäureclearance nach einmaliger oraler Gabe von 100 mg Benzbromaronum bei einer gesunden, männlichen Versuchsperson. (Nach ZÖLLNER et al., 1968)

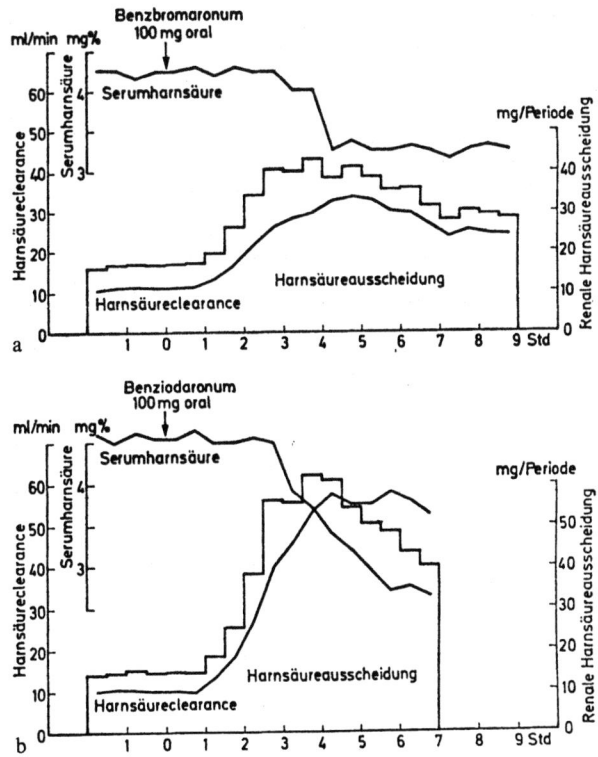

Abb. 16a u. b. Serumharnsäurespiegel, Harnsäureausscheidung und Harnsäureclearance nach einmaliger oraler Gabe von 100 mg Benzbromaronum (a) bzw. 100 mg Benziodaronum (b) bei einer gesunden Versuchsperson. (Nach ZÖLLNER et al., 1970)

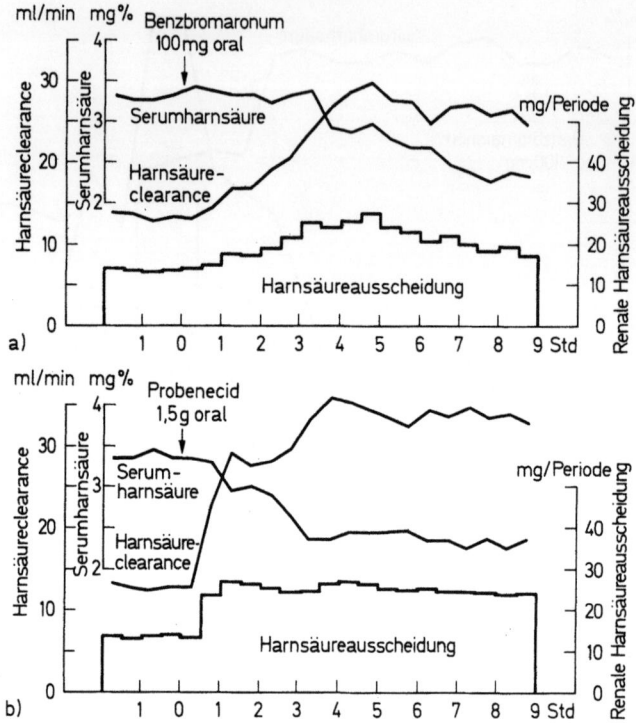

Abb. 17a u. b. Serumharnsäurespiegel, Harnsäureausscheidung und Harnsäureclearance nach einmaliger oraler Gabe von 100 mg Benzbromaronum (a) bzw. 1,5 g Probenecid (b) bei einer gesunden Versuchsperson. (Nach ZÖLLNER et al., 1970)

4. Tag wurde der Ausgangsspiegel wieder erreicht. Der Serumharnsäureabfall ging mit einem Anstieg der renalen Harnsäureausscheidung einher, wobei erst nach 4—5 Tagen die normale Ausscheidungsrate wieder erreicht wurde. Während des Wiederanstiegs der Plasmaharnsäure fand sich keine Verringerung der renalen Harnsäureausscheidung unter die Werte der Kontrollperiode (Abb. 18). Im Gegensatz zu STERNON (1967), der bei einigen Hyperuricämikern und Gichtkranken bei einem ausgeprägten Abfall des Serumharnsäurespiegels nur eine mäßige Vermehrung der renalen Harnsäureausscheidung beobachtete, sahen ZÖLLNER et al. (1970) bei allen Normalpersonen nach einmaliger Gabe von 100 mg Benzbromaronum per os innerhalb von 24 Std eine Harnsäuremehrausscheidung, die größer als die Abnahme des Harnsäurepools (berechnet nach ZÖLLNER, 1960) war. So betrug die Differenz zwischen Harnsäuremehrausscheidung und errechneter Poolabnahme im Mittel 186 mg, bei einer Versuchsperson z. B. 493 mg. Die wahrscheinlichste Erklärung ist die, daß bei abnehmendem Harnsäurespiegel die enterale Ausscheidung zugunsten der renalen Harnsäureausscheidung abnimmt (ZÖLLNER, 1960). Unter Umständen blockiert Benzbromaronum selbst noch zusätzlich die enterale Harnsäureelimination (ZÖLLNER et al., 1970). In diesem Sinne wäre auch die Konstanz der Serumharnsäure während der ersten 3 Std bei Zunahme der Harnsäureclearance zu erklären.

Die wirksamen Dosen von Benzbromaronum liegen bei 50—150 mg/tgl. Nur gelegentlich muß eine höhere Dosis gewählt werden. Patienten mit Hyperuricämie und solche, die längere Zeit mit Allopurinol vorbehandelt worden sind,

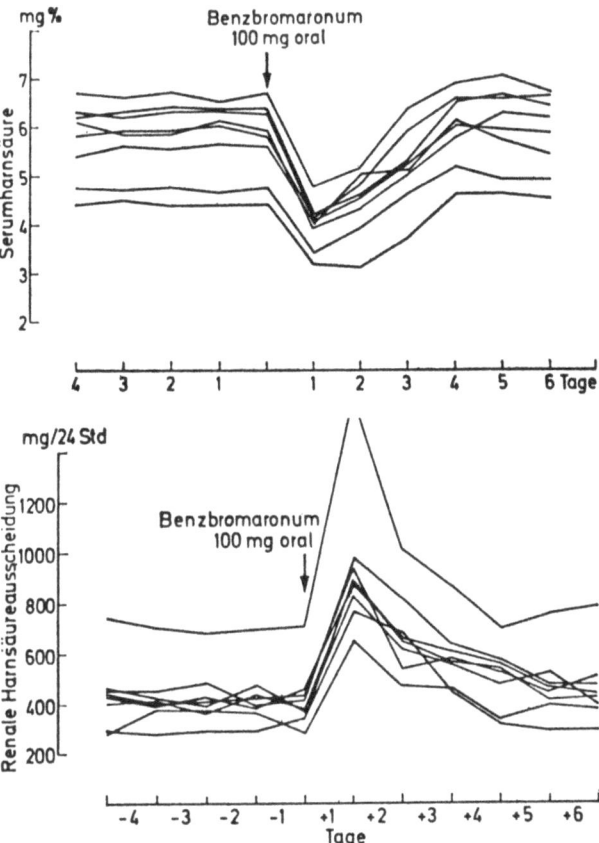

Abb. 18. Verlauf von Serumharnsäure und Harnsäureausscheidung im 24 Std-Urin bei 8 gesunden Versuchspersonen nach einmaliger oraler Gabe von 100 mg Benzbromaronum. Die täglich ausgeschiedene Harnsäuremenge wurde jeweils am Ende der Sammelperiode eingetragen. Zu diesem Zeitpunkt wurden auch die Serumharnsäurewerte bestimmt. (Nach ZÖLLNER et al., 1970)

reagieren grundsätzlich in gleicher Weise wie gesunde Kontrollpersonen, solange die Nierenfunktion nicht nennenswert eingeschränkt ist (MERTZ, 1969). Eine maximale Verminderung des Serumharnsäurespiegels während täglicher Zufuhr von 100 mg tritt nach etwa 5 Tagen ein. Die mittlere Abnahme beträgt dabei 46 ± 14% des Ausgangswertes (MERTZ, 1969), in Einzelfällen werden Senkungen von 60% beobachtet (ZÖLLNER et al., 1970; GROSS u. GIRARD, 1972).

Klinische Erfahrungen mit Benzbromaronum wurden von STERNON et al. (1967), KOTZAUREK u. HUEBER (1968), MASBERNARD u. FRANCOZ (1969), ZÖLLNER et al. (1970b), MERTZ et al. (1970) und anderen Autoren mitgeteilt. MASBERNARD u. FRANCOZ (1969), die 35 Patienten über insgesamt ein Jahr mit Benzbromaronum behandelten, berichteten über deutliche Besserungen des klinischen Zustandsbildes. ZÖLLNER et al. (1970b) therapierten 85 Patienten bis zu einem Jahr mit Benzbromaronum. 76 Patienten litten an Gicht. In 81 Fällen kam es unter 100 bzw. 50 mg Benzbromaronum tägl. zu einer Normalisierung der Plasmaharnsäure (Spiegel unter 6 mg/100 ml). Ein Patient benötigte hierzu 150 mg, bei 3 Patienten konnte die initiale Normalisierung mit 100 mg nicht aufrechterhalten werden; die hierfür notwendige Dosis betrug 150 mg.

Tabelle 9. Übersicht über die Ergebnisse einer uricosurischen Therapie mit Benzbromaronum. (Nach ZÖLLNER et al., 1970b)

Patienten Art	Zahl	Anfallsfrei unter Benzbromaronum	
		0—6 Monate	6 Monate und länger
Vorbehandelt	49		
Anfallsfrei	20	95% (19)	100% (18 v. 18)
Nicht anfallsfrei	29	82% (24)	81% (16 v. 19)
Nicht vorbehandelt	27		
Lange Anamnese	16	68% (11)	100% (6 v. 6)
Erstanfall	11	63% (7)	100% (4 v. 4)
	76	80% (61)	94% (44 v. 47)

Von den 76 Gichtkranken waren 20 Patienten durch Vorbehandlung anfallsfrei. Unter Benzbromaronum blieben bis auf einen alle anfallsfrei. 16 nicht vorbehandelte Patienten hatten eine längere Anfallsanamnese; unter Behandlung mit Benzbromaronum waren 11 Patienten sofort anfallsfrei, bei 5 Patienten bestanden noch Anfälle. Von den nach dem Erstanfall behandelten 11 Patienten blieben 7 anfallsfrei. Von 29 nicht ausreichend vorbehandelten Patienten wurden 80% rasch anfallsfrei. In dieser Gruppe besserten sich nicht alle Patienten, so daß sich hier vermutlich die besonders therapieresistenten Fälle befinden. Von 47 mehr als 6 Monate behandelten Patienten hatten nach dieser Zeit nur noch 3 einen Gichtanfall (Tab. 9). Eine Verkleinerung der bestehenden Tophi wurde während der Beobachtungszeit nicht festgestellt. Das gelegentliche Auftreten von Steinkoliken muß als Folge jeder uricosurischen Therapie betrachtet werden.

Nebenwirkungen nach Verabreichung von Benzbromaronum wurden bis jetzt selten gesehen. Am häufigsten treten gastrointestinale Störungen auf. Kopfschmerzen und vermehrter Harndrang sind vorübergehender Natur (MERTZ, 1969). Unter 85 Patienten beobachteten ZÖLLNER et al. (1970b) bei einem Patienten eine variable Eosinophilie sowie in 9 Fällen Übelkeit und Sodbrennen. Zwei Patienten gaben Muskelzuckungen in der Handmuskulatur an, 5 Patienten bemerkten eine Gewichtszunahme von 1—2 kg, 4 Patienten litten vorübergehend (4—6 Wochen) unter Impotenz. In keinem Fall mußte jedoch das Mittel abgesetzt werden. Bei 1—2 wöchiger Medikation konnten MERTZ et al. (1970) keine Veränderungen von Blutbild, Kohlenhydrat- und Lipidstoffwechsel, der Leber- und Nierenfunktion sowie des EKG und Blutdrucks registrieren. ZÖLLNER et al. (1970c) fanden während der Langzeitbehandlung mit Benzbromaronum eine unbedeutende Abnahme des Quickwertes.

Benzbromaronum ist ein Uricosuricum, das gegenüber den bisher üblichen den Vorzug hat, langsam zu wirken und deshalb nur einmal täglich in niederer Dosierung eingenommen werden zu müssen. Wegen dieser Eigenschaft, die den Patienten des Risikos eines Rebounds bei vergessener Einnahme entliebt, muß dieses Präparat als eine Bereicherung der Therapie der Hyperuricämie, speziell wenn sie sich als Gicht und nicht als Nierenkrankheit manifestiert, angesehen werden.

Cumarin- und Indandionderivate

Den Benzofuranderivaten strukturell nahe stehen eine Reihe weiterer Arzneimittel mit uricosurischer Wirkung (ZÖLLNER u. GRÖBNER, 1969; Abb. 19, Abb. 20). Über die Feststellung eines gemeinsamen pharmakologischen Wir-

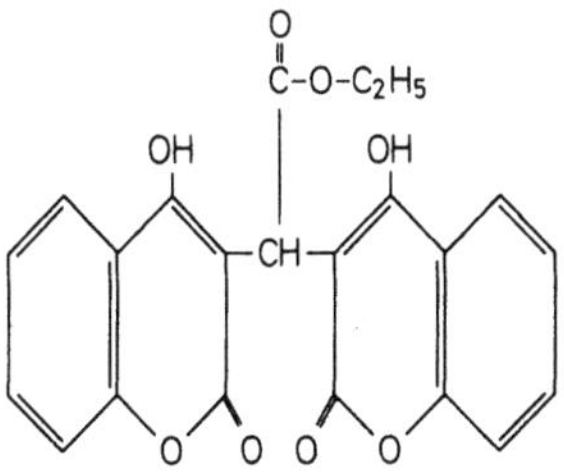

Äthylbiscumacetat

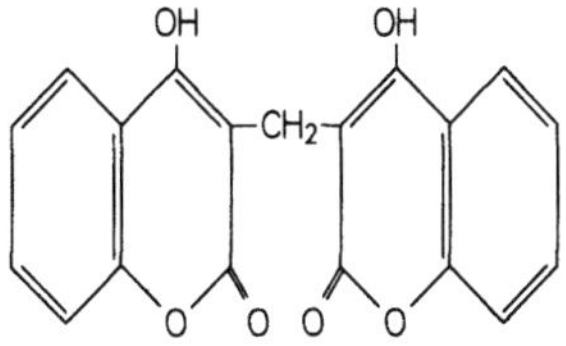

Bishydroxycumarin

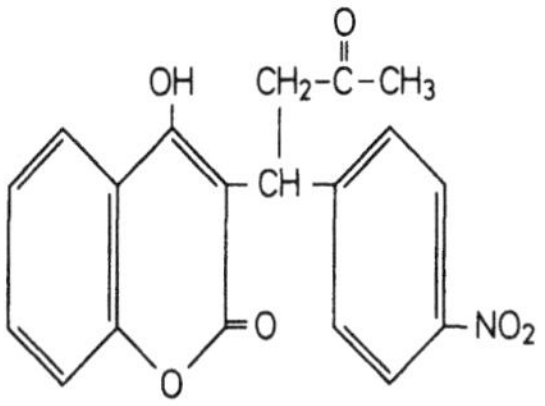

Acenocumarol

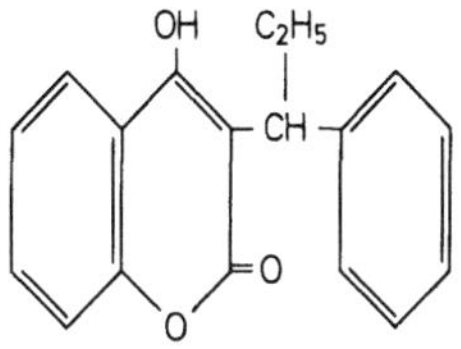

Phenprocumarol

Abb. 19. Strukturformeln einiger Cumarinderivate

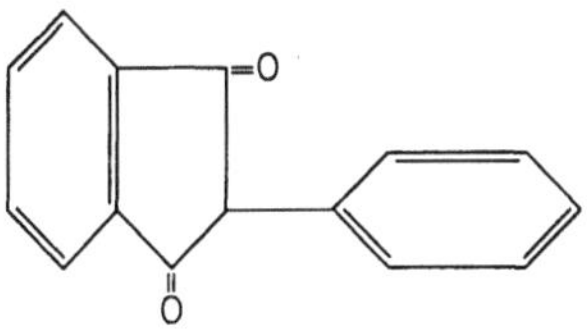

2-Phenylindandion (1,3)

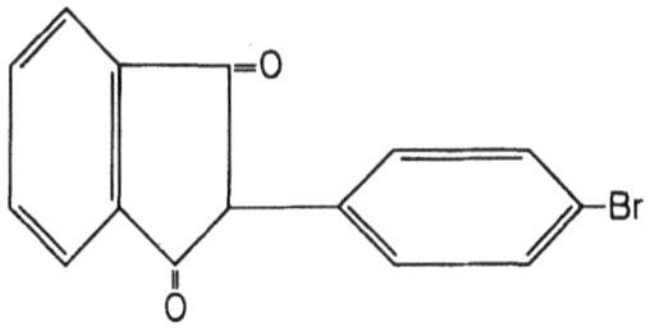

2-(4'-Bromphenyl)-indandion (1,3)

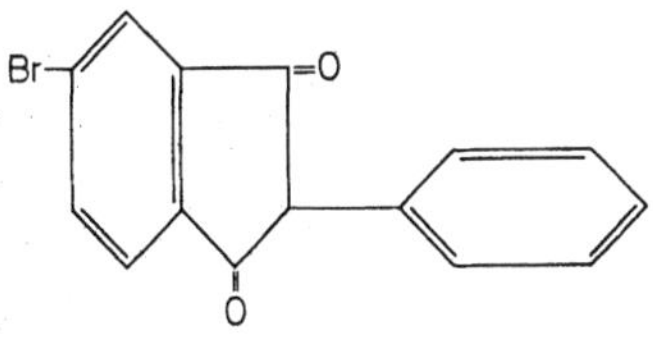

2-Phenyl-5-brom-indandion (1,3)

Abb. 20. Strukturformeln einiger Indandionderivate

kungsprinzips hinaus kommt den Stoffgruppen beträchtliches biochemisches Interesse zu, da einige der Verbindungen als Antagonisten des Vitamins K in der Prothrombinsynthese bekannt sind bzw. Vitamin K deren uricosurische Wirkung aufheben kann.

SOUGIN-MIBASHAN und HORWITZ beobachteten 1955 bei einem hyperuricämischen Patienten ein bis zwei Tage nach Einleitung einer Anticoagulantientherapie mit Äthylbiscumacetat (Tromexan®) eine Normalisierung der Serumharnsäurekonzentration. Eine nähere Überprüfung der Wirkung dieses Vitamin-K-

Antagonisten auf die Serumharnsäure ergab, daß eine einmalige orale Dosis von 1,2—1,8 g Äthylbiscumacetat schon ein bis zwei Std nach Verabreichung zu einem ausgeprägten Anstieg der Harnsäureclearance und Senkung des Serumharnsäurespiegels führt. Drei Jahre später berichteten HANSEN u. HOLTEN (1958) sowie DREYFUSS u. CZACZKES (1958) über die gleiche Beobachtung bei Medikation von Bishydroxycumarin (Dicumarol®). Die notwendigen Dosen zur Erzielung einer Harnsäuremehrausscheidung im Urin betrugen dabei 25—750 mg. Ein Anstieg der Harnsäureclearance wird auch nach Gabe von Acenocumarol (Sintrom®) (KUSUS, 1965) erreicht. Phenprocumarol (Marcumar®) dagegen besitzt nur einen geringen uricosurischen Effekt (PASERO, 1960).

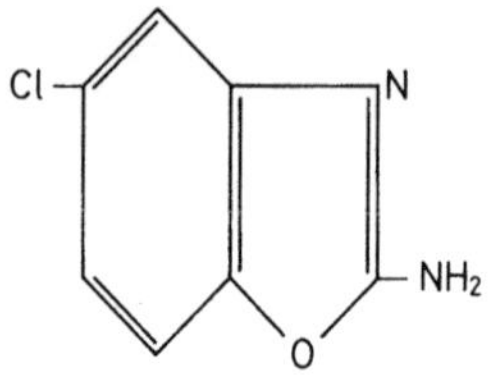

Zoxazolamin

Abb. 21. Zoxazolamin

Ausgehend von der uricosurischen Wirkung der Cumarinderivate haben PASERO u. MASINI (1957, 1958a) weitere Vitamin K-Antagonisten geprüft und gefunden, daß auch Indandionderivate die Harnsäureclearance steigern. Es zeigte sich deutlich, daß uricosurische und hypoprothrombinämische Wirkung nicht immer in gleicher Intensität auftreten. Strukturveränderungen, die zu einer stärkeren Senkung des Quick-Wertes führen, können den uricosurischen Effekt praktisch unbeeinflußt lassen. So fand PASERO (1960) 2 Std nach oraler Gabe von 200 mg 2-Phenylindandion eine Erhöhung der Harnsäureclearance von 10,31 ml/min auf 19,21 ml/min, während nach Einnahme von 7 mg Bromindion (2-(4-Bromphenyl)-indandion) bei gleicher hypoprothrombinämischer Wirksamkeit innerhalb derselben Zeit die Harnsäureclearance von 9,91 ml/min nur auf 12,0 ml/min anstieg. Wird das Brom in den Indandionkern (2-Phenyl-5-brom-indandion) eingeführt, so geht die hypoprothrombinämische Wirkung verloren, der uricosurische Effekt jedoch bleibt erhalten (PASERO u. MARINI, 1958).

Vitamin K hemmt die uricosurische Wirkung von Äthylbiscumacetat, 2-Phenylindandion, Acenocumarol und Phenprocumarol. 2-Phenyl-5-brom-indandion soll allerdings durch Vitamin K nicht beeinflußt werden (PASERO u. MARINI, 1958a). Bei den anderen genannten Verbindungen ist die Frage eines renalen Antagonismus noch nicht geprüft.

Zoxazolamin

Dem 2-Phenyl-5-brom-indandion strukturell ähnlich ist auch das Zoxazolamin (Abb. 21), dessen uricosurische Eigenschaften von REED et al. (1958) beschrieben wurden. Diese Autoren beobachteten bei einem Gichtkranken nach mehrtägiger oraler Einnahme von 500—750 mg Zoxazolamin einen Abfall der Serumharnsäure von 10,5 mg/100 ml auf 4,5 mg/100 ml. BURNS et al. (1958) konnten bereits mit einer Dosis von 15 mg einen uricosurischen Effekt herbeiführen. Renale Clearanceuntersuchungen derselben Autoren bei Gichtkranken, denen Einzeldosen von 100—1000 mg Zoxazolamin verabreicht wurden, zeigten 40—60 min nach Arzneimittelgabe einen mittleren Anstieg des Quotienten aus C_{HS}/C_{INULIN} um das Fünf- bis Sechsfache. Auf Grund von Berichten über hepato- und nephrotoxische Wirkungen des Zoxazolamins wurde das Präparat jedoch aus dem Handel gezogen.

Uricosurisch wirksame Pharmaka unterschiedlicher Struktur

Phenylchinolincarbonsäure (Atophan®)

Phenylchinolincarbonsäure (Abb. 22) wurde 1911 von WEINTRAUD (zitiert bei GUTMAN, 1966) auf Grund ihrer uricosurischen, analgetischen und entzündungshemmenden Eigenschaften in die Therapie der Gicht eingeführt. Der Autor berichtete, daß bei einem Gichtkranken unter wochenlanger Behandlung mit dieser

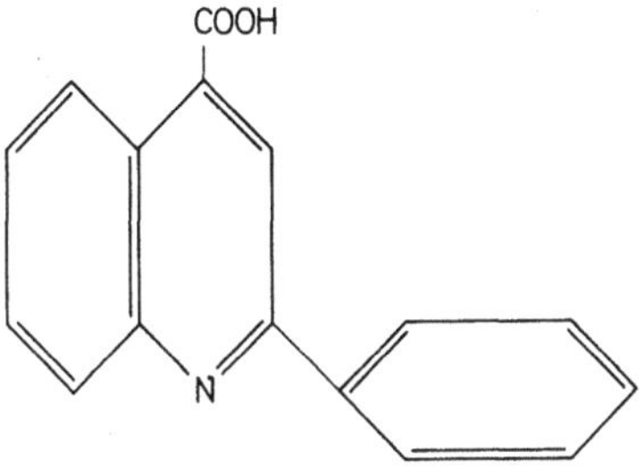

Abb. 22. Phenylchinolincarbonsäure

Verbindung Uratdepots kleiner geworden seien. Spätere Untersucher konnten diese Wirkung auf die Tophi zwar nicht bestätigen (CARRELL u. ELLIOTT, 1933 usw.), doch besteht kein Zweifel an den uricosurischen Eigenschaften dieses Pharmakons. Entscheidend gegen eine Therapie mit Phenylchinolincarbonsäure sprechen jedoch ihre Nebenwirkungen, unter denen die prognostisch sehr ernste Leberschädigung an erster Stelle steht. Selbst geringe Dosen können dabei das Bild des „Atophanikterus" hervorrufen (LÖFFLER u. KOLLER, 1955).

Niridazol

Auf die Senkung der Serumharnsäure durch Niridazol (Abb. 23), das seit Jahren in der Therapie der Bilharziose eingesetzt wird, wiesen erstmals PODEVIN et al. (1968) hin. Untersuchungen zur Frage des Wirkungsmechanismus ergaben, daß Niridazol zu einem Anstieg der renalen Harnsäureausscheidung führt, während die Oxypurinelimination konstant bleibt (GRÖBNER et al., 1971). Die gegenüber den gebräuchlichen Uricosurica nur geringe Wirkung, eine besonders ausgeprägte paradoxe Harnsäureretention nach Zufuhr niedriger Dosen sowie das Auftreten von toxischen Symptomen bei chronischer Anwendung machen dieses Arzneimittel für die Gichtbehandlung jedoch ungeeignet (GRÖBNER et al., 1971).

Clofibrat, MK-185, Röntgenkontrastmittel etc.

Eine mäßige uricosurische Wirkung wird auch dem Antihyperlipidämicum Clofibrat (p-Chlorphenoxyisobutyrat) (Abb. 24) zugeschrieben (HOWARD et al., 1963; BERKOWITZ, 1965). Dabei beobachtete BERKOWITZ (1965) eine Korrelation zwischen der Höhe des Serumtriglyceridspiegels und dem Ausmaß der Serumharnsäuresenkung durch Clofibrat. Bei Patienten mit normalen Lipidwerten war die uricosurische Wirkung am geringsten.

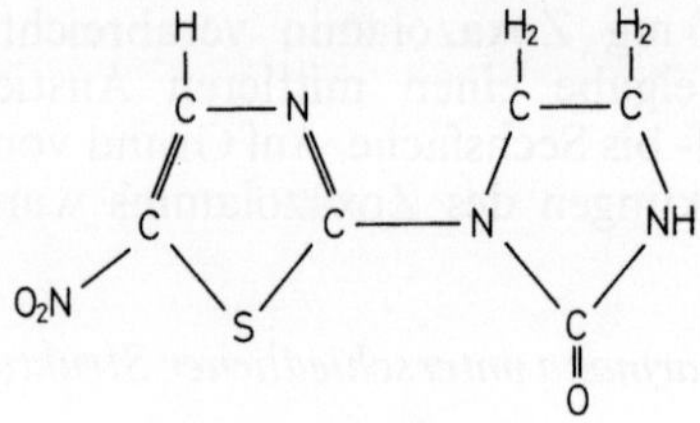

Abb. 23. Niridazol

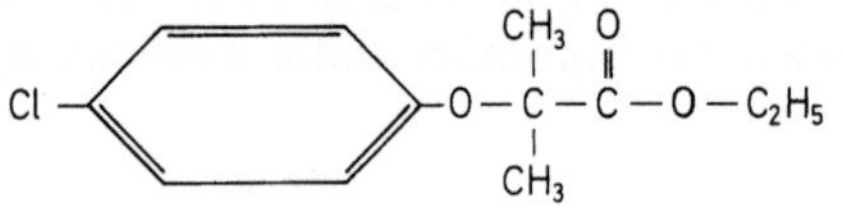

Clofibrat

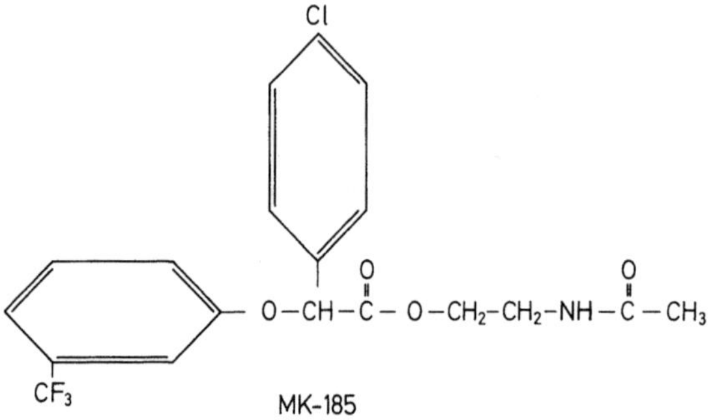

MK-185

Abb. 24. Clofibrat und MK-185

Dem Clofibrat strukturell nahe steht das MK-185 (Abb. 24), das sowohl erhöhte Serumlipoide als auch die Serumharnsäure senkt (JAIN et al., 1970; MORGAN et al., 1971; WOLFRAM et al., 1973). So stellten JAIN et al. (1970) bei 10 Patienten, die 4 Wochen lang täglich 10 mg MK-185/kg KG einnahmen, einen Abfall der Serumharnsäure um 27,6% des Ausgangswertes fest. Die dreitägige Verabreichung einer Dosis von 20 mg MK-185/kg KG führte zu einem Anstieg der renalen Harnsäureausscheidung sowie Verminderung der Oxypurinelimination im Urin. Eine signifikante Senkung der Serumharnsäure konnte während dieser kurzen Beobachtungsperiode nicht registriert werden. WOLFRAM et al. (1973) fanden, daß der uricosurische Effekt dieses Arzneimittels bei Dauerbehandlung dem des Probenecids entspricht.

Schließlich sollen noch eine Reihe weiterer Verbindungen, auf die an dieser Stelle nicht näher eingegangen wird, die renale Harnsäureausscheidung fördern. Sie umfassen das Cortison, ACTH, Phenacetin, Adrenalin, Theophyllin, Coffein, Salyrgan, Renin, Phenolrot, polyhydrische Alkohole, hypertone Glucoselösungen sowie Mannit (Zit. bei MERTZ, 1971). Eine uricosurische Wirkung wird auch einer Reihe von Röntgenkontrastmitteln zugeschrieben (POSTLETHWAITE u. KELLEY, 1971; KELLEY, 1971).

Komplikationen einer uricosurischen Therapie und deren Prophylaxe

Gichtanfälle

Zu Beginn einer uricosurischen oder Allopurinol-Therapie muß mit gehäuften Gichtanfällen gerechnet werden. Sie beruhen auf Ausfällungen von Uratkristallen infolge Schwankungen des Serumharnsäurespiegels. Sehr günstig hat sich hierbei die zusätzliche Verwendung kleiner Colchicindosen (0,5—1,5 mg/tgl.) erwiesen.

TALBOTT (1957) hat als erster systematisch festgestellt, daß die dauernde Zufuhr von Colchicin (zwischen 0,5 mg jeden zweiten Tag bei leichten Anfällen und 1,5 mg pro die bei schweren Attacken) die Anfallsbereitschaft stark herabsetzt. Zahlreiche Autoren konnten diese Erfahrung bestätigen (z.B. YÜ u. GUTMAN, 1961; GUTMAN, 1965). So beobachtete GUTMAN (1965) unter 734 Patienten vor der Anwendung von Colchicin bei 80% der Fälle Gichtattacken verschiedenen Schweregrades. Unter einer Colchicinprophylaxe dagegen — mit oder ohne gleichzeitige uricosurische Therapie — traten unter 260 Patienten, deren Behandlungsdauer sich im Mittel über 6,4 Jahre erstreckte, in 75% der Fälle keine oder nur noch milde Gichtanfälle auf.

In der Regel führen wir eine Colchicinprophylaxe (0,5—1,5 mg/tgl.) in Kombination mit einem Uricosuricum oder Allopurinol über insgesamt 3—6—12 Monate durch. Nach diesem Zeitraum kann im allgemeinen Colchicin abgesetzt werden, da bei der Mehrzahl der Patienten unter konsequenter Fortsetzung der uricosurischen Behandlung nur noch in Ausnahmefällen Gichtanfälle auftreten. TALBOTT (1967) empfiehlt eine längere Colchicintherapie. Patienten, denen zwei Jahrzehnte lang Colchicin in Kombination mit einem Uricosuricum verabreicht wurde, sind in seinem Krankengut keine Seltenheit.

Toxische Symptome scheinen unter einer Colchicinprophylaxe nicht aufzutreten. Im allgemeinen werden die kleinen Dosen gut toleriert. Bei chronischer Colchicin-Anwendung sollte jedoch die Möglichkeit von Änderungen der genetischen Information durch Chromosomenschädigung nicht außer acht gelassen werden (MERTZ, 1971).

In Ausnahmefällen kann statt Colchicin auch Indomethacin (2 × 25 mg/tgl.) zur Anfallsprophylaxe angewendet werden. Mit störenden Nebenwirkungen ist dabei in dieser Dosierung nicht zu rechnen.

Renale Komplikationen und deren Prophylaxe

Während der uricosurischen Wirkung eines Arzneimittels wird die Harnsäurekonzentration im Verlauf des Tubulussystems angehoben. Da Uricosurica durch Blockierung der Harnsäurerückresorption wirken, findet diese Konzentrationserhöhung bereits am Ort der tubulären Rückresorption statt und läßt sich bis in die Sammelröhrchen verfolgen. Es ist deshalb nicht verwunderlich, daß unter uricosurischer Therapie intratubuläre Harnsäureausfällungen, die zu Anurie führen, vorkommen können. Grundsätzlich dürfen Uricosurica deshalb nur einschleichend dosiert werden. Gleichzeitig sollte auf eine reichliche Flüssigkeitszufuhr geachtet sowie wenigstens zu Beginn der Therapie eine Neutralisierung des Harns angestrebt werden. Die minimale Harnmenge, die für eine nennenswerte Harnsäureverdünnung im Urin erzielt werden sollte, beträgt 1,5 Liter/tgl., weil bis zu dieser Größe der Harnausscheidung auch noch ein gewisser uricosurischer Effekt der Wasserzufuhr zum Tragen kommt. Im allgemeinen werden jedoch größere Harnmengen gefordert (2—2,5 Liter/tgl.). Dabei muß den Patienten die Messung des täglichen Harnvolumens, nicht der Trinkmenge, vorgeschrieben werden, da die letztere von vielen äußeren Umständen abhängt. Wichtig ist dabei, daß die Diurese auch nachts fortbesteht. ZÖLLNER (1968) verordnet deshalb reichliche Flüssigkeitszufuhr vor dem Schlafengehen sowie einen halben Liter Wasser in der Mitte der Schlafperiode. An die Notwendigkeit, einen Wecker zu stellen, sowie an die auftretende Nykturie gewöhnen sich die Patienten rasch.

Die Harnneutralisierung erfolgt mit Eisenbergscher Lösung (bestehend aus 40 g Citronensäure, 60 g Natriumcitrat, 66 g Kaliumcitrat, 6 g Pomeranzenextrakt, die in Sirup gelöst werden, Endvolumen 600 ml) oder dem zuckerfreien Uralyt-U®. Dabei muß bei Steinträgern die Harnneutralisierung über Monate durchgeführt werden. Der Harn-pH sollte vom Patienten selbst mittels eines Teststreifens kontrolliert werden und nicht unter 6,4 abfallen. Eine zu starke Alkalisierung ist jedoch ebenfalls zu vermeiden, da sie die Gefahr einer Phosphatausfällung in sich birgt. Als Kontraindikationen einer „alkalisierenden" Therapie gelten schwere Herz- und Niereninsuffizienz. Die Spätrisiken chronischer Alkalisierung dürften sich auch bei Behandlung der Harnsäurenephrolithiasis ergeben. ZÖLLNER (1968) betrachtet deshalb die Alkalisierung als Maßnahme zur Steinauflösung bzw. zur Verhinderung der Ausfällung von Harnsäure zu Beginn einer uricosurischen Therapie, während er als Dauerprophylaxe der Steinbildung diätetische Maßnahmen, Allopurinol sowie reichliche Flüssigkeitszufuhr empfiehlt.

Therapieverlauf

Unter konsequenter uricosurischer Behandlung bleiben nach einer kürzeren oder längeren Zeit, die durch das Ausmaß der Harnsäuredepots bestimmt wird, weitere Gichtanfälle aus. Tophi werden kleiner oder können ganz verschwinden. So konnte GUTMAN (1965) unter 140 Fällen, denen über mehr als 2 Jahre Probenecid oder Sulfinpyrazon bzw. eine Kombination beider Präparate verabreicht wurde, die Zahl der Patienten, die unter fortgeschrittener oder mäßig fortgeschrittener tophöser Gicht litten, von 66% auf 28% senken. Dieses Ziel wird jedoch meist erst nach Monaten oder Jahren erreicht. Knochentophi können sich unter Wiederherstellung des Gelenks zurückbilden, meist beobachtet man allerdings eine Defektheilung.

Die renalen Komplikationen sind ebenfalls zum Teil reversibel. So sind Steinauflösungen keine Seltenheit. Sicherer und einfacher ist es jedoch, Patienten mit Harnsäurenephrolithiasis oder eingeschränkter Nierenfunktion von Anfang an nicht mit Uricosurica, sondern mit Allopurinol zu behandeln. Keine verbindlichen Aussagen können bis jetzt bezüglich des Therapieerfolges bei der Gichtniere gemacht werden. Von PHILLIPS (1955) konnte während einer 34monatigen Probenecidbehandlung bei einem 31jährigen Gichtkranken eine wesentliche Besserung der Nierenfunktion beobachtet werden.

Trotz adäquater Behandlung ist der Therapieerfolg bei etwa $^1/_3$ aller Patienten, denen Uricosurica verordnet werden, unbefriedigend. So konnten GUTMAN u. YÜ (1957) bei 17% aller Patienten, die Probenecid erhielten, den Serumharnsäurespiegel nicht unter 7,0 mg-% senken. THOMPSON et al. (1962) berichteten über ähnliche Mißerfolge. Arzneimittelunverträglichkeit, gleichzeitige Salicylateinnahme und Niereninsuffizienz sind in erster Linie ursächlich anzuschuldigen. Nach den Erfahrungen von KUZELL et al. (1964) werden ungefähr zwei Drittel aller Patienten gegen Probenecid refraktär. Die Toleranz gegenüber Sulfinpyrazon soll besser sein (KUZELL, 1964).

Nicht selten empfiehlt es sich, uricosurische Arzneimittel kombiniert bzw. gleichzeitig mit Allopurinol zu verabreichen.

Literatur

AUSTRIAN, CH. R., BOGER, W. P.: Sensitization and subsequent desensitization to probenecid (benemid). Arch. intern. Med. **98**, 505—509 (1956).
BARTELS, E. C.: Gout — now amenable to control. Ann. intern. Med. **42**, 1—10 (1955).
BARTELS, E. C., MATOSSIAN, G. S.: Gout: Six-year follow-up on probenecid (benemid) therapy. Arthr. and Rheum. **2**, 193—202 (1959).
BAUER, W., KLEMPERER, F.: The treatment of gout. New Engl. J. Med. **231**, 681—685 (1944).
BAUER, W., SINGH, M. M.: Management of gout. New Engl. J. Med. **256**, 171—176 (1957).
BERKOWITZ, D.: The effects of chlorophenoxyisobutyrate with and without androsterone on the serum lipids, fat tolerance and uric acid. Metabolism **14**, 966—975 (1965).
BEYER, K. H., WIEBELHAUS, V. D., TILLSON, E. K., RUSSO, H. F., WILHOYTE, K. M.: "Benemid" -p-(di-n-propylsulfamyl)-benzoic-acid: Inhibition of glycine conjugative reactions. Proc. Soc. expt. Biol. (N. Y.) **74**, 772—775 (1950).
BEYER, K. H., RUSSO, H. F., TILLSON, E. K., MILLER, A. K., VERWEY, W. F., GASS, S. R.: "Benemid" p-(di-n-propylsulfamyl)-benzoic-acid: Its renal affinity and its elimination. Am. J. Physiol. **166**, 625—640 (1951).
BISHOP, C., RAND, R., TALBOTT, J. H., JR.: The effect of benemid (p-(di-n-propylsulfamyl)-benzoic acid) on uric acid metabolism in one normal and one gouty subject. J. clin. Invest. **30**, 889—895 (1951).
BISHOP, CH., BEYER, A., TALBOTT, J. H.: Isotopic uric acid in gouty and rheumatoid arthritis patients treated with probenecid and phenylbutazone. Proc. Soc. exp. Biol. (N.Y.) **86**, 760—762 (1954).
BLUESTONE, R., KIPPEN, J., KLINENBERG, J. R.: Effect of drugs on urate binding to plasma proteins. British med. J. **1969 IV**, 590—593.
BOGER, W. P., BEATTY, J. O., PITTS, F. W., FLIPPIN, H. F.: The influence of a new benzoic acid derivative on the metabolism of paraamino-salicylic acid (PAS) and penicillin. Ann. intern. Med. **33**, 18—31 (1950).
BOGER, W. P., STRICKLAND, S. C.: Probenecid (benemid)- its uses and sideeffects in 2502 patients. Arch. intern. Med. **95**, 83—92 (1955).
BRØCHNER-MORTENSEN, K.: Uric acid in blood and urine. Acta med. scand. Suppl. **134**, (1937).
BRØCHNER-MORTENSEN, K.: Gout. Ann. rheum. Dis. **17**, 1—15 (1958).
BRODIE, B. B., YU, T. F., BURNS, J. J., CHENKIN, T., PATON, B. C., STEELE, J. M., GUTMAN, A. B.: Observations on G-25671, a phenylbutazone analogue (4-(phenylthioethyl)-1,2-diphenyl-3,5-pyrazolidinedione). Proc. Soc. exptl. Biol. (N. Y.) **86**, 884—887 (1954).
BROEKHUYSEN, J., DELTOUR, G., BEKAERT, J.: Recherches dans la serie des benzofurannes IV. Transit et metabolisme de l' éthyl-2-(hydroxy-4- diiodo-3,5-benzoyl)-3-benzofuranne chez l' animal et chez l' homme. Arch. int. Pharmacodyn. **83**, 379—399 (1961).
BROEKHUYSEN, J., PACCO, M., SION, R., DEMENLENAESE, L., VAN HEE, M.: Metabolism of Benzbromarone in Man. Europ. J. clin. Pharmacol. **4**, 125—130 (1972).
BUCHBORN, E., WENK, M.: Harnsäureausscheidung unter Longacid beim Gesunden und bei chron. Gicht. Klin. Wschr. **32**, 564 (1954).
BURNS, J. J., ROSE, R. K., CHENKIN, TH., GOLDMAN, A., SCHUBERT, A., BRODIE, B. B.: The physiological disposition of phenylbutazone (butazolidin) in man and a method for its estimation in biological material. J. Pharmacol. exp. Ther. **109**, 346—357 (1953).
BURNS, J. J., YU, T. F., BERGER, L., GUTMAN, A. B.: Zoxazolamine, physiological disposition, uricosuric properties. Amer. J. Med. **25**, 401—408 (1958).
BURNS, J. J., YU, T. F., DAYTON, P., BERGER, L., GUTMAN, A. B., BRODIE, B. B.: Relationship between pka and uricosuric activity in phenylbutazone analogues. Nature **182**, 1162—1163 (1958a).
BURNS, J. J., YU, T. F., DAYTON, P. G., GUTMAN, A. B., BRODIE, B. B.: Biochemical pharmacological considerations of phenylbutazone and its analogues. Ann. N.J. Acad. Sci. **86**, 253—286 (1960).
BURNS, J. J., YU, T. F., RITTERBAND, A., PEREL, J. M., GUTMAN, A. B., BRODIE, B. B.: A potent new uricosuric agent, the sulfoxide metabolite of the phenylbutazone analogue, G-25671. J. Pharmacol. exp. Ther. **119**, 418—426 (1957).
CAMPBELL, H.: The salicylic treatment of gout, neuralgia and diabetes. London: Renshaw 1878.
CARREL, H. B., ELLIOTT, C. A.: Cinchophen poisoning. Med. Clin. N. Amer. **17**, 473—485 (1933).
COTTET, J., VITTU, CH.: Action de la benziodarone sur l'hyperuricémie goutteuse. Presse Méd. **75**, 1355—1356 (1967).
DANCHOT, J.: Dissertation, Paris 1968.

Dayton, P. G., Sicam, L. E., Landrau, M., Burns, J. J.: Metabolism of sulfinpyrazone (anturane) and other thio analogues of phenylbutazone in man. J. Pharmacol. exp. Ther. **132**, 287—290 (1961).

Dayton, P. G., Yu, T. F., Chen, W., Berger, L., West, L. A., Gutman, A. B.: The physiological disposition of probenecid, including renal clearance in man, studied by an improved method for its estimation in biological material. J. Pharmacol. exp. Ther. **140**, 278—286 (1963).

De Seze, S., Ryckewaert, A., Levernieux, J., Marteau, R.: Physiopathology, clinical manifestation and treatment of gout. Part. 2. Clinical and therapeutic studies. Ann. rheum. Dis. **17**, 15—22 (1958).

Delbarre, F., Auscher, C., Amor, B.: Action uricosurique de certains dérivés du benzofuranne. Soc. Méd. Hôp. Paris **116**, 1193—1196 (1965).

Delbarre, F., Auscher, C., Amor, B.: Action uricosurique et antigoutteuse de certains dérivés du benzofuranne. Presse Méd. **73**, 2725—2726 (1965a).

Delbarre, F., Auscher, C., Olivier, J. L., Rose, A.: Traitement des hyperuricémies et de la goutte par des dérivés du benzofuranne. Sem. Hôp. Paris **43**, 1127—1133 (1967).

Deltour, G., Broekhuysen, J., Ghislain, M., Bourgeois, F., Binon, F.: Recherches dans la série des benzofurannes. XXI. Effet inhibiteur de dérivés benzofuranniques phénoliques et de quelques analogues sur la xanthine oxidase hépatique du rat in vitro. Arch. int. Pharmacodyn. **161**, 25—30 (1967).

Dofel, W.: Über die Wirkung von Benzbromaronum auf die renale Harnsäureausscheidung Gesunder. Inaugural-Dissertation 1971.

Dreyfuss, F., Czaczkes, J. W.: The uricosuric action of bishydroxycoumarin (dicumarol). Arch. intern. Med. **102**, 389—391 (1958).

Emmerson, B. T.: A comparison of uricosuric agents in gout with special reference to sulphinpyrazone. Med. J. Aust. **1**, 839—844 (1963).

Ford, R. V., Spurr, C. L.: Metabolic and renal effects of probenecid (benemid). Clin. Res. Proc. **1**, 10 (1953).

Friend, D. G.: Uricosuric drugs. Practitioner **200**, 153—157 (1968).

Frost, H.: „Exzessive" Gicht bei einem jungen Mann. Behandlung mit Benemid und Indomethacin. Dtsch. med. Wschr. **90**, 1575—1578 (1965).

Gamp, A.: Zur medikamentösen Behandlung der chronischen Gicht. Ärztl. Wschr. **12**, 779—783 (1957).

Garcia, D. A., Yendt, E. R.: The effects of probenecid and thiazides and their combination on the urinary excretion of electrolytes and on acid-base equilibrium. Canad. med. Ass. J. **103**, 473—483 (1970).

Gerbaux, J. O.: Traitement de la goutte et de certains rhumatismes avec hyperuricémie par la benziodarone. Rev. Rhum. **35**, 98—115 (1968).

Goodman, L. S., Gilman, A.: The pharmacological basis of therapeutics, 4. Ed. 1970.

Greiling, H.: Zur klinischen Biochemie der Gicht. Dtsch. med. J. **10**, 336 (1969).

Griebsch, A., Zöllner, N.: Normalwerte der Plasmaharnsäure in Süddeutschland. Z. klin. Chem. **11**, 346—356 (1973).

Gröbner, W., Heimstädt, P., Zöllner, N.: Über die Wirkung von Niridazol (Ambilhar®) auf Serumharnsäure sowie renale Harnsäure- und Oxypurinausscheidung. Verh. dtsch. Ges. inn. Med. **77**, 183—185 (1971).

Gross, A., Girard, V.: Über die Wirkung von Benzbromaron auf Urikämie und Urikosurie. Med. Welt (Stuttg.) **23**, 133—136 (1972).

Gross, A., Girard, V., Gaultier, J.: Démonstration et étude de l'action uricosurique de la benziodarone. Thérapie **12**, 1097—1111 (1967).

Gutman, A. B.: Combined Staff Clinic: Uric acid metabolism and gout. Amer. J. Med. **9**, 799—817 (1950).

Gutman, A. B.: Treatment of primary gout: The present status. Arthr. and Rheum. **8**, 911—920 (1965).

Gutman, A. B.: Uricosuric drugs with special reference to probenecid and sulfinpyrazone. Advanc. Pharmacol. **4**, 91—142 (1966).

Gutman, A. B.: Recent developments in the therapy of gout. J. the Amer. Geriat. Soc. **16**, 499—504 (1968).

Gutman, A. B., Dayton, P. G., Yu, T. F., Berger, L., Chen, W., Sicam, L. E., Burns, J. J.: A study of the inverse relationship between pka and rate of renal excretion of phenylbutazone analogs in man and dog. Amer. J. Med. **29**, 1017—1033 (1960).

Gutman, A. B., Yu, T. F.: Benemid (p-(Di-n-propylsulfamyl)-benzoic acid) as uricosuric agent in chronic gouty arthritis. Trans. Ass. Amer. Phycns. **64**, 279—288 (1951).

GUTMAN, A. B., YU, T. F.: Current principles of management of gout. Amer. J. Med. 13, 744—759 (1952).
GUTMAN, A. B., YU, T. F.: Protracted uricosuric therapy in tophaceous gout. Lancet 1957 II, 1258—1260.
HALL, A. P., BARRY, P. E., DAWBER, T. R., MCNAMARA, P. M.: Epidemiology of gout and hyperuricemia. A long-term population study. Amer. J. Med. 42, 27—37 (1967).
HANSEN, O. E., HOLTEN, C.: Uricosuric effect of dicoumarol. Lancet 1958 I, 1047—1048.
HERTZ, PH., JAGER, H., RICHARDSON, J.: Probenecid-Induced Nephrotic Syndrome. Arch. Path. 94, 241—243 (1972).
HOWARD, R. P., ALAUPOVIC, P., BRUSCO, O. J., FURMAN, R. H.: Effects of ethylchlorophenoxyisobutyrate alone or with androsterone (Atromid) on serum lipids, lipoproteins and related metabolic parameters in normal and hyperlipidemic subjects. J. Atheroscler. Res. 3, 482—499 (1963).
JAIN, A., RYAN, J. R., HAGUE, D., MCMAHON, F. G.: The effect of MK-185 on some aspects of uric acid metabolism. Clinical Pharmacol. 11, 551—557 (1970).
JENNINGS, G. H.: The value of sodium salicylate in the treatment of gout. Rep. Chron. Rheum. Dis. 3, 106 (1937).
JOHNSON, H. P., JR., ENGLEMAN, E. P., FORSHAM, P. H., KRUPP, M. A., GREEN, T. W., GOLDFIEN, A.: Effects of phenylbutazone in gout. New. Engl. J. Med. 250, 665—670 (1954).
KELLEY, W. N., ROSENBLOOM, F. M., MILLER, J., SEEGMILLER, J. E.: An enzymatic basis for variation in response to allopurinol. Hypoxanthine-guanine-phosphoribosyltransferase deficiency. New Engl. J. Med. 278, 287—293 (1968).
KELLEY, W. N.: Uricosurica and X-Ray Contrast Agents. New Engl. J. Med. 284, 975—976 (1971).
KERSLEY, G. D., COOK. E, R., TOVEY, D. C. J.: Value of uricosuric agents and in particular of G-28315 in gout. Ann. Rheum. Dis. 17, 326—333 (1958).
KIDD, E. G., BOYCE, K. C., FREYBERG, R. H.: Clinical studies of phenylbutazone (Butazolidin) and butapyrin (Irgapyrin) in rheumatoid arthritis, rheumatoid spondylitis and gout. Ann. Rheum. Dis. 12, 20—24 (1953).
KOLB, F. O., RUKES, J. M.: Effects of benemid (probenecid) in the treatment of hypoparathyreoidism and pseudohypoparathyreoidism. J. Clin. Endocr. 14, 785 (1954).
KOTZAUREK, R., HUEBER, E. F.: Über klinische Erfahrungen mit 2-Äthyl-3-(4-hydroxy-3,5-dibrom-benzoyl)-benzofuran („Benzbromaron") bei der Behandlung der Gicht und Hyperurikämie. Wien. med. Wschr. 118, 1014—1018 (1968).
KUSUS, T.: Harnsäureclearance bei Leberkrankheiten und ihre Beeinflussung mit Vit. K. Inaugural-Dissertation, München 1965.
KUZELL, W. C., SCHAFFARZICK, R. W.: Phenylbutazone (Butazolidin) and Butapyrin: a study of clinical effects in arthritis and gout. Calif. Med. 77, 319 (1952).
KUZELL, W. C., GLOVER, R., GIBBS, J., BLAU, R.: Effect of anturane on serum uric acid and cholesterol in gout. A long-term study. Acta rheum. scand. Suppl. 8, 31—40 (1964).
KUZELL, W. C., SCHAFFARZICK, R. W., NAUGLER, W. E., GAUDIN, G., MANKLE, E. A., BROWN, B.: Phenylbutazone (Butazolidin) in gout. Amer. J. Med. 16, 212—217 (1954).
KUZELL, W. C., SCHAFFARZICK, R. W., NAUGLER, W. E., KOETS, P., MANKLE, E. A., BROWN, B., CHAMPLIN, B.: Some observations on 520 gouty patients. J. chron. Dis. 2, 645—669 (1955).
LAUDAT, M. H., RYCKEWAERT, A., LAGRUE, G., MILLIEZ, P., DE SEZE, S.: Le rôle de l'insuffisance rénale uricoéliminatoire dans la goutte primitive. Rev. franc. Etud. clin. biol. 7, 155 (1962).
LÖFFLER, W., KOLLER, F.: Die Gicht. In: Handbuch der inneren Medizin, 7. Band, 2. Teil: Stoffwechsel-Krankheiten, S. 435. Berlin-Göttingen-Heidelberg: Springer 1955.
MARSON, F. G. W.: Radiological evidence of value of treatment in gout. Brit. J. Radiol. 25, 539—541 (1952).
MARSON, F. G. W.: Studies in gout, with particular reference to the value of sodium salicylate in treatment. Quart. J. Med. 22, 331—346 (1953).
MARSON, F. G. W.: Sodium salicylate and probenecid in the treatment of chronic gout. Assessment of their relative effects in lowering serum uric acid levels. Ann. Rheum. Dis. 13, 233—245 (1954).
MASBERNARD, A., HILTENBRAND, C., MEMIN, Y., DECHELOTTE, J.: La benziodarone dans le traitement de fond de la maladie goutteuse. Rev. méd. Toulouse 4, 401—424 (1968).
MASBERNARD, A., FRANCOZ, P.: Zur uricosurischen Wirkung des Benzbromarons. Therapiewoche 19, 1553—1560 (1969).

MASBERNARD, A., HILTENBRAND, C., MEMIN, Y.: Benziodaron in the long-term management of gout. In: Progress of nephrology, p. 65—73. Berlin-Heidelberg-New York: Springer 1969.

MASBERNARD, A., VACCON, L.: Analyse comparative de l'action pharmacodynamique des dérivés bromés et iodés du benzofuranne chez les sujets sains et hyperuricémiques. Incidentes pratiques. Bull. Soc. Médicochir. Hôpit. γ Form. Sanit des Armées **2**, 605—622 (1970).

MCKINNEY, S. E., PECK, H. M., BOCHEY, J. M., BYHAN, B. B., SCHUCHARDT, G. S., BEYER, K. H.: Benemid (p-di-n-propylsulfamyl)-benzoic acid: Toxicologic properties. J. Pharmacol. exp. Ther. **102**, 208—214 (1951).

MEDVEDOWSKY, J. L., MARCOVICI, J.: Action de la benziodarone sur l'uricémie et l'uricosurie. Gazette médicale Fr. n° 13 (1966).

MELLINGHOFF, C. H., GROSS, R. H.: Erfahrungen über die Gicht, insbesondere über die uricosurische Therapie mit Anturan®. Z. Rheumaforsch. **21**, 42—50 (1962).

MERTZ, D. P.: Veränderungen der Serumkonzentration von Harnsäure unter der Wirkung von Benzbromaronum. Münch. med. Wschr. **111**, 491—495 (1969).

MERTZ, D. P.: Gicht; Grundlagen, Klinik und Therapie. Stuttgart: Thieme 1971.

MERTZ, D. P., SULZBERGER, I., KLÖPFER, M.: Diabetes mellitus, Hyperlipidämie, Fettleber, Hypertension bei primärer Gicht und deren Beeinflussung durch Benzbromaronum. Münch. med. Wschr. **112**, 241—247 (1970).

MIKKELSEN, W. M., DODGE, H. J., VALKENBURG, H.: The distribution of serum uric acid values in a population unselected as to gout or hyperuricemia. Amer. J. Med. **39**, 242 (1965).

MORGAN, J. P., BIANCHINE, J. R., TAH-HSIUNG, MARGOLIS, S.: Hypolipidemic, Uricosuric and Thyroxine-displacing Effects of MK-185 (Halofenate). Clin. Pharmacol. Ther. **12**, 517—524 (1971).

MÜLLER, M. M., BRESNIK, W.: Der Einfluß von Benziodaron auf den Purinstoffwechsel bei Gichtpatienten und Stoffwechselgesunden. Klin. Wschr. **50**, 1015—1016 (1972).

MUGLER, A.: Etude des effets de la benziodarone chez cent goutteux en cure de diurèse. Effets sur l'acide urique et l'acide oxalique. In: Rein et Foie: Maladies de la Nutrition, Tome X, p. 273—292 (1967).

MUGLER, A.: Effet uricosurique d'un dérivé de la phénylbutazone, la „cétophénylbutazone". Rev. Rhum. **38**, 33—39 (1971).

NIVET, M., MARCOVICI, J., COMPAGNON, P., LARUELLE, P.: Action hypo-uricémiante de la benziodarone per os. Sem. Hôp. Paris **43**, 135—138 (1967).

NIVET, M., MARCOVICI, J., LAURUELLE, P., MME FARAH: Note préliminaire sur l'action d'un benzofuranne sur l'uricémie. Soc. Méd. Hôp. Paris **116**, 1187—1192 (1965).

OGRYZLO, M. A., HARRISON, J.: Evaluation of uricosuric agents in chronic gout. Ann. rheum. Dis. **16**, 425—437 (1957).

OLMER, M., LAFON, J.: Action hypo-uricémiante de la benziodarone dans l'insufficance rénale chronique. Marseille-méd. **104**, 269—271 (1967).

PASCALE, L. R., DUBIN, A., HOFFMAN, W. S.: Therapeutic value of probenecid (Benemid) in gout. J. Amer. med. Ass. **149**, 1188—1194 (1952).

PASCALE, L. R., DUBIN, A., HOFFMAN, W. S.: Influence of benemid on urinary excretion of phosphate in hypoparathyreoidism. Metabolism **3**, 462—470 (1954).

PASERO, G.: Über die uricosurische Wirkung antiprothrombinämischer Substanzen und einiger neuer Indandionderivate. Dtsch. med. Wschr. **85**, 854 (1960).

PASERO, G., MASINI, G.: Sull 'azione uricurica degli antiprotrombinici di sintesi. Boll. Soc. med.-chir. Pisa **25**, 124 (1957).

PASERO, G., MARINI, N.: Sull 'azione uricurica del 2-fenil-5-bromo-1,3-indandione. Gazz. med. ital. **117**, 561—567 (1958).

PASERO, G., MARINI, N.: Influenza della vitamina K sull'azione uricurica del 2-fenil-5-bromo-1,3-indandione. Boll. Soc. med.-chir. Pisa **26**, 321 (1958a).

PASERO, G., MASINI, G.: L'ipouricemia negli itteri colurici. Minerva med. **49**, 3155 (1958).

PASERO, G., MASINI, G.: Sull'azione uricurica degli antiprotrombinici di sintesi. Arch. E. Maragliano Pat. Clin. **14**, 297 (1958a).

PEREL, J. M., CUNNINGHAN, R. F., FALES, H. M., DAYTON, P. G.: Identification and renal excretion of probenecid-metabolites in man. Life Sci. **9**, I, 1337—1343 (1970).

PEREL, J. M., DAYTON, P. G., MCMILLAN SNELL, M., YU, T. F., GUTMAN, A. B.: Studies of interactions among drugs in man at the renal level: Probenecid and sulfinpyrazone. Clin. Pharmacol. Ther. **10**, 834—840 (1969).

PERSELLIN, R. H., SCHMID, F. R.: The use of sulfinpyrazone in the treatment of gout. J. Amer. med. Ass. **175**, 971—975 (1961).
PETERS, J. P., VAN SLYKE, D. D.: Quantitative clinical chemistry interpretations, Vol. I. Baltimore: Williams & Wilkins 1946.
PHILLIPS, R. W.: Reversal of renal insufficiency in gout. Arch. intern. Med. **96**, 823—827 (1955).
PODEVIN, R., PAILLARD, F., AMIEL, C., RICHET, G.: Action de la benziodarone sur l'excrétion rénale de l'acide urique. Rev. franç. Etud. clin. biol. **12**, 361—367 (1967).
PODEVIN, R., PAILLARD, F., VOUDICLARI, S., RICHET, G.: Action du niridazol (Ciba 32.644 Ba) sur le métabolisme de l'acide urique chez l'homme. Rev. franç. Etud. clin. biol. **13**, 624—628 (1968).
POSTLETHWAITE, A. E., KELLEY, W. N.: Uricosuric Effect of Radiocontrast Agents. Ann. intern. Med. **74**, 845—852 (1971).
REED, E. B., FEICHTMEIER, T. V., WILLETT, F. M.: Zoxazolamine — a potent uricosuric agent. New Engl. J. Med. **258**, 894—896 (1958).
REYNOLDS, E. S., SCHLANT, R. C., GONICK, H. C., DAMMIN, G. J.: Fatal massive necrosis of the liver as a manifestation of hypersensitivity to probenecid. New Engl. J. Med. **256**, 592—596 (1957).
RICHET, G., COTTET, J., AMIEL, C., LEROUX-ROBERT, C., PODEVIN, R.: Traitement de l'hyperuricémie des gotteux et des insuffisants rénaux par la benziodarone. Presse Méd. **74**, 1247—1249 (1966a).
RICHET, G., LEROUX-ROBERT, C., PODEVIN, R., AMIEL, C.: Essais de traitement de l' hyperuricémie chez les insuffisants rénaux chroniques. Rev. Franç. Etud. clin. biol. **11**, 396—400 (1966).
RIZZUTO, V. J., INGLESBY, TH. V., GRACE, W. J.: Probenecid (Benemid) intoxication with status epilepticus. Amer. J. Med. **38**, 646—648 (1965).
RYCKEWAERT, A., KUNTZ, D., HENRARD, J. C., PUEL, M., DE SEZE, S.: Le traitement de fond de la goutte par la benziodarone. Presse Méd. **77**, 1157—1160 (1969).
SALA, G., BALLABIO, C. B., AMIRA, A., RATTI, G., CIRLA, E.: Renal mechanisms for urate excretion in normal and gouty subjects. Contemp. Rheum. 581 (1956).
SCOTT, J. T., O'BRIEN, P. K.: Probenecid, nephrotic syndrome and renal failure. Ann. rheum. Dis. **27**, 249—252 (1968).
SEE, G.: Etudes sur l'acide salicylique et les salicylates; traitement du rhumatisme aigu et chronique de la goutte et de diverses affections du système nerveux sensitif par les salicylates. Bull. Acad. Méd. (Paris) **6**, 689, 897 (1877).
SEEGMILLER, J. E., GRAYZEL, A. J.: Use of the newer uricosuric agents in the management of gout. J. Amer. med. Ass. **173**, 1076—1080 (1960).
SETAISHI, CH., HORIUCHI, Y., MASHIMO, K.: Increase of urinary insulin excretion following probenecid administration in man. Endocr. jap. **17**, 421—423 (1970).
SHORE, P. A., BRODIE, B. B., HOGBEN, C. A. M.: The gastric secretion of drugs: A pH partition hypothesis. J. Pharmacol. exp. Ther. **119**, 361—369 (1957).
SIROTA, J. H., YU, T. F., GUTMAN, A. B.: Effect of benemid (p-(di-n-propylsulfamyl-) benzoic acid) on urate clearance and other discrete renal functions in gouty subjects. J. clin. Invest. **31**, 692—701 (1952).
SOUGIN-MIBASHAN, R., HORWITZ, M.: The uricosuric action of ethylbiscoumacetate. Lancet **1955 I**, 1191—1197.
STERNON, J., KOCHELEFF, P., COUTURIER, E., BALASSE, E., VANDEN-ABEELE, P.: Effet hypo-uricémiant de la benzbromarone-étude de 24 cas. Acta clin. belg. **22**, 285—293 (1967).
TALBOTT, J. H.: Gout. New York-London: Grune & Stratton 1957.
TALBOTT, J. H.: The choice of a uricosuric drug in gout. Arthr. and Rheumat. **2**, 182—185 (1959).
TALBOTT, J. H.: Die Gicht. Stuttgart: Hippokrates-Verlag 1967.
TALBOTT, J. H., BISHOP, C., NORCROSS, B. M., LOCKIE, L. M.: The clinical and metabolic effects of benemid in patients with gout. Trans. Ass. Amer. Phycns **64**, 372 (1951).
THOMPSON, G. R., DUFF, J. F., ROBINSON, W. D., MIKKELSEN, W. M., GALINDEZ, H.: Long term uricosuric therapy in gout. Arthr. and Rheum. **5**, 384—395 (1962).
WEINER, J. M., MUDGE, G. H.: Renal tubular mechanisms for excretion of organic acids and basis. Amer. J. Med. **36**, 743—762 (1964).
WOLFRAM, G., KELLER, CH., KILANI, CH., ZÖLLNER, N.: Erste klinische Erfahrungen in der Behandlung von Hyperuricämie und Hyperlipidämie mit dem Clofibratderivat MK 185. 79. Tagung der dtsch. Ges. Inn. Medizin 1973.
WOLFSON, W. Q., COHN, C., LEVINE, R., HUDDLESTUN, B.: Transport and excretion of uric acid in man. III. Physiologic significance of the uricosuric effect of caronamide. Amer. J. Med. **4**, 774 (1948).

Wyngaarden, J. B.: The effect of phenylbutazone on uric acid metabolism in two normal subjects. J. clin. Invest. **34**, 256—262 (1955).

Yu, T. F., Burns, J. J., Gutman, A. B.: Results of clinical trial of G-28315, a sulfoxide analog of phenylbutazone, as a uricosuric agent in gouty subjects. Arthr. and Rheum. **1**, 532—543 (1958).

Yu, T. F., Dayton, P. G., Gutman, A. B.: Mutual suppression of the uricosuric effects of sulfinpyrazone and salicylate: A study in interactions between drugs. J. clinical Invest. **42**, 1330-1339 (1963).

Yu, T. F., Gutman, A. B.: Mobilisation of gouty tophi by protracted use of uricosuric agents. Amer. J. Med. **11**, 765—769 (1951).

Yu, T. F., Gutman, A. B.: Ultrafiltrability of plasma urate in man. Proc. Soc. exp. Biol. (N. Y.) **84**, 21—24 (1953).

Yu, T. F., Gutman, A. B.: Paradoxical retention of uric acid by uricosuric drugs in low dosage. Proc. Soc. exp. Biol. Med. **90**, 542—547 (1955).

Yu, T. F., Gutman, A. B.: Study of the paradoxical effects of salicylate in low, intermediate and high dosage on the renal mechanisms for excretion of urate in man. J. clin. Invest. **38**, 1298—1315 (1959).

Yu, T. F., Gutman, A. B.: Renal interaction of drugs affecting urate excretion in man. Pharmacologist **1**, 53 (1959a).

Yu, T. F., Gutman, A. B.: Efficacy of colchicine prophylaxis in gout: prevention of recurrent gouty arthritis over a mean period of five years in 208 gouty subjects. Ann. intern. Med. **55**, 179—192 (1961).

Yu, T. F., Gutman, A. B.: Principles of current management of primary gout. Amer. J. Med. Sci. **254**, 893—907 (1967).

Yu, T. F., Paton, B. C., Chenkin, Th., Burns, J. J., Brodie, B. B., Gutman, A. B.: Effect of a phenylbutazone analog (4-(phenyl-thioethyl)-1,2-diphenyl-3,5-pyrazolidinedione) on urate clearance and other discrete renal functions in gouty subjects. Evaluation as uricosuric agent. J. clin. Invest. **35**, 374—385 (1956).

Yu, T. F., Sirota, J. H., Gutman, A. B.: Effect of phenylbutazone (3,5 dioxo-1,2-diphenyl-4-n-butylpyrazolidine) on renal clearance of urate and other discrete renal functions in gouty subjects. J. clin. Invest. **32**, 1121—1132 (1953).

Zöllner, N.: Moderne Gichtprobleme. Ätiologie, Pathogenese, Klinik. Ergebn. inn. Med. Kinderheilk. **14**, 321 (1960).

Zöllner, N.: Eine einfache Modifikation der enzymatischen Harnsäurebestimmung. Normalwerte in der deutschen Bevölkerung. Z. klin. Chem. **1**, 178 (1963).

Zöllner, N.: Physiologie und Pathologie der Harnsäure. Praxis **53**, 1122 (1964).

Zöllner, N.: Die Gichtniere. In: Handbuch der inneren Medizin, 8. Band: Nierenkrankheiten, 3. Teil, S. 77. Berlin-Heidelberg-New York: Springer 1968.

Zöllner, N., Stern, G., Gröbner, W., Dofel, W.: Über die Senkung des Harnsäurespiegels im Plasma durch Benzbromaronum. Klin. Wschr. **46**, 1318 (1968).

Zöllner, N., Dofel, W., Gröbner, W.: Die Wirkung von Benzbromaronum auf die renale Harnsäureausscheidung Gesunder. Klin. Wschr. **48**, 426—432 (1970).

Zöllner, N., Griebsch, A., Fink, J. K.: Über die Wirkung von Benzbromaronum auf den Serumharnsäurespiegel und die Harnsäureausscheidung des Gichtkranken. Dtsch. med. Wschr. **95**, 2405—2412 (1970a).

Zöllner, N., Griebsch, A., Gröbner, W., Hector, G., Schattenkirchner, M.: Klinische Erfahrungen mit dem neuen Uricosuricum Benzbromaronum. Verh. dtsch. Ges. inn. Med. **76**, 853 (1970b).

Zöllner, N., Griebsch, A., Gröbner, W., Hector, G., Schattenkirchner, M.: Unveröffentlicht (1970c).

Zöllner, N., Gröbner, W.: Die Wirkung von Cumarin-, Indandion- und Benzofuranderivaten auf die renale Harnsäureausscheidung. Dtsch. med. Wschr. **94**, 2652—2654 (1969).

d) Diät einschließlich experimenteller Grundlagen

Von

A. GRIEBSCH

Mit 3 Abbildungen

Allgemeines

Die Ansichten über die Rolle der Diät bei der Behandlung von Gicht und Hyperuricämie waren bis in die letzten Jahre hinein widersprüchlich und divergent. Wie bereits im Kapitel über den Einfluß der exogenen Purine erwähnt, fehlte es speziell im anglo-amerikanischen Schrifttum nie an Vertretern der Ansicht, daß Diät, speziell purinarme Kost, keine oder eine nur ganz untergeordnete Rolle für die Gichttherapie spielt. Demgegenüber ist in Mitteleuropa, nicht zuletzt angesichts der Beobachtungen, daß die calorienarme und besonders fleischarme Kost in Notzeiten einen beachtlichen Rückgang der Häufigkeit der Gicht nach sich gezogen hat, stets die Meinung aufrechterhalten worden, daß die Ernährung, genauer die Zufuhr von Nahrungspurin, einen Umweltfaktor darstellt, der das genetisch determinierte Gichtleiden entweder unterdrücken (Notzeiten) oder stärker zum Tragen (Überflußgesellschaft) bringen kann.

In den letzten 20 Jahren, besonders seit GUTMAN und sein Arbeitskreis (1952) zeigen konnten, daß sich durch eine purinarme Kost der Harnsäurespiegel um durchschnittlich 1,2 mg/100 ml senken läßt, ist durch eine Reihe von experimentellen Beobachtungen, u.a. aus dem Arbeitskreis von SEEGMILLER et al. (1961), WASLIEN et al. (1968 u. 1970) und auch aus unserem Arbeitskreis (ZÖLLNER et al., 1972; GRIEBSCH u. ZÖLLNER, 1970a u. b., 1974) der Einfluß der Purinzufuhr auf die klinisch wichtigen Parameter des Harnsäurestoffwechsels, also auf Plasmaspiegel und Harnsäure-Ausscheidung quantitativ erfaßt worden. Damit ist der Einfluß der Diät auf diese Größen experimentell ausreichend belegt. Gleichzeitig ist neben der Rolle von Purinrestriktion und Purinzufuhr auf diese Parameter auch die Auswirkung anderer alimentärer Faktoren, wie der Zufuhr von Alkohol, Fett, Proteinen und Kohlenhydraten sowie des Fastens auf den Harnsäurestoffwechsel untersucht und quantitativ beschrieben worden.

Experimentelle Grundlagen

Verwendung von Standard- und Formeldiäten für Ernährungsexperimente über den Harnsäurestoffwechsel

Zweifellos läßt sich z.B. durch eine purinarme Standarddiät und noch eindeutiger durch purinfreie flüssige Formeldiät die Purinzufuhr vermindern oder ausschalten. Dies führt zu einem Abfall der Harnsäureausscheidung und des Harnsäurespiegels, wie bereits im Kapitel über exogene Purine beschrieben wurde. Bei diesen Ernährungsexperimenten kann die Größe von Harnsäureplasmaspiegel und renaler Harnsäureausscheidung durch Vermeidung von Schwankungen der Calorienzufuhr und der Anteile von Kohlenhydraten, Fett und Eiweiß um so exakter erfaßt werden, je genauer die experimentellen Diätformen kalkuliert sind.

Tabelle 1. Beispiel für die Calorienberechnung aus der Körperoberfläche von Versuchspersonen, für die Verteilung von Kohlenhydraten, Fett und Eiweiß (in g, kcal und in % der Calorien) sowie Purin-N-Gehalt bei Standarddiät (oben) und Formeldiät (unten)

Lfd. Nr.	Ge-schl. M/W	Alter Jahre	Größe (m)	Ge-wicht (kg)	Kör-perofl. (m²)	Grund-umsatz (Cal/m²)	Tages-Grund-umsatz (Cal/24 h)	Tages-Arbeits-umsatz (Cal/24 h)	Verab-folgte Kalorien (Cal/24 h)	Kohlenhydrat Menge (g)	Cal	%	Fette Menge (g)	Cal	%	Eiweiß Menge (g)	Cal	%	Purin-N mg/Tag
I. STANDARD-DIÄT																			
1	w	22	1,65	52,2	1,57	35,2	1326,3	2387,3	2018	285,4	1141	56,5	64,5	600	29,7	69,1	276,4	13,7	18,2
2	w	22	1,69	61,0	1,70	35,2	1436,2	2585,2	2102	280,5	1122	53,4	78,0	725	34,5	63,6	254,4	12,1	18,2
3	m	19	1,85	79,0	2,02	40,1	1944,0	3499,2	3670	464,2	1813	49,4	146,5	1372	37,4	110,2	440,8	12,0	32,0
4	m	30	1,78	65,0	1,81	37,6	1606,3	2940,0	3670	464,2	1813	49,4	146,5	1372	37,4	110,2	440,8	12,0	32,0
5	m	22	1,76	67,0	1,82	39,2	1712,5	3082,5	2730	341,2	1365	50,0	109,5	1008	36,9	89,2	356,8	13,0	32,0
6	m	22	1,76	66,5	1,81	39,2	1702,9	3065,2	2770	492,2	1969	71,0	62,0	567	20,5	58,6	234,3	8,5	18,2
7	m	20	1,72	68,5	1,81	39,8	1729,0	3112,2	2102	280,5	1122	53,4	78,0	725	34,5	63,6	254,4	12,1	18,2
Mittelwerte		23,8		65,6				2953	2723			54,7%			33,0%			12,3	24,1
II. FORMEL-DIÄT																			
1	m	32	1,82	85,6	2,06	37,2	1839	3310,4	3310,4	455,2	1820,7	55	106,8	993,1	30	117,4	496,5	15	0
2	w	22	1,59	48,0	1,47	35,2	1242	2235,2	2235,2	307,5	1229,4	55	72,1	670,6	30	83,8	335,3	15	0
3	m	22	1,84	76,5	2,00	39,2	1881	3386,1	3386,1	465,6	1862,4	55	109,2	1015,8	30	127,0	507,9	15	0
4	w	23	1,62	49,0	1,51	35,2	1275,6	2296,0	2296,0	315,2	1262,8	55	74,0	688,8	30	86,1	344,4	15	0
5	w	22	1,65	52,5	1,57	35,2	1326	2387,1	2387,1	328,2	1312,9	55	77,0	716,1	30	89,5	358,0	15	0
Mittelwerte		24,2		62,3				2723	2723			55%			30%			15%	

Tabelle 2. Beispiel für das Verhalten des Körpergewichts von acht Versuchspersonen unter freigewählter Kost (N.K.) sowie unter flüssiger Formeldiät mit verschiedenen Zusätzen von Purinvorläufern (0, I, II) während 35 Versuchstagen und mittleres Körpergewicht ($\bar{x}$)

Versuchstag	Belastungs- Stufe	1 NU	2 HU	3 NU	4 NU	5 NU	6 NU	7 NU	8 NU	Versuchsperson NU = Normourikämiker HU = Hyperurikämiker
1	NK	41,0	73,9	61,6	69,2	81,4	72,0	65,0	50,7	
4		41,3	74,0	60,5	69,1	83,0	72,0	64,0	50,4	
6		40,8	72,9	59,8	68,4	80,7	72,0	64,0	50,4	
8	0	41,0	73,0	60,0	68,3	80,6	72,5	63,0	49,7	
11		41,1	74,2	60,5	68,4	80,6	72,0	63,0	49,9	
12		41,3	74,2	60,5	68,6	80,6	72,0	62,7	50,1	
14		41,2	73,9	60,9	68,3	80,4	72,0	63,3	50,5	
16		41,4	73,4	60,7	68,5	80,1	72,0	63,0	50,5	Körpergewicht (kg)
18	I	41,6	73,9	60,7	68,9	80,2	71,6	63,3	50,7	
21		41,7	73,7	60,8	68,4	80,1	71,3	62,9	49,9	
22		41,6	73,7	60,4	68,0	80,0	71,2	62,4	50,3	
24		41,7	73,4	60,7	68,0	80,0	71,0	62,7	50,0	
26		41,8	73,6	61,1	67,5	80,5	71,2	62,0	49,2	
28	II	42,0	73,5	60,8	67,9	79,9	71,4	62,8	49,1	
31		41,8	73,7	60,0	67,5	79,9	71,1	62,0	49,1	
33		41,2	72,3	59,6	67,9	79,7	70,5	61,2	50,0	
35	NK	42,3	73,8	61,0	69,0	80,4	72,0	63,9	51,3	
$\bar{x}_{1-8}$		41,5	73,7	60,6	68,3	80,5	71,6	63,0	50,1	

Allgemeine Voraussetzung der Diätberechnung

Experimentelle Diätformen müssen eine Reihe von Voraussetzungen erfüllen, um die Einflüsse der Kost auf den Harnsäurestoffwechsel möglichst gering zu halten. Zur Erhaltung der Gewichtskonstanz müssen die Diäten isocalorisch sein; dazu muß zunächst der Calorienbedarf der Versuchsperson genau bestimmt werden. Da die Ermittlung des Grundumsatzes mittels Spirometrie — speziell bei größeren Gruppen von Versuchspersonen — technisch schwer durchführbar ist, hat sich bei uns die Kalkulation des Grundumsatzes auf Grund der Körperoberfläche mittels der Daten von BOOTHBY et al. (1936) oder nach FLEISCH (1951) bewährt (vgl. Tab. 1). Der so unter Berücksichtigung von Alter und Geschlecht errechnete Grundumsatz läßt sich nach Angaben von ZÖLLNER in THANNHAUSERS Lehrbuch (1957) auf den Tagesarbeitsumsatz in Abhängigkeit von der Schwere der körperlichen Tätigkeit umrechnen. Für leichte bis mittelschwere körperliche Arbeit, wie sie die meisten freiwilligen Versuchspersonen ausüben (Studenten/innen, leichte Schreibarbeit, Laborarbeiten), kommt meist ein Umrechnungsfaktor von 1,6 in Betracht, der zwischen dem Faktor für den Calorienverbrauch eines Patienten, der nicht bettlägerig ist (1,4) und dem für den Arbeitsaufwand einer Hausfrau oder bei Büroarbeit (1,7) liegt. Die Kontrolle darüber, ob der gewählte Faktor dem tatsächlichen Calorienbedarf entspricht, erfolgt durch tägliche Gewichtskontrolle (vgl. Tab. 2). Ein steady-state der beobachteten Parameter des Harnsäurestoffwechsels stellt sich erst nach 8—10 Tagen ein, was experimentelle Diätformen zeitlich recht aufwendig macht (vgl. Abb. 1).

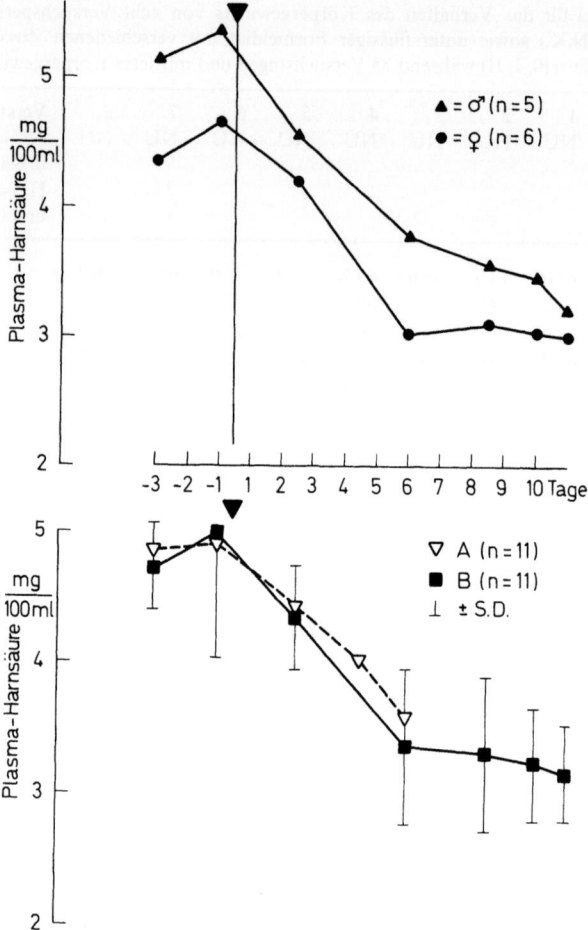

Abb. 1. Verhalten der Harnsäureplasmaspiegel unter purinfreier Formeldiät über 11 Tage bei 5 männlichen und 6 weiblichen Versuchspersonen (oben) sowie Verhalten dieser Größe nach 6 (gestrichelte Linie) und nach 11 (durchgezogene Linie) Versuchstagen (unten). Man beachte den Eintritt des steady state vom 8.—10. Versuchstag. (Nach Daten v. GRIEBSCH u. ZÖLLNER, 1970a/b, 1971 u. 1972)

Purinarme Standarddiät

Die meisten Autoren verwenden für das Studium der Wirkung der Purinrestriktion verschiedene Modifikationen einer purinarmen Standarddiät. Man versteht darunter eine durch schriftliche Speisepläne (vgl. Tab. 3) fixierte, aus purinarmen Nahrungsmitteln zusammengestellte Kost, deren Caloriengehalt meist durch Zugabe oder Weglassen praktisch purinfreier Bestandteile, meist von Kohlenhydraten, dem errechneten Calorienbedarf angepaßt wird. Da der Puringehalt jedoch nur mittels Nahrungsmitteltabellen kalkuliert werden kann, ergeben sich — trotz insgesamt niedrigen Puringehalts (vgl. Tab. 1) — doch Schwankungen von Tag zu Tag und von Versuchsperson zu Versuchsperson. Der Vorteil der Standarddiät liegt allerdings darin, daß sie abwechslungsreich und wohlschmeckend ist, so daß ihre Einhaltung den Versuchspersonen keine Mühe bereitet.

Tabelle 3. Beispiel für eine purinarme Standard-Diät mit einem Purin-N-Gehalt zwischen 18,6 und 32 mg/Tag. Die Pläne werden z.B. in zwei Calorienstufen von 2370 bzw. 2600 kcal erstellt und durch Zufügen oder Weglassen von purinfreien Nahrungsmitteln (z.B. Zwieback, Schokolade) an den individuellen Calorienbedarf angepaßt. Meist wird für jeden Wochentag ein eigener Plan aufgestellt und den Versuchspersonen ausgehändigt

Speisenplan A (niedrigere Calorienstufe, 2370 kcal) Dienstag

Frühstück:	Kaffee oder Tee mit Zucker nach Belieben und 2 Teel. Kondensmilch (7,5% Fett) 1 Scheibe Toastbrot (25 g), 1 Scheibe Mischbrot (40 g = von einem langen Brot eine Scheibe, ca. $^1/_2$ cm dick), 2 Scheiben Scheibletten Edamer Käse o. a. (40% Fett), 20 g Butter/Margarine, 1 EBl. Marmelade.
Mittagessen:	1 Brötchen bzw. Semmel, 1 Scheibe Pumpernickel, 10 g Butter/Margarine, 1 Gervais-Käse.
Zwischenmahlzeit:	1 gr. Apfel (ca. 200 g), $^1/_4$ l Trinkmilch, 50 g Zwieback, $^1/_2$ Tafel Vollmilch-Schokolade (50 g).
Abendessen:	Nudelomelette[a] von 60 g Nudeln, 1 Ei, $^1/_2$ Tasse Milch (50 g), 1 Teel. Öl, Kopfsalat (ca. 30 g) angemacht mit 1 Teel. Öl, Zucker nach Belieben.
Getränke:	Apfelsaft, Tee mit Zucker, Weißwein.

[a] Anleitung für Nudelomelette: Nudeln in Salzwasser weich kochen. Öl in der Pfanne erhitzen, Nudeln darin schwenken, das Ei mit der Milch und Gewürzen wie Salz, Muskat, Petersilie, Paprika verquirlen, über die Nudeln gießen und fest werden lassen.

Purinfreie Formeldiäten

Flüssige isocalorische Formeldiäten werden nach einem Vorschlag von AHRENS JR.(1951) für verschiedene Ernährungs-Experimente verwendet und sind seit 20 Jahren erprobt (AHRENS JR., 1970); auch in unserem Arbeitskreis liegen seit längerer Zeit Erfahrungen vor (WOLFRAM u. ZÖLLNER, 1971). Durch die halbsynthetische Formeldiät läßt sich eine völlig purinfreie, isocalorische Kostform verwirklichen. Dabei werden die individuellen Schwankungen sehr gering, so daß Ergebnisse, die unter einer freigewählten Kost mit der 100fachen Anzahl von Versuchspersonen gewonnen werden müßten, mittels purinarmer *Standard*-Diät mit dem entsprechenden Bruchteil bei kleiner Standardabweichung erzielt werden. Der Quotient aus Standard-Abweichung und Mittelwert, die sogenannte Varianz (oder die in bezug auf den Mittelwert korrigierte Standard-Abweichung) zeigt darüber hinaus, daß bei Verwendung von *purinfreien* flüssigen *Formel*diäten die Ergebnisse noch wesentlich genauer werden (vgl. Tab. 4).

Tabelle 4. Einfluß der Kostform auf die Standardabweichung (s bzw. S.D.) und die Varianz (s/x̄) der Plasmaharnsäure. s ist unter Standard-Diät nur ²/₃ so groß wie unter freigewählter Kost bei einem Hundertstel der Versuchspersonen; unter Formeldiät beträgt s nur noch ein Viertel des Werts unter freier Kost

Diät	Anzahl der Versuchspers.	Dauer (Tage)	Standard-Abweichung	Varianz
Freigewählte Kost	662	—	± 1,22	± 0,50
Purinarme Standard-Diät	6	7	± 0,81	± 0,35
Purinfreie Formeldiät	5	6	± 0,30	± 0,09

Auswirkungen der Purinrestriktion

Wirkung bei Normalpersonen

Die Basalwerte von Harnsäureplasmaspiegel und -ausscheidung, die sich durch weitgehende oder völlige Purinrestriktion erzielen lassen, sind bereits im Kapitel über exogene Purine dargestellt worden. Ergänzend sei hier darauf hingewiesen, daß die beobachteten Daten auch von Geschlecht der Versuchspersonen (vgl. Abb. 1 oben) und von der Dauer der Beobachtungszeit (Abb. 1 unten) abhängen. Die Harnsäureplasmaspiegel liegen für Männer schon unter freigewählter Kost höher als für Frauen, jedenfalls im geschlechtsreifen Alter der Frau (vgl. GRIEBSCH u. ZÖLLNER, 1973). Auch nach zehntägiger Purinrestriktion bleibt dieser Unterschied erhalten, wenngleich in geringerem Ausmaß. Er findet seine Erklärung nicht nur in durchschnittlich etwas höherem Körpergewicht (und damit Zellumsatz) des Mannes, sondern beruht auch auf der harnsäurespiegelsenkenden Wirkung der weiblichen Geschlechtshormone vor Eintritt der Menopause (vgl. MIKKELSEN et al., 1965; WOLFSON et al., 1949; GRIEBSCH u. ZÖLLNER, 1973). Ein neues Gleichgewicht der Harnsäurespiegel spielt sich erst nach acht bis zehn Tagen eines purinfreien Diätregimes ein, während bis zum sechsten Tag noch eine fallende Tendenz anhält; dieser Umstand erklärt divergierende Daten mancher Arbeitsgruppen.

Bei der Messung der Harnsäureausscheidung ist es wichtig, etwaige Sammelfehler bei der Sammlung des 24 Std-Urins zu erfassen. Dazu eignet sich die gleichzeitige Bestimmung der Kreatininausscheidung, die für jede Versuchsperson innerhalb eines 24 Std-Zeitraums bei gleichbleibender körperlicher Betätigung annähernd konstant ist. Zusammenfassend kann gesagt werden, daß sich der Harnsäureplasmaspiegel bei Gesunden durch völlige Purinrestriktion um 2 mg-% oder mehr als $1/3$ des Ausgangswertes unter freigewählter Kost senken läßt.

Wirkung der Purinrestriktion bei familiärer Hyperuricämie und bei Gicht (Normo- und Überproduktoren)

Die Auswirkung der Purinrestriktion hat bei *Normalpersonen* einen Abfall der Harnsäureplasmaspiegel von $4{,}97 \pm 0{,}97$ ($\bar{X} \pm s$) mg/100 ml nach elf Tagen auf $3{,}09 \pm 0{,}39$ mg/100 ml zur Folge, was einem Rückgang um 37,8% oder auf 62,2% des Ausgangswertes entspricht. *Familiäre Hyperuricämiker* zeigten in unseren Versuchen in neun Tagen einen Abfall von 6,70 auf 3,87 mg/100 ml, was prozentual eine vergleichbare große Reduktion um 42,2% oder auf 57,8% des Ausgangswertes bedeutet, doch findet unter sonst gleichen Bedingungen der Rückgang der Spiegel auf einem höheren Niveau statt. Daten von RIESELBACH et al. (1970) für

Gichtkranke, bei denen in Normo- und Überproduktoren[1] unterschieden worden war, lassen erkennen, daß eine fünftägige Purinrestriktion bei *Normoproduktoren* einen Rückgang von $9,65 \pm 1,79$ ($\bar{X} \pm s$) mg/100 ml auf $6,95 \pm 1,85$ mg/100 ml bewirken, was einen Rückgang um rund 18% oder auf 72% des Ausgangswertes bedeutet; der Effekt ist also geringer als bei Gesunden. *Hyperproduktoren* fallen dagegen unter derselben fünftägigen Purinrestriktion nur von $9,51 \pm 0,84$ mg/ 100 ml auf $9,10 \pm 1,99$ mg/100 ml ab, was nur noch eine Verringerung um 4% oder auf 96% des Ausgangswertes bedeutet. Obwohl diese Daten wegen der kürzeren Dauer der Purinrestriktion nicht direkt mit denen unserer Gesunden vergleichbar sind, so darf mit aller Vorsicht doch gefolgert werden, daß eine diätetische Purinbeschränkung zumindest bei den (seltenen) Hyperproduktoren nur von untergeordneter Bedeutung ist.

Auswirkungen einzelner Harnsäurepräkursoren

Einige wichtige Daten der Literatur einschließlich unserer eigenen Ergebnisse sind bereits im Kapitel über exogene Purine beschrieben worden. Dort sind auch die Unterschiede der Auswirkung einzelner Purinvorläufer anhand der verschiedenen Regressionen zwischen Zufuhr und Anstieg der Harnsäureplasmaspiegel graphisch dargestellt (vgl. Abb. 2). Im einzelnen ist die Auswirkung von RNS bisher am besten untersucht, so in den Arbeitsgruppen von NUGENT et al. (1959) und NUGENT (1965), von GUTMAN (YÜ et al., 1962), von SEEGMILLER et al. (1962) sowie von WASLIEN und ihrem Arbeitskreis (1968, 1970).

1970 konnten wir (GRIEBSCH u. ZÖLLNER, 1970b) erstmals über die unterschiedliche Auswirkung von DNS und RNS berichten, die für die Erstellung neuer Lebensmitteltabellen berücksichtigt werden sollte.

Auch Einzellerproteine, wie die der purinreichen Algen, wurden in ihren Effekten auf den Harnsäurestoffwechsel überprüft (WASLIEN et al., 1968, 1970; GRIEBSCH u. ZÖLLNER, 1971; ZÖLLNER et al., 1972).

Schließlich haben wir auch Ribonucleotide wie 5'-AMP und 5'-GMP daraufhin untersucht, wie sehr unter ihrer Zufuhr Harnsäurespiegel und -ausscheidung ansteigen (GRIEBSCH u. ZÖLLNER, 1974). Die wichtigsten Daten aller genannten Versuche unserer Arbeitsgruppe gehen aus Abb. 2 hervor. Zusammenfassend ergibt sich aus diesen Experimenten, daß RNS in einem weit höheren Maße als auf Grund der älteren Literatur vermutet, nämlich zu rund 50% in den Harnsäurestoffwechsel eingeht, während DNS sich nur halb so stark auswirkt.

Demgegenüber werden Ribonucleotide weit stärker, nämlich im Falle von 5'-AMP fast vollständig renal wieder eliminiert. Als Erklärung für die Beobachtung wird man die schwerere Hydrolysierbarkeit von DNS gegenüber RNS unter der Wirkung von nucleinsäurespaltenden Enzymen im Darm sowie die raschere Resorption der Mononucleotide, die nicht mehr hydrolysiert werden müssen, aus dem Darmlumen diskutieren müssen, die damit möglicherweise zum Teil der in den unteren Darmabschnitten in den Vordergrund tretenden bakteriellen Uricolyse entgehen.

Auswirkungen von Alkohol, Fasten, Fett, Eiweiß und Kohlenhydraten auf den Harnsäurestoffwechsel

Wirkung des Alkohols

Bereits 1863 sprach GARROD in seiner klassischen Publikation über die Gicht den Alkohol als die am stärksten wirksame unter den prädisponierenden Ursa-

---
[1] Dieses Synonym wird hier auch anstelle des Begriffes Hypersekretoren angewendet, obwohl in der Klinik meist nur die vermehrte Harnsäureausscheidung gemessen werden kann.

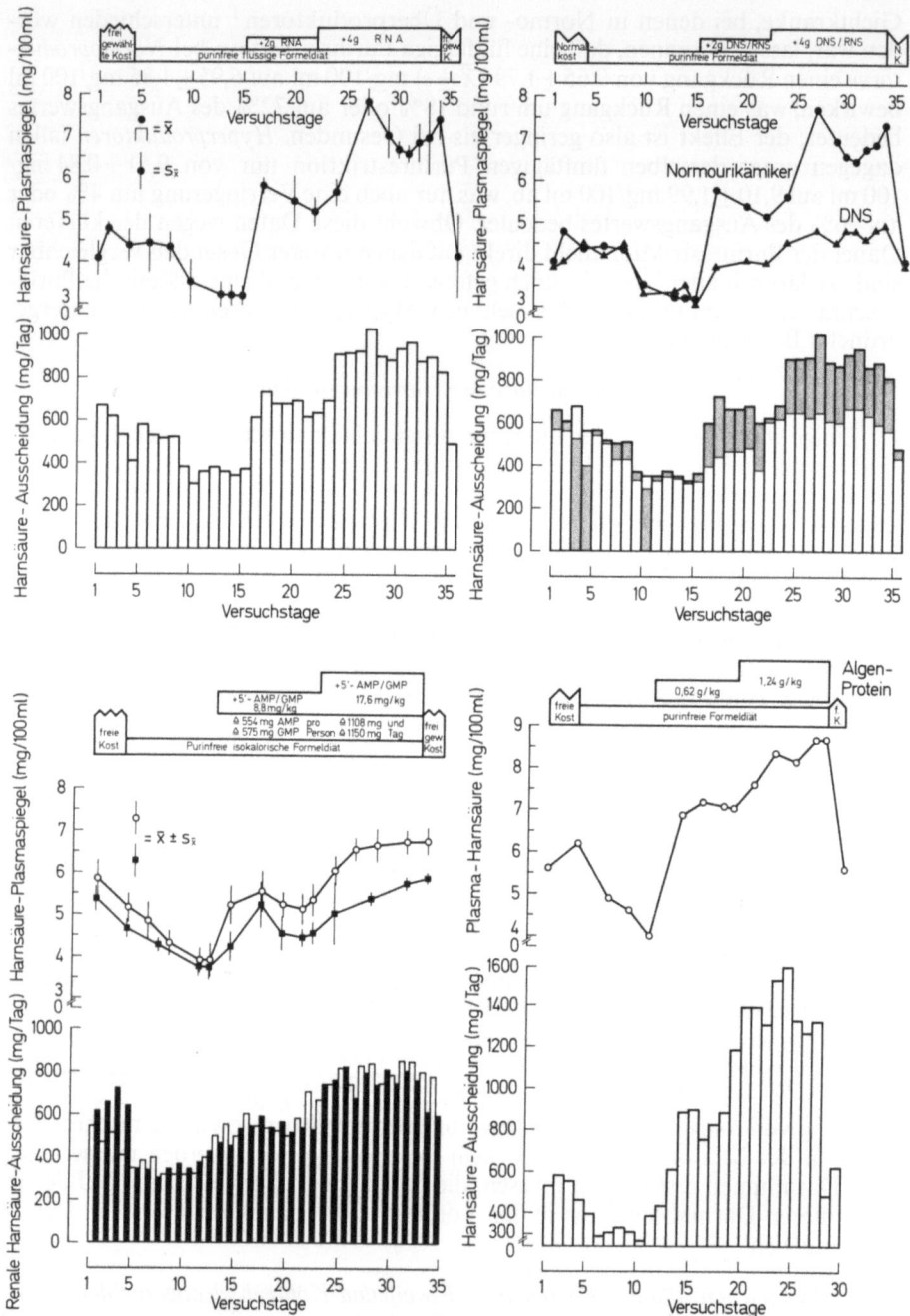

Abb. 2. Verhalten von Harnsäureplasmaspiegel und -ausscheidung unter RNS (links oben), RNS-DNS im Vergleich (rechts oben), 5'AMP u. 5'GMP (links unten) und bei Belastung mit Algen (rechts unten). Ordinate: Harnsäureplasmaspiegel (mg/100 ml) bzw. renale Harnsäureausscheidung (mg/24 h). Abszisse: Versuchstage. (Nach ZÖLLNER et al., 1972; sowie GRIEBSCH u. ZÖLLNER, 1974)

chen der Gicht an. LIEBER u. DAVIDSON (1962) begannen dann — unter dem Eindruck eines Patienten, der bei seinen Trinkexcessen lernte, prophylaktisch mit Colchicin den Gichtanfällen vorzubeugen — die Hyperuricämie von alkoholisierten Patienten zu messen und fanden bei diesen auch erhöhte Blutlactatspiegel; ebenso führten Infusionen von Äthanol zu Hyperuricämie und erhöhten Blutlactatspiegeln. Zur Erklärung wurde angenommen, daß bei der Reduktion von Äthanol zu Acetaldehyd NAD (früher DPN) zu $NADH_2$ reduziert wird, das seinerseits das Gleichgewicht zwischen Brenztraubensäure und Milchsäure auf die Seite der letzteren verschiebt.

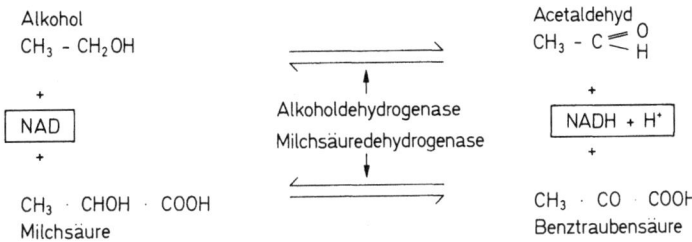

Die dabei beobachteten Blutlactatspiegel (LIEBER, 1965) sind ab Konzentrationen von 15—20 mg-% in der Lage, die renale Harnsäureausscheidung zu hemmen und bei 30 mg-% fast vollständig zu unterdrücken. Daraus resultiert der Begriff der „äthanolinduzierten Hyperuricämie". 1967 stellten dann MACLACHLAN und RODNAN fest, daß diese von der Höhe der Alkoholzufuhr abhängt und daß Zufuhrraten von 68—100 g Äthanol in zwei bis vier Stunden bei purinarmer Kost Spiegel und Ausscheidung der Harnsäure nur gering hemmen, die Zufuhr von 112—135 g dagegen signifikant Hyperlactatämie, Verringerung der Harnsäureausscheidung und Hyperuricämie bewirkt.

Die äthanolinduzierte Hyperuricämie wurde schließlich auch durch epidemiologische Studien von STAKER et al. (1967) an 157 Freiwilligen in Australien und von EVANS et al. (1968) an einer Population der Cook's-Inseln im Südpazifik bestätigt.

Rolle des Fastens und der Ketoacidose

Obwohl lange bekannt war, daß Fasten die Harnsäureausscheidung verringert und zur Hyperuricämie führt, konnten erst 1960 MCCARTHY und OGRYZLO zeigen, daß neuntägiges Fasten die Harnsäurespiegel auf Werte erhöht, die zwischen 53% und 171% über den Ausgangswerten lagen. Gleichzeitig ging die Harnsäureausscheidung (mg/Tag) auf 23—32% der Ausgangswerte zurück.

MACLACHLAN u. RODNAN (1967) stellten bei zweitägigem Fasten Anstiege der Serumharnsäurespiegel um 1,0—2,5 mg/100 ml bei Gichtpatienten und um 1,9—3,5 mg/100 ml bei nicht Gichtkranken fest, bei denen gleichzeitig Erhöhungen der Ketonkörper β-Hydroxybutyrat und der Acetessigsäure festgestellt wurden, die z.B. in einem Fall von 0,4 auf 5,5 bzw. von 0,0 auf 3,1 mg/100 ml anstiegen. Die Beobachtung wurde dahingehend erklärt, daß die erhöhten Spiegel der Ketonkörper eine Hemmung der renalen Harnsäuresekretion bewirken, was durch eine Verringerung der Harnsäureausscheidung zur Hyperuricämie führt.

Die Kombination von Alkoholzufuhr und Fasten zeigte einen additiven oder synergistischen Effekt, wobei sowohl die Blutlactatspiegel höher waren als bei

Alkohol mit normaler Ernährung als auch die β-Hydroxybutyratspiegel höher als unter Fasten allein. Schon 1923 hatten GIBSON und DOISY beobachtet, daß die orale Zufuhr von Natriumlactat die Harnsäureausscheidung hemmt. YÜ et al. aus dem GUTMANSCHEN Arbeitskreis berichteten 1957 über Clearancestudien, bei denen Na-D-Lactat-Infusionen zu ausgeprägter Verringerung der Harnsäureausscheidung bei Gichtkranken führte, wobei die Harnsäureclearance von 10,4 ml/min auf 1,4 ml/min zurückging.

GOLDFINGER et al. (1965) infundierten β-Hydroxybutyrat und Natrium-Acetoacetat und fanden die dabei beobachtete Harnsäureretention am besten mit den β-Hydroxybutyratspiegeln korreliert.

Die Befunde dienten ihnen auch als Erklärung für die harnsäureerhöhende Wirkung der diabetischen Ketoacidose und der Hyperuricämie bei den Personen, die unter fettreicher Diät stehen.

Einfluß einer fettreichen Kost

Über die Auswirkungen des Fastens auf die Harnsäureausscheidung lagen bereits um die Jahrhundertwende Beobachtungen vor (SCHREIBER u. WALDVOGEL, 1899; CATHCART, 1907; HIRSCHSTEIN, 1907). Ab 1924 wurde dann unter diesen Bedingungen auch ein entsprechender Anstieg der Serumharnsäurespiegel gezeigt (LENNOX, 1924). Vergleichbare Wirkungen unter Kostformen mit hohen Dosen von Fett wurden ebenfalls beschrieben (CATHCART, 1909; GRAHAM u. POULTON, 1913/14; HARDING et al., 1925 u. 1927 bei Schwangeren). Diese Ernährungsversuche — zunächst an nichtgichtkranken Personen — später durch LOKKIE u. HUBBARD (1925) auch an Gichtpatienten — zeigten, daß Fasten und jede Kostform, die hohe Fettutilisation mit dem Auftreten von „Acetonkörpern" im Urin hervorruft, zu einer gleichzeitigen Verminderung der renalen Harnsäureelimination führten. Wenn das Auftreten der Ketonkörper durch gleichzeitige Zufuhr adäquater Mengen von Kohlenhydraten oder Eiweiß verhindert wurde (vgl. LENNOX, 1924), blieb auch eine Verminderung der Harnsäureausscheidung aus. Damit waren Hinweise darauf gegeben, daß die Veränderungen der Harnsäureausscheidung parallel zur Ketose auftreten, gleichgültig, ob diese im Rahmen einer gesteigerten Fettutilisation von Nahrungsfett (fettreiche Kost) oder körpereigenem Fett (Fasten) auftrat. Allerdings war damals noch nicht klar, ob das Auftreten der Ketonkörper die einzige Erklärung für die Verminderung der Harnsäureausscheidung darstellte. Dazu haben allerdings neuere Untersuchungen über das Fasten und verschiedene Nahrungsfaktoren ausnahmslos gezeigt, daß die renale Harnsäureelimination während einer induzierten Ketose vermindert wurde (McCARTHY u. OGRYZLO, 1960; SCOTT et al., 1964). Dies wurde zusätzlich erhärtet durch die Hyperuricämie bei diabetischer Ketoacidose (PADOVA u. BENDERSKY, 1962) und die bereits erwähnten Versuche mit Infusionen von Na-Hydroxybutyrat (SCOTT et al., 1964; GOLDFINGER et al., 1965).

Genauere Daten legten erstmals ADLERSBERG u. ELLENBERG (1939) vor, aus denen hervorgeht, daß bei einer Versuchsperson die Erhöhung des Fettanteils einer Kost von 49% auf 70% — allerdings bei gleichzeitigem Anstieg der Gesamtcalorienzufuhr von 1845 auf 3195 kcal — zu einem Rückgang der Harnsäureausscheidung von (im Mittel) 532 mg/tgl. auf 408 mg/tgl. oder um 23% führte. Der durchschnittliche Abfall bei fünf Versuchspersonen betrug 21%. Gleichzeitig stieg der Harnsäurespiegel um 11,6% an. Als Erklärung für diesen Mechanismus zogen LECOCQ u. MCPHAUL JR. (1965) — basierend auf Beobachtungen von BONSNES u. DANA (1946) und von FRIEDMAN (1947) über die Konkurrenz von Glucose und Aminosäuren mit der Harnsäure um einen gemeinsamen renalen Transportmechanismus entlang der Tubulusepithel — das Postulat heran, daß Ketonkörper und Harnsäure ebenfalls um einen gemeinsamen tubulären Sekretionsmechanismus konkurrieren.

Die neuesten Beobachtungen von LECOCQ u. MCPHAUL, JR. (1965) und von OGRYZLO (1965) (von denen einige wichtige Daten über Kost und Veränderungen der Harnsäureparameter in unserer Tab. 5 umgerechnet wurden) zeigten, daß unter fettreicher Kost (90% bzw. 73% der Calorien) die Harnsäurespiegel um 43% bzw. 36% steigen, wobei die Ausscheidung, gemessen (OGRYZLO) um −46% bzw. die Harnsäureclearance um −33% bzw. −46% (LECOCQ) zurückgeht. Gleichzeitig stiegen die Ketonkörper im Serum von unter 2 mg-% auf etwa 8 mg-% an. Zusammenfassend beschreibt OGRYZLO die Auswirkung fettreicher Kost als „jener des Fastens vergleichbar, jedoch weniger dramatisch". In beiden Fällen kommt es zu einer excessiven Fettutilisation. Der Effekt läßt sich auch noch nachweisen, wenn die fettreiche Kost einer Periode des Fastens folgt. Er wird durch anschließende isocalorische Protein- und Zuckerzufuhr im Plasma und Urin, durch Purinzufuhr nur im Plasma (bei überschießender Urinausscheidung) normalisiert. Gleichzeitig reduzieren Kohlenhydrat- und Proteinzulagen in ausreichender Menge die Rate der produzierten und ausgeschiedenen Ketonkörper unter Fasten wieder auf normale Werte. Daraus wird geschlossen, daß es wichtiger sei, die Fettzufuhr des Gichtkranken zu kontrollieren als die Purinzufuhr, obwohl beiden eine wichtige Rolle eingeräumt wird.

Wirkung der Proteinzufuhr

Diese wurde aus didaktischen Gründen bereits im Kapitel über exogene Purine aufgeführt.

Einfluß der Kohlenhydrate auf den Harnsäurestoffwechsel

1939 zeigten ADLERSBERG u. ELLENBURG, daß eine kohlenhydratreiche Kost (500 g KH, 80 g Protein, 100 g Fett) über vier bis sechs Tage verabfolgt keine nennenswerte Erhöhung der Harnsäureausscheidung bewirkt. Die Ausscheidungsmengen stiegen von durchschnittlich 559 mg/tgl. auf 584 mg/tgl. oder um 25 mg bzw. um 4,5% an. PADOVA et al. fanden 1964, daß nach oraler Gabe von 100 g Glucose die Plasmaharnsäurespiegel bei vier von fünf Diabetikern um 9% abfielen, während die Harnsäureclearance um 56% anstieg; quantitativ vergleichbare Daten erhielten sie bei zehn nichtdiabetischen Vergleichspersonen. Als Ursache wird eine gesteigerte Insulinsekretion durch die Glucosebelastung diskutiert, da in früheren Beobachtungen von PADOVA et al. (1962) sich Hinweise auf uricosurische Effekte des Insulins ergeben hatten. Ausgehend von diesen Beobachtungen bestimmten 1967 SKEITH et al. die Harnsäureclearance unter Infusionen mit Glucose bzw. Mannit und fanden nur bei ersterem Anstiege der Harnsäureclearance in nennenswertem Ausmaß. So stieg unter Glucose (10%) (i.v.) die Clearance der Harnsäure von $9,7 \pm 1,1$ auf $19,3 \pm 2,0$ ml/min ($n = 7$) oder auf 199% bzw. fast das Doppelte an; unter Mannit zeigten dieselben Versuchspersonen mit Ausgangswerten von $10,4 \pm 0,9$ ml/min dagegen nicht signifikant veränderte Harnsäureclearancewerte ($9,2 \pm 1,0$ ml/min). Der Anstieg der Harnsäureclearance unter Glucose geht auf eine vermehrte Harnsäureausscheidung zurück, die unter Glucoseinfusion von 525 ± 62 g/min auf 962 g/min anstieg, während die Plasmaspiegel mit $5,4 \pm 0,3$ bzw. $5,0 \pm 0,3$ mg/100 ml nach Infusion praktisch gleichblieben. Gleichzeitige Messungen der osmolaren Clearance (C_{osm}) zeigten unter Mannit dreifach höhere Werte als unter Glucose, so daß die Autoren vermuten,

Tabelle 5. Auswirkungen einer fettreichen Kost (73 bzw. 90% Fett) gegenüber einer Kontroll-Diät (15,5% Fett) auf den Harnsäurespiegel (Steigerung um +36% bzw. +43%) und die Harnsäureausscheidung (Abfall um −46%) bzw. die Harnsäure-Clearance (Verringerung um −36% bzw. −46%) in den Versuchen von Ogryzlo (oben) und Lecocq u. Mc Phaul (unten)

Autor	Kostform	Anteil				Ges. Cal. (kcal)	Harnsäure-Plasmaspiegel (mg/100 ml)	Änderung	Harnsäure-Ausscheidung (mg/tgl.) bzw. Clearance (ml/min)	Änderung
			Kohlenhydrate	Eiweiß	Fett					
Ogryzlo (1965)	Kontroll-Diät	g kcal %	400 1604 57	190 779 27,5	50 450 15,5	2833	7,0	—	860 bzw. 7,5	—
	Fettreiche Kost	g kcal %	100 410 14,4	90 369 13	230 2070 73	2849	9,5	+36%	460 bzw. 5,0	−46% bzw. −33%
Lecocq u. Mc Phaul (1965)	Kontroll-Diät	g kcal %	? ? ?	? ? ?	? ? ?	3000	4,9	—	? bzw. 13	—
	Fettreiche Kost	g kcal %	? ? ?	? ? ?	300 2700 90	3000	7,0	+43%	? bzw. 7	−46%

daß die Wirkung der Glucose auf die Harnsäureausscheidung auf anderen als Faktoren der osmotischen Diurese beruht.

Neuerdings haben NARINS et al. die Einflüsse von Kohlenhydraten oral und parenteral, und zwar einerseits die der Glucosezufuhr (parenteral) sowie von Galaktose- und Fructoseinfusionen mit der Wirkung der oralen Fructosezufuhr in Ernährungsexperimenten (von 5 bzw. 8 Tagen Dauer) verglichen. Die Ergebnisse wurden dahingehend zusammengefaßt, daß eine *rasche* Fructoseinfusion im Gegensatz zu der von Glucose und Galaktose bei gesunden Freiwilligen einen etwa 30%igen Anstieg der Serumharnsäure bewirkt. In *Langzeitinfusionen* (4—6 Std) haben auch HEUCKENKAMP et al. (1971) einen Anstieg der Plasmaharnsäurespiegel unter Fructose um 26% nachweisen können, der allerdings erst bei Zufuhrraten von 1,5 g/kg *KG*/Std und mehr signifikant ist. NARINS et al. zeigten auch, daß die Anstiege mit einer gesteigerten renalen Harnsäureausscheidung (sowie der von PO_4^{---}, HCO_3^- und Glucose) einhergehen. Jedoch führt *nur* Fructose zu einer Steigerung der Harnsäureproduktion, während alle drei Hexosen die proximale Tubulusfunktion hemmen. Die Daten dieser Autoren sprechen dafür, daß Fructose-Infusionen die Umwandlung von präformierten Adenin-Nucleotiden in Harnsäure stimulieren, während sie die Neusynthese von Harnsäure hemmen. Auch FOX u. KELLEY (1972) nehmen einen gesteigerten Abbau von Purin-Nucleotiden für diese Erscheinung an.

Im Vergleich dazu wurde die Wirkung einer langdauernden *oralen Zufuhr* von Fructose an 8 Freiwilligen mittels 5- bzw. 8tägiger Zulage von 100 g Fructose zu einer freigewählten Kost (NARINS et al.) studiert; im Gegensatz zur parenteralen Zufuhr zeigte sich weder eine Veränderung der Plasmaspiegel noch der Ausscheidung der Harnsäure, im Gegensatz zu *rascher* oraler Zufuhr (vgl. RAIVIO et al., 1969; STIRPE et al., 1970). Daraus ergibt sich die Schlußfolgerung, daß fructosereiche Kost, zumindest beim Gesunden, *keine* Auswirkung auf den Harnsäurestoffwechsel hat. Die Empfehlung einer fructosearmen Kost aufgrund von Beobachtungen über Hyperuricämie unter Fructoseinfusionen zur Therapie der Gicht (SCHÖNTHAL et al., 1972) scheint somit noch nicht ausreichend begründet.

Auf Grund dieser Daten ergibt sich zusammenfassend, daß Alkohol, extremes Fasten, fettreiche Kost und die Zulage von Eiweiß (vgl. Kapitel exogene Purine) zur Erhöhung der Harnsäureplasmaspiegel führt.

Kohlenhydrate, speziell Fructose, haben dagegen bei oraler Zufuhr keine nennenswerte Wirkung.

Die Wirkung des Alkohols beruht auf der verminderten Harnsäureausscheidung bei erhöhten Lactatspiegeln, die des Fastens auf der verringerten Harnsäureelimination durch Ketonkörper; der Wirkung einer fettreichen Kost liegt dasselbe Prinzip zugrunde.

Für die Diätetik der Gicht ist somit insgesamt eine kohlenhydratreiche Kost mit mäßigem Anteil von Fett (bis höchstens ca. 30% der Calorien) und des Eiweißes (bis ca. 20% der Calorien) anzustreben; ferner die Vermeidung von Alkoholexzessen und von extremem Fasten.

Praktische Diätetik

Einfache Diätempfehlung bei Gicht

Die bisher beschriebenen Einflüsse verschiedener Nahrungsmittel, speziell von Kohlenhydraten, Fett und Eiweiß sowie der exogenen Purine (vgl. Kapitel III.2.b) sind zwar für das Verständnis der Stoffwechselvorgänge bei Hyperuricämie und Gicht von grundsätzlicher Bedeutung, haben aber für die praktische Durchführung der Diät bei diesen Krankheiten untergeordnete Bedeutung.

Tabelle 6. Praktische Anweisungen für Diät bei Gicht und Hyperuricämie

1. Kontrollieren Sie Ihr Gewicht und streben Sie das Normalgewicht an. Als grobe Faustregel kann dienen, daß Sie soviel kg wiegen sollen, wie Sie cm über 100 cm groß sind.
2. Beschränken Sie die Zufuhr von Purinen in der Nahrung. Das sind Stoffe aus Zellkernen, die vom Körper zu Harnsäure abgebaut werden.
 a) Vermeiden Sie Innereien, wie Leber, Niere, Milz, Bries, Herz usw., sowie bestimmte Fischsorten und -gerichte wie Sardellen, Kaviar, Ölsardinen sowie Fleischextrakt.
 b) Beschränken Sie die Zufuhr von purinhaltigem tierischem Eiweiß, indem Sie nicht mehr als eine Fleischmahlzeit pro Tag zu sich nehmen.
3. Decken Sie Ihren Eiweißbedarf vorwiegend aus Milch und Milchprodukten und Eiern.
4. Weitgehend arm an Purinen sind außerdem die meisten Gemüse und Salate, das Brot sowie alle Teigwaren, Kartoffeln, Mehl und Zucker sowie alle Fette und Öle.
5. Vermeiden Sie aber eine übermäßige Fettzufuhr; auch Alkohol in größeren Mengen kann die Harnsäureausscheidung hemmen. Kaffee und Tee können Sie dagegen unbedenklich trinken.

Die Wirksamkeit der für die Dauerbehandlung der Gicht heute verfügbaren Medikamente erlaubt es, die Diätvorschriften auf ein Minimum zu reduzieren. Außerdem sind Gichtkranke nicht selten lebensfrohe, gutem Essen und Trinken durchaus zugeneigte Menschen, unter denen man oft ausgesprochene Genießer und Gourmets findet. So werden zu detaillierte und strenge Diätvorschriften nicht oder nur von neurotisch strukturierten Patienten über längere Zeit exakt eingehalten. In der Praxis zeigt sich, daß einige wenige Faustregeln verläßlicher befolgt werden, als ausführliche Diätanweisungen. Die in Tab. 6 aufgeführten Regeln haben sich in der täglichen „Gicht-Sprechstunde" bewährt und reichen in den unkomplizierten Fällen, wenn der Patient gut auf Uricosurica oder Synthesehemmer anspricht, auch völlig aus. Die konsequente Einhaltung dieser einfachen Regeln hat hier — analog wie in der Therapie von Störungen des Kohlenhydrat- und Fettstoffwechsels — den Zweck, daß eine Basisbehandlung erfolgt, die es erlaubt, die Effekte der Arzneimittel besser, d.h. ohne grobe exogene Schwankungen, beobachten und diese dadurch besser dosieren zu können. Darüber hinaus kann dadurch unter Umständen die Dauertherapie mit etwas niedrigeren Dosen durchgeführt, d.h. es können Medikamente eingespart werden.

Neben diesen einfachen Regeln empfiehlt es sich, die Patienten von unnötigen Beschränkungen zu befreien und tiefverwurzelte Vorurteile in der Gichtdiätetik abzuschaffen. Dazu gehört das Verbot von „rotem Fleisch" gegenüber „weißem", von Tomaten, Rhabarber sowie von Methylpurinen in Form von Kaffee und Tee, die nicht in den Harnsäurestoffwechsel eingehen (THANNHAUSER-ZÖLLNER, 1957).

Diät bei asymptomatischer Hyperuricämie

Eine besondere Bedeutung hat die Diät für jene Gruppe von Hyperuricämikern, die wiederholt Harnsäurespiegel oberhalb der (statistischen) Normgrenze ($\bar{X} + s$) von z.Z. 7,2 mg/100 ml aufweisen. Gichtanfälle können einerseits schon bei Harnsäurespiegeln über 6,5 mg/100 ml auftreten, andererseits liegt in der deutschen Durchschnittsbevölkerung der durchschnittliche Harnsäurespiegel der Männer bei den heutigen Ernährungsgewohnheiten bei 6,0 mg/100 ml (vgl. GRIEBSCH u. ZÖLLNER, 1973). Die Häufigkeit von Gichtanfällen steigt mit der Höhe der Harnsäurespiegel, wie aus den Zahlen von FRAMINGHAM hervorgeht (HALL, 1967). Bei Spiegeln bei 6—6,9 mg/100 ml ($n = 790$) tritt die Gicht mit einer Häufigkeit von 1,9%, bei 7,0—7,9 mg/100 ml ($n = 162$) von 16,7%, bei solchen von 8,0—8,9 mg/100 ml ($n = 40$) sogar von 25% auf. Wegen dieses erhöhten

Risikos für Gichtanfälle werden Personen mit Harnsäurespiegeln über 8 mg/100 ml meist schon prophylaktisch medikamentös behandelt. Auf Grund dieser Überlegungen läßt sich eine Gruppe von „Hyperuricämikern" abtrennen. Es handelt sich dabei um Personen, die Harnsäurespiegel zwischen 6,5 bzw. 7,2 mg/100 ml und 8,0 mg/100 ml aufweisen. Von ihnen wird nach obigen epidemiologischen Beobachtungen etwa jeder Vierte bis Sechste innerhalb von zehn Jahren einen Gichtanfall erleiden; um diesem Risiko vorzubeugen, will man aber andererseits auch nicht ein neues Risiko eingehen, wie es die medikamentöse Therapie darstellen kann.

Für diesen Patientenkreis stellt eine purinarme Gicht- bzw. Hyperuricämiediät das Mittel der Wahl zur Behandlung dar. Je nach Dauer, seit der die Hyperuricämie besteht (und damit der Größe der Harnsäuremenge im Harnsäureraum des Körpers) wird man entweder eine *purinarme* Diät mit Mengen bis zu 300 mg Harnsäure ($\hat{=}$ 125 mg Purin-N) pro Tag oder 2000 mg Harnsäure ($\hat{=}$ 833 mg Purin-N) pro Woche einsetzen oder sogar eine *streng purinarme* Diät ($\hat{=}$ 120 mg Harnsäure pro Tag oder $\hat{=}$ 1000 mg Harnsäure pro Woche) anwenden.

Streng purinarme Diät

Eine völlig purinfreie Kostform läßt sich nur mittels der Anwendung flüssiger Formeldiät ermöglichen; diese ist in der praktischen Diätetik nicht verwendbar. Eine Standardkost kann andererseits aus ernährungsphysiologischen Gründen nicht ohne Fleisch und Gemüse längere Zeit aufrechterhalten werden, ist also immer nur purinarm. Bei der *streng* purinarmen Diät sind *bis zu* 120 mg Harnsäure pro Tag (50 mg Purin-N) erlaubt, jedoch soll in der Woche nicht mehr als 1000 mg Harnsäure (417 mg Purin-N) erreicht werden (ZÖLLNER, 1973).

Tabelle 7 zeigt ein Beispiel (Tab. 7a) für eine streng purinarme Kost sowie (Tab. 7b) die Verteilung von Purin, Eiweiß, Fett, Kohlenhydrat und Calorien im Wochenmittel (mit Standard-Abweichung).

Bei dieser Kost schwanken die Einzelwerte der Harnsäure- bzw. Purin-N-Zufuhr um weniger als 50% des Durchschnittswertes. Die Schwankung bzw. Standard-Abweichung im Eiweiß-Anteil und in der Gesamtcalorienzufuhr liegt sogar unter 10% des Mittelwertes.

Das Eiweiß wird bei dieser Kost überwiegend in Form von Pflanzeneiweiß zugeführt, wobei aber die purinreicheren Sorten, wie grüne und gelbe Erbsen, Linsen und weiße Bohnen in Wegfall kommen. Fleisch wird auf Portionen von maximal 100 g beschränkt und ist nur zwei- bis dreimal wöchentlich erlaubt. Dabei ist das Eiweißminimum von 1 g/kg KG oder rund 70 g/Tag im Wochenmittel fast eingehalten.

Diese Kostform wird nur in jenen seltenen Fällen anzuwenden sein, wo Allopurinol nicht wirksam ist und die Anwendung von Uricosurica durch renale Komplikationen sich verbietet (z. B. Nephrolithiasis, Zustand nach einseitiger Nephrektomie usw.), oder wo die Wirkung dieser Substanzen bei einer seit vielen Jahren oder Jahrzehnten unbehandelten Gicht durch die Größe der im Organismus angehäuften Harnsäurepools nicht ausreicht.

Purinarme Kost

Für die letztgenannten Fälle und für alle übrigen, speziell wenn man wegen der Seiteneffekte Medikamente einsparen möchte, reicht die *purinarme* Kost aus.

Diese ist definiert durch einen Anteil von bis zu 300 mg Harnsäure (125 mg Purin-N) pro Tag oder 2000 mg Harnsäure (833 mg Purin-N) pro Woche (vgl.

Tab. 8). Hierbei werden auch größere Zugeständnisse an die Schwankungen des Harnsäuregehalts von Tag zu Tag gemacht. Dabei ist im Mittel *eine* mittelgroße (120—140 g) *Fleischportion* pro Tag erlaubt, welches *gekocht* weniger Purine enthält, da diese teilweise ins Kochwasser übertreten. Für die praktische Durchführung kann man die Patienten auf die seriösen Diätbroschüren des Buchhandels verweisen, speziell wenn diese auf den Puringehalt bezogen auf die Calorienzufuhr und auf die üblichen Portionsgrößen eingehen (vgl. KORFMACHER u. ZÖLLNER, 1974; ZÖLLNER, 1974).

Wie sehr sich nämlich der Anteil an Purinen bzw. Harnsäure verschiebt, wenn man ihn statt auf 100 g des Nahrungsmittels auf 100 kcal berechnet, zeigt Abb. 3, wo nach dieser Umrechnung vor allem die Gemüse stärker ins Gewicht fallen.

Tabelle 7a. Beispiel für einen Tagesdiätplan für eine *streng* purinarme Kost (bis 1000 mg Harnsäure pro Woche) mit Angaben über die Verteilung von Eiweiß, Fett und Kohlenhydraten und Caloriengehalt (modifiziert nach ZÖLLNER, 1974)

	Harn-säure (mg)	Eiweiß (g)	Fett (g)	Kohlen-hydrate (g)	Calorien-gehalt (Kcal)
a) *1. Frühstück*					
Tee, Kaffee	—	—	—	—	—
$^1/_8$ l Milch	—	4,2	3,1	6,0	71
10 g Zucker	—	—	—	10,0	41
100 g Roggenbrot	40,0	6,0	—	41,0	250
10 g Butter	—	—	8,0	0,1	75
15 g Marmelade	—	0,1	—	9,7	41
Zwischensumme	40,0	10,3	11,1	66,8	478
b) *2. Frühstück*					
Buttermilchkaltschale	—	9,4	11,1	68,8	298
c) *Mittagessen*					
Ungar. Suppe	6,5	1,4	10,0	9,0	137
100 g Ochsenfleisch	120,0	20,6	3,5	0,6	123
Bechamelkartoffel	3,7	6,8	12,2	35,2	286
Gurkensalat (50 g) mit Rahm (20 g), Zitronensaft und Kräutern	10,0	1,7	2,0	0,8	34
Zwischensumme	140,2	30,5	27,7	75,6	580
d) *Nachmittags*					
100 g Blaubeeren	—	1,0	—	12,0	60
e) *Abendessen*					
Römischer Gries	—	16,1	21,2	38,5	424
Tomatensoße	12,5	2,5	8,7	12,6	147
	192,7	69,8	74,7	244,3	1987
Harnsäure (mg)	192,7				
Purin-N (mg)	80,3				
Eiweiß		69,8			
Fett			74,7		
Kohlenhydrate				244,3	
Calorien (kcal)					1987

Tabelle 7b. Der zweite Teil der Tabelle zeigt, wie diese Größen sich über eine Woche hin verteilen und enthält das Wochenmittel sowie die Standardabweichung desselben (Modifiziert nach Daten von ZÖLLNER, 1974)

Wochentag	Mo	Die	Mi	Do	Fr	Sa	So	Wochenmittel	s
Harnsäure (mg)	192,7	79,5	86,2	95,4	212,0	97,5	84,5	121,11	± 55,26
Purin-N (mg)	80,3	33,12	35,9	39,8	88,3	40,6	35,2	50,46	± 23,38
Eiweiß (g)	69,8	62,8	59,4	66,2	72,3	69,1	65,5	66,45	± 4,27
Fett (g)	74,7	67,5	79,1	75,3	58,7	63,8	65,8	69,27	± 7,31
KH (g)	244,3	241,4	220,9	231,2	240,8	247,8	206,0	233,20	± 15,04
Calorien (Kcal)	1987	1903	2076	1977	2000	1970	1882	1970,7	± 181,26

Tabelle 8. Beispiel für eine Tagesspeisenfolge für purinarme Kost (Aus ZÖLLNER, 1974)

1. Tag	Harnsäure mg	Eiweiß g	Fett g	Kohlenhydrate g	kcal
1. Frühstück					
Tee, Kaffee oder Malzkaffee	—	—	—	—	—
⅛ l Milch	—	4,2	3,1	6,0	71
10 g Zucker	—	—	—	10,0	41
50 g Pumpernickel	2,5	4,0	0,4	25,5	125
50 g Weißbrot	7,5	3,4	0,3	23,9	135
10 g Butter	—	—	8,0	—	75
15 g Marmelade	—	—	—	10,0	41
2. Frühstück					
100 g Joghurt	—	3,3	2,8	3,9	56
1 Knäckebrot (10 g)	1,0	1,0	—	7,0	35
10 g Butter	—	—	8,0	—	75
Mittagessen					
Kartoffelsuppe 5	1,3	2,6	2,2	23,2	126
Kalbskotelette in Aluminiumfolie gebraten 16	125,0	21,5	10,5	—	165
Kartoffelbrei 46	7,5	4,2	2,8	30,3	168
Gurkengemüse 27	20,0	2,9	10,5	6,5	136
Nachmittags					
100 g Pfirsiche	—	1,0	—	12,0	60
Abendessen					
150 g Spargel + 5 g Öl	45,0	3,0	10,0	2,5	114
50 g Schinken, gekocht	35,0	12,5	15,2	—	215
100 g Roggenbrot	40,0	6,0	—	40,0	250
10 g Butter	—	—	8,0	—	75
	284,8	69,6	81,8	200,8	1963

5, 16, 46 und 27 verweisen auf Rezepte im Anhang
5 = 100 g, 16 = 100 g, 46 = 212 g, 27 = 215 g

In Tab. 9 sind die wichtigsten Gruppen von Nahrungsmitteln mit je einigen typischen Vertretern aufgeführt und der Harnsäuregehalt pro 100 g, pro Portionsgröße und pro 100 kcal angegeben. In einer groben Unterteilung läßt sich eine Gruppe von purinreichen Nahrungsmitteln (Purin-N > 50 mg/100 g) (Innereien, Fleischextrakt, Fleisch, Fisch und purinreiche Gemüse) einer Gruppe von purinarmen Nahrungsmitteln (Purin-N < 50 mg/100 g) gegenüberstellen, zu denen die purinarmen Gemüsesorten, Obst, Mehl und Mehlprodukte und Zucker sowie Milch und Milchprodukte, Fette und verschiedene Getränke gehören.

Berücksichtigt man die üblichen Portionsgrößen, so wird der Unterschied zwischen beiden Gruppen eher noch ausgeprägter. Dabei darf aber nicht übersehen werden, daß Speisepläne für eine purinarme Kost *eine Deckung des Eiweißbedarfs* (Eiweißminimum) berücksichtigen müssen. Dies führt wegen des geringeren Gehalts an Eiweiß und der niedrigeren biologischen Wertigkeit von Pflanzeneiweiß dazu, daß pflanzliche Eiweißträger in größeren Mengen verabfolgt werden

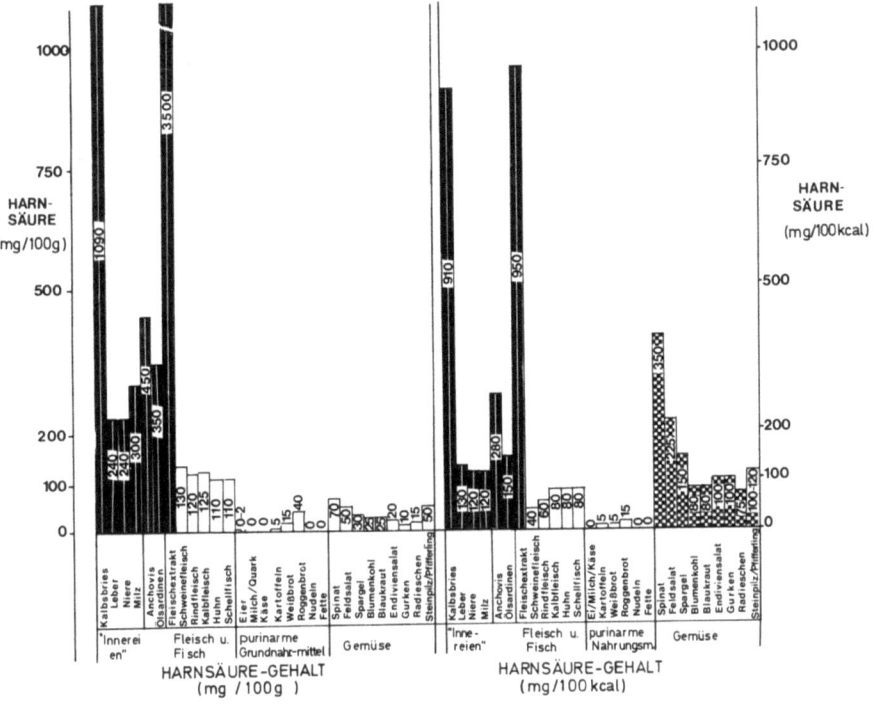

Abb. 3. Graphische Darstellung des Harnsäuregehaltes (nach Umrechnung von Purin-N auf Harnsäure mittels Faktor 2,4) einiger Nahrungsmittelgruppen. Bei Berechnung von mg Harnsäure *pro 100 g* Nahrungsmittel zeigen Fleisch und Fisch höhere, Gemüse niedrigere Werte als bezogen auf *100 kcal*; unter diesem Gesichtspunkt liegen die Werte der hier angeführten Gemüse ebenso hoch oder höher wie die von Fleisch oder Fisch

Tabelle 9. Übersicht über den Gehalt der wichtigsten Nahrungsmittelgruppen (und einzelne Beispiele dazu) an Purin-N und Umrechnung auf Harnsäure pro 100 g (frisch), über den Caloriengehalt, die üblichen Portionsgrößen und den Harnsäuregehalt bezogen auf Portion und auf 100 Calorien des Nahrungsmittels. Als Grenzwert zwischen purinreich (oberer Teil der Tabelle) und purinarm (unten) wurde ein Gehalt von 120 mg Harnsäure (50 mg Purin-N) pro 100 g angenommen, analog dazu einer von 80 mg Purin-N pro 100 kcal (vgl. Text)

	Purin-N-Gehalt (mg/100 g) kursiv: Werte ≥ 50 fett < 50	Harnsäure-Gehalt (mg/100 g) kursiv: Werte ≥ 120 fett < 120	Calorien-Gehalt (kcal/100 g)	Portionsgrößen (g)	Harnsäure-Gehalt pro Portion (mg/Port.)	Harnsäure-Gehalt pro kal. (mg/100 kcal) kursiv: Werte ≥ 80 fett Werte < 80
1) Innereien	*100—454*	*240—1098*	i.M. 125	125	300—1372	*185—915*
Leber	*100*	*240*	130	125	300	*185*
Niere	*100*	*240*	120	125	300	*185*
Bries	*454*	*1098*	120	125	1372	*915*
Herz	—	—	—	—	—	—
2a) Fleischextrakt	*i.M. 1460*	*3500*	370	10	146	*950*

Tabelle 9. (Fortsetzung)

	Purin-N-Gehalt (mg/100 g) *kursiv:* Werte ≥ 50 **fett < 50**	Harnsäure-Gehalt (mg/100 g) *kursiv:* Werte ≥ 120 **fett < 120**	Calorien-Gehalt (kcal/100 g)	Portionsgrößen (g)	Harnsäure-Gehalt pro *Portion* (mg/Port.)	Harnsäure-Gehalt pro kal. (mg/100 kcal) *kursiv:* Werte ≥ 80 **fett** Werte < 80
2b) Fleisch	*46—54*	*110—130*	130—300	i. M. 140	143—195	85—230
Schwein	*54,2*	*130*	300	130—150	170—195	**43**
Rind	*50,0*	*130*	200	130—150	156—180	**60**
Kalb	*52,1*	*125*	160	130—150	163—188	**78**
Huhn	**45,8**	**110**	130	130—150	143—165	*85*
3) Fisch	*50—146*	*120—350*	80—240	—	144—274	88—213
a) purinreiche Sort.	*88—146*	*211—350*	140—240	—	144—274	88—164
Salz- u. Matjesher.	—	—	—			
Sardellen	*95,8*	*230*	140	62,5	143,8	*164*
Ölsardine	*146,0*	*350*	240	125,0	437,5	*146*
Hering	*88*	*211*	240	150,0	274,3	*88*
b) purinarme Sort.	*50—71*	*120—170*	80	—	156—255	150—213
Kabeljau	*50,0*	*120*	80	130—150	156—180	*150*
Forelle	*71,0*	*170*	80	130—150	204—255	*212,5*
4) Gemüse u. Obst	**0,6—56**	*5—290*	—	—	—	—
a) purinreiche Sort.	**6,3—56**	*20—290*	20—340	—	140—580	100—850
Hülsenfr. getr.	*56,3*	*130—210*	320—340	125	162—262	**40—62**
Erbsen grün	*60,4*	*50—290*	80	200	100—580	62,5—362
Spinat	**24,2**	**70**	20	200	140	*350*
b) Steinpilze u. Pfifferlinge	**6,3—21,0**	**20—50**	30—50	200	40—100	**67—100**
c) purinärmere Gemüsesorten	**2,1—10,4**	**5—25**	20—100	200—300	10—75	**5—83**
Blumenkohl	**10,4**	**25**	30	200—300	50—75	*83,3*
Kopfsalat	**4,2**	**10**	20	200—300	20—30	**50**
Kartoffeln	**2,1**	**5**	100	200	10	**5**
d) Früchte u. Obst	**0—6,25**	**0—15**	20—80	125—200	0—30	**0—75**
e) Nüsse	**10,4—41,7**	**50—100**	190—680	60	30—60	**7,4—52,6**
5) Mehl u. Mehlprod. Kohlenhydrate	**6—16**	**5—90**	240—400	—		**2,1—26**
Schwarzbrot	**16,6**	**40**	250	25	10	**16**
Weißbrot	**6,25**	**5—25**	240	50	2,5—12,5	**2,1—10,4**
Mehl/Nudeln/Reis	**8,33/0/0**	**90/0/0**	350/360/360	—	90/0/0	**25,7/0/0**
Zucker + Süßigkeiten	**0**	**0**	400	—	0	**0**
6) Milch- u. Molkereiprodukte	**0—0,8**	**0—2**	60—930	—	—	**0—1,3**
Ei/57 g	**0,8**	**0—2**	157	57	2	**1,3**
Milch/Quark/Käse	**0**	**0**	60/100/400	—	0	**0**
Butter/Margar./Öl	**0**	**0**	750/750/930	—	0	**0**
7) Getränke	**0—6,7**	**0—16**	1—93	—		
Kaffee	**0**	**0**	5	250	0	**0**
Tee	**0**	**0**	< 1	250	0	**0**
Bier	**6,7**	**16**	31	500	80	**51,6**
Wein	**0**	**0**	63—93	250	0	**0**

Tabelle 10. Übersicht über den Puringehalt in mg Purin-N pro 100 g Nahrungsmittel für die wichtigsten Nahrungsmittelgruppen und Beispiele dazu (analog zu Tabelle 9) bei verschiedenen Autoren (a = vom Kalb, b = roh, c = fett, d = vom Rind, e = vom Schwein, f = vom Schaf). Man beachte die relativ gute Übereinstimmung älterer und neuerer Analysen, jedoch das Fehlen der Angaben zum Purin-N-Gehalt in einer Reihe von Nahrungsmitteltabellen

	Heupke u. Rost	Souci et al. (1967)	McCance u. Widdowson (1960)	Doc. Geigy (1968)	Zöllner, Korf u. Macher (1973, 1974)
1) „Innereien"	100—412	80—400	94—426	94—400	100—454
Leber	104,2[a]	95[a]	143	120[a]	100
Niere	100,0[d]	80	94[d]	94[d]	100[a]
Bries	412,5[a]	400[a]	426[d]	400[a]	454[a]
Herz	?	+ +	174[f]	94[d]	— —
2a) Fleischextrakt	—	—	—	—	(i.M. 833—1460 —2083)
2b) Fleisch	35—51	40—87	50—80	49—60	46—54
Schweinefleisch	51,2	48	50—66	49	54,2
Rindfleisch	46,25[b]	40	58	58	50
Kalbfleisch	47,5[b]	48	80	50	52,1
Huhn	35,4[c]	87	61	60	45,8
3) Fisch	50—792	40—790	—	—	50—146
a) purinreich:	83—792	69—790	—	—	87—146
Salz- od. Matjeshering	791,7	790	—	—	—
Sardellen	100,0	78	—	—	95,8
Ölsardinen	145,8	120	234	234	146
Hering	83,3	69	119[b]	119	87,5
b) purinarm:	50—71	40—56	50—92	61—92	50—71
Kabeljau	50,0	40	50—62	62	50,0
Forelle	70,83	56	92	92	70,8
4) Gemüse/Obst	1—50	1—80	—	—	0,6—56
a) purinreich:	21—50	5—80			6,3—56
Hülsenfrüchte tr.	37—50,0	45—54	—	—	56,3
Erbsen grün	20,83	80	—	—	60,4
Spinat	29,2	23,0	—	—	29,16
b) purinarm:	1—14	1—33			0,6—42
Blumenkohl	10,0	10,0	—	—	10,4
Kopfsalat	13,75	4,5	—	—	4,2
Kartoffeln	1,0	5,6	—	—	2,1
c) Pilze	6,25—20,8	5—18	—	—	6,3—21,0
d) Früchte/Obst	0	0,9—5,8	—	—	0—6,25
e) Nüsse	0	8,4—32,6	—	—	10,4—41,7
5) Mehl u. Mehlprodukte Kohlenhydrate	0	8—14	—	—	6—16
Schwarzbrot	0	14	—	—	16,6
Weißbrot	0	8	—	—	6,25
Mehl, Nudeln, Reis	0	0	—	—	8,33/0/0
Zucker u. Süßigkeiten	0	0	—	—	0

Tabelle 10. (Fortsetzung)

	Heupke u. Rost	Souci et al. (1967)	McCance u. Widdowson (1960)	Doc. Geigy (1968)	Zöllner, Korf u. Macher (1973, 1974)
6) Milch u. Molkereiprodukte	0	0—5	—	—	0—0,8
Ei	0	0	—	0	0,8
Milch, Quark, Käse	0	1,4/1—5	—	0	0
Butter, Margarine, Öl	0	0	—	0	0
7) Getränke	0	0	—	—	0—6,7
Kaffee	0	0	0	—	0
Tee	0	0	—	—	0
Bier	0	0	—	—	6,7
Wein	0	0	—	—	0

müssen. Dazu kommt, daß Gemüse und andere nichttierische Proteinträger wegen des höheren Anteils an Cellulose und Wasser weniger Calorien pro Gewichtseinheit aufweisen, also ebenfalls *zur Deckung des Calorienbedarfs* in größerer Menge zuzuführen sind. So wird es wichtig, den Purin-N- bzw. Harnsäuregehalt pro kcal eines Nahrungsmittels zu berücksichtigen. Wie die letzte Spalte der Tab. 9 zeigt, wird man unter diesem Gesichtspunkt einige Fleischsorten (Beispiele Schwein, Rind, Huhn) vorziehen, einige pflanzliche Nahrungsmittel (Beispiele Pilze, Blumenkohl) zurückstellen müssen, wenn man z.B. einen etwas willkürlich gewählten Grenzwert von 80 mg Harnsäure/100 kcal als Grenze zwischen purinreich und purinarm ansetzt.

Zusammenstellung von Diätplänen

In einigen Fällen wird die Diät bei Gicht und Hyperuricämie nicht allein den Purin-N-Gehalt berücksichtigen müssen, nämlich dann, wenn gleichzeitig eine Zweitkrankheit, speziell eine andere Stoffwechselkrankheit vorliegt. Dies gilt beispielsweise für die Kombination von Gicht und *latentem* Diabetes und für Fettstoffwechselstörungen. Für erstere Kombination wird eine Häufigkeit von 52 (35—70)%, für letztere von 92(56—100)% angegeben (Schilling, 1971).

Dann muß entweder ein vorgegebener Diätplan stark modifiziert oder ein spezieller Speiseplan ausgearbeitet werden. Dazu sind aber Nahrungsmitteltabellen erforderlich, die den Gehalt der Nahrungsmittel an Purin-N angeben. Tab. 10 zeigt solche Angaben für die wichtigsten Nahrungsmittel. Eine Reihe von Tabellen beruht allerdings auf älteren Analysen oder enthält für die meisten Nahrungsmittel keine Purin-N-Angaben. Diese Lücken sollten durch eine moderne Lebensmittelchemie ebenso geschlossen werden wie jene, die noch in der Kenntnis über den Gehalt der Nahrungsmittel an Ribo- und Desoxyribonucleinsäuren bestehen; gerade der letztere Gesichtspunkt würde die Aufstellung verläßlicherer Nahrungsmitteltabellen ermöglichen.

Literatur

Adlersberg, D., Ellenberg, M.: Effect of carbohydrate and fat in the diet on uric acid excretion. J. biol. Chem. **128**, 79 (1939).

Ahrens, E. H., Jr.: The use of liquid formula diet in metabolism studies. 15 years experience. Advanc. metabol. disorders **4**, 297—331 (1970).

AHRENS, E. H., JR., DOLE, V. P., BLANKENHORN, D. H.: Amer. J. clin. Nutr. **2**, 336 (1954). Zit. n. AHRENS 1970.
BONSNES, R. W., DANA, E. S.: On the increased uric acid clearance following intravenous infusion of hypertonic glucose solutions. J. clin. Invest. **25**, 386 (1946).
BOOTHBY, W. M., BERKSON, J., DUNN, J. E.: Amer. J. Physiol. **116**, 468 (1936). Zit. n. THANNHAUSERS Lehrbuch.
CATHCART, E. P.: On metabolism during starvation. I. nitrogenous. J. Physiol. (Lond.) **35**, 500 (1906/7). Zit. n. OGRYZLO.
CATHCART, E. P.: Über die Zusammensetzung des Hungerharns. Biochem. **6**, 109 (1907).
CATHCART, E. P.: The influence of carbohydrates and fats on protein metabolism. J. Physiol. (Lond.) **39**, 311—330 (1909/1910).
DOCUMENTA GEIGY: Wissenschaftl. Tabellen, 7. Aufl. Basel: Geigy 1968.
EVANS, J. G., PRIOR, I. A. M., HARVEY, H. P. B.: Relation of serum uric acid to body bulk. Haemoglobin and alkohol intake in two south-pacific polynesian populations. Ann. rheum. Dis. **27**, 319—325 (1965).
FLEISCH, A.: Helv. med. Acta **18**, 23 (1951). Zit. n. THANNHAUSER.
FOX, I. H., KELLEY, W. N.: Studies on the mechanism of fructose-induced hyperuricemic in man. Metabolism **21/8**, 713—721 (1972).
GARROD, A. B.: The nature and treatment of gout and rheumatic gout, p. 251. London: Walton and Moberly 1863.
GIBSON, H. V., DOISY, E. A.: J. biol. Chem. **55**, 605 (1923). Zit. n. YÜ et al. 1957.
GOLDFINGER, S., KLINGENBERG, J. R. SEEGMILLER, J. E.: Renal retention of uric acid induced by infusion of β-hydroxybutyrate and acetoacetate. New Engl. J. Med. **272**, 351—355 (1965).
GRAHAM, G., POULTON, E. P.: On the variations in the excretion of endogenous uric acid produced by changes in diet. Quart. J. Med. **7**, 13 (1913/14).
GRIEBSCH, A., ZÖLLNER, N.: Verhalten der Harnsäurespiegel im Plasma unter dosierter Zufuhr von Nucleinsäuren. Verh. Dtsch. Ges. inn. Med. **76**, 849—853 (1970a).
GRIEBSCH, A., ZÖLLNER, N.: Über die dosisabhängige Wirkung oral verabreichter DNA und RNA auf Harnsäurespiegel und Harnsäureausscheidung des Gesunden und des Hyperurikämikers. Hoppe-Seylers Z. physiol. Chem. **351**, 1297—1298 (1970b).
GRIEBSCH, A., ZÖLLNER, N.: Harnsäure-Plasmaspiegel und renale Harnsäureausscheidung bei Belastung mit Algen, einer purinreichen Eiweißquelle. Verh. Dtsch. Ges. inn. Med. **77**, 173—177 (1971).
GRIEBSCH, A., ZÖLLNER, N.: Normalwerte der Plasmaharnsäure in Süddeutschland. Vergleich mit Bestimmungen von zehn Jahren. Z. klin. Chem. **11**, 346—356 (1973).
GRIEBSCH, A., ZÖLLNER, N.: Effect of Ribonucleotides given orally on uric acid production in man. In: Advances in Experimental Medicine and Biology. Vol. 41 B: Purine metabolism in man (O. Sperling, A. de Vries, J. B. Wyngaarden, Eds.), p. 443. New York-London: Plenum Press 1974.
GUTMAN, A. B., YU, T. F.: Current principles of management in gout. Amer. J. Med. **13**, 744—759 (1952).
HARDING, V. J., ALLIN, K. D., EAGLES, B. A., VAN WYCK, H. B.: The effect of high fat diets on the content of uric acid in the blood. J. biol. Chem. **63**, 37 (1925).
HARDING, V. J., ALLIN, K. D., EAGLES, B. A.: Influence of fat and carbohydrate diets upon the level of blood uric acid. J. biol. Chem. **74**, 631 (1927).
HEUCKENKAMP, P. U., SCHILL, K., ZÖLLNER, N.: Zum Mechanismus des Serumharnsäureanstiegs unter konstanter Fructose-Infusion beim Menschen. Verh. Dtsch. Ges. inn. Med. **77**, 177—180 (1971).
HEUPKE, W., ROST, G.: Was enthalten unsere Nahrungsmittel? Ihre Zusammensetzung und ihr biologischer Wert. II. Aufl. Frankfurt: Umschau Verlag.
HIRSCHSTEIN, L.: Die Beziehungen der endogenen Harnsäure zur Verdauung. Arch. exp. Path. Pharmakol. **57**, 229 (1907).
KORFMACHER, I., ZÖLLNER, N.: Gicht — lebenslange Behandlung unerläßlich. Dtsch. Ärztebl. **17**, 1221—1230 (1974).
LECOCQ, F. R., McPHAUL, J. J., JR.: The effects of starvation, high fat diets and ketone infusions on uric acid balance. Metabolism **12/2**, 186—197 (1965).
LENNOX, W. G.: Increase of uric acid in the blood during prolonged starvation. J. Amer. med. Ass. **82**, 602 (1924).
LIEBER, CH. S.: Hyperuricemia induced by Alkohol. Arthr. and Rheum. **8**, 786—798 (1965).
LIEBER, CH. S., DAVIDSON, C. S.: Some metabolic effects of ethyl alcohol. Amer. J. Med. **33**, 319—327 (1962).

LIEBER, CH. S., JONES, D. P., LOSOWSKY, M. S., DAVIDSON, C. S.: Interrelation of uric acid and ethanol metabolism in man. J. clin. Invest. **41**, 1863 (1962).

LOCKIE, L. M., HUBBARD, R. S.: Gout: Changes in symptoms and purine metabolism produced by high fat diets in four gouty patients. J. Amer. med. Ass. **104**, 2072 (1935). Zit. n. OGRYZLO (1965).

MACLACHLAN, M. J., RODNAN, G. P.: Effects of food, fast and alcohol on serum uric acid and acute attacks of gout. Amer. J. Med. **42**, 38—57 (1967).

MACCANCE, R. A., WIDDOWSON, E. M.: The Composition of Foods. Vol. 267. Her Majesty's Stationary Office. London 1960.

MCCARTHY, D. D., OGRYZLO, M. A.: Effects of fasting on uric acid excretion by the kidney. Second Canadian Conference on Research in Rheumatic Diseases Toronto Oct. 28—29, 1960, p. 76.

MCCARTHY, D. D., OGRYZLO, M. A.: Effect of fasting on uric acid excretion by the kidney. Arthr. and Rheum. **3**, 280—281 (1960).

MIKKELSEN, W. M., DODGE, H. J., VALKENBURG, H.: Amer. J. Med. **39**, 242—251 (1965).

NARINS, R. G., WEISBERG, J. S., MYERS, A. R.: The effects of carbohydrates on uric acid metabolism. Metabolism **23**, 5, 455—466 (1974).

NUGENT, C. A.: Renal urate excretion in gout studied by feeding ribonucleic acid. Arthritis Rheumat. **8**, 671—685 (1965).

NUGENT, C. A., TYLER, F. H.: The renal excretion of uric acid in patients with gout and in nongouly subjects. J. clin. Invest. **39**, 1890—1898 (1959).

OGRYZLO, M. A.: Hyperuricemia induced by high fat diets and starvation. Arthritis Rheumat. **8**, 799—822 (1965).

PADOVA, J., BENDERSKY, G.: Hyperuricemia in diabetic ketoacidosis. New. Engl. J. Med. **267**, 530 (1962).

PADOVA, J., PATCHEFSKY, A., ONESTI, G., FALUDI, G., BENDERSKY, G.: The effect of glucose loads on renal uric acid excretion in diabetic patients. Metabolism **13/6**, 507—512 (1964).

RAIVIO, K. J., KEKOMÄKI, M. P., MÄENPÄÄ, P. H.: Depletion of liver adenin nucleotides induced by D-fructose. Biochem. Pharmacol. **18**, 2615 (1969).

SAKER, B. M., TOFLER, O. B., BURVILL, M. J., REILLY, K. A.: Alcohol consumption and gout. Med. J. Aust. **1**, 1213—1216 (1967).

SCHILLING, F.: Klinik und Therapie der Gicht. In: Fettsucht — Gicht. 6. Mergentheimer Stoffwechseltagung (W. Boecker, Hrsg.). Stuttgart: Thieme 1971.

SCHÖNTHAL, H., AL-HUJAJ, M., ELBRECHTER, J.: Zur Therapie der Gicht. Dtsch. med. Wschr. **32**, 1195 (1972).

SCHREIBER, WALDVOGEL: Beiträge z. Kenntnis der Harnsäureausscheidung unter physiologischen und pathologischen Verhältnissen. Arch. exp. Path. Pharmakol. **42**, 69—82 (1899).

SCOTT, J. T., MCCALLUM, F. M., HOLLOWAY, V. P.: Starvation, ketosis and uric acid excretion. Clin. Sci. **27**, 209—221 (1964).

SEEGMILLER, J. E., GRAYZEL, A. I., HOWELL, R. R., PLATO, C.: The renal excretion of uric acid in gout. J. clin. Invest. **41**, 1094—1098 (1962).

SEEGMILLER, J. E., GRAYZEL, A. I., LASTER, L., LIDDLE, L.: Uric acid production in man. J. clin. Invest. **40**, 1304—1314 (1961).

SKEITH, M. D., HEALEY, L. A., CUTLER, R. E.: Urate excretion during mannitol and glucose diuresis. J. Lab. clin. Med. **70**, 213—220 (1967).

SOUZI, S. W., FACHMANN, W., KRAUT, H.: Die Zusammensetzung der Lebensmittel. Stuttgart: Wissenschaftliche Verlags GmbH 1969.

STIRPE, F., DELLA CORTE, E., BONETTI, E., DE STEFANO, F.: Fructose induced Hyperuricemia. Lancet **1970**, 1310—1311.

WASLIEN, C. I., CALLOWAY, D. H., MARGEN, S.: Uric acid production of men fed graded amounts egg protein and nucleic acid. Amer. J. clin. Nutr. **21**, 892—897 (1968).

WASLIEN, C. I., CALLOWAY, D. H., MARGEN, S., COSTA, F.: Uric acid levels in men feed algae and yeast as protein sources. J. Food. Sci. **35**, 294—298 (1970).

WOLFRAM, G., ZÖLLNER, N.: Der Linolsäurebedarf des Menschen. Wiss. Veröff. der Dtsch. Ges. Ernährung **22**, 51—60 (1971).

WOLFSON, N. Q., UREVSKY, D., LEVINE, R., KADOTA, K., COHN, C.: Endocrine Factors in gout. J. clin. Endocr. **9**, 666 (1949).

YÜ, T. F., BERGER, L., GUTMAN, A. B.: Renal function in gout. Effect of Uric acid loading on renal excretion of uric acid. Amer. J. Med. **33**, 829—844 (1962).

Yü, T. F., Sirota, J. H., Berger, L., Halpern, M., Gutman, A. B.: Effect of Sodium Lactate Infusion on Urate Clearance in Man. Proc. Soc. exp. Biol. (N. Y.) **96**, 809—813 (1957).

Zöllner, N.: Gesamtstoffwechsel. In: Thannhausers Lehrbuch des Stoffwechsels. (Zöllner, N., Hrsg.). Stuttgart: Thieme 1957.

Zöllner, N.: Diät bei Gicht und Harnsäuresteinleiden. Thienemanns Diätkochbücher. Stuttgart: Thienemann 1974 (im Druck).

Zöllner, N., Griebsch, A.: Diet and gout. In: Advances in Experimental Medicine and Biology. Vol. 41 B: Purine metabolism in man (O. Sperling, A. de Vries, J. B. Wyngaarden, Eds.). New York: Plenum Press 1974.

Zöllner, N., Griebsch, A., Gröbner, W.: Einfluß verschiedener Purine auf den Harnsäure-Stoffwechsel. Ernährungs-Umschau **3**, 74—82 (1972).

e) Hyperuricämie durch therapeutische Maßnahmen

Von

D. P. Mertz

Mit 7 Abbildungen

Allgemeine Gesichtspunkte

Die Entwicklung einer sekundären oder nichtgichtigen Hyperuricämie, die mit primärer Gicht oder ihrer asymptomatischen Anlage nicht in Zusammenhang steht, beruht entweder auf einer vermehrten Bildung oder verminderten Ausscheidung von Harnsäure, bzw. auf einer Kombination beider Möglichkeiten (Mertz, 1966/67). Die Uratausscheidung erfolgt überwiegend über die Niere (Lucke, 1931; Sorensen, 1959, 1965). Normalerweise werden unabhängig von der Harnsäurekonzentration im Serum durchschnittlich weniger als 2% der glomerulär filtrierten Uratmenge im Endharn ausgeschieden. Anteilmäßig entspricht diese Quantität etwa 20% der mit dem Harn eliminierten Harnsäure (Steele u. Rieselbach, 1967). Zu 98% wird die filtrierte Harnsäure im proximalen Tubulussegment reabsorbiert (Mudge et al., 1968; Zins u. Weiner, 1968). Die dafür zuständigen Tubuluszellen können Harnsäure im Sinne eines bidirektionalen Transportes in den proximalen Tubulus sezernieren. Der Prozentsatz der Uratsekretion an der renalen Gesamtausscheidung ist bei sehr verschieden hohen Serumwerten mit über 80% recht stabil.

Im Hinblick auf die Ätiologie der sekundären Hyperuricämien können folgende Bedingungen (s. bei Mertz, 1966/67) bedeutsam sein: (1) Vermehrter Anfall von Harnsäure, beispielsweise bei gesteigertem Zellzerfall jeder Art oder experimentell unter der Wirkung von Äthylaminothiadiazol (Krakoff u. Balis, 1959); (2) verminderte renale Ausscheidung bei Niereninsuffizienz (Sarre u. Mertz, 1965); (3) verschiedene Störungen im Stoffwechsel wie CO-Vergiftung, Ketose, bei Akromegalie, Myxödem, Hypoparathyreoidismus, Hyperparathyreoidismus, essentieller Hypercholesterinämie, Glykogen-Speicherkrankheit vom Typ I, III und VI (Kelley et al., 1968), arterieller Hypertension (Breckenridge, 1966; Cannon et al., 1966); (5) Arzneimittel und verschiedene Diätvorschriften. Von diesen Möglichkeiten spielen die als Nebenwirkung von gewissen Medikamenten oder durch verschiedene diätetische Maßnahmen auftretenden sekundären Hyperuricämien eine wichtige Rolle. Ohne Frage trägt die weite und vielfach unkontrollierte Anwendung medikamentöser und diätetischer Therapieverfahren zu dem erschreckend hohen Prozentsatz von ätiologisch oft ungeklärten sekundären Hyperuricämien in der Allgemeinbevölkerung hochzivilisierter Staaten bei.

Die Häufigkeit, mit der Hyperuricämie in einem nach Gicht und Hyperuricämie unausgewählten Querschnitt der Allgemeinbevölkerung auftritt, wird auf 4,5—12% geschätzt (HAUGE u. HARVALD, 1955; SCHRADE et al., 1960; GRAYZEL et al., 1961; POPERT u. HEWITT, 1962; ITSKOVITZ u. SELLERS, 1963; TALBOTT, 1964). Nach Schätzungen von GRAYZEL et al. (1961) können Harnsäurekonzentrationen von über 6 mg/100 ml Serum bei 17% aller gesunden Männer und Werte von über 5 mg/100 ml Serum bei 16% gesunder Frauen erwartet werden. Dieses Ergebnis stimmt gut mit den Befunden der Tecumseh-Studie (MIKKELSEN et al., 1965) überein, wonach unter 2987 unausgewählten Männern aller Altersklassen über 4 Jahren in 20,8% Harnsäurekonzentrationen von 6 oder mehr mg/100 ml Serum und bei 21,9% von 3013 Frauen über 4 Jahre Harnsäurewerte von 5 und mehr mg/100 ml Serum vorgefunden wurden. Ähnliche Resultate lieferte die Framingham-Studie (HALL et al., 1967), wobei 22% von 2283 erwachsenen Männern der Allgemeinbevölkerung eine Harnsäurekonzentration von 6 und mehr mg/100 ml Serum hatten. Bei Bewertung derartiger Statistiken muß allerdings die willkürlich sehr unterschiedlich gezogene Grenze zwischen normaler und erhöhter Harnsäurekonzentration mit berücksichtigt werden. Es ist nicht einfach, bei einer Allgemeinbevölkerung einen so hohen Anteil einer bestimmten Stoffwechselstörung anzunehmen, schließt doch der Begriff Hyperuricämie eine Abnormität im Harnsäurestoffwechsel ein. Folgt man einem Vorschlag von BRØCHNER-MORTENSEN et al. (1963) und nimmt als obere Normgrenze für die Harnsäurekonzentration einen Wert von 7 mg/100 ml Serum bei Männern und von 6 mg/100 ml bei Frauen an, dann fand sich in der Tecumseh-Studie nur mehr bei 7,4% der untersuchten Männer und bei 7,2% der Frauen eine Hyperuricämie. Vergleichbare Werte erbrachte die Framingham-Studie (HALL et al., 1967). Von insgesamt 5127 erwachsenen Personen hatten 4,8% eine Harnsäurekonzentration von über 7 mg/100 ml Serum, und zwar 9,2% der Männer und 0,4% der Frauen. Das Risiko, mit dem sich Gicht innerhalb von 10 Jahren bei diesen Personen entwickelt, beträgt etwa 1:5. Gemessen an diesem Standard erscheinen die Angaben, wonach Männer in leitenden Positionen in 43% Harnsäurekonzentrationen von 6 und mehr mg/100 ml (POPERT u. HEWITT, 1962; DUNN et al., 1963) und in 16% (POPERT u. HEWITT, 1962) bzw. 19,5% (LANESE et al., 1969) ein Harnsäureniveau von mindestens 7 mg/100 ml aufweisen, als unerwartet hoch. Andererseits ist bekannt, daß Hypertoniker mit gut erhaltener Nierenfunktion unabhängig von Dauer und Schweregrad der Blutdruckerhöhung und von der Höhe der Serumkaliumkonzentration etwa fünfmal häufiger eine Hyperuricämie aufweisen, als bei der Gesamtbevölkerung gleicher Altersstufen zu erwarten ist (DOLLERY et al., 1960; KINSEY et al., 1961; BRECKENRIDGE, 1966; CANNON et al., 1966). CANNON et al. (1966) fanden bei 47% von 217 hypertensiven Patienten Serumharnsäurewerte von über 6,4 mg/100 ml bei Männern und von über 5,9 mg/100 ml bei Frauen. Im einzelnen fand sich Hyperuricämie bei 43% von 141 Patienten mit essentieller Hypertension, bei 44% von 52 Patienten mit renaler oder renovasculärer Hypertension und bei 75% von 24 Patienten mit maligner Hypertension. Wegen dieser großen Häufigkeit kann Hyperuricämie bei arterieller Hyertension unmöglich auf genetische Faktoren, wie etwa bei essentieller Hypertension, oder auf die Ätiologie des zugrundeliegenden Nierenleidens bezogen werden. Unbehandelte Hypertoniker hatten in 38%, behandelte Patienten in 58% Hyperuricämie. Diese Zahl stieg bei Patienten, die Thiazidsaluretica erhielten, auf 67% an!

Hyperuricämie birgt nicht nur die Gefahr einer Uratnephropathie in sich. Die Vermeidung oder Behandlungsbedürftigkeit einer Hyperuricämie ergibt sich auch im Hinblick auf eine Verminderung der Thrombosebereitschaft von hyperuricämischen Patienten. Bekanntlich haben Gichtkranke eine erhöhte Thrombocytenadhäsivität (MUSTARD et al., 1963). Für das Zusammentreffen von Hyperuricämie mit Thrombose der Coronarien (KAHN u. PROZAN, 1959; DREYFUSS, 1960; MOORE u. WEISS, 1963; GERTLER et al., 1964), der Gehirn- (HANSEN, 1965) und peripheren Arterien (KRAMER et al., 1958) wird teilweise die Hyperuricämie per se verantwortlich gemacht. Experimentelle Erhöhung der Harnsäurekonzentration stimuliert bei Ratten die durch ADP in vitro (GAARDER et al., 1961) und in vivo (NORDÖY u. CHANDLER, 1964) induzierte Thrombocytenaggregation (NEWLAND, 1968). Umgekehrt vermindert sich die Entwicklung einer Thrombose bei Hypouricämie signifikant. Bekanntlich ist die Aggregation von Thrombocyten eine der frühesten Stadien der Thrombose und wird unabhängig vom Reiz durch ADP vermittelt. Es ist möglich, daß Harnsäure als Metabolit der Adeninnucleotide einschließlich ADP den Abbau von ADP und damit die Stabilität der ADP-induzierten Plättchenthromben durch eine Wirkung auf die Abbaurate von ADP im Blut beeinflußt.

Hyperuricämie durch Saluretica

Der hyperuricämische Effekt von Thiazidderivaten wurde 1958 erstmals von LARAGH et al. am Beispiel von Chlorothiazid aufgezeigt. Eine Erhöhung des Harnsäurespiegels im Serum wurde unter anderem auch nach Gabe von Acetazolamid (GUTMAN et al., 1956), Hydrochlorothiazid (MERTZ, 1959), Chlorthalidon (BRYANT et al., 1962; REUTTER u. SCHAUB, 1964) und Furosemid (SCHIRMEISTER u. WILLMANN, 1964) beobachtet. Dabei verstärkt Acetazolamid die durch Hydrochlorothiazid bewirkte Hyperuricämie (AYVAZIAN u. AYVAZIAN, 1961). Die durch Saluretica bewirkte Zunahme der Serumharnsäurekonzentration wird als Folge einer Hemmung der tubulären Uratsekretion, die durch diese Mittel in therapeutischen Dosen bewirkt wird, angesehen (DEMARTINI et al., 1962). Auf der anderen Seite beeinflussen kalium-einsparende Diuretica den Harnsäurestoffwechsel im klinischen Sinne nicht signifikant. Hierzu zählen der Aldosteronantagonist Spironolacton (HOLLANDER u. WILKINS, 1966), Triamteren (HAVARD, 1962; HEATH u. FREIS, 1963; THOMPSON u. CROWLEY, 1965; MORIN et al., 1965) und Amilorid-HCl (HEIDLAND et al., 1967; HITZENBERGER et al., 1968).

Die Häufigkeit einer durch saluretische Therapie hervorgerufenen oder geförderten Hyperuricämie ist beträchtlich, läßt sich jedoch nicht genau angeben. Schätzungsweise liegt der Jahresverbrauch an Saluretica in der Bundesrepublik Deutschland in der Größenordnung von einer halben Milliarde Tabletten (JAHNECKE, 1967)! Nach REUTTER u. SCHAUB (1964) reagieren etwa 80% aller mit Thiazid- und verwandten Sulfonamidsaluretica behandelten Personen mit einem signifikanten Anstieg der Uratkonzentration im Serum. Harnsäurekonzentrationen von mehr als 7 mg/100 ml Serum finden sich bei 40 bis 50% der mit diesen Medikamenten behandelten Patienten (BORHANI, 1960; BRYANT et al., 1962). BERNHEIM (1968) fand unter 40 Nichtdiabetikern während der saluretischen Therapie über mehr als 6 Monate in 42,5% Hyperuricämie und in 20—30% Störungen der Zuckerregulation. Bei einem Vergleich von 55 Kranken mit primärer Gicht mit 17 Kranken, bei denen das Gelenkleiden durch saluretische Mittel ausgelöst worden war, konnten Störungen des Kohlenhydratstoffwechsels in 55—60% der Kranken mit primärer oder induzierter Gicht festgestellt werden. Akute Gichtanfälle (OREN et al., 1958; WARSHAW, 1960; ARONOFF, 1960) werden durchschnittlich 3,7 Jahre nach Beginn einer Thiazid-Therapie (Schwankungsbreite 8 Monate bis 7 Jahre) bei bis zu 5—10% hypertensiver Patienten beobachtet

(HOLLANDER u. WILKINS, 1966). OREN et al. (1958), TSALOFF u. LESTINA (1960) sowie ARONOFF u. BARKUM (1961) beobachteten die Entwicklung von arthritischen Symptomen während der Thiazidbehandlung sogar bei Patienten, deren Vorgeschichte keinen Anhalt für Gicht bot. Im Verlauf einer Langzeittherapie mit Saluretica wird nach etwa dreimonatiger Behandlung ein Maximum der Serumharnsäurekonzentration erreicht (HEIMSOTH u. HARTMANN, 1965).

Die genannten Thiazidsaluretica beeinflussen die renale Behandlung von Harnsäure biphasisch. Zunächst wirken sie uricosurisch und dann harnsäureretinierend (DEMARTINI, 1959; HEALEY et al., 1959; BRYANT et al., 1962; SCHIRMEISTER u. WILLMANN, 1964). Im Vergleich zur Zuwachsrate der Natriumausscheidung ist die anfängliche Steigerung der Harnsäureausscheidung jedoch gering. Sie ist etwa doppelt so hoch wie der Kontrollwert. Diese Wirkung bleibt jedoch, wie die Abb. 1 zeigt, beim Hypertoniker aus (MERTZ u. SCHWOERER, 1969). Vermutlich sind am Zustandekommen des initial uricosurischen Effektes von Saluretica die starke osmotische Diurese und kompetitive Wirkungen am gemeinsamen Transportsystem im proximalen Tubulus (WEINER u. MUDGE, 1964) beteiligt. Für die harnsäureretinierende Wirkung der Saluretica werden sowohl renale als auch extrarenale Momente verantwortlich gemacht. Die renale Komponente wird auf eine Hyperlactacidämie bezogen. Seit langer Zeit ist bekannt, daß eine Erhöhung der Milchsäurekonzentration im Serum zu einem sofortigen scharfen Abfall der Harnsäureausscheidung führt (GIBSON u. DOISY, 1923; QUICK, 1932). Eine Hyperlactacidämie kommt nach Gabe von Saluretica einmal durch eine initiale Verminderung der renalen Eliminierung von Lactat zustande (SCHIRMEISTER et al., 1967a). Die daraus resultierende Retention von Lactat reicht jedoch zur Erklärung der Hyperlactacidämie nach Gabe von Saluretica nicht aus. Vielmehr scheint der unter der Wirkung der Saluretica zu beobachtende Blutlactatanstieg hauptsächlich auf einer gesteigerten Lactatbildung in Folge von vermehrter Freisetzung von Catecholaminen durch Schrumpfung des Plasmavolumens zu beruhen (SCHIRMEISTER et al., 1968). Es ist anzunehmen, daß die bei hypertensiven Patienten festgestellte endogene Milchsäureakkumulation (CANNON et al., 1966) eine wesentliche Voraussetzung für das Ausbleiben der initial uricosurischen Wirkung der Saluretica bei solchen Kranken ist (MERTZ u. SCHWOERER, 1969).

Indessen stellten AYVAZIAN u. AYVAZIAN (1961) sowie REUTTER u. SCHAUB (1964) unter dem Einfluß der Saluretica bei normalen Kontrollpersonen und Gichtpatienten mit stark verminderter glomerulärer Filtratrate einen deutlichen Anstieg der Serumharnsäurekonzentration fest, obwohl Harnsäureausscheidung und Harnsäureclearance gleich zunahmen. Weiterhin stellten STANBURY et al. (1960) fest, daß kleine Dosen von Hydrochlorothiazid die renale Harnsäureausscheidung bei praktisch unveränderter Harnsäureclearance fördern. Dies ist nur durch die gleichzeitige Entwicklung einer Hyperuricämie möglich. Andererseits verändert sich die Serumharnsäurekonzentration während der initial uricosurischen Wirkung der Salureticaa nicht signifikant (SCHIRMEISTER u. WILLMANN, 1964; MERTZ u. SCHWOERER, 1969). Aus diesen Befunden wurde auf eine zusätzliche extrarenale Wirkung der Saluretica auf den Harnsäurestoffwechsel geschlossen. Zur Diskussion standen eine Veränderung der Harnsäuresynthese, eine Ausschwemmung von Harnsäure aus dem Harnsäurepool oder eine Verminderung der extrarenalen Ausscheidung von Harnsäure (STANBURY et al., 1960). SCHIRMEISTER et al. (1967b) fanden, daß Furosemid die unter Allopurinol allein zu beobachtende Verminderung der Serumharnsäurekonzentration beim Menschen deutlich abschwächt. Dieser Befund läßt sich nur im Sinne einer Mobilisation von Harnsäure aus dem Harnsäurepool erklären, wenn man von der kaum gegebenen Möglichkeit einer vermehrten Ausscheidung von Harnsäure durch den Gastro-

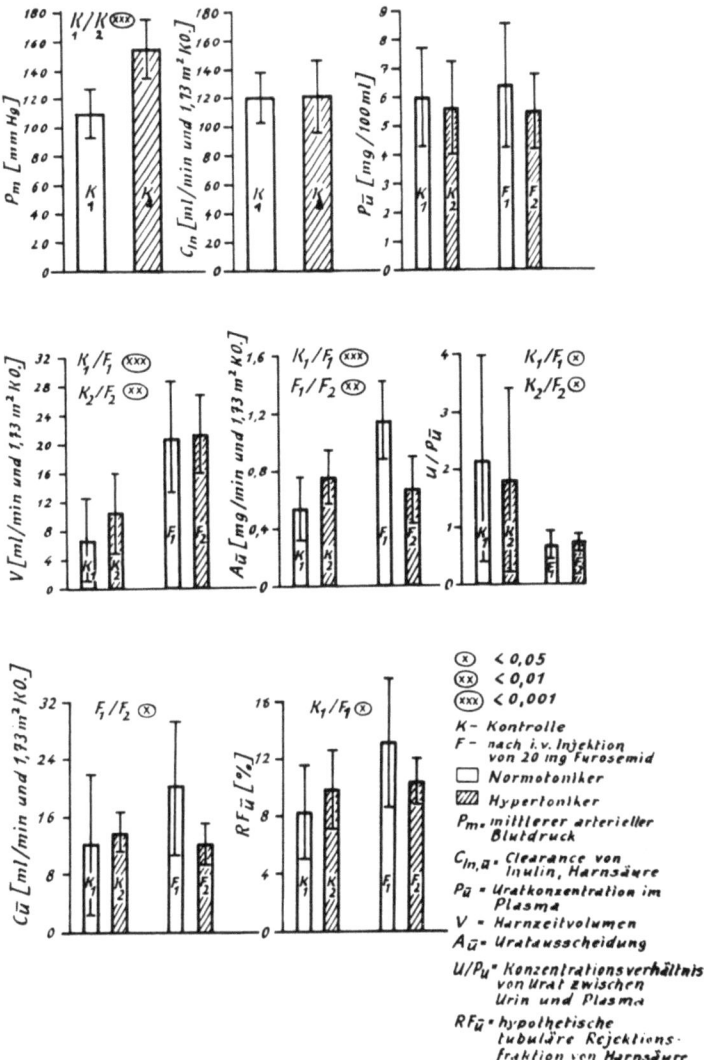

Abb. 1. Verhalten der renalen Ausscheidung von Harnsäure ($\overline{U}$) nach intravenöser Injektion von 20 mg Furosemid bei Normotonikern ($n = 8$) und Hypertonikern ($n = 7$)

intestinaltrakt absieht. So sind also für den unter Langzeitbehandlung mit Saluretica beobachteten Harnsäureanstieg im Serum renale und extrarenale Faktoren bedeutsam.

Die potentiell schädlichen Wirkungen einer chronischen Hyperuricämie, die durch Langzeitbehandlung mit Thiazidderivaten oder verwandten Substanzen hervorgerufen wird, können durch eine zusätzliche Behandlung mit Probenecid abgewendet werden (OREN et al., 1958; REUTTER u. SCHAUB, 1964; FREIS u. SAPPINGTON, 1966; BREST et al., 1966). In Gegenwart von Azotämie erweist sich Allopurinol als wirksameres Mittel gegen die Hyperuricämie als Probenecid (WYNGAARDEN et al., 1965; MERTZ, 1966/67). Ein Entzug der Saluretica bei zum

Beispiel antihypertensiver Therapie ist also nicht notwendig, zumal in etwa einem Drittel der Patienten trotz Absetzens der saluretischen Therapie gelegentlich noch Gichtanfälle auftreten (HOLLANDER u. WILKINS, 1966).

Sogenannte „Paradoxeffekte" uricosurischer Mittel

Von besonderem Interesse ist die Tatsache, daß Salicylate in einer Dosierung von 5—6 g täglich uricosurisch und bei Gabe von 1—2 g täglich harnsäureretinierend wirken (FAUVEL, 1907; KLEMPERER u. BAUER, 1944; YÜ u. GUTMAN 1959). In mittlerer Dosierung verändern Salicylate die Harnsäureausscheidung nicht. Sorgfältige Clearance-Untersuchungen haben gezeigt, daß die sogenannten „Paradoxeffekte" von Salicylat auf das Clearance-Verhältnis Urat/Inulin in der Hauptsache von der Konzentration von freiem Salicylat im Tubulusharn abhängig sind. YÜ u. GUTMAN (1959) nahmen an, daß niedrige Konzentrationen von freiem Salicylat im Tubulusharn die tubuläre Uratsekretion unterdrücken. Mittlere Konzentrationen von freiem Salicylat sollen sowohl die tubuläre Reabsorption als auch die tubuläre Sekretion in einem Ausmaß hemmen, daß keine oder nur geringe Nettoänderungen der Uratausscheidung resultieren. Vermutlich beeinträchtigt freies Salicylat in hoher Konzentration die tubuläre Reabsorption so stark, daß die gleichzeitige Hemmung der Sekretion quantitativ nicht mehr ins Gewicht fällt und sich daraus ein uricosurischer Nettoeffekt ergibt. Ähnliche „Paradoxeffekte" wurden nach Gabe von Probenecid, Phenylbutazon und Chlorothiazid beobachtet (YÜ u. GUTMAN, 1955; DEMARTINI et al., 1962). Aus diesem Grunde ist es wichtig, eine Dauerbehandlung der Gicht mit Uricosurica nicht in zu kleiner Dosierung durchzuführen. Kleine Dosen von Salicylat vermindern den uricosurischen Effekt von Probenecid (GUTMAN u. YÜ, 1951) und gewissen Phenylbutazon-Abkömmlingen (KERSLEY et al., 1958). Es ist daher nicht ratsam, verschiedene Uricosurica in Kombination mit Salicylaten zu geben. Die depressorische Wirkung von Probenecid auf die durch Salicylate hervorgerufene vermehrte Harnsäureausscheidung ist als Folge einer inhibitorischen Wirkung von Probenecid auf die tubuläre Sekretion von Salicylsäure zurückzuführen. In dieser Beziehung unterscheidet sich das harnsäuresenkende Benzofuran-Derivat Benzbromaronum (ZÖLLNER et al., 1968, 1970a, b; MERTZ, 1969), bei dem die paradoxe Wirkung der Harnsäureretention bei niedriger Dosierung fehlt (PODEVIN, 1967), und Salicylate in analgetischen Dosen den hypouricämischen Effekt nicht antagonistisch beeinflussen (GROSS u. GIRARD, 1972), von den anderen Uricosurica.

Urat wird über denselben sekretorischen Transportmechanismus wie andere organische Säuren (beispielsweise PAH) transportiert (WEINER u. MUDGE, 1964). Es ist daher zu erwarten, daß andere organische Anionen wie Salicylat und Chlorothiazid diesen Flux kompetitiv hemmen. Unter dieser Betrachtungsweise läßt sich die von YÜ u. GUTMAN (1959) begründete Anschauung von einer biphasischen Reaktion der Uratausscheidung auf Salicylat beim Menschen gut erklären. Unterschiede ergeben sich nur darin, daß Reabsorption und Sekretion in derselben Zelle des proximalen Tubulusepithels lokalisiert sind, und daß der Träger für den Einstrom derselbe oder ähnlich demjenigen ist, der beim PAH-Transport eine Rolle spielt. Offenbar ist der sekretorische Flux gegenüber gewissen Substanzen empfindlicher als der reabsorptive. Bei Anwendung anderer Substanzen kann die umgekehrte Situation vorliegen und daher eine biphasische Reaktion nicht nachweisbar sein (ZINS u. WEINER, 1968). Da die Sekretion und die Reabsorption von Urat durch einen spezifischen Träger bestimmt sind, spielt eine unspezifische Uratbewegung auf dem Wege einer nichtionalen Diffusion durch die Wand des proximalen Tubulus keine Rolle.

Hyperuricämie durch cytostatische Therapie

Eine Hyperuricämie bei neoplastischer Erkrankung spiegelt für gewöhnlich eine stark erhöhte Harnsäurebildung durch vermehrten Nucleinsäureumsatz von Seiten der Tumorzellen wider. Während der cytostatischen Therapie führt der vermehrte Untergang neoplastischer Zellen und der nachfolgende Katabolismus der Nucleinsäuren zu einer weiteren Erhöhung des Serumharnsäurespiegels. Auf diese Weise kann der Serumharnsäurewert, der vor einer cytostatischen Behandlung trotz signifikanter Erhöhung des Purinkatabolismus noch normal gewesen sein mag, auf deutlich erhöhte Werte ansteigen. Mit dem vermehrten Abbau von Nucleinsäuren infolge Tumoreinschmelzung nimmt die Komplikationsquote an Hyperuricämie zu. Eine Harnsäurenephropathie entwickelt sich besonders bei einer Chemotherapie der akuten Leukämie (KRITZLER, 1958). Bei cytostatischer Behandlung besteht Gefahr eines akuten Nierenversagens durch Harnsäureausfällungen (MUGGIA et al., 1967). Über eine Gichtauslösung durch Behandlung mit Amethopterin bei Psoriasis berichten MARTIN et al. (1967).

Hyperuricämie durch parenterale Infusionsbehandlung

Lactat

Nach Einnahme von 10—14 g Natriumlactat kommt es zu einer Verminderung der Harnsäureausscheidung durch die Nieren, verbunden mit einem Anstieg der Blutharnsäure (GIBSON u. DOISY, 1923). Die Annahme, Lactat wirke infolge einer Zunahme der tubulären Reabsorption von Harnsäure harnsäureretinierend (REEM u. VANAMEE, 1964), stützt sich auf Clearance-Untersuchungen am Hund. Die Tatsache, daß die Reabsorption von Harnsäure normalerweise nicht durch eine maximale Transportrate (Tm) reguliert wird, und die in der Zeiteinheit sezernierte Uratmenge von beträchtlicher Größenordnung ist (MUDGE et al., 1968), läßt diese Annahme fraglich erscheinen. Theoretisch ist sie allerdings nicht ausgeschlossen. Infundiert man gesunden Versuchspersonen während einer 60 min-Periode 1000 ml 1,75%ige racemische Natriumlactat-Lösung intravenös, dann vermindert sich die Harnsäureclearance bei einem gleichzeitigen Anstieg des Serumharnsäurespiegels beträchtlich (BURCH u. KURKE, 1968). An diese Wirkung sollte bei intravenöser Infusion von Lactat-Lösung bei gefährdeten Fällen stets gedacht werden.

Äthylalkohol

Nach Zufuhr von Äthylalkohol steigt der Serumharnsäurespiegel an (QUICK, 1935). Für die hyperuricämische Wirkung ist eine Verminderung der renalen Harnsäureausscheidung infolge einer Hyperlactacidämie durch Alkoholoxydation verantwortlich zu machen (LIEBER et al., 1962). Bei Zufuhr von Alkoholmengen unter 100 g innerhalb von vier Stunden nimmt jedoch der Serumlactatgehalt normalerweise nur wenig zu, so daß eine Konzentration, die für eine Hemmung der Uratausscheidung durch die Niere notwendig ist, nicht erreicht wird (MAC-LACHLAN u. RODNAN, 1967).

Der Alkoholumsatz zu Acetaldehyd und dann zu Acetat erfordert die Reduktion großer Mengen von NAD (Nicotinamid-Adenin-Dinucleotid) zu NADH. Wenn also Alkohol im Stoffwechsel verbrannt wird, beeinträchtigt der sich daraus ergebende Anstieg von NADH das Gleichgewicht aller NAD-NADH-abhängigen Reaktionen und somit auch die Überführung von Lactat in Pyruvat. In der Peripherie gebildetes Lactat wird aus der Zirkulation durch die Leber entfernt

(ALPERT, 1965). In der Leber wird Lactat entweder zu CO_2 über den Krebs-Cyclus abgebaut oder in Glucose über den Cori-Cyclus zurückverwandelt. Beim Lactatumsatz ist in jedem Falle die Überführung in Pyruvat notwendig. Diese Reaktion schließt die Reduktion von NAD zu NADH ein und erfordert zusätzlich die Gegenwart von Lactatdehydrogenase (LIEBER u. DAVIDSON, 1962).

Kombination von Fasten und Äthylalkohol wirkt sich additiv auf die Erhöhung des Serumharnsäurespiegels aus (MACLACHLAN u. RODNAN, 1967). Diese Veränderung geht mit einer stärkeren Zunahme der Serumlactatkonzentration, als nach Zufuhr von Alkohol mit Nahrung beobachtet wird, und der Serumkonzentration von β-Hydroxybuttersäure, als sie während einer äquivalenten Fastenperiode auftritt, einher. Wenn Gichtpatienten während einer Fastenperiode größere Alkoholmengen konsumieren, entwickeln sich akute Anfälle häufiger. Bedingung hierfür sind starke akute Schwankungen des Harnsäurespiegels. Probenecid kann den Harnsäureanstieg im Serum während Fastens mit oder ohne Alkoholkonsum nicht verhindern (MACLACHLAN u. RODNAN, 1967). Ähnliche Beobachtungen machten MCCARTHY u. OGRYZLO (1961) mit Sulfinpyrazon, das bei gefasteten Personen keinen Einfluß auf die Serumwerte von Urat oder Ketonkörpern hat.

In diesem Zusammenhang sei vermerkt, daß Phenformin den Lactatanstieg bei diabetischen Personen nach Gabe von Glucose oder Alkohol verstärkt und verlängert (JOHNSON u. WATERHOUSE, 1968).

Fructose

Infusion von Fructose ruft ebenfalls einen Anstieg der Serumkonzentration von Milchsäure und Harnsäure hervor (PERHEENTUPA u. RAIVIO, 1967; MEHNERT et al., 1967). Durch die Hyperlactacidämie wird die renale Eliminierung von Harnsäure beim gesunden Menschen ohne Veränderung der Clearancewerte von Inulin und PAH (YÜ et al., 1957) herabgesetzt.

Trotzdem steigt jedoch die Serumharnsäurekonzentration nach hochdosierter rascher Infusion (1,5 g/kg Körpergewicht in 20%iger Lösung innerhalb von 20—25 min) der vorwiegend in der Leber verwerteten Kohlenhydrate Sorbit, Xylit und Fructose vorübergehend an (FÖRSTER et al., 1970). Der nach Fructoseinfusion auftretende Anstieg der Serumharnsäurekonzentration ist durch Allopurinol hemmbar, also auf erhöhte Harnsäureproduktion zurückzuführen (FÖRSTER u. MEHNERT, 1967).

Während einer intravenösen Infusion von 5 ml/min einer 10%igen *Xylit*lösung steigt die Serumharnsäurekonzentration von jungen gesunden Versuchspersonen beiderlei Geschlechts um etwa 30% über das Ausgangsniveau an (vgl. Abb. 2) und bleibt nach 100 min langer Infusion in einer Nachbeobachtungsperiode von weiteren 140 min erhöht (MERTZ et al., 1972a). Da sich keine zeitliche Parallelität zwischen den Veränderungen der Serumharnsäurewerte und dem Blutlactatgehalt nachweisen läßt (vgl. Abb. 2 u. 3), ist die Annahme unwahrscheinlich, daß die hyperuricämisierende Wirkung einer akuten Belastung mit Xylit auf einer Hyperlactacidämie mit konsekutiver renaler Harnsäureretention beruht. In den Fructoseversuchen von FÖRSTER et al. (1970) ergab sich ebenfalls ein vorübergehender Anstieg der Serumharnsäurekonzentration um durchschnittlich 30% des Ausgangswertes. Eine Zunahme der Serumharnsäurekonzentration mit gleichbleibender oder konsekutiv erhöhter renaler Harnsäureexkretion wurde nach oraler oder *parenteraler Verabreichung leberaffiner Kohlenhydrate* wiederholt beobachtet (PERHEENTUPA u. RAIVIO, 1967; MEHNERT u. FÖRSTER, 1967; FÖRSTER et al., 1967, 1970; MÄENPÄÄ et al., 1968; RAIVIO et al., 1969).

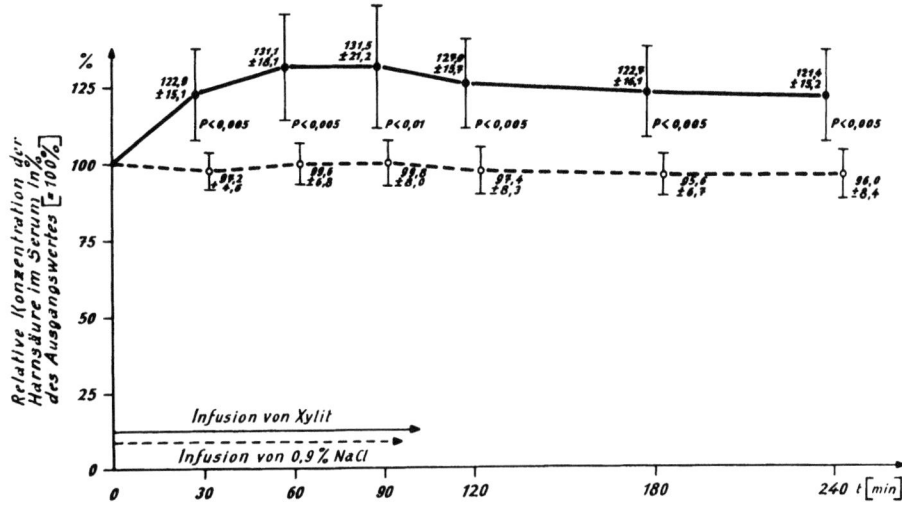

Abb. 2. Verhalten der Serumkonzentration von Harnsäure unter der akuten Wirkung einer i.v. Infusion von 5 ml/min einer 10%igen Xylitlösung. (Nach MERTZ et al., 1972a)

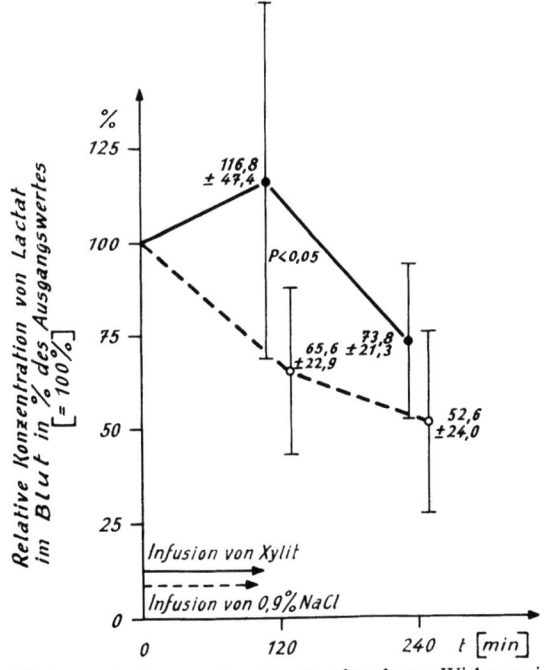

Abb. 3. Verhalten der Blutkonzentration von Lactat unter der akuten Wirkung einer i.v. Infusion von 5 ml/min einer 10%igen Xylitlösung. (Nach MERTZ et al., 1972a)

Der innerhalb weniger Minuten prompt einsetzende Anstieg der Serumharnsäurekonzentration ist von der in der Zeiteinheit infundierten Kohlenhydratmenge abhängig (HEUCKENKAMP et al., 1971; SAHEBJAMI u. SCALETTAR, 1971). Mit Zufuhrmengen von 1,5 g/kg Körpergewicht in der Stunde kommt es bereits 90 min nach Infusionsbeginn von Fructose zu einem signifikanten Anstieg der Serum-

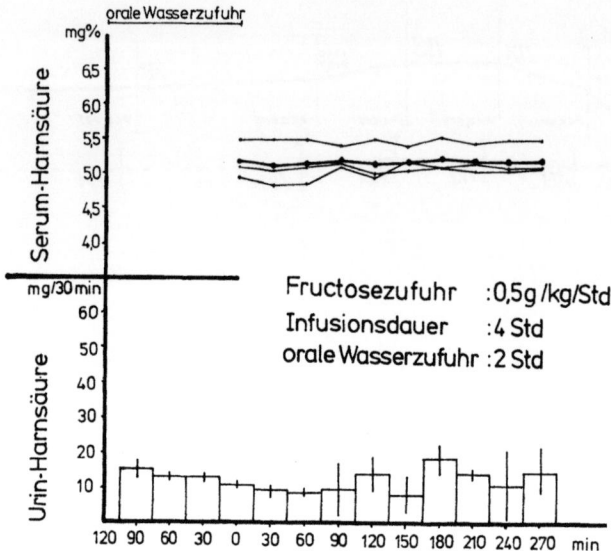

Abb. 4. Verhalten von Serumharnsäurekonzentration und Harnsäureausscheidung im Urin während i.v. Infusion von 0,5 g Fructose/kg Körpergewicht und Std. (Nach HEUCKENKAMP et al., 1971)

harnsäurekonzentration von $5,03 \pm 0,25$ mg/100 ml nüchtern auf $6,35 \pm 0,20$ mg/100 ml (Mittelwert mit Standardabweichung) (HEUCKENKAMP et al., 1971). In Abb. 4 u. 5 sind diese Veränderungen graphisch dargestellt.

Bei gesunden Personen stellten HEUCKENKAMP u. ZÖLLNER (1972) unter konstanter intravenöser Dauerinfusion von 0,5 g Xylit/kg Körpergewicht und Std einen Anstieg der Harnsäurekonzentration (mit Standardabweichung) von $4,65 \pm 0,78$ mg/100 ml Serum auf $7,16 \pm 0,92$ mg/100 ml Serum nach der 165. Infusionsminute fest. Xylit steigert demnach die Serumharnsäurekonzentration wesentlich stärker als Fructose und in Zufuhrraten, bei denen Fructose den Serumharnsäurewert noch nicht verändert.

Normalerweise verhalten sich die Serumkonzentrationen von Harnsäure und anorganischem Phosphat während einer mehrstündigen intravenösen Infusion von 1,5 g/kg und Std Fructose spiegelbildlich: Einem anfänglichen Harnsäureanstieg entspricht ein Phosphatabfall. Am Ende der Infusion fällt die Harnsäurekonzentration ab, und der Phosphatspiegel steigt an. Ein derartiges Verhalten kann aber nur bei einem Teil der Gichtpatienten beobachtet werden (HEUCKENKAMP et al., 1972), selbst wenn die Harnsäureausscheidung der Gichtiker nicht unterschiedlich von derjenigen Gesunder ist. Die Serumkonzentration von anorganischem Phosphat ändert sich während der Fructoseinfusion bei Gichtkranken nicht, und bei ausgeprägter Hyperuricämie zeigt auch der Harnsäurewert keine Änderung. — Bis 30 min nach Beendigung einer Infusion von 5 ml/min einer 10%igen Xylitlösung fällt die Serumkonzentration von anorganischem Phosphor gegenüber den Kontrollen ab, um sich anschließend zu normalisieren (vgl. Abb. 6). Diese Reaktion spiegelt wahrscheinlich ein vorübergehendes Festlegen von Phosphat in phosphorylierten Zwischenstufen und danach eine zur Aufrechterhaltung der Homoiostase reaktiv einsetzende Freisetzung von anorganischem Phosphat aus dem gebundenen Zustand wider (MERTZ et al., 1972a).

Da renale Mechanismen oder eine Ausschwemmung von Harnsäure vom intra- in den extracellulären Raum ausscheiden (PERHEENTUPA u. RAIVIO, 1967),

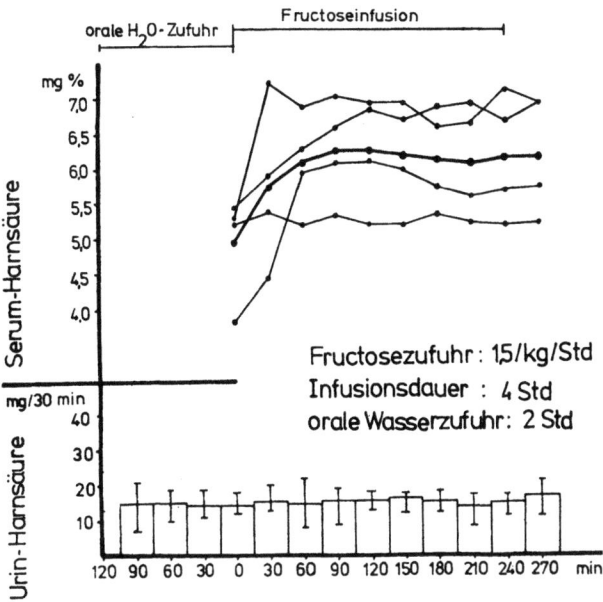

Abb. 5. Verhalten von Serumharnsäurekonzentration und Harnsäureausscheidung im Urin während i.v. Infusion von 1,5 g Fructose/kg Körpergewicht und Std. (Nach HEUCKENKAMP et al., 1971)

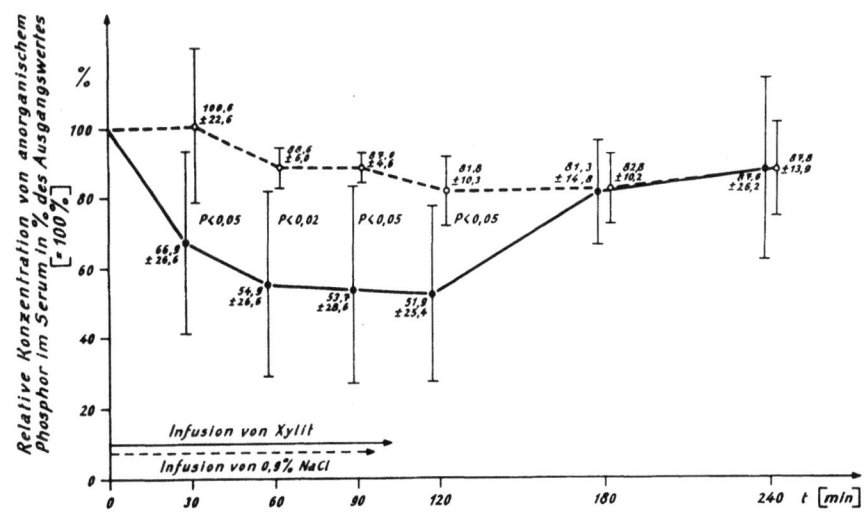

Abb. 6. Verhalten der Serumkonzentration von anorganischem Phosphor unter der akuten Wirkung einer i.v. Infusion von 5 ml/min einer 10%igen Xylitlösung. (Nach MERTZ et al., 1972a)

kommt hierfür eine Mehrproduktion von Harnsäure in Betracht. Aus einem Abfall der ATP-Konzentration, der Menge an Adeninnucleotiden und des anorganischen Phosphatgehaltes in der Leber von Ratten nach Fructosebelastung wurde auf einen beschleunigten Abbau von präformierten Purinkörpern geschlossen. MÄENPÄÄ et al. (1968) sowie RAIVIO et al. (1969) machten dafür eine Enthemmung der Adenyldesaminase durch einen intracellulär stark absinkenden anorganischen Phosphatspiegel und eine von Inosin aus weitergehende Spaltung und Oxy-

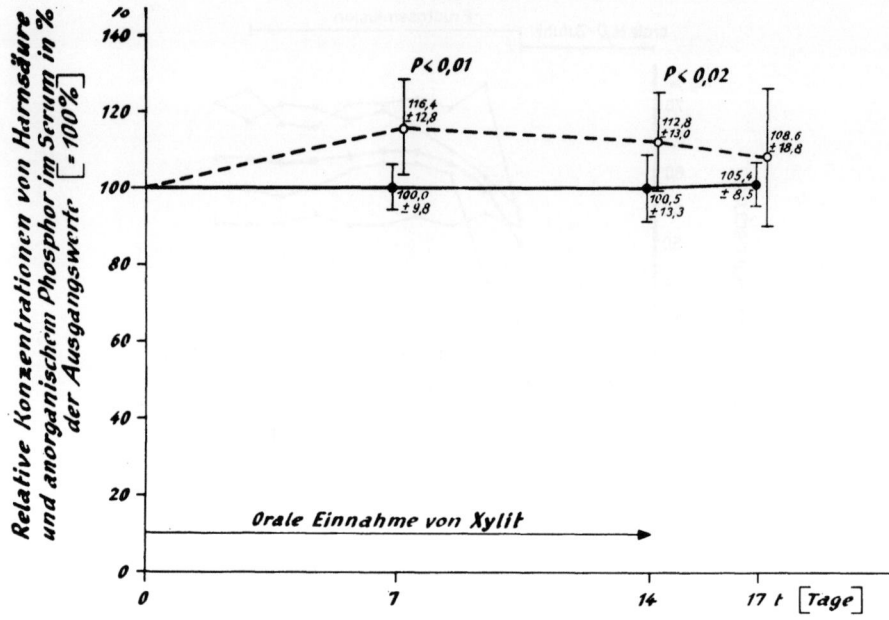

Abb. 7. Verhalten der Serumkonzentrationen von Harnsäure (———) und anorganischem Phosphor (- - - -) unter der Wirkung einer oralen Gabe von 15—50 g/Tag Xylit. (Nach MERTZ et al., 1972b) (Nach MERTZ u. SCHWOERER, 1969)

dation von Purinnucleotiden verantwortlich. Diese Deutung hat jedoch an Tragfähigkeit verloren. Zumindest stehen dieser Theorie die adaptiv gestiegenen Serumkonzentrationen von anorganischem Phosphat (vgl. Abb. 7) gegenüber (MERTZ et al., 1972b). Vielmehr ist einer Deutung im Sinne einer vermehrten De-novo-Synthese der Vorzug zu geben, wonach die während Fructose- (vgl. Abb. 5) oder Xylitbelastung auftretende Hyperuricämie durch einen erhöhten Nucleinsäurenumsatz in der Leber induziert wird (HEUCKENKAMP et al., 1971). Möglicherweise kommt es bei Gabe von Xylit und in geringerem Maße unter der Zufuhr von Fructose zu einer Anhäufung von Ribosephosphat, wodurch die Neubildung von Harnsäure über einen vermehrten Anfall von Phosphoribosylphosphat gesteigert wird.

Ein akuter Anstieg der Serumharnsäurekonzentration kann auch durch *orale Applikation von Fructose, Sorbit und Xylit* sowie von *Saccharose*, dagegen nicht durch Zufuhr von Glucose oder Galaktose (auch bei intravenöser Infusion) hervorgerufen werden (FÖRSTER, 1972), wobei sich Xylit am wirksamsten erweist (FÖRSTER u. ZIEGE, 1971). Schon nach einer oralen Gabe von nur 12,5 g Xylit wurde eine Steigerung der Serumharnsäurekonzentration festgestellt, während hierzu 25—50 g Fructose oder Sorbit bzw. mehr als 100 g Saccharose als Einzeldosis erforderlich waren. Umgekehrt nimmt die Serumharnsäurekonzentration unter saccharosearmer Ernährung etwa um 0,5 mg/100 ml ab. Der akute Serumharnsäureanstieg nach Verabreichung der Zuckeraustauschstoffe ist nicht besorgniserregend (ausgenommen bei Gichtkranken, die unbehandelt sind), der er nach oraler Applikation nur bei Dosierungen auftritt, die ohnehin bei Verwendung als Süßungsmittel oder Zuckeraustauschmittel kaum angewandt werden. Während mittellangfristiger oraler Aufnahme von 50 g Xylit täglich unter Konstanthaltung des Körpergewichtes blieb dagegen die Serumharnsäurekonzentration unverändert (MERTZ et al., 1972b). Hierbei muß die Tatsache berücksichtigt werden, daß eine intakte renale Harnsäureausscheidung eine Rolle spielt und ein Kohlenhydrataustausch, jedoch keine absolute Xylit-Wirkung eingetreten ist (vgl. Abb. 7). Im akuten Experiment erfolgt nach oraler Verabreichung von 50 g Xylit in 400 ml Leitungswasser innerhalb von 30 min ein signifikanter Anstieg der Serumharnsäurekonzentration um 0,5—2,5 mg/100 ml, der bis 4 Std nach Zufuhr nachweisbar ist (FÖRSTER u. ZIEGE, 1971). Die von FÖRSTER u. ZIEGE vorgelegten Befunde stehen zu den Ergebnissen von MERTZ et al. (1972b) keineswegs im Widerspruch, da sich die hyperuricämisierende Wirkung von tagsüber verzehrtem Xylit über Nacht wieder ausgleicht und somit im morgens abgenommenen Nüchternserum nicht mehr in Erscheinung tritt.

FOX u. KELLEY (1972) sahen die durch Fructose induzierte Hyperuricämie und Zunahme der renalen Ausscheidung von Harnsäure und Oxypurinen als Ergebnis eines gesteigerten Abbaus von Purinnucleotiden an. Als hauptsächliche Stütze ihrer Auffassung diente der Nachweis, daß es beim Menschen unter rascher intravenöser Infusion von Fructose zu einem Abfall der in den Erythrocyten bestimmten Konzentrationen von PRPP und Ribose-5-Phosphat ohne meßbare Änderung der ATP-Konzentration kommt. Im Falle einer vermehrten Neubildung von Harnsäure hätten die Konzentrationen von PRPP und des Präkursors Ribose-5-Phosphat ansteigen müssen. Die genannte These kann jedoch keineswegs auf die durch Xylit induzierte Hyperuricämie, die noch rascher als diejenige nach Fructose auftritt, übertragen werden, da Xylit im Gegensatz zu Fructose (MÄENPÄÄ et al., 1968; RAIVIO et al., 1969) den Katabolismus von Purinnucleotiden nicht beschleunigt.

Bekanntlich kontrollieren Adenyl- und Guanylribonucleotide sowie Ribonucleotide der Inosinsäure auf dem Wege einer Rückkopplung (WYNGAARDEN u. ASHTON, 1959) die Aktivität des Schlüsselenzyms der Purinneubildung, nämlich von PRPP-Amidotransferase (=Glutamin-PP-Ribose-P-Amidotransferase). Stehen diese Ribonucleotide in verminderter Konzentration zur Verfügung, dann ergibt sich eine vermehrte De-novo-Biosynthese von Purinen. Dieser Rückkopplungsmechanismus spielt auch bezüglich der durch Fructose induzierten Hyperuricämie eine Rolle. Neuere Untersuchungen von NARINS et al. (1974) bestätigen die Ansicht, daß Fructose beim Menschen eine Hyperuricämie durch Erhöhung der Umwandlung von vorgebildeten Purinnucleotiden in Harnsäure hervorruft und gleichzeitig die De-novo-Biosynthese von Purin hemmt. Tierexperimente zeigen, daß die rasche Phosphorylierung der Fructose durch die Rattenleber zu einer Verarmung des Gewebes an ATP und anorganischem Phosphat führt (RAIVIO et al., 1969; WOODS et al., 1970). Es kommt zu einer frühzeitigen und anhaltenden Erhöhung des Gehaltes an IMP und einem späteren Anstieg der Konzentration von anorganischem Phosphat in der Leber. Beide Stoffe sind als Inhibitoren von PRPP-Amidotransferase bekannt (WYNGAARDEN u. ASHTON, 1959; HOLMES et al., 1973). Die auf Grund eines Mangels an ATP und anorganischem Phosphat auftretende Enthemmung der 5'-Nucleotidase und Adenosindesaminase befähigt die Leber, mehr Harnsäure aus präformierten Purinnucleotiden zu bilden. Gegen die Möglichkeit einer vermehrten Harnsäurebildung durch Fructose spricht auch der rasche Anstieg der Serumharnsäurekonzentration innerhalb von 15 Minuten nach Beginn einer Fructosebelastung.

Hyperuricämie durch diätetische Maßnahmen

Bei totalem Fasten nimmt die Harnsäurekonzentration im Serum infolge einer Verminderung der renalen Clearance progressiv zu (LENNOX, 1924, 1925; MORGULIS u. EDWARDS, 1924; MURPHY u. SHIPMAN, 1963; CRISTOFORI u. DUN-

CAN, 1964). Die Retention von Harnsäure verschwindet nach Unterbrechung des Fastens, so daß CRISTOFORI u. DUNCAN (1964) Gicht nicht als Kontraindikation für eine 14tägige totale Fastenkur ansahen. THOMPSON et al. (1966) berichteten über Erfolge mit einer totalen Fastenkur bis zu 249 Tagen, wobei lediglich unbegrenzte Mengen kalorienfreier Getränke (Wasser, Tee, Kaffee) und ein Multivitamin-Präparat eingenommen werden durften. Die mit dem totalen Fasten erzielte Gewichtsabnahme betrug maximal 44 kg in 236 Tagen. Die Fastenkur wurde gut toleriert. Bei allen Kranken stellten sich eine Ketonurie von schwankender Größenordnung sowie ein Anstieg der Serumharnsäurekonzentration ein, ohne daß es zu manifesten Erscheinungen einer Gicht gekommen wäre. Eine gestörte Glucosetoleranz während längeren Fastens findet sich bei über 20jährigen Kranken (SUSSMAN, 1966). Diese Störung der Glucosetoleranz beruht aller Wahrscheinlichkeit nach auf einem peripheren Antagonismus gegenüber der Glucoseverwertung im Muskel und nicht auf einer unzureichenden Insulinsekretion. Nach der Fastenkur wurden erhöhte Serumwerte für unveresterte Fettsäuren gefunden.

Als verantwortlicher Faktor für die Harnsäureretention kommt eine metabolische Acidose vermutlich nicht in Betracht, da fastende Personen durch Zufuhr von Bicarbonat nicht vermehrt Harnsäure ausscheiden (LENNOX, 1925). Wichtig erscheint die Ketose (LENNOX, 1925; MURPHY u. SHIPMAN, 1963). Bei experimenteller Ketonämie besteht eine umgekehrte Beziehung zwischen der renalen Harnsäureausscheidung und der Plasmakonzentration von Ketonkörpern (QUICK, 1932; SCOTT et al., 1964; CHEIFETZ, 1965). Die Tatsache, daß die bei Fasten (MORGULIS u. EDWARDS, 1924; LENNOX, 1924; CRISTOFORI u. DUNCAN, 1964) sowie bei fettreicher und kohlenhydratarmer Kost (LOCKIE u. HUBBARD, 1935) auftretende Hyperuricämie durch Zufuhr von Glucose beseitigt werden kann, zeigt die Bedeutung des Kohlenhydratstoffwechsels bei diesen Veränderungen auf.

Unter ketogener Diät steigt der Serumharnsäurewert wesentlich stärker als bei Fasten an. SCHMIDT et al. (1969) stellten nach mehrtägiger Verabfolgung einer ketogenen 1000 Calorien-Diät bei acht adipösen Patienten eine Zunahme der Harnsäurekonzentration von $7{,}71 \pm 1{,}40$ mg/100 ml Serum in der Vorperiode auf $15{,}75 \pm 4{,}24$ mg/100 ml Serum fest. Gleichzeitig stieg die Serumkonzentration von β-Hydroxybuttersäure um mehr als das Zwölffache ($11{,}3 \pm 2{,}6$ gegenüber $0{,}9 \pm 0{,}1$ mg/100 ml) und diejenige von Acetessigsäure um mehr als das Fünffache ($2{,}45 \pm 0{,}71$ gegenüber $0{,}47 \pm 0{,}24$ mg/100 ml) ihres Ausgangswertes. Eine Korrelation zwischen dem Anstieg der Ketosäuren und der Gewichtsabnahme ließ sich nicht nachweisen. Verglichen mit einer 1000 Calorien-Mischkost unter Einhaltung von zwei Fastentagen wöchentlich bot eine isocalorische ketogene Diät keine Vorteile hinsichtlich Schnelligkeit und Dauerhaftigkeit einer Gewichtsabnahme.

ARKY u. FREINKEL (1964) fanden einen Rückgang der Ketoacidose bei jugendlichen Diabetikern unter der Wirkung von Äthylalkohol und vermuten als Ursache eine Hemmung der Gluconeogenese und Ketogenese durch den Alkohol. Es handelt sich dabei offenbar um eine kurzdauernde Erscheinung. MACLACHLAN u. RODNAN (1967) beobachteten bei Fasten am Morgen des zweiten Tages eine Hemmung des Konzentrationsanstieges von β-Hydroxybuttersäure im Serum, wenn Alkohol getrunken wurde. Bei fortgesetztem Fasten stieg die Serumkonzentration von β-Hydroxybuttersäure übermäßig schnell an, so daß am Morgen des folgenden Fastentages der Serumgehalt dieses Stoffes höher als am Ende eines zweitägigen Fastens ohne Alkoholzufuhr war. Entsprechend verhielten sich die Harnsäurewerte. Wenn Alkohol die Gluconeogenese tatsächlich hemmen sollte, dann ist die Vermehrung der Serumkonzentration von β-Hydroxybuttersäure als Ergebnis eines vermehrten Fettabbaues nach Verarmung an Leberglykogen aufzufassen.

Hyperurikämie durch respiratorische Acidose

Therapeutische Maßnahmen, die eine respiratorische Acidose hervorrufen können, wie Narkose, führen ebenfalls zu einer beträchtlichen Hyperurikämie (Isomäki u. Kreus, 1968) infolge verminderter renaler Ausscheidung von Harnsäure. Nach den bis jetzt vorliegenden Untersuchungen kann die Möglichkeit einer Mehrproduktion von Harnsäure allerdings nicht sicher ausgeschlossen werden. Bei einer Kohlensäurespannung (pCO_2) von 106 mm Hg wurde ein Harnsäurespiegel von 11,2 mg/100 ml Serum beobachtet. Nach Abfall der Kohlensäurespannung im Blut nahm die Harnsäureausscheidung zu, und die Hyperurikämie verschwand im Verlaufe weniger Tage völlig. Respiratorische Acidose selber führt — unabhängig von ihrer Genese — zu Hyperurikämie.

Verschiedenes

Pyrazinamid (Yü et al., 1961) und Benzoesäure (Quick, 1932) können ebenfalls eine Hyperurikämie durch verminderte renale Harnsäureexkretion hervorrufen. Aus tierexperimentellen Studien (Davis et al., 1965) wird geschlossen, daß Pyrazinamid die tubuläre Sekretion von Harnsäure hemmt.

Literatur

Alpert, N. R.: Lactate production and removal and the regulation of metabolism. Ann. N.Y. Acad. Sci. **119**, 995 (1965).
Arky, R. A., Freinkel, N.: Alcohol hypoglycemia. Arch. intern. Med. **114**, 501 (1964).
Aronoff, A.: Acute gouty arthritis precipitated by chlorothiazide. New Engl. J. Med. **262**, 767 (1960).
Aronoff, A., Barkum, H.: Hyperuricemia and acute gouty arthritis precipitated by thiazide derivates. Canad. med. Ass. J. **84**, 1181 (1961).
Ayvazian, J. H., Ayvazian, L. F.: A study of the hyperuricemia induced by hydrochlorothiazide and acetazolamide separately and in combination. J. clin. Invest. **40**, 1961 (1961).
Bernheim, C.: Goutte et diabète. Schweiz. med. Wschr. **98**, 327 (1968).
Borhani, N. O.: Chlorothiazide and hydrochlorothiazide: A comparative study of their hypotensive, saluretic, and hyperuricemic action. Ann. intern. Med. **53**, 342 (1960).
Breckenridge, A.: Hypertension and hyperuricaemia. Lancet **1966 I**, 15.
Brest, A. N., Heider, C., Mehbod, H., Onesti, G.: Drug control of diuretic-induced hyperuricemia. J. Amer. med. Ass. **195**, 42 (1966).
Brøchner-Mortensen, K., Cobb, S., Rose, B. S.: Report subcommittee on criteria for the diagnosis of gout in surveys. In: Kellgren, J. H., Jeffrey, M. R., Ball, J. (Eds.): The epidemiology of chronic rheumatism, Vol. 1, pp. 295—297. Philadelphia: F. A. Davis 1963.
Bryant, J. M., Yu, T. F., Berger, L., Schvartz, N., Torosdag, S., Fletcher, L., Fertig, H., Schwartz, S., Quan, R. B. F.: Hyperuricemia induced by the administration of chlorthalidone and other sulfonamide diuretics. Amer. J. Med. **33**, 408 (1962).
Burch, R. E., Kurke, N.: The effect of lactate infusion on serum uric acid. Proc. Soc. exp. Biol. (N.Y.) **127**, 17 (1968).
Cannon, P. J., Stason, W. B., Demartini, F. E., Sommers, S. C., Laragh, J. H.: Hyperuricemia in primary and renal hypertension. New Engl. J. Med. **275**, 457 (1966).
Cheifetz, P. N.: Uric acid excretion and ketosis in fasting. Metabolism **14**, 1267 (1965).
Cristofori, F. C., Duncan, G. G.: Uric acid excretion in obese subjects during periods of total fasting. Metabolism **13**, 303 (1964).
Davis, B. B., Field, J. B., Rodnan, G. P., Kedes, L. H.: Localization and pyrazinamide inhibition of distal transtubular movement of uric acid-2-C^{14} with a modified stop-flow technique. J. clin. Invest. **44**, 716 (1965).

DEMARTINI, F. E.: Effect of chlorothiazide on uric acid excretion. Bull. rheum. Dis. **10**, 195 (1959).
DEMARTINI, F. E., WHEATON, E. A., HEALEY, L. A., LARAGH, J. H.: Effect of chlorothiazide on the renal excretion of uric acid. Amer. J. Med. **32**, 572 (1962).
DOLLERY, C. T., DUNCAN, H., SCHUMER, B.: Hyperuricaemia related to treatment of hypertension. Brit. med. J. **1960 II**, 832.
DREYFUSS, F.: The role of hyperuricemia in coronary heart disease. Dis. Chest **38**, 332 (1960).
DUNN, J. P., BROOKS, G. W., MAUSNER, J., RODNAN, G. P., COBB, S.: Social class gradient of serum uric acid levels in males. J. Amer. med. Ass. **185**, 431 (1963).
FAUVEL, P.: Mode d'action du salicylate de soude sur l'excretion urique. C. R. Acad. Sci. (Paris) **144**, 932 (1907).
FÖRSTER, H.: Grundlagen für die Verwendung der drei Zuckeraustauschstoffe Fructose, Sorbit und Xylit. Medizin u. Ernähr. **13**, 7 (1972).
FÖRSTER, H., MEHNERT, H.: Fructose induced hyperuricemia. Lancet **1967 II**, 1205.
FÖRSTER, H., MEHNERT, H., ALHOUG, I.: Anstieg der Serumharnsäure nach Fructose. Klin. Wschr. **45**, 436 (1967).
FÖRSTER, H., MEYER, E., ZIEGE, M.: Erhöhung von Serumharnsäure und Serumbilirubin nach hochdosierten Infusionen von Sorbit, Xylit und Fructose. Klin. Wschr. **48**, 878 (1970).
FÖRSTER, H., ZIEGE, M.: Anstieg der Serumharnsäurekonzentration nach oraler Zufuhr von Fructose, Sorbit und Xylit. Z. Ernährungsw. **10**, 394 (1971).
FOX, I. H., KELLEY, W. N.: Studies on the mechanism of fructose-induced hyperuricemia in man. Metabolism **21**, 713 (1972).
FREIS, E. D., SAPPINGTON, R. F.: Long-term effect of probenecid on diuretic-induced hyperuricemia. J. Amer. med. Ass. **198**, 127 (1966).
GAARDER, A. M., JONSEN, J., LALAND, S., HELLEM, A. J., OWREN, P. A.: Adenosine diphosphate in red cells as a factor in the adhesiveness of human blood platelets. Nature **192**, 531 (1961).
GERTLER, M. M., WHITE, P. D., CADY, L. D., WHITIER, H. H.: Coronary heart disease, a prospective study. Amer. J. med. Sci. **248**, 377 (1964).
GIBSON, H. V., DOISY, E. A.: A note on the effect of some organic acids upon the uric acid excretion of man. J. biol. Chem. **55**, 605 (1923).
GRAYZEL, A. I., LIDDLE, L., SEEGMILLER, J. E.: Diagnostic significance of hyperuricemia in arthritis. New Engl. J. Med. **265**, 763 (1961).
GROSS, A., GIRARD, V.: Über die Wirkung von Benzbromaron auf Urikämie und Urikosurie. Med. Welt (Stuttg.) **23**, 133 (1972).
GUTMAN, A. B., YU, T. F.: Benemid(p-[di-n-propylsulfamyl]-benzoic acid) as uricosuric agent in chronic gouty arthritis. Trans. Ass. Amer. Phycns. **64**, 279 (1951).
GUTMAN, A. B., YU, T. F., SIROTA, J. H.: Contrasting effects of bicarbonate and diamox, with equivalent alkalinization of the urine, on salicylate uricosuria in man. Fed. Proc. **15**, 85 (1956).
HALL, A. P., BARRY, P. E., DAWBER, T. R., MCNAMARA, P. M.: Epidemiology of gout and hyperuricemia. Amer. J. Med. **42**, 27 (1967).
HANSEN, O. E.: Acute gouty arthritis provoked by cerebrovascular disease. Acta med. scand. **178**, 423 (1965).
HAUGE, M., HARVALD, B.: Heredity in gout and hyperuricemia. Acta med. scand. **152**, 247 (1955).
HAVARD, C. W. H.: Diuretic action of triamterene in man. Minerva med. **54** (81, Suppl.), 2997 (1962).
HEALEY, L. A., MAGID, G. J., DECKER, J. L.: Uric acid retention due to hydrochlorothiazide. New Engl. J. Med. **261**, 1358 (1959).
HEATH, W. C., FREIS, E. D.: Triamterene with hydrochlorothiazide in the treatment of hypertension. J. Amer. med. Ass. **186**, 119 (1963).
HEIDLAND, A., KLÜTSCH, K., MOORMANN, A.: Zur renalen Kalium-Retention nach Verabfolgung von Amilorid-HCl. Arzneimittel-Forsch. **17**, 1314 (1967).
HEIMSOTH, V., HARTMANN, F.: Untersuchungen zur Störung des Harnsäurestoffwechsels nach Saluretica-Verabreichung. Dtsch. med. Wschr. **90**, 1905 (1965).
HEUCKENKAMP, P.-U., HAGEN, K., MAHRENHOLZ, U., ZÖLLNER, N.: Vergleichende Untersuchungen des Harnsäure- und Phosphatspiegels bei Gesunden und Patienten mit manifester Gicht während mehrstündiger i.v. Fructosezufuhr. Verh. dtsch. Ges. inn. Med. **78**, 1326 (1972).
HEUCKENKAMP, P.-U., SCHILL, K., ZÖLLNER, N.: Zum Mechanismus des Serumharnsäureanstiegs unter konstanter Fructoseinfusion beim Menschen. Verh. dtsch. Ges. inn. Med. **77**, 177 (1971).
HEUCKENKAMP, P.-U., ZÖLLNER, N.: Xylitbilanz während mehrstündiger Infusionen mit konstanten Zufuhrraten bei gesunden Menschen. Klin. Wschr. **50**, 1063 (1972).

HITZENBERGER, G., KAMPFFMEYER, H., CONWAY, J.: The diuretic effect of desmethyl-pipazuroyl-guanidine (MK-870) in man. Clin. Pharmacol. Ther. **9**, 71 (1968).
HOLLANDER, W., WILKINS, R. W.: The pharmacology and clinical use of rauwolfia, hydralazine, thiazides, and aldosterone antagonists in arterial hypertension. Progr. cardiovasc. Dis. **8**, 291 (1966).
HOLMES, E. W., MCDONALD, J. A., MCCORD, J. M., WYNGAARDEN, J. B., KELLEY, W. N.: Human glutamine phosphoribosylpyrophosphate amidotransferase. J. biol. Chem. **248**, 144 (1973).
MIsomäki, H., Kreus, K.-E.: Serum and urinary uric acid in respiratory acidosis. Acta med. scand. **184**, 293 (1968).
ITSKOVITZ, H. D., SELLERS, A. M.: Gout and hyperuricemia after adrenalectomy for hypertension. New Engl. J. Med. **268**, 1105 (1963).
JAHNECKE, J.: Hochdruck, Saluretica und Glucosetoleranz. Dtsch. med. Wschr. **92**, 1270 (1967).
JOHNSON, H. K., WATERHOUSE, C.: Relationship of alcohol and hyperlactatemia in diabetic subjects treated with phenformin. Amer. J. Med. **45**, 98 (1968).
KAHN, P. M., PROZAN, G. B.: Hyperuricemia-relationship to hypercholesterinemia and acute myocardial infarction. J. Amer. med. Ass. **170**, 1909 (1959).
KELLEY, W. N., ROSENBLOOM, F. M., SEEGMILLER, J. E., HOWELL, R.: Excessive production of uric acid in type I glycogen storage disease. J. Pediat. **72**, 488 (1968).
KERSLEY, G. D., COOK, E. R., TOVEY, D. C. J.: Value of uricosuric agents and in particular of G-28315 in gout. Ann. rheum. Dis. **17**, 326 (1958).
KINSEY, D., WALTHER, R., SISE, H. S., WITHLAW, G., SMITHWICK, R.: Incidence of hyperuricemia in 400 hypertensive patients. Circulation **24**, 972 (1961).
KLEMPERER, F., BAUER, W.: Influence of aspirin on urate excretion. J. clin. Invest. **23**, 950 (1944).
KRAKOFF, J. H., BALIS, M. E.: Studies of the uricogenic effect of 2-substituted thiadiazoles in man. J. clin. Invest. **38**, 907 (1959).
KRAMER, D. W., PERILSTEIN, P. K., DE MEDEIROS, A.: Metabolic influences in vascular disorders with particular reference to cholesterol determinations in comparison with uric acid levels. Angiology **9**, 162 (1958).
KRITZLER, R. A.: Anuria complicating treatment of leukemia. Amer. J. Med. **25**, 532 (1958).
LANESE, R. R., GRESHAM, G. E., KELLER, M. D.: Behavioral and physiological characteristics in hyperuricemia. J. Amer. med. Ass. **207**, 1878 (1969).
LARAGH, J. H., HEINEMANN, H. O., DEMARTINI, F. E.: Effect of chlorothiazide on electrolyte transport in man. Its use in the treatment of edema in congestive heart failure, nephrosis, and cirrhosis. J. Amer. med. Ass. **166**, 145 (1958).
LENNOX, W. G.: Increase of uric acid in the blood during prolonged starvation. J. Amer. med. Ass. **82**, 602 (1924).
LENNOX, W. G.: A study of the retention of uric acid during fasting. J. biol. Chem. **66**, 521 (1925).
LIEBER, S. L., DAVIDSON, C. S.: Some metabolic effects of ethyl alcohol. Amer. J. Med. **33**, 319 (1962).
LIEBER, S. L., JONES, D. P., LOSOWSKY, M. S., DAVIDSON, C. S.: Interrelation of uric acid and ethanol metabolism in man. J. clin. Invest. **41**, 1863 (1962).
LOCKIE, L. M., HUBBARD, R. S.: Gout: Changes in symptoms and purine metabolism produced in high fat diets in four gouty patients. J. Amer. med. Ass. **104**, 2072 (1935).
LUCKE, H.: Beiträge zur Physiologie und Pathologie des menschlichen Harnsäurestoffwechsels. IX. Die Bewertung der enterotropischen Harnsäure für die Regulation des menschlichen endogenen Harnsäure-Stoffwechsels. Z. ges. exp. Med. **76**, 188 (1931).
MACLACHLAN, M. J., RODNAN, G. P.: Effects of food, fast and alcohol on serum uric acid and acute attacks of gout. Amer. J. Med. **42**, 38 (1967).
MARTIN, J. H., GORDON, M., WALLACE, R.: Methotrexate in psoriasis. Precipitation of gout. Arch. Derm. **96**, 431 (1967).
MCCARTHY, D. D., OGRYZLO, M. A.: Effects of fasting on uric acid excretion by the kidney. In: Proc. of the second Canadian conf. on research in rheumatic diseases, pp. 76—79. Toronto 1961. The Canadian arthritis and rheumatism Soc.
MÄENPÄÄ, P. H., RAIVIO, K. O., KEKOMÄKI, M. P.: Liver adenine nucleotides: Fructose-induced depletion and its effect on protein synthesis. Science **161**, 1253 (1968).
MERTZ, D. P.: Pharmakologische Eigenschaften von Hydrochlorothiazid im Vergleich zur Wirkung anderer Diuretica. Naunyn Schmiedebergs Arch. exp. Path. Pharmak. **237**, 71 (1959).
MERTZ, D. P.: Gicht und Hyperuricämie. Arch. klin. Med. **212**, 143 (1966). — Erweiterte und überarbeitete Fassung. Boehringer/Mannheim 1967.

Mertz, D. P.: Veränderungen der Serumkonzentration von Harnsäure unter der Wirkung von Benzbromaronum. Münch. med. Wschr. **111**, 491 (1969).

Mertz, D. P., Kaiser, V., Klöpfer-Zaar, M., Beisbarth, H.: Fett- und Harnsäurestoffwechsel unter der akuten Wirkung von Xylit. Klin. Wschr. **50**, 1097 (1972a).

Mertz, D. P., Kaiser, V., Klöpfer-Zaar, M., Beisbarth, H.: Serumkonzentrationen verschiedener Lipide und von Harnsäure während 2wöchiger Verabreichung von Xylit. Klin. Wschr. **50**, 1107 (1972b).

Mertz, D. P., Schwoerer, P.: Renale Ausscheidung von Natrium und Harnsäure bei arterieller Hypertonie unter der akuten Wirkung von Saluretica. Klin. Wschr. **47**, 109 (1969).

Mikkelsen, W. M., Dodge, H. J., Valkenburg, H.: The distribution of serum uric acid values in a population unselected as to gout or hyperuricemia. Amer. J. Med. **39**, 242 (1965).

Moore, C. B., Weiss, T. E.: Uric acid metabolism and myocardial infarction. In: James, T. N., Keyes, W. (Eds.): The etiology of myocardial infarction. Henry Ford Hospital international symposium, p. 459. Boston: Little, Brown 1963.

Morgulis, S., Edwards, A. C.: Chemical changes in the blood during fasting and subsequent refeeding. Amer. J. Physiol. **68**, 477 (1924).

Morin, Y., Turmel, L., Fortier, J.: Triamterene: Clinical studies in arterial hypertension. Amer. Heart J. **69**, 195 (1965).

Mudge, G. H., Cucchi, J., Platts, M., Brian O'Connell, J. M., Berndt, W. O.: Renal excretion of uric acid in the dog. Amer. J. Physiol. **215**, 404 (1968).

Muggia, F. M., Ball, T. J., Ultmann, J. E.: Allopurinol in the treatment of neoplastic disease complicated by hyperuricemia. Arch. intern. Med. **120**, 12 (1967).

Murphy, R., Shipman, K. H.: Hyperuricemia during total fasting. Arch. intern. Med. **112**, 954 (1963).

Mustard, J. F., Murphy, E. A., Ogryzlo, M. A., Smythe, H. A.: Blood coagulation and platelet economy in subjects with primary gout. Canad. med. Ass. J. **89**, 1207 (1963).

Narins, R. G., Weisberg, J. S., Myers, A. R.: Effects of carbohydrates on uric acid metabolism. Metaboslism **23**, 455 (1974).

Newland, H.: AntagonismAmer. J. med. Sci. **256**, 44 (1968).

Nordöy, A., Chandler, A. B.: Platelet thrombosis induced by adenosine diphosphate in the rat. Scand. J. Haemat. **1**, 16 (1964).

Oren, B. G., Rich, M., Belle, M. S.: Chlorothiazide (diuril) as a hyperuricacidemic agent. J. Amer. med. Ass. **168**, 2128 (1958).

Perheentupa, J., Raivio, K.: Fructose-induced hyperuricemia. Lancet **1967 II**, 528.

Podevin, R., Paillard, F., Amiel, C., Richet, G.: Action de la benziodarone sur l'excrétion rénale de l'acide urique. Rev. franç. Étud. clin. biol. **12**, 361 (1967).

Popert, A. J., Hewitt, J. V.: Gout and hyperuricemia in rural and urban populations. Ann. rheum. Dis. **21**, 154 (1962).

Quick, A. J.: The relationship between chemical structure and physiological response. III. Factors influencing the excretion of uric acid. J. biol. Chem. **98**, 157 (1932).

Quick, A. J.: The effect of exercise on the excretion of uric acid with a note on the influence of benzoic acid on uric acid elimination in liver diseases J. biol. Chem. **110**, 107 (1935).

Raivio, K. O., Kekomäki, M. P., Mäenpää, P. H.: Depletion of liver adenine nucleotides induced by D-fructose. Dose-dependence and specifity of the fructose effect. Biochem. Pharmacol. **18**, 2615 (1969).

Reem, G. H., Vanamee, P.: Effect of sodium lactate on urate clearance in the Dalmatian and in the mongrel. Amer. J. Physiol. **207**, 113 (1964).

Reutter, F., Schaub, F.: Harnsäurestoffwechsel und Salidiuretika. Dtsch. med. Wschr. **89**, 1101 (1964).

Sahebjami, H., Scalettar, R.: Effects of fructose infusion on lactate and uric acid metabolism. Lancet **1971 I**, 366.

Sarre, H., Mertz, D. P.: Sekundäre Gicht bei Niereninsuffizienz. Klin. Wschr. **43**, 1134 (1965).

Schirmeister, J., Man, N. K., Hallauer, W.: Lactat- und Harnsäureretention nach oralen Diuretikagaben beim Menschen. Klin. Wschr. **45**, 1219 (1967a).

Schirmeister, J., Man, N. K., Hallauer, W.: Zum Mechanismus des Blutlactatanstiegs nach Diuretikagaben. Klin. Wschr. **46**, 1062 (1968).

Schirmeister, J., Man, N. K., Warning, D., Hallauer, W.: Zur Frage der extrarenalen Ursache einer Harnsäureretention nach Furosemid. Verh. Dtsch. Ges. inn. Med. **73**, 1025 (1967b).

SCHIRMEISTER, J., WILLMANN, H.: Über die Harnsäure- und andere Clearances nach intravenöser Gabe von Furosemid beim Menschen. Klin. Wschr. **42**, 623 (1964).

SCHMIDT, H., JANIK, I., VOIGT, K.-D.: Auswirkungen einer ketogenen Kost auf das Körpergewicht, den Intermediär- und Elektrolytstoffwechsel von Adipösen. Dtsch. med. Wschr. **94**, 78 (1969).

SCHRADE, W., BÖHLE, E., BIEGLER, R.: Humoral changes in arteriosclerosis. Lancet **1960 II**, 1409.

SCOTT, J. T., MCCALLUM, F. M., HOLLOWAY, V. P.: Starvation, ketosis and uric acid excretion. Clin. Sci. **27**, 209 (1964).

SORENSEN, L. B.: Degradation of uric acid in man. Metabolism **8**, 687 (1959).

SORENSEN, L. B.: Role of the intestinal tract in the elimination of uric acid. Arthr. and Rheum. **8**, 694 (1965).

STANBURY, J. G., WYNGAARDEN, J. B., FRERICKSON, D. S.: The metabolic basis of inherited disease, p. 725. New York: Mc Graw-Hill 1960.

STEELE, T. H., RIESELBACH, R. E.: The renal mechanism for urate homeostasis in normal man. Amer. J. Med. **43**, 868 (1967).

SUSSMAN, K. E.: Effect of prolonged fasting on glucose and insulin metabolism in exogenous obesity. Arch. intern. Med. **117**, 343 (1966).

TALBOTT, J. H.: Gout, 2nd Ed. New York: Grune & Stratton 1964.

THOMPSON, R. A., CROWLEY, M. F.: Trial of a triamterene-benzthiazide combination (Dytide). Postgrad. med. J. **41**, 706 (1965).

THOMPSON, T. J., RUNCIE, J., MILLER, V.: Treatment of obesity by total fasting for up to 249 days. Lancet **1966 II**, 992.

TSALOFF, V., LESTINA, F.: Gout after chlorothiazide therapy. Quart. Bull. Northw. Univ. med. Sch. **34**, 254 (1960).

WARSHAW, L. J.: Acute attacks of gout precipitated by chlorothiazide-induced diuresis. J. Amer. med. Ass. **172**, 802 (1960).

WEINER, I. M., MUDGE, G. H.: Renal tubular mechanisms for excretion of organic acids and bases. Amer. J. Med. **36**, 743 (1964).

WOODS, H. F., EGGLESTON, L. V., KREBS, H. A.: The cause of hepatic accumulation of fructose 1-phosphate on fructose loading. Biochem. J. **119**, 501 (1970).

WYNGAARDEN, J. B., ASHTON, D. M.: The regulation of activity of phosphoribosylpyrophosphate amidotransferase by purine nucleotides: a potential feedback control of purine biosynthesis. J. biol. Chem. **234**, 1492 (1959).

WYNGAARDEN, J. B., RUNDLES, E. W., METZ, E. N.: Allopurinol of the treatment of gout. Arch. intern. Med. **62**, 842 (1965).

YU, T. F., BERGER, L., GUTMAN, A. B.: Suppression of tubular secretion of urate by pyrazinamide in the dog. Proc. Soc. exp. Biol. (N.Y.) **107**, 905 (1961).

YU, T. F., GUTMAN, A. B.: Paradoxical retention of uric acid by uricosuric drugs in low dosage. Proc. Soc. exp. Biol. (N.Y.) **90**, 542 (1955).

YU, T. F., SIROTAM, J. H., BERGER, L., HALPERN, M., GUTMAN, A. B.: Effect of sodium lactate infusion on urate clearance in man. Proc. Soc. exp. Biol. (N.Y.) **96**, 809 (1957).

YU, T. F., GUTMAN, A. B.: A study of the paradoxical effects of salicylate in low, intermediate and high dosage on the renal mechanisms for excretion of urate in man. J. clin. Invest. **38**, 1298 (1959).

ZINS, G. R., WEINER, I. M.: Bidirectional urate transport limited to the proximal tubule in dogs. Amer. J. Physiol. **215**, 411 (1968).

ZÖLLNER, N., DOFEL, W., GRÖBNER, W.: Die Wirkung von Benzbromaronum auf die renale Harnsäureausscheidung Gesunder. Klin. Wschr. **48**, 426 (1970a).

ZÖLLNER, N., GRIEBSCH, A., FINK, J. K.: Über die Wirkung von Benzbromaron auf den Serumharnsäurespiegel und die Harnsäureausscheidung des Gichtkranken. Dtsch. med. Wschr. **95**, 2405 (1970b).

ZÖLLNER, N., STERN, G., GRÖBNER, W., DOFEL, W.: Über die Senkung des Harnsäurespiegels im Plasma durch Benzbromaronum. Klin. Wschr. **46**, 1318 (1968).

4. Die chirurgische Behandlung der Gicht

Von

A. GÖB

Mit 8 Abbildungen

Die chirurgische Behandlung der fortgeschrittenen knotigen Gicht wird oft empfohlen und mit gutem Erfolg ausgeführt. Es kommt im wesentlichen darauf an, zu vermeiden, daß die Gichtknoten perforieren und sich infizieren. Bei guter Hautdeckung können auch größere subcutane Knoten, aber auch solche, die von Knochen und Gelenkenden ausgehen, operativ erfolgreich angegangen werden.

Die Indikation zur Operation wird aber bedauerlicherweise meist erst dann gestellt, wenn das Tragen von Schuhen oder Handschuhen nicht mehr möglich ist, wenn an Füßen und Händen die Gelenke sehr stark aufgetrieben und deformiert erscheinen, oder wenn die Tophi perforieren. Es wäre zweckmäßiger, die knotige Gicht dann anzugehen, wenn die Haut noch intakt und die Zerstörung des Knochens noch nicht sehr fortgeschritten ist. Eine Indikation zur Operation ist bei dieser Art von gichtiger Gelenkverformung gegeben, wenn die medikamentöse Therapie nicht in dem gewünschten Ausmaße wirksam ist und somit die Wiederherstellung zu lange dauern würde.

Die operative Behandlung ist also angezeigt:

1. a) Bei großen Gichtknoten in Schleimbeuteln an exponierten Stellungen, besonders an Olecranon, Patella und Ferse, da bei zunehmender Spannung der Haut Ulcerationen mit anschließender Infektion entstehen können.

b) Bei kleineren Gichtknoten an den Finger- und Zehengelenken, die zur Ulceration neigen. Die Haut ist hier meist unter einer gewissen Spannung und perforiert leicht.

2. Zur Korrektur von Finger-, Zehen- bzw. Fußdeformitäten.

3. Zur Stabilisierung schmerzhafter körperbelasteter Gelenke des Fußes bzw. des Beines.

4. Zur Entlastung von Nerven, die von Tophi eingeengt sind.

Schleimbeuteltophi an vorspringenden Körperregionen

Tophi, die an vorspringenden Gegenden des Körpers, wie am Olecranon, an der Patella, an Fersen oder an den darunterliegenden Schleimbeuteln sich lokalisieren, sind operativ leicht zu beherrschen. Der Olecranontophus und der an der Patella wird insgesamt ausgeschält. Das kalkige, bröckelige Gewebe ist meist von Bindegewebe durchzogen, liegt im Schleimbeutel selbst oder hat diesen bereits perforiert. Entfernt man den Schleimbeutel mitsamt seinem Inhalt, so hat man den ausgeweiteten Hautbeutel zu verkleinern und dafür zu sorgen, daß sich nicht ein großer Bluterguß bildet. Letzteres ist durch eine Naht der Haut an die Unterlage und durch einen Druckverband zu vermeiden.

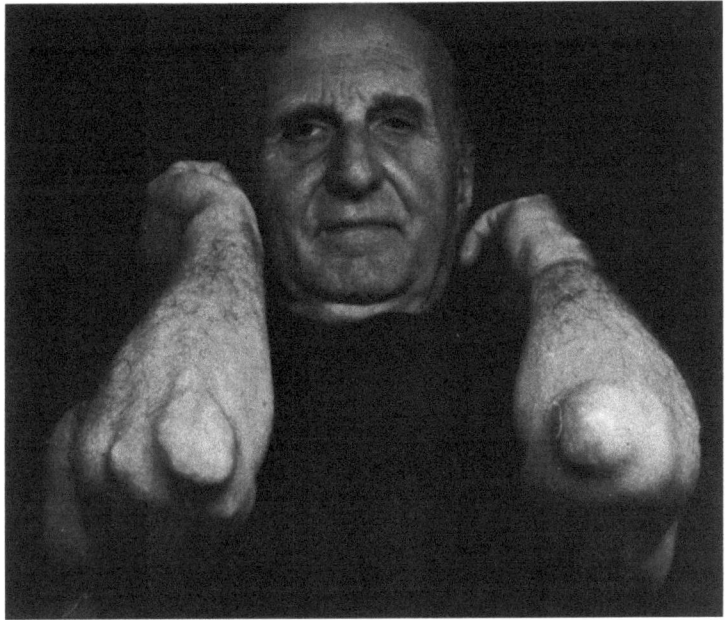

Abb. 1.: Entzündliche, mit Uraten gefüllte Schleimbeutel an beiden Ellbogengelenken

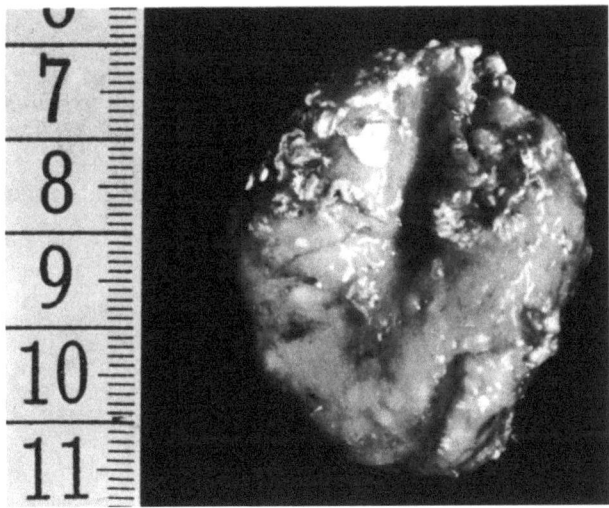

Abb. 2. Präparat des rechten Schleimbeutels

Die Schleimbeutel im Bereich des Ansatzes der Achillessehne am Calcaneus erfordern mehr Beachtung. Die Haut im Fersenbereich wird durch einen oder mehrere vorspringende Tophi, die sich in den Schleimbeuteln über und unter der Achillessehne entwickeln, noch zusätzlich dünner, als sie schon ist. Gelegentlich ist die Achillessehne selbst in die kalkigen Veränderungen mit einbezogen.

Bei der Entfernung der kalkigen Massen sollte man die Achillessehne allerdings nicht unter Hintanstellung ihrer Stabilität auch von den letzten Kalkmas-

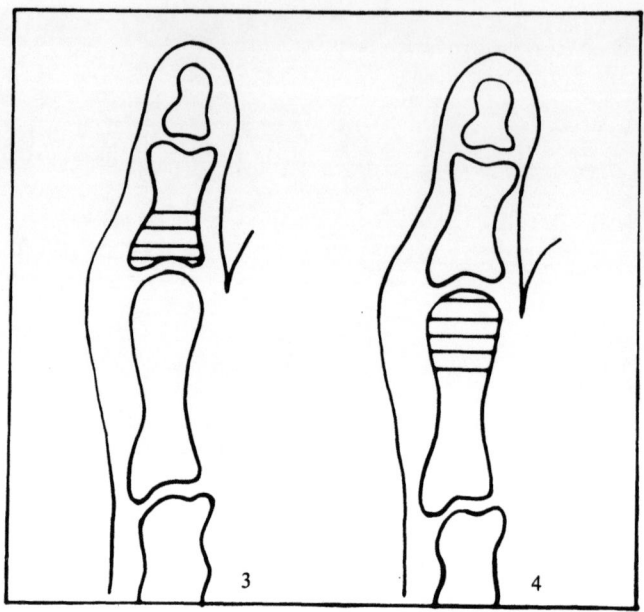

Abb. 3. Resektion der Basis der Grundphalanx I, modifiziert nach BRANDES

Abb. 4. Resektion des Metatarsalköpfchens nach HUETER-MAYO

sen befreien. Nach der Entfernung der größeren Tophi heilen selbst die kleineren Defekte der Sehnenansätze schnell, und es bildet sich auch in dem teilverkalkten Sehnengewebe wieder eine gute bindegewebige Stabilität.

Deformierungen an Finger- und Zehengelenken

Im Bereich der Finger- und der Zehengelenke, aber auch im Bereich des Fußes kann die Gicht groteske Deformierungen verursachen. Meist hängt das Auftreten dieser gichtigen Veränderungen vom Alter des Patienten und von der Dauer und der Schwere der Erkrankung ab.

Es lassen sich dabei an den Fingern und Zehen sowie an der Mittelhand und am Mittelfuß
1. destruierende, zur Gelenkversteifung neigende Formen und
2. osteolytische Formen

erkennen.

Die erste Form weist bei der operativen Revision Kalkdepots auf den Gelenkflächen sowie arthrotische Veränderungen auf.

Operationen am Großzehengrundgelenk

Operation nach Brandes modifiziert

Am Fuß ist das Großzehengrundgelenk das häufigst veränderte Gelenk. Das operative Vorgehen lehnt sich an das bei der Behandlung des Hallux valgus an. Die Brandessche Operation mit Resektion der Basis der Grundphalanx wird allerdings um die Resektion der Gelenkkapsel erweitert. Sie wird im allgemeinen schnell die schmerzhafte Versteifung des Großzehengrundgelenks beseitigen.

Operation nach Hueter-Mayo

Gelegentlich können ausgedehnte entzündliche Gelenkveränderungen vorherrschen, wobei die Synovialmembran stets stärker entzündlich verändert und der Knorpel besonders im Bereich des Mittelfußköpfchens destruiert ist. In weiter fortgeschrittenen Fällen weist auch das Mittelfußköpfchen Kalkdepots mit entzündlichen Granulationen auf.

Die Kapselresektion sowie die Operation nach HUETER-MAYO, also die Resektion des Mittelfußköpfchens, dürfte sich hier als zweckmäßig erweisen.

Gelegentlich greifen die Veränderungen von der Gelenkkapsel des Großzehengrundgelenks auf die Sehnenscheiden und die Sehnen über. Das Granulationsgewebe und die kalkigen Infiltrationen müssen dann neben der operativen Versorgung der Gelenkanteile auch aus den Sehnenscheiden entfernt werden. Bei völliger Auflösung von wichtigen Sehnen, meist handelt es sich um die Strecksehnen, muß eine Sehnenverlagerung vorgenommen werden, sofern sich eine benachbarte Sehne anbietet.

Operation an den Fingergelenken

Tophi an den Fingern lokalisieren sich gerne am Daumenendgelenk oder an den Mittelgelenken der Finger im Bereich der Strecksehne. Sie haben mit der Gelenkkapsel Beziehung und breiten sich sowohl ins Gelenk wie auch auf die Strecksehne aus. Kleinere Veränderungen bringen das Gelenk in seiner Form und Beweglichkeit nicht in Gefahr.

Die Tophi mit ihren erkrankten Teilen der Kapsel und der Strecksehne können reseziert werden.

Schwerere Formveränderungen mit Deformierungen, die auf Osteolysen der Gelenkenden zurückzuführen sind, sind sowohl an der Hand wie am Fuß problematisch.

Operationen bei Gelenkveränderungen mit Osteolysen an Fingern und Zehen, an Hand und Fuß

In fortgeschrittenen Fällen entwickeln sich an den Gelenkenden im Knochen durch Uratablagerung Defekte, die zusätzlich eine entzündliche Komponente haben. Es können sich dabei die Gelenkanteile völlig auflösen. Im Röntgenbild findet sich eine blasige Auftreibung der Gelenkenden mit nur noch angedeuteten Strukturen und becherförmigen Defekten. Der noch bestehende Knochen ist stark osteoporotisch. Die Veränderungen können sich über mehrere Gelenke erstrecken, so daß man auch röntgenologisch mehr den Eindruck einer Arthritis mutilans hat.

Die Veränderungen beschränken sich schließlich nicht nur auf die Gelenke der Finger und der Zehen, sondern sie greifen auch über auf die Gelenke des Mittelfußes und der Hand.

Am Fuß werden zumeist die Grundgelenke der Zehen zuerst angegriffen, und dann schließlich auch die Mittelfußgelenke mit ihren spongiösen Anteilen des Knochens zerstört. Erhalten bleiben meistens die Diaphysen der Mittelfußknochen. Über die Gelenkkapsel werden schnell die Strecksehnen, die Sehnenscheiden und die übrigen Weichteile einschließlich der Muskulatur in die Erkrankung mit einbezogen.

In ähnlicher Weise ergeben sich auch Veränderungen an den Fingergelenken, die auch auf die Hand übergreifen.

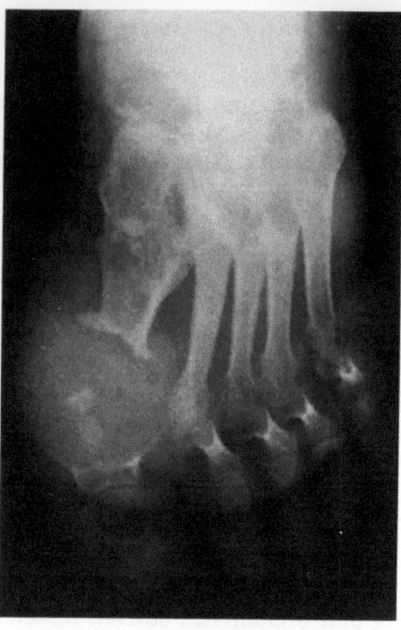

Abb. 5. Schwerste Osteolysen bei starker Anreicherung von Uraten im Bereich der Grundgelenke der Großzehe links und im Bereich der Kleinzehe

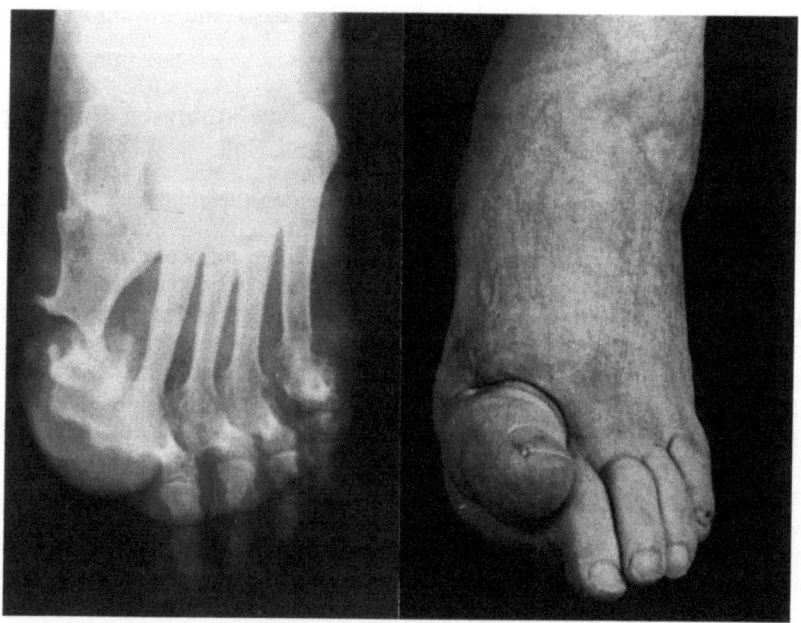

Abb. 6. Postoperativer Zustand

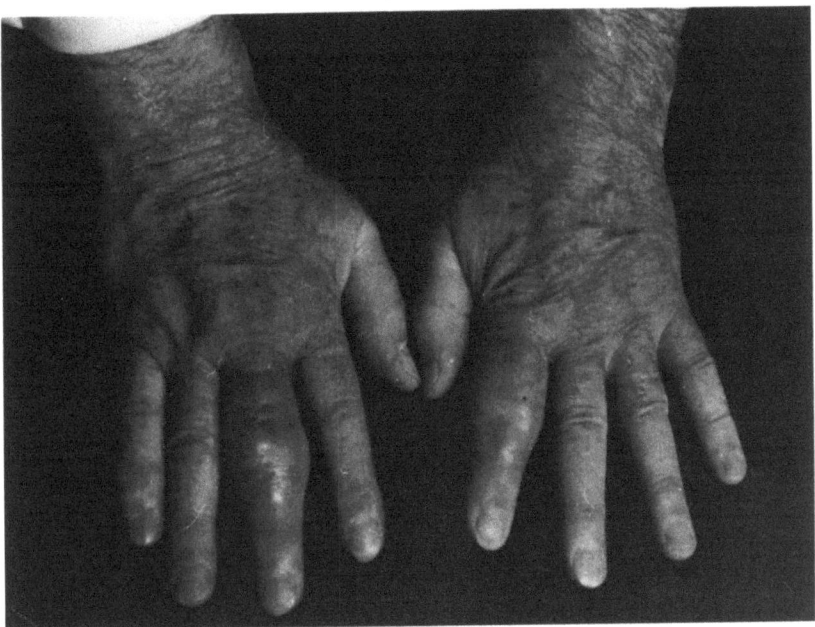

Abb. 7. Gichtige Auftreibung und Deformierung der Mittelgelenke am 3. Finger rechts und am 2. Finger links

Die Behandlung am Fuß bei schweren Osteolysen mit schweren Deformierungen und Verformungen des Fußes zielt darauf hin, daß der Fuß wieder in einen Schuh, der einigermaßen den allgemeinen Anforderungen genügt, gebracht werden kann. Man versucht dabei die Kalkdepots, die in den osteolysierten Anteilen des Knochens liegen, zu entfernen, aber doch so viel von knöchernen Anteilen zu erhalten, daß die Stabilität gesichert ist. Es wird aber trotzdem vom Rest des Skeletts nur eine sehr fragwürdige Stabilität in fortgeschrittenen Fällen zu erwarten sein. Die Nachversorgung mit entsprechendem orthopädischem Schuhwerk ist in jedem Falle gegeben.

Die operative Behandlung der gichtigen Fingerdeformitäten bei Osteolysen ist dankbarer, als es zunächst scheinen mag. Es lassen sich an den Gelenkenden selbst größere Kalkdepots ausräumen, ohne daß die Gelenkstabilität zu sehr gefährdet wird. Man sollte die Gelenkkapsel resezieren, aber den seitlichen Bandapparat möglichst erhalten. Strecksehnen sind meist so geschädigt, daß sich oft eine Umkipp-Plastik als nötig erweist. Zur Schnittführung hat sich auf der Strecksehne ein doppelter Winkelschnitt als zweckmäßig erwiesen.

Die postoperative Versorgung ist für den Fuß der Unterschenkel- oder der Fußgips, je nachdem wie ausgedehnt der operative Eingriff oder die Zerstörung war. Für die Hand ist es die Fingerschiene.

Sobald die Wundheilung abgeschlossen ist, hat sich uns eine *postoperative Röntgentiefenbestrahlung* zur Entzündungshemmung als wertvoll erwiesen. Die Narben werden reizloser, und die überschießenden postoperativen Reaktionen an Knochen und Sehnen halten sich in Grenzen.

Eine entscheidende Bedeutung hat in der postoperativen Phase die interne Gichtbehandlung mit Colchicin für die ersten Tage sowie die Weiterbehandlung mit Probenecid oder Allopurinol. Die Dauerbehandlung sollte exakt weiterge-

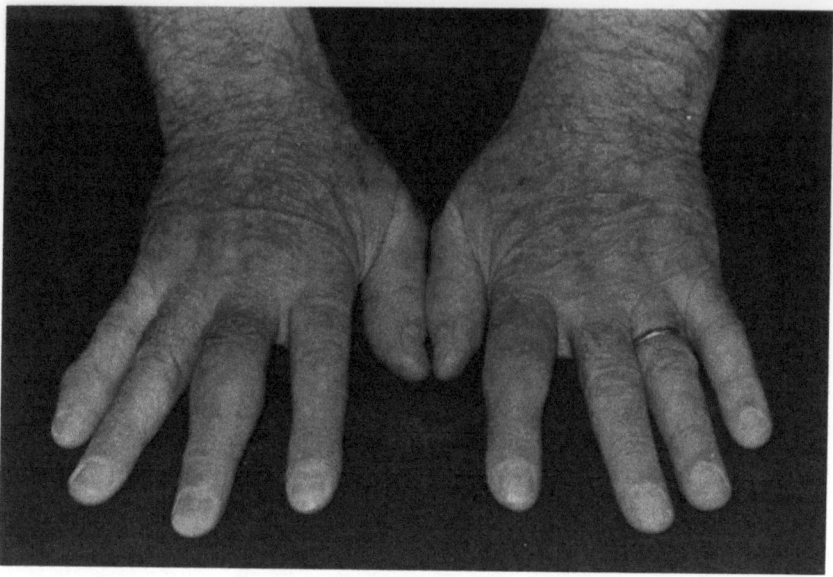

Abb. 8. Postoperativer Zustand nach einem Vierteljahr, freie Beweglichkeit der operierten Fingergelenke

führt werden, obwohl nach allgemeiner Erfahrung die Gicht an den operierten Gelenken sich nicht wieder in derselben Weise manifestiert. Die Lokalisation an anderen Gelenken ist aber dabei nicht ausgeschlossen.

Gicht an anderen Gelenken und ihre Behandlung

Die Gicht greift klinisch mit zunehmender Krankheitsdauer von den kleinen auf die größeren Gelenke über und erreicht zunächst das Kniegelenk. Wahrscheinlich sind jedoch alle Gelenke ergriffen und die kleineren Gelenke weisen lediglich frühere Manifestationen auf.

Operationen am Kniegelenk

Am Kniegelenk äußert sich die Erkrankung zunächst in der Form der chronischen Synovitis mit arthrotischen Veränderungen. Oft wird die Erkrankung nicht richtig gedeutet, da die arthrotischen Zeichen sowohl klinisch wie röntgenologisch im Vordergrund stehen. Die operative Behandlung im Bereich des Kniegelenks wird im allgemeinen die Entfernung der synovialen Gelenkkapsel, die Synovektomie, oder die Entfernung degenerierter, abgerissener Menisci sein. Beläge mit Uraten auf den Gelenkflächen oder kleinere Uratdepots in den Gelenkflächen selbst können ausgekratzt werden. Bei stark veränderten Gelenkkapseln sollte allerdings darauf geachtet werden, daß die gesamte synoviale Kapsel entfernt wird. Wenn die Menisci stark verkrustet sind, müssen auch diese mit herausgenommen werden.

Postoperativ muß die Mobilisation bei entsprechender Extension am Tibiakopf mit einer Kirschner-Drahtextension möglichst bald aufgenommen werden. Es müssen auch Redon-Drainagen zum Absaugen von Blutergüssen eingelegt werden, um der Neigung zur Gelenkversteifung entgegenzuwirken.

Der Befall größerer Gelenke wird nicht sehr häufig beobachtet. Man sollte der Zerstörung größerer Gelenke unbedingt durch interne Behandlung vorbeugen. Sollten solche Zerstörungen eingetreten sein, so käme hier nur der Ersatz mit Gelenkprothesen in Frage.

Infizierte Tophi und Gelenkgicht

Sind durch Ulcerationen der Haut Tophi oder deformierte Gelenke bereits infiziert, so muß je nach dem Stand der Infektion der Tophus oder das Gelenk eröffnet und drainiert werden. Gichtige Schleimbeutel sind dabei leichter zu beherrschen als gichtige Gelenke. Die Abdeckung mit Antibiotica bei vorheriger Resistenzbestimmung ist selbstverständlich.

Infektionen an den Gelenken lassen sich im allgemeinen aber gut beherrschen, und man sollte sich nicht zu schnell zur Amputation entschließen.

Schluß

Manche Gichterkrankung verläuft so ungünstig, daß trotz medikamentöser Behandlung Gelenkdeformitäten und Schleimbeutelbefall auftreten. Unregelmäßige Einnahme der Gichtmittel ist oft die Ursache einer schnellen Entwicklung von Tophi und Gelenkdeformitäten. Man sollte in solchen Fällen auch kleinere Veränderungen operativ angehen, wenn sich eine schnelle Größenzunahme von Tophi in Gelenknähe zeigt, oder wenn Gichttophi an exponierten Stellen schnell an Größe zunehmen und sich entzünden. Die operative Behandlung vermeidet dann die Deformierung des Gelenks und wirkt ganz allgemein durch die Entfernung der Uratdepots auf den Stoffwechsel entlastend.

Literatur

BACKMANN, L.: Chirurgische Behandlungsmöglichkeit der Gicht. Therapiewoche 22, 140—142 (1972).
BACKMANN, L., BÄUMER, A.: Harnsäuregehalt chirurgisch entfernter Gichtknoten und gichtig veränderter Schleimbeutel. Münch. med. Wschr. 111, 1620—1622 (1969).
KUZELL, W.C., GAUDIN, G.-P.: Studiengruppe f. rheumat. Krankheiten, Instit. f. Pharmakologie u. Therapie, Med. Fak. d. Univ. Stanford, San Francisco.
MERTZ, D.P.: Gicht und Hyperuricämie. Arch. klin. Med. 212, 143—190 (1966).
TALBOTT, J.H.: Gout. 3rd ed. New York-London: Grune & Stratton 1967.

5. Therapie der Gichtniere

Von

D. P. Mertz

Veränderungen im Sinne einer Gichtnephropathie lassen sich bei den meisten Gichtpatienten histologisch nachweisen. Klinisch kann man allerdings nur in etwa der Hälfte aller Fälle Anzeichen einer Nierenschädigung finden (Mertz u. Babucke, 1971). Die klinischen Symptome einer Nierenbeteiligung bei Gicht bestehen in einer gelegentlichen leichten bis mäßigen Proteinurie mit Zylindrurie, einer mehr oder weniger ausgeprägten Leukocyturie, Uratkristallen im Harnsediment und einer Einschränkung der Konzentrationsfähigkeit. Außer Nierensteinkoliken können sich Kreuzschmerzen einstellen. Mikrohämaturie mit Proteinurie besteht klinisch meist dann, wenn die Glomeruli primär oder sekundär in stärkerem Umfang in die Nephropathie einbezogen sind. Die Blutdruckerhöhung ist dabei nahezu konstant.

Die meisten pathologischen Befunde bei Gichtnephropathie sind unspezifisch (Reubi, 1962; Zöllner, 1968; Mertz, 1968, 1971). Gefäßveränderungen im Sinne einer unspezifischen Glomerulosklerose, Arteriosklerose und Arteriolosklerose (Zollinger, 1962), chronische interstitielle Nephritis, die an eine Pyelonephritis erinnert, und Nephrolithiasis sind die häufigsten Befunde bei Gichtnephropathie. Nach Zollinger (1962) sind die mikroskopisch bestätigten Gichttophi in den Nierenpapillen als pathognomonisch für Gicht zu bezeichnen. Bei Würdigung aller verfügbaren Literaturangaben finden sich Uratablagerungen in der Niere schätzungsweise bei vier Fünftel, interstitielle Entzündungen bei drei Viertel, davon Pyelonephritis in zwei Drittel aller Fälle, vasculäre Veränderungen bei etwa der Hälfte und Nephrolithiasis bei etwa zwei Zehntel aller Gichtpatienten (Mertz, 1968, 1971). Normalerweise erübrigt sich eine percutane Nierenpunktion bei Gichtpatienten, da die Nierenbiopsie keine therapeutischen Konsequenzen nach sich zieht. Um so mehr wird die Bedeutung der Röntgendiagnostik einer Gichtniere durch deren Besonderheiten unterstrichen.

Die Röntgendiagnostik einer Gichtniere ist durch die Besonderheiten einer diffusen interstitiellen Fibrosierung des Organs gekennzeichnet. Typisch sind die im Hilusbereich um die Kelche verlaufenden, bis zur Rindenregion reichenden, unregelmäßig begrenzten rinnenförmigen Aufhellungsbezirke (Kröpelin u. Mertz, 1972). Diesem Phänomen entspricht pathologisch-anatomisch eine besonders im inneren Markraum vorhandene diffuse zellarme Sklerose. Eindeutige röntgenologisch faßbare Veränderungen ruft die chronisch sklerosierende interstitielle Gichtnephritis erst nach Herabsetzung der glomerulären Filtratrate auf weniger als die Hälfte des Normalwertes hervor. Die röntgenologisch erkennbaren makroskopischen Veränderungen einer Gichtniere sind unspezifisch. Eine Spezifität liegt nur für die Läsionen einer chronisch sklerosierenden interstitiellen Nephritis vor, die jedoch viele Ursachen hat.

Die Behandlung einer Gichtnephropathie schließt vier Maßnahmen ein:
1. Die Behandlung der Gicht als Gelenk- und Allgemeinerkrankung.
2. Die Behandlung und Prophylaxe der Harnsäuresteinbildung.
3. Die Behandlung einer arteriellen Hypertension.
4. Die Behandlung einer Harnwegsinfektion.

Auf Grund der für uns heute möglichen prophylaktischen Behandlung während der interkritischen Phasen und im chronischen Stadium läßt sich die Gicht erfolgreicher beeinflussen als alle anderen Gelenkerkrankungen. Vor allem hat die große Gefahr einer Uratlithiasis bei Gicht viel von ihrem Schrecken eingebüßt. Liegt eine ausgesprochene Uratnephropathie mit Harnsäureausfällungen oder eine Niereninsuffizienz vor, dann ist Allopurinol als Basistherapeuticum das Mittel der Wahl. Wichtig ist die Forderung nach einer konsequenten Dauerbehandlung bis ans Lebensende. Bei Niereninsuffizienz oder Urolithiasis ist auf Uricosurica zu verzichten. In der üblichen Dosierung von 300—400 mg täglich wirkt Allopurinol weder nephrotoxisch noch hämatotoxisch oder hepatotoxisch. Im Gegenteil können bei Niereninsuffizienz im Verlauf einer primären Gicht durch Dauermedikation von 100—200 mg Allopurinol täglich sogar gewisse durch Uratablagerungen bedingte funktionelle Nierenstörungen beseitigt werden. Da Allopurinol und sein Hauptmetabolit Oxypurinol vorwiegend auf renalem Wege ausgeschieden wird, ist bei Niereninsuffizienz die Dosis auf die Hälfte bis ein Drittel der üblichen Menge zu beschränken (MERTZ, 1973a). Möglicherweise zu Beginn der Allopurinol-Therapie auftretende Gelenksensationen lassen sich durch subklinische Dosen von Colchicin (jeden 2. Tag etwa 0,5 mg) oder ersatzweise von Indometacin (25 mg 1—2 × täglich) verhindern. Die hypouricämisierende Wirkung von Allopurinol steht in direkter Abhängigkeit vom Ausgangsniveau der Serum-Harnsäurewerte. Anzustreben ist eine Serum-Harnsäurekonzentration von weniger als 6 mg/100 ml. Bei nur geringer Nierenbeteiligung (ohne Nephrolithiasis oder Tendenz zur Nephrolithiasis) mit Filtratwerten über 75 ml pro Minute ist eine Dauerbehandlung mit Uricosurica durchaus möglich, wobei die Kautelen für eine uricosurische Therapie (Trinken von mindestens 2000 ml Flüssigkeit täglich zusätzlich und Alkalisierung des Harns) zu beachten sind. Nach Ausschwemmung der Harnsäuredepots, also nach Herbeiführung eines Gleichgewichtes zwischen Anfall und Ausscheidung von Harnsäure, genügt als zusätzliche Therapie meist reichliches Trinken von Flüssigkeit. Unter den Uricosurica hat sich Benzbromaronum wegen seiner raschen, kräftigen, langfristigen und zuverlässigen Wirkung in geringer Dosierung am besten bewährt. Bei guter Nierenfunktion und geringer Überproduktion von Harnsäure reicht eine einmalige Dosierung von 50 mg täglich, in allen anderen Fällen von maximal 100 mg täglich zur Erzielung einer Harnsäurekonzentration von weniger als 6 mg/100 ml Serum aus (MERTZ, 1969). Da jedoch die Niere in den meisten Gichtfällen deutlich mitbetroffen ist, nehmen die Uricosurica heute zugunsten der Uricostatica nur noch eine Ersatzposition ein.

Bei Gichtpatienten unter 35 Jahren manifestiert sich die Erkrankung in einem Drittel der Fälle zunächst an den Nieren und erst später an den Gelenken (HENNINGES u. MERTZ, 1971). Bei abakterieller interstitieller Uratnephropathie mit oder ohne arterielle Hypertension besteht im Frühstadium grundsätzlich die Möglichkeit, Nierenbeteiligung und Blutdruckerhöhung durch alleinige Verordnung von Allopurinol zu beseitigen.

Die Dauerbehandlung mit Allopurinol stellt bis zu einem gewissen Grade schon eine Behandlung und Prophylaxe der Harnsäuresteinbildung dar. Verschiedentlich wurde beobachtet, daß Allopurinol in der Lage ist, eine Uratlithiasis durch Auflösung der Steine zu beseitigen (ZÖLLNER u. SCHATTENKIRCHNER, 1967). Unterstützt wird diese Therapie durch Alkalisierung des Harnes. Hierbei haben sich Citratgemische besser bewährt als Natriumbicarbonat. Neuere Befunde zeigen, daß eine Alkalisierung des Harnes offenbar nicht ausreicht, eine Steinbildung zu verhindern. Sowohl in kurativer als auch in prophylaktischer Hinsicht haben Citronensäure-Citrat-Gemische (Uralyt®-U) deutliche Vorteile vor Natriumbicarbonat: Durch Zufuhr von dreimal täglich 3 g eines Citronensäure-Citrat-Gemisches per os kann man innerhalb von Wochen oder Monaten reine Uratsteine bis zur Größe eines Nierenkelchausgußsteines auflösen. Die Citrat-Therapie kann aber auch eine Nierensteinbildung verhindern. In therapeutischer Hinsicht ist wichtig, daß der Harn-pH-Wert bei dreimaliger Kontrolle am Tag nicht unter 6,4 liegt. Werte zwischen 6,4 und 6,8 werden als optimal angesehen, da in diesem Bereich noch keine Gefahr einer Phosphatausfällung oder der Aktivierung einer Infektion besteht. Überdies scheint ein Urin-pH-Wert von 7 und mehr zur Auflösung oder Prophylaxe von Harnsäuresteinen gar nicht notwendig zu sein (MERTZ, 1968). Bei Neigung zu Harnsäureausfällungen ist zudem ein Wasserstoß ein- oder zweimal wöchentlich etwa im Sinne eines Volhardschen Verdünnungsversuches nützlich (MERTZ, 1972).

Die Behandlung einer arteriellen Hypertension, die bei Gichtpatienten meist nierenbedingt ist (MERTZ, 1968, 1971), und einer Pyelonephritis erfolgt nach den allseits bekannten Richtlinien, wobei in beiden Fällen eine Dauertherapie mit laufender Kontrolle erforderlich ist. Im Falle einer Hochdruckbehandlung von Gichtpatienten mit Medikamenten, die Thiazid-Saluretica enthalten, muß die Allopurinol-Dosis erhöht werden, da mit Allopurinol dauerbehandelte Gichtiker wie gesunde Personen mit einem signifikanten Anstieg der Serum-Harnsäurewerte reagieren (MERTZ, 1973b). Verabreichung von Spironolacton beeinflußt die Serum-Harnsäurekonzentration weder bei gesunden Personen noch bei mit Allopurinol dauerbehandelten Gichtkranken. Bei kombinierter Anwendung von Spironolacton mit einem mittellangfristig wirkenden Thiazid-Salureticum entspricht die Erhöhung der Serum-Harnsäurekonzentration derjenigen, die unter der Wirkung des Thiazid-Saluretikums allein zustandekommt. Grundsätzlich besteht die medikamentöse Behandlung der arteriellen Hypertension bei Gichtnephropathie aus Allgemeinmaßnahmen, Natriumentzug und Sympathicushemmung. Die Allgemeinmaßnahmen umfassen Fragen der Lebensführung, der Freizeitgestaltung, des Urlaubs, der Berufsausübung. Seit vielen Jahren empfehlen wir intelligenten hochdruckkranken Gichtpatienten mit Erfolg die Selbstmessung des Blutdruckes zu Hause. Bei fortgeschrittener Azotämie (Niereninsuffizienz) und Auftreten von Nebenerscheinungen, wie plötzliche Verschlechterung der Nierenfunktion mit Nachlassen der Diurese oder cerebrale Ausfallserscheinungen, sollte auf eine antihypertensive Therapie entweder verzichtet oder nur zur Vermeidung von Blutdruckkrisen bzw. von Zuständen mit excessiver Blutdrucksteigerung zurückgegriffen werden. Bei Reststickstoff-Konzentrationen von mehr als 80—100 mg/100 ml Serum oder Kreatininwerten über 8—10 mg/100 ml Serum ist jede antihypertensive Therapie wegen der Gefahr einer raschen Verschlechterung der Nierenfunktion relativ kontraindiziert. Liegen die Reststickstoffwerte zwischen 60 und 80 mg/100 ml Serum (entsprechend einer Kreatininämie von 4—8 mg/100 ml), dann setzt man die Blutdruckwerte nicht unter 180/110 mm Hg herab. Das Vermeiden von Blutdruckspitzen kann sich in solchen Fällen bereits vorteilhaft auswirken. Eine Blutdrucksenkung ist bei hypertensiven Gichtpatienten, deren glomeruläre Reserve durch diätetische Maßnahmen schon voll ausgeschöpft ist und die immer noch eine Retention harnpflichtiger Substanzen aufweisen, vorsichtig einzuleiten. Sehr stark erhöhte Blutdruckwerte sollten dann nicht unter ein Niveau von weniger als 180 mm Hg systolisch vermindert werden, da sonst nach allgemeiner ärztlicher Erfahrung die Retention harnpflichtiger Substanzen infolge einer, wenn auch nur vorübergehenden, Abnahme der glomerulären Filtratrate enorm zunehmen kann.

Es besteht kein Zweifel an der Notwendigkeit, auch die Pyelonephritis bei Gicht energisch zu behandeln, um die Entwicklung oder das weitere Fortschreiten einer Hochdruckerkrankung zu verhindern. Bei chronisch-rezidivierender Pyelonephritis ist neben einer gichtspezifischen Therapie eine oft über Jahre sich erstreckende Dauer-Langzeittherapie anzustreben. Die Erfahrung hat gezeigt, daß diese Therapie zweckmäßig mit Gaben eines Breitband-Antibioticums über 2—3 Wochen in ausreichender Dosierung (initiale Stoßtherapie) eingeleitet wird (MERTZ, 1973c). Zur Fortsetzung der Behandlung über Wochen oder Monate, je nach Lage des Falles (unter bakteriologischer Harnkontrolle), eignen sich Sulfonamide (mit hohen Blut- und Gewebespiegeln) oder Nitrofuranderivate. Solche „Kuren" müssen in entsprechenden Intervallen über viele Monate bis Jahre wiederholt werden. Dieses Behandlungsschema ist einer intermittierenden Langzeittherapie (eine Woche/Monat) oder einer Kurzzeittherapie mit Rücksicht auf die Gefahr einer Resistenzentwicklung, eines Rezidivs oder einer Reinfektion vorzuziehen. Auf diese Weise gelingt es vielfach, das Leiden am Fortschreiten zu hindern und die Ausgangslage für eine Behandlung einer pyelonephritischen Hypertension zu verbessern. Manchmal kann die Hypertension völlig beseitigt werden.

Bei Einhaltung dieser therapeutischen Empfehlungen können Diätvorschriften weitgehend gelockert werden. Empfehlenswert sind eine vernünftige Diät, wie sie prophylaktisch und therapeutisch bei Atherosklerose und Diabetes mellitus angewandt wird, sowie eine Einschränkung des Alkoholkonsums. Im Vordergrund steht eine Normalisierung des Körpergewichtes durch Verabfolgung einer calorien- und kohlenhydratarmen Kost, wobei auf die Gabe von reinen monomeren oder dimeren Zuckerarten zugunsten von polymeren Kohlenhydraten verzichtet werden sollte, durch Verabreichung bis etwa 25% der Calorien als Eiweiß und 40—50% als Fett unter Bevorzugung hochungesättigter Fettsäuren (MERTZ, 1973c). Bei Entwicklung einer schweren Niereninsuffizienz ist auf eine Kartoffel-Ei-Diät (KLUTHE u. QUIRIN, 1971) umzustellen. Im Falle einer arteriellen Hypertension empfiehlt sich eine diätetische Kochsalzrestriktion.

Prognose

In Anbetracht der heute verfügbaren Therapiemöglichkeiten bei Hyperuricämie wird das *Risiko* von Gichttophi in den Nieren selbst bei ungenügend behandelten Gichtpatienten mit leicht erhöhten Serum-Harnsäurewerten meist überschätzt. Die jetzt zu beobachtenden Nierenschäden beziehen sich weit mehr auf Gefäßveränderungen als auf große Gichttophi oder chronisch sklerosierende abakterielle interstitielle Entzündungen in den Nieren. Nach meiner Erfahrung befindet sich die glomeruläre Filtratrate bei den meisten Gichtpatienten im altersüblichen Normbereich, wohingegen der Nierenplasmastrom in der Regel leicht eingeschränkt ist. Scheidet man jedoch alle Fälle mit arterieller Hypertension aus, dann liegt die PAH-Clearance bei Gichtkranken nicht signifikant unter dem für das betreffende Lebensalter normalen Vergleichswert. Aus diesem Grund ist die Kontrolle einer arteriellen Hypertension bei primärer Gicht zur Verhinderung einer Gichtnephropathie ebenso wichtig wie die Kontrolle der Hyperuricämie oder wie die Verhütung eines Nierenschadens bei der hypertensiven, nicht-gichtigen Bevölkerung.

Literatur

HENNINGES, D., MERTZ, D. P.: Urikopathie von Jugendlichen. Besonderheiten im klinischen Bild. Münch. med. Wschr. **113**, 458 (1971).
KLUTHE, R., QUIRIN, H.: Diätbuch für Nierenkranke, 2. Aufl., Stuttgart: Thieme 1971.
KRÖPELIN, T., MERTZ, D. P.: Zur Röntgendiagnostik der Gichtniere. Dtsch. med. Wschr. **97**, 71 (1972).
MERTZ, D. P.: Gichtniere und Nierengicht. Dtsch. med. J. **19**, 413 (1968).
MERTZ, D. P.: Veränderungen der Serumkonzentration von Harnsäure unter der Wirkung von Benzbromaronum. Münch. med. Wschr. **111**, 491 (1969).
MERTZ, D. P.: Gicht. Grundlagen, Klinik und Therapie. Stuttgart: Thieme 1971.
MERTZ, D. P.: Therapie der Gichtnephropathie. Dtsch. med. Wschr. **97**, 982 (1972).
MERTZ, D. P.: Krankheitskatastrophen: Niereninsuffizienz. Münch. med. Wschr. **115**, 747 (1973a).
MERTZ, D. P.: Wirkung von Spironolacton und Thiabutazid auf die Serumkonzentrationen von Harnsäure und Lipiden bei Gichtkranken und Stoffwechselgesunden. Dtsch. med. Wschr. **98**, 11 (1973b).
MERTZ, D. P.: Risikofaktor Gicht. Mannheim: Boehringer 1973c.
MERTZ, D. P., BABUCKE, G.: Epidemiologie und klinisches Bild der primären Gicht. Beobachtungen zwischen 1948 und 1968. Münch. med. Wschr. **113**, 617 (1971).
REUBI, F., VORBURGER, C.: Die Gichtniere. Münch. med. Wschr. **104**, 2152 (1062).
ZOLLINGER, H. U.: Pathologisch-anatomische Untersuchungen über die Gicht. In: Rheumatismus in Klinik und Forschung (Hrsg. W. Belart). Bern-Stuttgart: H. Huber 1962.
ZÖLLNER, N.: Die Gichtniere. In: Handbuch der Inneren Medizin, 5. Aufl., Bd. VIII/3 (Hrsg. H. SCHWIEGK), S. 77ff. Berlin-Heidelberg-New York: Springer 1968.
ZÖLLNER, N., SCHATTENKIRCHNER, M.: Allopurinol in der Behandlung der Gicht und der Harnsäure-Nephrolithiasis. Dtsch. med. Wschr. **92**, 654 (1967).

VIII. Prognose der Gicht

Prognose der Gicht

Von

A. RAUCH-JANSSEN und A. GRIEBSCH

Über die Prognose der Gicht gibt es — von wenigen Einzelarbeiten abgesehen — keine umfangreichen Publikationen. Auch die wenigen Lehrbücher der Prognostik (CURSCHMANN, 1948; WINTER, 1950) enthalten keine verwertbaren Angaben zum Thema Gicht. Die Auswertung der Weltliteratur von 1964—1974 ergab zwar 182 Arbeiten, die sich mit dieser Fragestellung befassen, jedoch nur sieben davon enthalten vergleichbare Ergebnisse zur Prognose; alle diese Arbeiten sind in den letzten Jahren erschienen (Tab. 1), wohl im Hinblick auf die zunehmende Häufigkeit der Gicht, die eine prognostische Beurteilung immer dringlicher macht.

Über Morbidität und Mortalität der Gicht führten selbst die großen deutschen Lebensversicherungsunternehmen kein ausreichendes Zahlenmaterial (BURKHARDT, 1970)[1]. Prospektive Studien über Lebenserwartung und Todesursache bei Gicht wurden in den letzten Jahren durchgeführt; das Zahlenmaterial war allerdings entweder zu klein (KLEMM, 1970) oder die medizinischen Angaben erwiesen sich als unzureichend (Münchner Rückversicherungsgesellschaft, 1970). Die bisher geringe Bedeutung der Gicht als Todesursache geht auch daraus hervor, daß im Jahrbuch des Statistischen Bundesamtes diese Erkrankung nicht als Todesursache aufgeführt wird (RAESTRUP, 1968; Münchner Rückversicherungsgesellschaft, 1970). Auch die Aufzeichnungen des Bayerischen Statistischen Landesamtes über die Jahre 1930—1960 vermitteln keine wesentlichen Erkenntnisse.

Dokumentationen über Erkrankungshäufigkeit und Sterblichkeit an Gicht wurden zwar von großen kommunalen Krankenhäusern durchgeführt (Amt für Kommunale Grundlagenforschung und Statistik München, 1971), repräsentieren jedoch lediglich ein ausgelesenes Kollektiv von Krankenhauspatienten und sind somit nicht auf die Allgemeinbevölkerung übertragbar (RAESTRUP, 1968). Die Prognose der Gicht beinhaltet jedoch sowohl die individuelle Prognose als auch die einer Population. Voraussetzung für die gerechte Risikobeurteilung sind genaue Kenntnisse über Ätiologie, Pathogenese, Diagnose und Therapie der Gicht — Forderungen, die durch den heutigen Wissenstand weitgehend erfüllt werden.

Bei der prognostischen Begutachtung der Gicht müssen drei Aspekte herangezogen werden: die Häufigkeit der zu erwartenden Anfälle, die Arbeitsfähigkeit und die Lebenserwartung (ZÖLLNER, 1970, 1974).

Prognose der Arthritis urica und der Uratnephrolithiasis

Epidemiologische Untersuchungen an auslesefreiem Material in Framingham (HALL u. Mitarb., 1967) haben ergeben, daß mit steigendem Serumharnsäurespiegel das Risiko der Entwicklung eines Gichtanfalles zunimmt. So entwickelte jeder

---

[1] In den Sterbefallregistern wurden Gichtkranke unter der Rubrik ihrer „Sekundärleiden" erfaßt (DOLL, 1959).

Tabelle 1. Zahl der Publikationen in der Weltliteratur von 1964—1974 zum Thema Prognose der Gicht

Jahre	Anzahl der Publikationen	davon verwertbar	%
1964/65	32	0	0
1966/67	32	0	0
1968/70	42	1	2,4
1971—1974	54	3	5,1
1974	17	3	17,6
Insgesamt	182	7	3,85

53. Patient mit maximalen Serumharnsäurewerten zwischen 6,0 bis 6,9 mg-% einen Gichtanfall. Diese Relation verringerte sich auf 1:6 bei Werten zwischen 7,0 bis 7,9 mg-% und auf 1:4 bei Werten zwischen 8,0 bis 8,9 mg-%. Bei einem Serumharnsäurespiegel von 9,0 mg-% und darüber konnte das Auftreten eines Gichtanfalles als sicher angesehen werden. Prognostisch bedeuten diese Ergebnisse, daß bei Feststellung eines Serumharnsäurespiegels von unter 7,0 mg-% nur selten mit der Entwicklung einer Gicht zu rechnen ist, bei einer Serumharnsäure von 9,0 mg-% und darüber die Gicht jedoch nahezu gewiß ist. Eine dauerhafte Senkung des Serumharnsäurespiegels vermindert die Anfallsbereitschaft. Zwar werden zu Beginn der Behandlung noch vereinzelt Anfälle beobachtet (ZÖLLNER u. SCHATTENKIRCHNER, 1967; KORFMACHER, 1973; ZÖLLNER, 1973; GRIEBSCH u. KORFMACHER, 1975), nach etwa 6 Monaten bleiben jedoch weitere Gichtanfälle aus (ZÖLLNER, 1966).

Bereits bestehende Uratablagerungen werden unter konsequenter Therapie abgebaut, Weichteiltophi bilden sich zurück und anstelle der Knochentophi tritt normale Bälkchenstruktur (ZÖLLNER, 1970; SCHILLING, 1971; MERTZ, 1973). Bei fortgeschrittener Gicht beobachtet man jedoch Defektheilung.

Nierensteine wurden in Framingham bei insgesamt 13,3% aller Personen mit Harnsäurespiegeln über 7,0 mg-% bzw. bei 40% aller mit Maximalwerten über 9,0 mg-% beobachtet. Mit steigendem Harnsäurespiegel nimmt somit das Risiko der Entwicklung einer Nephrolithiasis zu. Unter konsequenter Therapie gelingt es meist, Harnsäuresteine wieder aufzulösen.

Zusammenfassend kann somit die Prognose der Arthritis urica sowie der Uratnephrolithiasis bei rechtzeitiger Diagnosestellung und konsequenter Therapie (purinarme Diät und Arzneimittel) als günstig bezeichnet werden (ZÖLLNER u. GRÖBNER, 1971), Heilung ist die Regel.

Die Beurteilung der Berufsfähigkeit

Die Berufsfähigkeit des Gichtkranken richtet sich weitgehend nach dem Ausmaß der Arthritis (ZÖLLNER, 1970; ZÖLLNER u. GRÖBNER, 1971). Unter den bereits beschriebenen Voraussetzungen der rechtzeitigen Diagnose und konsequenten Therapie ist der Patient vor einer vorzeitigen Einschränkung der Berufsfähigkeit weitgehend geschützt (KORFMACHER, 1973). Da zwischen Erstbefall und deformierendem Stadium in der Regel mehrere Jahrzehnte vergehen, entwickeln sich chronisch deformierende Gelenkentzündungen mit nachfolgenden Versteifungen und Kontrakturen selten (TALBOTT, 1967). Eine vorzeitige Invalidisierung bei Gicht ist heutzutage eine Ausnahme (MERTZ, 1975). Schwerwiegende operative oder orthopädische Maßnahmen stellen ebenfalls eine Seltenheit dar. Die Arbeitsleistung des Gichtkranken richtet sich nach Ausmaß, Dauer und Häufigkeit der Anfälle, Lokalisation der Funktionsstörung und schließlich der Manifestation als schweres Allgemeinleiden und ist somit wiederum eine Frage der konsequenten und sachgerechten Therapie (SCHILLING, 1968).

Die Prognose der Gicht quoad vitam

Die primäre Gicht ist — zumindest unzureichend behandelt — ein progressiv verlaufendes Leiden (LIPSON u. SLOCUMB, 1965). Dies ist bei der Fragestellung der Lebenserwartung zu berücksichtigen. Zwar hat sich durch Einführung der Uricosurica und der Harnsäure-Synthesehemmer die Prognose der Gichtanfälle und der Uratnephrolithiasis entscheidend verbessert, ob jedoch durch diese Behandlung auch die Gichtniere, sowie die bei Gicht häufig beobachteten cardiovasculären Erkrankungen verhütet werden, bedarf noch weiterer Untersuchungen (ZÖLLNER, 1974). Darüber hinaus ist darauf hingewiesen worden (RAESTRUP, 1968), daß wir von den beschriebenen Arzneimitteln noch nicht sicher wissen, ob sie ohne nennenswerte Nebenwirkungen quoad vitam über jahrzehntelange Zeiträume eingenommen werden können.

Die Todesursachen von Gichtkranken wurden schon seit langem diskutiert, besonders im Hinblick auf die bisher in der Literatur beschriebenen möglichen Zusammenhänge zwischen Gicht bzw. Hyperurikämie und anderen Krankheiten (vgl. Kapitel WOLFRAM). Angaben über die Lebenserwartung von Gichtkranken waren bisher jedoch nur unter allen Vorbehalten möglich (HALL, 1965). Erste nähere Angaben zur Todesursache bei Gicht machte BRØCHNER-MORTENSEN (1941), der unter 77 autoptisch untersuchten Gichtikern 28,6% fand, deren Tod cardiovasculär bedingt war. Die Untersuchungen von TALBOTT und LILIENFIELD (1959) an zwei ähnlich großen Kollektiven Gichtkranker ergaben, daß bei 43,5 bzw. 61% der Tod auf cardiovasculäre Ursachen zurückzuführen war. Zu einem vergleichbar hohen Anteil der Herz- und Gefäßbeteiligung kamen HALL u. Mitarb. (1967) mit 56% cardiovasculär bedingten Todesfällen. Diese Autoren stimmten demnach darin überein, daß unter den Todesursachen der Gichtpatienten die cardiovasculären Erkrankungen — speziell Herzinfarkt und Herzinsuffizienz — weit vor den renalen Störungen liegen (Tab. 2). TALBOTT und TERPLAN (1960)

Tabelle 2. Todesursachen Gichtkranker aus 3 Kollektiven nach Angaben von TALBOTT u. LILIENFIELD (1959) bzw. HALL u. Mitarb. (1967)

Autor	TALBOTT u. LILIENFIELD		HALL u. Mitarb.
Beobachtungszeitraum	1938—1942	1946—1958	1955—1967
Anzahl des Gesamtkollektivs	64	118	5127
Anzahl der ausgewerteten Fälle Gichtkranker	54	114	76
Todesfälle	23 (42,6%)	13 (11,4%)	9 (11,8%)
Todesursachen			
Cardiovasculär bedingt	10 (43,5%)	8 (61%)	5 (56%)
Renal bedingt	1	0	2
Malignome	4	2	0
Sonstige Erkrankungen	5	1	2
Ursache unbekannt	3	2	0

Tabelle 3. Todesursachen Gichtkranker sowie Durchschnittsalter bei Tod, Erkrankungsbeginn und durchschnittliche Krankheitsdauer. Angaben nach TALBOTT u. TERPLAN (1960) bzw. KAGAMI u. Mitarb. (1970)

Todesursachen	Anzahl (%)		Durchschnittsalter bei Tod		Durchschnittsalter bei Erkrankungsbeginn		durchschnittliche Krankheitsdauer (Jahre)	
	Talbott/ Terplan	Kagami u. Mitarb.	Talbott/ Terplan	Kagami u. Mitarb.	Talbott/ Terplan	Kagami u. Mitarb.	Talbott/ Terplan	Kagami u. Mitarb.
Urämie	49 (29,9)	56 (45,5)	56,1	52,5	39,8	42,8	16,3	9,7
cardiale Erkrankungen	37 (22,6)	25 (20,3)	65,5	63,4	47,1	53,2	18,4	10,2
Apoplexie	7 (4,3)	12 (9,8)	61,4	65,7	43,0	58,3	18,4	7,4
Malignome	20 (12,2)	13 (10,6)	67,7	65,0	52,8	55,2	14,9	9,8
Andere Erkrankungen	51 (31,1)	17 (13,8)	65,7	58,1	50,8	47,0	14,9	11,1
Gesamtanzahl beobachteter Gichtkranker	164 (100)	123 (100)	62,8	58,2	46,5	48,4	16,3	9,8

ermittelten unter 164 Gichtkranken 26,9%, die an cardialen Erkrankungen bzw. Apoplexie verstarben und 29,9%, deren Tod durch Urämie hervorgerufen wurde. Die übrigen Gichtpatienten verstarben an den Folgen von Malignomen und nicht näher definierten Erkrankungen. Die Autoren beschrieben in insgesamt 82% ihrer Fälle Uratablagerungen in der Niere und in 80% pyelonephritische Veränderungen; die prognostische Beurteilung dieser Befunde quoad vitam war jedoch zum Beobachtungszeitpunkt schwer abzusehen. Dies stellt auch heute noch ein Problem dar. Ungelöst ist noch weitgehend, ob sich die vasculären — speziell cardiovasculären — Begleitkrankheiten, auf dem Weg über Gichtniere — Hochdruck — allgemeine Gefäßsklerose ausprägen (KOLLER u. ZOLLINGER, 1945).

Über die Bedeutung der Urämie als häufigste Todesursache bei Gicht berichten andere Autoren (BAUER u. CALKINI, 1959; RAKIC u. Mitarb., 1964; REASTRUP, 1968). Auch ZÖLLNER u. Mitarb. (1970, 1971, 1973, 1974) halten die renalen Komplikationen für die Ursache vorzeitiger Todesfälle bei Gicht. Diese Meinung wird bestätigt durch eine neuere, umfangreiche statistische Analyse der Todesursachen von primärer Gicht in Japan (KAGAMI u. Mitarb., 1970). Von 123 ausgewerteten Gichtkranken verstarben 45,5% an Urämie und 30,1% an cardialen Erkrankungen und Apoplexie. Die an Urämie Verstorbenen wiesen ein relativ niedriges Erkrankungs- und Todeszeitalter bei durchschnittlich kurzer Krankheitsdauer auf. Tabelle 3 zeigt die Daten dieser Untersuchung, verglichen mit denen von TALBOTT und TERPLAN (1960).

Zusammenfassend kann man feststellen, daß die Prognose von Patienten mit Gicht zunächst gut ist. Bedenkt man allerdings, daß bereits beim ersten Gichtanfall meist Veränderungen in der Niere vorliegen, so ist es zweifellos die Niere, die die Lebenserwartung des Gichtikers einschränkt (ZÖLLNER, 1971; ZÖLLNER u. KORFMACHER, 1974). Dabei scheint das Ausmaß der Nierenschädigung bestimmend für die Prognose zu sein (KAGAMI u. Mitarb., 1970). Frühzeitige Diagnosestellung, konsequente Therapie und sorgfältige Überwachung des Patienten verhindern jedoch bis zu einem gewissen Grad ein Fortschreiten der Erkrankung.

Die Altersprognose des Gichtkranken richtet sich nach dem Manifestationsalter der Gicht, dem Schweregrad und der Krankheitsdauer sowie eventuell auftretenden Begleitkrankheiten. Untersuchungen haben ergeben, daß bei einem Drittel der an Gicht Erkrankten die ersten Symptome im Alter von 60—69 Jahren auftreten. Darüber hinaus wurde seit 1965 — dank der Fortentwicklung von Diagnose und Therapie — eine kontinuierliche Zunahme der Lebenserwartung bei Gicht und ihrer möglichen Begleitkrankheiten registriert (KAGAMI u. Mitarb., 1970). Auch die Altersprognose der Gicht kann daher als günstig bezeichnet werden.

Literatur

Amt für kommunale Grundlagenforschung und Statistik München: Persönliche Mitteilung, München 1971.
BAUER, W., CHALKINS, E.: Gout. In: Diseases of Metabolism, 4th ed. Philadelphia: Saunders 1959.
BRØCHNER-MORTENSEN, K.: Hundred gouty patients. Acta med. scand. **106**, 81 (1941).
BURKHARDT, H.: Verband der Lebensversicherungsunternehmen. Persönliche Mitteilung. Bonn 1970.
CURSCHMANN, H.: Lehrbuch der speziellen Prognostik innerer Krankheiten, 3. Aufl. Stuttgart: Ehnke 1942.
DOLL, H.: Lehrbuch der Lebensversicherungsmedizin. Karlsruhe: Braun 1959.
GRIEBSCH, A., ZÖLLNER, N.: Diagnostik und Therapie des Gichtleidens. Medizin heute **13**, 4 (1972).
GRIEBSCH, A., KORFMACHER, I.: Diät bei Hyperurikämie. Münch. med. Wschr. **16**, 1373 (1975).
HALL, A. P.: Correlations among hyperuricemia, hypercholesterolemia, coronary disease and hypertension. Arthr. Rheum. **8**, 846 (1965).
HALL, A. P., BARRY, P. E., DAWBER, T. R., MC NAMARA, P. M.: Epidemiology of gout and hyperuricemia. A long-term population study. Amer. J. Med. **42**, 27 (1967).
HEIDELMANN, G., THIELE, P.: Das Gichtsyndrom. Dresden: Steinkopff 1973.
KAGAMI, T., NOMURA, T., OGINO, K.: Statistische Analyse der Todesursachen nach primärer Gicht in Japan. Naika **26**, 1099 (1970).
KLEMM, A.: Allianz Lebensversicherungs AG. Persönliche Mitteilung. Stuttgart 1970.
KOLLER, F., ZOLLINGER, H. U.: Gichtische Glomerulosklerose. Schweiz. med. Wschr. **75**, 97 (1945).
KORFMACHER, I.: Langzeittherapie der Gicht. Der Praktische Arzt. Dortmund: Krüger 1973.
KORFMACHER, I., ZÖLLNER, N.: Gicht — lebenslange Behandlung unerläßlich. Dtsch. Ärztebl. **17**, 1221 (1974).
LIPSON, R. L., SLOCUMB, C. H.: The progressive nature of gout with inadequate therapy. Arth. Rheum. **8**, 80 (1965).
MERTZ, D. P.: Gicht. Stuttgart: Thieme 1973.
MERTZ, D. P.: Sozialmedizinische Aspekte der Gicht. Dtsch. Ärztebl. **43**, 2982 (1975).
Münchner Rückversicherungsgesellschaft: Persönliche Mitteilung. München 1970.
RAESTRUP, O.: Die Prognostik der Gicht. Münch. med. Wschr. **110**, 1249 (1968).
RAKIC, M. T., VAKENBURG, H. A., DAVIDSON, R. T., ENGELS, J. P., MIKKELSEN, W. M., NEEL, J. N., DUFF, J. F.: Observations of the natural history of hyperuricemia and gout. Amer. J. Med. **37**, 862 (1964).
SCHILLING, F.: Klinik und Therapie der Gicht und deren Abgrenzung von der Pseudogicht. In: Fettsucht-Gicht. Stuttgart: Thieme 1971.
SCHILLING, F.: Rehabilitation chronisch entzündlich rheumatischer Krankheiten. Ärzteblatt Rheinland-Pfalz **21**, 844 (1968).
TALBOTT, J. H., LILIENFIELD, A.: Longevity in gout. Geriatrics **14**, 409 (1959).

TALBOTT, J. H., TERPLAN, K. L.: The kidney in gout. Medicine **39**, 405 (1960).
TALBOTT, J. H.: Gout, 3th. ed. New York: Grune and Stratton 1967.
WINTER, H.: Die Individualprognose in der Inneren Medizin. Wien 1950.
WOLFRAM, G., ZÖLLNER, N.: Die Gicht als Stoffwechselproblem in der Praxis. Ärztl. Fortbild. **19** (1971).
ZÖLLNER, N.: Behandlung der Gicht und der Uratnephrolithiasis mit Allopurinol. Verh. dtsch. Ges. inn. Med. **72**, 781 (1966).
ZÖLLNER, N., SCHATTENKIRCHNER, M.: Allopurinol in der Behandlung der Gicht und der Harnsäure-Nephrolithiasis. Dtsch. med. Wschr. **14**, 654 (1967).
ZÖLLNER, N.: Erfolgsbeurteilung bei der Gichtbehandlung. Therapiewoche **20**, 1655 (1970).
ZÖLLNER, N., GRÖBNER, W.: Prognoseverbesserung der Gicht durch geeignete Therapie. Lebensversicherungsmedizin **6** (1971).
ZÖLLNER, N.: Lehrbuch der Inneren Medizin. 3. Aufl. Stuttgart-New York: Schattauer 1973.
ZÖLLNER, N.: Grundlagen der Gichtforschung. Münch. med. Wschr. **116**, 865 (1974).

IX. The Lesch-Nyhan Syndrome and Adult X-Linked Hyperuricaciduria

The Lesch-Nyhan Syndrome and Adult X-Linked Hyperuricaciduria

Von

W. N. KELLEY and J. B. WYNGAARDEN

With 9 Figures

Introduction

Well over a century ago GARROD, A. B. demonstrated that an elevated serum urate concentration was a characteristic chemical feature of gout (GARROD, 1848). Over the past twenty years, a series of studies have established that a number of distinct metabolic abnormalities, both familial and acquired, may be responsible for the development of hyperuricemia (SEEGMILLER et al., 1963; GUTMAN and YU, 1965; WYNGAARDEN, 1966). Thus, even inherited hyperuricemia is heterogeneous, and not the result of an alteration at only a single genetic locus. Elucidation of the molecular bases of hyperuricemia can best be accomplished by the recognition and study of specific diseases within the hyperuricemic population.

In 1967, SEEGMILLER et al. described a virtually complete deficiency of an enzyme of purine metabolism, hypoxanthine-guanine phosphoribosyltransferase, in erythrocyte lysates from 3 patients and in cultured skin fibroblasts from a fourth patient with Lesch-Nyhan syndrome (SEEGMILLER et al., 1967). This is a disorder characterized by choreoathetosis, striking growth and mental retardation, spasticity, self-mutilation, and marked hyperuricemia, with excessive uric acid production (LESCH and NYHAN, 1964). The enzyme defect was subsequently confirmed in other tissues as well as in cultured skin fibroblasts and erythrocytes from many similarly affected patients (KELLEY, 1968a).

A number of patients have now been described with a "partial" rather than a "complete" deficiency of hypoxanthine-guanine phosphoribosyltransferase (KELLEY et al., 1967a; KELLEY et al., 1969; KOGUT et al., 1970; SPERLING et al., 1970; DELBARRE et al., 1970). These patients usually present with gouty arthritis or uric acid calculi and do not have the devastating neurological and behavioral features characteristic of the functionally complete enzyme defect (KELLEY et al., 1969).

The etiology of a deficiency of hypoxanthine-guanine phosphoribosyltransferase is a mutation of the DNA in the X chromosome at the locus which codes for this enzyme. These disorders comprise a well-defined segment of the hyperuricacidurias. The syndrome associated with a functionally complete deficiency of this enzyme is of special interest in that it provides the first example of a specific enzyme defect associated with a reproducible pattern of abnormal behavior. The partial deficiency of this enzyme represented the first enzyme abnormality found in patients with adult-onset gout. Both are well-defined at the clinical and molecular levels.

Enzyme Defect

Hypoxanthine-guanine phosphoribosyltransferase (PRT) catalyzes the conversion of hypoxanthine to inosinic acid and guanine to guanylic acid in the presence of phosphoribosylpyrophosphate (PP-ribose-P) (KORNBERG et al., 1955, KORN et al., 1955). The natural purine base, xanthine, and several purine analogs, including 6-mercaptopurine, allopurinol, 8-azaguanine and 6-thioguanine, are also substrates (KRENITSKY et al., 1969a; BROCKMAN, 1965) (Fig. 1). The enzyme is activated by magnesium and is inhibited by the products of the reaction. Guanylic acid and its di- and triphosphates are much stronger inhibitors than inosinic or xanthylic acid (KRENITSKY et al., 1969a).

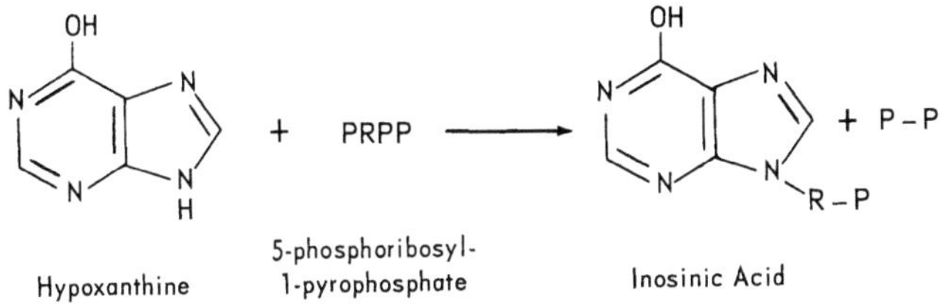

Fig. 1. The reaction catalyzed by hypoxanthine-guanine phosphoribosyltransferase, illustrated with hypoxanthine as substrate

Patients with the Lesch-Nyhan syndrome usually have very little or no detectable hypoxanthine-guanine phosphoribosyltransferase activity in erythrocytes or in other tissues obtained at the time of autopsy (Table 1). One patient with this syndrome has been found to have a mutant form of hypoxanthine-guanine phosphoribosyltransferase with altered kinetic constants for both PP-ribose-P and purine substrates (MCDONALD and KELLEY, 1971) (Table 2). Erythrocytes from this patient have normal hypoxanthine-guanine phosphoribosyltransferase activity when assayed at very high concentrations of substrates; however, at the usual concentrations employed for the assay *in vitro* there is essentially no activity. It seems unlikely, on the basis of the known intracellular concentration of these substrates, that this mutant enzyme exhibits any function *in vivo*. This mutant form of the enzyme also differs from the normal in exhibiting sigmoidal kinetics with PP-ribose-P as the variable substrate (Fig. 2). Very low levels of activity ranging from 0.005 to 5% of normal have recently been reported in several other patients with the classic syndrome (SORENSEN, 1970; MIZUNO et al., 1970; ARNOLD and KELLEY, 1972). Despite the absence of detectable enzyme activity in hemolysates from most patients with this disease, all so far examined appear to have a protein which exhibits cross-reactivity (CRM+) with an antibody to the normal enzyme (RUBIN et al., 1971; ARNOLD and KELLEY, 1972). The amount of this protein is equal to the amount of enzyme found in normal subjects. This indicates that the mutations responsible for the development of functionally complete deficiencies of this enzyme are on the structural gene coding for the enzyme.

Fibroblasts cultured from many patients with Lesch-Nyhan syndrome have uniformly been shown to have low but detectable levels of PRT activity (FUJIMOTO and SEEGMILLER, 1970; KELLEY and MEADE, 1971a) (Table 3). Detailed examination of the mutant enzyme in fibroblasts cultured from 10 patients with the Lesch-Nyhan syndrome revealed at least 3 different phenotypes (Table 4). These studies provide additional evidence that the mutations are on the structural gene for the PRT enzyme. In addition, they indicate that the mutations are

Table 1. Specific activity of phosphoribosyltransferase of erythrocyte hemolysates from subjects with Lesch-Nyhan syndrome

Subjects	Phosphoribosyltransferase activity µmoles/mg protein per hour		
	Hypoxanthine, mean ± SD	Guanine, mean ± SD	Adenine, mean ± SD
Normal (32)[a]	103 ± 18	103 ± 21	31 ± 6
Lesch-Nyhan Syndrome			
JW	< 0.01	< 0.004	58
TS	< 0.01	< 0.004	39
DF	< 0.01	< 0.004	53
BM	< 0.01	< 0.004	49
MB	< 0.01	< 0.004	56
SM	< 0.01	< 0.004	51
FH	< 0.01	< 0.004	94
MW	< 0.01	< 0.004	65
JS	< 0.01	< 0.004	71

[a] Number of subjects studied. (From KELLEY, 1968a)

Table 2. Comparison of the kinetic properties of the normal and a mutant hypoxanthine-guanine phosphoribosyltransferase (PRT) enzyme

Enzyme source		Phosphoribosyltransferase Activity (nmole mg^{-1} hr^{-1})		Apparent K_m(MgPP-ribose-P)		Apparent K_m (Guanine) (M)	Apparent K_m (Hypoxanthine) (M)
Cell	Type	Guanine	Hypoxanthine	Guanine	Hypoxanthine		
Erythrocyte	Normal	98 ± 14	97 ± 19[a]	2.5 × 10^{-4}		5.0 × 10^{-6}	1.7 × 10^{-5}
	Mutant	8.2 (12.1)	33.7 (94.4)	3.2 × 10^{-3b}	2.8 × 10^{-3b}	4.8 × 10^{-5}	1.8 × 10^{-4}
Fibroblast	Normal	141 ± 17		1.0 × 10^{-4}			
	Mutant	10.4		2.0 × 10^{-3b}			

[a] Mean ± S.D. in 119 subjects. Numbers in parentheses represent V_{max} of the mutant enzyme for each purine substrate calculated from the Michaelis-Menten formula ($V_{max} = (K_m + S)/S$). Mean ± S.D. in normal cell strains.
[b] Values depict $S_{0.5}$ rather than K_m. (From MCDONALD and KELLEY, 1971)

probably not large deletions, or frame shift or nonsense mutations. They are most likely either point mutations causing a change in a single amino acid or very small deletions. It is clear that a striking degree of genetic heterogeneity exists in the mutations leading to the Lesch-Nyhan syndrome.

Patients with the "partial" enzyme defect exhibit levels of PRT activity in erythrocytes ranging from 0.01% to nearly 30% of normal (KELLEY et al., 1969; KOGUT et al., 1970; SPERLING et al., 1970; DELBARRE et al., 1970) (Table 5). PRT activity in leukocytes and in fibroblasts cultured from these patients is similar to that observed in erythrocytes. The level of PRT activity is generally the same within one family but often differs between families. In addition, in two members of one family there was substantially more activity with hypoxanthine (10% of normal) than with guanine as substrate (0.5% of normal) (KELLEY et al., 1967a). These observations suggested that the mutations leading to partial loss of enzyme

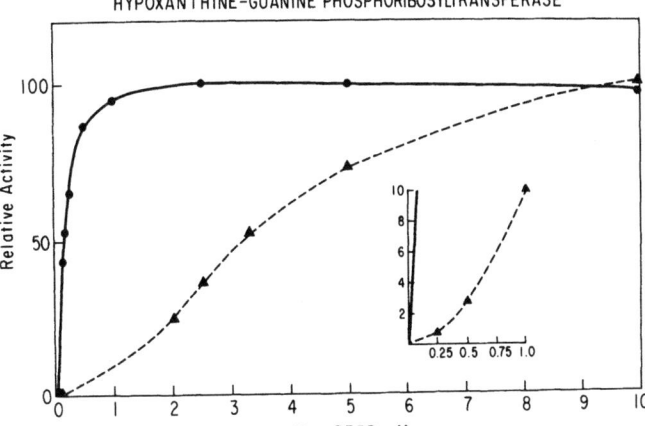

Fig. 2. Effect of Mg PP-ribose-P concentration on GMP synthesis by normal and a mutant PRT enzyme (From McDonald and Kelley, 1971)

activity may be different among the families studied. Substantial evidence for this was obtained by study of thermal inactivation of the PRT enzymes obtained from 6 patients in 3 families. The PRT enzyme obtained from two members of the L. Family was very heat-resistant; that from 3 members of the J. Family was very sensitive to heat, and that from Patient T.S. was slightly more heat-sensitive than the normal enzyme (Kelley et al., 1969) (Fig. 3). A mixture of the dialyzed hemolysates from members of the J. and L. Families showed the expected intermediate sensitivity of the enzyme mixture to heat, demonstrating that no labilizing or

Table 3. Phosphoribosyltransferase activity in fibroblasts cultured from hyperuricemic patients

Cell strain	No. of Assays	Passage	Hypoxanthine-guanine phosphoribosyltransferase Activity (nmoles/mg protein/hr)	
			Mean	Range
Normal	13[a]	3—11	141 ± 17[b]	95—190
Lesch-Nyhan syndrome				
121	17[c]	4—17	0.6	0.1—2.0
123	26	4—29	0.7	0.1—2.9
S.M.	4	13—24	1.0	0.1—2.4
J.R.	4	15—16	1.1	0.1—1.7
M.W.	3	13—17	1.3	0.1—2.0
182	9	5—16	0.6	0.1—3.0
193	8	5—13	11.0	5.4—15.2
197	9	7—11	2.0	0.9—6.1
198	10	4— 8	2.7	1.4—3.6
199	10	4— 7	2.9	1.9—4.9
200	10	4— 9	4.0	0.1—9.0
"Partial" PRT Deficiency				
C.N.	2	—	11.0	—
E.S.	2	—	26.0	—

[a] Different cell strains.
[b] Standard deviation.
[c] Number of different preparations.
(Modified from Kelley and Meade, 1971a).

Table 4. Genetic heterogeneity of hypoxanthine-guanine phosphoribosyltransferase deficiency in fibroblasts derived from patients with Lesch-Nyhan syndrome

	Product Inhibition[a]	Thermal Stability	Prototype (cell strain)
Normal	+	+	
Mutant			
Type 1	+	+	193
Type 2	+	−	182, 197, 198, 199
Type 3	−	−	121

[a] +, normal; −, abnormal. (From KELLEY and MEADE, 1971a.)

Table 5. Specific activity of phosphoribosyltransferase (PRT) in erythrocyte hemolysates in hyperuricemic subjects

Subject[a]	PRT activity (μmole/mg protein/hr)		
	Hypoxanthine	Guanine	Adenine
Normal (32), mean ±SD	103±18	103±21	31.1±6.0
Hyperuricemia, mean ±SD			
Normal uric acid production (6)	99±13	106±10	31.2±6.9
Excessive uric acid production, mean ±SD			
Normal enzyme (10)	103±18	104±22	30.4±5.3
Partial Deficiency (18)			
J. Family			
F.J.	1.3	0.6	46
R.J.	1.5	0.8	43
T.J.	1.8	0.8	56
L. Family			
F.L.	11.8	0.5	74
M.L.	8.7	0.5	64
S. Family			
T.S.	9.9	9.5	39
D. Family			
A.D.	12.2	17.3	33
G. Family			
J.G.	9.4	8.8	32
R.G.	9.2	7.5	38
S_2 Family			
G.S.	0.03	0.009	58
I. Family			
T.I.	0.06	0.09	32
R. Family			
A.R.	0.9	0.5	48
M. Family			
C.M.	2.7	3.7	26
T. Family			
R.T.	0.06	0.07	36
M.W.	0.06	0.05	29
R.L.	0.09	0.10	44
N. Family			
C.N.	0.3	0.3	35
E.S.	0.4	0.3	39

[a] Number of subjects in parentheses. (From KELLEY et al., 1969.)

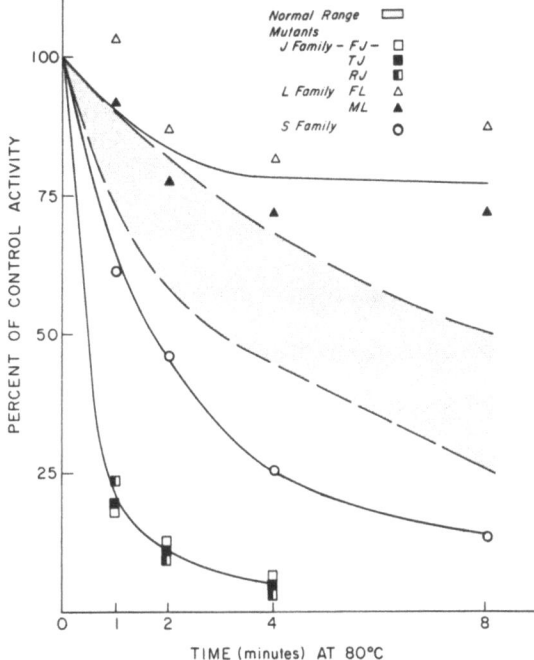

Fig. 3. Inactivation of normal and mutant phosphoribosyltransferase when heated at 80° C for the time indicated. (From KELLEY et al., 1969)

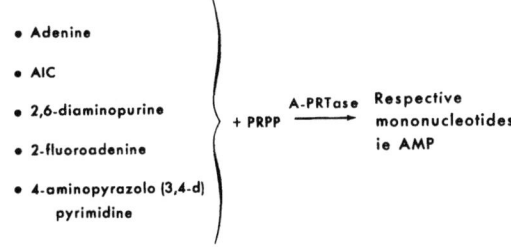

Fig. 4. Reactions catalyzed by adenine phosphoribosyltransferase

stabilizing factors were present in the J. or L. hemolysates. These findings suggested, therefore, that separate structural gene mutations were responsible for the partial enzyme defect observed in each of these 3 families.

The activity of a closely related enzyme, adenine phosphoribosyltransferase, which catalyzes the synthesis of adenylic acid from adenine and PP-ribose-P (Fig. 4), is elevated in erythrocytes from patients with the "functionally complete" deficiency of PRT (SEEGMILLER et al., 1967; KELLEY, 1968a). Many patients with a partial deficiency of PRT also show increased activity of erythrocyte APRT (KELLEY et al., 1969). GREENE et al. have recently demonstrated that PP-ribose-P stabilizes purified adenine phosphoribosyltransferase *in vitro*. In addition, PP-ribose-P levels are increased in erythrocytes from patients lacking PRT who exhibit increased erythrocyte adenine phosphoribosyltransferase activity (GREENE et al., 1970; FOX and KELLEY, 1971). GREENE and colleagues have suggested that increased PP-ribose-P levels stabilize the adenine phosphoribosyltransferase enzyme *in vivo* and that stabilization leads to a diminished rate of degradation of the enzyme and thus to an increased specific activity (GREENE et al., 1970). GREENE et al. (1970) and RUBIN and co-workers (1969) reported that APRT was more stable in circulating erythrocytes from patients with Lesch-Nyhan syndrome than from normal subjects. This does not appear to be the case in cultured fibroblasts despite the increased PP-ribose-P levels in this cell type as well (KELLEY, 1971 b).

Excessive Uric Acid Production

Clinical description

The excessive production of uric acid characteristic of both the "complete" and "partial" PRT deficiency syndromes results from an accelerated rate of purine biosynthesis *de novo*. Glycine-1-^{14}C is very rapidly incorporated into uric acid in such patients. The cumulative incorporation of this compound into urinary uric acid over a 7-day period is as much as 20 times normal in some cases (LESCH and NYHAN, 1964; NYHAN et al., 1965; KELLEY et al., 1967b).

The excessive production of uric acid is reflected in its increased excretion in the urine. The daily excretion of uric acid in patients with the "complete" enzyme defect is extremely high when one considers the small size of these patients. Excretion values range from 25 to 143 mg/kg/day in patients with the "complete" defect (MICHENER, 1967; ROSENBERG et al., 1968) and from 10 to 36 mg/kg/day in patients with "partial" deficiency of PRT (KELLEY et al., 1969). The upper limits of normal in adults and children are 10 and 18 mg/kg/day respectively (MICHENER, 1967). The excretion of uric acid can also be expressed in relation to creatinine excretion, another index of body mass. The ratio of uric acid to creatinine concentration in urine samples obtained from patients with both "partial" and "complete" PRT deficiency is uniformly greater than in age-matched controls (Fig. 5). The consistency of this elevated ratio, the ease of collecting random urine samples, and the simplicity of the chemical determinations make the uric acid-to-creatinine ratio in urine a good (though nonspecific) screening test for this disorder (KAUFMAN et al., 1968). Several other disorders also associated with excessive uric acid production, such as type I glycogen storage disease and certain lymphoproliferative disorders, will cause an occasional false-positive test result.

Because of the increased quantity of uric acid in the urine, most patients experience uric acid crystaluria at some time. Occasionally the first sign noted by the mother is the presence of orange crystals on a diaper during the first few weeks of life (HOEFNAGEL et al., 1965). Unfortunately, this is rarely brought to the physician's attention except in retrospect, and even when recognized, such crystals are easily mistaken for some other urinary constituent such as cystine. Many patients go on to develop symptomatic uric acid nephrolithiasis which may lead to obstructive uropathy with severe and unrelenting azotemia. Nineteen of the 28 patients with the "partial" PRT deficiency have had uric acid calculi. In at least 9 of these patients, this was the initial symptom prompting the patient to seek medical care.

The excessive production of uric acid leads to the development of hyperuricemia. The serum urate concentration may range from 7 mg/100 ml to as high as 18 mg/100 ml in the absence of renal insufficiency. In an occasional patient, a random value falls within the normal range (VAN BOGOERT et al., 1966; RILEY, 1960; BERMAN et al., 1969). The serum urate concentration may provide an initial

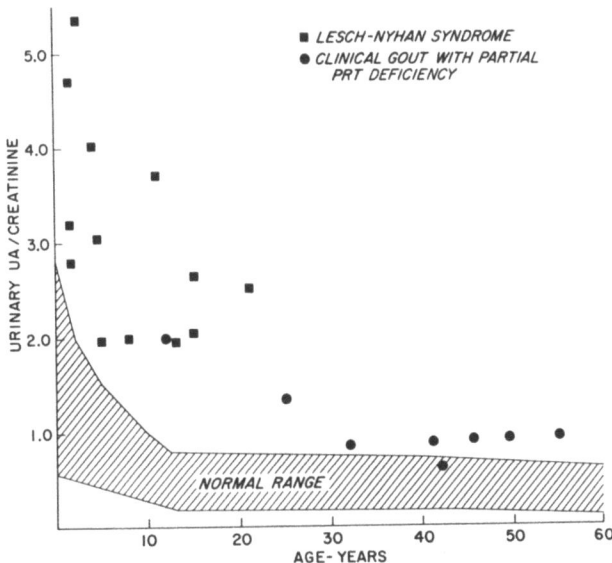

Fig. 5. Ratio of uric acid to creatinine concentration in urine samples obtained from patients with the Lesch-Nyhan syndrome ("complete" PRT deficiency) and those with gout and a "partial" deficiency of PRT. The normal range represents the mean ± 2 standard deviations in a total of 284 control subjects of various ages. (From Kaufman et al., 1968)

clue to the diagnosis, but it is not an infallible screening test, because of its variability, especially in the younger patient.

Only an occasional patient with the "complete" enzyme defect has developed classic gouty arthritis and tophaceous deposits of monosodium urate (Sass et al., 1965; Riley, 1960). By contrast, a history of gouty arthritis was present in 20 of the 23 patients with the "partial" defect who were older than 13 before effective hypouricemic therapy was instituted. Over one half of this latter group have developed tophi.

Hypoxanthine and xanthine, the immediate precursors of uric acid, are readily converted to uric acid by the ample quantities of xanthine oxidase present in the liver, so that only a moderate increase in the total urinary excretion of these compounds occurs. In normal individuals xanthine is usually excreted in excess of hypoxanthine, due to the reutilization of hypoxanthine to inosinic acid. In patients deficient in hypoxanthine-guanine phosphoribosyltransferase the inability to convert hypoxanthine to inosinic acid leads to a substantial increase in the excretion of hypoxanthine over that of xanthine (Balis et al., 1967; Balis, 1968).

Pathogenesis

There are several possible mechanisms by which a deficiency of hypoxanthine-guanine phosphoribosyltransferase activity could lead to excessive purine synthesis. A deficiency of this enzyme might lead to an increase in purine synthesis *de novo* by virtue of decreased synthesis of IMP or GMP since these nucleotides are normally important inhibitors of purine biosynthesis *de novo*. Attempts to measure intracellular levels of IMP and GMP have been of only limited value because of the very low intracellular concentration of these compounds under normal conditions (Rosenbloom et al., 1968).

Table 6. Erythrocyte PP-ribose-P levels hemizygotes and heterozygotes for "complete" PRT deficiency

	Erythrocyte PP-ribose-P (nmole/ml)
Normal values	4.4 ± 1.8
Hypoxanthine-guanine phosphoribosyltransferase deficiency	
Hemizygote	
E.S.	39.4
J.K.	20.5
W.E.	49.5
Heterozygote	
M.S.	6.5
M.E.	4.5
H.K.	1.5

The concentration of PP-ribose-P is elevated in erythrocytes (GREENE and SEEGMILLER, 1969a; FOX and KELLEY, 1971) and in cultured fibroblasts (ROSENBLOOM et al., 1968) from patients with both the "partial" and "complete" enzyme defect (Table 6). In fibroblasts the elevated concentration is attributable to decreased utilization of the compound rather than to increased synthesis (ROSENBLOOM et al., 1968). An increased concentration of PP-ribose-P could stimulate purine biosynthesis *de novo* by providing more substrate for the limiting step of this pathway, PP-ribose-P amidotransferase. The increased synthesis of purines in patients with type I glycogen storage disease due to a deficiency of glucose-6-phosphatase has also been attributed on theoretical grounds to an increased concentration of PP-ribose-P (ALEPA et al., 1967; JAKOVCIC and SORENSEN, 1967; KELLEY et al., 1968b). In order for PP-ribose-P to stimulate purine synthesis *de novo* in either of these conditions, however, the normal concentration of PP-ribose-P would need to be substantially less than that required for saturation of the enzyme. The concentration of PP-ribose-P in normal human erythrocytes ranges from 1 to 5×10^{-6}M, which is well below its Km for PP-ribose-P amidotransferase in mammalian adenocarcinoma cells (4.7×10^{-4}M) (HILL and BENNETT, 1969). The Michaelis constants for this enzyme in normal human tissue are not known, and the intracellular concentration of PP-ribose-P has not been established in tissues other than the mature erythrocyte. Recent data from a study of the effects of orotic acid on purine synthesis in cultured human cells and in intact man provide strong evidence that intracellular levels of PP-ribose-P are important in the regulation of purine biosynthesis *de novo* (KELLEY et al., 1970a; KELLEY et al., 1970b). It thus seems likely that increased levels of PP-ribose-P are at least partly responsible for the increased purine biosynthesis *de novo* in patients with "complete" or "partial" PRT deficiency.

Central Nervous System Dysfunction

Clinical description

Patients with the "complete" PRT deficiency generally appear normal at birth. Although hypotonia, recurrent vomiting, and difficulty with secretions are noted in some patients during the first three months of life (NYHAN, 1968a), the earliest consistent abnormality is a delay in motor development noted at three or four

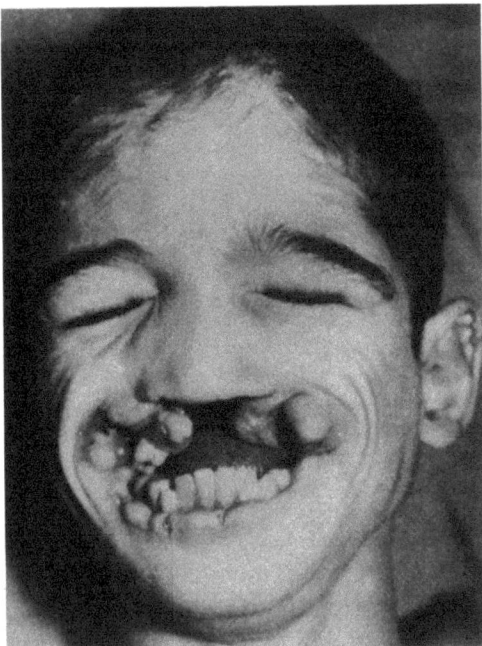

Fig. 6. Evidence of severe mutilation of lips in a patient with the "complete" deficiency of hypoxanthine-guanine phosphoribosyltransferase. (From NYHAN, 1968a)

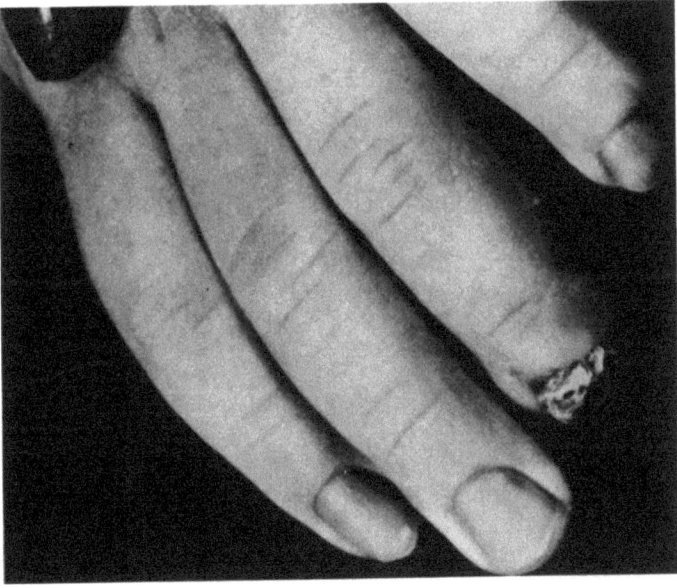

Fig. 7. Evidence of autoamputation of a distal phalanx in a patient with "complete" hypoxanthine-guanine phosphoribosyltransferase deficiency. (NYHAN, 1968a)

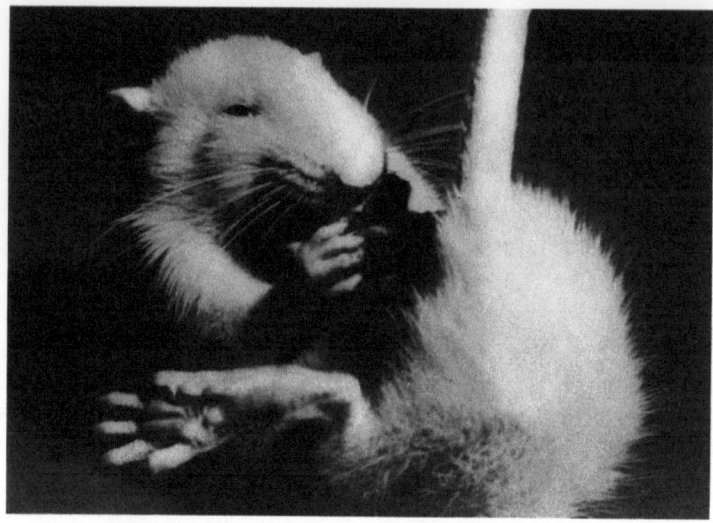

Fig. 8. Automutilation observed in a rat after the administration of large doses (185 mg/kg) of caffeine (1,3,7-tri methyl xanthine) for 12 days. (Courtesy of F. M. ROSENBLOOM, M.D.)

months of age. Between eight months and one year, extrapyramidal signs develop, characterized by fine athetoid movements of the hands and feet, dystonia, and chorea. The athetosis, which is similar to that noted with asphyxia, birth injury, and hyperbilirubinemia, accounts at least in part for the dysarthria noted later in life (DREIFUSS et al., 1968). At about one year, signs of pyramidal tract involvement develop, such as hyperreflexia, sustained ankle clonus, extensor plantar responses, and scissoring of the legs. These findings are so marked that they preclude ambulation in the older patient.

The most striking neurological feature of the Lesch-Nyhan syndrome is compulsive self-destructive behavior. At two or three years of age, most children affected begin to bite their fingers, lips, and buccal mucosa (Figs. 7 and 8). This compulsion for self-mutilation becomes so extreme that it may be necessary to keep the elbows in extension with splints or the hands wrapped with gauze. In several patients mutilation of lips has only been controlled by extraction of teeth.

Retarded children with a variety of other disorders will often exhibit finger biting, as well as other types of self-destructive behavior, although the occurrence of lip biting seems to be almost unique to the Lesch-Nyhan syndrome. Severe self-biting also occurs in a number of neurological disorders characterized by loss of pain sensation (GILLESPIE and PERUCCA, 1960); however, detailed study of patients with PRT deficiency has failed to reveal any sensory abnormalities.

Patients with the "complete" enzyme defect attempt to injure themselves by a variety of maneuvers in addition to self-biting, and typically exhibit unusual aggressiveness toward others. They respond to stressful situations with increased agitation, episodes of opisthotonic posturing, and attempts at self-mutilation. As an affected individual becomes older, an internal struggle develops between the apparent desire to inflict injury and attempts to control this urge.

Most patients with the Lesch-Nyhan syndrome appear to be mentally deficient. When attempted by routine methods, IQ testing usually results in values ranging from 30 to 65. However, the poor performance on formal testing is in part related to dysarthria and choreoathetosis. One patient appeared to have normal intelligence when testing was designed to minimize these factors (SCHERZER and ILSON, 1969). Approximately 50% of patients reported in the literature have had seizures. In some patients these have been interpreted as decerebrate cerebellar fits (HOEFNAGEL, 1967).

Routine studies of cerebrospinal fluid are normal. Electromyograms and nerve conduction velocities are also normal (BERMAN et al., 1969). Electroencephalograms may reveal diffuse slowing.

Six of the 28 patients described with a "partial" deficiency of PRT have had evidence of neurologic dysfunction (KELLEY et al., 1969; KOGUT et al., 1970; SPERLING et al., 1970; DELBARRE et al., 1970). In 4 of these, the neurological features suggested a forme fruste relationship to the devastating neurological disease found in patients with the "complete" enzyme defect. Patients M. L. and F. L. are siblings who have a spinocerebellar syndrome characterized by nystagmus, hyperreflexia, and an inability to perform heel-to-toe walking. One patient, G. S., had a delayed onset of speech as a child and a lifelong history of spasticity. The fourth patient has a long history of a seizure disorder. Three of these 4 patients (all except F. L.) are mildly retarded with IQ values ranging from 67 to 75 by formal testing.

Pathology

There was no distinctive pathology in the central nervous system in 8 patients with "complete" PRT deficiency that have come to autopsy. The findings described by SASS et al. of demyelinative and vascular lesions of the cerebral and cerebellar white matter, degeneration of the granules in Purkinje cells, multiple small chronic infarcts, and the presence of de Galantha staining material, can probably be attributed to the severe uremia preceding death (SASS et al., 1965). PARTINGTON and HENNEN (1967) noted nonurate perivascular birefringent crystals in the alcoholfixed brain from one of their patients. One of the 2 original cases reported by LESCH and NYHAN (1964) was autopsied at the NIH in 1966. A brownish pigmentation was noted over the cerebral cortex, although this could not be detected histologically (ROSENBLUM et al., 1971). RILEY's patient (1960) was found at autopsy to have thinning of the cerebellar cortex and loss of cells in the granular layer (SEEGMILLER, 1968). Autopsies of 4 additional cases have failed to reveal any significant changes in the central nervous system (HOEFNAGEL et al., 1965; CRUSSI et al., 1969; RENUART, 1971).

Pathogenesis

The mechanism by which a decrease in PRT activity might produce the neurological disorder observed in all patients with a functionally complete deficiency of the enzyme and in some with its "partial" absence is still obscure. The most compelling arguments against a causal role of uric acid in the central nervous dysfunction are the demonstration of normal concentrations of uric acid in the cerebrospinal fluid (CSF) of all patients examined (ROSENBLOOM et al., 1967) and the failure of hypouricemic therapy to alter central nervous system function. The absence of xanthine oxidase in the central nervous system (AL-KHALIDI and CHAGLASSIAN, 1965) suggests that the oxypurine precursors of uric acid, hypoxanthine and xanthine, might accumulate if the tissues of the brain participated in the excessive synthesis of purines. An elevated concentration of oxypurines was found in patients with "partial" or "complete" deficiency of PRT (ROSENBLOOM et al., 1967). The higher CSF plasma concentration ratio of oxypurines in affected than in normal individuals is suggestive evidence of excessive purine synthesis within

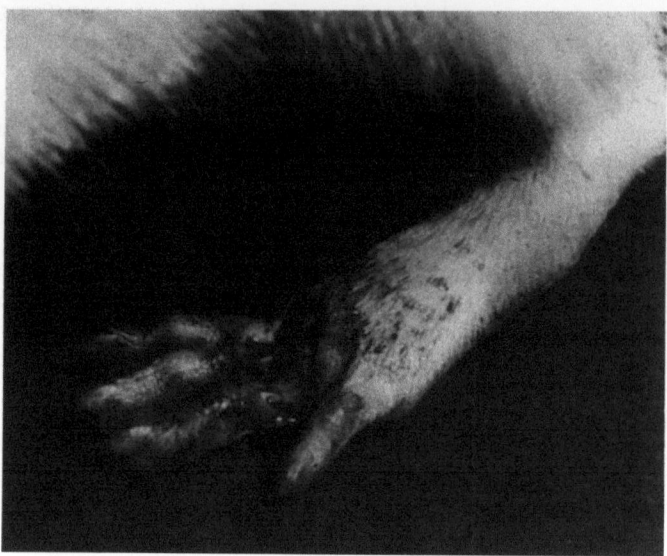

Fig. 9. Close-up view of a self-inflicted injury in a rat receiving large doses of caffeine as described in Fig. 6. (Courtesy of F. M. ROSENBLOOM, M.D.)

the central nervous system of PRT deficient subjects. The administration of caffeine, a methylated xanthine, produces self-mutilation in rats (BOYD et al., 1965; SEEGMILLER, 1968) (Fig. 9). However, the finding of an elevated CSF concentration of hypoxanthine and xanthine in two patients with a "partial" deficiency of PRT who showed no evidence of central nervous system dysfunction suggests that these compounds are not in themselves responsible for the central nervous system disease (KELLEY et al., 1969).

Table 7. Specific activity of phosphoribosyltransferase (PRT) in human necropsy tissue

Tissue	PRT		
	Hypoxanthine	Guanine	Adenine
Brain			
Frontal lobe	497	736	12
Basal ganglia	843	1137	43
Spinal cord	42	57	4
Cerebellum	463	660	68
Liver	41	66	155
Spleen	36	60	50
Kidney	28	48	11
Muscle	0.1	5	15
Ovary	143	194	46
Pancreas	42	41	5
Jejunum	18	27	9
Adrenal	35	58	31
Erythrocytes	103	103	31
Leukocytes	128	183	221

(From KELLEY et al., 1969)

It is possible that a toxic product may accumulate or that a compound necessary for normal central nervous system function may be deficient as a direct result of the enzyme defect. The observations in man (ROSENBLOOM et al., 1967a) and the Rhesus monkey (KRENITSKY, 1969b) that hypoxanthine-guanine phosphoribosyltransferase activity is normally higher in the central nervous system than in any other tissue (Table 7), and that the activity of PP-ribose-P amidotransferase, the rate-limiting step in the *de novo* pathway, is low in the CNS (HOWARD et al., 1970), suggest that the brain may be unusually dependent on the salvage pathway for the synthesis of IMP and GMP. The possibility exists, therefore, that in the absence of hypoxanthine-guanine phosphoribosyltransferase the central nervous system may be unable to maintain intracellular concentrations of GMP or IMP necessary for normal function. In the absence of hypoxanthine-guanine phosphoribosyltransferase activity, these purine nucleotides must be synthesized entirely by the *de novo* pathway. The increased activity of this pathway could lead to depletion of certain co-factors, such as ATP or folic acid, and deficiencies of these critical substances could impair normal development or limit normal function. There are no data currently available which would allow further consideration of these possibilities.

Hematologic Abnormalities

At least 10 of the reported patients with the "complete" PRT deficiency were anemic prior to the onset of renal insufficiency (CATEL and SCHMIDT, 1959; RILEY, 1960; PARTINGTON and HENNEN, 1967; ROSENBERG et al., 1968; LABRUNE et al., 1968; MARIE et al., 1967; MANZKE, 1967). CATEL and SCHMIDT (1959) described the anemia in their patient as megaloblastic in character. A number of investigators have confirmed the presence of macrocytic erythrocytes in the peripheral blood and megaloblastic changes in the bone marrow in patients with the "complete" and "partial" PRT deficiency (MARIE et al., 1967; MANZKE, 1967; VAN DER ZEE et al., 1968). Such changes may be present even in the absence of overt anemia.

Several patients with megaloblastic changes in the bone marrow and macrocytic erythrocytes have had a low serum folate concentration (KELLEY et al., 1969). Fibroblasts derived from similar individuals show an increased growth requirement for adenine which can be overcome by high concentrations of folic acid (FELIX and DE MARS, 1969). These findings suggest that the accelerated rate of purine synthesis *de novo* leads to an increased utilization of folate, an essential cofactor at 2 sites in the *de novo* pathway. Adenine is readily converted to AMP and then to IMP and GMP. These purine nucleotides inhibit PP-ribose-P amidotransferase and thereby reduce the rate of *de novo* synthesis and presumably the rate of folate utilization. It is not known, however, whether the low serum folate levels occasionally observed are due to increased utilization or are in fact related to the anemia. The finding by VAN DER ZEE et al., (1968) that the megaloblastic anemia failed to respond to exogenous folate but did respond to adenine indicates that additional factors may be important *in vivo*.

Genetics

The familial nature of this syndrome was recognized by LESCH and NYHAN (1964) in their original report. No particular ethnic background is apparent. Although most patients are Caucasians, the disease has been described in at least 5 oriental (MIZUNO et al., 1970) and 2 Negro families.

Major clinical manifestations occur only in affected males, with evidence of transmission through carrier females. In all large pedigrees the pattern of inheritance is consistent with either an X-linked or a sex-limited mode of transmission (SHAPIRO et al., 1966; NYHAN et al., 1967). The absence of male-to-male transmission, a critical test of X-linked inheritance, could not be evaluated because patients with the "complete" enzyme defect do not reproduce. The finding of patients with a "partial" deficiency of the same enzyme was particularly valuable in this regard since they have a milder disease and do produce offspring. No male-to-male transmission of the defect has been observed in this latter group (KELLEY et al., 1969), which is consistent with the enzyme being coded by DNA on the X chromosome. X-linked inheritance would also account for the striking absence of parental consanguinity despite the rarity of the disease.

The use of fibroblasts in culture has made it possible to demonstrate that the obligate heterozygotes for the "complete" enzyme defect are mosaics in terms of hypoxanthine-guanine phosphoribosyltransferase activity. When an autoradiographic technique was used 60% of the cells from an obligate heterozygote appeared to have normal activity, whereas the remaining 40% had none (ROSENBLOOM et al., 1967b). The two cell populations have been separated by cloning techniques and by selective chemical treatment (MIGEON et al., 1968; SALZMAN et al., 1968; MIGON, 1970; FELIX and DE MARS, 1971). These findings provide substantial support for the X-linked mode of inheritance and are consistent with the Lyon hypothesis (LYON, 1961).

Several observations indicate that heterozygotes for a deficiency of hypoxanthine-guanine phosphoribosyltransferase exhibit subtle biochemical abnormalities *in vivo*, even though they are generally asymptomatic clinically. An elevated serum urate concentration has been noted in at least 3 such patients (KELLEY et al., 1969) and one was reported to have recurrent monoarticular arthritis thought clinically to represent gout. In addition, several obligate heterozygotes have been noted to excrete greater than normal quantities of uric acid in their urine (HOEFNAGEL et al., 1965; SHAPIRO et al., 1966). Finally, studies on the incorporation of glycine-1-^{14}C into urinary uric acid in 5 heterozygous individuals have demonstrated that there is a moderate increase in the rate of *de novo* purine synthesis (KELLEY et al., 1969; EMMERSON and WYNGAARDEN, 1970).

Obligate heterozygotes for the "complete" enzyme defect cannot be reliably detected by assay of the enzyme in erythrocytes lysates. Several studies have demonstrated both directly (MCDONALD and KELLEY, 1972) and indirectly (NYHAN et al., 1970) that the mutant enzyme is not present in circulating erythrocytes from proved heterozygotes; in most cases enzyme activity has been within the normal range (KELLEY, 1968a; DANCIS et al., 1968). In addition, efforts to detect mosaicism in circulating lymphocytes have been unsuccessful (DANCIS et al., 1968). It has recently been suggested that assay of PRT activity in hair follicles may provide a simple method for the detection of heterozygosity at the PRT locus (GARTLER et al., 1971; GOLDSTEIN et al., 1971). Cultured fibroblasts provide another means of detection of mutants heterozygous for this enzyme defect. Culture of cells obtained from amniotic fluid has allowed the heterozygous as well as the hemizygous state to be diagnosed in utero (FUJIMOTO et al., 1968; DE MARS et al., 1969).

Pharmacogenetics

In addition to the naturally occurring substrates for hypoxanthine-guanine phosphoribosyltransferase, which include hypoxanthine, guanine, and xanthine, a number of purine analogs are converted to their nucleotide derivatives by this enzyme. Several of these analogs, including 6-mercaptopurine, its nitroimidazole derivative azathioprine, and allopurinol, are used clinically. The deficiency of hypoxanthine-guanine phosphoribosyltransferase is associated with in altered response to certain effects of these drugs both *in vivo* and *in vitro*.

Administration of azathioprine to individuals with normal hypoxanthine-guanine phosphoribosyltransferase activity leads to a striking reduction in the novo purine synthesis which may be accompanied by a decline in both serum and urinary uric acid. This is presumably due to the conversion of azathioprine to 6-mercaptopurine, which is then converted to its ribonucleotide by hypoxanthine-guanine phosphoribosyltransferase. The ribonucleotide derivative of 6-mercaptopurine is a potent inhibitor of PP-ribose-P amidotransferase, the rate-limiting step in the *de novo* pathway (McCollister et al., 1964). In patients lacking hypoxanthine-guanine phosphoribosyltransferase, azathioprine has no effect on the synthesis of purines *de novo* (Kelley et al., 1967b; Sorensen and Benke, 1967; Nyhan et al., 1968b). In addition, the absence of this enzyme in lymphocytes obtained from these patients is associated with a loss of the ability of azathioprine to suppress phytohemagglutinin-induced transformation of these cells as measured by incorporation of tritiated thymidine into DNA (Brown et al., 1968). Resistance to the potential inhibitory effects of 6-mercaptopurine on *de novo* purine synthesis has also been demonstrated in cultured fibroblasts derived from such patients (Seegmiller et al., 1967).

The effects of administration of allopurinol to patients deficient in hypoxanthine-guanine phosphoribosyltransferase differ in several distinctive ways from the effects in normal individuals. In patients lacking PRT allopurinol does not have its usual inhibitory effect on purine biosynthesis *de novo* (Newcombe et al., 1966; Sweetman and Nyhan, 1967a; Kelley et al., 1968c) and a normally occurring ribonucleoside derivative of allopurinol does not appear in the urine (Sweetman, 1967b); PP-ribose-P depletion does not occur (Fox et al., 1970), and the drug appears to produce an even more striking inhibitory effect on xanthine oxidase (Kelley et al., 1969). Each of these observations can readily be attributed to the deficiency of hypoxanthine-guanine phosphoribosyltransferase.

Treatment

Through its effect upon xanthine oxidase, allopurinol lowers the uric acid content of both serum and urine in patients with X-linked hyperuricaciduria. This drug can be used to prevent uric acid stone formation, uric acid and urate nephropathy, gouty arthritis, and development of tophi. When these findings are already present, progression can be stopped and some reversal possibly achieved. For this reason, every patient with "partial" or "complete" PRT deficiency should be treated with allopurinol. Because of the extremely large load of uric acid already supplied to the kidney, uricosuric therapy should probably not be used unless allopurinol is also administered. In most patients without tophi, allopurinol will be adequate by itself to maintain a normal serum urate concentration. The possibility of xanthine stone formation during allopurinol treatment does exist (Sorensen, 1968; Greene et al., 1969b) but can be minimized by increasing urine flow and raising urine pH. This potential complication should not deter physicians from using allopurinol in this disease. Allopurinol has not been shown to affect the progression of central nervous system dysfunction, but only a few patients with the "complete" enzyme defect have been treated with allopurinol from birth.

Approaches toward prevention or correction of the central nervous system dysfunction remain experimental. The observations that these children have no apparent abnormalities in central nervous system function at birth and that no distinctive pathological changes are noted at postmortem examination provide encouragement that the CNS disease may be preventable or treatable.

A major experimental approach to the central nervous system dysfunction has been replacement of the presumed deficiency of GMP or IMP. This has been attempted by administration of GMP (ROSENBERG et al., 1968), guanosine (KELLEY et al., 1969), inosine (BERMAN et al., 1969), adenine (VAN DER ZEE et al., 1968; BENKE and ANDERSON, 1969; VAN DER ZEE et al., 1970), 2,6-diaminopurine (BERMAN et al., 1969), or folic acid (BENKE and ANDERSON, 1969) without well-documented improvement. Glutamate has also been tried without convincing success (GHADIMI et al., 1970).

Although approaches to therapy have so far been directed almost entirely at correcting possible consequences of the enzyme defect, it may be possible in the future to design means of increasing the levels of enzyme activity *in vivo*. Since most patients with a "partial" rather than a "complete" deficiency of the enzyme have little if any neurological disease, one might reason that such an approach would be helpful in terms of the neurologic dysfunction even if only low levels of activity of the enzyme were achieved. Studies are now proceeding in a number of laboratories, in which cultured fibroblasts or lymphoblasts are being used as a model system to test possibilities which might be of therapeutic benefit. Such possibilities include stabilization of the mutant enzyme by chemical agents or induction by viral transformation. In the patient with a mutant form of the PRT which exhibits altered Michaelis constants, it is possible that some degree of enzyme function may be achieved *in vivo* by increasing the concentration of substrates (MCDONALD and KELLEY, 1971). Perhaps fibroblasts or lymphoblast transplants could be used as a source of enzyme if conditions were such that they could survive *in vivo*.

References

ALEPA, F.P., HOWELL, R.R., KLINENBERG, J.R., SEEGMILLER, J.E.: Relationships between glycogen storage disease and tophaceous gout. Amer. J. Med. **42**, 58—66 (1967).

AL-KHALIDI, U.A., CHAGLASSIAN, T.H.: The species distribution of xanthine oxidase. Biochem. J. **97**, 318—320 (1965).

ARNOLD, W.J., KELLEY, W.N.: Human hypoxanthine-guanine phosphoribosyltransferase: Purification and subunit structure. J. biol. Chem. **246**, 7398—7404, 1971.

ARNOLD, W.J., KELLEY, W.N.: In preparation (1972).

BALIS, M.E.: Aspects of purine metabolism. Fed. Proc. **27**, 1067—1074 (1968).

BALIS, M.E., KRAKOSS, I.H., BERMAN, P.H., DANCIS, J.: Urinary metabolites in congenital hyperuricosuria. Science **156**, 1122—1123 (1967).

BENKE, P.J., ANDERSON, J.: Use of folic acid, adenine and biocarbonate in newborn twins with the Lesch-Nyhan syndrome (abstract). Pediat. Res. **3**, 356 (1969).

BERMAN, P.H., BALIS, M.E., DANCIS, J.: Congenital hyperuricemia an inborn error of purine metabolism associated with psychomotor retardation, athetosis, and self mutilation. Arch. Neurol. (Chic.) **20**, 44—53 (1969).

BOYD, E.M., DOLMAN, M., KNIGHT, L.M., SHEPPARD, E.P.: The chronic oral toxicity of caffeine. Canad. J. Physiol. Pharmacol. **43**, 995—1007 (1965).

BROCKMAN, R.W.: Resistance to purine antagonists in experimental leukemia systems. Cancer Res. **25**, 1596—1605 (1965).

BROWN, R.S., KELLEY, W.N., SEEGMILLER, J.E., CARBONE, P.P.: The action of thiopurines in lymphocytes lacking hypoxanthine guanine phosphoribosyltransferase (abstract). J. clin. Invest. **47**, 12a (1968).

BUCHANAN, J.M.: The enzymatic synthesis of the purine nucleotides. Harvey Lect. **54**, 104—130 (1960).

BUCHANAN, J. M., HARTMAN, S. C.: Enzymatic reactions in synthesis of the purines. Advances Enzymol. **21**, 199—261 (1959).

CASKEY, C. T., ASHTON, D. M., WYNGAARDEN, J. B.: The enzymology of feedback inhibition of glutamine phosphoribosylpyrophosphate amidotransferase by purine ribonucleotides. J. biol. Chem. **239**, 2570—2579 (1964).

CATEL, W., SCHMIDT, J.: Über familiäre gichtische Diathese in Verbindung mit zerebralen und renalen Symptomen bei einem Kleinkind. Dtsch. med. Wschr. **84**, 2145—2147 (1959).

CRUSSI, F. G., ROBERTSON, D. M., HISCOX, J. L.: The pathological condition of the Lesch-Nyhan syndrome. Report of two cases. Amer. J. Dis. Child. **118**, 501—506 (1969).

DANCIS, J., BERMAN, P. H., JANSEN, V., BALIS, M. E.: Absence of mosaicism in the lymphocyte in X-linked congenital hyperuricosuria. Life Sci. **7**, 587—591 (1968).

DELBARRE, F., CARTIER, P., AUSCHER, C., DEGERY, A., HAMET, M.: Gouttes Enzymopathiques: Dyspurinies par deficit en hypoxanthine-guanine-phosphoribosyl-transferase frequence et caracteres cliniques de l'anenzymose. Presse méd. **78**, 729—733 (1970).

DEMARS, R., SARTO, G., FELIX, J. S., BENKE, P.: Lesch-Nyhan mutation: prenatal detection with amniotic fluid cells. **164**, 1303—1305 (1969).

DREIFUSS, F. E., NEWCOMBE, D. S., SHAPIRO, S. L., SHEPPARD, G. L.: X-linked primary hyperuricemia (Hypoxanthine-guanine phosphoribosyl-transferase deficiency encephalopathy). J. ment. Defic. Res. **12**, 100—107 (1968).

EMMERSON, B. T., WYNGAARDEN, J. B.: Purine metabolism in heterozygous carriers of hypoxanthine-guanine phosphoribosyltransferase deficiency. Science **166**, 1533—1535 (1969).

FELIX, J. S., DEMARS, R.: Purine requirement of cells cultured from humans affected with Lesch-Nyhan syndrome (Hypoxanthine-guanine phosphoribosyltransferase deficiency). Proc. nat. Acad. Sci. (Wash.) **62**, 536—543 (1969).

FELIX, J. S., DEMARS, R.: Detection of females heterozygous for the Lesch-Nyhan mutation by 8-azaguanine-resistant growth of cultured fibroblasts. J. Lab. clin. Med. **77**, 596—604 (1971).

FOX, I. H., KELLEY, W. N.: Phosphoribosylpyrophosphate in man: Biochemical and clinical significance. Ann. intern. Med. **74**, 424—433 (1971).

FOX, I. H., WYNGAARDEN, J. B., KELLEY, W. N.: Depletion of erythrocyte phosphoribosylpyrophosphate in man, a newly observed effect of allopurinol. New Engl. J. Med. **283**, 1177—1182 (1970).

FUJIMOTO, W. Y., SEEGMILLER, J. E.: Hypoxanthine-guanine phosphoribosyltransferase deficiency: Activity in normal, mutant, and heterozygote-cultured human skin fibroblasts. Proc. nat. Acad. Sci. (Wash.) **65**, 577—584 (1970).

FUJIMOTO, W. Y., SEEGMILLER, J. E., ULENDORF, B. W., JACOBSON, C. B.: Biochemical diagnosis of an X-linked disease in utero. Lancet **1968 II**, 511—512.

GARROD, A. B.: Observations on certain pathological conditions of the blood and urine in gout, rheumatism and Bright's Disease. Tr. med.-chir. Soc. Edinb. **31**, 83 (1848).

GARTLER, S. M., SCOTT, R. C., GOLDSTEIN, J. L., CAMPBELL, B., SPARKES, R.: Lesch-Nyhan syndrome: Rapid detection of heterozygotes by the use of hair follicles. Science **172**, 572—574 (1971).

GHADIMI, H., BHALLA, C. K., KIRCHENBAUM, D. M.: The significance the deficiency state in Lesch-Nyhan disease. Acta paediat. scand. **59**, 233—240 (1970).

GILLESPIE, J. B., PERRUCA, L. G.: Congenital generalized indifference to pain (Congenital analgia). Amer. J. Dis. Child. **100**, 124—126 (1960).

GOLDSTEIN, J. L., MARKS, J. F., GARTLER, S. M.: Expression of two x-linked genes in human hair follicles of double heterozygotes. Proc. nat. Acad. Sci. In press, 1971.

GREENE, M. L., BOYLE, J. A., SEEGMILLER, J. E.: Substrate stabilization: Genetically controlled reciprocal relationship of 2 human enzymes. Science **167**, 337—339 (1970).

GREENE, M. L., FUJIMOTO, W. Y., SEEGMILLER, J. E.: Urinary xanthine stones — a rare complication of allopurinol therapy. New Engl. J. Med. **280**, 426—427 (1969 b).

GREENE, M. L., SEEGMILLER, J. E.: Erythrocyte 5-phosphoribosyl-l-pyrophosphate (PRPP) in gout: Importance of PRPP in the regulation of human purine synthesis. Arthrit. and Rheum. (abstract) **12**, 666—667 (1969 a).

GUTMAN, A. B., YU, T. F.: Uric acid metabolism in normal man and in primary gout. New Engl. J. Med. **273**, 252—260, 313—321 (1965).

HENDERSON, J. F.: Feedback inhibition of purine biosynthesis in ascites tumor cells. J. biol. Chem. **237**, 2631—2635 (1962).

HENDERSON, J. F., MILLER, H. R., KELLEY, W. N., ROSENBLOOM, F. M., SEEGMILLER, J. E.: Kinetic studies of mutant human erythrocyte adenine phosphoribosyltransferases. Canad. J. Biochem. **46**, 703—706 (1968).
HILL, D. L., BENNETT, L. L.: Purification and properties of 5-phosphoribosyl pyrophosphate amidotransferase from adenocarcinoma 755 cells. Biochemistry **8**, 122—130 (1969).
HOEFNAGEL, D.: Seminars on the Lesch-Nyhan syndrome: Discussion. Fed. Proc. **27**, 1045 (1967).
HOEFNAGEL, D., ANDREW, E. D., MIREAULT, N. G., BERNDT, W. O.: Hereditary choreoathetosis, self mutilation, and hyperuricemia in young males. New Engl. J. Med. **273**, 130—135 (1965).
HOWARD, W. J., APPEL, S. H.: Control of purine biosynthesis: FGAR amidotransferase (abstract). Clin. Res. **16**, 344 (1968).
HOWARD, W. J., KERSON, L. A., APPEL, S. H.: Synthesis *de novo* of purines in slices of rat brain and liver. J. Neurochem. **17**, 121—123 (1970).
JAKOVCIC, S., SORENSEN, L. B.: Studies of uric acid metabolism in glycogen storage disease associated with gouty arthritis. Arthrit. and Rheum. **10**, 129—134 (1967).
KAUFMAN, J. M., GREENE, M. L., SEEGMILLER, J. E.: Urine uric acid to creatinine ratio—screening test for inherited disorders of purine metabolism. J. Pediat. **73**, 583—592 (1968).
KELLEY, W. N., ROSENBLOOM, F. M., HENDERSON, J. F., SEEGMILLER, J. E.: A specific enzyme defect in gout associated with overproduction of uric acid. Proc. nat. Acad. Sci. (Wash.) **57**, 1735—1739 (1967a).
KELLEY, W. N., ROSENBLOOM, F. M., SEEGMILLER, J. E.: The effect of azathioprine (imuran) on purine synthesis in clinical disorders of purine metabolism. J. clin. Invest. **46**, 1518—1529 (1967b).
KELLEY, W. N.: Hypoxanthine-guanine phosphoribosyltransferase deficiency in the Lesch-Nyhan syndrome and gout. Fed. Proc. **27**, 1047—1052 (1968a).
KELLEY, W. N.: Studies on the adenine phosphoribosyltransferase enzyme in human fibroblasts lacking hypoxanthine-guanine phosphoribosyltransferase. J. Lab. clin. Med. **77**, 33—38 (1971b).
KELLEY, W. N., FOX, I. H., WYNGAARDEN, J. B.: Regulation of purine biosynthesis in cultured human cells. I. Effects of orotic acid. Biochim. biophys. Acta (Amst.) **215**, 512—516 (1970b).
KELLEY, W. N., GREENE, M. L., FOX, I. H., ROSENBLOOM, F. M., LEVY, R. I., SEEGMILLER, J. E.: Effects of orotic acid on purine and lipoprotein metabolism in man. Metabolism **19**, 1025—1035 (1970a).
KELLEY, W. N., GREENE, M. L., ROSENBLOOM, F. M., HENDERSON, J. F., SEEGMILLER, J. E.: Hypoxanthine-guanine phosphoribosyltransferase deficiency in gout. Ann. intern. Med. **70**, 155—206 (1969).
KELLEY, W. N., MEADE, J. C.: Studies on hypoxanthine-guanine phosphoribosyltransferase in fibroblasts from patients with the Lesch-Nyhan syndrome: Evidence for genetic heterogeneity. J. biol. Chem. **246**, 2953—2958 (1971a).
KELLEY, W. N., ROSENBLOOM, F. M., MILLER, J., SEEGMILLER, J. E.: An enzymatic basis for variation in response to allopurinol hypoxanthine-guanine phosphoribosyltransferase deficiency. New Engl. J. Med. **278**, 287—293 (1968c).
KELLEY, W. N., ROSENBLOOM, F. M., SEEGMILLER, J. E., HOWELL, R. R.: Excessive production of uric acid in type I glycogen storage disease. J. Pediat. **72**, 488—496 (1968b).
KOGUT, M. D., DONNELL, G. N., NYHAN, W. L., SWEETMAN, L.: Disorder of purine metabolism due to partial deficiency of hypoxanthine-guanine phosphoribosyltransferase: A study of a family. Amer. J. Med. **48**, 148—161 (1970).
KORN, E. D., REMY, C. N., WASILEJKO, H. C., BUCHANAN, J. M.: Biosynthesis of nucleotides from bases by partially purified enzymes. J. biol. Chem. **217**, 875—883 (1955).
KORNBERG, A., LIEBERMAN, I., SIMMS, E. S.: Enzymatic synthesis of purine nucleotides. J. biol. Chem. **215**, 417—427 (1955).
KRENITSKY, T. A.: Tissue distribution of purine ribosyl- and phosphoribosyltransferase in the Rhesus monkey. Biochim. biophys. Acta (Amst.) **179**, 506—509 (1969b).
KRENITSKY, T. A., PAPAIOANNOU, R., ELION, G. B.: Human hypoxanthine phosphoribosyltransferase I. Purification, properties and specificity. J. biol. Chem. **244**, 1263—1270 (1969a).
LABRUNE, B., CARTIER, M., HAMET, M. M., BONNENFANT, F., VELIN, J., RIBIERRE, M., MALLET, R.: Encephalopathie familiale avec hyperuricemie. Presse méd. **76**, 2337—2340 (1968).
LESCH, M., NYHAN, W. L.: A familial disorder of uric acid metabolism and central nervous system function. Amer. J. Med. **36**, 561—570 (1964).
LYON, M. F.: Gene action in the X-chromosome of the mouse (Mus musculus L.). Nature **190**, 372—373 (1961).
MAGASANIK, B., KARIBIAN, D.: Purine nucleotide cycles and their metabolic role. J. biol. Chem. **235**, 2672—2681 (1960).

MAGER, J., MAGASANIK, B.: Guanosine 5'-phosphate reductase and its role in the interconversion of purine nucleotides. J. biol. Chem. **235**, 1474—1478 (1960).

MANZKE, H.: Hyperuricämie mit Cerebralparese, Syndrome eines hereditären Purinstoffwechselleidens. Helv. paediat. Acta **22**, 258—270 (1967).

MARIE, J., ROYER, P., RAPPAPORT, R.: Hyperuricemie congenitale avec troubles neurologiques, renaux et sanguins. Arch franç. Pédiat. **24**, 501—510 (1967).

MCCOLLISTER, R. J., GILBERT, W. R., JR., ASHTON, D. M., WYNGAARDEN, J. B.: Pseudofeedback inhibition of purine synthesis by 6-mercaptopurine ribonucleotide and other purine analogues. J. biol. Chem. **239**, 1560—1563 (1964).

MCDONALD, J. A., KELLEY, W. N.: LESCH-NYHAN syndrome: Altered kinetic properties of mutant enzyme. Science **171**, 689—691 (1971).

MCDONALD, J. A., KELLEY, W. N.: LESCH-NYHAN syndrome: Absence of the mutant enzyme in erythrocytes of a heterozygote for both normal and mutant hypoxanthine-guanine phosphoribosyltransferase. Biochem. Genet. (in press).

MICHENER, W. M.: Hyperuricemia and mental retardation with athetosis and self-mutilation. Amer. J. Dis. Child. **113**, 195—206 (1967).

MIGEON, B. R.: X-linked hypoxanthine-guanine phosphoribosyltransferase deficiency: Detection of heterozygotes by selective medium. Biochem. Genet. **4**, 377—383 (1970).

MIGEON, B. R., DER KALOUSTIAN, V. M., NYHAN, W. L., YOUNG, W. J., CHILDS, B.: X-linked hypoxanthine-guanine phosphoribosyltransferase deficiency: heterozygote has two clonal populations. Science **160**, 425—427 (1968).

MIZUNO, T., SEGAWA, M., KURIMADA, T., MARUYAMA, H., ONISAWA, J.: Clinical and therapeutic aspects of the LESCH-NYHAN syndrome in JAPANESE children. Neuropädiatrie **2**, 38—52 (1970).

MOMOSE, H., NISHIKAWA, H., KATSUJJA, N.: Genetic and biochemical studies of 5' nucleotide fermentation. II. Repression of enzyme formation in purine nucleotide biosynthesis in Bacillus subtilis and derivation of derepressed mutants. J. gen. Microbiol. **11**, 211—220 (1965).

NEWCOMBE, D. S., SHAPIRO, S. L., SHEPPARD, G. L., DREIFUSS, F. E.: Treatment of X-linked primary hyperuricemia with allopurinol. J. Amer. med. Ass. **198**, 315—317 (1966).

NIERLICH, D. P., MAGASANIK, B.: Control by repression of purine biosynthetic enzymes in Aerobacter aerogenes. Fed. Proc. **22**, 476 (1963).

NIERLICH, D. P., MAGASANIK, B.: Regulation of purine ribonucleotide synthesis by end product inhibition. The effect of adenine and guanine ribonucleotides on the 5'-phosphoribosylpyrophosphate amidotransferase of *Aerobacter aerogenes*. J. biol. Chem. **240**, 358—365 (1965).

NYHAN, W. L.: LESCH-NYHAN syndrome. Summary of clinical features. Fed. Proc. **27**, 1034—1041 (1968a).

NYHAN, W. L., BAKAY, B., CONNOR, J. D., MARKS, J. F., KEELE, D. K.: Hemizygous expression of glucose-6-phosphate dehydrogenase in erythrocytes of heterozygotes for the LESCH-NYHAN SYNDROME. Proc. nat. Acad. Sci. (Wash.) **65**, 214—218 (1970).

NYHAN, W. L., OLIVER, W. J., LESCH, M.: A familial disorder of uric acid metabolism and central nervous system function. II. J. Pediat. **67**, 257—263 (1965).

NYHAN, W. L., PESEK, J., SWEETMAN, L., CARPENTER, D. G., CARTER, C. H.: Genetics of an X-linked disorder of uric acid metabolism and cerebral function. Pediat. Res. **1**, 5—13 (1967).

NYHAN, W. L., SWEETMAN, L., CARPENTER, D. G., CARTER, C. H., HOEFNAGEL, D.: Effects of a azathioprine in a disorder of uric acid metabolism and cerebral function. J. Pediat. **72**, 111—118 (1968b).

PARTINGTON, W. M., HENNEN, B. K. E.: The LESCH-NYHAN syndrome: Self-destructive biting, mental retardation, neurological disorder and hyperuricemia. Develop. Med. Child. Neurol. **9**, 563—572 (1967).

RILEY, J. D.: Gout and cerebral palsy in three-year-old boy. Arch. Dis. Childh. **35**, 293—295 (1960).

ROSENBERG, D., MONNET, P., MAMELLE, J. L., COLOMBEL, M., SALLE, B., BOVIER-LAPIERRE, M.: Encephalopathie avec troubles du metabolisme des purines. Presse méd. **76**, 2333—2336 (1968).

ROSENBLOOM, F. M., HENDERSON, J. F., CALDWELL, I. C., KELLEY, W. N., SEEGMILLER, J. E.: Biochemical bases of accelerated purine biosynthesis de novo in human fibroblasts lacking hypoxanthine-guanine phosphoribosyltransferase. J. biol. Chem. **243**, 1166—1173 (1968).

ROSENBLOOM, F. M., KELLEY, W. N., HENDERSON, J. F., SEEGMILLER, J. E.: Lyon hypothesis and X-linked disease. Lancet **2**, 305—306 (1967b); **1967 b II**, 305—306.

ROSENBLOOM, F. M., KELLEY, W. N., MILLER, J., HENDERSON, J. F., SEEGMILLER, J. E.: Inherited disorders of purine metabolism: correlation between central nervous system dysfunction and biochemical defects. J. Amer. med. Ass. **202**, 175—177 (1967a).

Rosenblum, W. I., Rosenbloom, F. M., Seegmiller, J. E.: Unpublished results.

Rubin, C. S., Balis, M. E., Piomelli, S., Berman, P. H., Dancis, J.: Elevated AMP pyrophosphorylase activity in congenital IMP pyrophosphorylase deficiency (Lesch-Nyhan disease). J. Lab. clin. Med. **74**, 732—741 (1969).

Rubin, C. S., Dancis, J., Yip, L. C., Nowinski, R. C., Balis, M. E.: Purification of IMP: Pyrophosphate phosphoribosyltransferases, catalytically incompetent enzymes in Lesch-Nyhan disease. Proc. nat. Acad. Sci. (Wash.) **68**, 1461—1464 (1971).

Salzmann, J., de Mars, R., Benke, P.: Single allele expression at an X-linked hyperuricemia locus in heterozygous human cells. Proc. nat. Acad. Sci. (Wash.) **60**, 545—552 (1968).

Sass, J. K., Itabashi, H. H., Dexter, R. A.: Juvenile gout with brain involvement. Arch. Neurol. (Chic.) **13**, 639—655 (1965).

Scherzer, A. L., Ilson, J. B.: Normal intelligence in the Lesch-Nyhan syndrome. Pediatrics **44**, 116—119 (1969).

Seegmiller, J. E.: Pathology and pathologic physiology. Summary: Discussion. Fed. Proc. **27**, 1044—1046 (1968).

Seegmiller, J. E., Laster, L., Howell, R. R.: Biochemistry of uric acid and its relation to gout. New Engl. J. Med. **268**, 712—716, 764—773, 821—827 (1963).

Seegmiller, J. E., Rosenbloom, F. M., Kelley, W. N.: An enzyme defect associated with a sex-linked human neurological disorder and excessive purine synthesis. Science **155**, 1682—1684 (1967).

Shapiro, S. L., Sheppard, G. L., Jr., Dreifuss, F. E., Newcombe, D. S.: X-linked recessive inheritance of a syndrome of mental retardation with hyperuricemia. Proc. Soc. exp. Biol. (N.Y.) **122**, 609—611 (1966).

Sorensen, L. B.: Seminars on the Lesch-Nyhan syndrome: Management and treatment: Discussion. Fed. Proc. **27**, 1099 (1968).

Sorensen, L. B.: Mechanism of excessive purine biosynthesis in hypoxanthine-guanine phosphoribosyltransferase deficiency. J. clin. Invest. **49**, 968—978 (1970).

Sorensen, L. B., Benke, P. J.: Biochemical evidence for a distinct type of primary gout. Nature **213**, 1122—1123 (1967).

Sperling, O., Frank, M., Ophir, R., Lieberman, U. A., Adam, A., de Vries, A.: Partial deficiency of hypoxanthine-guanine phosphoribosyltransferase associated with gout and uric acid lithiasis. Europ. J. Clin. Biol. Res. **15**, 942—947 (1970).

Sweetman, L.: Urinary and cerebrospinal fluid oxypurine levels and allopurinol metabolism in the Lesch-Nyhan syndrome. Fed. Proc. **27**, 1055—1059 (1967b).

Sweetman, L., Nyhan, W. L.: Excretion of hypoxanthine and xanthine in genetic disease of purine metabolism. Nature **215**, 859—860 (1967a).

van Bogaert, L., Damme, J. V., Verschueren, M.: Sur un syndrome professif d'hypertonie extrapyramidale avec osteoarthropathies goutteuses chez deux freres. Rev. Neurol. **114**, 15—32 (1966).

van der Zee, S. P. M., Lommen, E. J. P., Trijbels, J. M. F., Schretlen, E. D. A. M.: The influence of adenine on the clinical features and purine metabolism in the Lesch-Nyhan syndrome. Acta paediat. scand. **59**, 259—264 (1970).

van der Zee, S. P. M., Schretlen, E. D. A. M., Monnens, L. A. H.: Megaloblastic anemia in the Lesch-Nyhan syndrome. Lancet **1968 I**, 1427.

Wyngaarden, J. B.: Gout. In: The Metabolic Basis of Inherited Disease, 2nd Ed. (Stanbury, J. B., Wyngaarden, J. B., Fredrickson, D. S., (Eds.): pp. 667—728. New York: McGraw-Hill 1966.

Wyngaarden, J. B., Ashton, D. M.: The regulation of activity of phosphoribosylpyrophosphate amidotransferase by purine ribonucleotides; a potential feedback control of purine biosynthesis. J. biol. Chem. **234**, 1492—1496 (1959).

Wyngaarden, J. B., Greenland, R. A.: The inhibition of succinoadenylate kinosynthetase of *Escherichia coli* by adenosine and guanosine 5'-monophosphates. J. biol. Chem. **238**, 1054—1057 (1963)

X. Xanthinuria

1. Xanthinuria

By

E. W. HOLMES and W. N. KELLEY

With 1 Figure

Xanthinuria is a disorder of purine metabolism that results from a marked deficiency of xanthine oxidase activity. While a number of patients with this disorder are asymptomatic, others have nephrolithiasis and myopathy as a consequence of the derangement in purine metabolism. Since some individuals with this disorder are only discovered incidently through the finding of hypouricemia and because the available data suggest the disorder is inherited in an autosomal recessive manner, it is impossible to estimate the prevalence of the mutant gene in the general population. However, xanthinuria must be very uncommon since one prospective survey for hypouricemia in a large general hospital failed to detect a single case in 6629 consecutive uric acid determinations (RAMSDELL and KELLEY, 1973). To date, only 19 cases of xanthinuria have been reported. Interest in this disorder has not been stiffled by its rarity, however, because the absence of xanthine oxidase provides a unique opportunity to understand several aspects of purine metabolism in man.

Clinical Features

As pointed out earlier 47% of the individuals with this disorder are totally asymptomatic and they are discovered through the incidental finding of hypouricemia. Of the 19 cases of xanthinuria which have been documented in the literature only 2 individuals have had a myopathy and 7 have had urolithiasis (DENT and PHILPOT, 1954; DICKINSON and SMELLIE, 1959; ENGLEMAN et al., 1964; AYVAZIAN, 1964; DELATTE and MENDOZA, 1967; FREZAL et al., 1967; BRADFORD et al., 1968; CHALMERS et al., 1969; SPERLING et al., 1971; CURNOW et al., 1971; SORENSEN et al., 1972; FRAYHA et al., 1973; HOLMES et al., 1974; MENDOZA et al., 1972). Since crystalline deposits of hypoxanthine and xanthine have been found in the muscle tissue and renal stones from these patients, it would appear that these clinical findings are a direct result of the derangement in purine metabolism. Xanthinuria has also been reported in one patient with a pheochromocytoma (ENGLEMAN et al., 1964) and another with hemochromatosis (AYVAZIAN, 1964). However the later two findings are probably coincidental, since hypouricemia is not a common feature of pheochromocytoma (ENGLEMAN et al., 1964) or hemochromatosis (AYVAZIAN, 1964). In addition in one xanthinuric patient in whom iron metabolism has been examined, it was found to be normal (SEEGMILLER et al., 1964).

The myopathy has been described as a "tight sensation" or distension and likened to muscle cramps. These symptoms are usually present in the muscles of the lower extremities and they are aggravated by exercise. There is no weakness or tenderness, but electromyograms were consistent with a myopathic process (ENGLEMAN et al., 1964; CHALMERS et al., 1969). Muscle biopsy revealed fibers of increased diameter and numerous hypoxanthine and xanthine crystals were identified (CHALMERS et al., 1969; PARKER et al., 1969). In addition the muscle tissue from the two patients with the myopathy revealed increased concentrations of hypoxanthine and xanthine when compared to control specimens (PARKER et al., 1970).

Nephrolithiasis is a more common finding in these patients and may be the symptom which brings the xanthinuric patient to the doctors attention. These patients may have the typical symptoms of renal colic and may develop obstructive uropathy. The stones vary in size from a few millimeters to several centimeters. The pure xanthine stone is brownish in color, smooth in texture, and friable (KRETSCHMER, 1937). The pure stone is radiolucent unless calcium is entrapped.

In general xanthine stones are a rare cause of nephrolithiasis, and only about 50 cases have been reported. Oxypurine excretion and serum urate were not recorded in many of these patients so that it is impossible to ascertain how many of these individuals had xanthine oxidase deficiency. Certainly not all patients with xanthine stones have hereditary xanthinuria (WYNGAARDEN, 1972).

One other possible clinical manifestation of xanthinuria is arthritis. One patient presented with polyarthritis and it has been suggested that this was the result of a crystal-induced arthritis (BRADFORD et al., 1968; SEEGMILLER et al., 1964). However, hypoxanthine and xanthine crystals were not demonstrated in the synovial fluid.

Enzyme Defect

Xanthine oxidase catalyzes the oxidation of hypoxanthine to xanthine and xanthine to uric acid (Fig. 1). The enzyme may function as an oxidase in which case molecular oxygen is the immediate electron acceptor or as a dehydrogenase in which case a number of different compounds may be the electron acceptor. The human enzyme obtained from liver is more active *in vitro* as the dehydrogenase (SEEGMILLER, 1969). Xanthine oxidase from bovine milk has been purified and found to contain molybdenum, FAD and nonheme iron (MASSEY et al., 1969). The mechanism of action is probably a two-step dehydrogenation in which hypoxanthine is converted to xanthine, xanthine is released from the enzyme and subsequently bound in a different orientation before it is oxidized to uric acid (BERGMANN and DIKSTEIN, 1956).

In Xanthinuria the deficiency of xanthine oxidase varies from 0% to 25% of control. Hepatic tissue (AYVAZIAN, 1964; FREZAL et al., 1967; BRADFORD et al., 1968; FRAYHA et al., 1973; WATTS et al., 1964), small intestinal mucosa (BRADFORD et al., 1968; CHALMERS et al., 1969; SPERLING et al., 1971; WATTS et al., 1964) rectal mucosa (HOLMES et al., 1974), and colostrum (OLIVER et al., 1971) obtained from xanthinuric subjects have all been reported to be deficient in xanthine oxidase activity. When studied, both the oxidase and dehydrogenase activities of the enzyme were comparably reduced (WATTS et al., 1964). In addition, activity could not be restored by the *in vitro* addition of molybdenum, FAD or iron. The variability in enzyme activity from different individuals with xanthinuria may represent different mutations or simply a difference in methodology. There is some preliminary data that suggest there may be different mutations which result in xanthine oxidase deficiency (see below).

The molecular basis for the observed decrease in xanthine oxidase activity in xanthinuria is not known. This condition could result from a mutation on the structural gene coding for xanthine oxidase with the consequent production of normal amounts of enzyme protein that is catalytically ineffective or the mutation could be in a gene that controls the rate of synthesis or degradation of a structurally normal xanthine oxidase. To date the human enzyme has not been purified, nor has an antibody been produced against it; therefore these possibilities remain to be examined. It is interesting to note that hepatic xanthine oxidase is an inducible enzyme in rats when dietary protein is varied (ROWE and WYNGAARDEN, 1966). There are also some data in man that suggest hepatic, but not small—intestinal, xanthine oxidase activity is increased when the rate of purine biosynthesis is increased (MARCOLONGO et al., 1973).

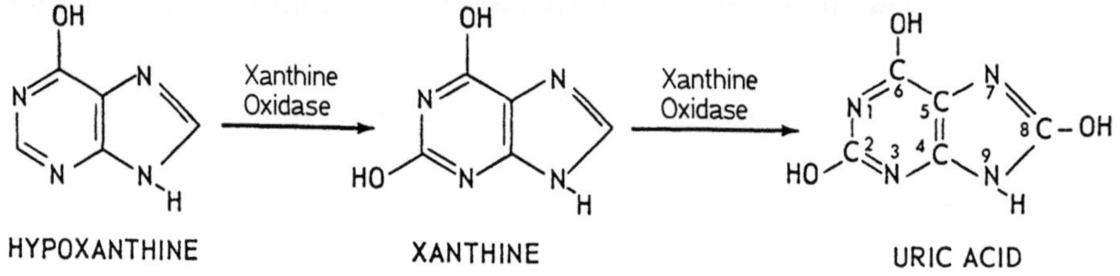

Fig. 1. Reaction catalyzed by xanthine oxidase

Metabolic Alterations

As a consequence of the xanthine oxidase deficiency, several alterations in purine metabolism are observed. The "problem" that usually brings these individuals to the attention of the physician is hypouricemia. Serum uric acid is usually less than 1 mg/100 ml, but may range from 0.05 to 1.6. Likewise, urinary uric acid excretion is very low with values ranging from 0 to 40 mg per 24 hrs on a purine free diet (DENT and PHILPOT, 1954; DICKINSON and SMELLIE, 1959; ENGLEMAN et al., 1964; AYVAZIAN, 1964; DELATTE and MENDOZA, 1967; FREZAL et al., 1967; BRADFORD et al., 1968; CHALMERS et al., 1969; SPERLING et al., 1971; CURNOW et al., 1971; SORENSEN et al., 1972; FRAYHA et al., 1973; HOLMES et al., 1974; MENDOZA et al., 1972). On the other hand, serum oxypurines (hypoxanthine plus xanthine) are usually elevated (DICKINSON and SMELLIE, 1969; DELATTE and MENDOZA, 1967; CHALMERS et al., 1969; SPERLING et al., 1971; CURNOW et al., 1971; SORENSEN et al., 1972; HOLMES et al., 1974) and urinary oxypurines are always strikingly increased (DENT and PHILPOT, 1954; DICKINSON and SMELLIE, 1959; ENGLEMAN et al., 1964; AYVAZIAN, 1964; DELATTE and MENDOZA, 1967; FREZAL et al., 1967; BRADFORD et al., 1968; CHALMERS et al., 1969; SPERLING et al., 1971; CURNOW et al., 1971; SORENSEN et al., 1972; FRAYHA et al., 1973; HOLMES et al., 1974; MENDOZA et al., 1972). However, total purine excretion (the sum of hypoxanthine, xanthine and uric acid) is normal or slightly decreased in these individuals.

When urinary oxypurines have been quantitated as hypoxanthine and xanthine, individuals with xanthinuria have been shown to excrete much more xanthine relative to hypoxanthine than normal individuals (DICKINSON and SMELLIE, 1959; AYVAZIAN, 1964; DELATTE and MENDOZA, 1967; FREZAL et al., 1967; BRADFORD et al., 1968; CHALMERS et al., 1969; SPERLING et al., 1971; SORENSEN et al., 1972; HOLMES et al., 1974; MENDOZA et al., 1972). The mechanism responsible for this is not certain, but two explanations have been offered. Since individuals with xanthinuria have some xanthine oxidase activity demonstrable *in vitro* (ENGLEMAN et al., 1964; AYVAZIAN, 1964; BRADFORD et al., 1968; SPERLING et al., 1971; HOLMES et al., 1974) and *in vivo* (ENGLEMAN et al., 1964; BRADFORD et al., 1968), the relative excess of xanthine may be a result of the residual xanthine oxidase activity. Another explanation derives from the experiments in normal and xanthinuric subjects that have demonstrated extensive reutilization of hypoxanthine by hypoxanthine-guanine phosphoribosyltransferase while little of the xanthine is reutilized (ENGLEMAN et al., 1964; BRADFORD et al., 1968; AYVAZIAN and SKUPP, 1965). In fact, one study of a xanthinuric subject has suggested that hypoxanthine-guanine phosphoribosyltransferase may be virtually saturated *in vivo* by purine bases (HOLMES et al., 1974). In xanthinuric subjects the xanthine that is produced endogenously is not converted to uric acid and only small amounts are reutilized; consequently most of the xanthine is excreted in the urine. However, the hypoxanthine that is produced endogenously is not converted to xanthine at the usual rate, but it is extensively reutilized in the synthesis of inosinic acid.

Genetics

Only subjects who are homozygous for the deficiency of xanthine oxidase exhibit abnormalities which are detectable clinically. In the cases where family studies are available, no parents of affected subjects have been demonstrated to have xanthine oxidase deficiency (DENT and PHILPOT, 1954; ENGLEMAN et al., 1964; FRAYHA et al., 1973; HOLMES et al., 1974; MENDOZA et al., 1972). Likewise unaffected sibs have had normal uric acid and oxypurine excretion except in one case (DENT and PHILPOT, 1954; ENGLEMAN et al., 1964; AYVAZIAN, 1964; DELATTE and MENDOZA, 1967; SPERLING et al., 1971; FRAYHA et al., 1973; SEEGMILLER, 1969). Therefore, it appears that the heterozygote is phenotypically normal. Of the reported cases 6 have been female and 13 have been male (DENT and PHILPOT, 1954; DICKINSON and SMELLIE, 1959; ENGLEMAN et al., 1964; AYVAZIAN, 1964; DELATTE and MENDOZA, 1967; FREZAL et al., 1967; BRADFORD et al., 1968; CHALMERS et al., 1969; SPERLING et al., 1971; CURNOW et al., 1971; SORENSEN et al., 1972; FRAYHA et al., 1973; HOLMES et al., 1974; MENDOZA et al., 1972). Since this disorder shows no predilection for either sex, the mutation is probably on an autosomal gene. This pattern of inheritance is consistant with an autosomal recessive disorder.

There are several lines of evidence that suggest the genetic defect in xanthinuria is not homogeneous. As already mentioned there is a wide variation in the amount of xanthine oxidase activity measured *in vitro* in patients from different families (AYVAZIAN, 1964; FREZAL et al., 1967; BRADFORD et al., 1968; CHALMERS et al., 1969; SPERLING et al., 1971; FRAYHA et al., 1973; HOLMES et al., 1974; WATTS et al., 1964; OLIVER et al., 1971). These data are difficult to interpret since the assay methods were not comparable in all cases. Another observation that suggests genetic heterogeneity is the report of a potential heterozygote with an increased urinary excretion of oxypurines (DELATTE and MENDOZA, 1967; SEEGMILLER, 1969). As pointed out above, all other obligate heterozygotes (parents of affected individuals) studied have had normal oxypurine excretion.

Treatment

Treatment for xanthinuria is usually not necessary since the majority of individuals with this disorder are asymptomatic. In those patients with renal stones, it is necessary to ensure the usual measures of adequate hydration and relief of any obstructing lesions. Alkalinization of the urine may be necessary on occasion, but continued and prophalytic use is not recommended since increasing the urine pH from 5 to 7 has relatively little effect on the solubility of xanthine and produces no significant change in the solubility of hypoxanthine (KLINENBERG et al., 1965). A role for allopurinol in treating xanthine stones has been suggested because in one patient it decreased the ratio of xanthine to hypoxanthine in the urine (ENGLEMAN et al., 1964). The increase in hypoxanthine relative to xanthine would be of potential benefit since hypoxanthine is approximately 10 times more soluble than xanthine (KLINENBERG et al., 1965). However, this may not be of benefit in all patients since allopurinol increased xanthine excretion relative to hypoxanthine in another patient (HOLMES et al., 1974).

The myopathy observed in the patients with xanthinuria has been relatively mild and no specific therapy has been recommended. Allopurinol would probably not be of benefit for this complication of xanthinuria since xanthine and hypoxanthine crystals have also been observed in muscle tissue from gouty subjects on allopurinol therapy (WATTS et al., 1971).

References

AUSCHER, C., PASQUIER, C., MERCIER, N., DELBARRE, F.: Oxidation of pyrazolo 3,4-d-pyrimidine in a xanthinuric man. Proceedings of the International Symposium on purine metabolism in man, (eds.) A. DE UZIES, O. SPERLING, J. B. WYNGAARDEN. New York: Plenum Publishing Co. 1974.

AYVAZIAN, J. H.: Xanthinuria and hemochromatosis. New Engl. J. Med. 270, 18 (1964).

AYVAZIAN, J. H., SKUPP, S.: Purine utilization and excretion in xanthinuria. J. clin. Invest. 44, 1248 (1965).

BERGMANN, F., DIKSTEIN, S.: Studies on uric acid and related compounds. III. Observations on the specificity on mammalian xanthine oxidases. J. biol. Chem. 223, 765 (1956).

BRADFORD, M. J., KRAKOFF, I. H., LEEPER, R., BALIS, M. E.: Study of purine metabolism in a xanthinuric female. J. clin. Invest. 47, 1325 (1968).

CASTRO-MENDOZA, H. J., DELATTE, L. C., ERRAZTI, R. A. R.: Una neuva observacion de xanthinuaia familiar. Rev. clín. esp. 124, 341 (1972).

CHALMERS, R. A., JOHNSON, M., PALLIS, C., WATTS, R. W. E.: Xanthinuria with myopathy. Quart. J. Med., New Series 38, 493 (1969).

CURNOW, D. H., MASAREL, J. R., CULLEN, K. J., MCCALL, M. G.: Xanthinuria discovered in population screening. Brit. med. J. 1, 403 (1971). 1971 I, 1971.

DELATTE, C. L., CASTRO-MENDOZA, H.: Xanthinuria familiar. Rev. clin. esp. 107, 244 (1967).

DENT, C. E., PHILPOT, G. R.: Xanthinuria, an inborn error (or deviation) of metabolism. Lancet 1954 I, 182.

DICKINSON, C. J., SMELLIE, J. M.: Xanthinuria. Brit. med. J. 1959 II, 1217.

ENGLEMAN, K., WATTS, R. W. E., KLINENBERG, J. R., SJOERDSMA, A., SEEGMILLER, J. E.: Clinical, physiological and biochemical studies of a patient with xanthinuria and pheochromocytoma. Amer. J. Med. 37, 839 (1964).

FRAYHA, R. A., SALTI, I. S., HAICLAR, G. I. A., AL-KHALIDI, U., HEMADY, K.: Hereditary xanthinuria and xanthine urolithiasis: an additional 3 case. J. Urol. (Baltimore, Md.) 109, 871 (1973).

FREZAL, J., MALASSENET, R., CARTIER, R., FESSARD, C., ROY, C., REY, J., LAMY, M.: Sur un cas de xanthinurie. Arch. franc. Pédiat. 24, 129 (1967).

HOLMES, E. W., MASON, D. H., GOLDSTEIN, L. I., BLOUNT, R. E., JR., KELLEY, W. N.: Xanthine oxidase deficiency: Studies in a previously unreported case. Clin. Chem. 20, 1076 (1974).

KELLEY, W. N., WYNGAARDEN, J. B.: Effect of dietary purine restriction, allopurinol and oxipurinol on urinary excretion of ultraviolet-absorbing compounds. Clin. Chem. 16, 707 (1970).

KELLEY, W. N., BEARDMORE, T. D.: Allopurinol: Alteration in pyrimidine metabolism in man. Science 169, 388 (1970).

KLINENBERG, J. R., GOLDFINGER, S., MILLER, J., SEEGMILLER, J. E.: The effectiveness of a xanthine oxidase inhibitor on the treatment of gout. Ann. intern. Med. 62, 639 (1965).

KRETSCHMER, H. L.: Xanthine calculi: Report of a case and a review of the literature. J. Urol. (Baltimore, Md.) 38, 183 (1937).

MARCOLONGO, R., MARINELLO, E., POMPUCCI, G., PAGANI, R.: The role of xanthine oxidase in hyperuricemic states. Arthrit. and Rheum. 17, 430 (1974).

MASSEY, V., BRUMBY, P. E., KOMAI, H., PALMER, G.: Studies on milk xanthine oxidase. Some spectral and kinetic properties. J. biol. Chem. 244, 1682 (1969).

OLIVER, I., SPERLING, O., LIBERMAN, U. A., FRANK, M., DEVRIES, A.: Deficiency of xanthine oxidase activity in colostrum of a xanthinuric female. Biochem. Med. **5**, 279 (1971).
PARKER, R., SNEDDEN, W., WATTS, R. W. E.: The quantitative determination of hypoxanthine and xanthine ("oxypurines") in skeletal muscle from two patients with congenital xanthine oxidase deficiency (xanthinuria). Biochem. J. **116**, 317 (1970).
PARKER, R., SNEDDEN, W., WATTS, R. W. E.: The mass-spectrometric identification of hypoxanthine and xanthine ("oxypurines") in skeletal muscle from two patients with congenital xanthine oxidase deficiency (xanthinuria). Biochem. J. **115**, 103 (1969).
RAMSDELL, C. M., KELLEY, W. N.: The clinical significance of hypouricemia. Ann. intern. Med. **78**, 239 (1973).
ROWE, P. B., WYNGAARDEN, J. B.: The mechanism of dietary alterations in rat hepatic xanthine oxidase levels. J. Biol. Chem. **241**, 5571 (1966).
RUNDLES, R. W., WYNGAARDEN, J. B., HITCHINGS, G. H., ELION, G. B.: Drugs and uric acid. Ann. Rev. Pharmacol. **9**, 345 (1969).
SEEGMILLER, J. E., ENGLEMAN, K., KLINENBERG, J. R., WATTS, R. W. E., SJOERDSMA, A.: Xanthine oxidase and iron. New Engl. J. Med. **270**, 534 (1964).
SEEGMILLER, J. E.: Hereditary xanthinuria, in Duncan's Diseases of Metabolism, 6th Ed. (Eds. BONDY, P. K., ROSENBERG, L. E.), p. 581. Philadelphia: Saunders 1969.
SORENSEN, L. B., TESAR, J. T., ELLMAN, M. H., COLWELL, J.: A new case of xanthinuria. Amer. J. Med. **53**, 690 (1972).
SPERLING, O., LIBERMAN, U. A., FRANK, M., DEVRIES, A.: Xanthinuria. An additional case with demonstration of xanthine oxidase deficiency. Amer. J. clin. Path. **55**, 351 (1971).
WATTS, R. W. E., ENGLEMAN, K., KLINENBERG, J. R., SEEGMILLER, J. E., SJOERDSMA, A.: The enzyme defect in a case of xanthinuria. Biochem. J. **90**, 4 (1964).
WATTS, R. W. E., SNEDDEN, W., PARKER, R. A.: A quantitative study of skeletal-muscle purines and pyrazolo(3,4-d)pyrimidines in gout patients treated with allopurinol. Clin. Sci. **41**, 153 (1971).
WYNGAARDEN, J. B.: Xanthinuria. In: The Metabolic Basis of Inherited Disease, 3rd Ed. (STANBURY, J. B., WYNGAARDEN, J. B., FREDRICKSON, D. S., EDS.), p. 992. NEW YORK: MCGRAW-HILL 1973.

XI. Hereditary Orotic Aciduria

Hereditary Orotic Aciduria

By

R. R. HOWELL*

With 7 Figures

Hereditary orotic aciduria is a rare, genetically transmitted disease which presents in children with a refractory megaloblastic anemia, the excretion of large quantities of the pyrimidine orotic acid in the urine, and retardation of physical growth and development. Although only seven cases have been reported, there is already considerable variation in the clinical and laboratory presentations in this disease.

The fact that this disorder is the only known genetic defect in man involving pyrimidine biosynthesis and the occurrence of well-documented dual enzyme deficiencies has attracted considerably more attention to this rare disease than its incidence would warrant.

Clinical Studies

The clinical presentation of the original patient reported by HUGULEY et al. (1959) is summarized below. Their study of this first patient is an exquisite example of clinical investigation.

Case Report (from HUGULEY et al., 1959)

J.M.R., a white male infant, was born on June 19, 1954, at term. Delivery was normal, and birth weight was 3884 g. He was put on SMA formula, and his general development seemed quite normal, except that he appeared to his mother to be less active and more somnolent than his older siblings. At three months of age his mother noted pallor. At four months he developed a persistent cough. At five months diarrhea began with large, loose, pale, foul-smelling stools. He was hospitalized and found to have severe anemia with a hemoglobin of 6.0 g/100 ml. He was given antibiotics and blood transfusions. At age nine months, after persistent diarrhea, cough, and anemia he was admitted to Emory University Hospital (Atlanta, Georgia, U.S.A.) for the first time. The infections had been treated with sulfisoxazole, penicillin, and tetracycline. He had never received chloramphenicol or anticonvulsant drugs.

The parents were living and well. The parents had a common ancestor, believed to be French in origin, who was the grandfather of the father and the great-grandfather of the mother. All other ancestors were English or Scots. Neither parent nor any of the three siblings had anemia or any abnormalities of the erythrocytes (see Fig. 1 for family pedigree).

---

* JOSEPH P. KENNEDY, JR.: Memorial Foundation Senior Research Scholar in Mental Retardation. Certain of the author's studies cited were supported by Grant AMO 9251 from the National Institutes of Health.

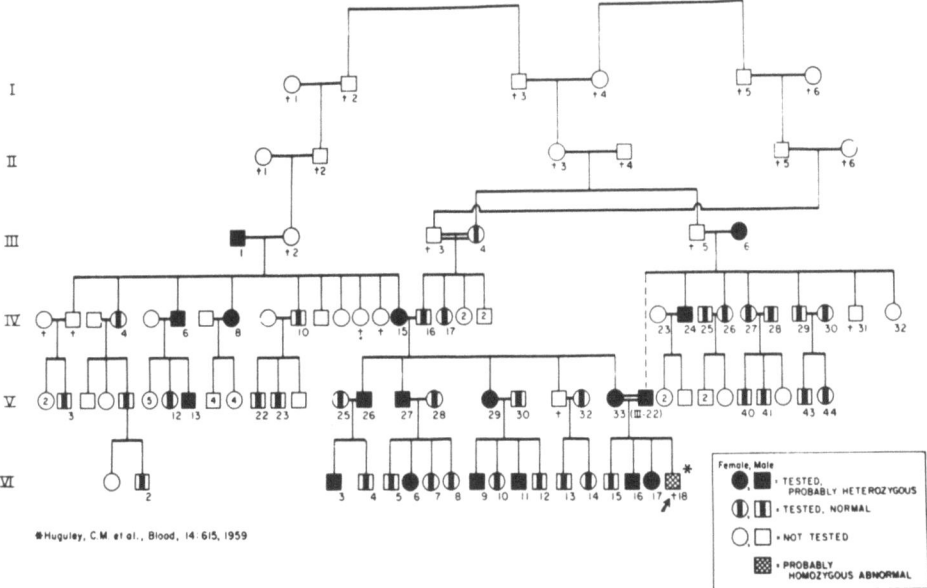

Fig. 1. Pedigree of the family in which the first infant was reported to have orotic aciduria. Erythrocyte enzyme data are the basis for identifying some family members as probable heterozygotes. (From FALLON et al., 1964, with permission)

On physical examination the child was pale and weak, but well-developed and well-nourished. The sclerae were blue, but there was no jaundice. The skin was clear except for a few petechiae about the neck. The tongue was normal. There was no enlargement of the lymph nodes. A few rales and rhonchi were scattered through the lung fields. The heart was normal except for a soft apical systolic murmur. The edge of the liver was palpable. The tip of the spleen descended 1 to 2 cm on inspiration. No neurologic abnormalities were noted. There was torsion of the left tibia outward. There were no other skeletal abnormalities.

Laboratory findings included the following: erythrocytes, 2.80 million per mm^3, hemoglobin, 6.7 g/100 ml; reticulocytes, 2.2%; platelets 260400/mm^3; WBC, 2050/mm^3. Differential white blood cell count revealed 44% segmented neutrophils, 29% lymphocytes, and 27% monocytes. The appearance of the erythrocytes was strikingly abnormal. There was pronounced anisocytosis with many macrocytes and many microcytes. The cells were quite hypochromic, and there was a considerable degree of poikilocytosis. There were two nucleated RBC per 100 WBC. Mean corpuscular hemoglobin averaged 21.3 pg.

The marrow was hypercellular with striking abnormalities of the pernicious anemia type in cells of both granulocytic and rubricytic series.

Serum iron was 200 μg/100 ml. The serum direct bilirubin was 0.25 mg/100 ml and the total bilirubin 1.3 mg/100 ml. Coomb's test was negative. Serum protein was 5.4 g/100 ml with 3.7% albumin.

A specimen of urine had a pH of 5.5 and specific gravity of 1.021; albumin and sugar were absent. Microscopic examination of the urine sediment revealed an occasional white blood cell and a moderate number of nonspecific, fine crystals.

Roentgenograms of the chest (including fluoroscopy) and of the gastrointestinal tract were normal.

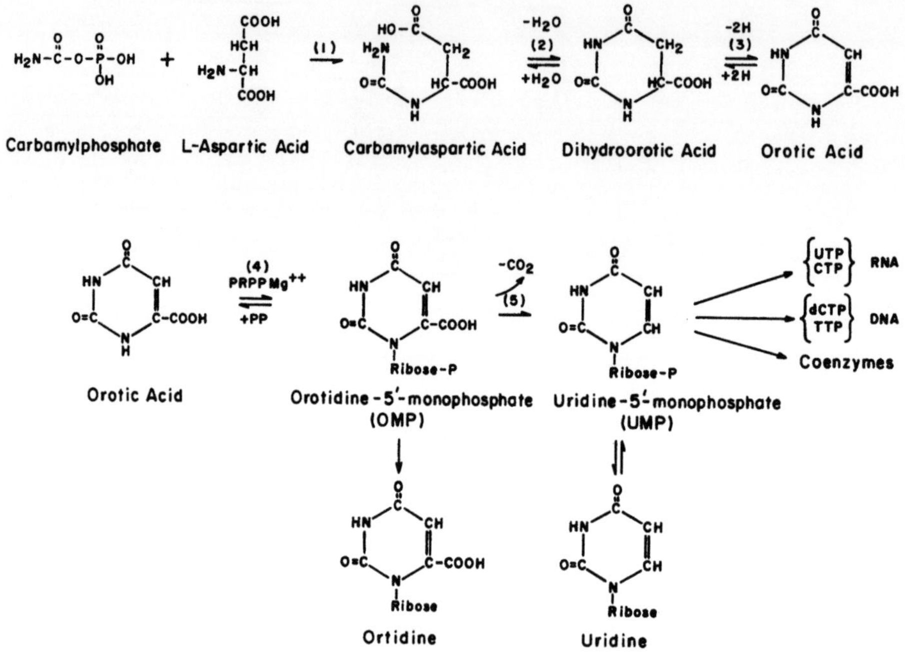

Fig. 2. The major pathways in mammalian *de novo* pyrimidine biosynthesis. The enzymes catalyzing various reactions are indicated by the numbers in brackets: (1) Aspartate transcarbamylase; (2) Dihydroorotase; (3) Dihydroorotic acid dehydrogenase; (4) Orotidine-5'-monophosphate (OMP) pyrophosphorylase; (5) Orotidine-5'-monophosphate (OMP) decarboxylase. Enzymes (4) and (5) are deficient in most patients with hereditary orotic aciduria. In one patient only enzyme (5) is deficient

A gastric analysis showed no free hydrochloric acid during fasting, but 17.5° of free acid appeared after histamine stimulation. A paper electrophoresis study of the patient's hemoglobin on September 20, 1955, was normal. Fetal hemoglobin concentration was 6.1%. Schilling tests were made on August 21, 1956, with an excretion in the urine of 5.8% of the administered B_{12}, and on December 19, 1956, with an excretion of 4.8%. Following the addition of intrinsic factor, he excreted 7.6% on December 26, 1956.

Crystalluria

A prominent feature of the child's course throughout this period was the presence of crystals in the urine. With a good urine output the freshly voided urine did not contain visible crystals, but large numbers of crystals appeared when urine was left to stand. When his intake of fluids was reduced by illness, his urine volume was small and crystals precipitated in his bladder. On several occasions he developed urethral obstruction, and on one occasion right ureteral obstruction. Fortunately, the obstructions cleared each time after fluid intake was increased.

It was then found that the ultraviolet absorption spectra of the crystals at both acid and alkaline pH were identical to those of an authentic sample of the pyrimidine orotic acid (Fig. 2). Paper chromatography using four different solvent systems revealed that the R_f's for the dissolved crystals were identical with those for authentic orotic acid. Melting point studies on the crystals and two derivatives of

Table 1. Clinical features in hereditary orotic aciduria

Case no.	Authors	Sex	Age at diagnosis (months)	Birth weight (g)	Gestation	Megalo-blastic anemia	Remission of hematologic abnormalities on pyrimidines	Mental retardation	Growth retardation	Gross hematuria with crystalluria	Other significant physical findings
1.	Huguley et al. (1959)	M	30	3884	Full term	+	+	+	+	+	Died with varicella pneumonia and heart failure
2.	Becroft et al. (1965)	M	17	4150	Full term	+	+	+	+	+	Unusual hair and strabismus
3.	Haggard et al. (1967)	M	20	1800	35 weeks	+	+	+	+	+	Strabismus
4.	Fox et al. (1969)	M	4	1500	32 weeks	+	+	+	+	+	Unusual hair; multiple abnormalities; died
5.	Rogers et al. (1968)	F	11	2950	Full term	+	+	0	+	+	Strabismus and VSD (probable).
6.	Tubergen et al. (1969)	F	7½ years	2950	Full term	+	+	0	0	+	None
7.	Soutter et al. (1970)	M	5	3175	Full term	+	+	+	+	+	Eczema and unusual hair

the crystals also revealed similar values to those for orotic acid. Column chromatography using a Dowex-1-chloride resin was used to identify and measure orotic acid in the urine.

Summary of Clinical Features

Certain key clinical features of this patient and the other six reported patients are presented in Table 1 (HUGULEY et al., 1959; BECROFT and PHILLIPS, 1965; HAGGARD and LOCKHART, 1967; ROGERS et al., 1968; FOX et al., 1969; TUBERGEN et al., 1969; SOUTTER et al., 1970).

Fetal growth has been normal and in all instances weight has been appropriate for gestational age, but two of the affected infants have been born prematurely.

Most infants have failed to thrive; six of the seven have had retardation of growth and five of the seven appear to be developmentally retarded (see Table 1).

Severe anemia with megaloblastic changes in the marrow has been a consistent feature. During evaluation of the anemia, crystalluria, sometimes with hematuria and/or urinary tract obstruction, has been observed.

The study of these urinary crystals by chromatography (both paper and ion-exchange), ultraviolet spectroscopy, isotope dilution, and chemical (colorimetric) methods has produced data consistent with the crystals being orotic acid. Excretion of orotic acid, not during treatment, has varied around 1500 mm per day.

Photomicrographs of the peripheral blood smear and bone marrow of the typical patient reported by HAGGARD and LOCKHART (1967) are shown in Fig. 3 and 4.

These patients have improved modestly with steroids but have improved dramatically with nucleotide mixtures, or more recently with uridine. Growth has accelerated dramatically, as illustrated in the patient reported by BECROFT and PHILLIPS (1965) (Fig. 5).

Nature of the Defect in Orotic Aciduria

HUGULEY et al. (1959) postulated a "localized" defect in pyrimidine biosynthesis so that the patient was unable to progress beyond orotic acid; they made the analogy between their patient and certain bacterial mutants in pyrimidine biosynthesis reported by YATES and PARDEE (1956). If the enzyme defect were complete, this would make it impossible for the patient to synthesize ribonucleic acid (RNA) and desoxyribonucleic acid (DNA). Needless to say, this would dramatically impair not only cell division but the machinery required for protein synthesis, as the turnover of mammalian ribosomes is rapid compared to the cell's lifespan (LOEB et al., 1965).

The first patient described died of varicella before specific enzymatic studies could be performed (HUGULEY et al., 1959). SMITH et al. (1961) cleverly studied the erythrocytes of the parents and siblings of the original patient and showed reduced activities of both orotidine-5'-monophosphate (OMP) pyrophosphorylase (E.C. 2.4.2.10: orotidine-5'-phosphate: pyrophosphate phosphoribosyltransferase) and OMP decarboxylase (E.C. 4.1.1.23: orotidine-5'-phosphate carboxy-lyase) in certain family members (the parents and two siblings). Their studies were based on the correct assumption that the disorder would be transmitted in an autosomal recessive fashion and that parents and possibly certain family members would show reduced activity of the enzyme in question due to their being obligate heterozygotes. No inhibitor was revealed when this family's erythrocytes were mixed with controls. Erythrocyte enzymes which catalyze the formation of orotic acid (aspartate carbamyltransferase and dihydroorotase) were normal in this fam-

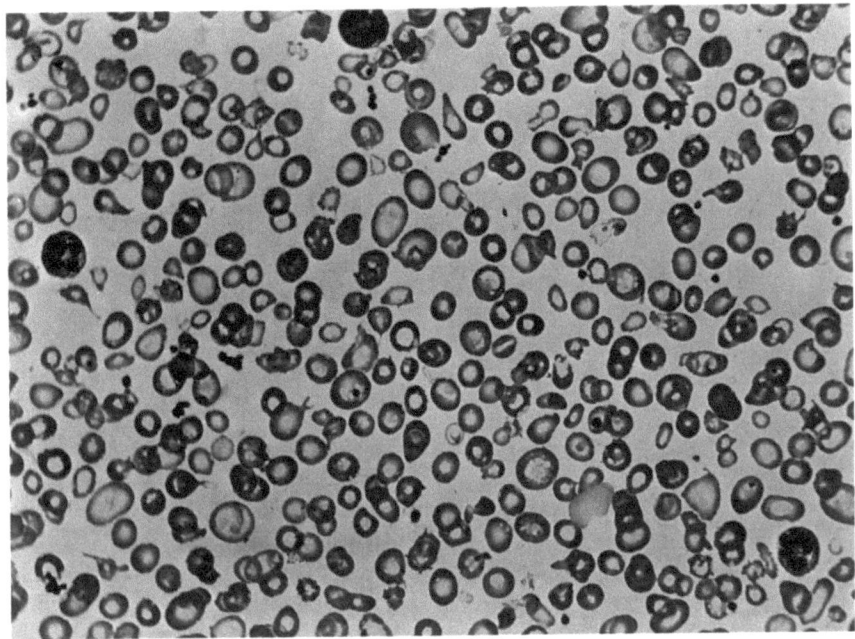

Fig. 3. Peripheral blood smear of patient with hereditary orotic acidura (reported by HAGGARD and LOCKHART, 1967). Dramatic anisocytosis and poikilocytosis is evident. Hypersegmented polymorphonuclear leukocytes are also present (x 850)

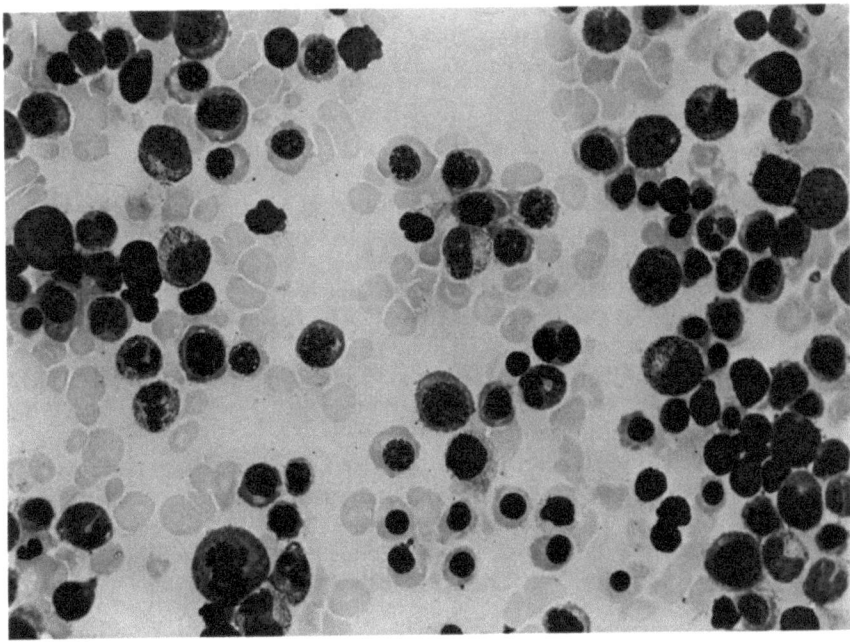

Fig. 4. Bone marrow of patient with hereditary orotic aciduria reported by HAGGARD and LOCKHART (1967). Distinct megaloblastic changes are present (x 850)

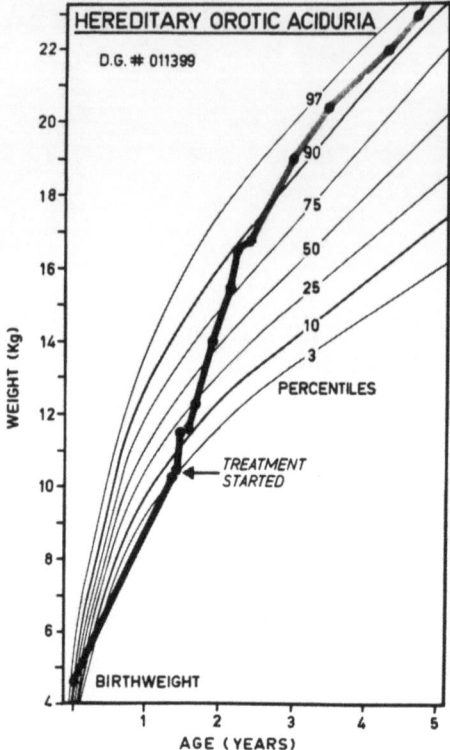

Fig. 5. Effect of uridine treatment on patient D.G. reported by BECROFT and PHILLIPS (1965). The patient's weight rose rapidly from near the third percentile to almost the ninetyseventh percentile with the institution of uridine therapy

ily. It was suggested that deficiencies of these two enzymes were responsible for the patient's inability to convert orotic acid to uridine-5'-phosphate (SMITH et al., 1961) (Fig. 2). Subsequent assays on the red blood cells of homozygous patients have revealed, as predicted, no activity for either of these enzymes. In addition, both these enzyme activities have been shown to be deficient in leukocytes, saliva, and liver in one or more of the affected patients.

One of the seven known patients is, however, deficient only in OMP decarboxylase activity. The activities of other enzymes in *de novo* pyrimidine biosynthesis appear to be normal in these patients.

Fibroblasts were developed from two patients with hereditary orotic aciduria and a single carrier, and the activities of the pyrimidine enzymes compared to those in controls (HOWELL et al., 1967; KROOTH, 1964). When the cells were grown *in vitro* in a controlled environment it was clear that there was a dual enzyme deficiency in this condition, as had previously been shown in hemic cells (see Table 2). Dihydroorotase activity was normal, as in the erythrocytes.

The concurrent deficiency of two enzymes which catalyze sequential reactions can be explained in several ways (HOWELL, 1970). For instance, a single enzyme could catalyze both reactions. This is ruled out by the fact that the enzyme

Table 2. Orotidylic pyrophosphorylase activity of normal and mutant cell strains[a]

Cell strain	Presumed genotype	Orotidylic pyrophosphorylase mµM $C^{14}O_2$/h/mg protein
RU	RR	6.05, 6.20, 6.02
OFR[b]	Rr*	3.02, 2.05
AUC[c]	r*r*	0.039, 0.012
PIE[d]	r*r*	0.038, 0.011, 0.012 |//
Orotidylic decarboxylase activity of the several cell strains[a]		
CD	RR	3.00
ACA	RR	3.90 2.70
JDU	RR	5.14
RU	RR	4.47, 4.68, 5.24, 4.60
OFR[b]	Rr*	1.55, 2.06
AUC[c]	r*r*	0.091, 0.027, 0.026, 0.019
PIE[d]	r*r*	0.109, 0.131

[a] Data from Howell et al. (1967). All studies in this chart were carried out on fibroblasts developed from skin biopsies and growing *in vitro*.
[b] Heterozygous sibling of original patient reported by Huguley et al. (1959).
[c] Patient reported by Becroft and Phillips (1965).
[d] Patient reported by Haggard and Lockhart (1967).

activities can be separated during purification from mammalian tissues and also by the fact that one patient lacks only OMP decarboxylase activity (Fox et al., 1969).

It has been suggested that this condition might represent a mutation at a controller (regulator or operator) locus and that these two enzymes reside in a single operon (Krooth, 1964; Smith et al., 1966). Although this hypothesis is attractive, it is not at present susceptible to a direct experimental test.

Treatment

Vitamins, Iron

Deficiency of Vitamin B_{12} and folic acid is the usual cause of megaloblastic anemias but they have been uniformly ineffective in the treatment of hereditary orotic aciduria. Neimann's case, discussed in detail elsewhere, (Neimann et al., 1965) responded to folic acid but it seems very likely to me that this infant had a different disorder. There has not been evidence for iron deficiency and iron therapy has not been useful. Nor have pyridoxine, alpha tocopherol, or liver extract produced any beneficial effects (Huguley et al., 1959; Smith et al., 1966; Haggard and Lockhart, 1967).

Steroids

A partial hematologic remission has been seen in the patients where this drug was administered (see Fig. 6). In the first patient described, 75 mg cortisone per day produced brisk reticulocytosis and a significant increase in the hemoglobin. The white blood cell count and differential count also returned to normal. Haggard's patient also responded to steroids but megaloblastic changes persisted in the marrow (Haggard and Lockhardt, 1967).

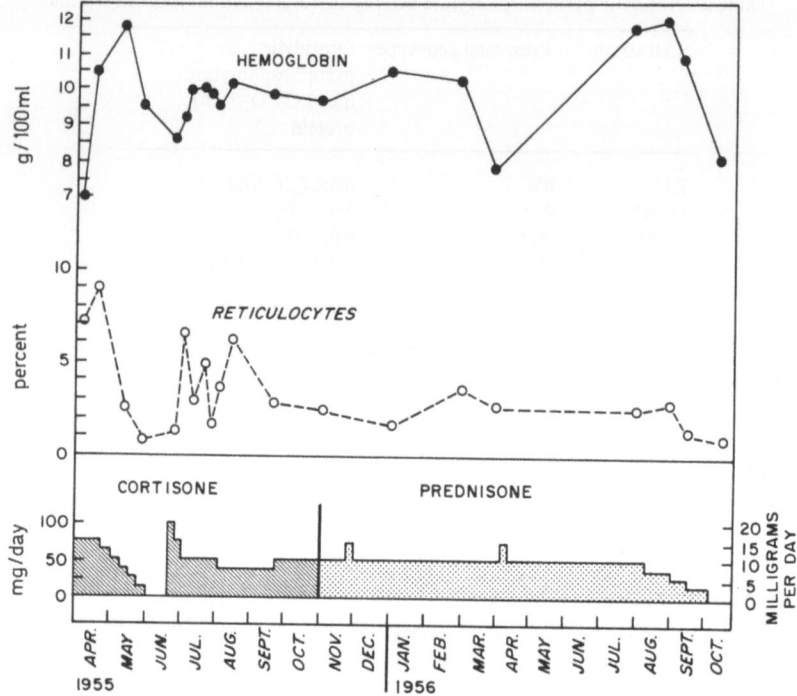

Fig. 6. The response of the patient reported by HUGULEY et al. to steroid treatment. The partial, but distinct, hematologic remission following cortisone and prednisone is seen. (From HUGULEY et al., 1959, with permission)

In view of our information on the nature of the enzyme defect, it is interesting to speculate about the nature of the effect of steroids. There is a small amount of residual enzyme activity (about 1 to 4%) present in skin fibroblasts derived from patients with hereditary orotic aciduria (HOWELL et al., 1967). The fact that there are dual, sequential enzymes which are deficient with detectable (albeit small) activities of these enzymes has been widely interpreted as suggesting a possible regulatory disorder (SMITH, 1966). Additionally, it has been shown that 6-azauridine can increase dramatically the activities of OMP-pyrophosphorylase and coordinately OMP decarboxylase in mutant fibroblasts growing *in vitro* (PINSKY and KROOTH, 1967). Steroids might exert their beneficial effect *in vivo* by increasing the activity of these enzymes. Hydrocortisone and related steroids are known to be potent enzyme inducers in many mammalian systems (TOMKINS et al., 1965).

Uridine and Pyrimidine Nucleotides

The megaloblastic anemia in all patients has responded completely to replacement therapy with pyrimidines. In the first patient, a remission was induced by a nucleotide mix extracted from yeast.

Diarrhea accompanied this treatment and was thought to be related to the high phosphate content in the nucleotides. Uridine (the nucleoside of uracil, see Fig. 2) has been therapeutically effective in the remaining patients.

BECROFT has reported six years' experience with uridine therapy in his patient (BECROFT et al., 1969). Uridine in a dose of 150 mg/kg/day has induced and

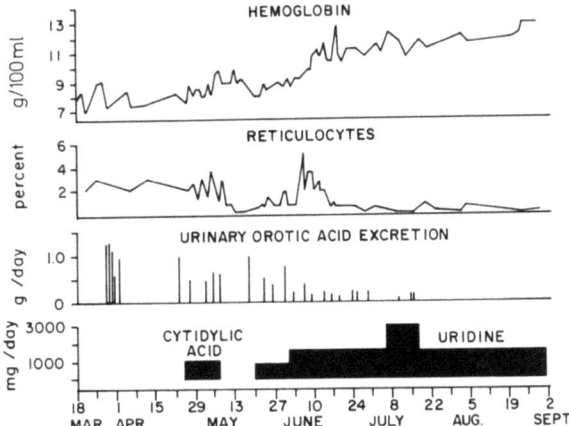

Fig. 7. The response of the patient reported by BECROFT et al. (1965) to oral uridine therapy. There was not only a complete hematologic remission but a striking reduction in the urinary excretion of orotic acid occurred. (From BECROFT et al., 1965, with permission)

maintained a complete hematologic remission. Pysical growth and development has been excellent. The patient has developed intellectually but remains mildly retarded (I.Q. measured by Wechsler Intelligence Scale, 73 to 81 at age seven years).

Uracil, the pyrimidine base (whose nucleoside is uridine) has not been effective in producing a hematologic remission. It is, therefore, apparent that the conversion of uracil to uridine is slow in man and it is thus not possible to replace the more expensive uridine with uracil for therapy.

Another consistent and dramatic effect of uridine (or nucleotide) therapy has been the reduction of excretion of orotic acid in urine (Fig. 7) (HUGULEY et al., 1959; BECROFT and PHILLIPS, 1965). Patients with untreated orotic aciduria usually excrete around 1,000 times the normal amount (which averages 1.4 mg/24 hrs of orotic acid. Treatment with uridine (around 1.5 g/day) reduces this by about 60%. This reduction in orotic acid excretion seems to be a clear indication of the existence of feedback inhibition in man.

It is well established that the *de novo* synthesis of pyrimidines is under metabolic control involving both control of the rate of synthesis of enzymes and control of this enzyme activity by end products (SMITH et al., 1966). In this situation, the primary site of control is the enzyme aspartate transcarbamylase. In E. coli there is evidence that all five enzymes involved in the synthesis of uridine-5'-phosphate are controlled as a unit. The exact type of regulation varies with the source of the enzyme; for example in E. coli, CMP is a potent inhibitor, but in P. fluorescens UTP is the strongest inhibitor, and in lettuce, UMP.

The dramatic reduction in orotic acid excretion after the administration of uridine (or other compounds beyond the genetic-metabolic block) strongly suggests that very similar metabolic feedback control exists in man. Additionally, the activities of aspartate transcarbamylase and dihydroortase activities were markedly increased in the red cells of at least one untreated patient (SMITH et al., 1966). Also, the patient reported by Fox et al. (1969), who was deficient only in OMP decarboxylase, had highly elevated OMP pyrophosphorylase activity in the red cells prior to treatment with uridine. Therefore, in the person unable to synthesize pyrimidine nucleotides (e.g. the patient with hereditary orotic aciduria), inhibition is removed at the aspartate transcarbamylase and maximum orotic acid production ensues.

When intracellular nucleotide levels are reestablished by feeding pyrimidines, feedback regulation is reestablished and orotic acid production is reduced.

Orotic acid overproduction occurs in a mutant of Brevibacterium ammoniagenes (SKODOVA and SKODA, 1969) which is deficient in OMP pyrophosphorylase activity. The mechanism here is also felt to be the lack of feedback inhibition at the level of aspartate transcarbamylase.

Genetics

Hereditary orotic aciduria is transmitted in an autosomal recessive fashion. FALLON et al. (1964) studied 45 relatives of the original proband and 33 unrelated controls, assessing erythrocyte orotidylic (OMP) decarboxylase activity. They found a normal range of 13.2 ± 3.3 units of enzyme activity (one unit equals one millimicromole of orotidylic acid decarboxylated per 10^9 erythrocytes per hour). In the family members there were two distinct populations; one group of 27 persons had a mean activity of 14.4 (s.d. 4.8 units). A second group of 18 persons had values with a 3.0 mean (s.d. 0.89). These data, illustrated by the pedigree shown in Fig. 1, are highly supportive of an autosomal recessive inheritance and with the heterozygote individual having reduced erythrocyte enzyme activity. Three cases of male-to-male transmission and four of nontransmission from male-to-female were noted, excluding an X-linked genetic defect.

In at least six patients with hereditary orotic aciduria, parents and/or other family members have had reduced erythrocyte OMP decarboxylase and/or OMP pyrophosphorylase activity (BECROFT and PHILLIPS, 1965; HAGGARD and LOCKHART, 1967; ROGERS et al., 1968; FOX et al., 1969; TUBERGEN et al., 1969; SOUTTER et al., 1970).

Two studies have detected single individuals heterozygous for hereditary orotic aciduria while examining rather small control populations. This would suggest (but far from prove) that the carrier frequency for the disease is considerably higher than its great rarity of the affected homozygote would suggest (SMITH et al., 1961; ROGERS et al., 1968). One possibility is that the condition may be fatal *in utero* or in infancy (SMITH et al., 1961). The fact that fetal development is normal in these patients with enzymatic defects in *de-novo* pyrimidine biosynthesis provides undisputable evidence for the placental transfer of pyrimidines (either free or as nucleosides or nucleotides). This would thereby bypass the genetic defect and provide substrates for vital nucleic acid synthesis in the rapidly growing fetus. Experimental evidence has been obtained in animals which shows placental transfer of orotic acid, UMP, and uridine. UMP is transferred moderately across the placenta from the seventeenth through the nineteenth day of pregnancy (in rats) although it remains phosphorylated (HAYASHI et al., 1968). Uridine in these studies was selectively taken up by fetal tissues.

In view of all this, *in-utero* death appears most unlikely to me. It would seem highly likely, however, that death of these children in infancy might be a major problem, without the diagnosis ever having been made. SMITH (1965) has called this situation properly pyrimidine auxotrophism in man.

At least one other distinct possibility exists, as suggested by TUBERGEN et al. (1969). These authors described a seven-year-old girl with completely normal growth and development. It is quite possible that the condition might go unrecognized, and considered anemia of unknown cause in a patient like this. As mentioned previously, crystalluria is not an overt problem unless it accompanies dehydration.

Heterozygous carriers for this disorder, as for many other recessively inherited enzyme disorders, are clinically normal. Heterozygosity can be shown by enzyme assays using erythrocytes, leukocytes, and fibroblasts.

ROGERS and PORTER (1968) have used a simple colorimetric method to estimate urinary orotic acid. Using this technique, they confirm the findings of LOTZ et al. (1963) that heterozygotes for this condition excrete elevated amounts of orotic acid in the urine. They feel this is a reliable, and certainly simple, test for heterozygosity. FOX et al. (1970) point out that orotidine gives equally as positive a reaction as does orotic acid in the urine; this does not detract from, and perhaps enhances the usefulness of the method. With this method they detected the orotidinemia produced by allopurinol.

The Possible Relationship of Orotic Aciduria and Gout

The father and one brother of the first known patient with hereditary orotic aciduria had hyperuricemia and typical gouty arthritis. The occurrence of these two diseases in the same family intrigued SMITH et al. (1961) but no relationship was apparent, and a group of gouty subjects had normal activities of OMP pyrophosphorylase and OMP decarboxylase in their red cells. Equally intriguing to me was the fact that the mother of the second known patient (BECROFT and PHILLIPS, 1965) is a three-quarter caste Maori. The Maori as a group are known to have significantly higher serum urate concentrations than most Americans (SEEGMILLER et al., 1963).

It may be random chance, but these observations could be related. Carriers for orotic aciduria might well have increased intracellular concentrations of PRPP since they have reduced OMP pyrophosphorylase and might use reduced PRPP utilization in the pyrimidine pathway. This excess PRPP, a substrate for *de novo* uric acid production can lead to *de novo* overproduction of uric acid. Such a situation exists in the Lesch-Nyhan syndrome (see Chapter IX). Conversely, when orotic acid is added to cultured human cells, *de novo* purine synthesis is markedly reduced (KELLEY et al., 1970). It is felt this effect is mediated by depletion of intracellular PRPP by the pyrophosphorylation of orotic acid.

The fact that these children grow at all probably indicates that they are "leaky" mutants (SMITH et al., 1966); the enzyme data indeed indicates that small amounts of enzyme activity are present. In one of the patients reported by TUBERGEN et al. (1969) growth and development were normal, and she had slightly greater enzyme activities in fibroblasts than the other patients. This very modest difference may account for her very different (normal) growth and development. It is quite possible that total deficiency of these enzymes would be fatal in the newborn period. Small amounts of nucleotides are present in human and cow's milk which might permit marginal survival (KOBATA et al., 1962). Cow's milk (but not human milk) contains about 400 μmoles orotic acid per liter. This, of course, would not benefit the patient.

Other Conditions Associated with Orotic Aciduria

NEIMANN et al. (1965) have reported a three-month infant who presented with severe anemia with distinct megaloblastic changes in the bone marrow. The leukocyte count, unlike the low white blood cell count seen in most of the patients reported with orotic aciduria, was normal. In NEIMANN's patient significant crystalluria was well documented and the crystals were shown to be orotic acid. In addition, the patient's tissues were unable to metabolize aspartic acid to CO_2. No direct enzyme assays were performed in this patient, however.

This patient's hematologic problems responded completely to folic acid, which clearly differentiated him from any other patient with hereditary orotic aciduria. It seems plausible that this patient had a defect in the folic acid-requiring enzyme that catalyzes the conversion of uridylic to thymidylic acid (thymidylate synthetase). It could be postulated that a defect of thymidylate synthetase (for example with altered binding of tetrahydrofolate) would produce a megaloblastic anemia. A defect of this nature might cause increased excretion of orotic acid and other pyrimidines (e.g., uridine, orotidine) by reducing the conversion of uridylic to thymidylic acid. An examination of urine from this patient with the aid of one of the newly developed high-resolution ultraviolet analyzers currently in use in the author's laboratory (VAVICH and HOWELL, 1970) would be most informative. Along these same lines, it would also be of interest to quantitate urinary pyrimidines in the more common type of folic acid deficiency.

Orotic Aciduria Secondary to Other Genetic Defects

The excretion of large amounts of orotic acid in the urine of patients with primary genetic defects in the urea cycle has been recognized several times. Patients with reductions of hepatic ornithine transcarbamylase activity have been found to have urinary orotic acid excretions around 190—240 mg/24 hrs while on a normal protein intake (LEVIN et al., 1969b; CORBEEL et al., 1969). In addition, uridine and uracil excretion has been substantially above normal (LEVIN et al., 1969a). The pattern of pyrimidine excretion is therefore distinct from hereditary orotic aciduria. This excessive pyrimidine excretion, unlike that seen in hereditary orotic aciduria, can be reduced by a low protein intake. The reduction in the utilization of carbamylphosphate by the urea cycle is thought to result in a shunting of this compound into *de novo* pyrimidine biosynthesis.

We have recently studied the urine of a patient thought (but not yet proved) to have a defect in urea synthesis. We used the Mark II, Oak Ridge ultraviolet high-resolution analyzer and found large amounts of orotic acid, uridine, and uracil. It is possible that patients with other defects in urea synthesis distal to the synthesis of carbamylphosphate, e.g. arginosuccinic aciduria (secondary to a deficiency of arginosuccinase) (CARTON et al., 1969), may produce excessive orotic acid excretion through a similar mechanism.

Drug-Induced Orotic Aciduria

6-Azauridine

The pyrimidine analogue, 6-azauridine, after its biological conversions to 6-azauridine-5'-phosphate is a potent inhibitor of orotidylic decarboxylase. This drug has been used in the experimental treatment of human leukemia and solid tumors. Pronounced crystalluria was observed during therapy with 6-azauridine in man. Extensive studies of this situation showed that orotic aciduria developed soon after 6-azauridine therapy was begun and orotidine was present soon thereafter in the urine. These patients were found to have a pronounced increase in the urinary excretion of uric acid, which was due in part to a direct action of 6-azauridine but also secondary to the uricosuric effect of orotic acid in man (FALLON et al., 1961).

Allopurinol

Allopurinol (4-hydroxy-pyrazolopyrimidine) is a drug widely used for the management of hyperuricemia. Its urate-lowering effect is mediated by way of its potent inhibition of the enzyme xanthine oxidase and also very probably through a feedback mechanism involving *de novo* purine biosynthesis. Fox et al. (1970) have recently shown that in patients receiving allopurinol there is a marked increase in the urinary excretion of orotidine. KELLEY and BEARDMORE (1970) have shown that allopurinol ribonucleotide is a potent inhibitor of orotidylic acid (OMP) decarboxylase and that patients receiving allopurinol have markedly increased urinary excretion of orotic acid and orotidine consistent with OMP decarboxylase inhibition *in vivo*.

The Possibility of Prenatal Diagnosis

We demonstrated in early studies (HOWELL et al., 1967) that both OMP pyrophosphorylase and OMP decarboxylase were deficient in fibroblasts derived from skin biopsies of affected patients. In addition, activities of these enzymes in fibroblasts derived from a family member of the first patient reported were intermediate, suggesting heterozygotes might be detected by this means.

Although OMP pyrophosphorylase and OMP decarboxylase have not yet to my knowledge been studied in fibroblasts derived from amniotic fluid cells, it seems possible that study of these enzyme activities in amniotic fluid cell fibroblasts derived from the mother at risk for having children with orotic aciduria would permit prenatal detection of this disorder. Necessary control studies could be accomplished quickly should a family at risk require counseling.

Summary

1. Hereditary orotic aciduria is characterized by refractory megaloblastic anemia and the excretion of large amounts of orotic acid in the urine. Growth and development are usually but not always retarded.

2. Six of the seven known patients have been deficient in both orotidine-5'-monophosphate (OMP) pyrophosphorylase and OMP decarboxylase activity. A single patient is known who is deficient only in OMP decarboxylase.

3. The disease is transmitted as an autosomal recessive trait and heterozygous individuals have intermediate enzyme activities.

4. Orotic aciduria occurs secondary to certain drug therapy as well as when genetic defects in urea biosynthesis result in the shunting of carbamylphosphate into *de novo* pyrimidine biosynthesis.

5. The enzyme defect has been clearly shown in skin fibroblasts growing *in vitro*. By analogy with other situations one would expect fibroblasts developed from amniotic fluid cells normally to contain these enzymes and thereby permit prenatal diagnosis of this disease.

Acknowledgement

The author is very grateful to Dr. Mary Ellen Haggard, who generously loaned slides of the bone marrow and peripheral smear of the patient she has reported. Figures 3 and 4 were made from these slides.

References

BECROFT, D. M. O., PHILLIPS, L. I.: Hereditary orotic aciduria and megaloblastic anaemia: A second case, with response to uridine. Brit. med. J. **1965 1**, 547—552.

BECROFT, D. M. O., PHILLIPS, L. I., SIMMONDS, A.: Hereditary orotic aciduria: Long-term therapy with uridine and a trial of uracil. J. Pediat. **75** (5), 885—891 (1969).

CARTON, D., DE SCHRIJVER, F., KINT, J., VAN DURME, J., HOOFT, C.: Case report: Arginiosuccinic aciduria. Acta paediat. scand. **58**, 528—534 (1969).

CORBEEL, L. M., COLOMBO, J. P., VAN SANDE, M., WEBER, A.: Periodic attacks of lethargy in a baby with ammonia intoxication due to a congenital defect in ureogenesis. Arch. Dis. Childh. **44**, 681—687 (1969).

FALLON, H. J., FREI, E., BLOCK, J., SEEGMILLER, J. E.: The uricosuria and orotic aciduria induced by 6-azauridine. J. clin. Invest. **40**, 1906—1914 (1961).

FALLON, H. J., SMITH, L. H., GRAHAM, J. B., BURNETT, C. H.: A genetic study of hereditary orotic aciduria. New Engl. J. Med. **270**, 878—881 (1964).

FOX, R. M., O'SULLIVAN, W. J., FIRKIN, B. G.: Orotic aciduria. Amer. J. Med. **47**, 332—336 (1969).

FOX, R. M., ROYSE-SMITH, D., O'SULLIVAN, W. J.: Orotidinuria induced by allopurinol. Science **168**, 861—862 (1970).

HAGGARD, M. E., LOCKHART, L. H.: Megaloblastic anemia and orotic aciduria. Amer. J. Dis. Child. **113**, 733—740 (1967).

HAYASHI, T. T., SHIN, D. H., WIAND, S.: Placental transfer of orotic acid, uridine, and UMP. Amer. J. Obstet. Gynec. **102** (8), 1144—1153 (1968).

HOWELL, R. R.: Commentary: Inborn errors of metabolism: Some thoughts about their basic mechanisms. Pediatrics **45** (6), 901—905 (1970).

HOWELL, R. R., KLINENBERG, J. R., KROOTH, R. S.: Enzyme studies on diploid cell strains developed from patients with hereditary orotic aciduria. Johns Hopk. med. J. **120** (2), 81—88 (1967).

HUGULEY, C. M., JR., BAIN, J. A., RIVERS, S. L., SCOGGINS, R. B.: Refractory megaloblastic anemia associated with excretion of orotic acid. Blood **14** (6) 615—634 (1959).

KELLEY, W. N., BEARDMORE, T. D.: Allopurinol: Alteration in pyrimidine metabolism in man. Science **169**, 388—390 (1970).

KELLEY, W. N., FOX, I. H., WYNGAARDEN, J. B.: Regulation of purine biosynthesis in cultured human cells. I. Effects of orotic acid. Biochim. biophys. Acta (Amst.) **215**, 512—516 (1970).

KOBATA, A., SUZUOKI-ZIRO, KIDA, M.: The acid-soluble nucleotides of milk. I. Quantitative and qualitative differences of nucleotides constituents in human and cow's milk. J. Biochem. **51** (4), 277—287 (1962).

KROOTH, R. S.: Properties of diploid cell strains developed from patients with an inherited abnormality of uridine biosynthesis. Sympos. quant. Biol. **29**, 189—212 (1964).

LEVIN, B., ABRAHAM, J. M., OBERHOLZER, V. G., BURGESS, E. A.: Hyperammonaemia: A deficiency of liver ornithine transcarbamylase. Arch. Dis. Childh. **44**, 152—161 (1969a).

LEVIN, B., OBERHOLZER, V. G., SINCLAIR, L.: Biochemical investigations of hyperammonaemia. Lancet **1969 2**, 170—174.

LOEB, J. N., HOWELL, R. R., TOMKINS, G. M.: Turnover of ribosomal RNA in rat liver. Science **149** (3688), 1093—1095 (1965).

LOTZ, M., FALLON, H. J., SMITH, L. H., JR.: Excretion of orotic acid and orotidine in heterozygotes of congenital orotic aciduria. Nature (Lond.) **197**, 194—195 (1963).

NEIMANN, N., NAJEAN, Y., SCIALOM, C., BOULARD, M., PIERSON, M., BERNARD, J.: Etude d'un cas d'anemia megaloblastique de l'enfant avec excretion anormale d'acide orotique. Nouv. Rev. franç. hemat. **5** (3), 445—458 (1965).

PINSKY, L., KROOTH, R. S.: Studies on the control of pyrimidine biosynthesis in human diploid cell strains, I. Effect of 6-azauridine on cellular phenotype. Proc. nat. Acad. Sci. (Wash.) **57**, 925—932 (1967).

ROGERS, L. E., PORTER, F. S.: Hereditary orotic aciduria. II. A urinary screening test. Pediatrics **42** (3), 423—428 (1968).

ROGERS, L. E., WARFORD, L. R., PATTERSON, R. B., PORTER, F. S.: Hereditary orotic aciduria. I. A new case with family studies. Pediatrics **42** (3), 415—422 (1968).

SEEGMILLER, J. E., LASTER, L., HOWELL, R. R.: Biochemistry of uric acid and its relation to gout. New Engl. J. Med. **268**, 712—716, 764—773, 821—827 (1963).

Skodova, H., Skoda, J.: Mechanism of overproduction of orotic acid by a mutant of *Brevibacterium ammoniagenes*. Appl. Microbiol. **17** (1), 188—189 (1969).

Smith, L. H., Jr.: Hereditary orotic aciduria-pyrimidine auxotrophism in man (Editorial). Amer. J. Med. **38** (1), 1—6 (1965).

Smith, L. H., Jr., Huguley, C. M., Jr., Bain, J. A.: Hereditary orotic aciduria. In: The Metabolic Basis of Inherited Disease, 2nd Edit., p. 739—758. New York: McGraw-Hill 1966.

Smith, L. H., Jr., Sullivan, M., Huguley, C. M., Jr.: Pyrimidine metabolism in man. IV. The enzymatic defect of orotic aciduria. J. clin. Invest. **40**, 656—664 (1961).

Soutter, G. G., Yu, J. S., Lovric, A., Stapleton, T.: Hereditary orotic aciduria. Australian paediat. J. **6** (1), 47—52 (1970).

Tomkins, G. M., Garren, L. D., Howell, R. R., Peterkofsky, B.: The regulation of enzyme synthesis by steroid hormones: The role of translation. J. cell. comp. Physiol. **66**, 137—152 (1965).

Tubergen, D. G., Krooth, R. S., Heyn, R. M.: Hereditary orotic aciduria with normal growth and development. Amer. J. Dis. Child. **118**, 864—870 (1969).

Yates, R. A., Pardee, A. B.: Control of pyrimidine biosynthesis in Escherichia Coli by a feedback mechanism. J. biol. Chem. **221**, 757—770 (1956).

Vavich, J. M., Howell, R. R.: Ultraviolet-absorbing compounds in urine of normal newborns and young children. Clin. Chem. **16**, 702—706 (1970).

Sachregister

Abbauprodukte der Harnsäure 140
Acenocumarol 525
Acetazolamid 172, 414, 562
acetoacetate 11
Achillessehne bei Gicht 260
Acidose, metabolische 573
Acrodermatitis chronica atrophicans 315
ACTH 201
Adenin 60, 484
adenine phosphoribosyltransferase 31, 608
— — deficiency 51
adenosine-5'-monophosphate 56
Adenylcyclase 453
Adjuvans-Arthritis 451
Akromegalie 560
alcoholism, acute 11
Alkalisierung 367, 385
Alkalisierungstherapie 400
Alkoholika 199, 200
Alkoholismus 167
Alkoholkonsum 239, 243, 244
Alkoholspiegel, hoher 173
allantoic acid 156
allantoin 156
Allopurinol 462, 618, 648
— -Behandlung 191, 380, 383f., 416, 468ff., 588
— -Metabolismus 471
— -Nebenwirkungen 480
— -Pharmakokinetik 472
Alpha$_1$-Alpha$_2$ urate binding globuline 51
Alpha-Methyl-Dopa 417
Altersprognose der Gicht 599
Amethopterin 466
amino acids in gout 83
Aminopterin 466
ammonium-^{15}N 71
AMP 128, 165
— -Spaltung 130
Anämie, perniziöse 169
Anaphylatoxin 198
anemia 616
Angiopathien, periphere, obliterierende 247
angiotensin 151
Ankylose 268
Antacida 446
antihypertensive Behandlung 416

Antileukozytenserum 190
Antiphlogistica-Wirkungsmechanismus 453
Antirheumatica 445 ff.
Antistreptolysintiter 291
A-PRT 57, 79
Äquilibriumdialyse 183
Arteriolonekrose 230
arthritis 628
Arthritis, akute 194
—, chronische 303 ff.
—, pseudo-guttöse bei Psoriasis 295, 297
— psoriatica 262, 348
—, rheumatoide 197
— urica 167, 197, 266
— —, Prognose 595 f.
— — der Sacroiliacalgelenke 214
— — der Schultergelenke 214
— — an traumatisch vorgeschädigten Gelenken 333
— — der Wirbelsäule 214
Arthrose, aktivierte 299
Arthrosen 299, 308 ff.
—, sekundäre 265
Äthylalkohol 566, 573
Äthylaminothiadiazol 560
Äthylbiscumacetat 524
Atrophie, hypertrophe 331
Ausscheidungstheorie 396
Aussparungseffekt 399
Auswertung der Röntgenaufnahmen 325
8-Azaguanin 484
Azaserin 465
Azathioprin 483, 618
6-Azauridine 647

Basen, freie 130
Basisinformationen für die RD der Gicht 324 f.
Becken-Kelchsystem, Engstellung 342
Befallmuster der Gelenke 343 f.
— der Gichtarthritis 304, 306
Begleitkrankheiten der Gicht 599
—, vasculäre 598
Benzaronum 516
Benzbromaronum 378
Benziodaronum 514, 517
Benzobromaronum 516, 588

Benzoesäure 574
— -Derivate 493, 498
Benzofuranderivate 493, 513
Berufsfähigkeit bei Gicht 596
Berylliose 172
Beta-Hydroxybuttersäure 573
— -hydroxybutyrate 11
— -Receptorenblocker 417
Bilanz, energetische der Purine 135
Bildanalyse, systematische 325
biosynthesis of purines 53
Bishydroxycumarin 525
Bleigicht 172
Bleivergiftung 164
Blutgerinnungssystem 193
Blutkrankheiten und Gicht 169f.
Bradykinin 192, 194, 196, 197, 198
Brandessche Operation 581
breakdown of uric acid 157
Bromindion 525
Bromsulphaleinretention 238
Bromsulphaleintest bei Diabetikern 241
Bursa-Tophi 311
Bursitiden 301f.
Bursitis olecrani 301
— urica olecrani 257

C_1-Esterase 198
cadmium intoxication 156
Calcaneus-Exostosen 334
Calcinosis interstitialis 313
Calciumoxalat-Kristalle 188
—, Steinbildung 402
Calciumphosphatkristalle 188
Calciumpyrophosphatdihydratkristalle 188
Calciumpyrophosphatkristalle 187, 284
cancer of the lung 11
carbon dioxide 156
carboxylase activities for the keta acids of leucine
    isoleucine and valine 32
Carboxypeptidase B 196
— N 194
Carcinome 201
Carinamid 498ff.
Carpaltunnel-Syndrom 265
central nervous system dysfunction
    (Lesch-Nyhan) 611ff.
chemotaktische Eigenschaften der Uratkristalle
    199
Chemotaxis 196, 439
Chlorothiazid 562, 565
chlorprothixene 150
Chlorthalidon 172, 562
Cholesterin 203
Cholografin 150
Chondrocalcinose 280f., 308
Chondrocalcinosis 187

Chondrocalcinosis polyarticularis 354
Chondroitinsulfat 182
chronic lead intoxication 96
— renal disease 16
— — — disease, excretion of uric acid in 152
Citronensäure-Citrat-Gemische 589
Clofibrat 246, 526
Clonidin 417
CO-Vergiftung 560
Colcemid 434
Colchicein 435
Colchicin 186, 189, 199, 423ff., 433ff., 588
— -Dosis 426f.
— -Nebenwirkungen 425
— -Prophylaxe 496, 504, 528
— -Test 286, 424
— -Überempfindlichkeit 425
— -Vergiftung 444
Complement, Bedeutung des 198
— -Fraktionen 199
— -System 198
Coronarangiographie 248
coronare Herzkrankheit 248
Coronarkrankheit 247
Coronarrisiko bei Hyperuricämie 249
correlation of serum uric acid with other
    population characteristics 14
Cortison 201
cotton pellet-Granulom 451
Coxsackie-Viren 262
cross-reactivity with antibody 604
crystalluria 637
Cumarinderivate 493, 523
Cylindrurie 374
Cytochrom P 450 447
Cytoplasma der Neutrophilen 192

Dactylitis psoriatica 296
Dauer-Langzeittherapie der chron.
    Pyelonephritis 590
Defektheilung bei Gicht 596
degeneration, hepatolenticular 11
degradation products of uric acid 156
Dehydroepiandrosteron 202
Diabetes 173, 244, 247
— und Spondylosis hyperostotica 341
— mellitus 15, 232, 290, 414
diabetic acidosis 11
diabetische Arthropathie 354
Diagnose einer Gichtniere 375
diagnostic criteria for gout 18
Diamantstaub 188
Diät bei asymptomatischer Hyperuricämie 549
—, experimentelle Grundlagen 536ff.
— und Harnsäurespiegel 377
—, streng purinarme 550
Diätbehandlung 462, 536

Diätempfehlung bei Gicht 548
Diätetik, praktische 548
Diätpläne 557
Diätvorschriften bei Gichtniere 590
Diazoxid 417
Dicoumarine 172
diet, high fat 11
dietary factors in primary gout 95
Differentialdiagnose der chronischen Gicht 302 ff.
— der extraarticulären Gichtanfälle 299 f.
— der Fingerendgelenkarthritis 296
— der Fingermittelgelenkarthrose 310
— der Gicht 276 ff.
— des Gichtanfalls 262 f., 277 f.
— bei der Röntgendiagnostik 344 ff.
disorder, autosomal recessive 630
distribution of serum uric acid values 12
Diuretica, kaliumeinsparende 562
diuretics 98, 150
dizygotic twins 30
DON (Diazo-Oxo-Norleucin) 465
Dorsalcyste 316
Down-Syndrom 167
drug-induced hyperuricemia 98
Durchschnittsalter bei Gicht 598

effect of drugs and intermediary metabolites on the renal excretion of uric acid 149 ff.
Eisenbergsche Lösung 385, 503, 529
Eiweißgehalt der Nahrung 129
Elektrolytpool, verarmter 173
elektronenmikroskopische Untersuchungen 191
Ellbogen-Tophi 311
enchondrale Dysostose, cystoide Form 354
Enchondrome 354
endogenous nucleic acids, increased breakdown 155
Endopeptidase 192, 195
Energieeinsparung bei Purinen 135
Energieentfaltung, glykolytische 188
Entzündungsmediatoren 454
Entzündungsmodelle 451
enzymatic spectrophotometric methods 9
enzyme defect 604 ff.
Enzyminduktion 448
Epicondylitis humeri 300
epidemiologische Studien 238, 243, 247, 249
Erkrankungshäufigkeit bei Gicht 595
Ernährungsexperiment, chronisches 166
Ernährungsexperimente über den Harnsäurestoffwechsel 536
Erythrämie 171
Erythrocyten 135
Etacrynsäure 172, 414

Etagen-Differentialdiagnose der chronischen Polyarthritis 305
ethanol 93
ethnic differences in serum uric acid levels and gout 19
excretion of uric acid into the intestinal tract 156
— — — — in sweat 157
extracellular fluid, changes in the volume 151

Faktor XI 195
— XII 192, 193, 195, 197, 198
Fanconi syndrome 11, 156
family studies of gout and hyperuricemia 29
Fasten 173, 544, 567, 572
Femurkopfinfarkt 231
Ferse bei Gicht 300
Fettleber und Hyperuricämie 238
fettreiche Kost 545
Fettsucht 200
Fibrinolyse 193
fibroblasts 604
Filtrations-Rückresorptions-Theorie 361
Fingergelenke bei Gicht 259
Fingerknöchelpolster 316
Folsäureanaloge 465
Formeldiät, purinfreie 125, 536, 540
Framingham-Studie 248
Fructose 166, 201, 567, 571 f.
Furosemid 414, 562

Gaspedal-Gicht 257
Gefäßdilatation 196
Gefäßpermeabilität 198
Gefäßveränderungen 415
—, hypertone 413
Gefäßverkalkungen 340
Gelenkgicht 255 ff., 586
—, chondrale Form 214
—, synoviale Form 216
Gelenkkapsel-Resektion 581
genetic aspects of gout 29
— — — hyperuricemia 29
— heterogeneity 605
genetics (Lesch-Nyhan) 616
Genetik der Gicht 115 ff.
Gen-Koppelung 244
Gentisinsäure 496
geographic differences in serum uric acid levels and gout 19
Gerinnungssystem 193
Gerinnungszeit 195
Geschlechtsprädominanz 344
— -verteilung der Harnsäurekonzentration 561
— bei primärer Gicht 170

Gicht   179, 181, 182, 183, 185, 237
Gicht, akute   187, 188
— bei Alkoholikern   164
— bei Blutkrankheiten   164
—, chirurgische Behandlung   579ff.
—, chronische   264ff.
— und Diabetes   241
—, familiäre   166
—, hereditäre   164
— und Hochdruck   412ff.
— und Hypercholesterinämie   243
— und Hyperlipidämie   243
— und Leukämie   165, 201
— der Patella   214
—, primäre   164, 167
—, — konstitutionelle   164
—, Prognose   599
—, rechtzeitige Diagnosestellung   596
— der Schleimbeutel   221
—, sekundäre   164ff., 359
— und Spondylosis hyperostotica   341
Gichtanfall   180, 181, 185, 196, 528, 595
—, akuter   185, 186, 187, 190, 191, 192, 194, 197, 198, 199, 200, 201, 202, 255, 277
Gichtanfälle, extraarticuläre   299
—, Prognose   597
—, pseudo-phlegmonöse   302
Gichtarthritis   267
—, chronische   303
Gichtbehandlung, postoperative   584
Gicht-Dauertherapie   461f.
Gichterkrankung   391
Gichtformen, atypische   268
Gichtknoten   269f.
Gichtkranke   187, 188, 190, 196, 201
Gichtniere   180, 182, 223ff., 356ff., 597f.
— -Behandlung   377ff., 587ff.
—, Prognose   376f.
—, Prophylaxe   386
—, Therapie   377ff., 587ff.
—, Verlauf   370, 376f.
Gichtperlen   270
Gicht-Prophylaxe   422ff.
— -Therapie   422ff., 462ff.
— -Verlauf   255ff.
Glomerulumsklerose   228, 415
glucose-6-phosphatase   32
— — — deficiency   50, 74
— — — -Mangel   167
glutamic acid dehydrogenase hypothesis   84
Glutamin-Analoge   465
glutaminase hypothesis   84
glutamine metabolism in primary gout   84
— phosphoribosylpyrophosphate amidotransferase   54, 64
— -PP-ribose-P amidotransferase   88
glutathione reductase variants   50

— — — and gout   88
Glycin, markiertes   171
glycine-1-^{14}C   69
— -^{15}N   69
—, incorporation into uric acid   68
glycogen storage disease type I   74
glycopyrrolate   92
Glykogen-Speicherkrankheit   560
Glykogenose   164, 166
— I   167
Glykolyse   184
Glykoneogenese   200
GMP   128
Gonokokken-Arthritis   262
gout associated with specific enzymatic defects   74
—, chemical feature   603
—, epidemiology   9
—, genetics   45
—, primary   82
—, secondary   96
gouty arthritis, acute   25
— kidney   356
— nephropathy   156
Granularatrophie, rote (benigne)   229
Granulocyten   187, 188, 189, 190, 191, 192, 194, 195, 202
— -Schnitte   192
Großzehengrundgelenk bei Gicht   184, 213
—, Operation   581
Guanethidin   417
guanine   60
guanosine   60
— -5'-monophosphate   56

Hageman-Faktor   192, 193, 194, 195, 196, 197, 198
— — -Mangel   195
Hallux rigidus   308
hämatopoetische Krankheiten   186
Hämaturie   373
Hämochromatose   290
Hämodialyse   289
Harnacidität   400
— neutralisierung   496
Harnsäure   131, 165, 180, 181, 182, 183, 185, 186, 199
— im Tophus   269
Harnsäureabbau   138
Harnsäureausfällung   369
—, intratubuläre   383, 528
—, tubuläre   495
Harnsäure-Ausscheidung   129, 165, 190, 200, 201, 395
—, enterale   364
—, extrarenale   139

Sachregister

— bei famil. Hyperuricämie 492
—, renale 358 f.
—, saliväre 359
Harnsäurebildung bei famil. Hyperuricämie 492
—, vermehrte 165
Harnsäureclearance 169, 361, 492
Harnsäure-Eigenschaften 179
Harnsäuregehalt der Gelenkflüssigkeit 213
Harnsäureinfarkt 360
Harnsäure-Infusionen 186
Harnsäure-Konzentration 185
— im Endharn 395
—, tubuläre 382
Harnsäurekristalle 180
Harnsäure-Lithiasis 391 ff.
— -Löslichkeit 365, 385
Harnsäuremehrausscheidung 494 f., 501 f., 507
Harnsäuremikrokristalle 167
Harnsäurepool 494, 501
Harnsäurepräcursoren 542
Harnsäurequote, endogene 384
Harnsäureretention, paradoxe 493, 497, 501, 515 f.
Harnsäurerückresorption, tubuläre 493
Harnsäuresekretion, tubuläre 362, 493
Harnsäurespiegel 129
Harnsäuresteinbildung 395
—, Prophylaxe 588
Harnsäuresteindiathese, idiopathische 400
Harnsäuresynthese 462 ff.
Harnsäuretransport, tubulärer 365
Harnsäureverschlußstein 402
Harnsteinbildung 391
Hartnup disease 11
Hautgicht, chronische 310
heart disease, coronary 28
Heberden-Arthrose 308
— -Knötchen 309, 316, 351
hematologic abnormalities (Lesch-Nyhan) 616
Hemmstoffe der Purin- und Harnsäuresynthese 465
Herzinfarkt 247
Hexadimethinbromid 196
HG-PRT 57
high fat diet 11
Hinweis-Symptome, radiologische 339 ff.
Histopathologie der Chondrocalcinose 282
Hodgkin's disease 11
Hüftkopfnekrose 308
—, idiopathische 344
Hydralazin 416
Hydrochlorothiazid 562
Hydrolase 191
Hydrops intermittens 294
Hydroxylapatit-Kristalle 289
3'-Hydroxyphenylbutazon 505, 508

p-Hydroxysulfinpyrazon 511, 513
Hypercalcämie 402
Hypercalcurie 402
Hypercholesterinämie 243, 248
—, essentielle 560
— bei Gicht 249, 414
hypercholesterolemia 16
Hyperlactat-Acidämie 172 f., 201
hyperlactic acid 149
Hyperlipidämie 239, 244, 247, 414
—, sekundäre 246
Hyperlipoproteinämie 244, 414
hyperlipoproteinemia 16, 52
Hyperostose, senile ankylosierende 340
Hyperostosis frontalis interna 231
hyperparathyroidism 11
Hyperparathyreoidismus 173, 560
—, primärer 232
—, sekundärer 287
Hypertension 16
—, arterielle 560, 588 f.
—, essentielle 561
—, renale 561
—, renovasculäre 561
Hypertonie 228, 249, 375
Hypertoniehäufigkeit 412
Hypertonus 247
Hypertriglyceridämie 243, 248, 415
hypertriglyceridemia 16
hyperuricaciduria, adult X-linked 603 ff.
Hyperuricämie 181, 183, 184, 186, 189, 199, 200, 214, 237, 241, 396
—, arzneimittelbedingte 171
—, Belastung mit RNS 128
— durch cytostatische Therapie 566 ff.
— und Diabetes 242
— durch diätetische Maßnahmen 572
—, familiäre 357, 492
— und Gicht 248, 276 f.
— -Häufigkeit 561
— und Hyperlipidämie 243 ff.
— und Hypertonie 412 ff.
—, nicht gichtige 560
—, primäre 167 f.
— durch respiratorische Acidose 574
— durch Saluretica 562
—, sekundäre 164 ff., 168, 359, 395, 560
—, symptomlose 237, 239, 248
— durch therapeutische Maßnahmen 560 ff.
— -Therapie 462 ff.
hyperuricemia 11, 627
—, asymptomatic 32, 45
—, classification 44
—, definition 43
—, development 603, 609
—, epidemiology 9
—, population studies 47

hyperuricemia, secondary 96
—, X-linked 49
Hypoparathyreoidismus 560
hypoxanthine 60, 627
Hypoxanthin-Guanin-Phosphoribosyltransferase 31, 492
hypoxanthine, guanine phosphoribosyltransferase 603, 630
—, — — deficiency 49
—, — — deficiency in gout 76

Ikterus, familiärer, hämolytischer und Gicht 169
Indandionderivate 493, 523, 525
Indometacin 199, 428, 449, 450
Injektion, interartikuläre von Natriumurat 195
inosine 60
inosine-5'-monophosphate 56
Insertionstendopathien 299f.
Insulinresistenz bei Hypertriglyceridämie 242
Insulinwirkung 246
Inulin-Clearance 201
Invalidisierung bei Gicht 596
iodipamide 150
iodopyracet 150
iopanoic acid 150
iron in treatment 642

Kalk-Bursitis 302
Kalk-Gicht 289, 313
Kallidin 198
Kallikrein 192, 193, 194, 196, 198
— -Inhibitor 197
Kallikreinogen 196
Kapseltaschen, paraossäre bei Gicht 219
Ketoacidose 173, 544
—, diabetische 243
Ketonämie 573
ketonemia 149
Ketonkörper 246
Ketophenylbutazon 508
Ketose 560
kinetic constants, altered 604
Kininase 194, 195, 197
Kinine 192, 194, 195, 196, 197, 198
Kininogenase 192, 193
Kininogene 192, 193, 196
Kinin-System 192
Kniegelenk bei Gicht 213
Knochentophi 265f., 596
Kochsalzrestriktion 414
Kohlenhydrate, Einfluß auf Harnsäure-
  stoffwechsel 546
—, leberaffine 567
Kohlenhydratstoffwechsel 415
Kolik von Devonshire 164
kolikauslösende Faktoren 397
Koliken 396

Kolloidtheorie 393
Komplementsystem 192, 193
Kostformen, ketogene 199
Krankheitsdauer der Gicht 598
Kristallgröße 187
Kristallisationstheorie 393
Kristallisationszentrum 393
Kristallmorphologie 284
Kristallographie 180

L-glutamine 63
— in gout 83
Lactat 199, 200, 246, 566
Lactat-Acidämie 200
Lactatanstieg 199
Lactatbildung 188
lactate 11
Lactat-Produktion 200
lead intoxication, chronic 96
— nephropathy 11
Lebenserwartung bei Gicht 595, 597, 599
Lebergröße 239, 241
Lebersarkoidose und Hyperuricämie 232
Lesch-Nyhan-Syndrom 31, 49, 76, 119, 357, 416, 602ff.
leukemia 97
Leukocyturie 373
Leukämien 165, 201
Leukocyten 187, 189, 191f., 194, 196, 199
— -Austritt 196
Leukopenie 190
Leukose 166
leukotaktische Wirkung der Uratkristalle 197, 198
Leukotaxis 197, 198
Lipoid-Dermato-Arthritis 314, 315
Lipoid-Gicht 312
Liposomen 203
lithiasis, idiopathic uric acid 27
Lochdefekte an den Zehen 330
Lokalisation des Erstanfalls der Gicht 277
Longacid 504
Lumicolchicin 434
Lupus erythematodes 298
Lymphoblastenleukämie 169
Lysosomen 191, 202, 203, 455

Magenschleimhautproduktion 449
Manifestationsalter der Gicht 599
maple syrup urine disease 32
Marktophi 224
Matrixuntersuchungen 394
measurement of uric acid 9
Mechanismus der akuten Arhtritis urica 281
Medikamente zur Hemmung der Harnsäure-
  bildung 380f.
Megakaryocyten 171
Meniscusverkalkungen 283, 286, 288

Sachregister

mental deficiency (Lesch-Nyhan) 613
6-Mercaptopurin 482
Mesangiumsklerose 228
metabolic alterations 629
Metabolisierung von Indometacin 450
— der Purinbasen 132
Metaplasie, myeloische 171
6-Methylmercaptopurin-Ribonucleosid 483
Mikrofilamente 440
Mikrotrauma als lokalisierender Faktor 257
Mikrotubuli 436f.
Milchsäure 184, 189
Mitoserate 448
MK-185 526
Mobilisation, postoperative 585
mongolism 11
Mononatriumurat 179, 183
— -Kristalle 187f., 191, 202, 279
Mononatriumuratmonohydrat 179, 269
— -Kristalle 179
mononucleosis, infectious 11, 98
Monoribonucleotide 128
monozygotic twins 30
Morbidität der Gicht 595
Mortalität an Gicht 595
mosaics (enzyme defect) 617
Mucopolysaccharid 184
Mucopolysaccharidbiosynthese 454
multiple myeloma 97
Myelocyten 171
myeloid metaplasia 96
myeloische Metaplasie 170
myeloproliferative disease 155
— disorders 11
Myelose, subleukämische 171
myopathy 627
myxedema 11
Myxödem 560

NADH/NAD$^+$-Quotient 173
Nahrungspurine, Resorption von 129
Natriummonourat 184
Natriummonouratkristalle 188
Natriumorotat-Kristalle 188
Natriumurat 188
Nephritis, interstitielle 225
Nephrocalcinose 232
Nephrolithiasis 27, 391, 596, 627
— bei Gicht 371f.
— bei Polycythämie 171
Nephropathie 413, 587
—, glomeruläre 225, 228
nephropathy 28
—, acid obstructive 156
Nephrosklerose 415
Neutralisierung der Harnsäure 385, 528f.
Nieren bei Hyperurikämie 183

Nierenbiopsie 376
Nierenerkrankungen 188
Nierenfunktionseinschränkung 412, 413
Nierenfunktionsproben 374
Niereninsuffizienz 412, 560
—, chronische 181, 186
Nierenkrankheiten, entzündliche 164
Nierenpunktion 369, 587
Nierensteinbildung 169
Nierensteine 341
Niridazol 526
normal range of distribution of serum acid values 14
Nucleasen der intestinalen Mucosa 130
— des Pankreas 130
Nucleoproteide 130
nucleoside-5-phosphatase 59
Nucleotidbildung, Präcursor 134

Oberflächenspannung 188
Ödeme 427
Ohrtophi 311
Onychopathia psoriatica 296f.
Operation nach Hueter-Mayo 582
Operationen am Kniegelenk 585
operative Steinentfernung 400
Orotat-Kristalle 189
orotic aciduria, clinical features 639
— —, conditions associated with 646
— —, drug-induced 647
— —, genetics 645
— — and gout 646
— —, hereditary 635ff.
— —, nature of defect 639
— —, prenatal diagnosis 648
— — secondary to other genetic defects 647
Orotsäure 484
Osteolysen der Gelenkenden, Operation 582
Osteomyeloreticulose 171
Osteomyelosklerose 171
Ostitis deformans Paget 231
Oxyphenbutazon 445, 505, 507
oxypurines 629
Oxypurinol 471

Paraarthritis urica 302
Paradoxeffekte uricosurischer Mittel 565
Parahydroxysulfinpyrazon 503
Parathormon-Resistenz 289
Passage intestinaler Membranen 131
Pathogenese der Harnsäureablagerungen 179
pathologische Anatomie der Gicht 213ff.
Periarthritiden 300f.
Periarthritis calcarea 301
Periostitis urica 302
Peritendinitis calcarea 297, 301, 313
Permeabilitätsfaktor 196

Peroxydase 190
pH-Abfall 188, 197
— -Optimum 197
— -Verschiebung 184
Phagocytose 189, 191, 438
— von Uratkristallen durch Leukocyten 186
Phagocytosetätigkeit 188, 190
Phagolysosomen 202
Phagosomen 190, 202
Phalangen bei Gicht 219
Pharmakokinetik 435ff.
pathogenesis (Lesch-Nyhan) 614
— of primary gout, role of the kidney 153f.
pathology (Lesch-Nyhan) 614
pharmacogenetics (Lesch-Nyhan) 617
Phenformin 567
Phenprocumarol 525
Phenylbutazon 149, 201, 445, 493, 504, 565
Phenylbutazonderivate 497
Phenylchinolincarbonsäure 526
Phenylindandion 172, 525
Phlebitis urica 302
5-Phosphoribosyl-1-Amin 53, 62, 492
5-Phosphoribosyl-1-Pyrophosphat 53, 62, 492
phosphoribosylpyrophosphate in gout 86
— concentrations in gout 87
— synthetase 32
— turnover in gout 86
phosphoribosyltransferase 57
Phosphorylasen 131
Pied hérissé 334
pinephrine 151
Plasmahalbwertszeit 447
Plasmaharnsäure, Normalwerte 127
Plasmaharnsäurespiegel 165
Plasmathromboplastinantecedent 195
Plasmauratbindung 183
Pneumonien 201
Polarisation 280, 284f.
Polarisationsmikroskop 187
polarisiertes Licht 187
Polyarthritis, chronische 187, 189, 194, 263, 305f.
—, — rheumatische 344
—, primär-chronische 184
— psoriatica 307
—, subakute 292
— und Uratgicht 232
Polyarthrose 308, 351
—, destruierende 309, 351
polyartikulärer Beginn der Gicht 268
Polycythaemia vera 164, 170f., 181
polycythemia vera 96
Polysaccharid-Gehalt 182
population studies of gout and hyperuricemia 30

PP-ribose-P concentration 611
— synthetase activity in gout 81
Prädiabetes 243
prevention of gout 32
Probenecid 149, 172, 186, 378, 497f., 518, 564f.
Prodromastadium der Gicht 259
Prognose der Gicht 595ff.
— bei Gichtniere 590
Prostaglandine 454
protein binding of urate 143
Proteinbindung 446
Proteinpolysaccharid 182, 183
Proteinurie 372
Proteinzufuhr 546
PRT deficiency, adult 76
Pseudogicht 263, 280, 289, 291, 424
Pseudogichtsyndrom-Einteilung 283
pseudogout 19
Psoriasis 11, 173
— arthropathica 294
— und Hyperuricämie 232
— vulgaris 262
psychosocial factors 17
purinarme Kost 550ff.
Purin-Basen 132
Purinbelastung 165
— der Bevölkerung 166
Purinbiosynthese-Stimulation durch Medikamente 485
Purindefizit 381
purine bases in gout 93
Purine, exogene — Einfluß auf den Harnsäurestoffwechsel 123ff.
—, — Einfluß auf Normalpersonen 127ff.
— der Nahrung 130
purine metabolism 603, 627
— nucleoside phosphorylase 58
Purinkörper 190
Purinmetabolismus 186
Purinnucleoside 130
Purinnucleotide 130
Purinrestriktion 541
Purinstoffwechsel, de novo 134
Purinsynthese 357, 462ff.
—, de novo-Hemmung 135, 475, 482ff.
Purinumsatz 165
Pyelonephritis 375, 415, 590
—, Behandlung 589
Pyralolidinderivate 504
Pyrazinamid 166, 172, 363, 574
pyrazinamide 90, 92
— suppression 146
pyrazinoic acid 149
Pyrazolidinderivate 493
pyrimidine nucleotides 643
Pyrimidinnucleoside 130
Pyrimidinnucleotide 130

Pyrophosphat-Arthropathie 280
PZA suppression test 92

Quantität der Resorption von Purinbasen 135

random motility 439
Rassen-Studien 238
reabsorption, tubular of urate 144
Redoxgleichgewicht 173
Reflexdystrophie an den Vorfüßen 331
Reitersche Krankheit 292f.
renal disease, chronic 11, 16
— excretion, in man normal mechanism 143
— —, of urate 10
Renin-Angiotensin-Aldosteron-System 416
Reserpin 417
Reticulohistiocytosis 315
Rezirkulation der Purinkörper 132
Reutilisationsstoffwechsel der Purinbasen 134
Rheumafaktor 290, 305, 307
Rheumaknoten 311
rheumatisches Fieber 291f.
Rheumatismus, palindromer 263, 298
rheumatoide Arthritis 344
Ribomononucleotid 165
Riesenzell-Granulome 315
Risikofaktor Hyperuricämie und Gicht 246ff.
risk factor in coronary heart disease 28
RNS-Belastung 128
Röntgenbefunde 326
Röntgenbild bei Gicht 219
Röntgendiagnostik: Differentialdiagnose 344ff.
— der Ellenbogengelenke 338
— der Finger- und Handgelenke 333f.
— des Fuß-Skeletts 334
— der Gicht 322ff.
— der Hüftgelenke 335
— der Iliosacralgelenke 339
— der Kniegelenke 335
— der Schultergelenke 338
— der Sesambeine der Großzehengrundgelenke 332f.
—, taktische und technische Hinweise 325ff.
— der Wirbelsäule 338
— der Zehengelenke 328ff.
Röntgenkontrastmittel 526
Röntgenspektrographie 269
Röntgensymptome 326
Röntgentiefenbestrahlung, postoperative 584
Röntgenuntersuchung der Harnwege 398f.

Saccharose 571
Salicylate 149, 172, 201, 380, 493, 496, 512, 515f., 565
Salicylismus 497f.
Saluretica 166, 171f.
—, harnsäureretinierende Wirkung 563
—, Jahresverbrauch 562

Salzhaushalt 449
Sarkoid-Arthritis 354
Sarkoidose 172, 263, 424
saturnine gout 99
Säureproduktion 448
Säurestarre des Urins 399
Schleimbeutel an Achillessehne 580
Schleimbeuteltophi 579
Schrumpfniere 164
—, arteriosklerotische 413
—, maligne, weiße 231
—, vasculäre 228
secretion, tubular of urate 145
Sehnengicht 221
Sekundärinfekte 313
self-destructive behavior (Lesch-Nyhan) 613
serum uric acid, effects of disease states 11
— triglyceride 149
Serumharnsäure-Konzentration 180
—, renale Harnsäureausscheidung 167
Serumharnsäurespiegel 186, 201, 203, 491, 595
Serumlactatspiegel 413
sickle cell anemia 11
— — disease 98
Sorbit 571
Spätstadium der Gicht 265
Spirituosen 199
Spironolacton 562
Spondylitis ancylopoetica 308, 348
Spondylosis hyperostotica 340
Standarddiäten, purinarme 125, 536, 539
starvation 11
Steinanalyse 398
steroids in treatment 642
Stoffwechselweg, "do it yourself" der Nucleotide 134
strumigene Wirkung 449
Subluxationsstellung der Zehen 330
Sulfinpyrazon 149, 378, 502, 510
Synovektomie 585
Synovia-Analyse 278
Synovialflüssigkeit bei Gicht 261
Synovitis, kristallinduzierte 188
—, mikrokristallin induzierte 279

Telepaque 149
Tendosynovitis 302
Tendovaginitis 302
Thalassämie 166, 170
thalassemia 11
Therapie der Gicht 462ff.
— der Hyperuricämie 462ff.
— der Steinkrankheit 399ff.
—, uricosurische Komplikationen 528
Therapieverlauf 529
Thiacide 172
Thiacid-Saluretica 412, 561
6-Thioguanin 483

Thorax, breiter 340
Thrombocytenadhäsivität 562
— -Aggregation 249
Thrombosebereitschaft 562
Tietze-Syndrom 219
Todesursachen bei Gicht 595, 597f.
Tomogramme 325
tophaceous deposits 26
Tophi 32, 180, 181, 183, 185, 216, 268f., 587
— am Daumenendgelenk, Operation 582
—, infizierte 586
— innerhalb der Gelenkknorpel 186
— -Rückbildung 272
Tophusbildung 180, 181, 184
— -Entstehung 185
— -Gicht 302ff.
toxemia of pregnancy 11
Transferase-Mangel 167
Transportdefekt, tubulärer 167
Transportmechanismus 565
Transportsystem der Purinbasen 132
Trasylol K 197
treatment (Lesch-Nyhan) 618
Triamteren 562
Triglycerid 414
Trimethylcolchicinsäure 434
twin studies 30f.

Überernährung 415
Übergewicht und Gicht 414
— und Hyperurikämie 237, 239, 242
Überproduktionstheorie 128, 396
Ulcerationen 313
ulcerogene Wirkung 448
Umgebungsfaktoren der Gicht 115ff., 120
Umwandlung, intrazelluläre der Nucleoside 130
Umweltfaktoren 166
Uralyt-U® 385, 400, 529
Urämie 598
Uratablagerungen 181, 184, 185, 186, 596
— in den Gefäßen 223
—, periarticuläre 266
Urate 181, 182, 183, 186, 189
—, amorphe 187
— homeostasis 146
Uratgicht 289
Uratkristallablagerungen 182
Uratkristalle 180, 181, 182, 185, 187, 188, 189, 190, 194, 196
Uratkristall-Injektion 189, 190, 196, 199
Uratkristallphygozytose 198, 202
Uratnephrolithiasis 165
—, Prognose 595f.
Uratphagocytose 439, 443
Uratquote, endogene 124, 126
Uratsalze 182, 186

Uratsekretion, tubuläre 562
Uratsteine 223
Urattophi 223
urea 156
uric acid, colorimetric procedures 9
— — crystaluria 609
— —, drug ingestion 10
— —, effects of drugs 10
— — excessive production 609
— — excretion in gout 90
— —, extrarenal elimination 156
— — in feces 157
— — in gastric juice 157
— — in gout, extrarenal disposal 94
— — in gout, overproduction 73
— — in gout, production 65
— — in hepatic bile 157
— —, measurement 9
— —, miscible pool 66
— — in mixed saliva 157
— — nephrolithiasis 52
— —, renal excretion 142
— —, normal values 142
— — ribonucleoside 61
— —, turnover 66
Uricase 59, 199
— -Injektion, therapeutische 484
Uricaseverdauung 187
Uricolyse 140, 190
—, intestinale 133, 140
uricolysis 45
uricolytic activity in human tissues 156f.
Uricosurica 272, 378, 383, 416, 462, 491f., 588, 597
uricosurisch wirksame Verbindungen 493
— Substanzen 172
— Wirkung 449
Uricurie 501
uridine nucleotides 643
Urin-pH-Wert 401
urinary ammonia production in gout 83
— flow 151
— uric acid 65, 68
Urolithiasis 391

Vererbungsmodus der Gicht 116
Verknöcherungen an den Sehnenansätzen 340
Verteilung der Gelenkgicht 213
Vitamin K-Antagonisten 365, 525
vitamins in treatment 642

Wasserdiurese 378, 492
Wasserhaushalt 449
Weichteiltophi 270, 310, 596
—, Häufigkeit 273
—, Verteilung 304

Weichteilverformungen der Finger 344
Wilson's disease 156
Wurstfinger 295
Wurstzeh 295

xanthine 60, 627
— oxidase 61, 627
— — activity in gout 89
— stones 628

Xanthin-Oxydase-Hemmung 474
Xanthinsteine 381
xanthinuria 11, 626 ff.
—, treatment 630
Xanthome 312
Xylit 569, 571

Zoxazolamin 493, 497, 525
Zuckerguß-Wirbelsäule 340

Handbuch der inneren Medizin

9 Bände
Begründet von L. Mohr, R. Staehelin
Herausgeber: H. Schwiegk
Subskriptionspreise gelten bei
Abnahme des gesamten Werkes

1. Band: **Infektionskrankheiten**
2 Teile. 4. Aufl. 1952
Gebunden zus. DM 450,–; US $ 184.50
Subskriptionspreis
Gebunden DM 360,–; US $ 147.60
ISBN 3-540-01632-5

*2. Band: **Blut und Blutkrankheiten**
6 Teile. 5. völlig neubearb. u. erw. Aufl.

1. Teil: **Allgemeine Hämatologie und Physiopathologie des erythrocytären Systems**
Herausgeber: L. Heilmeyer. 1968
Gebunden DM 290,–; US $ 118.90
Subskriptionspreis
Gebunden DM 232,–; US $ 95.20
ISBN 3-540-04151-6

2. Teil: **Klinik des erythrocytären Systems**
Herausgeber: L. Heilmeyer. 1970
Gebunden DM 320,–; US $ 131.20
Subskriptionspreis
Gebunden DM 256,–; US $ 105.00
ISBN 3-540-04849-9

3. Teil: **Leukocytäres und retikuläres System**
Herausgeber: H. Begemann
In Vorbereitung

4. Teil: **Leukocytäres und retikuläres System 2**
Herausgeber: H. Begemann. 1974
Gebunden DM 268,–; US $ 109.90
Subskriptionspreis
Gebunden DM 214,40; US $ 88.00
ISBN 3-540-06355-2

5. Teil: **Krankheiten des lymphocytären Systems**
Herausgeber: H. Begemann. 1974
Gebunden DM 248,–; US $ 101.70
Subskriptionspreis
Gebunden DM 198,40; US $ 81.40
ISBN 3-540-06254-8

6. Teil: **Blutgerinnung und hämorrhagisches System**
In Vorbereitung

*3. Band: **Verdauungsorgane**
6 Teile. 5. völlig neubearb. u. erw. Aufl.

1. Teil: **Diseases of the Esophagus**
By G. Vantrappen, J. Hellemans. 1974
Cloth DM 390,–; US $ 159.90
Subscription price
Cloth DM 312,–; US $ 128.00
ISBN 3-540-06694-2

2. Teil: **Magen**
Herausgeber: L. Demling. 1974
Gebunden DM 390,–; US $ 159.90
Subskriptionspreis
Gebunden DM 312,–; US $ 128.00
ISBN 3-540-06788-4

3. Teil: **Dünndarm**
Herausgeber: G. Strohmeyer
In Vorbereitung

4. Teil: **Dickdarm**
Herausgeber: K. Müller-Wieland
In Vorbereitung

5. Teil: **Leber und Gallenwege**
Herausgeber: G. A. Martini, H. Thaler
In Vorbereitung

6. Teil: **Pankreas**
Herausgeber: M. M. Forell. 1976
Gebunden DM 480,–; US $ 196.80
Subskriptionspreis
Gebunden DM 384,–; US $ 157.50
ISBN 3-540-07257-8

*4. Band: **Erkrankungen der Atmungsorgane**
4 Teile. 5. völlig neubearb. u. erw. Aufl.

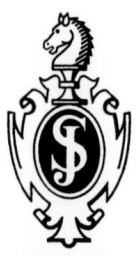

**Springer-Verlag
Berlin
Heidelberg
New York**

Fortsetzung

1. Teil: **Pneumokoniosen**
Herausgeber: W. T. Ulmer, G. Reichel. 1976
Gebunden DM 390,–; US $ 159.90
Subskriptionspreis
Gebunden DM 312,–; US $ 128.00
ISBN 3-540-07507-0

5. Band: **Neurologie**
3 Teile. Redigiert von R. Jung. 4. Aufl. 1953
Gebunden zus. DM 790,–; US $ 323.90
Subskriptionspreis
Gebunden DM 632,–; US $ 259.20
ISBN 3-540-01714-3

6. Band: **Konstitution. Allergische Krankheiten. Krankheiten der Knochen, Gelenke und Muskeln. Krankheiten aus äußeren physikalischen Ursachen. Ernährungskrankheiten. Vitamine und Vitaminkrankheiten.**
2 Teile. 4. Aufl. 1954
Gebunden zus. DM 390,–; US $ 159.90
Subskriptionspreis
Gebunden DM 312,–; US $ 128.00
ISBN 3-540-01809-3

*7. Band: **Stoffwechselkrankheiten**
4 Teile. 5. völlig neubearb. u. erw. Aufl.

1. Teil: **Erbliche Defekte des Kohlenhydrat-, Aminosäuren- und Proteinstoffwechsels**
Herausgeber: F. Linneweh. 1974
Gebunden DM 348,–; US $ 142.70
Subskriptionspreis
Gebunden DM 278,40; US $ 114.20
ISBN 3-540-06313-7

2. Teil a: **Diabetes mellitus A**
Herausgeber: K. Oberdisse. 1975
Gebunden DM 360,–; US $ 147.60
Subskriptionspreis
Gebunden DM 288,–; US $ 118.10
ISBN 3-540-07062-1

2. Teil b: In Vorbereitung

3. Teil: **Gicht**
Herausgeber: N. Zöllner. 1976
Gebunden DM 290,–; US $ 118.90
Subskriptionspreis
Gebunden DM 232,–; US $ 95.20
ISBN 3-540-07258-6

4. Teil: **Fettstoffwechsel**
Herausgeber: G. Schettler, H. Greten, G. Schlierf, D. Seidel. 1976
In Vorbereitung
ISBN 3-540-07585-2

8. Band: **Nierenkrankheiten**
3 Teile. Herausgeber: H. Schwiegk
5. völlig neubearb. u. erw. Aufl. 1968
Gebunden zus. DM 780,–; US $ 319.80
Subskriptionspreis
Gebunden DM 624,–; US $ 255.90
ISBN 3-540-04152-4

9. Band: **Herz und Kreislauf**
6 Teile. 4. Aufl. 1960
Gebunden zus. DM 1500,–; US $ 615.00
Subskriptionspreis
Gebunden DM 1200,–; US $ 492.00
ISBN 3-540-02542-1

1. Teil: 1960
Gebunden DM 305,–; US $ 125.10
ISBN 3-540-02536-7

2. Teil: 1960
Gebunden DM 395,–; US $ 162.00
ISBN 3-540-02537-5

3. Teil: 1960
Gebunden DM 460,–; US $ 188.60
ISBN 3-540-02538-3

4. Teil: 1960
Gebunden DM 235,–; US $ 96.40
ISBN 3-540-02539-1

5. Teil: 1960
Gebunden DM 270,–; US $ 110.70
ISBN 3-540-02540-5

6. Teil: 1960
Gebunden DM 335,–; US $ 137.40
ISBN 3-540-02541-3

*Subskriptionspreise werden gewährt bei Verpflichtung zur Abnahme aller Teilbände bis zum Erscheinen des gesamten Bandes.

Preisänderungen vorbehalten

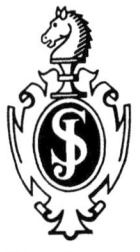

**Springer-Verlag
Berlin
Heidelberg
New York**

MIX
Papier aus verantwortungsvollen Quellen
Paper from responsible sources
FSC® C105338

If you have any concerns about our products,
you can contact us on
ProductSafety@springernature.com

In case Publisher is established outside the EU,
the EU authorized representative is:
**Springer Nature Customer Service Center GmbH
Europaplatz 3, 69115 Heidelberg, Germany**

Printed by Libri Plureos GmbH
in Hamburg, Germany